Primary
Care
Medicine

J. B. LIPPINCOTT COMPANY

Philadelphia / Toronto

Primary Care Medicine

ALLAN H. GOROLL, M.D.

Assistant Professor of Medicine
Harvard Medical School;
Faculty Member, Primary Care Program; and
Assistant in Medicine
Massachusetts General Hospital
Boston, Massachusetts

LAWRENCE A. MAY, M.D.

Assistant Clinical Professor of Medicine
UCLA School of Medicine
University of California, Los Angeles and
Consultant for General Internal Medicine and
Geriatrics
Wadsworth Veterans Administration Hospital
Los Angeles, California

ALBERT G. MULLEY, M.D.

Instructor in Medicine and Associate Director
Kaiser Fellowship Program in General Internal
Medicine
Harvard Medical School; and
Assistant in Medicine and Associate Director of
Medical Practices Evaluation Unit
Massachusetts General Hospital
Boston, Massachusetts

With 34 Contributors

Goroll, Allan H
  Primary care medicine.
  Includes bibliographies and index.
  1. Family medicine. I. May, Lawrence A., joint author. II. Mulley, Albert G., joint author. III. Title.
RC46.G56   616   80-27142
ISBN 0-397-50421-7

5 6

To JOHN D. STOECKLE, M.D.

Contents

4. Respiratory Problems

Contributors

ANN B. BARNES, M.D.
Assistant Clinical Professor of Obstetrics and
Gynecology
Harvard Medical School; and
Assistant Gynecologist
Massachusetts General Hospital
Boston, Massachusetts

ARTHUR J. BARSKY, M.D.
Assistant Professor of Psychiatry
Harvard Medical School; and
Chief, Acute Psychiatry Service
Massachusetts General Hospital
Boston, Massachusetts

ROBERT J. BOYD, M.D.
Assistant Clinical Professor of Orthopedic
Surgery
Harvard Medical School; and
Associate Orthopedic Surgeon and
Director, Problem Back Clinic
Massachusetts General Hospital
Boston, Massachusetts

DAVID C. BREWSTER, M.D.
Assistant Professor of Surgery
Harvard Medical School; and
Assistant Surgeon
Massachusetts General Hospital
Boston, Massachusetts

LESLIE S.-T. FANG, M.D.
Instructor in Medicine
Harvard Medical School; and
Assistant in Medicine
Massachusetts General Hospital
Boston, Massachusetts

LEE GOLDMAN, M.D.
Assistant Professor of Medicine
Harvard Medical School; and
Associate in Medicine
Peter Bent Brigham Hospital
Boston, Massachusetts

ELLIE J.C. GOLDSTEIN, M.D.
Assistant Professor of Medicine
State University of New York
Downstate Medical Center College of
Medicine
Brooklyn, New York

JOHN D. GOODSON, M.D.
Instructor in Medicine
Harvard Medical School; and
Faculty, Primary Care Program and
Assistant in Medicine
Massachusetts General Hospital
Boston, Massachusetts

ALLAN H. GOROLL, M.D.

Assistant Professor of Medicine
Harvard Medical School;
Faculty, Primary Care Program; and
Assistant in Medicine
Massachusetts General Hospital
Boston, Massachusetts

DAVID A. GREENBERG, O.D., M.P.H.

Assistant Professor and Director
Division of Community Optometry
New England College of Optometry
Boston, Massachusetts

FREDERICK G. GUGGENHEIM, M.D.

Associate Professor of Psychiatry and
Chief, Psychiatric Consultation Liaison Division
Southwestern Medical School
University of Texas Health Sciences Center
Dallas, Texas

JOHN P. KELLY, D.M.D., M.D.

Assistant Clinical Professor of Oral and
    Maxillofacial Surgery
Harvard School of Dental Medicine; and
Assistant Oral and Maxillofacial Surgeon
Massachusetts General Hospital
Boston, Massachusetts

WILLIAM KIVETT, M.D.

Dermatology Consultant
United States Public Health Service
San Pedro, California

STEVEN R. LEVISOHN, M.D.

Instructor in Medicine
Harvard Medical School; and
Assistant in Medicine
Massachusetts General Hospital
Boston, Massachusetts

JACOB J. LOKICH, M.D.

Assistant Professor of Medicine
Harvard Medical School; and
Chief, Medical Oncology
New England Deaconess Hospital
Boston, Massachusetts

MICHAEL N. MARGOLIES, M.D.

Assistant Professor of Surgery
Harvard Medical School; and
Assistant Surgeon
Massachusetts General Hospital
Boston, Massachusetts

LAWRENCE A. MAY, M.D.

Assistant Clinical Professor of Medicine
UCLA School of Medicine
University of California, Los Angeles and
Consultant for General Internal Medicine and
    Geriatrics
Wadsworth Veterans Administration Hospital
Los Angeles, California

ROBERT M. MILLER, M.D.

Assistant Clinical Professor of Medicine
UCLA School of Medicine
University of California, Los Angeles
Los Angeles, California

ALBERT G. MULLEY, M.D.

Instructor in Medicine and Associate Director
Kaiser Fellowship Program in General Internal
    Medicine
Harvard Medical School; and
Assistant in Medicine and Associate Director
Medical Practices Evaluation Unit
Massachusetts General Hospital
Boston, Massachusetts

SAMUEL R. NUSSBAUM, M.D.

Research Fellow in Medicine
Harvard Medical School; and
Clinical Assistant in Medicine
Massachusetts General Hospital
Boston, Massachusetts

AMY A. PRUITT, M.D.

Instructor in Neurology
Harvard Medical School; and
Assistant in Neurology and Assistant Director of
    Outpatient Neurology Unit
Massachusetts General Hospital
Boston, Massachusetts

MARVIN J. RAPAPORT, M.D.

Assistant Clinical Professor of Medicine
UCLA School of Medicine
University of California, Los Angeles
Los Angeles, California

RONALD M. REISNER, M.D.

Professor and Chairman, Department of
    Dermatology
University of California, Los Angeles
Los Angeles, California

CLAUDIA U. RICHTER, M.D.

Clinical Fellow in Ophthalmology
Harvard Medical School; and
Resident in Ophthalmology
Massachusetts Eye and Ear Infirmary
Boston, Massachusetts

JAMES M. RICHTER, M.D.

Research Fellow in Medicine
Harvard Medical School; and
Clinical and Research Fellow
Massachusetts General Hospital
Boston, Massachusetts

NANCY A. RIGOTTI, M.D.

Clinical Fellow in Medicine
Harvard Medical School; and
Resident in Medicine
Massachusetts General Hospital
Boston, Massachusetts

DAVID C. RISH, M.D.

Assistant Clinical Professor of Medicine
University of California, Los Angeles
Los Angeles, California

ERIC J. SACKNOFF, M.D.

Adult and Pediatric Urologist
Mount Auburn Hospital
Cambridge, and
Emerson Hospital
Concord, Massachusetts

RICHARD M. SALIT, M.D.

Assistant Clinical Professor of Medicine
UCLA School of Medicine
University of California, Los Angeles
Los Angeles, California

WILLIAM V.R. SHELLOW, M.D.

Assistant Clinical Professor of Dermatology
UCLA School of Medicine
University of California; and
Chief, Dermatology Outpatient Service
Wadsworth Veterans Administration Hospital
Los Angeles, California

HARVEY B. SIMON, M.D.

Assistant Professor of Medicine
Harvard Medical School; and
Associate Physician
Massachusetts General Hospital
Boston, Massachusetts

DANIEL E. SINGER, M.D.

Clinical and Research Fellow
Harvard Medical School; and
Clinical Fellow
Massachusetts General Hospital
Boston, Massachusetts

EVE E. SLATER, M.D.

Assistant Professor of Medicine
Harvard Medical School; and
Assistant in Medicine and
Chief, Hypertension Unit
Massachusetts General Hospital
Boston, Massachusetts

ARTHUR J. SOBER, M.D.

Associate Professor in Dermatology
Harvard Medical School; and
Assistant Dermatologist
Massachusetts General Hospital
Boston, Massachusetts

ROGER F. STEINERT, M.D.

Clinical Fellow in Ophthalmology
Harvard Medical School; and
Resident in Ophthalmology
Massachusetts Eye and Ear Infirmary
Boston, Massachusetts

JOHN D. STOECKLE, M.D.

Associate Professor of Medicine
Harvard Medical School;
Chief, Medical Clinics;
Associate Director, Primary Care Program and
Physician, Massachusetts General Hospital
Boston, Massachusetts

BEVERLY WOO, M.D.

Instructor in Medicine
Harvard Medical School; and
Junior Associate in Medicine
Peter Bent Brigham Hospital
Boston, Massachusetts

Foreword

Physicians have traditionally provided direct, initial, comprehensive care for patients as well as continuity of care. In the past two decades the growing proportion of specialist physicians has endangered this traditional role of the physician. The development of highly technologic, tertiary, inpatient medical care has preoccupied the attention of our teaching institutions. Coping with the increased armamentarium of diagnostic and therapeutic interventions has distracted some physicians from traditional roles in patient care. The primary care movement has been a national response to this situation aimed at providing more physicians skilled in dealing wisely and humanely with illness in their patients and providing the overall supervision and continuity of medical care that we expect of good generalists. It encourages these physicians to know their patients as human and social beings as well as bearers of organ pathology. Promotion of prevention as well as the practice of curing is an important part of primary care.

The concerns which have led to renewed attention of the medical profession to primary care medicine have had a very salutory effect on our teaching institutions. There has been a resurgence of training in the ambulatory setting. Medical students and residents have learned that many illnesses formerly thought to require hospitalization can be effectively managed in the ambulatory setting. As usual, this is not an original discovery; rather, it is a return to the emphasis that was very much a part of training programs in the earlier decades of this century.

Primary Care Medicine has grown out of the experiences of a group of young physicians who have pioneered in the rebirth of primary care medicine within the Harvard medical community. They have organized primary care practices which have served as training sites for other physicians and health workers. They have examined their own practices, as well as the published experience of others, in order to provide within this text a synthesis of the best available information for ambulatory management of adult medical patients. Their discussions are brief and practical rather than exhaustive, but the interested reader is provided with a key annotated bibliography which directs him to further sources of information. This book is not meant to compete with the traditional exhaustive textbook of Medicine. Rather, its brief, clear discussions and analyses of current knowledge are prepared for the busy practitioner who daily encounters many problems for which he needs to quickly know the best available answers.

To whom is the book addressed? To the primary care physician, of course. It will be his bible—a valuable source of guidance and of solace in innumerable management situations. But it is becoming increasingly evident that the medical subspecialist devotes a considerable portion of his practice time to the provision of first contact and continuous care of the medical needs of his patients. This book will, therefore, find a welcome place on the desk of both the medical subspecialist and the medical generalist and is addressed to everyone engaged in the clinical practice of adult Medicine.

Alexander Leaf, M.D.
Jackson Professor of Medicine
Harvard Medical School; and
Chief, Medical Services
Massachusetts General Hospital
Boston, Massachusetts

Preface

Primary Care Medicine is designed to be of help to those who provide primary care to adults. It attempts to delineate rational approaches to the screening, evaluation, and management of common and important clinical problems encountered in office practice. Because optimal primary care is coordinated, comprehensive, continuous and personal, the tasks of such care must include not only accurate diagnosis and technically sound treatment, but also personal support, patient education, skillful use of consultants, prevention, and health maintenance. These important components of primary care are addressed and incorporated into discussions of screening, workup, and management strategies.

Chapters in Part 1 of *Primary Care Medicine* define the scope and tasks of primary care, and introduce fundamental concepts pertinent to screening and the use and interpretation of tests. Subsequent chapters focus on individual clinical problems. The book is problem-oriented to facilitate its use in everyday care. In each instance, epidemiology, natural history, pathophysiology, and the value of clinical findings and laboratory tests are considered in terms of their contribution to decision-making. The objective is to use pertinent information from the literature and from our practice in a logical and practical manner to define effective and efficient approaches to common clinical problems. Each chapter concludes with an annotated bibliography of pertinent references for more detailed reading.

This book is an outgrowth of our practice and teaching activities in the Primary Care Program at Massachusetts General Hospital. We are indebted to our patients, teachers, and students for their assistance, particularly in defining the content of a textbook of primary care medicine. We are especially grateful to the following colleagues for their encouragement and invaluable consultation: Lloyd Axelrod, M.D.; Mark Clarke, M.D.; William Crowley,

M.D.; Jeffrey Galpin, M.D.; Neil Goldberg, M.D.; Stephen Goldfinger, M.D.; David Greenblatt, M.D.; Timothy Guiney, M.D.; David Kanarek, M.D.; Edward Kirshen, M.D.; William Seaman, M.D.; Jack Wands, M.D.; Robert Weinrib, M.D.; Edwin Wheeler, M.D.; William Wilson, M.D.; Lee Witters, M.D.; and Peter Yurchak, M.D.

We are also grateful to William Shellow, M.D., for coordinating the material relevant to dermatology.

Preparation of the manuscript would not have been possible without the help of Carol Scola and Sarah Bollinger.

We are indebted to J. Stuart Freeman and his colleagues at Lippincott/ Harper & Row without whose guidance and forbearance this long-evolving project could not have come to fruition.

Finally, extra special thanks are due to Kati Tims for the many hours she devoted to the preparation of this book.

Allan H. Goroll, M.D.
Lawrence A. May, M.D.
Albert G. Mulley, M.D.

Primary
Care
Medicine

1

Principles of Primary Care

1

Tasks of Primary Care
JOHN D. STOECKLE, M.D.

DEFINITION OF PRIMARY CARE

Primary care is coordinated, comprehensive and personal care, available on both a first contact and continuous basis. It incorporates several tasks: medical diagnosis and treatment, psychological assessment and management, personal support, communication of information about illness, prevention, and health maintenance.

This book addresses the clinical problems encountered by primary care physicians in office practice of adult medicine. In this setting, the physician's responsibilities and tasks extend beyond the narrow technological confines of medical diagnosis and treatment. Although a great deal of effort must be focused on accurate diagnosis and technically sound therapy, the other clinical tasks that complete the very definition of primary care also assume major importance.

Alongside this clinical definition of primary care stands a plethora of other definitions; these derive from organizational, functional, professional and academic perspectives. For example, policy planners have defined primary care as a *level of medical services,* one that is provided outside the hospital. Presumably, primary care (community-based services) is, then, a less technical practice compared to secondary care (consultant or specialty services) and tertiary care (hospital services). This organizational definition provides a scheme for the allocation of public resources among these health services, each of which has a distinct professional, economic, institutional and political structure. For another definition, Alpert and Charney have looked at important *patient care functions* of doctors, namely, to provide access, continuity and integration. While this view is useful in describing the functions performed by practitioners for their patients within organized health services, it does not define the content of their clinical work. From the standpoint of professionalism, primary care has been defined as a *specialty* concentrating on humanistic medicine practiced outside the hospital, but devoid of the special procedures and technology that typically characterize medical specialization. This definition has been useful in organizing a segment of the profession, for example, family practice, and in providing a new curriculum for the education and training of doctors. From the university comes still another definition of primary care as an *academic discipline* concerned with the expansion of knowledge unique of primary practice and to personal care, a definition that contains the promise of a departmental position for primary care in the medical school.

While each of these definitions presents a particular perspective about primary care and serves some special purpose, none explains the primary care physician's day-to-day work with patients.

By taking the perspective of the doctor's practice, primary care can be defined by several tasks: (1) medical diagnosis and treatment; (2) psychological diagnosis and treatment; (3) personal support of pa-

1

tients of all backgrounds, in all stages of illness; (4) communication of information about diagnosis, treatment, prevention and prognosis; (5) maintenance of patients with chronic illness; (6) prevention of disability and disease through detection, education, persuasion and preventive treatment. These tasks comprise the clinical work of doctors providing primary care. They not only restate medicine's central mandate of patient care, but also constitute a clinical definition of primary care to which the information in this text is applied.

CONTRIBUTION OF
SOCIAL SCIENCE RESEARCH

Except for medical diagnosis and treatment, the tasks which define primary care may seem merely vocational, i.e., practical but not scientifically based. However, social science research has provided a logical and rational basis for the clinical work of primary care. The data derived from these studies concern the patient's illness rather than the doctor's definition of disease; they are contained in the cognitive, communicative and behavioral processes by which the patient defines being ill; and they are found in the clinical and social science literature on such topics as the patient's emotional reactions, personality, expectations, requests, attributions, views of treatment and social networks, to mention but a few. Knowledge concerning such aspects of care in conjunction with statistical thinking contributes a rational framework for the work of primary care.

Medical diagnosis and treatment remains a central task, although it is by no means the end point of care. As the patient's first contact with medical services, the primary doctor must not only be knowledgeable about disease, but must exercise critical judgment in determining the scope, site and pace of the medical workup and management. In organizing diagnosis and management, the physician needs to know the clinical presentation and natural history of illness, the uses and limits of the laboratory, and the indications for and shortcomings of invasive tests and therapeutic measures. In continuing care, the issues are the same. The doctor's critical attitude to the use of technology and to the referral of patients for special therapies or diagnostic techniques remains essential. Chapter 2 considers methods developed in clinical epidemiology and decision analysis which promise to help the clinician rationally choose among a sometimes bewildering array of diagnostic and therapeutic options.

Psychological diagnosis and treatment and *personal support* complement the medical components of care. Studies documenting the relationship between emotional reactions and illness, coupled with surveys showing a high frequency of such reactions in office practice, underscore their importance in patients seeking medical help. Recognition of anxiety, depression, sexual dysfunction, personality disturbance and psychosis is necessary for the interpretation of bodily complaints, the communication of personal feelings, and the joint decision of doctor and patient on acceptable and effective treatment plans.

Recognition of emotional reactions alone is insufficient. The doctor's response to the normal patient's psychological defenses is essential to securing cooperation and relieving anxiety. Understanding the patient's defenses and personality style allows the clinician to provide meaningful support and to respond appropriately to the patient's emotional needs. The care rendered is then likely to be perceived as personal and psychologically acceptable. Much of this analysis of the psychological aspects of clinical practice derives from contributions by Kahana and Bibring, Lipsett, Balaint, and Zaborenko.

Information about the patient's expectations and requests is also important. *Expectations* often play a major part in seeking help, complying with treatment, and feeling satisfied with care. In their studies of illness behavior and patients' use of doctors, Zola and Mechanic viewed expectations as explanations of patients' decisions to go to see the doctor. If attention was not paid to the patient's reason for coming, the corollary was clear: the patient would not stay in treatment. In health centers in Israel, Shuval found specific expectations of visits to doctors: status enhancement in seeing socially important professionals; catharsis of grief, anger and despair; sanctioning of failure to cope; and understanding and control of illness through medical "scientific" explanations. This brief list is by no means complete, for along with these so-called "latent" expectations are traditional or "real" medical ones—for example, that the doctor is a healer of disease and possesses techniques for its control, relief or cure. Such expectations not only explain the decision to seek medical care but are, in fact, elements of the clinical tasks of personal support and communication of information about illness.

Newer clinical studies by Lazare and colleagues have separated *requests* from expectations. Requests are specific and concrete helping actions and behaviors identified by patients. These studies identified some fourteen requests and demonstrated that their prompt recognition and negotiation benefited both patient and doctor. The doctor's interest in ascertaining what treatment the patient wants indicates a reciprocity that is associated with greater satisfaction and adherence to medical advice. These efforts are part of the task of personal support and management. Still other elements of the management task, such as decisions about continued care, referral and discharge, are also realized through an understanding of requests; thus physicians need both to elicit and to respond to them.

The communication of information about illness—the need to inform, explain, reassure and advise patients—is essential to primary care. This task is often dependent on a knowledge of the patient's *attributions,* i.e., what the patient thinks is the cause of illness. If the patient's attributions differ from the doctor's and are not uncovered, his anxieties may not be relieved, nor will the doctor's explanation be accepted. Knowing how and what to tell the patient about his illness is often difficult, especially if his interpretation of the illness has not been elicited.

Mechanic, for example, suggests that patients with bodily complaints may go to the primary care doctor not for relief of physical discomfort but rather to learn what causes their complaints and sometimes to obtain reassurance that their complaints have less serious causes than they thought. Such confirmation or correction of the patient's attributions is a kind of "attribution therapy." From a broader perspective, Kleinman assigns to attributions a major function in all medical care systems, namely, the control of illness through the explanation of its cause. In effect, the doctor's clinical or scientific explanations of illness provide labels, names and models so that the patient feels his illness can be understood and controlled, regardless of its technical treatment. In essence, the patient's beliefs about illness need to be elicited so that they can be used in explanation, education and reassurance.

Maintenance of the chronically ill requires continuous, long-term treatment and is a distinct task of primary care. Here, obtaining patient compliance is essential because most long-term treatment now takes place without daily medical supervision, and most of that treatment requires the self-administration of drugs. To improve adherence to therapy, it has become increasingly important to learn about the *patient's views of treatment* and actual self-treatment. So far the record on adherence to treatment has not been good. A wide discrepancy between what is prescribed and what is done typifies the literature of "following the doctor's orders," and the problem seems to be as much the doctor's as the patient's.

Knowledge about patients' views and behaviors can be used to design more effective therapeutic regimens and to alter therapeutic directions. Moreover, the act of eliciting information may improve communication between doctor and patient, thus strengthening their relationship and further promoting therapeutic efforts. More studies of patient views of treatment and of the dynamics of the doctor-patient relationship should provide new knowledge that can be used to enhance compliance.

Prevention of disease and disability, another modern component of primary care, emphasizes screening and reduction in risk factors in order to avoid the more elaborate technologies sometimes necessary for cure. The primary physician needs to know which conditions and risk factors are worth screening for and how best to detect and effectively manage them; thus it is hoped that some potential causes of morbidity and mortality will be foreseen and prevented. (See Chapter 3.)

A less commonly considered but no less important aspect of prevention involves attention to the patient's *social network,* since illness is often precipitated by disruption of interpersonal relationships. For example, Parkes and others have noted an increased mortality and morbidity among recent widows, while Zola has reported that interpersonal crises were among the most frequent of five common circumstances that spurred the individual to come for medical attention. Knowledge of patients' social situations can help in prevention of illness and visits to the doctor by focusing attention on stresses which might be precipitants. Attention to social networks is important for personal treatment. If significant loss or separation occurs, a major part of treatment can involve helping the patient reestablish his social network, thus lessening his dependence on professional help from doctor, nurse or social worker.

THE PROMISE OF
PRIMARY CARE MEDICINE

So far the clinical tasks of primary care have been proposed as a perspective from which readers might view the information in this text, but, in fact, the tasks also promise changes—in our ideas about standards of treatment, professional relations, organization, prevention, clinical excellence and clinical effectiveness.

Treatment. The ideal of personal treatment is revived and reemphasized. Though it has not been entirely dead, the increasing size, specialization and organization of practice has often made personal, patient-centered treatment a luxury rather than a medical care necessity. Patient-centered treatment also means that specific therapeutic regimens must be not only technically correct, but designed to be acceptable to patients, especially when more patients are maintained outside the hospital.

Professional relations. The general functions of the physician as applied to access, integration and continuity are enhanced and made central. One consequence would be that decision-making would now systematically include and be coordinated by the generalist, when, so often in the past, it has not.

Organization. Since the goals of primary care include not only cure but also prevention and maintenance, ambulatory care is now the major mode for these health services.

Prevention. The ideal of prevention in practice has been to deal with the individual patient seeking help. Primary care medicine would also examine the epidemiology of the entire practice, perhaps its community base, and implement those preventive practices which have a rationale for easy detection and effective preventive intervention.

Clinical excellence. Skills in medical diagnosis and treatment have often been the only measure of clinical excellence. That ideal of excellence is now more broadly based to include skills in all the clinical tasks. Moreover, the value of a carefully performed history and physical examination receives renewed emphasis as concerns about overuse of the laboratory and excessive costs grow in importance.

Clinical effectiveness. The usual objective criteria for efficacy of diagnostic and treatment processes have been derived from the standards of clinical science. Consideration of subjective parameters such as patient acceptance and sense of well-being becomes mandatory in the primary care setting and must be added to the assessment of clinical efficacy.

These themes on the clinical tasks and promises of primary care run through the chapters that follow, sometimes explicitly, sometimes in latent fashion, but always central to the provision of personalized help to patients.

ANNOTATED BIBLIOGRAPHY

Alpert, J.J., and Charney, E.: The Education of Physicians for Primary Care. DHEW Publication No. 74–31B. U.S. Government Printing Office, 1975. *(Functional definition of primary care.)*

Balaint, M.: The Doctor, the Patient and the Illness. New York: International Universities Press, 1957. *(A classic study of the British general practitioner's negotiations with patients about diagnosis and treatment.)*

Davis, M.S.: Variations in patient's compliance with doctor's orders: Medical practice and doctor-patient interaction. Psychiatry Med., 2:31. *(An analysis of the importance of doctor-patient relationship in compliance.)*

Hicks, D.: Primary Health Care, a Review, Commissioned by the Department of Health and Social Security, London. Her Majesty's Stationery Office, 1976. *(Organizational definition of primary care.)*

Kahana, R.J., and Bibring, G.L.: Personality types in medical management. In N.E. Zinberg (ed.): Psychiatry and Medical Practice in a General Hospital. New York: International Universities Press, 1965, pp. 108–123. *(Discusses the use of defense mechanisms derived from personality assessment in treatment.)*

Kasl, S.V., and Cobb, S.: Health behavior, illness behavior and sick role behavior. I: Health and illness. Arch. Environ. Health, 12:245, 1966. *(A thorough review of sociological and psychiatric studies on the factors that lead to a decision to seek help.)*

Kleinman, A.M.: Toward a comparative study of medical systems: An integrated approach to the study of the relationship of medicine and culture. Sci. Med. and Man, 1:55, 1973. *(A study that examines the specific and general significance of attributions.)*

Lazare, A., Cohen, F., Mignone, R., et al.: The walk-in patient as a customer: A key dimension in evaluation and treatment. Am. J. Orthopsychiatry, 42:872, 1972.

Lazare, A., Eisenthal, S., Frank, A., and Stoeckle, J.D.: Studies on a negotiated approach to patienthood. The doctor-patient relation. In E. Gallagher (ed.): Fogarty International Center Series on the Teaching of Preventive Medicine, Vol. 4. Washington, D.C.: DHEW, 1977. *(Two studies that systematically examine requests of patients in a psychiatric clinic.)*

Lindemann, E.: Symptomatology and management of acute grief. Am. J. Psychiatry, 101:141, 1944.

(A classic paper on the symptoms in medical patients.)

Lipsett, D.: Medical and psychological characteristics of "crocks." Psychiatry Med., *15*:293, 1970. *(Describes the patient who needs to have bodily complaints and suggests a means of management that takes this need into account.)*

McDill, M.S.: Structure of social systems determining attitudes, knowledge and behavior toward disease. *In* A.J. Enelow and J.B. Henderson (eds): Applying Behavioral Sciences to Cardiovascular Risk. New York: American Heart Association, 1975. *(Reviews the potential use of networks in prevention of cardiovascular disease.)*

McKinlay, J.B.: Social networks, lay consultation and help-seeking behavior. Social Forces, *51*:275, 1973. *(Uses networks to explain differences in help-seeking behavior.)*

McWhinney, I.R.: General practice as an academic discipline. Lancet, *1*:419, 1966. *(Defines primary care from an academic perspective.)*

Mechanic, D.: Medical Sociology. New York: Free Press, 1968. *(A classic text detailing the interaction of social factors and illness.)*

Mechanic, D.: Social psychologic factors affecting the presentation of bodily complaints. N. Engl. J. Med., *286*:1132, 1972. *(A sociological study that examines the factors influencing the patient's decision to seek medical help.)*

Parkes, C.M.: Effects of bereavement on physical and mental health—A study of medical records of widows. Br. Med. J. *2*:274, 1964. *(One of a number of studies documenting increased morbidity and mortality among widows shortly after the death of their husbands.)*

Proger, S.: Doctor of primary medicine. (editorial) JAMA, *220*:410, 1972. *(Defines primary care as a specialty rather than as a function.)*

Schmale, A.H.: Relationship of separation and depression to disease. Psychosom. Med., *20*:259, 1958. (From the University of Rochester's Department of Psychiatry, a statement on the hypothesis of and evidence for the etiologic significance of affect, hopelessness and helplessness in the onset of illness.)

Shuval, J.T., Antonovsky, A., and Davies, A.M.: Social Function of Medical Practice: Doctor–patient Relationship in Israel. San Francisco: Jossey–Bass, 1970. *(An analysis of the rates and reasons for medical visits; provides a typology of the uses of medical visits.)*

Stimson, G.V.: Obeying the doctor's orders: A view from the other side. Soc. Sci. Med., *8*:97, 1974. *(A study that details what patients think after they have left the doctor's office.)*

Stoeckle, J.D., Zola, I.K., and Davidson, G.E.: On going to see the doctor. The contributions of the patient to the decision to seek medical aid. J. Chronic Dis., *16*:975, 1963. *(An analysis of patients' expectations in medical practice.)*

Stoeckle, J.D., Zola, I.K., and Davidson, G.E.: The quality and significance of psychological distress in medical patients. J. Chronic Dis., *17*:959, 1964. *(A review of the many studies of the psychological distress found in medical patients.)*

Waitzkin, H., and Stoeckle, J.D.: The communication of information about illness: Clinical, sociological and methodological considerations. *In* Z. J. Lipowski (ed.): Advances in Psychosomatic Medicine: Psychosocial Aspects of Physical Illness, Vol. 8. Basel: S. Karger, 1972, pp. 180–216. *(A review of the significance of and research on communication in medical practice.)*

Zabarenko, R.N., Zabarenko, L., and Hengea, R.A.: The psychodynamics of physicianhood. Psychiatry, *33*:102, 1970. *(This study is illustrative of the importance of understanding patients' defenses and personalities and the uses this knowledge may have in the treatment relationship.)*

Zola, I.K.: Studying the decision to see a doctor. *In* Z.J. Lipowski (ed.): Advances in Psychosomatic Medicine: Psychosocial Aspects of Physical Illness, Vol. 8. Basel: S. Karger, 1972, pp. 216–236. *(The paper describes the typology of decisions and their dynamics.)*

2

The Selection and Interpretation
of Diagnostic Tests

The diagnostic process often involves difficult decisions regarding the utilization of laboratory tests and the interpretation of their results. The amount of information likely to be provided by the test and the importance of making a specific diagnosis at that time must be weighed against any associated risks and costs. Appropriate use and interpretation of diagnostic tests requires an appreciation of the probabilistic nature of test results and an understanding of the measures of test validity. Since diagnostic classification is most important when it influences patient management, knowledge of the natural history of the disease considered and of the effectiveness of available therapies is also necessary to optimally choose among diagnostic strategies.

"Diagnostic" tests are used for purposes other than making a specific diagnosis in a patient known to be sick. Prognosis may be the important question if a specific disease has already been identified. Alternatively, the test may be used to screen for the presence of subclinical disease or to identify risk factors related to the subsequent development of disease. More simply, the test may be used to monitor the results of ongoing therapy.

The diagnostic process requires consideration of numerous diseases and their likelihoods. Upon completion of the history and physical examination, informal probabilities are assigned, and the diagnoses under consideration are ranked. The probability estimates are based on the physician's previous experience with similar patients and familiarity with relevant medical literature. The epidemiology and natural history of the case are implicitly incorporated into the assessments of likelihood. The purpose of subsequent laboratory testing is to refine initial probability estimates and, in the process, to revise and reorder the differential diagnosis. Although it is obvious that proper selection and interpretation of tests are critical to accurate diagnosis, errors in use of the laboratory are frequently made, often unknowingly.

DIAGNOSTIC TESTS AND
THE PROBABILITY OF DISEASE

A test that is perfectly *sensitive* for the disease considered will always be positive if the disease is actually present. A negative test in this situation "rules out" the disease. A test that is perfectly *specific* for the disease considered will always be negative if the disease is not present. Therefore a positive finding "rules in" the disease.

However, commonly used tests are rarely perfect. More often, sensitivity and specificity are also matters of probability. For example, if a screening test for glaucoma such as Schiotz tonometry has a sensitivity of 70 per cent and a specificity of 80 per cent, it will correctly diagnose 70 per cent of those with glaucoma and correctly give a negative result in 80 per cent of those who do not have the disease. But the test will be falsely negative in 30 per cent of those with disease and falsely positive in 20 per cent of those who are actually disease-free—the false-negative rate and false-positive rate of the test will be 30 per cent and 20 per cent respectively.

The clinician can often estimate the sensitivity and specificity of tests that he commonly uses based on his own experience. Values for sensitivity and specificity can be derived from evaluation studies among individuals with the disease in question and among individuals without the disease. But the probability that a test is positive when the disease is present (*sensitivity*) and the probability the test is negative if the disease is not present (*specificity*) are not the principal concerns. Both the physician and patient are more concerned with the implications of test results. What is the probability of disease if a test is positive (called the *predictive value positive*)? What is the probability of nondisease if the test is negative (called the *predictive value negative*)?

In order to estimate the predictive value of a positive or negative test, the clinician needs more information than simply the sensitivity and specificity of the test. He must also know the probability of disease before the test is performed (called the *prior probability* or, in the screening situation, the *prevalence*).

This dependence on prior probability or prevalence can be illustrated by returning to the glaucoma example. Given the hypothesized sensitivity of 70 per cent and specificity of 80 per cent, there are two ways any individual can have a positive test. Seventy per cent of those with glaucoma and 20 per cent of those without will be screened positive. If 1,000 patients are screened, only 20 of whom have glaucoma, one could expect 14 (.70 x 20) patients with glaucoma to have positive tests *and* 196 (.20 x 980) individuals without glaucoma to have positive tests. Since only 14 of 210 patients with positive tests have glaucoma, without additional diagnostic information, the probability of glaucoma in any individual with a positive test is less than 7 per cent! If the test was used in another population of 1,000 individuals of whom 100 actually had disease, 70 (.70 x 100) would have true-positive results and 180 (.20 x 900) would have false positive results. The predictive value of a positive result would be 70÷250 or 28 per cent. Similar calculations can be made for negative test results.

The revision of diagnostic probabilities is sometimes counterintuitive; it has been shown that most physicians rely too heavily on positive test results when the disease prevalence or prior probability is low. Not uncommonly, a test that has a high predictive value positive when patients are already likely to have the disease in question, such as an exercise stress test of a patient with typical angina, is erroneously assumed to be equally predictive when applied as a screening test to individuals much less likely to have disease.

The relationship between a test's validity, as defined by its sensitivity and specificity, and its predictive value, dependent on disease prevalence or prior probability, is illustrated in Table 2–1. Patients with and without disease are indicated by row entries and test results are indicated by column entries. Note that when the prior probability (or prevalence) of the disease and the sensitivity and specificity of the test are known, the table can be completed and predictive values can be calculated.

CHARACTERISTICS OF TESTS AND OF POPULATIONS

As noted, sensitivity and specificity are theoretically characteristics of the test and therefore can be considered measures of test validity independent of the patients tested. In fact, while sensitivity and specificity are independent of disease prevalence, they still may vary from one population to another if criteria for the presence of disease are not precisely defined or if the prevalence of other conditions that affect test results varies in the populations tested. For example, if disease is more readily detected in later stages, test sensitivity (for the entire spectrum of disease) will appear higher in a population with a greater proportion of advanced disease when compared with sensitivity in a population with the same disease prevalence but with earlier, less detectable disease. The presence of another disease may make a false-positive test for the disease in question more likely. Such co-morbidity, if concentrated in the population tested, can decrease test specificity.

The predictive value of test results always depends on the prior probability or prevalence as well as on the sensitivity and specificity. Knowledge of test validity alone is insufficient for the calculation of

Table 2–1. Sensitivity, Specificity and Predictive Values

	POSITIVE TEST RESULT	NEGATIVE TEST RESULT	TOTALS
Disease Present	TP	FN	TP + FN
Disease Not Present	FP	TN	FP + TN
Totals	TP + FP	FN + TN	TP + FP + FN + TN

TP = Patients with True-Positive Results
FN = Patients with False-Negative Results
FP = Patients with False-Positive Results
TN = Patients with True-Negative Results

Sensitivity $= \dfrac{TP}{TP + FN}$ (and False-Negative Rate* $= \dfrac{FN}{TP + FN}$)

Specificity $= \dfrac{TN}{FP + TN}$ (and False-Positive Rate* $= \dfrac{FP}{FP + TN}$)

Predictive Value Positive $= \dfrac{TP}{TP + FP}$

Predictive Value Negative $= \dfrac{TN}{FN + TN}$

*These terms are often used ambiguously in the literature with some authors confusing $\dfrac{FN}{TP + FN}$ with $\dfrac{FN}{FN + TN}$ and $\dfrac{FP}{FP + TN}$ with $\dfrac{FP}{TP + FP}$.

Table 2–2. Effect of Prior Probability (Prevalence) on Predictive Value of Positive Test Results

PRIOR PROBABILITY (PREVALENCE)	PREDICTIVE VALUE OF POSITIVE TEST		
	SENSITIVITY 90% SPECIFICITY 90%	SENSITIVITY 95% SPECIFICITY 95%	SENSITIVITY 99% SPECIFICITY 99%
0.1%	0.9%	1.9%	9.0%
1%	8.3%	16.1%	50.0%
2%	15.5%	27.9%	66.9%
5%	32.1%	50.0%	83.9%
50%	90.0%	95.0%	99.0%

predictive values. This relationship is further illustrated by the results of the examples in Table 2–2.

The physician frequently has some choice about the sensitivity and specificity of a test. Obviously, alternative tests, usually those which are more costly or invasive, may be more sensitive *and* more specific. A new technology or an improved skill in interpretation may improve both measures. Often, however, the physician can increase sensitivity only by accepting a decrease in specificity. The most graphic examples involve tests that provide quantitative results, such as the measurement of intraocular pressure in glaucoma screening. Population studies indicate that a sensitivity of 70 per cent and specificity of 80 per cent are reasonable estimates for Schiotz tonometry if the cutoff point for a positive test is 21.9 mm. of mercury. Raising the discrimination value to 25.6 mm. of mercury increases specificity to 95 per cent, but decreases sensitivity to 50 per cent. The physician must trade one against the other. The general case is illustrated in Figure 2–1. Note that the usual "normal" values for the test results are derived from frequency distributions of results among apparently well individuals; the potential trade-off between sensitivity and specificity is not considered.

Which is more important, sensitivity or specificity? In general, the answer depends on the cost—including patient inconvenience, morbidity, and mortality as well as dollars—of false-negative results compared with false-positive results. Sensitive tests or less stringent criteria for disease and the resulting low false-negative rate should be favored when effective treatment for the condition exists and the cost of lost opportunity is great. High specificity or more stringent criteria for disease and the resulting low false-positive rate are most important when a positive diagnosis does not significantly change therapy or outcome but may be a burden for the patient.

Rarely is the physician aware of the population distribution of disease and nondisease or the precise trade-off between sensitivity and specificity when he interprets a test result. The technical precision and accuracy of laboratory results must also be considered. Nevertheless, appropriate test interpretation requires an understanding of the effect of prior probabilities on the predictive value of results and careful weighing of the costs of false-positive and false-negative conclusions.

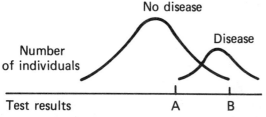

Fig. 2–1. Hypothetical distributions of test results (e.g., intraocular pressure measured by Schiotz tonometry) among patients with disease (e.g., glaucoma) and without disease. Because the test is not perfect, the distributions overlap. If all patients with values to the right of A are said to have "positive" results, the test will be 100% sensitive but will have a low specificity. If all patients with values to the right of B are said to have "positive" results, the test will be 100% specific but will have a low sensitivity. The choice of a cutoff value between A and B depends on the relative importance of false-positive and false-negative results (see text).

APPENDIX: BAYES' THEOREM

The revision of a prior probability on the basis of test results is an example of Bayes' theorem of conditional probability. Using the notation of probability theory, the simple case (disease is present or not) of Bayes' theorem can be expressed as:

$$P(D|T) = \frac{P(D) \cdot P(T|D)}{P(D) \cdot (T|D) + P(\bar{D}) \cdot P(T|\bar{D})}$$

Where: P (D) is the probability of disease (prior probability or prevalence);

P (T|D) is the probability of a positive test given that disease is present (sensitivity);

P (D̄) is the probability of no disease (1-prevalence);

P (T|D̄) is the probability of a positive test given that disease is not present (1-specificity); and

P (D|T) is the probability of disease given a positive test (predictive value positive).

Bayes' theorem can also be expressed using the terms introduced:

Predictive value positive =

$$\frac{\text{prevalence} \times \text{sensitivity}}{\text{prevalence} \times \text{sensitivity} + (1 - \text{prevalence}) \times (1 - \text{specificity})}$$

ANNOTATED BIBLIOGRAPHY

Elstein, A.S.: Clinical judgment: Psychological research and medical practice. Science, *194*:696, 1976. *(Discusses clinical and statistical models of medical decision-making.)*

Galen, R.S., and Gambino, S.R: Beyond Normality: The Predictive Value and Efficiency of Medical Diagnosis. New York: John Wiley & Sons, 1975. *(Application of concepts of sensitivity, specificity and predictive value to illustrate clinical problems.)*

McNeil, B.J., Keeler, E., and Adelstein, S.J.: Primer on certain elements of medical decision-making. N. Engl. J. Med., *293*:211, 1975. *(Concise review of applications of decision theory and information theory to the diagnostic process.)*

Ransohoff, D.F., and Feinstein, A.R.: Problems of spectrum and bias in evaluating the efficacy of diagnostic tests. N. Engl. J. Med., *299*:926, 1975. *(Reviews problems in disease definition and population selection that may affect evaluations of diagnostic tests.)*

Vecchio, T.J.: Predictive value of a single diagnostic test in unselected populations. N. Engl. J. Med., *274*:1171, 1966. *(Early paper pointing out the importance of prevalence to predictive value.)*

3

Health Maintenance and the Role of Screening

Public interest in health maintenance or, more positively, health enhancement has grown dramatically in recent years. Many Americans have demonstrated their interest in exercise, good dietary habits, maintenance of appropriate body weight, and stress reduction. Increased enthusiasm stems from growing awareness of associations between elements of lifestyle and health. Despite reliable evidence and public acceptance of these associations, however, many people continue to indulge in self-destructive habits such as smoking, overeating, and alcohol abuse. Efforts to alter such behavior are often frustratingly ineffective. Patients who seek reassurance from physician visits that include routine screening procedures often persist in behavior that greatly increases their risk of morbidity.

Physicians must acknowledge their primary role in prevention as that of educators. Accurate information regarding risk factors is most likely to reinforce health-enhancing behavior and alter self-destructive behavior. The physician must appreciate the potential for behavior modification and familiarize himself with local resources. Routine screening for specific diseases, the health maintenance activities most closely identified with the physician, should be performed selectively. The limits of screening tests as well as their potential health benefits should be clearly understood by every primary physician.

Specific risk factors and screening tests are discussed in subsequent chapters. This chapter will focus on the question, "What makes a disease or risk factor worth screening for?" The relationship between prevalence and predictive value of a test is particularly important in the screening situation (see Chapter 2). Because the physician is more interested in improving health outcomes for patients rather than simply providing them with diagnoses, elements of the natural history of the disease and of the effectiveness of therapy are critically important.

CRITERIA FOR SCREENING

Whether or not a screening policy results in improved health outcomes depends on characteristics of

Table 3–1.   Criteria for Screening

Characteristics of the Disease
1. Significant effect on the quality or length of life
2. Prevalence sufficiently high to justify costs
3. Acceptable methods of treatment available
4. Asymptomatic period during which detection and treatment significantly reduce morbidity and/or mortality
5. Treatment in the asymptomatic phase yields a better therapeutic result than treatment delayed until symptoms appear

Characteristics of the Test
1. Sufficiently sensitive to detect disease during the asymptomatic period
2. Sufficiently specific to provide acceptable predictive value positive
3. Acceptable to patients

Characteristics of the Population Screened
1. Sufficiently high disease prevalence
2. Accessibility
3. Compliance with subsequent diagnostic tests and necessary therapy

the disease(s), characteristics of the test(s) and characteristics of the patient population. These are summarized in Table 3–1.

NATURAL HISTORY OF THE DISEASE AND EFFECTIVENESS OF THERAPY

Screening tests are performed to identify asymptomatic disease. The alternative is to wait until the patient presents with symptoms and then make a diagnosis. The question is then, "What makes a disease worth diagnosing early?" The practical objective of screening is prevention of morbidity and mortality—not simply early diagnosis. There is little benefit to the patient, and perhaps considerable harm, in advancing the time of diagnosis of a disease for which earlier treatment does not influence outcome.

The importance of the natural history of the disease and effectiveness of therapy can be illustrated by considering Figure 3–1. As schematically shown, some variable time after the biological onset of a disease, a diagnosis is possible using a screening test. This is followed by another variable time period during which the patient has no symptoms. Usually, a short time after symptoms appear, the clinical diagnosis is made. Eventually, after the course of therapy has been selected and completed, there is an identifiable clinical outcome that can range from cure and complete health to death.

Often, outcome depends somewhat on the point during the natural history of the disease at which therapy is initiated. This is most clear in the case of localized versus metastatic cancer. Many tumors can be readily excised, and the patient cured of the disease, during early stages. The opportunity for cure is often lost when tumor spread makes excision or other local therapy impractical. The "escape from cure" may not be as dramatic as the point of tumor metastasis; a disease may simply become more refractory to therapy, increasing the likelihood of morbid complications. The practical purpose of screening is to advance the time of the diagnosis to a point in the natural history of the disease when a relative or absolute "escape from cure" is less likely to have occurred.

While the natural history of any disease varies a great deal among individuals afflicted, some generalizations are worthwhile. If an "escape from cure" generally occurs at point A in Figure 3–1 or at any point before available screening tests can detect the disease in question, the value of screening must be

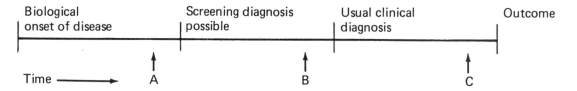

"Escape from cure" at point A: Screening may not affect outcome

"Escape from cure" at point B: High priority for screening

"Escape from cure" at point C: Education and improved access to care may be more efficient than screening tests

Fig. 3–1.   Relationships between screening and natural history of disease.

questioned. The most frequent result will be bad news sooner for the patient but no difference in outcome. If "escape from cure" routinely occurs after symptoms appear (for example at point C), screening may be valuable, but could likely be supplanted by patient and professional education programs aimed at insuring early presentation and prompt diagnosis. Diseases in which "escape from cure" generally occurs after the disease is detectable but while it remains asymptomatic (for example at point B) are the most appropriate targets of screening efforts.

Several points about the evaluation of screening programs can also be made with reference to Figure 3–1. Critics of indiscriminate screening point out that the benefits of a screening program can easily be overestimated if the relationship between time of diagnosis and natural history is not understood. One fallacy is to neglect the importance of *lead time* when evaluating the effect of screening on subsequent survival. Since screening has the potential to advance the time of diagnosis from one point in the natural history to another and since survival is by necessity measured from the time of diagnosis rather than onset, the survival of patients whose diseases are detected by screening should be expected to be longer than that of patients who present symptomatically. Extensive follow-up data on many patients allow approximation of the average length of time by which the diagnosis is advanced by screening. This illusory gain in survival, the lead time, can then be subtracted from any measured difference in survival duration to learn the true benefits of the screening program.

The second fallacy that can lead to overestimation of screening benefits depends on the variability in natural history among individual cases of the same disease. Individuals who have less aggressive disease and thereby spend more time in a detectable but asymptomatic stage are, other things being equal, more likely to be detected by a screening test than are patients with more aggressive disease. If patients with indolent asymptomatic disease are more likely to have an indolent clinical course after diagnosis, patients diagnosed by screening should be expected to have longer survival rates than patients who present symptomatically. Arguments about the impact of such biological determinism rather than advancing the time of diagnosis have most frequently been raised with regard to breast cancer. They apply generally to questions of screening, however. This potential bias toward prolonged survival among patients detected by screening tests has been called *time-linked bias sampling.*

Neither of these arguments is meant to deny the value of screening for treatable disease. They simply advise caution in interpreting apparently favorable results based on unsophisticated measures of effectiveness.

VALIDITY OF AVAILABLE SCREENING TESTS AND POPULATION SCREENED

Diseases worth identifying usually have a relatively low prevalence in the asymptomatic population. As a result, the specificity of the diagnostic test used is the principal determinant of the predictive value positive of the test. Tests that may be very useful in diagnosis when the prior probability of disease is 10 or 20 per cent may have an unacceptable rate of false-positive results when used in a screening situation. Such nonspecificity has been referred to as the *cost* of a screening test. The costs, including morbidity and patient concern, of diagnostic evaluations among patients with false-positive screens can far outweigh other costs of a screening program. The sensitivity and specificity of the screening test, costs, and patient acceptability are critical considerations in the decision to screen for disease.

The importance of disease prevalence in determining the predictive value positive is one basis for the use of risk factors in screening policy. By limiting screening to a high-risk population, the physician in effect increases the prevalence of the disease in the population tested (and alternatively increases the prior probability of the disease in any individual), thereby increasing the predictive value positive and decreasing the number of false-positive results.

HEALTH MAINTENANCE— WHAT IS APPROPRIATE?

Periodic health evaluation has been recommended with varying degrees of enthusiasm throughout the 20th century. Many patients believe in its value; the majority of Americans feel that more health resources should be expended on preventive efforts. Recently, however, the value of periodic examinations and specific preventive measures has been questioned. Evidence regarding the effectiveness of periodic examinations, measured in terms of decreased morbidity and mortality, is fragmentary. Supporters argue that there are additional benefits of regular physician contact that result in a greater sense of well-being. Such contact provides opportunities for appropriate patient education.

Routine examinations should be tailored to the risks of the individual patient. The use of indiscriminate laboratory screening has been shown to increase consumption of health care resources without evidence of benefit. The importance of characteristics of the patient, the disease, and the test in determining the appropriateness of specific attempts to identify asymptomatic disease has been reviewed in this chapter. The screening and health maintenance chapters that follow review available information about such characteristics and apply it to specific diseases or risk factors. It should be noted that uncertainty about test sensitivity and specificity, risk factors, and particularly natural history rarely, if ever, allows proof of the effectiveness of a screening procedure. Conclusions and recommendations based on the sometimes contradictory or highly speculative data available are therefore controversial.

ANNOTATED BIBLIOGRAPHY

Breslow, L., and Somer, A.R.: The lifetime health-monitoring program. N. Engl. J. Med., *296*:60, 1977. *(Specific screening prescriptions by age group.)*

Canadian Taskforce on the Periodic Health Examination: The periodic health examination. Can. Med. Assoc. J., *121*:1193, 1979. *(Provides recommendations for screening and health maintenance; based on very thorough study.)*

Cole, P.: What should the physician ask? Cancer, *37*:434, 1976. *(Part of a valuable collection of articles in the same issue on screening for cancer. Focuses on importance of directed history-taking to identify special risks of patients.)*

Feinleb, M., and Zelen, M.: Some pitfalls in the evaluation of screening programs. Arch. Eviron, Health, *19*:412, 1969. *(Reviews problems with predictive value positive, lead time, and time-linked bias sampling.)*

Frame, P.S., and Carlson, S.J.: A critical review of periodic health screening using specific screening criteria. J. Fam. Pract., *2*:29; 123; 189; 283; 1975. *(Considers 36 diseases. Screening recommended for only a few based on specific criteria.)*

Screening for Disease. Lancet, October 5 to December 21, 1974 (18-part series). *(A review of screening with unenthusiastic conclusions.)*

Spitzer, W.O., and Brown, B.P.: Unanswered questions about the periodic health examination. Ann. Intern. Med., *83*:257, 1975. *(Reviews the issue in terms of impact on health and effect on doctor-patient relationship.)*

4

Immunization
HARVEY B. SIMON, M.D.

Immunizations are an effective and important means of controlling many communicable diseases through primary prevention. The power of immunization programs is nowhere more evident than in the case of smallpox, which is now on the verge of total eradication as a result of an aggressive worldwide vaccination program. But if smallpox vaccine has been rendered obsolete through its own effectiveness, the other immunizing agents have not. An appalling number of Americans have not received their recommended immunizations. In large part, this is a failure of public education and of access to health care delivery. But while the pediatrician has been traditionally effective in immunizing individual patients, the primary care internist too often overlooks the importance of immunization.

Except for travelers, patients rarely request immunizations. It is up to the physician, then, to initiate consideration of immunization. The first step is to take a detailed immunization history. In addition, a history of prior adverse reactions to vaccines and of egg allergy should be sought. Finally, it is important to be aware of the current prevalence of infectious diseases in the local community, and, in the case of the traveler, in other parts of the world.

GENERAL PRINCIPLES OF IMMUNIZATION

In general, live attenuated vaccines (Table 4–1) provide more complete and longer lasting immunity than inactivated agents. However, because live vac-

Table 4-1. Immunizing Agents

Live Attenuated Vaccines
1. Viral
   a. Polio
   b. Measles
   c. Rubella
   d. Mumps
   e. Yellow fever
   f. Vaccinia

Inactivated Agents
1. Viral
   a. Influenza
   b. Rabies
2. Bacterial
   a. Pneumococcus
   b. Meningococcus
   c. Diphtheria (toxoid)
   d. Tetanus (toxoid)
   e. Pertussis
   f. Typhoid
   g. Cholera

Vaccines Prepared from Egg Media
1. Influenza
2. Rabies
3. Rocky Mountain spotted fever
4. Typhus
5. Yellow fever

Immunoglobulin Preparations for Passive Immunization
1. Human
   a. Immune serum globulin
   b. Tetanus immune globulin
   c. Measles immune globulin
   d. Vaccinia immune globulin
   e. Rabies immune globulin
   f. Zoster immune globulin
2. Equine
   a. Diphtheria antitoxin
   b. Botulism antitoxin

In pregnancy, rubella vaccine is absolutely contraindicated because of its potential teratogenicity. In general, other live virus vaccines should be avoided in pregnancy unless the risk of exposure and illness clearly outweighs the possible risks of the vaccine itself. Inactivated vaccines are safe in pregnancy.

Because passive immunity can interfere with active immunity, it is best to defer immunizations until 3 months have elapsed following administration of gamma globulin, blood, or plasma. Travelers requiring both vaccines and gamma globulin should receive the immune serum globulin 2 weeks after completing the vaccinations, if possible.

Patients who have exhibited hypersensitivity reactions to a vaccine should not receive that product again. Individuals with egg allergies should not be given vaccines prepared in egg cultures (Table 4–1). If multiple-dose immunization schedules are delayed or interrupted, they should be resumed without administering additional doses, no matter how long the interval between doses. In general, immunization should be avoided during significant febrile illnesses. Mild upper respiratory infections, however, need not preclude immunizations.

The decision to immunize must include consideration of the frequency of the condition, chances of exposure, risks and benefits of immunization, and cost.

cines can produce serious disseminated disease in the immunosuppressed host, these preparations should be avoided in patients who are immunologically deficient (leukemia or lymphoma patients, steroid and cancer chemotherapy recipients, patients with agammaglobulinemia, etc.). Inactivated vaccines (Table 4–1) are safe in these patients.

Two inactivated vaccines can be given simultaneously at separate injection sites, as can an inactivated vaccine and a live vaccine. However, if significant local or systemic reactions are anticipated, as is often the case with cholera or typhoid vaccines for example, it may be best to administer the vaccines on separate days. On theoretical grounds, it is desirable to separate vaccination with live virus vaccines by at least 1 month. However, studies have shown that a combination of measles, mumps, and rubella vaccines can be given to children along with the trivalent oral polio vaccine without adverse reactions or loss of effectiveness.

SPECIFIC IMMUNIZING AGENTS

Diphtheria and Tetanus Toxoid and Pertussis Vaccine

Although both diphtheria and tetanus are now uncommon in the United States, all individuals should receive the excellent protection afforded by the toxoids which are prepared by formaldehyde treatment of the bacterial toxins. Pertussis vaccine is indicated in all children below age 6, but older individuals are not nearly as susceptible to pertussis and should not receive the vaccine. Children between 6 weeks and 6 years of age should be given the combined diphtheria, pertussis, and tetanus (DPT) product. For patients first receiving immunization after age 6, three tetanus-diphtheria (Td) injections should be administered, with the second dose 1 to 2 months after the initial dose and the third dose 6 to 12 months later. A booster should be administered every 10 years.

Tetanus-diphtheria immunization is the only immunization universally indicated in adults (Table 4–

2), but is frequently overlooked. Immigrants and elderly individuals, particularly women and men who have not served in the military, are especially likely never to have been immunized.

If a patient has received a full primary tetanus series and boosters at regular 10-year intervals, additional boosters are not necessary at the time of injury. Other individuals should receive tetanus-diphtheria toxoids for minor wounds and both tetanus-diphtheria toxoids and tetanus immune globulin (TIG) for more serious wounds (Table 4-3).

Polio Vaccine

Although all children should receive polio vaccine, the very low incidence of poliomyelitis in the United States makes the routine immunization of adults unnecessary. Travelers who have never been immunized against polio and who are anticipating

Table 4-2. Indications for Immunization in Adults

Primary Immunization or Booster in All Adults
  Tetanus-diphtheria
Immunization in Selected, Vulnerable Individuals
  Influenza (the elderly and debilitated)
  Pneumococcus (sickle cell disease, splenectomy, elderly and debilitated)
  Rubella (women of childbearing age who are antibody-negative; must avoid pregnancy for 3 months)
Immunizations in Certain Epidemiologic Situations
  Immune serum globulin (for household exposures to hepatitis A and possibly hepatitis B)
  Meningococcus (epidemics; possibly household contacts; only types A and C available)
  BCG (selected tuberculin-negative individuals expecting intense exposure to tuberculosis)
Immunizations for International Travel (Depending on Area)
  Typhoid (two injections plus booster)
  Cholera (within two months of departure)
  Yellow Fever (Africa, South America)
  Polio (tropical or developing areas; booster or primary series if never immunized)
  Smallpox (Somalia, and where required by law)
  Plague (rural Vietnam, Cambodia, Laos)
  Typhus (rarely necessary)
  Immune Serum Globulin (for hepatitis A)
Passive Immunizations After Exposure
  Rabies Immune Globulin (plus vaccine)
  Tetanus Immune Globulin (plus toxoid)
  Diphtheria Antitoxin (plus toxoid)
  Botulism Antitoxin
  Immune Serum Globulin (for hepatitis A and possibly hepatitis B)
  Vaccinia Immune Globulin (for complications of smallpox vaccination)
  Zoster Immune Globulin (for certain vulnerable individuals after exposure; available only from CDC)
  Measles Immune Globulin (for certain vulnerable individuals after exposure)

Table 4-3.   Guide to Tetanus Prophylaxis

HISTORY OF TETANUS IMMUNIZATION (DOSES)	CLEAN MINOR WOUNDS		ALL OTHER WOUNDS	
	Td	TIG	Td	TIG
Uncertain	Yes	No	Yes	No
0-1	Yes	No	Yes	Yes
2	Yes	No	Yes	No*
3 or more	No†	No	No‡	No

Td = Tetanus-Diphtheria Toxoids
TIG = Tetanus Immune Globulin (human)

*Unless wound more than 24 hours old
†Unless more than 10 years since last dose
‡Unless more than 5 years since last dose
Source: Morbidity and Mortality Weekly Reports, 26:49, p. 407 (12/9/77)

visits to rural areas of developing countries should receive a full series of trivalent oral polio vaccine (TOPV) with the second dose 6 to 8 weeks after the first, and the final dose 8 to 12 months later. Previously immunized travelers should receive a single booster dose. An inactivated vaccine is available for use in immunosuppressed patients.

Measles, Mumps and Rubella Vaccines

These three live attenuated virus vaccines are available in a combined preparation for use in children at age 15 months or older. Measles and mump vaccines, however, are rarely indicated in adults. Nonimmune adult males are at risk for mumps orchitis. However, susceptibility is difficult to predict, since many adults with no history of clinical mumps are nevertheless immune as a result of subclinical childhood infection, and the mumps skin test is not a reliable predictor of immunity. Hence, routine mumps vaccination of adult males cannot be recommended. Immune serum globulin is not of proven value in post-exposure prophylaxis. Rubella vaccine is recommended for adolescent and adult women if serological tests for rubella antibody are negative, and if they are able to avoid pregnancy for 3 months following immunization. The most common side effects of rubella vaccination are arthralgias.

Smallpox Vaccine

Universal smallpox immunization in the United States was abandoned in 1971 because of the disappearance of the disease. Smallpox is on the verge of extinction, and vaccination is recommended only for travelers to any region in which it reappears, or to countries requiring an International Certificate of Vaccination.

Influenza Vaccine

Influenza remains a major worldwide problem because of frequent antigenic shifts in the virus. New vaccines are prepared in anticipation of the viral strains which are expected to prevail during the winter flu season. Indications for vaccination vary from year to year, depending on vaccine availability, the likelihood of influenza epidemics, and vaccine toxicity. In general, the elderly and debilitated, particularly those with cardiopulmonary disease, should receive influenza vaccine in the autumn prior to the flu season. Unlike other viral infections, a chemical agent, amantadine, is available to prevent clinical disease in patients exposed to influenza A_2. Amantadine is particulary useful in elderly patients directly exposed to the flu, as in nursing home outbreaks.

Meningococcus Vaccine

Vaccines prepared from the cell wall polysaccharides of types A and C meningococcus are now licensed and are available as monovalent A, monovalent C, or bivalent A-C vaccines. These are not recommended for general use, but are indicated for control of epidemics as in the military and for travelers to areas experiencing outbreaks of meningococcal meningitis. Meningococcal vaccine may be of some benefit in household contacts of patients with meningococcal disease.

Pneumococcus Vaccine

A multivalent vaccine prepared from pneumococcal capsular polysaccharides was licensed in this country from 1945 to 1947, but was withdrawn because of lack of use. Despite the use of penicillin and other antibiotics, however, pneumococcal pneumonia has remained a major cause of morbidity and mortality in the United States, with an estimated 500,000 cases annually and a case fatality rate of 5 to 10 per cent. A new vaccine released in 1978 contains 14 polysaccharide types which are responsible for about 80 per cent of pneumococcal disease. The vaccine appears to be at least 80 per cent effective in preventing pneumonia caused by these serotypes, and has been safe and well-tolerated thus far. Pneumococcal vaccine is indicated in individuals with increased susceptibility to pneumococcal infection, including splenectomized patients and those with sickle cell disease, nephrotic syndrome, cirrhosis, and chronic cardiopulmonary disease. Because mortality from pneumococcal pneumonia increases with age beyond age 50, the elderly can be expected to benefit from the vaccine as well; it is not clear, however, if age alone should be an indication for vaccination in the absence of underlying disease, or at what age such routine vaccination should be considered. Antibody response to pneumococcal vaccine has been poor below age 2.

Rabies Vaccine and Rabies Immune Globulin

Preexposure rabies vaccination is recommended only for people with occupational exposure to rabies virus. Both active immunization with vaccine and passive immunization with rabies immune globulin may be indicated after animal bites. Table 4–4 presents the United States Public Health Service guidelines for postexposure prophylaxis.

BCG Vaccine

Bacillus Calmette-Guerin vaccine is a live attenuated strain of *Mycobacterium bovis* which is up to 80 per cent effective in preventing tuberculosis. However, because of the sharp decline in new cases of primary tuberculosis in the United States, BCG, is recommended only in selected tuberculin-negative individuals with unavoidable intense exposure to tuberculosis, such as children of mothers with active tuberculosis. BCG may be useful in travelers anticipating close contact with people infected with tuberculosis, but an alternate approach is tuberculin skin-testing before and after travel, with administration of isoniazid in the event of skin-test conversion.

Immune Serum Globulin for Viral Hepatitis

Commercially available pooled human gamma globulin is of proven benefit in preventing or clinically modifying type A hepatitis ("infectious hepatitis"), particularly if given within 2 weeks of exposure to the virus. Individuals closely exposed to patients with hepatitis should be given gamma globulin, especially household contacts. The recommended dosage is .02 ml. per kg. body weight, or about 2 ml. in adults. Immune serum globulin is also useful in preventing hepatitis A in travelers to underdeveloped areas where hepatitis is endemic; the dose is 2 ml. for brief travel, and 5 ml. for travel of longer than 3 months, with repeat doses every 4 to 6 months if needed.

The use of gamma globulin for prevention of hepatitis B ("serum hepatitis") is under active study. Commercially available pooled gamma globulin is not effective in preventing parenterally transmitted hepa-

Table 4–4.   Guide to Postexposure Rabies Prophylaxis*

ANIMAL SPECIES	CONDITION OF ANIMAL AT TIME OF ATTACK	TREATMENT OF EXPOSED HUMAN
Wild		
Skunk		
Fox		
Coyote	Regard as rabid	RIG† + DEV‡
Raccoon		
Bat		
Domestic		
Cat or dog	Healthy	None§
	Unknown (escaped)	RIG + DEV
	Rabid or suspected rabid	RIG + DEV
Other		Consider individually

*These recommendations are only a guide. They should be applied in conjunction with knowledge of the animal species involved, circumstances of the bite or other exposure, vaccination status of the animal, and presence of rabies in the region.

†RIG (rabies immune globulin, human) is administered only once, at the beginning of therapy. Dose is 20 IU/kg., one-half muscularly in the buttocks and one-half thoroughly infiltrated around the wound. Equine anti-rabies serum should be used only if RIG is not available.

‡DEV (duck embryo vaccine) is administered in 23 1-ml. doses, starting the day that RIG is given. DEV may be given as 21 daily doses or as 2 doses/day for the first 7 days followed by 7 daily doses. A 1-ml. booster dose should be injected subcutaneously in the abdomen, lower back, or lateral aspect of the thigh; rotation of sites is recommended. Serum should be collected from all patients for rabies antibody testing at the time of the second booster dose.

Vaccine should be discontinued if fluorescent antibody test of animal killed at time of attack are negative.

§RIG and DEV should be started at first sign of rabies in biting dog or cat during 10-day holding period.

Modified with permission from *Recommendation of the Public Health Service Advisory Committee on Immunization Practices: Rabies.* U.S. Department of Health, Education, and Welfare, Public Health Service, Center for Disease Control, Atlanta, Georgia, April 1977.

titis B, but may be helpful in dealing with nonparenterally transmitted hepatitis B, as in household contacts. Special hyperimmune globulin is available for needle-stick exposure to hepatitis. (See Chapter 70.)

Typhoid Fever Vaccine

Although typhoid vaccination is not required, it is recommended for people traveling to parts of Africa, Asia, and Central and South America where the disease is endemic. The immunization series consists of two subcutaneous injections separated by at least 1 month, with boosters every 3 years if needed for additional travel. Typhoid vaccine is only about 70 per cent effective in preventing infection with *Salmonella typhi;* travelers should maintain vigilance with regard to food and water. Febrile reactions to the vaccine are relatively common.

Cholera Vaccine

Although cholera vaccine is incompletely effective, and the risk of cholera in Americans traveling abroad is low, cholera vaccination is required for travel to certain countries. One injection of vaccine prior to departure is sufficient for travel certification; a full primary series for individuals traveling to areas in which the disease is endemic includes a second injection at least a week after the first, with a booster every 6 months if indicated.

Yellow Fever Vaccine

This live attenuated viral vaccine is available only at designated yellow fever vaccination centers. Yellow fever is endemic in parts of tropical South America and Africa, and vaccination is required for travelers to these areas.

Typhus and Plague Vaccines

These vaccines are seldom indicated in American travelers, except for the occasional individual anticipating prolonged exposure in rural areas of Southeast Asia and scattered other remote regions.

Additional Prophylactic Measures for International Travel

In addition to ascertaining and obtaining appropriate immunizations, the traveler faces a number of potential health problems. All travelers should be evaluated medically before a long or difficult trip and should be fully informed about their medical status. The patient with chronic illness may find it useful to take along medical summaries and copies of electrocardiograms. An adequate supply of medication is essential. Patients with potentially serious illnesses might best be advised to avoid medically unsophisticated areas of the world.

Travelers to areas where malaria transmission might occur should be advised to take *malaria prophylaxis*. In most instances, the recommended drug is chloroquine phosphate, which is administered once weekly beginning at least 1 week prior to departure and continuing for 6 weeks after return. The drug is generally well-tolerated and serious toxicity on this schedule is rare, even if it is continued for prolonged periods. The dose of chloroquine is 5 mg. per kg. of body weight up to the full adult dose of 300 mg. base (500 mg. of chloroquine phosphate). The prophylaxis of chloroquine-resistant *P. falciparum* malaria is a difficult problem. Chloroquine-resistant strains are found in parts of Southeast Asia, Central America (including Panama), and northern South America. Malaria prophylaxis for travel to these regions remains controversial, and physicians faced with this problem should call the Center for Disease Control in Atlanta, Georgia, for the latest recommendations.

Travelers to tropical and underdeveloped areas should be cautioned to avoid potentially contaminated water and ice. Carbonated beverages, boiled water, and tea and coffee made with boiled water are generally safe. Chemical treatment of water with chlorine or iodine is also helpful, but while most pathogenic viruses and bacteria are killed, cysts capable of causing amebiasis or giardiasis may survive. Foods must also be selected with care. Most well-cooked hot food is safe, but raw fruits and vegetables should be avoided and dairy products should be consumed only if hygienic preparation and proper refrigeration are assured.

Although *traveler's diarrhea* is an extremely common problem, guidelines for its management remain imperfect. Mild self-limited diarrhea should remain untreated, except for appropriate fluid replacement. Widely used obstipating agents such as diphenoxylate (Lomotil) may provide symptomatic relief, but can actually prolong the course of bacterial diarrheas. Many cases of traveler's diarrhea are caused by enteropathogenic strains of *E. coli*. The role of antibiotics such as ampicillin in managing these infections is unclear. A recent study suggests that the prophylactic administration of doxycycline may help prevent traveler's diarrhea, but more studies are needed. Travelers should be advised to seek medical attention if they develop severe or protracted diarrhea, especially if accompanied by passages of blood or mucus, or if high fever is present. However, medical care may be unavailable in some areas, and "empirical" self-medication with ampicillin may be the only practical, if imperfect, alternative.

Further Information

An authoritative source of additional information on vaccinations and travel is the Center for Disease Control, 1600 Clifton Road, N.E., Atlanta, Georgia 30333. Useful publications available to physicians on request to the CDC include the *Morbidity and Mortality Weekly Reports* and the annual booklet, *Health Information for International Travel*.

ANNOTATED BIBLIOGRAPHY

Rimland, David, McGowan, J.E., Jr., Shulman, J.A.: Immunization for the internist. Ann. Intern. Med., 85:622, 1976. *(A comprehensive review of the role of the internist in immunization of adults.)*

Sack, D.A., Kaminsky, D.C., Sack, R.B., *et al.*: Prophylactic doxycycline for traveler's diarrhea. Results of a prospective—blind study of Peace Corps volunteers in Kenya. N. Engl. J. Med., 298:758, 1978. *(A double-blind clinical trial demonstrating that prophylactic administration of doxycycline can reduce the incidence of "turista.")*

U.S. Department of Health, Education and Welfare/ Public Health Service: Pneumococcal polysaccharide vaccine. Morbidity and Mortality Weekly Report; *27*(4):25, 1978. *(Recent CDC recommendations for the use of this important new vaccine.)*

U.S. Department of Health, Education and Welfare/ Public Health Service: Chemoprophylaxis of malaria. Morbidity and Mortality Weekly Report; *27*:10, Supplement, 1978. *(A detailed discussion of the chemoprophylaxis of malaria, including the difficult problem of chloroquine-resistant malaria.)*

U.S. Department of Health, Education and Welfare/ Public Health Service: Health information for international travel, 1977. Morbidity and Mortality Weekly Report, *26,* Supplement, 1977. *(These CDC reports are released annually and provide authoritative information on the health requirements of international travel.)*

Wolfe, M.S.: Management of the traveler to exotic places. Milit. Med.: *141*:831, 1976. *(A useful review of practical medical advice for the traveler.)*

2

Constitutional Problems

5

Evaluation of Chronic Fatigue

Chronic fatigue is a frustrating problem to assess because it is so vague. Nevertheless, it is one of the most frequent complaints seen in the office setting and is important because it is a sensitive though nonspecific indicator of underlying medical and/or emotional pathology. Regardless of cause, the patient typically reports a lack of energy, listlessness and generalized disinterest in family, work and leisure activities. Some patients inappropriately use the term "weakness" to describe their problem, though motor function remains intact. Many speculate that they have vitamin deficiencies, low iron or anemia. Self-treatment with vitamin and iron supplements is frequent.

Many people bothered by fatigue come to the primary physician looking for an organic cause; few initially admit to an emotional problem, even though most studies of fatigue report psychological etiologies in the vast majority of cases. The primary physician has the task of determining whether the problem is mainly a physiological or an emotional one; sometimes both mechanisms coexist.

PATHOPHYSIOLOGY AND CLINICAL PRESENTATIONS

Almost all illnesses are capable of causing fatigue; however, a few are noteworthy for the prominence of the symptom in the clinical presentation.

Fatigue is an important somatic symptom of *depression*, often coexisting with early morning awakening, appetite disturbances and multiple bodily complaints. Changes in central nervous system catecholamine metabolism are believed to play a major role in the pathogenesis of depression (see Chapter 215). *Chronic anxiety* may result in generalized fatigue, due in part to difficulty in obtaining adequate physical and psychological rest. Patients report trouble falling asleep and a host of associated bodily complaints. Many maintain their neck muscles in constantly tensed states, giving rise to occipital-nuchal headaches. Palpitations, difficulty breathing, chest tightness, and gastrointestinal troubles add to the clinical picture (see Chapter 214).

Some of the medications used to treat anxiety and depression have substantial sedating effects; when used in excess, they may actually worsen the patient's sense of fatigue rather than alleviate it. Of the *tricyclic antidepressants,* amitriptyline (Elavil) is among the more sedating, which makes it useful when agitation is a problem, but it can cause some patients to feel "knocked out" in the morning (see Chapter 215). Chronic use of *hypnotics* may aggravate difficulty in falling asleep and contribute to fatigue (see Chapter 220). *Minor tranquilizers* such as diazepam (Valium) can cause tiredness when taken daily in frequent doses sufficient to result in accumulation of high serum levels of the drug and its active metabolites (see Chapter 214). *Reserpine* may precipitate depression, especially when used in daily doses exceeding 0.5 mg; patients with a previous history of depression are at greater risk. The effect is believed to be due to depletion of norepinephrine stores. *Propranolol* has been implicated in the causation of fatigue and depression. In a series of 390 hypertensives, fatigue was the major reason for having to limit the dose of the drug.

Endocrine disturbances are treatable precipitants. Dysfunction of the thyroid, adrenal, pituitary, parathyroid or endocrine pancreas can be subtle in onset, starting out inconspicuously as fatigue. For example, *hypothyroidism* may begin with fatigue, often in association with weight gain, dry skin, mild hoarseness, cold intolerance, etc. (see Chapter 100). Patients with *Addison's disease* manifest insidious onset of fatigue in conjunction with weight loss, vague gastrointestinal upset, postural hypotension and, eventually hyperpigmentation. *Panhypopituitarism* may result from postpartum hemorrhage or a tumor of the sellar region. The patient with postpartum disease (Sheehan's syndrome) fails to lactate or menstruate; lassitude, decreased libido, and loss of axillary and pubic hair slowly develop. Later, symptoms of hypothyroidism may ensue.

Diabetes with marked glycosuria is another endocrinologic etiology of fatigue. When glycosuria is severe enough to produce caloric wasting and fatigue, there is usually polyphagia, polyuria and polydipsia (see Chapter 98). *Hyperparathyroidism* as well as other causes of hypercalcemia may present with fatigue and weakness. In an NIH series of 57 cases of primary hyperparathyroidism, fatigue was the most frequent symptom, occurring in 24 per cent. *Apathetic hyperthyroidism* is an uncommon but important source of fatigue in the elderly. Presentation includes profound weight loss and unexplained atrial fibrillation, in addition to apathy and extreme fatigue (see Chapter 99).

The correlation between iron deficiency anemia and fatigue is often poor, especially when the anemia is mild (see Chapter 83). In a double-blind study of menstruating women with mild anemia due to iron deficiency, there was no significant difference between the effects of iron and placebo on fatigue. The relation between severe anemia (hematocrit<20) and fatigue is more direct. Lassitude prevails, at times in association with exertional dyspnea or with postural hypotension when blood loss is acute.

Chronic congestive heart failure and *chronic lung disease* are sometimes heralded by lassitude, but dyspnea is a prominent feature, along with other obvious signs of heart and lung disease (see Chapters 27, 36, and 44).

Most *chronic inflammatory, infectious* or *neoplastic* processes are capable of precipitating fatigue; general malaise may even be the initial symptom. Fever, night sweats, weight loss, or pain often contribute to the clinical picture. Fatigue may precede the joint symptoms of rheumatoid disease (see Chapter 147). Marked fatigue and lymphadenopathy are the hallmarks of infectious mononucleosis (see Chapter 80).

Chronic renal failure may present inconspicuously with fatigue and few localizing symptoms or signs aside from laboratory findings of azotemia, mild anemia, impaired renal concentrating ability, and an abnormal urinary sediment (see Chapter 135). *Hepatocellular failure* is an important source of lassitude. Jaundice, ascites, petechiae, asterixis, spider angiomata and other signs of hepatic insufficiency usually contribute to the clinical picture. However, in chronic hepatitis, jaundice may be minimal while fatigue is prominent; the same holds for the prodromal phase of acute viral hepatitis (see Chapters 70 and 71).

DIFFERENTIAL DIAGNOSIS

Although the list of conditions which may present with fatigue is extensive, most cases have a strong overlay of anxiety and/or depression, even when the etiology is medical. Fatigue, of course, may accompany any illness, but those listed in Table 5–1 are notable for the prominence of lassitude in the clinical presentation. In a series of 300 cases of fatigue evaluated at the Lahey Clinic, 80 per cent were due to an emotional problem, 4 per cent to chronic infection, 3 per cent to heart disease, 2 per cent to anemia, and 1 per cent to nephritis.

WORK-UP

In most instances, the evaluation of fatigue can be conveniently performed in the office. Two or three visits may be needed to establish the underlying etiology; at times the patient may insist that medical illness be ruled out before agreeing to discuss psychosocial matters.

History should begin with a thorough description of the fatigue to be sure that the patient is not confusing focal neuromuscular disease with general-

Table 5-1. Some Conditions Presenting as Chronic Fatigue

1. Psychologic
   a. Depression
   b. Anxiety
2. Endocrine-Metabolic
   a. Hypothyroidism
   b. Diabetes mellitus
   c. Apathetic hyperthyroidism of the elderly
   d. Pituitary insufficiency
   e. Hyperparathyroidism or hypercalcemia of any origin
   f. Addison's disease
   g. Chronic renal failure
   h. Hepatocellular failure
3. Pharmacologic
   a. Hypnotics
   b. Antihypertensives
   c. Antidepressants
   d. Tranquilizers
4. Infections
   a. Endocarditis
   b. Tuberculosis
   c. Mononucleosis
   d. Hepatitis
   e. Parasitic disease
5. Neoplastic-Hematologic
   a. Occult malignancy
   b. Severe anemia
6. Cardiopulmonary
   a. Chronic congestive heart failure
   b. Chronic obstructive pulmonary disease

ized lassitude. Because depression underlies many cases of fatigue, it is essential to check for its somatic manifestations, such as early morning awakening, alteration of appetite, and multisystem functional complaints. It is also important to ask about significant losses, low self-esteem, and occurrence of crying spells and suicidal thoughts. Anxiety is suggested by unresolved conflict, persistent nervousness, recurrent bouts of excessive uneasiness, and trouble falling asleep. Any abuse of hypnotics or tranquilizers need to be ascertained and considered as a cause of disturbed sleep and resultant fatigue.

Fever, sweats, weight loss, change in bowel habits and adenopathy point toward smoldering infection or occult neoplasm. Weight loss can also be found in depression, Addison's disease and apathetic hyperthyroidism. Symptoms suggesting metabolic and endocrinologic causes include polyuria, polydipsia, changes in skin pigmentation and texture, hoarseness, cold intolerance, nausea, abdominal discomfort, etc. Also, any history of anemia, blood loss. renal disease, jaundice, urinary tract infections, or exposure to tuberculosis, hepatitis, or infectious mononucleosis

should be elicited. Epidemiologic considerations include travel in areas where parasitic infections are endemic and work in meat-packing industries or on a farm. Recent dental work and a known heart murmur may be clues to endocarditis. Symmetrical joint pain and morning stiffness suggest rheumatoid disease.

A full listing of all the patient's medications should be obtained. Of particular importance are over-the-counter antihistamine preparations used for allergies, nasal congestion and sleep, as well as any psychotropic agents, antihypertensives and other centrally acting drugs which may have been prescribed.

Physical examination should include rectal temperature and postural blood pressure determinations. If there is no fever on examination in the office, but fever is still a consideration, the patient should be instructed to take and record his temperature at home at 10:00 p.m. nightly when fever is likely to be maximal. Skin is assessed for change in pigmentation, purpura, dryness, rash, jaundice and pallor. Endocarditis may first be suggested by the finding of splinter hemorrhages or petechiae. Fundoscopic examination may reveal Roth's spots, diabetic retinopathy, or even, in rare instances, a tuberculoma. The sclerae are observed for icterus. If examination of the pharynx reveals petechiae at the junction of the hard and soft palate, mononucleosis ought to be considered. Tender lymphadenopathy may be a sign of infection or rapidly growing tumor; painless, firm glands require that tumor be·ruled out (see Chapter 80). The thyroid is checked for goiter; the lungs for rales, consolidation or effusion; and the heart for murmurs, gallops and rhythm disturbances. Unexplained atrial fibrillation in the elderly patient may be a manifestation of apathetic hyperthyrodism.

The abdomen is palpated for organomegaly, masses, ascites and hepatic tenderness. Rectal masses, prostatic enlargement and occult blood in the stool are looked for. Joint examination includes assessment for effusion, synovial thickening and deformity. Limbs are palpated for tenderness, tested for strength and observed for fasciculations indicative of a neuromuscular disease.

Laboratory studies. In the patient with a completely normal history and physical exam, and strong evidence for depression, there is no need to proceed with further laboratory investigation. In the patient with no evidence of depression, yet a normal history and physical, it may be useful to obtain a few simple blood tests: serum calcium, electrolytes, BUN,

SGOT and blood sugar in search of sub-rosa endocrinologic, hepatic or renal disease. Rarely is a T_4 or TSH helpful in the absence of other evidence suggesting hypothyroidism. If the patient is elderly, free thyroxine and total T_3 determinations may detect the occasional case of apathetic hyperthyroidism. In most patients with a normal history and physical exam, an in-depth evaluation of the emotional and social matrix is more likely to yield information with regard to the cause of fatigue than is a blind search for an occult medical condition.

SYMPTOMATIC RELIEF

When the cause of fatigue is endocrinologic, metabolic or infectious, treatment needs to be specific and aimed at the underlying condition. Malignancy is often accompanied by a reactive depression which can be helped by development of a strong, supportive doctor-patient relationship (see Chapter 90). The fatigue of endogenous depression can be treated with support and tricyclic antidepressants; imipramine may be less sedating than amitriptyline (starting dose is 25 to 50 mg. at bedtime, increased by 25 to 50 mg. at a time). The sleep disorder caused by depression may respond well to small doses, with the fatigue dissipating as the patient gets a good night's sleep. Affective changes may not occur at low doses (see Chapter 215).

Anxiety-related fatigue can be difficult to treat. Prescribing anti-anxiety agents can lead to excessive use and worsening of symptoms (see Chapter 214); however, a brief and limited trial of benzodiazepine therapy at bedtime is worth an attempt; e.g., 5 mg. of chlordiazepoxide can help the patient to fall asleep and get much-needed rest. There is no evidence that any one benzodiazepine is superior to any other for sleep, although flurazepam is widely promoted and prescribed, often in conjunction with another benzodiazepine. (This can sometimes lead to excessive benzodiazepine intake.) Once symptomatic control of anxiety is accomplished, work can begin on helping the patient to deal with his problems.

ANNOTATED BIBLIOGRAPHY

Allan, F.N.: Differential diagnosis of weakness and fatigue. N. Engl. J. Med., *231*:414, 1944. *(A classic study of 300 patients presenting to the Lahey Clinic with fatigue; an emotional etiology was present in 80 per cent.)*

Aurbach, G., Mallette, L., Patten, B., *et al.*: Hyperparathyroidism: Recent studies. NIH conference. *Ann. Intern. Med., 79*:566, 1973. *(Fatigue headed the list of symptoms reported in 57 cases of primary hyperparathyroidism; 24 per cent reported the problem.)*

Kales, A., Bixler, E., Tan, T., *et al.*: Chronic hypnotic use: Ineffectiveness, drug withdrawal, insomnia, and hypnotic drug dependence. JAMA, *227*:513, 1974. *(Chronic hypnotic use may actually worsen the problem of sleeplessness and its attendant difficulties.)*

Severe depression caused by reserpine. Medical Letter, *18*:17, 1976. *(Reviews the evidence linking reserpine with depression, and advises against using doses in excess of 0.25 mg. per day or prescribing to depressed patients.)*

Thomas, F., Mazzaferri, E., and Skillman, T.: Apathetic thyrotoxicosis: A distinctive clinical and laboratory entity. Ann. Intern. Med., *72*:679, 1970. *(These patients are typically elderly, are depressed in appearance, and have marked weight loss. In this small series, 7 of 9 had atrial fibrillation and many presented with cardiac complaints.)*

Wood, M., and Elwood, P.: Symptoms of iron deficiency anemia: A community survey. Br. J. Prev. Soc. Med., *20*:117, 1966. *(Correlation between hemoglobin concentration and symptoms was poor. Iron therapy produced no statistically significant improvement in symptoms.)*

Zacharias, F.: Patient acceptability of propranolol and occurrence of side effects. Post Grad. Med. J.: *52*(4):87, 1976. *(In a series of 390 hypertensives on propranolol, fatigue was reported as the most common side effect, which limited dose; the incidence of the problem was less than 5 per cent.)*

6
Evaluation of Fever
HARVEY B. SIMON, M.D.

Since antiquity, fever has been recognized as a cardinal manifestation of disease. Indeed, people identify fever as a sign of illness more readily than they recognize the importance of most other symptoms. In addition to causing concern, the presence of fever usually raises high therapeutic expectations. Even in the preantibiotic era, John Milton observed that "the feaver is to the Physitians, the eternal reproach" (1641); in the popular mind today, fever is equated with infection, and infections are expected to respond to the administration of "wonder drugs." As a result, the physician is faced with the challenge of defining the etiology of the fever, instituting appropriate therapy, and explaining the reasons for limiting antibiotic usage to bacterial infections.

PATHOPHYSIOLOGY AND CLINICAL PRESENTATION

Popular lore notwithstanding, 98.6°F (37°C) is *not* normal body temperature. In fact, there is no single normal value; like so many other biological functions, body temperature displays a circadian rhythmicity. In healthy individuals, mean rectal temperatures vary from a low of about 97°F (36.1°C) in early morning to a high of about 99.3°F (37.4°C) in late afternoon. In children, the normal range may be even greater. Moreover, physiological factors such as exercise and the menstrual cycle can further alter body temperature. In practical terms, understanding the diurnal rhythm of body temperature is important for two reasons. First, many patients have been unnecessarily subjected to extensive workups and even psychologically invalided in erroneous quest of a cause for deviation from the mythical "normal" of 98.6°F. Second, the fever of disease states is superimposed upon the normal cycle, so that fevers are generally highest in the evenings and lowest in the mornings. As a result, frequent temperature recordings throughout the day are required to monitor fever in sick patients; the absence of fever in a single office visit does not exclude a febrile illness.

The presenting complaints of the febrile patient may be explained by the fever itself or by the underlying disease process. The signs and symptoms caused by fever *per se* vary tremendously. Some patients with fever are otherwise asymptomatic. More common is a sensation of warmth or flushing, usually with malaise and fatigue. Myalgias are common and may be severe. These are probably best explained by the fact that in order to raise body temperature to its new set point, the hypothalamus, via somatic efferents, increases muscle tone, and this may be painful. These same factors account for one of the most dramatic manifestations of fever: the shaking chill or rigor. It is taught that rigor is a manifestation of bacteremia, but in fact any stimulus which raises the hypothalamic setpoint rapidly may produce a rigor. Patients experiencing a rigor exhibit uncontrolled violent shaking and trembling and characteristically heap themselves with blankets even as their temperatures are shooting up. This phenomenon also has a physiological basis. Despite the high central or core temperature, these patients subjectively feel cold because surface temperature is reduced: in order to generate fever in response to hypothalamic stimuli, cutaneous vasoconstriction occurs, skin temperature falls, and cold receptors in the skin sense this as cold. Quite the reverse occurs during defervescence; body temperature falls in response to cutaneous vasodilatation, and drenching sweats typically terminate an episode of fever.

Other manifestations of temperature elevation include central nervous system symptoms ranging from a mild inability to concentrate to confusion, delirium or even stupor, especially in the elderly or debilitated patient. High fevers (104°-106°F) may produce convulsions in infants and young children without any primary neurologic disorder. Increased cardiac output is an invariable consequence of fever, and tachycardia typically accompanies fever. Tachycardia is so usual that its absence should lead one to suspect uncommon problems such as typhoid fever, in which relative bradycardia is typical (for unknown reasons), or even to think of factitious fever. Patients with underlying heart disease may respond to the high output stress of fever with angina or heart failure.

Another sign of fever may be the so-called fever blister—labial herpes simplex. The problem is probably not precipitated by fever *per se*, for it is much more common in some infections, such as pneumococcal pneumonia and meningococcal meningitis, than in other febrile states.

Because fever accompanies infection so frequently, numerous investigators have tried to determine if fever has any protective or beneficial role. There are a few circumstances, such as central nervous system syphilis, in which elevations of body temperature may exceed the thermal tolerance of the infectious agent. In fact, induced fever was once a form of therapy for syphilis. Aside from a few other exceptions, fever has no known role in host defense, except insofar as it impels the patient to seek medical attention.

Is fever detrimental? Most otherwise healthy individuals can tolerate temperatures up to 105°F (40.5°C) without ill effects, although even in these individuals symptoms often warrant therapy. In children, high fevers should be suppressed because convulsions may occur. Patients with heart disease should also receive antipyretic therapy. Each 1°F of temperature increases the basal metabolic rate by 7 per cent, resulting in increased demands on the heart which may precipitate myocardial ischemia, failure or even shock. In addition, extreme hyperthermia beyond 108°F (42.1°C) can cause direct cellular damage, probably by denaturing protein. Vascular endothelium seems particularly susceptible to such damage, and disseminated intravascular coagulation frequently accompanies extreme hyperthermia. Other structures which may be directly damaged include brain, muscle and heart. Finally, metabolic derangements such as hypoxia, acidosis, and sometimes hyperkalemia can result from extreme pyrexia, and in turn further contribute to coma, seizures, arrhythmias or hypotension, which may be lethal. Nevertheless, patients have survived temperatures of up to 108° without demonstrable organ damage, but mortality in this temperature range is appreciable. Body temperatures as high as 113° been demonstrated in man, but these have been uniformly lethal.

Table 6–1. Causes of Fever of Undetermined Origin

"THE BIG THREE"

I. Infections: 40%
   A. Systemic
      1. Tuberculosis (miliary)
      2. Infective endocarditis (subacute)
      3. Miscellaneous infections: cytomegalovirus infection, toxoplasmosis, brucellosis, psittacosis, gonococcemia, chronic meningococcemia, disseminated mycoses
   B. Localized
      1. Hepatic infections (liver abscess, cholangitis)
      2. Other visceral infections (pancreatic, tuboovarian, and pericholecystic abscesses, and empyema of gallbladder)
      3. Intraperitoneal infections (subhepatic, subphrenic, paracolic, appendiceal, pelvic and other abscesses
      4. Urinary tract infections (pyelonephritis, renal carbuncle, perinephric abscess, prostatic abscess)
II. Neoplasms: 20%. Especially lymphomas, leukemias, renal cell carcinoma, atrial myomas, and cancers metastatic to bone or liver
III. Collagen-vascular disease: 15%. Including temporal arteritis and juvenile rheumatoid arthritis as well as systemic lupus erythematosus, rheumatoid arthritis, polyarteritis nodosa, Wegener's granulomatosis, and mixed connective tissue disease

LESS COMMON CAUSES

I. Noninfectious granulomatous diseases (especially sarcoidosis and granulomatous hepatitis)
II. Inflammatory bowel disease
III. Pulmonary embolization
IV. Drug fever
V. Factitious fever
VI. Hepatic cirrhosis with active hepatocellular necrosis
VII. Miscellaneous uncommon diseases (familial Mediterranean fever, Whipple's disease, etc.)
VIII. Undiagnosed

Modified from Jacoby, G. A., and Swartz, M. N., N. Engl. J. Med., *289*:1407, 1973.

weeks, exceeding temperatures of 101°F, and eluding 1 week of intensive diagnostic study.

DIFFERENTIAL DIAGNOSIS

Many inflammatory, infectious, neoplastic or hypersensitivity processes may produce fever. Most acute fevers are accompanied by obvious signs and symptoms of the underlying cause, such as upper respiratory infection, cystitis, gastroenteritis. However, unexplained persistent fever can be a major diagnostic challenge. Table 6–1 lists causes of "fevers of unknown origin," defined as those persisting for 3

WORKUP

The febrile patient presents a common but demanding problem in differential diagnosis. In most cases, a careful history and physical exam will provide important clues, so that laboratory studies can be utilized selectively. In addition, the initial office evaluation should help determine the proper pace of diagnostic tests and of therapeutic intervention. If the illness is insidious in onset and only slowly pro-

Table 6–2. Febrile Patients Requiring
Special Attention

1. Vulnerable Hosts
   a. Age (very young or very old)
   b. Corticosteroid or immunosuppressive therapy
   c. Serious underlying diseases (neutropenia, sickle
      cell anemia, diabetes, cirrhosis, advanced COPD,
      renal failure, malignancies, etc.)
   d. Implanted prosthetic devices (heart valves, joint
      prostheses, etc.)
2. Toxic Patients
   a. Rigors, prostration, extreme pyrexia
   b. Hypotension, oliguria
   c. CNS abnormalities
   d. Cardiorespiratory compromise
   e. New significant cardiac murmurs
   f. Petechial eruption
   g. Marked leukocytosis or leukopenia

gressive, or if the patient is nontoxic and clinically
stable, one may proceed with the workup in a deliberate manner on an ambulatory basis, utilizing serial
clinical observations and time as key diagnostic tools.
On the other hand, if the patient is a compromised
host, or if he is acutely ill and toxic, several immediate diagnostic studies are mandatory, and treatment
may even be required before all results are available;
hospitalization is usually necessary in such cases. Table 6–2 lists some factors which should prompt an
aggressive approach to diagnosis and therapy.

Febrile illnesses are most commonly acute processes which are either readily diagnosed and treated
(common bacterial infections) or are self-limited despite the lack of a specific diagnosis (viral infections,
allergic reactions). However, occasionally patients
will present with undiagnosed fevers fulfilling the
classic criteria for "fever of unknown origin." In both
situations, the key to diagnosis is often a meticulous
history and physical exam.

History. The infectious disease history should
stress several items not routinely emphasized: (1)
host factors, (2) epidemiology, (3) symptomatology,
(4) drug history. In regard to *host factors,* one
should determine if the patient is basically healthy,
or if he has an underlying disease which may render
him unusually susceptible to infection. Patients with
hematologic and other malignancies, diabetes mellitus, neutropenia or sickle cell anemia may become
infected with unusual opportunistic pathogens or
may fail to respond normally to common infectious
agents. Patients taking corticosteroids or other immunosuppressive agents are especially vulnerable to
infection. Individuals with implanted prosthetic devices such as artificial heart valves or hip prostheses

are also at increased risk of serious infection. Finally,
patients with past histories of certain infectious processes such as pyelonephritis may be prone to relapses or recurrences of similar problems.

Turning to *epidemiology,* it is helpful to ask if
the patient has traveled to places where he may have
been exposed to "exotic" infections such as typhoid
fever or malaria. Less obvious factors such as exposure to animals may be of great importance. Vectors
of infection may be found even among household
pets, such as cats (cat-scratch disease and *Pasteurella multocida* cellulitis from bites or scratches, and
toxoplasmosis from fecal contamination), parakeets
(psittacosis) and turtles (salmonellosis). A history of
bites by stray dogs, skunks or bats may suggest the
possibility of rabies. More commonly, exposure to
someone with a communicable disease such as tuberculosis or influenza can provide the central clue to
diagnosis. An inquiry into what is "going around" in
the community may be helpful. The patient's occupational history is sometimes revealing as well; for example, abatoir workers may be exposed to brucellosis, leather workers to anthrax, and gardeners to
sporotrichosis.

Attention to *symptomatology* may serve to pinpoint the site of infection. Localizing symptoms such
as headache, alterations of consciousness, cough,
dyspnea, flank pain, dysuria, or abdominal pain, are
particularly useful in focusing diagnostic studies. Finally, history should include a careful inquiry into
any *drugs* used. Has the patient been taking antibiotics which may alter his susceptibility to infection by
favoring drug-resistant organisms or mask infection
by rendering him culture-negative? Does he have
drug allergies or underlying problems such as renal
failure which may alter the choice of therapeutic
agents? Is the patient taking any medications which
may be responsible for fever as a manifestation of
hypersensitivity?

Physical examination. Unlike other conditions in
which the physical examination is only confirmatory,
essential clues may be uncovered by a detailed examination of the febrile patient. Vital signs should be
determined in all cases. Fever is an important but
nonspecific sign of infection; some patients with infections are afebrile while others may have a fever
resulting from noninfectious causes such as hypersensitivity states and lymphoreticular malignancies. The
shaking chill or rigor may suggest bacteremia but is
also not specific. In the neonate or in occasional
adults with overwhelming sepsis, hypothermia may
be present. Respiratory distress may signal pulmo-

nary infection or septic shock, and hypotension may be the presenting finding leading to a diagnosis of sepsis.

The skin and mucous membranes may provide crucial information. To cite a few examples: petechial eruptions suggest meningococcemia or Rocky Mountain spotted fever; pustular lesions, gonococcemia (see Chapter 113) or staphylococcal endocarditis; splinter hemorrhages and conjunctival petechiae, endocarditis; ecthyma gangrenosa, *Pseudomonas* septicemia; macular or vesicular eruptions, viral infections. Similarly, the optic fundi should be examined. Roth spots suggest endocarditis. Choroidal tubercles may be the only positive finding in miliary tuberculosis, and similar lesions may result from *Candida* septicemia.

Enlarged lymph nodes should be carefully sought and their distribution noted (see Chapter 80). Examination of the chest includes a search for signs of pneumonia and empyema, and the heart is auscultated for murmurs and rubs. Abdominal examination may reveal hepatomegaly, splenomegaly or signs of biliary sepsis, abscess formation or peritonitis. The rectal and pelvic examinations are essential for the diagnosis of prostatic or pelvic infections (see Chapters 133 and 113). Musculoskeletal examination may suggest septic arthritis or osteomyelitis (see Chapter 138). Neurologic evaluation may raise the possibility of meningitis or encephalitis.

Laboratory studies. If the history and physical examination provide strong indications of an infectious process, laboratory studies can be used selectively to confirm or refute the clinical diagnosis. For example, in the patient with an obvious viral upper respiratory infection, no studies are necessary. In patients with bronchitis, a sputum smear and culture may be all that are required, but if pneumonia is a possibility, a chest radiograph and CBC are minimal additional requirements (see Chapter 43). In the patient with probable cystitis, a urinalysis and culture are sufficient, but if pyelonephritis is likely, a CBC, blood cultures and renal function tests should be added, and an IVP may be very helpful (see Chapter 129).

In other patients, however, more extensive tests are needed to establish a diagnosis when the cause of fever remains unknown. While such studies must be individualized, the approach to diagnosis of an obscure fever should include:

COMPLETE BLOOD COUNTS AND DIFFERENTIAL.

Leukocytosis and a "shift to the left" suggest but do not prove bacterial infection. Toxic granulations, Döhle bodies and vacuoles in polymorphonuclear leukocytes are suggestive of bacterial sepsis, but are not entirely specific. While the erythrocyte sedimentation rate is very nonspecific, it may be helpful in occasional patients. A normal erythrocyte sedimentation rate (ESR) can provide reassurance and obviate further studies if the patient appears well, while a very elevated ESR is an invitation to additional testing and may even be a clue to a specific process such as temporal arteritis (see Chapter 150).

URINALYSIS. Pyuria strongly suggests urinary tract infection. Gram stain of the unspun urine specimen can be diagnostic (see Chapter 129).

RADIOGRAPHIC STUDIES. Chest radiographs may detect infiltrates or effusions even in the absence of abnormalities on physical examination, while KUB and upright abdominal films can disclose air-fluid levels in the bowel. Contrast studies and scans may be needed if there is suspicion of abscess, tumor or other mass lesions. (See below.)

BLOOD CHEMISTRIES. The blood sugar determination is helpful in search of previously unsuspected diabetes mellitus. The test is also important in evaluating the significance of the sugar concentration in various body fluids. Liver function tests are useful in helping to define obscure sources of fever. For example, transaminase elevation suggests hepatitis, and isolated rises in alkaline phosphatase point to infiltration of the liver.

EXAMINATION OF BODY FLUIDS. If there is any possibility of meningitis, a lumbar puncture is mandatory. Aspiration and study of pleural effusions, ascitic fluid or joint effusions may be diagnostic. Such specimens should be examined directly by cell counts and stains (see below). Sugar and protein determinations help differentiate etiologies; in general, bacterial, mycobacterial and fungal infections produce low sugar and high protein levels in body fluid.

CULTURES. If the patient has a heart murmur, or a prosthetic heart valve, or appears seriously ill, cultures of blood should be obtained (having at least two blood cultures from separate venipunctures is preferred). Most patients should have cultures taken of urine (clean catch or catheterized specimen), and sputum. If other body fluids are obtainable, they should likewise be cultured. Special mycobacterial and fungal media are required if these agents are suspected, especially if the patient is a compromised host. Anaerobic cultures are important when one is dealing with a possible abscess or other infection of the pulmonary, gastrointestinal pelvic regions.

MICROSCOPIC EVALUATION. Any body fluid which can be obtained should be examined by the Gram stain technique. Sputum, urine, wound exudates, cerebrospinal fluid, pleural fluid, ascitic fluid and joint fluid often reveal the cause of infection on Gram stain. Even Gram stains of the stool may be helpful in certain specific situations, such as acute diarrhea with suspicion of staphylococcal enterocolitis. The presence of bacteria in a specimen of body fluid which is normally sterile is presumptive evidence of infection. This is particularly true when one is examining the spun sediment obtained from cerebrospinal fluid. Likewise, bacteria are not found in normal ascitic, joint or pleural fluid. Bacteria in unspun urine correlates well with the presence of a significant urinary tract infection. However, Gram stains must be examined and interpreted with a certain amount of caution. For example, if one sees epithelial cells in a sputum specimen, one can be certain that the specimen contains mouth organisms and is not representative of conditions in the tracheobronchial tree. In such instances, one should obtain a better sputum sample, either by reexpectoration or by an invasive technique such as transtracheal aspiration. In the presence of bacterial pneumonia, the sputum usually contains many polymorphonuclear leukocytes and a large number of bacteria. Acid-fast stains are required to visualize mycobacteria (see Chapter 43), and specially stained wet mounts of body fluids can be useful in uncovering numerous types of fungal infections.

IMMUNOLOGIC STUDIES. Serological tests (e.g., Widal titers for salmonella, ASLO titers for streptococcal infections and acute rheumatic fever, the heterophil for infectious mononucleosis) and skin tests (especially the tuberculin test) need to be considered in the workup. Testing for antinuclear antibody and rheumatoid factor may help in the diagnosis of a vasculitis. The presence of rheumatoid factor or immune complexes (Raji cell assay) can be clues to "culture-negative" endocarditis or underlying rheumatoid disease (see Chapter 139). In the diagnosis of obscure fevers, it is often useful to freeze and save an "acute phase serum" for later comparison with a "convalescent serum."

OTHER STUDIES. Needless to say, an enormous number of studies are available for the evaluation of undiagnosed febrile illnesses. It is important to proceed with these in a logical, step-by-step fashion in-stead of subjecting the patient to a random series of expensive, time-consuming, uncomfortable or even hazardous studies. The first step in the subsequent workup is to document fever by measuring rectal temperatures every 4 hours. If fever is documented, further testing should be directed to the most common causes of fever of unknown origin, as listed in Table 6–1. Obviously, the order of testing should be determined by clues present in the individual patient, beginning with the simplest, least expensive studies. Radiographic studies which may be revealing when carefully selected include a barium enema, an upper GI series with small bowel follow-through, an intravenous pyelogram (with lateral views for retroperitoneal nodes), abdominal ultrasound, liver-spleen scan, lung scan, and possibly gallium scanning or lymphangiography. Bone marrow or liver biopsy may be very helpful. A lumbar puncture is unlikely to help unless nuchal rigidity neurologic abnormalities are present. A blind laparotomy should not be performed unless there are clear-cut clues to intra-abdominal abnormalities which cannot be evaluated with less-invasive procedures.

THERAPEUTIC TRIALS. In the acutely ill patient it may be necessary to begin broad antibiotic coverage before the diagnosis is established. It is essential, though commonly forgotten, to obtain cultures of blood, urine and other pertinent fluids prior to initiating treatment so that rational decisions can be made later concerning therapy. In the patient with a true "FUO," blind therapeutic trials are rarely helpful, and are often confusing or even harmful. In this context it is useful to remember one definition of empiric therapy, i.e., that which the ignorant do to the helpless. In occasional patients with fever of unknown origin, therapeutic trials may be necessary, including intravenous antibiotics for suspected culture-negative endocarditis, combined chemotherapy for occult tuberculosis, or salicylates or steroids for noninfectious inflammatory disease. Such trials should always be conducted with a specific end point or time limit in mind, carefully planned observations, patient consent, and a mixture of humility and trepidation.

THE SECOND LOOK. Despite the array of sophisticated technology available for the study of febrile illnesses, the history and physical examination remain the keys to diagnosis in most cases. Time can be a most valuable diagnostic tool. Unless the patient is progressively deteriorating, it may be advisable to interrupt the workup for a period of clinical observation, possibly with the aid of symptomatic therapy such as antipyretics. A second look, beginning with the history and physical examination, may then be fruitful.

SYMPTOMATIC THERAPY

The best therapy is obviously to treat the underlying cause. However, antipyretic therapy may provide comfort and prevent complications. The first issue, of course, is to determine if fever should be treated. Elevated temperature itself does not necessarily call for therapy. But if unpleasant symptoms are present, if the patient has limited cardiac reserve, or if the complications of fever are imminent, antipyretics should be administered.

Antipyretic therapy depends upon the use of both chemical agents and physical methods. The most effective antipyretic drugs are the salicylates and acetaminophen; both appear to act on the hypothalamus to lower the thermal set point. Although parenteral salicylates are available, oral or rectal administration of either aspirin or acetaminophen is preferable. Doses of up to 1.2 grams of either drug may be given to adults to initiate antipyretic therapy. In addition to intrinsic toxicities, it must be remembered that both aspirin and acetaminophen may occasionally produce an overresponse, with hypothermia and even dangerous hypotension. Patients with typhoid fever or Hodgkin's disease, and the elderly and debilitated seem to be at somewhat greater risk for this uncommon complication. Other drugs which may be considered in special circumstances are the phenothiazines, which also act directly on the hypothalamus. However, phenothiazine therapy of fever has a substantial toxic potential, and must be considered experimental.

Physical cooling is also extremely effective. At the simplest level, undressing the patient and exposing him to a cool ambient temperature will allow cooling by radiation; a bedside fan will promote cooling by convection, as well. Sponging with cool water or alcohol is also helpful, promoting evaporation. With extreme elevations (greater than 106°F), more drastic measures are necessary and hospitalization urgent. Immersion in an ice water bath is the most efficient of these methods and may be indicated in hyperthermic emergencies such as heat stroke. All methods of physical cooling present the risk of hypothermic over-response and should, therefore, be discontinued when body temperature begins to fall below critical levels.

Hyperthermic emergencies are rare, but fever is common, and most often presents as an unpleasant symptom rather than a medical crisis. It seems appropriate, therefore, to conclude with a comment about patient comfort. Although fever causes discomfort in most patients, use of physical cooling produces discomfort in virtually all individuals; often the treatment is remembered as far worse than the illness itself. As a result, these measures should be employed only when fever itself presents medical problems. The same is true to a lesser extent of aspirin and acetaminophen. In particular, many patients find rapid rises and falls of temperature very distressing; therefore, administering antipyretics every 4 hours for the first day or two of treatment may be preferable to waiting for the height of the fever spike.

INDICATIONS FOR ADMISSION

When temperature reaches 105°F, hospitalization needs to be considered. The very toxic or vulnerable patient (see Table 6–2) should be admitted promptly for aggressive study, monitoring and control of temperature. When there is weight loss and debilitation, early hospitalization should also be considered. Moreover, when fever remains elevated beyond 101°F for weeks and ambulatory diagnostic efforts have been unsuccessful, it is often beneficial to bring the patient into the hospital for closer evaluation and documentation of fever; the advice of an infectious disease consultant can be helpful.

PATIENT EDUCATION

Whenever fever is suspected in the ambulatory setting, the patient should be instructed to keep a record of temperatures, preferably rectal, taken each evening, when elevations are most likely to occur. The patient needs to be assured that there is nothing abnormal about temperatures in the range of 97.0°F to 99.3°F.

ANNOTATED BIBLIOGRAPHY

Deal, W.B., and Cluff, L.E.: Fever. *In* L.E. Cluff and J.E. Johnson (eds.), Clinical Concepts of Infectious Diseases. Baltimore: Williams & Wilkins Co., 1972, p. 111. *(A useful overview of clinical aspects of fever.)*

Dinarello, C.A., and Wolff, S.M.: Pathogenesis of fever in man. N. Engl. J. Med., *298*:607, 1978. *(A* comprehensive basic science review of recent advances in the understanding of the pathogenesis of fever.)

Jacoby, G.A., and Swartz, M.N.: Fever of undetermined origin. N. Engl. J. Med., *289*:1407, 1973. *(A concise clinical update on the etiologic considerations which should be undertaken in the patient with FUO.)*

Petersdorf, R.G., and Beeson, P.B.: Fever of unexplained origin: Report on 100 cases. Medicine, *40*:1, 1961. *(A classic paper which defines the etiologies of FUO and details a logical diagnostic approach.)*

Simon, H.B.: Extreme pyrexia. JAMA, *236*:2419, 1976. *(A study of the etiologies and consequences of temperatures of 106° F and above.)*

7

Evaluation of Weight Loss

Involuntary weight loss is a very sensitive, though nonspecific, indicator of underlying illness. In many instances accompanying symptoms readily suggest the cause, but when a marked fall in weight is the sole or predominant complaint, the assessment can be difficult since the list of etiologies is extensive. Identifying the principal mechanism(s) of weight loss on clinical grounds helps to limit the range of possibilities and focus laboratory testing.

PATHOPHYSIOLOGY AND CLINICAL PRESENTATION

When the number of calories available for utilization falls below daily needs, weight is lost; 1 pound of fat is consumed for every 3500-calorie deficit. The principal mechanisms resulting in caloric deficits are reduced food intake, malabsorption, excess nutrient loss and increased caloric requirements. Loss of fluid will also register as a fall in weight, with about 1 kg. (2.2 pounds) lost for every liter removed.

Although more than one mechanism may be operating in a given case, each mechanism has a few characteristic clinical features. Anorexia or disinterest in food typifies causes of *reduced intake.* Foul-smelling, bulky, greasy stools are seen in the later stages of *malabsorption;* subtle changes in stool consistency and frequency are noted earlier (see Chapter 58). Recurrent vomiting, profuse diarrhea, polyuria or fistulous drainage can lead to *excessive loss.* Increased food intake, hyperactivity or fever are prominent in cases of *increased demand.*

Many conditions associated with weight loss are clinically obvious and require little discussion, but others may be subtle in presentation with few obvious manifestations beyond substantial fall in weight. Anorexia nervosa, carcinoma of the pancreas, early malabsorption, apathetic hyperthyroidism of the elderly, and diabetes are examples of illnesses which sometimes fall into the latter category and deserve further elaboration.

The patient suffering from *anorexia nervosa* may deny any disturbance of appetite, yet persist in restricting food intake to the point of cachexia. The condition occurs predominately among adolescent girls and young women. They decide to diet to an extreme degree, are preoccupied with a phobic concern about being fat and are motivated by a relentless pursuit of thinness. Dieting persists because its psychological gratifications outweigh those derived from intake of food. Paradoxically, the patient often reports feeling well and initially appears bright and undisturbed by the weight loss; anorexia is usually denied. At times, a few specific foods are the only ones consumed, e.g., vegetable juices. Amenorrhea is invariable and appears shortly after weight loss begins. A variant of anorexia nervosa consists of surreptitiously induced vomiting which follows engorgement with food; hypokalemic alkalosis results.

Carcinoma of the pancreas is the archetypal neoplasm associated with dramatic weight loss. Mean age of onset is 55; males outnumber females by 2 to 1. There are about 9.5 cases per 100,000 population. Weight loss is found in 79 to 90 per cent at time of diagnosis, and averages 15 to 20 pounds. The degree of weight loss does not seem to correlate with size, location or extent of disease. For example, in a series of 100 cases, eight patients had resectable tumors; of the eight, two had weight losses of 25 to 40 pounds respectively. Aversion to food is more typical of this malignancy than is true anorexia. In many instances,

Table 7-1.   Some Important Causes of
Weight Loss

1. Decreased Intake
   a. Anorexia nervosa
   b. Depression
   c. Anxiety
   d. Poor dentition
   e. Esophageal disease
   f. Gastrointestinal disease worsened by food
   g. Drugs (e.g., digitalis excess, amphetamines, anti-tumor agents)
   h. Hypercalcemia
   i. Alcoholism
   j. Prodrome of viral hepatitis
   k. Hypokalemia
   l. Uremia
   m. Malignancy
   n. Chronic congestive heart failure
   o. Chronic inflammatory disease
2. Impaired Absorption
   a. Cholestasis
   b. Pancreatic insufficiency
   c. Postgastrectomy
   d. Small bowel disease
   e. Parasitic infection (e.g., giardiasis)
   f. Blind loop syndrome
   g. Drugs (e.g., cholestyramine, cathartics)
3. Increased Nutrient Loss
   a. Uncontrolled diabetes mellitus
   b. Persistent diarrhea
   c. Recurrent vomiting
   d. Drainage from a fistulous tract
4. Excess demand
   a. Hyperthyroidism
   b. Fever
   c. Malignancy
   d. Emotional states (e.g., manic disease)
   e. Amphetamine abuse

weight loss precedes all other symptoms; once jaundice and abdominal pain supervene, the tumor is usually far advanced. Many other gastrointestinal malignances follow a similar clinical course.

In addition to occult malignancy, a host of other conditions may present predominently with weight loss due to an appetite disturbance and are described elsewhere: depression (see Chapter 215), alcoholism (see Chapter 216), the prodrome of viral hepatitis (see Chapter 70), hypercalcemia (see Chapter 94), uremia (see Chapter 135), hypokalemia, and digitalis excess (see Chapter 27).

Marked weight loss is a late sign of *malabsorption,* but modest reductions can occur in the early stages of illness when stools are noted to be a bit softer and more frequent than usual. Steatorrhea, abdominal discomfort, bloating and pain accompany more dramatic falls in weight when disease is farther

advanced. Early *Crohn's disease* in adolescents has been noted on occasion to begin inconspicuously with anorexia predominating. For example, in a small series of eleven adolescent girls labeled as having anorexia nervosa, three turned out to have Crohn's disease when barium studies were obtained. *Blind loop syndrome* and *giardiasis* may also have indolent presentations with weight loss and vague abdominal discomfort; however, changes in stools are usually present as well, with patients reporting of mushy, foulsmelling bowel movements (see Chapter 58).

Increased caloric demand due to hyperthyroidism is usually obvious; however, *apathetic hyperthyroidism* of the elderly may be mistaken for malignancy because weight loss is profound and the patient appears listless. The typical symptoms of excess thyroid hormone are absent, and unexplained atrial fibrillation is often present (see Chapter 99).

Although diabetes mellitus is commonly found in overweight adults, it may be the cause of weight loss when there is substantial wasting of calories due to a poorly controlled glycosuria. Young male insulin-dependent diabetics are sometimes plagued by diarrhea, exacerbating fluid and nutrient losses; true malabsorption has been noted in a few (see Chapter 98).

DIFFERENTIAL DIAGNOSIS

The extensive number of causes of weight loss can be grouped pathophysiologically. Decreased intake, impaired absorption, increased loss and excess demand are the principle mechanisms around which the differential can be organized (Table 7–1). Almost any illness can cause weight loss; the table emphasizes those conditions seen in the ambulatory setting which have weight loss as a prominent feature of the clinical presentation. Data are scarce on the frequency of the various etiologies in cases where weight loss is the principal complaint.

WORKUP

History. The first tasks are to document that weight loss has indeed occurred and to determine its extent. Some patients will need to begin recording weights on a regular basis; others will have already made the necessary quantitative observations or present with obvious cachxia. History can be used to help identify the mechanism(s) responsible for the decline in weight by obtaining the details of daily food intake (including a calorie count), and inquiring into the presence of any appetite disturbance, steatorrhea, diarrhea, vomiting, polyuria, or symptoms of a hypermetabolic state.

When decreased intake is suspected, one needs to check for somatic symptoms of depression (see Chapter 215), excessive use of alcoholism (see Chapter 216), poor dentition, fever, dysphagia, discomfort induced by eating, drug use, history of renal disease, symptoms of heart failure, melena, abdominal pain, anxiety, and exposure to hepatitis. If the patient is a young woman, anorexia nervosa should be considered, and inquiry is worthwhile into eating habits, self-image and attitudes about weight. Family members should be questioned as well.

When impairment of absorption is suspected, inquiries are made into previous gastrointestinal surgery, the character of the stools, jaundice, history of pancreatitis, travel to an area known for giardiasis or other parasites, symptoms of inflammatory bowel disease, (see Chapter 65), easy bruising, paresthesias, and sore tongue. Increased nutrient loss is assessed historically by ascertaining the quality and quantity of material lost, as well as the frequency and duration of the condition. Of major importance is checking for symptoms of diabetes such as polyuria and diarrhea. When excess demand is under consideration, the patient needs to be questioned about fever, malignancy, symptoms of hyperthyroidism and apathetic hyperthyroidism (see Chapter 99), amphetamine and thyroxine use, chronic anxiety (see Chapter 214) and manic states.

Physical examination should begin with an accurate weight determination. One then needs to check for wasting, apathetic appearance, fever, tachycardia, pallor, ecchymoses, jaundice, stigmata of hyperthyroidism, glossitis, poor dentition, goiter, adenopathy, signs of congestive heart failure, organomegaly, hyperactive bowel sounds, ascites, and abdominal and rectal masses. Stool should be obtained for gross and microscopic observation and guaiac testing. Position and vibration sense are tested for evidence of subacute combined degeneration and peripheral neuropathy.

Laboratory testing must be selective in order to avoid being wasteful and burdensome, for the number of potential investigations is enormous. History and physical examination will usually serve to identify the basic mechanism(s) of weight loss and suggest specific causes which can be confirmed or ruled out by further investigation.

DECREASED INTAKE. The serum calcium, potassium, SGOT, BUN and creatinine are worth ordering when the precise etiology of decreased intake remains obscure. Any patient taking a digitalis preparation should have a serum drug level obtained.

IMPAIRED ABSORPTION. The stool should be examined for fat. A simple initial test is the *qualitative stool fat examination* using the Sudan III stain. With the patient on his usual diet, a small amount of stool is mixed with saline on a glass slide. A drop of Sudan III and acetic acid are added and covered with a cover slip. After heating briefly, the slide is examined under the microscope with the high-dry magnification. Fat will appear as yellow-orange globules; more than one or two globules per field is abnormal and indicative of malabsorption.

If the qualitative study is abnormal or if malabsorption is a serious consideration, a *72-hour stool collection* with the patient on a 100-gram fat diet should be obtained and analyzed *quantitatively* for fat. The test is the most sensitive indicator of malabsorption, though nonspecific. A finding greater than 6 grams per day of fecal fat is two standard deviations from the mean when a person takes in 60 to 100 grams of fat daily, and correlates well with probability of underlying pathology. A normal quantitative stool fat is strong evidence against clinically significant malabsorption.

If the stool fat test is abnormal, an *upper GI series* with small bowel follow-through and a *d-xylose* test can be ordered to provide anatomic detail and functional assessment of the small bowel. In the d-xylose test at least 4 grams of xylose should be detected in the urine over 5 hours in normal subjects after intake of 25 grams of xylose. Renal function and hydration need to be maintained at optimal levels during the test, but if that is impossible, serum xylose levels can be checked at 2 hours and should be 20 mg per 100 ml or more. The test is a sensitive indicator of small bowel absorption. A *Schilling test* with intrinsic factor is a sensitive measure of small bowel absorptive capacity in the terminal ileum where B_{12} uptake occurs. More than 7 per cent of labeled B_{12} should be excreted in the urine over 24 hours. If blind loop syndrome is present, the test may be falsely positive for malabsorption since bacterial overgrowth will consume the B_{12} and lead to decreased absorption.

Should the d-xylose test be normal, there is a good chance the problem is one of pancreatic insufficiency rather than small bowel disease. A serum *amylase* may reveal pancreatitis (see Chapter 70) but a *secretin stimulation* test should be ordered to best assess exocrine function. The test requires placing a tube in the proximal small bowel to sample pancreatic secretions for volume and concentration. Normal bicarbonate concentration is 90 mEq per liter or more. It is necessary to chill the sample promptly after collection to prevent degradation of unstable pancreatic enzymes.

If x-ray reveals blind loops, a C^{14} *glycyl choline test* will help document bacterial overgrowth. Normally, conjugated bile salts are taken up unchanged into the enterohepatic circulation, but with excessive numbers of bacteria, bile salts will be metabolized to $C^{14}O_2$ which readily diffuses across the luminal wall and eventually is exhaled and detected by a counter. The test may also be positive in the presence of a diseased or resected terminal ileum.

For diagnosis of giardiasis, a stool sample suffices in many instances. Since parasites are passed intermittently, three or more stools on alternate days should be examined. Because the cysts are hardy, a fresh stool specimen is not required. Trophozoites are more likely to be found in acute cases. Examination of a duodenal aspirate or jejunal biopsy is resorted to when suspicion is high but stools are negative. Although these tests are more productive, they are cumbersome; some clinicians advocate a diagnostic trial of an anti-giardial drug such as metronidazole instead.

INCREASED NUTRIENT LOSS. Laboratory assessment should include testing for significant glycosuria in quantifying volume losses.

EXCESS DEMAND. Suspicion of hyperthyroidism necessitates free T_4 and total T_3 determinations, especially in the elderly apathetic patient with unexplained atrial fibrillation and weight loss. There are some data suggesting that a TRH stimulation test is a more sensitive means of detecting apathetic hyperthyroidism.

One of the most difficult diagnostic issues encountered in workup of weight loss concerns the possibility of *occult malignancy*. Deciding when to embark on a search for tumor requires an estimate not only of the likelihood of finding a malignancy, but also of the chances it will be treatable. Unfortunately, by the time weight loss has occurred, most gastrointestinal malignancies are rather far advanced. When weight loss is the only symptom pancreatic carcinoma may still be resectable if no other symptoms have appeared. There is hope that abdominal ultrasound and computerized axial tomography will improve case detection and early identification of resectable tumors (see Chapter 53).

SYMPTOMATIC THERAPY

Most causes of weight loss require correction of the etiology and cannot be readily treated symptomatically. However, there are important exceptions to this generalization. Sometimes the severe anorexia associated with malignancy or use of antitumor agents can be overcome by use of phenothiazines or even tetrahydrocannabinol (see Chapter 74). The poor intake seen with hepatitis can be improved by providing small frequent feedings, especially in the morning when nausea is less severe (see Chapter 70). Appetite disturbances associated with depression are often amenable to tricyclic therapy (see Chapter 215). Maldigestion due to pancreatic insufficiency can be compensated for by use of oral pancreatic enzyme preparations (see Chapter 72). The bacterial overgrowth of blind loop syndrome responds to oral broad-spectrum antibiotic therapy such as tetracycline 250 mg four times daily for multiple 10-day courses or for 3 or 4 days each week indefinitely. Caloric supplements in the form of medium chain triglyceride and dextrose preparations can provide marked improvement when there is severe fat and carbohydrate maldigestion or malabsorption. Initially, 3 ounces are given with each meal and gradually increased to 6 ounces, including supplements between meals.

Fat-soluble vitamin supplements are also needed in cases of malabsorption to prevent malnutrition, even though caloric intake may be replenished. The fat-soluble Vitamins A, D and K are most the likely to be depleted. Dosage requirements in such cases are 25,000 to 50,000 units per day for vitamin A, 30,000 units for vitamin D, and 4 to 12 mg for oral vitamin K. Monthly B_{12} injections of 1000 mcg are needed for terminal ileal disease presenting with megaloblastic anemia (see Chapter 77). Control of excessive vomiting and diarrhea is discussed in Chapters 54 and 58 respectively.

INDICATIONS FOR REFERRAL AND ADMISSION

Any patient suspected of having anorexia nervosa should be admitted to the hospital and seen by a psychiatrist experienced in dealing with the problem. When malabsorption is documented by 72-hour stool fat assessment, consultation with a gastroenterologist should coincide with proceeding to further assessment.

ANNOTATED BIBLIOGRAPHY

Finlay, J.M., Hogarth, J., and Wightman, K.J.: A clinical evaluation of the d-xylose tolerance test. Ann. Intern. Med., *61*:411, 1964. *(Detailed description of the test.)*

Gullick, H.: Carcinoma of the pancreas. Medicine, *38*:47, 1959. *(A review of 100 cases. Weight loss occurred in 85.7 per cent. Of eight patients with resectable neoplasms, weight loss was a notable and early symptom in two. There was no correlation between weight loss and site of disease.)*

Gryboski, J., Katz, J., Sangree, H., and Herskovic, T.: Eleven adolescent girls with severe anorexia. Clin. Pediatr., *7*:684, 1968. *(Three of the eleven thought to have anorexia nervosa proved to have Crohn's disease.)*

Kamath, K.R., and Murugasu, R.: A comparative study of four methods of detecting *Giardia*. Gastroenterology, *66*:16, 1974. *(Mucosal biopsy was most sensitive, followed by duodenal aspiration and stool examination.)*

Kanis, J.A.: Anorexia nervosa: A clinical psychiatric and laboratory study. Q. J. Med., *43*:321, 1974. *(A detailed analysis of 24 patients and review of literature; 64 refs.)*

Sherr, H.P., Sasaki, Y., Newman, A., et al.: Detection of bacterial deconjugation of bile salts by a convenient breath-analysis technic. N. Engl. J. Med., *285*:656, 1971. *(A controlled study of the C^{14} cholyl glycine test for diagnosis of blind loop syndrome.)*

Thomas, F.B., Massaferri, E.L., and Skillman, T.G.: Apathetic thyrotoxicosis: A destinctive clinical and laboratory entity. Ann. Intern. Med., *72*:679, 1970. *(Classic article describing this syndrome, which is characterized by marked weight loss, apathy and atrial fibrillation in the elderly.)*

Wolfe, M.: Giardiasis. JAMA, *233*:1362, 1975. *(Terse review of clinical presentation, diagnosis and therapy; 21 refs.)*

3

Cardiovascular Problems

8
Screening for Hypertension

Hypertension can justifiably be considered the most significant condition the practitioner concerned with health maintenance will meet in clinical practice. The size of the affected population is staggering—20 per cent of adults in the United States have systolic pressures greater than 160 mm. of mercury or diastolic pressure greater than 95 mm. of mercury, including more than one third of people over age 70. Excess morbidity and mortality caused by hypertension have been documented. The benefits of treatment for many, if not all, hypertensives have been proven. Nevertheless, despite improvement in hypertension management in recent years, many who should be treated remain either unaware of their elevated blood pressure, not treated, or not controlled.

Evaluation and management of the identified hypertensive patient are presented in Chapters 13 and 21. This chapter will briefly review the epidemiology of high blood pressure, its importance as a risk factor, and the evidence for the effectiveness of therapy.

EPIDEMIOLOGY AND RISK FACTORS

Most estimates of the prevalence of hypertension derive from the Public Health Service National Health Examination Survey conducted during the early 1960s. Subsequent smaller surveys have substantiated both its prevalence (approximately 20 per cent among all adults), and the importance of age, race, and sex as epidemiologic correlates.

Age. The prevalence rate of systolic hypertension rises steadily with age: diastolic pressures rise less steeply after the fifth or sixth decade. It is not clear whether this increase is limited to a subset of the population with a tendency toward hypertension or, more likely, whether a rise in blood pressure is part of aging. The prevalence of hypertension (using the rather stringent definition of systolic greater than or equal to 160 mm. of mercury or diastolic greater than or equal to 95 mm. of mercury) among persons aged 25 to 34 is approximately 5 percent. By age 55 to 64, it has risen to 35 to 40 per cent.

Sex. Males in all age groups have a higher incidence of hypertension. In the third and fourth decades, it is more than twice as common among men than among women. The ratio decreases with advancing age, but a significant male predominance persists.

Race. A marked increase in prevalence has been documented among black men and women in all age groups. The overall prevalence ratio is 2:1, but it is higher in younger age groups and lower in older ones. Hypertension is also more severe among blacks. The relative rate of diastolic pressure greater than 115 mm. of mercury is nearly five times higher for blacks than whites.

Other factors. Hypertension is more likely if there is a positive family history. There is a positive association between obesity and hypertension that appears to be independent of technical problems as-

Table 8–1. Results of Veterans Administration
Cooperative Study

| | DIASTOLIC 115–129 MM. HG* | | DIASTOLIC 90–114 MM. HG† | |
	CONTROL (N=70)	TREATED (N=73)	CONTROL (N=194)	TREATED (N=186)
Death	4	0	19	8
Other Morbid Events	23	2	57	14

*Veterans Administration Cooperative Study Group on Antihypertensive Agents, JAMA, *202*:1028, 1967 (*Average follow-up 18 months.*)

†————, JAMA, *213*:1143, 1970 (*Average follow-up 40 months.*)

sociated with sphygmomanometer cuff size. Increased salt intake has been incriminated; while crude linear relationships between average salt intake and hypertension prevalence have been described in populations, an individual's prior or current salt intake is not a predictor of blood pressure level. The role of psychological stress and resulting sympathetic stimulation appears to be variable. Blood pressure levels have been correlated with subjective estimates of increased stress in population studies. Cigarette smoking, an important risk factor in its own right, is not positively associated with increased blood pressure, but hypertensive smokers are at significantly greater risk than are hypertensive nonsmokers. Other forms of hypertension, including that associated with renal disease, are discussed in Chapter 13.

HYPERTENSION AS A RISK FACTOR FOR CARDIOVASCULAR MORBIDITY AND MORTALITY

That hypertensives have a dramatically increased risk of cardiovascular morbidity and mortality is indisputable. The combined results of epidemiologic studies indicate that middle-aged males with diastolic blood pressures of 95 to 104 mm. of mercury have a twofold increase in mortality due to coronary disease during a 10-year follow-up. If the diastolic level is 105 mm. of mercury of greater, the risk is threefold. Death rates from all causes were 60 per cent and 200 per cent greater in the respective hypertensive groups than among normotensive men. A 60 per cent increase was also evident among men with diastolic blood pressures of 85 to 94 mm. of mercury, when compared with men with lower pressures.

Epidemiologic studies have clearly demonstrated the additive effects of multiple risk factors in predicting coronary heart disease. The presence of hyperlipidemia, smoking or diabetes in association with hypertension is an indication for more aggressive risk factor reduction.

Systolic hypertension has been shown to be the most powerful predictor of nonhemorrhagic and hemorrhagic stroke in males and females. Hypertensives have a fourfold risk of brain infarction when compared with normotensives. The Framingham study has also shown hypertension to be the dominant predictor of congestive heart failure, with a sixfold increase in incidence among hypertensives.

NATURAL HISTORY OF HYPERTENSION AND EFFECTIVENESS OF THERAPY

With rare exceptions, hypertension is an asymptomatic disease. The natural history is one of insidious damage that is most often clinically silent for a decade or more. Consequently, it is a more ominous finding, and, in particular, a potent predictor of coronary disease, in younger age groups.

Arguments for the vigorous early treatment of moderately and severely elevated blood pressure rest on the convincing results of the Veterans Administration Cooperative Study. The data are summarized in Table 8–1. Among those treated, the rate of major nonfatal events and of cardiovascular death was reduced more than tenfold among severely hypertensive men and threefold among moderately hypertensive men. Treatment was most effective in reducing risks of stroke and congestive heart failure. There was no significant reduction in coronary events among patients with lowered levels of hypertension. A reduction in subsequent coronary events and death in patients with known coronary disease has been reported, but the available data are fragmentary. Middle-aged hypertensive men treated in a Swedish primary prevention trial have had lower incidences of fatal and nonfatal coronary events than their untreated counterparts. Little is known about the benefits derived from treatment of mild hypertension, particularly in women. Practicing clinicians are forced to generalize from available data and weigh presumed benefits against the cost, inconvenience, and largely unknown risks of prolonged antihypertensive therapy.

SCREENING METHODS

The process of identifying patients with high blood pressure in the primary care setting is straightforward. Blood pressure determination should be a routine component of patient evaluation regardless of the presenting complaint. Reliable equipment is important. Aneroid manometers, if used, should be checked regularly. All personnel recording blood pressures should be aware of sources of measurement error, such as inappropriate cuff size. Variability of blood pressure may be related to recent physical activity, emotional state, or body position. While such factors must be kept in mind, the predictive value of the "casual" blood pressure determination has been validated.

CONCLUSIONS AND RECOMMENDATIONS

Hypertension is an extraordinarily common condition and the strongest predictor of subsequent cardiovascular and cerebrovascular morbidity and mortality. It is essentially asymptomatic, and end-organ damage is insidious. Benefits of antihypertensive therapy for a large segment of the population have been conclusively proven. The detection and appropriate management of hypertension is one of the foremost responsibilities of the practitioner. Specific recommendations regarding the evaluation and selection of patients for treatment are discussed in Chapter 21.

ANNOTATED BIBLIOGRAPHY

Berglund, G., Sannerstedt, R., Andersson, O., et al.: Coronary heart disease after treatment of hypertension. Lancet, *1*:1, 1978. *(Middle-aged hypertensive men treated with hypotensive drugs [usually starting with propranolol] had significantly lower incidences of fatal and nonfatal coronary events than untreated men. Data from the Goteborg primary prevention trial; controls were not randomized.)*

Burch, G.E., and Shewey, L.: Sphygmomanometric cuff size and blood pressure recordings. JAMA, *225*:1215, 1973. *(Use of wrong size cuff can lead to erroneous reading.)*

Paul, O.: Risks of mild hypertension: A ten-year report. Br. Heart J., *33*:116, 1971. *(Reviews the data of 6 prospective studies in the United States. The increased risk of morbid and mortal cerebrovascular and cardiovascular events for men with diastolic pressures of 85 to 90 is evident.)*

Veterans Administration Cooperative Study Group on Antihypertensive Agents: Effects of treatment on morbidity in hypertension. Results in patients with diastolic blood pressures averaging 115 through 129 mm. Hg. JAMA, *202*:1028, 1967.

Veterans Administration Cooperative Study Group on, Antihypertensive Agents: Effects of treatment on morbidity in hypertension II. Results in patients with diastolic blood pressure averaging 90 through 114 mm Hg. JAMA, *213*:1143, 1970.

Veterans Administration Cooperative Study Group on Antihypertensive Agents: Effects of treatment on morbidity in hypertension III. Influence of age, diastolic pressure, and prior cardiovascular disease. Further analysis of side effects. Circulation, *45*:901, 1972. *(The studies described in these papers are the basis for the current approach to antihypertensive therapy. They are required reading for the primary care provider.)*

Weiss, N.S.: Relation of high blood pressure to headache, epistaxis, and selected other symptoms. The United States Health Examination Survey of Adults. N Engl. J. Med, *287*:631, 1972. *(No clear relationship was shown between these symptoms and level of blood pressure. They may be better indicators of retinopathy in both normotensive and hypertensive patients.)*

9
Screening for Hyperlipidemia

Elevated serum levels of cholesterol and triglycerides are exceedingly common. While hyperlipidemia may be a manifestation of an underlying illness, it is most often the result of genetic and dietary determinants and of significance because of its association with atherosclerosis.

In deciding whether or not to screen for hyperlipidemia, the physician must consider several questions. Do elevated levels of cholesterol or triglycerides increase coronary risk? How effectively can these levels be lowered by diet and drugs? Most important, will lowering these levels reduce the risk of a coronary event? This chapter considers these issues. The heterogeneity of hyperlipidemia and classification schemes based on lipoprotein type and pattern of inheritance, as well as specific management recommendations, are reviewed in Chapter 22.

EPIDEMIOLOGY AND RISK FACTORS

Prevalence estimates of hyperlipidemia are based on rather arbitrary definitions of serum lipid elevations. More than 5 per cent of American adults have cholesterol levels greater than 275 mg. per 100 ml., and approximately 5 per cent have triglyceride levels greater than 220 mg. per 100 ml. While such levels may be considered upper limits of normal in the statistical sense, they should not be considered healthy. Coronary risk has been shown to increase continuously with cholesterol levels even within the American "normal" range. The two thirds of American adult males with serum cholesterol levels greater than 200 mg. per 100 ml. have an increased probability of developing atherosclerotic heart disease.

A review of the many factors that influence blood lipid levels, particularly cholesterol, provides a basis for identifying patients likely to benefit from lipid screening.

Genetic factors. The genetic influence on serum lipid levels is important, but has been clearly defined for only a fraction of patients with hyperlipidemia. Primary disorders inherited by means of a simple genetic mechanism (discussed in Chapter 22), account for only a fraction of patients with hyperlipidemia.

Nevertheless, these disorders are among the most common of the inherited errors of metabolism. Polygenic inheritance is far more common. Polygenic hypercholesterolemia affects 5 per cent of the general population.

Age. Cholesterol and triglyceride levels increase with age; serum cholesterol goes up by more than 2 mg./100 ml. per year on the average during early adulthood.

Sex. In general, men have higher cholesterol levels than women until age 50. Significantly, before menopause, women carry a higher proportion of cholesterol in the form of high-density lipoproteins, which have been inversely associated with coronary risk.

Diet. It is well established that a diet high in saturated fats raises the serum cholesterol level and that unsaturated fats lower it. Blood cholesterol is influenced somewhat by dietary cholesterol, but the effect is smaller than that of saturated fat intake. Caloric excess resulting in obesity is the most important dietary determinant of triglyceride level. Alcohol has little effect on cholesterol levels, but it can cause an acute rise in triglyceride level among people with hypertriglyceridemia.

Other factors. Epidemiologic data suggest that regular physical exercise lowers total cholesterol and triglyceride levels and raises high-density lipoprotein levels, but studies are not conclusive. Some authors have suggested that chronic anxiety, smoking and coffee consumption are associated with elevated cholesterol levels, but the evidence is fragmentary. Exogenous estrogens can cause extreme increases in triglyceride levels among patients with hypertriglyceridemia.

HYPERLIPIDEMIA AS A RISK FACTOR FOR CORONARY ARTERY DISEASE

A number of large, prospective studies, including those from Framingham and the University of Minnesota, have demonstrated cholesterol level to be an

Table 9-1. Probability of Developing Coronary Heart Disease in 6 Years Based on Age and Cholesterol Level in the Absence of Other Risk Factors (Expressed as Number of Cases per 100 Male Patients)*

CHOLESTEROL LEVEL	AGE						
	35	40	45	50	55	60	65
185	0.4	0.9	1.8	3.0	4.5	5.7	6.4
210	0.5	1.2	2.2	3.6	5.1	6.2	6.6
235	0.8	1.6	2.9	4.4	5.8	6.8	6.9
260	1.1	2.2	3.6	5.3	6.7	7.4	7.1
285	1.6	2.9	4.6	6.4	7.6	8.0	7.4
310	2.2	3.8	5.8	7.6	8.7	8.7	7.6
335	3.1	5.1	7.3	9.1	9.9	9.5	7.9

*Based on data from the Framingham Study.

independent predictor of coronary heart disease. In the Framingham study of men and women ages 35 to 64, the risk of a coronary event rose linearly with the cholesterol level, even within the American "normal" range. The strength of the association between total cholesterol level and coronary risk decreased with advancing age, and it was no longer significant after age 65. Studies in Air Force personnel have confirmed the decreased prognostic importance of cholesterol level in older men.

More recent studies from Framingham and elsewhere have focused on an inverse correlation between high-density lipoprotein (HDL) cholesterol and coronary risk. It has been suggested that measurement of HDL cholesterol and estimation of low-density lipoprotein (LDL) cholesterol will provide more accurate prediction of risk, particularly for older individuals. While the epidemiologic data are consistent with laboratory evidence that HDL may serve as a vehicle for the transport of cholesterol from cells to plasma, it is too soon to draw definite conclusions about the protective role of HDL.

The Framingham data can be used to demonstrate the importance of cholesterol level to the individual patient. Table 9-1 estimates the risk of developing coronary artery disease within 6 years for men of different ages with various cholesterol levels in the absence of other known risk factors (hypertension, electrocardiographic evidence of left ventricular hypertrophy and cigarette smoking).

None of the American prospective studies to date have found an independent contribution of triglyceride level to coronary risk when other factors such as cholesterol, blood pressure, smoking, glucose intolerance, ECG abnormalities and personality were corrected for. A prospective study conducted in Stockholm claimed that fasting triglyceride level was independent of cholesterol level in predicting coronary disease, but other risk factors except smoking were not considered. Increased coronary risk for patients with familial hypertriglyceridemia has not been demonstrated.

EFFECTIVENESS OF TREATMENT

The validity of screening for and treating hyperlipidemia depends on the effectiveness of dietary and drug therapy in lowering lipid levels and the efficacy of lowered levels in reducing morbidity and mortality.

Diet and drug therapy administered to hospitalized patients can lower the cholesterol level by a maximum of 30 per cent and can lower triglyceride levels from 15 per cent (in primarily hypercholesterolemic patients) to 200 per cent (in patients whose triglyceride levels are elevated out of proportion to cholesterol). In more relevant studies of ambulatory patients, cholesterol levels have been reduced by 6 to 15 per cent.

Diet and drug intervention trials have not yet demonstrated reduction in coronary morbidity or mortality with reduction of elevated serum lipids. There is experimental evidence in animal models indicating that lowering cholesterol intake and serum levels will lead to regression of atherosclerotic plaques, but data in humans are inconclusive. Though several early clinical studies of antilipid therapy suggest that clofibrate might prolong life in postinfarct patients, the Coronary Drug Project study group found no benefit from clofibrate therapy. The nicotinic acid group in the same study had fewer nonfatal reinfarctions, but mortality was unchanged. Unfortunately, patients in the Coronary Drug Project study were not preselected for hyperlipidemia, and, in fact, only about one half had elevated cholesterol levels. The effects of clofibrate in men with elevated cholesterol have been measured in a primary prevention trial recently completed in Europe. The incidence of nonfatal myocardial infarctions was significantly lower in the clofibrate group, but there was no difference in fatal infarctions, sudden deaths or the incidence of angina. Furthermore, there were significantly more deaths from all causes in the clofibrate group than in the high-cholesterol control group.

Additional clinical trials, some including interventions aimed at other coronary risk factors as well, are underway. The literature should be watched for their results.

It must be kept in mind that little if anything is known about the time required for lipid-lowering therapy to have an effect on the atheromatous process. What is known about the long asymptomatic period in the natural history of coronary disease suggests that primary prevention, if undertaken, should be initiated early.

SCREENING METHODS

Since an independent relationship to coronary disease (or to stroke and claudication in the Framingham Study) has been demonstrated for cholesterol but not for triglycerides, serum cholesterol level is the most appropriate screening test for the general population. Cholesterol is not acutely affected by diet; therefore, fasting samples are not necessary. Following an acute myocardial infarction (or other similar stress), cholesterol levels will gradually fall by as much as 20 per cent, but at the time of hospitalization the level may not be substantially different from baseline. A significant drop in cholesterol and triglyceride levels has been demonstrated when a patient assumes a recumbent position; this occurs within 5 minutes and reaches a maximum of 10 to 12 per cent within 20 to 30 minutes. Many automated cholesterol determinations give values 5 to 15 per cent higher than the standard Abell-Kendall method used in Framingham and other studies.

For screening purposes, measurement of triglyceride can be reserved for individuals with elevated cholesterol. Triglyceride measurement requires a 12- to 16-hour fast including omission of alcohol. Levels gradually increase following myocardial infarction.

Not long ago, lipoprotein electrophoresis was touted as a necessary test for the evaluation and treatment of hyperlipidemia. It has since been recognized that electrophoresis rarely adds to clinical decision-making.

At present, it is too early to recommend HDL determinations for screening purposes. The therapeutic implications of the inverse relationship between HDL cholesterol and coronary risk remain to be defined. Moreover, the mean difference between HDL levels in patients with low and with high coronary risk is approximately the same as the error of many available HDL assays. Calculation of individual risk of coronary disease should not be based on these imprecise measurements.

CONCLUSIONS AND RECOMMENDATIONS

- Epidemiologic studies have demonstrated that an elevated cholesterol level is an independent risk factor for the development of coronary artery disease. Risk is correlated with cholesterol levels even within the American normal range. Both genetic and dietary factors influence cholesterol level.
- Though hypertriglyceridemia is associated clinically with accelerated atherogenesis, its contribution to coronary risk has not been shown in epidemiologic study to be independent of cholesterol level and other risk factors.
- Diet and drug therapy effectively reduce serum lipid concentrations.
- Decreased mortality following the reduction of serum lipid levels has not as yet been demonstrated. Large-scale studies addressing this question are currently in progress.
- The most appropriate screening test for the general population is random serum cholesterol level. Fasting triglyceride levels can be reserved for patients with elevated cholesterol levels. Lipoprotein electrophoresis has no role in screening. The literature should be followed for developments in HDL study; at present, routine HDL measurement is not recommended.
- Serum cholesterol measurement is recommended for individuals under 55 years of age. Because of greater prognostic significance and increased likeli-

hood of benefit from early intervention, screening should be performed during early adulthood when possible. This is particularly important when there is a family history of hyperlipidemia or premature coronary disease.

ANNOTATED BIBLIOGRAPHY

Ahrens, E.H., Jr.: The management of hyperlipidemia: Whether, rather than how. Ann. Intern. Med., 85:87, 1973. *(A critical review of the "lipid hypothesis.")*

Barndt, R., Blankenhorn, D.H., *et al.*: Regression and progression of early femoral atherosclerosis in treated hyperlipoproteinemia patients. Ann. Intern. Med., 86:139, 1977. *(Though the question is a difficult one to approach experimentally, this paper suggests that at least early atherosclerotic lesions can be reversed by treatment of Type II and Type IV hyperlipoproteinemia.)*

Bortz, W.M.: The pathogenesis of hypercholesterolemia. Ann. Intern. Med., 80:738, 1974. *(A comprehensive review of factors that influence serum cholesterol levels.)*

Castelli, W.P., Doyle, J.T., Gordon, T., *et al.*: HDL cholesterol and other lipids in coronary heart disease. The cooperative lipoprotein phenotyping study. Circulation, 55:767, 1977. *(A small [3-4 mg./dl.] but consistent and statistically significant difference in HDL cholesterol level when measured in patients with and without coronary disease was evident in a total population of nearly 7,000 people. The apparent excess coronary disease held up when adjustments for levels of LDL cholesterol and triglycerides were made.)*

Cohn, P.F., Gabbay, S.I., and Weglicki, W.B.: Serum lipid levels in angiographically determined coronary artery disease. Ann. Intern. Med., 84:241, 1976. *(Significantly higher levels of cholesterol and triglycerides were found in those with coronary artery disease when compared with controls with normal coronaries. The association with coronary disease was stronger for cholesterol than triglycerides.)*

Kannel, W.B., Castelli, W.P., Gordon, T., *et al*: Serum cholesterol, lipoproteins and the risk of coronary heart disease: The Framingham Study. Ann. Intern. Med., 74:1, 1971. *(Demonstrates the predictive power of cholesterol levels; measurement of LDL and VLDL lipoproteins did not improve prediction, except in older women among whom VLDL measurement seemed most valuable. The most often quoted prospective study.)*

Miller, G.J., and Miller, N.E.: Plasma high-density lipoprotein concentration and development of ischemic heart disease. Lancet, 1:16, 19, 1975. *(Proposes that HDL is a transport protein essential to the catabolism and excretion of cholesterol.)*

Stamler, J.: The Coronary Drug Project (clofibrate and niacin in coronary heart disease). JAMA, 231:360, 1975. *(No demonstrable benefit of clofibrate in secondary prevention was shown, while fewer infarctions but no reduction in mortality were noted in those treated with nicotinic acid.)*

Committee of Principal Investigators: A cooperative trial in the primary prevention of ischemic heart disease using clofibrate. Br. Heart. J., 40:1069, 1978. *(Fewer nonfatal infarctions with clofibrate but no difference in fatal infarctions, sudden deaths or new angina; more deaths from all causes with clofibrate.)*

Kannel, W.B., Castelli, W.P., and Gordon, T.: Cholesterol in the prediction of atherosclerotic disease. Ann. Intern. Med., 90:85, 1979. *(Reviews the associations between total cholesterol, LDL cholesterol and HDL cholesterol and coronary risk.)*

Witztum, J., and Schonfeld, G.: High density lipoproteins. Diabetes, 28:326, 1979. *(Detailed but concise review of HDL as a risk factor, measurement techniques and factors that affect HDL levels. Well referenced [147 citations] and followed by abstracts of important articles.)*

10
Exercise and
Cardiovascular Disease

HARVEY B. SIMON, M.D.
STEVEN R. LEVISOHN, M.D.

In the past decade, exercise has become an American growth industry. An estimated 20 to 40 million Americans jog regularly, making it the most popular participant sport. In addition, other active sports such as tennis and racquetball, cross-country skiing, and biking have grown in popularity. Unlike other recreational activities, these sports attract participants not only for their intrinsic pleasures but because they are widely believed to be beneficial to health. In the case of jogging, the public has been exposed to conflicting claims ranging from the hypothesis that marathon running helps prevent myocardial infarctions to warnings that long distance running is a health hazard. Because of these controversies, the primary care physician is increasingly called upon to advise his patients about the effects of exercise on health and to prescribe an effective and safe exercise program.

PHYSIOLOGY AND CLINICAL IMPLICATIONS OF EXERCISE

Physical work may involve either aerobic or anaerobic metabolism, and may rely upon either isotonic or isometric muscular activity. The concept of aerobic exercise provides the foundation for endurance training. The total amount of stored energy available to muscle groups in the form of preformed ATP and phosphocreatine is sufficient to sustain less than 10 seconds of maximal exertion. Clearly, energy must be generated continuously during exercise, and the majority of this energy comes from the metabolism of muscle glycogen. The availability of oxygen determines whether this metabolism will be aerobic or anaerobic. When oxygen supply is adequate, metabolism is aerobic and glycogen is completely metabolized to pyruvate and then to water and CO_2 via the Krebs cycle. With increasing exercise, the ability of the lungs to take up oxygen and of the heart and blood vessels to deliver it to muscle cells is exceeded, and metabolism becomes anaerobic. The costs of an-

aerobic metabolism are substantial. Anaerobic metabolism is inefficient; it generates only one third as much energy from each gram of glycogen, and increases production of lactic acid, resulting in muscle cramps, fatigue, and dyspnea. Lactic acid is buffered by bicarbonate, resulting in increased CO_2 production and hyperventilation. Clinically, an abrupt rise in respiratory rate indicates that the anaerobic threshold has been crossed. Endurance training can be expected to increase the anaerobic threshold, thus allowing more work to be performed under favorable aerobic conditions.

The goal of training is to improve cardiopulmonary function and muscular efficiency. The type of exercise is critical. While maximal exertion or anaerobic training may be of some benefit to certain competitive athletes, the cornerstone of training for fitness is endurance or *aerobic exercise* using large muscle groups in continuous rhythmic activity for prolonged periods. Jogging and brisk walking are ideal for this. Other good training activities include biking, swimming, cross-country skiing, rowing and rope jumping. These activities provide *isotonic exercise* whereby skeletal muscle fibers change in length with little change in tension. Heart rate and cardiac output increase but peripheral vascular resistance falls. In contrast, sports depending on very brief bursts of intense activity such as weight lifting provide *isometric exercise* in which muscle tension increases with little change in fiber length. Such exercise produces a marked increase in peripheral vascular resistance and blood pressure with little increase in cardiac output. Aerobic power does not increase with isometric exercising, and the hypertensive response can be hazardous to patients with cardiovascular disease. Because arm work has a greater tendency to produce tachycardia and hypertension than does an equivalent degree of leg work, it is particularly important to limit the resistance level in arm exercises for patients with hypertension or heart disease. Sports which allow prolonged periods of inactivity such as baseball or golf are poor for cardiopulmonary conditioning. Similarly, while activities providing sustained but gentle muscular effort such as yoga can be important parts of a fitness program because they are excellent for promoting flexibility and strength, they are in themselves poor tools when used for the attainment of cardiopulmonary fitness.

The effects of regular exercise can be classified in terms of cardiovascular, musculoskeletal, metabolic, and psychological functions. The most thoroughly documented results of aerobic exercise concern changes in *cardiopulmonary performance.* Exercise requires an increase in the body's oxygen consumption, which is made possible by increased oxygen uptake by pulmonary ventilation, increased oxygen delivery by the heart and the peripheral circulation, and increased oxygen extraction by muscle. Endurance training enhances the efficiency of these processes by both central and peripheral mechanisms. At rest and at submaximal work loads, the fit individual has a slower heart rate than does the untrained person. Stroke volume is increased so that cardiac output for a given work load is unchanged. While the achievable maximum heart rate is not increased by training, the maximum cardiac output and maximum oxygen consumption are greatly enhanced so that the well-trained individual can both attain higher work loads and sustain them for prolonged periods before exhaustion.

Although there is little firm evidence that exercise increases myocardial oxygen supply or produces collateral vascularization in man, myocardial oxygen demands for a given work load decrease. This diminution in myocardial oxygen consumption is made possible by the lower heart rate and lower systolic blood pressure which accompany exercise in the fit individual. This can be of particular benefit to the patient with angina, since this "double product" of HR x BP determines the angina threshold (see postmyocardial infarction rehabilitation, Chapter 26). In addition, animal studies have demonstrated increased coronary artery cross sectional area, increased myocardial capillary density, and myocardial hypertrophy in rats and dogs forced to exercise.

The *peripheral effects* of exercise are of great importance in endurance training. Capillary blood flow to muscle is increased. Muscle fibers increase in volume, and muscle strength and endurance are enhanced. Muscle mitochondria increase in size and number, and respiratory enzymes increase. As a result, muscle oxygen extraction is improved. Training also improves neuromuscular coordination and musculoskeletal efficiency.

Another important cardiovascular effect of exercise is on the *blood pressure.* Systolic pressure normally rises during exercise, but this rise tends to be slightly less in the fit individual. More important, total peripheral resistance falls as result of improved muscle blood flow and decreased circulating catecholamine levels. The net result in trained individuals is lower blood pressure, both during exercise and at rest. Because this effect is actually more prominent in hypertensive subjects, endurance training can be an important nonpharmacologic adjunct for the control of mild to moderate hypertension. Only small numbers of hypertensive patients have been studied, and while preliminary results are encouraging, additional trials will be needed before exercise can be firmly recommended in the treatment of hypertension.

Less well-established cardiovascular benefits of exercise training include a possible diminution of arrhythmias, perhaps due to lower catecholamine levels. In addition, exercise increases fibrolytic activity and decreases platelet adhesiveness; these hematologic effects may, to some degree, protect against atherogenesis. In these areas, too, the data are preliminary.

The *metabolic benefits* of exercise are well documented. *Weight control* is an important motivating factor for many runners. An average jogger can be expected to consume about 600 calories in an hour of running. Other endurance activities have similar effects (Table 10–1). While exercise alone will produce only a slow reduction in total body weight, the percentage of body fat falls more rapidly, resulting in visible increases in muscle tone. Perhaps most important, runners become motivated to adhere to dietary patterns which will permit sustained weight control.

Another metabolic effect of great interest is that of regular exercise on the blood lipids. In many runners, serum *triglyceride* levels fall dramatically without changes in the dietary intake of fats or carbohydrates. The total *cholesterol* level changes less predictably, but *high-density-lipoprotein* levels tend to rise in runners, and these higher levels appear to be statistically linked to a lower risk for coronary artery disease (see Chapter 9).

The *psychological effects* of regular exercise are receiving a great deal of attention. Most individuals who engage in regular exercise develop an improved self-image. This can be of great importance in the rehabilitation of patients with ischemic heart disease (see Chapter 26), and can also be used to help motivate healthy individuals to modify other risk factors by following a prudent diet and discontinuing smok-

Table 10-1. Approximate Metabolic Expenditures Associated with Selected Activities

Energy outputs are expressed in mets. One met is the energy expended at rest, and equals 3.5 ml O_2/kg. body weight/minute. (Calorie consumption values are for a 70-kg. person.)

AVERAGE ENERGY OUTPUT	ACTIVITY
1 met	Rest
1½-2 mets 2-2½ Kcal./min.	Desk work Standing Strolling (1 mile/hr.)
2-3 mets 2½-4 Kcal./min.	Level walking (2 miles/hr.) Level biking (5 miles/hr.) Golf (power cart)
3-4 mets 4-5 Kcal./min.	Walking (3 miles/hr.) Biking (6 miles/hr.) Badminton Housework
4-5 mets 5-6 Kcal./min.	Golf (carrying clubs) Dancing Tennis (doubles) Raking leaves Calisthenics
5-6 mets 6-7 Kcal./min.	Walking (4 miles/hr.) Cycling (10 miles/hr.) Skating Shoveling garden soil Average sexual activity
6-7 mets 7-8 Kcal./min.	Brisk walking (5 miles/hr.) Tennis (singles) Snow shoveling Downhill skiing Water skiing
7-8 mets 8-10 Kcal./min.	Jogging (5 miles/hr.) Biking (12 miles/hr.) Basketball Canoeing Mountain climbing Ditch digging Touch football
8-9 mets 10-11 Kcal./min.	Jogging (6 miles/hr.) Cross-country skiing Squash or handball (recreational)
Over 10 mets Over 11 Kcal./min.	Squash or handball (competitive) Running 6 miles/hr.: 10 mets 8 miles/hr.: 13½ mets 10 miles/hr.: 17 mets

Modified from Fox, S. M., Naughty, J. P., and Gorman, D. A.: Physical activity and cardiovascular health. III. The exercise prescription; frequency and type of activity. Mod. Concepts Cardiovasc. Dis., *41*:6, 1972.

ing. The recreational aspects of exercise tend to lessen anxiety and depression. Running is being studied as a tool for the treatment of depression, and early results in small groups of patients are encouraging.

Nevertheless, the so-called runner's high proves elusive or illusionary for many joggers. While exercise has many psychological benefits, it is hardly a panacea. Patients can be encouraged to exercise for both psychological and physical gains, but they must have realistic expectations.

In sum, regular endurance-type exercise improves cardiopulmonary performance and tends to lower blood pressure, body weight and fat, and serum triglycerides while elevating serum high-density lipoproteins. Physical fitness may also assist in the psychological response to stress. Because of the amelioration in all of these risk factors, it would seem reasonable to expect that regular exercise would lessen morbidity and mortality from cardiovascular disease. Many epidemiologic investigators have explored the effects of exercise on longevity. In evaluating these studies, it must be remembered that attention to inactivity as a risk factor is relatively recent, with most work being done in the last decade. In addition, there are many intrinsic difficulties in population studies of this type. Perhaps the greatest problem is that of potential bias introduced by self-selection: if healthier people tend to exercise more, then improved mortality in active people may relate to underlying factors rather than to exercise *per se.* Additional difficulties include problems in quantifying exercise and small sample sizes. Finally, there are numerous confounding variables such as psychosocial factors, diet, alcohol consumption, smoking, genetic background, body build, lipid levels, and blood pressure.

In light of these many problems, it is not surprising that there is some divergence in the results of studies, as well as some controversy about the interpretation of the results. Nevertheless, the majority of investigations suggest that regular physical activity does indeed have a favorable effect on morbidity and mortality from cardiovascular disease. Perhaps the best known studies in this country are those of Paffenbarger and his co-workers. In a 22-year cohort analysis of 3686 San Francisco longshoremen who underwent multiphasic screening, it was found that high energy output at work reduced the risk of fatal myocardial infarction, especially in younger subjects. As expected, smoking and hypertension were independently associated with cardiac mortality. It was estimated that if low energy output, smoking and hypertension could have been eliminated, this population might have had an 88 per cent reduction in fatal myocardial infarctions over the 22 years of the study. In a retrospective study of 16,936 male Harvard graduates, the risk of first myocardial infarction was found to be inversely related to energy expenditure. Sedentary men were at 64 per cent higher risk than were classmates who expended an extra 2,000 or more kilocalories per week. Peak exertion in the form of strenuous sports enhanced the effect of total energy expenditure. Interestingly, varsity sports participation in college had no protective effect unless athletic activity was continued into subsequent adult years, implying that self-selection based on initial fitness or genetic endowment is not sufficient to explain these results. In this study the protective effects of adult exercise were found to be independent of other risk factors.

While these studies concentrate on the role of exercise in the prevention of cardiovascular disease, attention is also being directed to the role of physical training in the treatment of patients with established atherosclerotic heart disease. Data from these trials are statistically inconclusive because of problems with sample size and patient compliance, and because of the relative newness of these studies. Nevertheless, studies in this field demonstrate subjective improvement in exercising patients and indicate a trend toward a decrease in coronary events (see Chapter 26 on postmyocardial infarction rehabilitation).

MEDICAL SCREENING OF POTENTIAL EXERCISERS

The physician can and should play a central role in promoting physical fitness. An important goal is providing patient motivation through education: when the benefits and techniques of endurance training are understood clearly, compliance is enhanced. Medical screening of the prospective participant and prescription of an appropriate exercise program are essential for the person who has been inactive.

The first step in medical screening is obtaining a detailed personal and family history. Of particular importance in the family history is the presence of coronary heart disease, peripheral vascular disease, hypertension, stroke, diabetes or sudden death. Each patient should be carefully questioned about symptoms which suggest cardiovascular disease, including chest pain, palpitations, dyspnea, undue fatigue, syncope, and claudication. It is very important to review health habits in detail, with special attention to previous exercise patterns, smoking, diet, and the use of oral contraceptive agents.

A complete physical examination is also vital to the medical screening of the prospective exerciser.

Height and weight should be recorded and ideal lean body weight estimated. The blood pressure should be taken at rest with the patient supine and standing, and the heart rate and blood pressure recorded after mild exercise (stair climbing or sit-ups are satisfactory for this purpose). The chest is examined for rales, wheezes and rhonchi, and the heart for cardiomegaly, gallops, murmurs and rhythm disturbances. The peripheral pulses and abdomen need to be palpated to exclude the presence of peripheral vascular diseases or an aortic aneurysm. The musculoskeletal system should be evaluated both to exclude significant pathology and to determine if specific flexibility or strengthening exercises are required as part of the training program.

Several laboratory studies are helpful in the screening process. Most patients ought to have a CBC, urinalysis, and determinations of blood sugar, creatinine and cholesterol. For patients over the age of 35 who have been sedentary, a resting electrocardiogram should be performed to look for evidence of ischemia, left ventricular hypertrophy and disturbances of rhythm or conduction. A baseline chest roentgenogram will provide information on heart size, pulmonary parenchyma and vasculature.

If any of these screening procedures discloses evidence of overt cardiopulmonary disease, *exercise stress testing* is mandatory before an exercise program is initiated. Even if preliminary screening is negative, stress testing may be helpful for high risk individuals, including those with positive family histories, hypertension, diabetes, or hyperlipidemia. Obesity, cigarette smoking, and a previously sedentary life-style are further indications for stress testing. Because atherosclerotic heart disease is so prevalent in our society, stress testing is probably a prudent precursor to vigorous exercise programs in all males above age 40 and in all females above age 50, even if they are asymptomatic and apparently healthy. Although recent analyses of exercise stress testing is asymptomatic populations have cast doubt on the ability of the test to help identify underlying coronary disease in patients free of angina (see Chapter 31), the test is useful for uncovering exercise-induced arrhythmias and hypotension, evaluating the individual's exercise capacity and establishing the maximal and target heart rate for use in the exercise prescription (see Chapter 26).

In special cases, additional studies may be desirable, such as an FEV1, vital capacity and arterial blood gases in patients with subjective dyspnea or suspected pulmonary disease. Specialized ergometric testing can determine maximal oxygen consumption, total work capacity, and other physiological parameters. Another powerful tool is 24-hour ambulatory monitoring for arrhythmias using the Holter monitor (see Chapter 24). Finally, telemetry can enable constant monitoring of heart rate and rhythm during actual jogging.

Medical screening and exercise testing should allow the physician to assign each patient to one of three categories: (1) Individuals with normal studies can undertake exercise programs without medical supervision. Even in these healthy individuals, however, individualized exercise prescriptions and guidance regarding training techniques and safety precautions will be of great value. (2) Patients with ischemic heart disease, moderate hypertension, or moderate chronic obstructive lung disease will benefit from graded exercise programs, but it is best that they be referred to specialized exercise rehabilitation programs which provide medical supervision and facilities for emergency treatment. People taking digitalis, nitrates, or propanolol should be included in this supervised exercise group. However, if structured rehabilitation programs are not accessible, milder forms of exercise such as walking or stationary bicycling can still be recommended with appropriate precautions. (3) Physical exertion is contraindicated in the presence of congestive heart failure, ventricular irritability, unstable angina, uncontrolled hypertension, unstable diabetes, or uncontrolled epilepsy, although patients with these conditions can sometimes be enrolled in supervised programs if they respond to medical therapy. Patients with AV block, sick sinus syndrome, left ventricular or aortic aneurysms, and aortic valve disease should be excluded from exercise programs.

THE EXERCISE PRESCRIPTION

A fitness program depends on three elements: *frequency, intensity,* and *duration* of exercise. It is well established that at least three exercise sessions per week are required to develop and maintain fitness, and five sessions per week probably provide maximum benefit. Hence, the exercise prescription should call for at least three workouts each week. Many individuals prefer a routine of daily activity; this is certainly an excellent regimen but, especially during the first few months of training, it is advisable to schedule easier and harder workouts on alternate days in order to prevent injuries and allow the muscles to recover.

The intensity and duration of training are intimately related. Equal degrees of fitness can be attained through less intense exercise sustained over a long period or through more vigorous effort for shorter periods. Maximum cardiopulmonary fitness can be attained via 15 to 60 minutes of continuous aerobic exercises, strenuous enough to raise the heart rate to 60 to 80 per cent of maximum or the oxygen uptake to 50 to 85 per cent of maximum.

Obviously these optimal fitness goals must be attained very slowly and gradually, and the physician's exercise prescription should provide a practical means of attaining them. Both the starting point and the rate of progression depend on the health, age and fitness of the participant. As a rule of thumb, the beginner should plan to jog for a daily duration of 10 to 12 minutes at a pace sufficient to increase his heart rate to 60 to 80 per cent of maximum without producing breathlessness.

Each running session should include a 5- to 10-minute *warm-up period.* At the beginning of exercise, even the well-conditioned athlete experiences some degree of dyspnea due to anaerobic metabolism, because it takes 45 to 90 seconds for cardiac output to increase enough to meet the new work load, thus providing the "second wind." A warm-up period will minimize this initial anaerobic period and also allow muscles to loosen and stretch out, which prevents many injuries. For the runner, the warm-up period should consist of stretching exercise, calisthenics, and a gradual progression from walking to slow jogging to running.

The actual *training period* should initially consist of a total of 10 to 12 minutes of exercise. At first, it is best to alternate periods of effort with periods of recovery. This is easily accomplished by alternately walking and jogging. For example, an unfit or older individual might alternate 1 minute of jogging with 1 minute of walking, repeating this cycle 10 to 12 times during each training day. When this can be accomplished with comfort, perhaps at the end of 10 to 20 sessions over 2 to 3 weeks, the schedule can be changed to 2 minutes of jogging alternating with 2 minutes of walking, with 6 cycles in each session. When this is mastered, the jogging ritual can be extended to 3 or 4 minutes with only 1 or 2 minutes of rest for 3 or 4 cycles, and then to two 6-minute runs with 1 or 2 minutes of walking in between. By the end of 1 to 2 months, most individuals should expect to be able to jog for 10 to 20 minutes continuously, and to cover 1 to 2 miles during this period.

Obviously, the young and athletic individual will progress more rapidly than the older or unfit one; but it is important to urge restraint on even the athletic individual—one of the most common causes of orthopedic injuries is attempting too much too quickly. Once a base of 10 to 20 minutes of jogging is well established, further progress should be encouraged. It is reasonable to increase running time or distance by a rate of about 10 per cent per week; this can be accomplished by extending one or two sessions while preserving some short-distance days, or by gradually extending each session. At the end of 4 to 6 months, 3 to 4 miles of jogging 3 to 5 days per week will provide maximal conditioning. However, this level of activity must be maintained to sustain the cardiopulmonary benefits of running. Feelings of accomplishmentand well-being usually provide motivation for sustained participation, often at even higher levels.

In addition to the duration of running, it is important to consider the intensity or *pace* of the exercise. The most precise guide available is the heart rate. Patients should jog at a pace sufficient to raise the pulse to 60 to 80 per cent of maximum. When exercise testing has been performed, an observed maximal heart rate can be used for this calculation. In the absence of these data, the maximal heart rate can be predicted for healthy individuals by subtracting the age from 220. As a rough guide, the target of 60 to 80 per cent of this maximum translates to 130-150 beats/minute for younger people and to 110-125 beats/minute for older ones. The patient can be taught to take his carotid or radial pulse just before and immediately after exercise, and to adjust his pace to attain and maintain the target heart rate. It can be very helpful to have the patient keep a daily record of these figures together with the time and approximate distance covered. As training progresses, a more rapid pace will be required to achieve the target heart rate.

Many people find it difficult or unpleasant to take their pulses. In such cases, intensity of effort can be roughly gauged by the "talking pace"—the individual should go fast enough to feel that he or she is working hard while still being able to talk to a companion without a sensation of dyspnea. For most people, this will translate to a 10- to 12-minute mile at first with progression to 7- to 9-minute miles when fitness is attained.

The final element of the exercise prescription is the *cool-down period*. Following each training session, a period of 5 to 10 minutes of walking and stretching exercises is desirable. Very hot or very cold showers should be avoided.

PATIENT EDUCATION

It is clear that long-term prospective studies of large population groups will be needed to establish firmly the role of exercise in the prevention and treatment of cardiovascular disease. But primary care physicians need not await the results of these studies before advising their patients to exercise. Although smoking (see Chapter 32), hypertension (see Chapter 8), and hypercholesterolemia (see Chapter 9), are probably the most important treatable risk factors, physical inactivity appears to rank next. While patients should be told that exercise has not been proven conclusively to reduce mortality, initial studies are encouraging. Moreover, most people who exercise regularly will feel better, look better, and have enhanced capacities for work and recreation. These factors alone provide sufficient justification for the physician to encourage endurance-type exercise.

However, exercise is not without potential adverse effects, and patients should be educated about these factors as well. There is no question that exercise can precipitate cardiac arrhythmias or myocardial ischemia in individuals with coronary artery disease. Sudden death is a tragic if infrequent complication of exercise. Careful medical screening of potential exercisers, an individualized exercise prescription, and meticulous supervision of high-risk patients can minimize complications. Closely controlled conditioning programs have even enabled survivors of myocardial infarctions to engage safely in marathon running (see Chapter 26). Some runners encounter exercise-induced asthma, particularly during periods of cold weather. Advising use of a face mask that warms inspired air often suffices, but sometimes a mild bronchodilator (see Chapter 45) is necessary. Extreme environmental conditions may also produce thermal stress ranging from frostbite to heat stroke. Here, too, prevention is the best treatment; the physician should be able to advise the runner about appropriate fluid intake, clothing, acclimatization, and safe duration of exposure. Similar advice can prevent dehydration and electrolyte imbalance.

Musculoskeletal injuries are very common and result from overuse, inflexibility and muscle imbalance (see Chapters 144–145). Overuse is prevented by advising gradual increases in exercise; inflexibility and imbalance are avoided by stretching and strengthening exercises (see below). Providing advice about running shoes and running surfaces can also help lessen risk of injury.

PRACTICAL ADVICE
FOR THE BEGINNING RUNNER

Food and fluid intake. It is best to avoid running within 2 hours of a substantial meal. Despite many claims to the contrary, no specific dietary programs are required for running. The obese runner should restrict calories to reduce, while the lean individual may require increased caloric intake to maintain weight. Competitive runners feel that increased carbohydrate intake during the three days prior to a race helps increase endurance, and there is some experimental evidence suggesting that such "carbohydrate loading" does increase muscle glycogen content. Adequate fluid intake is essential, particularly in warm weather. While thirst will dictate the need for fluid replacement, it is best to begin drinking small amounts before thirst becomes overt, so that large volumes will not be needed at any one time. Water itself is excellent, though some runners prefer balanced electrolyte solutions or even carbonated beverages.

Climate. Thermal stress presents a great threat to the runner. When confronted with an abrupt change in climate, the runner should sharply reduce distance and speed for several days until acclimatization is achieved. In warm, humid weather, jogging should be confined to early morning or evening hours or shady locations, distances and speed should be reduced, fluids should be taken at frequent intervals during the run, and clothing should be light colored and light weight. Environmental temperatures between 50 and 60°F are ideal for running in shorts and T-shirts. Between 40 and 50°F warm-up suit is generally sufficient; below 40°F, gloves or mittens and a hat are important. Multiple layers of thin flexible clothing are better than a single bulky garment. Woolen fabrics are ideal but a soft cotton layer should be next to the skin. An extra layer of thermal underwear is vital for temperatures below 30°F, and if winds are strong or temperatures drop below 15°F, an additional layer such as a turtleneck, extra shorts and possibly a ski mask are required. Again, distances should be reduced in bitter cold, and it is particularly important to avoid wet conditions which can lead to frostbite, especially of the feet.

Air pollutants may cause irritation of the upper and lower respiratory tract and carbon monoxide can impair oxygenation and precipitate angina. One should avoid running on heavily traveled roads, during rush hours, and on days when temperature inversions increase air pollution.

Safety is of utmost importance. The runner should run facing the flow of cars. Sidewalks are preferred when possible. While country roads are ideal, it is desirable to run with a companion in isolated areas in case of injury. Daytime running is safer both because the runner is more visable to cars and because he can see road hazards more easily. Bright colored clothing should be encouraged, and at night reflectorized vests are mandatory. Dogs are best avoided by means of an impromptu detour, but if this is not possible they can generally be intimidated by a firm command to "go home" or by the threat of a stick or stone.

Equipment. One of the pleasures of running is that elaborate equipment is not required. However, good running shoes are essential. Many excellent shoes are available; the choice should be dictated by fit, comfort, and support rather than by endorsements or ratings. The toe box should provide enough room for dorsiflexion during takeoff, the sole should be flexible, and provide adequate cushioning, and the heel should be fairly snug without exerting pressure on the Achilles tendon. Most good running shoes are costly but can be expected to last for up to 1000 miles. Often, they can be resoled. While shoes are important, other items ranging from stopwatches to designer sweat suits are optional to say the least. Good shoes will help prevent musculoskeletal injuries. In addition, a relatively soft running surface is helpful; grass and turf are best if they are smooth and level, asphalt is preferable to concrete.

Orthotics and other orthopedic devices are sometimes helpful for refractory problems. Patients with overuse injuries who fail to limit their activity may require a splint or cast to enforce inactivity, even if immobilization is not actually necessary for healing. The use of such devices requires referral to an orthopedist or podiatrist skilled in treating runners' musculoskeletal problems.

Stretching. Regular running produces asymmetric muscular development. The calf, hamstring and Achilles can become overdeveloped and/or shortened and tight. Hill running and sprinting may produce similar effects on the quadriceps and hip flexors. A regular program of stretching exercises is essential to promote flexibility and balanced muscular development. These exercises are ideal for the warm-up and cool-down periods before and after running.

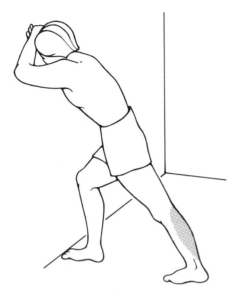

Fig. 10–1. Calf, Achilles, and soleus stretch. Stand 3 feet from a wall with one foot forward, leaning forward to support your upper body by resting your forearms against the wall. Bend the forward leg at the knee. Keep the rear leg straight with the heel on the floor and slowly press your hips forward until you feel the calf stretch. Hold for 15 seconds. Relax and then repeat with the rear knee slightly bent so that you feel the Achilles stretch. Repeat with the other leg forward.

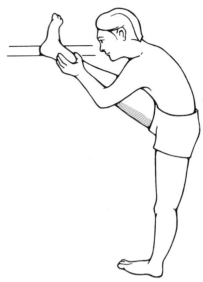

Fig. 10–2. Hamstring stretch. Rest one leg on a sturdy table or desk. Keeping both legs straight, slowly bend forward at the waist so that you feel the hamstring stretch. Hold 30 seconds. Repeat with the other leg up.

Stretching routines are almost as numerous and varied as runners themselves. Four exercises are of particular value: the Achilles, and soleus stretch (Fig. 10–1), the hamstring stretch (Fig. 10–2), the quadriceps stretch (Fig. 10–3), and the hip and side stretch (Fig. 10–4).

With increased running, it will be necessary to add more stretching. In addition to flexibility, balanced muscular strength can be important. Bent knee sit-ups are particularly valuable in strengthening abdominal muscles and preventing "side-stitches." Upper extremity strength is surprisingly important for runners. Push-ups are the simplest upper extremity exercise, but advanced runners often include limited weight lifting or isometrics as well.

Running is not a panacea, but it has many cardiopulmonary, metabolic and psychological benefits. The physician has a crucial role in the medical screening of potential runners, and he can prevent most problems with simple instructions. Periodic return visits may be necessary for dealing with various running-related problems. These visits afford the opportunity for the physician to counsel patience and

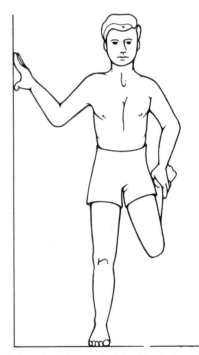

Fig. 10–3. Quadriceps stretch. Stand at arm's length from a wall with your feet parallel to the wall. Rest your hand on the wall for support. Hold your ankle in your free hand and pull the foot back and up until the heel touches the buttocks, while leaning slightly forward from the waist. Repeat with the other leg.

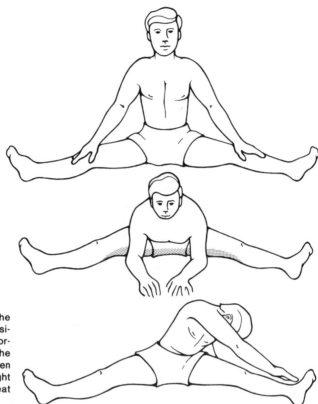

Fig. 10–4. Hip and side stretch. Sit on the floor and spread your legs as far apart as possible. With your legs and back straight, bend forward from the waist until you feel a stretch at the inner thighs. Hold for 20 seconds. Relax. Then twist at the waist and lean to touch your right hand to your left foot. Hold 20 seconds. Repeat on the other side.

persistence. Joggers who get through the difficult 2 or 3 months at the beginning of training are likely to develop running habits that are both enjoyable and healthful.

ANNOTATED BIBLIOGRAPHY

Books and symposia *(These three works provide comprehensive overviews of cardiovascular and metabolic aspects of exercise.)*

Amsterdam, E.A., Wilmore, J.H., and DeMaria, A.N., (eds.): Symposium on exercise in cardiovascular health and disease. Am. J. Cardiol, *33*:713, 1974.

Milvy P. (ed.): The marathon: Physiological, medical, epidemiological and psychological studies. Ann. N.Y. Acad. Sci., *301*:1, 1977.

Wenger, N.K. (ed.): Exercise and the Heart, Philadelphia: F.A. Davis Co., 1978.

Individual Papers

Cooper, K.H., Pollock, M.L., Martin R.P., White, S.R., Linnerud. A.C., and Jackson, A.: Physical fitness levels vs. selected coronary risk factors. A cross-sectional study. JAMA, *236*:116, 1976. *(A prevalence study of nearly 3000 men showing an inverse relationship between physical fitness and resting heart rate, blood presure, body weight, percent body fat, and serum levels of cholesterol, triglycerides and glucose.)*

Paffenbarger, R.S., Hale, W.E., Brand, R.J., and Hyde, R.T.: Work-energy level, personal characteristics, and fatal heart attack: A birth-cohort effect. Am. J. Epidemiol., *105*:200, 1977. *(A recent report on the 22-year cohort analysis of 3686 San Francisco longshoremen.)*

Paffenbarger, R.S., Wing, A.L., and Hyde, R.T.: Physical activity as an index of heart attack risk in college alumni. Am. J. Epidemiol., *108*:161, 1978. *(A survey of the effects of exercise on coronary risk in 16,936 Harvard graduates.)*

Pickering, T.G.: Jogging, marathon running and the heart Am. J. Med., *66*:717, 1979. *(An excellent editorial and terse summary of the proven and as yet unproven effects of jogging on the heart and risk of cardiovascular disease.)*

Scheuer, J., and Tipton, C.M.: Cardiovascular adaptation to physical training. Annu. Rev. Physiol., *39*:221, 1975. (*A scholarly review on the cardiovascular effects of exercise in man and animals.*)

11

Bacterial Endocarditis Prophylaxis

Once universally fatal, bacterial endocarditis remains a serious disease, with a mortality rate of about 25 per cent. Despite the now widespread availability of antibiotics, the incidence of this infection has not changed dramatically. Although controlled data are lacking, logic and pathogenesis of endocarditis argue that individual infections might be prevented by judicious use of prophylactic antibiotics. The primary care provider must be able to assess risks in individual patients. In addition, an understanding of the basis for prophylaxis recommendations is necessary if individuals likely to benefit from preventive measures are to be instructed effectively.

EPIDEMIOLOGY AND RISK FACTORS

Over the past several decades there has been a shift in the incidence of endocarditis to older age groups; the current mean age is about 50, males predominate among patients over 50, but the sex ratio is more nearly equal among those under 50.

The risk of endocarditis in an individual patient is partially a function of the predisposing cardiac lesion and of the occurrence of procedures likely to induce bacteremia. However, as many as 30 to 40 per cent of cases of endocarditis occur in the absence of underlying heart disease, and transient bacteremia is common. Additionally, the intensity of bacteremia, the characteristics of the blood-borne organisms, and host factors all play important roles. Since these additional determinants cannot be readily estimated, individual risk must be based on the diagnosis of predisposing lesion and the likelihood of bacteremia.

Chronic rheumatic heart disease was the underlying lesion in 80 to 90 per cent of cases of endocarditis in the preantibiotic era. Currently, rheumatic heart disease is present in approximately 40 per cent of patients with endocarditis. Congenital heart disease, undiagnosed murmurs, and atherosclerotic disease each account for 10 per cent of underlying lesions. The remaining 30 to 40 per cent of infections occur without known predisposing cardiac disease. In one series of 25 autopsies, 8 patients had no underlying heart disease.

Clearly, all individuals have some finite risk of developing endocarditis. Relative risks cannot be accurately estimated for specific heart lesions because of a lack of epidemiologic data. Since approximately 40 per cent of endocarditis cases occur in the presence of rheumatic heart disease (which has a prevalence of slightly more than 1 per cent in the adult population) and another 40 per cent occur in the absence of heart disease, the risk of endocarditis is increased a hundredfold in the rheumatic heart as opposed to the normal heart.

Risk in congenital heart disease seems comparable. Patent ductus arteriosus, ventricular septal defect, and tetralogy of Fallot are the congenital lesions most commonly associated with endocarditis. Pulmonary and aortic stenoses constitute lesser risks. Atrial septal defect is very rarely responsible for endocarditis.

Idiopathic hypertrophic subaortic stenosis (IHSS) confers significant risk of endocarditis. In a series of 126 IHSS patients followed for varying periods up to 12 years, there were three definite cases and three suspected cases. Nine cases were reported in three other series, with a combined total of 158 patients with IHSS followed for varying periods. The risk of endocarditis with mitral prolapse is unknown. In light of recent high estimates of prevalence of prolapsing mitral valve, endocarditis risk needs to be determined. One natural history study reported five cases in 855 patient-years of follow-up, an incidence higher than in patients free of valvular heart disease.

Prosthetic valves involve special risks. Prosthetic valve endocarditis has been divided into two groups: (1) early, associated with surgery and most often involving nosocomial pathogens such as staphylococci, and (2) late, often following procedures that induce

Table 11-1. Cardiac Risk Factors
for Endocarditis

1. High Risk
   a. Prosthetic heart valve(s)
   b. History of endocarditis
2. Moderate Risk
   a. Rheumatic or other acquired valvular disease
   b. Congenital heart disease (excluding atrial septal defect of the secundum type)
   c. Idiopathic hypertrophic subaortic stenosis
3. Probable Moderate Risk
   a. Mitral valve prolapse
   b. Undiagnosed murmurs

Table 11-2. Events Predisposing to Bacteremia

EVENT	PERCENTAGE OF INSTANCES IN WHICH BACTEREMIA OCCURS
Dental extraction	75%
Tooth brushing, flossing or irrigation	
Normal gingiva	20%
Gingivitis	50%
Bronchoscopy	
Fiberoptic	less than 1%
Rigid	15%
Fiberoptic endoscopy	10%
Sigmoidoscopy	5%
Barium enema	10%
Liver biopsy	5%
Transurethral resection of prostate	
Sterile urine	10%
Infected urine	50%

bacteremia and frequently associated with bacteria of low virulence. Late prosthetic valve endocarditis deserves special attention for two reasons: (1) organisms that are rarely able to infect damaged natural valves are more apt to infect prosthetic valves, and (2) when one deals with prosthetic valve endocarditis, the stakes are higher; treatment often involves valve replacement, and even with medical and surgical treatment overall mortality is significantly higher.

Another particularly high-risk group includes those who have previously had endocarditis. Recurrence rates as high as 10 per cent have been cited, and third infections have been reported in some individuals. Table 11-1 summarizes known predisposing lesions in approximate order of risk. It must be kept in mind that the absolute chance of endocarditis, even for the patient at risk, is extremely low, on the order of 1 case per 500 tooth extractions.

The association of bacteremia with various events is shown in Table 11-2. Leading the list are dental

procedures, rigid bronchoscopy and GU manipulations in the presence of urinary infection.

NATURAL HISTORY OF ENDOCARDITIS AND EFFECTIVENESS OF THERAPY

Untreated endocarditis is uniformly fatal. Current mortality rates are about 10 per cent with natural valves and 25 to 50 per cent with prosthetic valves. Death is often associated with congestive heart failure, arterial emboli, myocardial infarction, myocardial abscesses or other complications.

The efficacy of antibiotics used prophylactically has not been demonstrated. The large number of patients needed for such a study and the difficulties identifying patients at risk and of diagnosing episodes of potential bacteremia practically preclude such proof. Recommendations for prophylactic antibiotic regimens are based on an experimental animal model.

IDENTIFYING PATIENTS AT RISK

As discussed previously, a rough estimate of risk can be made by identifying the underlying heart disease and estimating the likelihood that bacteremia will occur. Predisposing cardiac disease is detected by history and physical examination. A history of congenital or rheumatic heart disease and presence of a murmur indicate substantial risk. Documentation of IHSS or the presence of valve calcification can also be considered indication for prophylaxis. All individuals with diastolic murmurs should be considered to be at risk. Difficulty arises when there is an isolated systolic murmur without a helpful history of other cardiac findings (see Chapter 15 on systolic murmurs). If the murmur is not easily identifiable, prophylaxis for high-risk procedures is the most reasonable course. These procedures include dental work, rigid bronchoscopy, prostate surgery and urinary catheter manipulation in the presence of infected urine.

RISK OF PROPHYLACTIC THERAPY

In the absence of previous sensitivity, the risk of serious reaction to penicillin prophylaxis is very small. No deaths were associated with the administration of benzathine penicillin G to over 300,000 Navy recruits for rheumatic fever prophylaxis. The largest studies have shown the incidence of all types of reactions to both intramuscularly and orally administered penicillin to be less than 1 per cent. Approximately half of these reactions were considered serious.

Less information is available concerning risks associated with other prophylactic antibiotics. However, the rate of allergic reactions is probably significantly lower and, even with aminoglycosides, there is little toxicity when the drug is given for the brief period necessary for adequate prophylaxis.

CONCLUSIONS AND RECOMMENDATIONS

- Clinical efficacy of endocarditis prophylaxis is difficult to demonstrate definitively. However, when the extreme degrees of morbidity and mortality associated with the disease are weighed against the negligible risk associated with prophylaxis, vigorous preventive efforts are justified. It is estimated that about half of cases occur in patients with known predisposing heart disease following an anticipated episode of bacteremia, and thus may be preventable.
- Identifiable risk varies with the type of heart abnormality and the event responsible for bacteremia, as summarized in Tables 11–1 and 11–2.
- Because patients with prosthetic valves are especially susceptible, they should receive vigorous prophylaxis for any procedure—oral, genitourinary or gastrointestinal—known to cause bacteremia. Similar vigorous therapy might also be applied to patients with a history of endocarditis. Specific recommendations for these *high-risk patients* are as follows:

For dental procedures or surgery of the respiratory tract:

1. Aqueous crystalline penicillin G (1,000,000 units I.M.) *mixed with* procaine penicillin G (600,000 units IM), *plus*
2. Streptomycin (1 gm. IM)

All of the above given 30 minutes before the procedure, followed by penicillin V (500 mg. PO) given every 6 hours for 8 doses.

For patients allergic to penicillin:

1. Vancomycin (1 gm. IV infused over 30 to 60 minutes), before the procedure, *followed by*
2. Erythromycin (500 mg. PO) given every 6 hours for 8 doses.

For GU or GI tract procedures:

1. Aqueous crystalline penicillin G (2,000,000 units IM or IV) *or* ampicillin (1.0 gm. IM or IV), *plus*
2. Gentamicin (1.5 mg./kg., not to exceed 80 mg. IM or IV) *or* streptomycin (1.0 gm. IM).

Initial doses are to be given 30 to 60 minutes before the procedure. Ampicillin or penicillin doses are repeated every 6 hours for 3 to 4 doses. If gentamicin is used, the same dose is given every 8 hours for 2 additional doses. If streptomycin is used, the same dose is given every 12 hours for 2 additional doses. Additional doses may be necessary for prolonged procedures. On the other hand, a single dose may be sufficient for simple outpatient procedures. Longer intervals between doses may be appropriate in patients with significantly compromised renal function.

- Patients with congenital or acquired valvular disease or with undiagnosed murmurs thought to reflect an anatomic abnormality should receive prophylaxis for all dental and upper respiratory tract procedures. Genitourinary and gastrointestinal procedures associated with a high frequency of bacteremia (including GU procedures in the presence of infected urine or prostate) should be done with antibiotic coverage. Endoscopy, barium enema, sigmoidoscopy, D & C and IUD insertion do not require antibiotic coverage.

Specific recommendations for these moderate-risk patients include:

1. Aqueous crystalline penicillin G (1,000,000 units IM) *mixed with* procaine penicillin G (600,000 units IM), both given 30 to 60 minutes before the procedure, *followed by* penicillin V (500 mg. PO) every 6 hours for 8 doses
2. Alternative when parenteral therapy is not feasible: Penicillin V (2.0 gm. PO) 30 to 60 minutes before the procedure, *followed by* penicillin V (500 mg. PO) every 6 hours for 8 doses

For patients allergic to penicillin:

1. Vancomycin as recommended for high-risk patients with penicillin sensitivity, *or*
2. Erythromycin (1.0 gm. PO), 90 to 120 minutes prior to the procedure, *followed by* erythromycin (500 mg. PO) every 6 hours for 8 doses

This regimen may also be preferred to oral penicillin for patients taking penicillin continuously for rheumatic fever prophylaxis. While endocarditis caused by penicillin-resistant organisms has not been a significant problem in such patients, it remains a theoretical concern.

- As in all preventive efforts, patient education is extremely important. All patients with identifiable risk should be urged to maintain a high level of oral health to minimize the potential for recurrent bacteremia. Patients receiving rheumatic fever prophylaxis must understand that their continuous therapy will *not* protect them from endocarditis.

ANNOTATED BIBLIOGRAPHY

Allen, H.A., Leatham, A., et al.: Significance and prognosis of an isolated late systolic murmur: A 9- to 22-year follow-up. Br. Heart J., *36*:525, 1974. *(Sixty-two patients with isolated late systolic murmur [33 also had a click] were followed for minimum of 9 years [mean 13.8]. Bacterial endocarditis occurred in 5 patients.)*

Dismukes, W.E., Karchmer, W.E., Buckley, M., et al.: Prosthetic valve endocarditis. Analysis of 38 cases. Circulation, *48*:365, 1973. *(Includes 19 cases of "late" endocarditis. Predisposing factors were identified in 12 cases, with dental or GU procedures incriminated in 7.)*

Doyle, E.F., Spagnuolo, M., Taranta, A., et al.: The risk of bacterial endocarditis during antirheumatic prophylaxis. JAMA, *201*:807, 1967. *(Sixteen cases of endocarditis were reported during 3615 patient-years of antirheumatic prophylaxis. No controls, but calculated incidence was not statistically different from that in historical control group. Four of the 16 organisms were penicillin-resistant.)*

Durack, D.T., and Petersdorf, R.G.: Chemotherapy of experimental streptococcal endocarditis. I. Comparison of commonly recommended prophylactic regimens. J. Clin. Invest., *52*:592, 1973. *(Experimental infections in the rabbit model demonstrate that administration of penicillin in high doses, for short durations alone or in low doses for long durations alone is not efficacious.)*

Epstein, E.J., and Coulshed, N.: Bacterial endocarditis in idiopathic hypertrophic subaortic stenosis. Cardiologica, *54*:30, 1969. *(This paper reviews reported cases of endocarditis in a combined series of 158 patients with IHSS.)*

Everett, E.D., and Hirschman, J.V.: Transient bacteremia and endocarditis prophylaxis. A review. Medicine, *56*:61, 1977. *(Incidence data for bacteremia associated with relevant clinical procedures gathered from the literature are reviewed.)*

Hilson, G.R.F.: Is chemoprophylaxis necessary? Proc. R. Soc. Med., *63*:267, 1970. *(A critical review of the prophylaxis rationale ends with a plea for a controlled trial.)*

Kaplan, E.L., Anthony, B.F., Bisno, A., et al.: Prevention of bacterial endocarditis. Circulation, *56*:39A, 1977. *(Summarizes the rationale and most recent AHA recommendations and recognizes the special risk of patients with prosthetic valves.)*

Lerner, P.I., and Weinstein, L.: Infectious endocarditis in the antibiotic era. N. Engl. J. Med., *274*:199, 1966. *(One hundred cases plus an extensive literature review.)*

Prophylaxis of bacterial endocarditis: Faith, hope and charitable interpretation. (Editorial.) Lancet, *1*:519, 1976. *(Argues the infeasibility of any clinical trial and the importance of experimental models.)*

Weinstein, L., and Rubin R.H.: Infectious endocarditis—1973. Prog. Cardiovasc. Dis., *16*:239, 1973. *(An update. Some information about susceptibility and predisposing events.)*

Wilson, W.R., Javmin, D.M., Danielson, G.K., et al.: Prosthetic valve endocarditis. Ann. Intern. Med., *82*:751, 1975. *(Gram-negative rods were found in 31 per cent of late cases.)*

12
Rheumatic Fever Prophylaxis

Despite a decline in incidence that began before the availability of antibiotics, rheumatic fever and rheumatic heart disease remain significant causes of preventable morbidity. Primary prevention depends on appropriate diagnosis and effective treatment of Group A streptococcal pharyngitis, discussed in Chapter 210. The prophylactic use of antibiotics has been shown to be effective for primary prevention during epidemics among closed populations. The major role of antibiotic prophylaxis, however, is in pre-

Table 12–1. Risk of Recurrent Rheumatic Fever
After Group A Streptococcal Infection

	PERCENT RECURRENCES OF STREPTOCOCCAL INFECTION
Interval since onset of last rheumatic episode	
Up to two years	28%
Two to five years	15%
Five years and over	10%
Number of previous attacks of rheumatic fever	
Two or more	27%
One	14%
Rheumatic heart disease	
Not present	13%
Present	26%

Modified from Spagnuolo, M., *et al.*, N. Engl. J. Med., *285*:641, 1971.

vention of second attacks. The risk of recurrence following streptococcal infection is especially high in patients with evidence of carditis. Continuous streptococcal prophylaxis in patients with prior rheumatic fever is the major means of preventing the cardiac sequelae of rheumatic fever recurrences. It is the task of the primary physician to identify patients who would benefit from such prophylaxis and to provide the instruction necessary for long-term compliance.

EPIDEMIOLOGY AND RISK FACTORS

The epidemiology of rheumatic fever parallels that of streptococcal infection. Rare below age 5, it is most common in older children and adolescents. Incidence decreases after adolescence; cases after age 40 are very rare. There is no clear predilection for either sex. A genetic predisposition has not been proven. Racial differences in incidence disappear when socioeconomic status is considered; crowded living conditions are an important variable. Crowding may also explain the high incidence in cold climates and during winter months in temperate climates.

All demographic risk factors are heavily outweighed by a previous history of rheumatic fever. The likelihood of an attack following streptococcal infection is at least five times higher among individuals with previous rheumatic fever.

NATURAL HISTORY OF RHEUMATIC FEVER AND EFFECTIVENESS OF THERAPY

Rheumatic fever follows between 0.5 per cent and 3.0 per cent of ineffectively treated cases of Group A streptococcal upper respiratory infections. Diagnosis and appropriate antibiotic therapy will prevent rheumatic fever in the individual case, but such efforts cannot be expected to eliminate rheumatic disease because of the high proportion of streptococcal infections that are subclinical. Approximately one third of patients with primary rheumatic fever have no history of preceding respiratory infections. Another one third have symptoms but do not seek medical care. The remainder are ineffectively diagnosed or treated.

Among all patients with Group A streptococcal infection and a history of previous rheumatic fever, the recurrence rate is 15 per cent. More specific rates can be estimated for subgroups depending on (1) the number of previous rheumatic attacks, (2) the interval since the last attack, and (3) whether or not there was evidence of carditis. Specific attack rates are summarized in Table 12–1.

Because of these high secondary attack rates and the ubiquity of the streptococcus, *continuous* antibiotic prophylaxis of streptococcal infection is the only feasible method of preventing rheumatic fever recurrences. Three antibiotic regimens have gained general acceptance:

1. Benzathine penicillin G, 1,200,000 units IM every 4 weeks
2. Sulfadiazine, 1 gm. PO q.d. (500 mg. for patients under 60 lbs.)
3. Penicillin G, 250,000 units PO b.i.d.

While the effectiveness of erythromycin (250 mg. PO b.i.d.) has not been studied, it is recommended for the rare patient allergic to both penicillin and sulfonamides. The classic study comparing the effectiveness of these three regimens in preventing streptococcal infection and rheumatic fever is summarized in Table 12–2.

There are no firm guidelines regarding the duration of continuous antibiotic prophylaxis following an episode of rheumatic fever. Factors that influence the

Table 12–2. Prophylaxis and Attack Rates of Streptococcal
Infection and Rheumatic Fever Recurrences

	ORAL SULFADIAZINE (1 GM. DAILY)	ORAL PENICILLIN G (200,000 UNITS DAILY)	IM BENZATHINE PENICILLIN G (1.2 MILLION UNITS EVERY 4 WEEKS)
Number of patient-years	576	545	560
Number of streptococcal infections (rate/100 patient-years)	138 (24.0)	113 (20.7)	34 (6.1)
Number of rheumatic fever recurrences (rate/100 patient-years)	16 (2.8)	30 (5.5)	2 (0.4)

Modified from Wood, H. F., *et al.*, Ann. Intern. Med., *60*:31, 1964.

likelihood of rheumatic recurrence following infection have already been reviewed. Within limits, the physician can estimate the risk of exposure of a particular patient to streptococcal infection. For example, parents of young children, teachers and other school personnel, health care providers and military personnel are at high risk.

RISKS OF ANTIBIOTIC PROPHYLAXIS

The risks of penicillin administration are discussed in Chapter 11 on endocarditis prophylaxis. It should be emphasized that, in a large series, reactions following parenteral administration were no more common than those following oral therapy.

CONCLUSIONS AND RECOMMENDATIONS

- Primary prevention of rheumatic fever depends on accurate diagnosis and treatment of symptomatic streptococcal upper respiratory infections. Prevention of rheumatic fever recurrences depends on continuous streptococcal prophylaxis of the patients at risk.
- Monthly injections of benzathine penicillin G (1,200,000 units IM) provide the most effective prophylaxis and are recommended in patients with both a high risk of streptococcal exposure and a high risk of rheumatic recurrence after infection. Acceptable oral regimens in patients at lower risk include:

    Sulfadiazine, 1 gm. PO q.d., *or*
    Penicillin G, 250,000 units PO b.i.d., *or*
    Erythromycin, 250 mg. PO b.i.d. (in patients allergic to both penicillin and sulfa drugs)

- The duration of prophylaxis should be based on the risk incurred by the particular patient.
- All patients with rheumatic fever should be treated

until age 25 or for 5 years following an episode (whichever is longer). In those with two or more previous attacks or with rheumatic heart disease, therapy should be continued until age 40 or for 10 years following the last episode. Prophylaxis in patients with rheumatic heart disease at high risk of streptococcal exposure should be continued indefinitely.

ANNOTATED BIBLIOGRAPHY

Breese, B.B., and Disney, F.A.: Penicillin in the treatment of streptococcal infections. A comparison of effectiveness of five different oral and one parenteral form. N. Engl. J. Med., *259*:57, 1958. *(No difference was found in reaction rates between I.M. and PO use.)*

Kaplan, E.L., Bisno, A., Derrick, W. et. al.: Prevention of rheumatic fever: AHA Committee Report. Circulation, *55*:1, 1977. *(Summary of argument for prophylaxis with recommendations.)*

Sellers, T.F.: An epidemiologic view of rheumatic fever. Prog. Cardiovasc. Dis., *16*:303, 1973. *(Reviews epidemiology.)*

Spagnuolo, M., Pasternack, B. and Taranta, A.: Risk of rheumatic fever recurrences after streptococcal infections. N. Engl. J. Med., *285*:641, 1971. *(Data are reviewed in Table 12–1.)*

McFarland, R.B.: Reactions to benzathine penicillin. N. Engl. J. Med., *259*:62, 1958. *(Reaction rate of 1.3 percent following single injection in 12,858 naval recruits.)*

Wood, H.F., Feinstein, A.R., Taranta, A. et al.: Rheumatic fever in children and adolescents. III. Comparative effectiveness of three prophylaxis regimens in preventing streptococcal infections and rheumatic recurrences. Ann. Intern. Med., *60*:31, 1964. *(Data are reviewed in Table 12–2.)*

13

Evaluation of Hypertension

EVE E. SLATER, M.D.

Most hypertensives are not even aware that they are being stalked by a quiet killer that often produces no symptoms until it is too late.

TIME Magazine
January 13, 1975, p. 60

High blood pressure, if unrecognized or untreated, leads to the development of heart failure, renal failure and stroke, and is considered the most significant cardiovascular risk factor. In the majority of cases, the cause of hypertension is unknown. Moreover, the disease is usually asymptomatic prior to the advent of complications. The silent nature of hypertension, ignorance regarding its pathogenesis, and frustration caused by the long-term, empiric therapy required have fostered apathy in physician and patient alike. Blood pressure measurements are commonly omitted during routine physical examinations or emergency room visits. Follow-up for patients with high blood pressure is often limited or nonexistent, and even when patients keep their appointments faithfully, they may not be taking their medications as prescribed. Of the estimated 35 million Americans with hypertension, only about half have been discovered, and of these, far fewer are receiving adequate therapy.

Adequate therapy of high blood pressure has been shown to reduce morbidity and mortality. Even partial correction can reduce complications significantly. In light of the clearly demonstrated benefits of treatment, apathy toward high blood pressure cannot be justified.

DEFINITION

The definition of high blood pressure is arbitrary. Actuarial data have shown that morbidity and mortality related to complications of hypertension increase linearly with increasing levels of either systolic or diastolic blood pressure. Hence, no critical level of blood pressure exists beyond which risk becomes highly magnified. For the sake of definition, we identify as hypertensive those blood pressure levels associated with a greater than 50 per cent increase in mortality. These are as follows: for men below age 45, 130/90 mm. Hg; for men over age 45, 140/95 mm. Hg; for women of all ages, 160/95 mm. Hg.

Primary or *essential hypertension,* which accounts for over 90 per cent of cases, is as yet without identifiable cause. Onset of disease is usually between ages 30 and 50, and a history of familial hypertension can often be elicited. *Secondary hypertension* has a definable etiology (Table 13–1), occurs within a wide age range, and is often abrupt in onset and severe in magnitude; family history is commonly negative. *Borderline hypertension* is blood pressure that intermittently rises above the normal levels for each given age group and sex. Established hypertension has been shown to develop more commonly in patients with borderline hypertension.

It is becoming increasingly apparent that the definition of hypertension must be individualized for each patient. The diagnosis derives not only from the absolute level of blood pressure, but also from the presence or absence of other *cardiovascular risk factors.* Factors identified by the Framingham study as significant contributors to cardiovascular risk are hypertension, cigarette smoking, elevated serum cholesterol levels, glucose intolerance and electrocardiographic evidence of left ventricular hypertrophy with strain. Thus the patient with borderline hypertension, a moderately elevated serum cholesterol level and a history of smoking has fivefold higher risk of incurring cardiovascular disease than the patient with borderline hypertension alone. Clearly, the patient at higher risk should be considered a candidate for prompt reduction of blood pressure and risk factor modification. A probability profile based upon these risk factors is available (see Kannel, 1976) and can be extremely useful in predicting whether therapeutic intervention is advisable.

PATHOGENESIS

Understanding the renin-angiotensin-aldosterone system has provided an explanation for certain forms of secondary hypertension as well as a framework for classifying patients with essential hypertension. Renin is released by the kidneys and acts within the

Table 13–1. Primary vs. Secondary Hypertension: Specific Screening Protocols

CAUSE	SCREEN	CONFIRMATION
Coarctation	PE: arm and leg BPs, chest x-ray ($33)	Angiography (approx. $200-$500)
Cushing's syndrome	PE, *Dexamethasone suppression* ($30) (1 mg. dexamethasone midnight, 8 a.m. cortisol)	Endo evaluation
Drug-induced hypertension	History: amphetamines, oral contraceptives, estrogens, corticosteroids, licorice, thyroid	
↑Intracranial pressure	Neurologic evaluation	
Pheochromocytoma	History of paroxysmal hypertension, headache, perspiration, palpitations *or* fixed diastolic $\geq$ 130 mm. Hg, *Urinary metanephrine* ($13.50) VMA ($7.50)	Catecholamine levels ($100), angiography (approx. $200-$500), CAT scan
Primary aldosteronism (Conn's or idiopathic)	*Serum K+* ($2.00), *urine K+* ($2.00), *stim. PRA* ($25.00)	Aldosterone levels ($50), venography with differential level (approx. $150), ? adrenal scan
Renal disease	Congenital, diabetes, glomerulonephritis, gout, interstitial or polycystic pyelonephritis, obstruction, vasculitis	
Renovascular disease	Suspect in young female or elderly patient with arteriosclerosis, especially if abrupt onset, negative family history, and abdominal bruit present, *Stim. PRA* ($25), IVP ($103), *? renal scan* ($225) .	Angiography with differential venous renins (approx. $500)

PE = physical examination

bloodstream to yield angiotensin II, a potent vasoconstrictor and primary stimulus for aldosterone release. Renin production is inversely proportional to effective blood volume: anything that increases effective blood volume suppresses renin; anything that decreases effective blood volume stimulates renin. Thus, in primary aldosteronism, autonomous production of the salt-retaining hormone aldosterone by an adrenal adenoma results in intravascular volume expansion and renin suppression. Conversely, in renal artery stenosis, decreased renal perfusion on the affected side is perceived by that kidney as decreased effective blood volume. Renin is secreted, and increases in angiotensin II and aldosterone result, thereby creating systemic hypertension and volume expansion. While renin initiates this form of hypertension, it is maintained in different patients by a varying ratio of elevated angiotensin II and aldosterone. Similarly, patients with essential hypertension can be placed in high, normal or low renin groups. Unlike patients with primary aldosteronism or renal artery stenosis, however, a pathogenetic lesion responsible for these different renin levels has not yet been identified.

The role of the central nervous system in the pathogenesis of essential hypertension is becoming increasingly appreciated. Studies on patients with borderline hypertension have allowed clear identification of subgroups in which a defect in autonomic nervous system controls exists, resulting in excessive sympathetic and reduced parasympathetic activity. Certainly pheochromocytoma provides a model for secondary hypertension based upon excessive catecholamines.

Dietary sodium has long been implicated in the pathogenesis of hypertension. In cultures in which salt intake is nonexistent, hypertension is an exceedingly rare disease. Interest is currently being focused upon the renal threshold of sodium excretion as a possible factor in the development of hypertension.

Lastly, cardiogenic factors appear to be important in the development of hypertension. In certain strains of rats in which hypertension develops spontaneously and is eventually fatal, cardiac hypertrophy occurs long before elevation of blood pressure.

CLINICAL PRESENTATION

Hypertension is usually asymptomatic until the development of substantial blood pressure elevation, in which case fatigue, headache, light-headedness, flushing or epistaxis may be reported. The rare syndrome of hypertensive encephalopathy, seen when diastolic blood pressure rises rapidly above 130 mm. Hg, is characterized by restlessness, confusion, somnolence, blurred vision, and nausea or vomiting; all these symptoms are related to increased intracranial pressure.

Certain forms of secondary hypertension may be characterized by specific symptoms. Thus the patient with coarctation of the aorta may experience leg claudication as a result of lower extremity ischemia; the patient with Cushing's syndrome may complain of hirsutism or easy bruising; the patient with pheochromocytoma may experience excessive perspiration, severe paroxysmal headaches or palpitations; and the patient with primary aldosteronism will be prone to symptoms of hypokalemia, i.e., muscle cramps, weakness and polyuria.

Once end-organ damage develops, symptoms will be related to congestive failure, renal failure, cerebrovascular insufficiency, peripheral vascular disease, or ischemic heart disease.

DIFFERENTIAL DIAGNOSIS

Over 95 per cent of cases are essential and can be subdivided into high, normal and low renin varieties. Secondary causes account for the remainder and are listed in Table 13–1.

WORKUP

History. Patient evaluation includes a careful interview with emphasis on family history of hypertension, diabetes or cardiovascular disease; patient's age at onset of elevated blood pressure; diet, especially with regard to salt intake; presence of other cardiovascular risk factors (smoking, diabetes, lipid abnormalities); symptoms of cardiovascular disease (angina, dyspnea, claudication, etc.); use of agents that can cause hypertension (birth control pills, steroids, thyroid, amphetamines in diet pills or cold capsules, large quantities of licorice); symptoms of secondary hypertension as summarized above; and history of renal disease or flank trauma.

Physical examination emphasizes weight measurement; funduscopy; thyroid examination; general cardiopulmonary examination; evaluation of peripheral vasculature including bilateral arm and leg pressure measurements, simultaneous radial and femoral pulse palpation and auscultation for bruits; abdominal palpation and auscultation; observation for the stigmata of Cushing's syndrome, chronic renal failure, or neurofibromatosis; and complete neurologic evaluation.

Several commonly held beliefs regarding the diagnosis of high blood pressure have been challenged recently by epidemiologic data such as those generated by the Framingham study. First, casual blood pressure determinations appear to be as reliable as basal levels in predicting long-term cardiovascular risk. This is not surprising if we accept the fact that a person capable of anxiety-provoked hypertension in

the setting of a physician's office is equally apt to respond to the stresses of daily life with labile hypertension. Second, risk appears directly proportional to systolic or diastolic blood pressure, elevation of either equally predisposing to the complications of hypertension.

Blood pressure is properly measured in both arms while the patient is seated comfortably. The cuff should be placed at heart level and as high as possible on the arm. The average of two successive measurements in each arm is recorded. Diastolic pressure is taken at the point at which sound disappears (Korotkoff 5) rather than when it changes in quality (Korotkoff 4). Cuff size must be adequate to avoid falsely elevated readings (cuff width $> \frac{2}{3}$ arm width, length of inflatable portion $> \frac{2}{3}$ arm circumference).

Laboratory studies. Recently, extensive laboratory evaluation of patients with high blood pressure has come under a great deal of criticism. The yield of curable cases of hypertension is small, and with increasing costs, extensive evaluation for all hypertensive patients would put undue stress upon health resources.

Laboratory evaluation of high blood pressure has three purposes: (1) to ascertain the degree of end-organ damage resulting from hypertension, (2) to identify patients at high risk for the development of cardiovascular complications, and (3) to screen for secondary, possibly reversible forms of the disease. Despite the wide array of sophisticated diagnostic techniques now readily available, there is increasing evidence that the diagnosis of secondary hypertension can be made accurately and economically by the alert physician on the basis of a careful history, a physical examination, and only a few simple diagnostic tests.

Tests considered essential in the evaluation of high blood pressure include: complete blood count, urinalysis, serum BUN or creatinine, serum K^+, fasting blood sugar, serum cholesterol, and electrocardiogram. The urinalysis provides evidence of primary renal disease. The extent of renal compromise due to renal disease or secondary to the hypertension itself is indicated by the BUN or creatinine. Fasting blood sugar, serum cholesterol, and ECG supply data regarding cardiovascular risk and ECG changes resulting from hypertension. Serum potassium is a valuable screening test for primary aldosteronism and should be known prior to the institution of diuretic therapy. Total cost of these determinations is reasonable. In most patients, evaluation should stop here.

Patients at somewhat higher risk for secondary

hypertension include (1) those under 35, (2) those with rapid onset of elevated blood pressure and a negative family history, (3) those with severe hypertension, and (4) those who have failed to respond to empirical therapy despite compliance. Fortunately, in a majority of patients at high risk for secondary hypertension, a specific diagnosis will be suggested by history and physical examination. Thus the patient with Cushing's syndrome should be easily identified by appearance; the patient with coarctation can be diagnosed by measurement of arm and leg blood pressure and simultaneous radial–femoral pulse palpation; patients with pheochromocytoma or drug-induced hypertension (e.g., due to oral contraceptives, decongestants, or diet pills) can often be identified in an interview; primary aldosteronism is almost always apparent from serum K^+; and renovascular disease is most common in young patients and in older ones in whom onset of hypertension is abrupt, especially if a flank bruit or diffuse vascular disease is detected. When doubt still exists, the workup should be expanded to include screening for pheochromocytoma; i.e., a 24-hour urinary metanephrine or vanillylmandelic acid (VMA); and, for renovascular hypertension, a plasma renin activity (PRA) and hypertensive IVP, since clinical evaluation alone is not completely reliable in identifying these forms of hypertension.

When a specific form of hypertension is suspected, each possibility can be accurately screened as follows: Cushing's syndrome: 1 mg. dexamethasone suppression (cost: $30); coarctation: chest x-ray (cost: $33); pheochromocytoma: 24-hour urinary metanephrine (cost: $13.50) or VMA (cost: $7.50); primary aldosteronism: stimulated plasma renin activity (cost: $25) and urinary K^+: creatinine (cost: $3.50); renovascular hypertension: stimulated plasma renin activity (cost: $25) and IVP (cost: $103). Should these tests return positive, diagnosis can then be confirmed by more extensive evaluation in patients considered good surgical candidates.

It should be remembered that the screening protocols given in Table 13–1 are not entirely reliable. For example normal PRA and hypertensive IVP tests do not completely exclude the possibility of renovascular hypertension, diagnosis of which may require venography with differential renal venous renin sampling and arteriography. These more costly and invasive procedures must be resorted to when, despite negative screening, the clinical presentation strongly indicates the diagnosis or when hypertension is severe and difficult to control

Two questions often asked regarding the routine

evaluation of hypertensive patients are, What are the current indications for obtaining a plasma renin level? and What is the proper way to measure renin?

As a diagnostic tool, plasma renin activity (PRA) is essential in the initial evaluation of patients suspected of having a renin-related form of secondary hypertension, specifically primary aldosteronism or renovascular hypertension. Differential renal venous renins are necessary to establish the diagnosis of renovascular hypertension, to lateralize the lesion and to predict surgical result. We do not, however, recommend that PRA be measured routinely. While subgroups of essential hypertensives have been derived from differences in PRA, the clinical characteristics of each group with regard to both prognosis and therapeutic response have not proved sufficiently different to warrant the routine measurement of PRA in all patients.

Knowledge of renin status may provide help in management. Patients with high levels of PRA tend to respond preferentially to sympatholytic agents, and patients with low PRA tend to benefit from diuretics. Nevertheless, most patients with mild hypertension can be treated effectively regardless of knowledge of the renin status. When two or three drug combinations are required in the management of moderate or severe hypertension, renin typing often facilitates drug selection, especially for patients who have responded poorly to empirical therapy, or for those who require rapid control, e.g., patients with unstable angina (see Chapter 21 on blood pressure management).

Renin measurement is performed easily in the outpatient setting. Since most of the commonly used antihypertensive medications (with the exception of methyldopa) are known to affect PRA, these medications should be withdrawn at least 2 weeks prior to testing for secondary hypertension. As a guide to therapy, renin determination can be helpful regardless of concurrent antihypertensive treatment. Parenthetically, the measurement of PRA within 6 months of oral contraceptive use is meaningless due to pill-induced vagaries in PRA levels. A high sodium diet, common to most patients, can obscure differences in PRA.

To render determination more accurate, mild stimulation of renin prior to measurement is recommended. Stimulated PRA is properly performed after the administration of a diuretic and after standing. Simple protocols are as follows: 40 to 80 mg. of furosemide PO followed by 4 hours of standing, or 40 mg. furosemide IV followed by one-half hour of standing. Such testing can easily be performed in the office. Since renin levels and their diagnostic significance vary depending upon the type of assay procedure performed, it is often necessary to seek local advice for interpretation of results. In our own laboratory, a stimulated PRA of less than 1.0 ng./ml./hr. suggests excessive salt intake, low-renin essential hypertension, or the possibility of mineralocorticoid secondary hypertension. A stimulated PRA of greater than 5.0 ng./ml./hr. indicates renin-dependent hypertension and suggests that a search for renovascular disease be undertaken.

ANNOTATED BIBLIOGRAPHY

Brunner, H.R., *et al.*: Essential hypertension: Renin and aldosterone, heart attack and stroke. N.Eng. J.Med., *286*:441, 1972. *(This is now a classic report describing renin typing in essential hypertension and proposing that renin relates to cardiovascular risk.)*

Ferguson, R.K.: Cost and yield of the hypertensive evaluation: Experience of a community-based referral clinic. Ann.Intern.Med., *82*:761, 1975. *(This paper emphasizes that secondary hypertension can be detected on the basis of a careful examination and only a few simple diagnostic tests.)*

Julius, S., and Esler, M.: Autonomic nervous cardiovascular regulation in borderline hypertension. Am.J.Cardiol., *36*:685, 1975. *(Summarizes current thoughts regarding the role of the central nervous system in initiation of high blood pressure.)*

Kannel, W.B.: Some lessons in cardiovascular epidemiology from Framingham. Am.J.Cardiol. *37*:269, 1976. *(This is required reading for practicing physicians. It provides guidelines for predicting cardiovascular risk.)*

Kaplan, N.M., *et al.*: The intravenous furosemide test: A simple way to evaluate renin responsiveness. Ann.Intern.Med., *84*:639, 1976. *(This paper describes the method of stimulated renin determination.)*

Laragh, J.H.: Symposium on hypertension: The use of renin and aldosterone profiles. Am.J.Med., *55*:261, 1973. *(This is an excellent description of the vasoconstrictor-volume models for hypertension.)*

Melby, J.D., and Finnerty, F.A., Jr.: Debates in medicine: Extensive hypertensive workup. JAMA, *231*:399, 1975. *(This article typifies the arguements regarding extensive workup for hypertension.)*

Wallach, L., Nyarai, I., and Dawson, K.G.: Stimulated renin: A screening test for hypertension. Ann.Intern.Med., *82*:27, 1975. *(This paper describes the method of stimulated renin determination.)*

14
Evaluation of Chest Pain

Chest pain is among the most frequent causes of unscheduled office visits. Concerns about heart and lung disease are uppermost in the minds of many who come for evaluation. Although many chest pains prove to be harmless, the primary physician must be skilled in accurately recognizing the signs of serious etiologies in the office, where one is limited to a careful history, physical examination, ECG, and perhaps chest x-ray. Of particular challenge are evaluating pleuritic chest pain and determining when atypical pain represents angina.

PATHOPHYSIOLOGY AND CLINICAL PRESENTATION

Most structures within, surrounding, or adjacent to the thorax are capable of producing chest pain. Pain originating from the *chest wall* is predominantly musculoskeletal in origin. It may last from a few seconds to several days and can be sharp, aching or dull. The discomfort is characteristically aggravated by deep inspiration, cough, direct palpation and movement. Sometimes the patient complains of chest tightness. Vigorous and unaccustomed exertion can lead to muscular and ligamentous strain. Common sites of involvement are the costochondral and chondrosternal junctions. *Precordial catch syndrome,* which is believed to result from muscle spasm, causes acute sharp pain worsened by breathing and terminated by stretching or taking a very deep breath. It occurs mostly in young adults. *Costochondritis (Tietze's syndrome)* causes localized swelling, erythema, warmth and tenderness at the costochondral junction. *Rib fracture* is usually preceded by a history of trauma or evidence of underlying malignancy. Of interest is the observation that musculoskeletal pain appears to occur with increased frequency in patients with angina, leading to considerable diagnostic confusion.

Other components of the chest wall are sometimes responsible for pain. For example, nerve irritation from a flare-up of *herpes zoster* causes discomfort in a dermatomal distribution. The neurologic complaints range from hypoesthesia to dysesthesia and hyperesthesia. Pain may precede the appearance of the vesicular rash by 3 to 5 days and, especially in the elderly, persist long after the rash resolves (see Chapter 185). Nerve injury from root compression due to *cervical spine disease* or a *thoracic outlet syndrome* can lead to pain in the chest and upper arm, superficially resembling angina. In the outlet syndrome, a cervical rib may compress part of the brachial plexus, resulting in motor and sensory deficits that occur in the arm in an ulnar distribution; at the same time, there is discomfort in the chest and upper arm (see Chapter 155).

Inflammation or distention of the *pleura* also produces pain worsened by deep inspiration and cough, but movement and palpation have little or no effect. A host of etiologies can trigger the inflammatory process, including infection, pulmonary infarction, neoplasm, uremia and connective tissue disease. The more florid the inflammation, the greater the pain; and infectious etiology is more likely to present with considerable pleuritic pain than is a low-grade serositis associated with connective tissue disease. Stretching of the pleura following a *spontaneous pneumothorax* results in the acute onset of pleuritic pain and dyspnea. The condition often accompanies emphysema, in which there can be rupture of a bleb being responsible. When the pneumothorax is large, deviation of the trachea may be noted as mediastinal shift occurs. *Pleurodynia* is a self-limited source of pleuritic pain. It is most common in children and young adults and associated with Coxsackie B infection. Usually there is a typical viral prodrome followed by acute onset of chest pain.

Pericarditis may also be a source of pleuritic pain, due to spread of the inflammatory process from the relatively insensitive pericardium to the adjacent parietal pleura. The pain is sharp, aggravated by respiratory motion and sometimes precipitated by swallowing if the posterior aspect of the heart is involved. When the diaphragmatic surface of the pericardium is involved, pain will be referred to the tip of the shoulder. Change in position may alter the pain; patients often note lessening of the pain upon sitting up and leaning forward. Pericarditis can also produce a second type of pain that mimics angina. The most important physical finding associated with pericarditis is a 2 or 3 component rub.

Chest pain can be produced by disease of the *pulmonary parenchyma* if the process extends into the pleura or another pain-sensitive structure in the chest. Consequently, the pain is usually pleuritic in quality. Among the most important etiologies are *pneumococcal pneumonia* (see Chapter 43), *acute pulmonary tuberculosis* (see Chapter 47), and *pulmonary embolization with infarction.* Most pulmonary emboli do not cause pleuritic pain, because the major sources of pain—infarction and congestive atelectasis—occur only in the context of marked embolic obstruction to blood flow to the lung. It is estimated by some that fewer than 10 per cent of embolic episodes are associated with pain. The most common manifestation of embolization is dyspnea, which is seen in virtually every case, though it may be transient. Tachypnea and tachycardia are the only consistently observed physical findings; they too may be evanescent. Pleural rub, effusion, fever, or hemoptysis suggests the presence of infarction.

Angina pectoris is the most important cardiac source of chest pain. Typically it is brought on by exertion, eating a large meal, or emotional stress and is relieved by rest or nitroglycerin. Sexual intercourse is a particularly frequent precipitant. Patients usually report a squeezing or pressure sensation and sometimes do not even refer to the discomfort as a pain. Descriptions of sharp pain are atypical. Radiation of the pain to the jaw, neck, shoulder, arm, back or upper abdomen is common, and some patients experience pain in one of these locations without having any chest symptoms. At times the arm is reported to feel numb. The duration of symptoms ranges from 2 to 20 minutes. Pain lasting longer is suggestive of acute coronary insufficiency or myocardial infarction; fleeting pains of a few seconds duration are not anginal in origin. Prompt response to nitroglycerin is characteristic of mild angina; relief is usually obtained within 5 minutes.

Other forms of angina include *nocturnal angina* or *angina decubitus*, in which the patient experiences pain while lying down, often awakening with typical anginal pain in the middle of the night. It is postulated that this might be a manifestation of pump failure, with the heart unable to handle the increased intravascular volume load resulting from recumbency. Another suspicion is that the increased physiological activity associated with REM sleep increases myocardial oxygen demand and triggers angina. *Variant angina* as described originally by Prinzmetal is characterized by anginal pain occurring exclusively at rest in conjunction wtih transient ST segment elevation on the electrocardiogram. Patients with this form of angina seem to have increased incidences of coronary artery spasm and major obstruction of a single vessel. Another form of variant angina has been described in which pain occurs both at rest and with exertion. Such patients have been found to have a high incidence of 2 and 3 vessel disease.

Atypical angina is a nonspecific term used to denote chest pain that differs in location or quality from the more typical form, yet is suggestive of angina in having similar precipitants, timing or other features. As many as 50 per cent of such patients prove to have coronary disease. Anginal pain is seen occasionally in *mitral valve prolapse*; however, most patients with prolapse and chest pain describe symptoms that are nonanginal in quality; i.e. poorly correlated with exertion or emotion and unrelieved by nitroglycerin.

Aortic and esophageal problems are important etiologies of chest pain. *Acute aortic dissection* produces a tearing, severe, sudden pain that often radiates to the back between the shoulder blades. *Esophageal reflux* of gastric contents gives a retrosternal burning sensation brought on by consuming a large meal, lying down, or bending over, it is lessened by antacids. *Esophageal spasm* may simulate ischemic pain in that it is substernal, may radiate to the neck, shoulder or arm, and is often relieved by nitroglycerin. It may occur with meals, acid reflux or come on spontaneously. Atypical pain due to *biliary tract disease* may also mimic angina, for it can present substernally and respond to nitroglycerin. On rare occasions, pancreatitis or peptic ulcer disease produces substernal chest pain.

Anxiety, depression, cardiac neurosis and malingering are the major psychogenic sources of chest pain. Patients with *anxiety* or *depression* describe a "heaviness" or "tightness" in the chest that lasts for hours to days. This sensation may be accompanied by a feeling of inability to take a deep breath. When there is associated hyperventilation, the resulting hypocapnia leaves the patient light-headed and tingling. *Cardiac neurosis* sometimes leads to reports of pain that are hard to distinguish from genuine angina; at other times the patient misinterprets a noncardiac chest pain. *Malingering* is characterized by a conscious effort to feign illness for the sake of obtaining secondary gain. Although other forms of psychogenic chest pain may bring secondary benefits to the patient, there is no premeditated attempt to deceive.

DIFFERENTIAL DIAGNOSIS

The differential diagnosis of chest pain can be organized along anatomic lines, as outlined in Table 14–1.

WORKUP

A careful history remains a most effective means of determining the cause of the patient's chest complaint. For example, in a study detailing the prevalence of angiographically confirmed coronary artery disease in almost 5000 patients, the prevalence of disease in persons who gave a history of typical angina was 89 per cent, whereas in people with nonanginal chest pain, the prevalence of coronary disease was 16 per cent. Questioning should emphasize timing and precipitating and alleviating factors. Quality, location and intensity of pain are notoriously misleading; for example, there is nothing pathognomonic about precordial pain radiating down the left arm. A common pitfall is to provide classic descriptions to the patient who cannot give a crisp account of the complaint. All too often patients will agree to neat descriptions under the duress of a physician's interrogation. Their initial vagueness may have been more useful diagnostically.

A few of the more important pain patterns are worth mentioning in terms of the differentials they suggest and how one separates one cause from another. Pain brought on by exertion and relieved by rest is indicative of angina; but psychogenic chest pain may also behave in this fashion. However, with the latter, chest complaints are usually accompanied by a host of other noncardiac signs and symptoms

Table 14-1.   Differential Diagnosis of Chest Pain

I. Chest Wall
  A. Muscular disorders
    1. Muscle spasm (precordial catch syndrome)
    2. Pleurodynia
    3. Muscle strain
  B. Skeletal disorders
    1. Costochondritis (Tietze's syndrome)
    2. Rib fracture
    3. Metastatic disease of bone
    4. Cervical or thoracic spine disease
  C. Neurovascular disorders
    1. Herpes zoster infection or postherpetic pain
    2. Nerve root compression
II. Cardiopulmonary
  A. Cardiac disorders
    1. Pericarditis
    2. Myocardial ischemia
    3. Prolapsed mitral valve
  B. Pleuropulmonary disorders
    1. Pleurisy of any etiology
    2. Pneumothorax
    3. Pulmonary embolization with infarction
    4. Pneumonitis
III. Aortic
  A. Dissecting aortic aneurysm
IV. Gastrointestinal
  A. Esophageal disorders
    1. Reflux
    2. Spasm
  B. Others
    1. Cholecystitis
    2. Peptic ulcer disease
    3. Pancreatitis
V. Psychogenic
  A. Anxiety (with or without hyperventilation)
  B. Cardiac neurosis
  C. Malingering
  D. Depression

(headache, light-headedness, nervousness, hyperventilation, weakness, sighing, fatigue), and coronary risk factors are often absent. Episodes may come on at rest, as with variant angina, but, unlike angina, are likely to last from hours to days. Prompt response (within 5 minutes) to sublingual nitroglycerin is not usually seen in psychogenic illness and can be a helpful distinguishing point.

Pain that worsens upon deep inspiration or cough suggests a pleural, pericardial and chest wall source. Focal tenderness at the site of pain narrows the differential to chest wall disease. Tenderness and swelling at the costochondral or sternochondral junction are characteristic of costochondritis (Tietze's syndrome). Coexistent viral illness and clustering of cases argues for pleurodynia due to Coxsackie infection. In young adults, acute pleuritic pain that resolves upon stretching or taking a very deep breath is virtually diagnostic of the precordial catch syndrome.

Pleuritic pain relieved by leaning forward and occurring in the context of a recent transmural infarction, viral illness, uremia, tuberculosis or collagen disease points to pericarditis. Pneumothorax comes into question when pleuritic pain is sudden in onset and accompanied by dyspnea in a patient with emphysema or previous history of pneumothorax. Such pain also requires consideration of pulmonary embolization, especially in a patient at risk for thrombophlebitis (recent surgery, past history of embolization, unilateral leg edema, oral contraceptive use). Pleuritic pain with cough and sputum production may be an indication of pneumonitis with pleural involvement, as in tuberculosis or pneumococcal pneumonia.

Onset of a sudden, maximally severe, tearing chest pain in a patient with hypertension, history of blunt trauma, coarctation, Marfan's syndrome, extensive atherosclerosis or known thoracic aneurysm should suggest dissecting aneurysm. Pain may radiate to the back with descending aortic involvement. In such cases, a high index of suspicion may be life-saving.

Chest pain brought on by eating may be due to angina, but esophageal, biliary, pancreatic and peptic diseases should also enter into consideration. Response to nitroglycerin lessens the likelihood of pancreatic and peptic problems, but esophageal and cystic duct spasms as well as angina are relieved by nitroglycerin. Physical examination and contrast studies are often necessary to identify gastrointestinal causes of chest pain.

Physical examination deserves careful attention. General appearance can be telling. An anxious, sighing, hyperventilating individual should be readily noticeable, as should the person in respiratory distress or extreme pain. Vital signs must be checked for fever, tachypnea, and tachycardia. Pressure needs to be taken in both arms in a patient with a suspected aortic dissection. Skin should be noted for cyanosis, herpetic rash, pallor, jaundice and xanthomas. Examination of the fundi may provide evidence of atherosclerotic, diabetic or hypertensive disease. Carotid pulse is palpated for delay in upstroke, suggesting hemodynamically significant aortic stenosis, a treatable cause of angina (see Chapter 25).

The chest wall is examined for signs of herpes and trauma, as well as for focal tenderness and swelling. If pain is elicited, it is important to ascertain that the pain on palpation is identical to that complained of previously. One listens for a pleural rub on inspiration and expiration and observes for signs of consolidation and effusion. Hyperresonance, absent breath sounds, and tracheal deviation from the mid-line point to a large pneumothorax that requires immediate attention.

In the cardiac examination, a three-component rub is indicative of pericarditis, but it is often evanescent. An S_4 and paradoxically split S_2 may accompany the chest pain of angina. A midsystolic click and late systolic murmur are evidence of a prolapsed mitral valve. Abdominal examination should focus on palpation of the right upper quadrant and epigastrium for tenderness and masses. Legs require careful examination for unilateral edema and other signs of phlebitis (see Chapter 30). Neurologic examination needs to include a careful look at the cervical and thoracic spine and extremities for focal tenderness and motor and sensory deficits.

Test selection should be based on the working differential diagnosis constructed from history and physical; routinely ordering a chest x-ray and an ECG on every patient with chest pain is wasteful and potentially misleading. However, if a patient insists on having an x-ray or ECG, the test is probably worth obtaining for the reassurance it may provide.

SUSPECTED ANGINA. It is important to keep in mind that the resting ECG and even the exercise stress test are often normal in patients with coronary disease (see Chapter 31). Moreover, there is a high incidence of false-positive stress tests among women who complain of chest pain; many have normal coronary vessels. The recent advent of the thallium cardiac scan may improve the sensitivity and specificity of exercise stress testing; the literature should be followed for developments in this area. In the occasional instance when noninvasive testing and clinical data are inconclusive and coronary disease must be ruled out, it may be necessary to resort to angiography. If no occlusive disease is noted on the angiogram, one might ask the angiographer to test for vasospasm, particularly if the patient has variant angina *and* the angiographer has experience in inducing coronary vasoconstriction. Attempts to induce vasospasm are not without risk and should be performed only in the catheterization laboratory by those skilled in the technique. Short of coronary angiography, the best means of diagnosing coronary disease remains a good history.

PLEURITIC PAIN. Patients with pleuritic pain should have a chest x-ray. In a study of 97 young patients (ages 18 to 40) with pleuritic chest pain, the combination of history, physical examination and chest film identified 95 per cent of cases of proven embolization. The most frequent x-ray finding in

cases of embolization was a unilateral effusion. When history and physical findings were used alone, the detection rate for embolization was 80 per cent. When lung scan was added after the chest x-ray, there was only a 5 per cent improvement in detection rate, but the scan did substantially reduce the number of false-positive diagnoses from 39 per cent after history, physical and x-ray to 16 per cent after scan. Other studies have shown that a normal scan virtually rules out the diagnosis of embolism, but high false-positive rates have been reported, especially in those with preexisting lung disease and in the elderly. The addition of ventilation scanning has not resolved the problem. Arterial blood gases were of no help in determining those who were likely to have embolization.

Thus, history, physical examination, and chest x-ray can be used to identify patients who might have an embolism and require further assessment. In whom embolism is highly likely to be present. If the patient is young and free of underlying lung disease, a scan can reduce the number of false-positive diagnoses. If the patient is elderly or has underlying lung disease, the scan is unlikely to be sufficiently specific; angiography without prior scanning is urged by some experts, especially if the considerable risk of anticoagulant therapy is high and a definitive diagnosis is needed before commencing treatment. The utility of an ECG in patients with suspected embolus is marginal. The electrocardiographic findings of acute right heart strain, $S_1Q_3T_3$, are helpful if present, but a normal ECG certainly does not rule out the diagnosis. Serum enzymes are of little use.

The chest x-ray may also reveal pneumonitis. Pneumococcal pneumonia and tuberculosis can present with acute pleuritic chest pain and may be mistaken clinically for pulmonary embolism. Consequently, any patient with pleuritic pain and sputum production should have Gram and acid-fast stain made. A pleural effusion may also be detected on chest film. Any nonloculated pleural effusion of unknown etiology should be tapped, Gram-stained, cultured, examined microscopically and sent for cell count, glucose, LDH and protein determinations (see Chapter 39).

Suspicion of pneumothorax is an indication for a chest film, but if x-ray is not immediately available and the patient is in respiratory distress, decompression should not be delayed. Chest x-ray is also helpful in the diagnosis of aortic dissection; but if this condition is suspected, emergency admission is indicated; delaying admission in order to obtain a chest film is unwise.

When pericarditis is under consideration, an ECG is essential. However, the ECG changes of early repolarization, a harmless finding seen in young men, may closely resemble those of acute pericarditis. The presence of concave ST segment elevations in both limb and precordial leads and presence of PR segment depressions in the precordial leads, if they occur in the limb leads, distinguish pericarditis from early repolarization. Cardiac ultrasonography may reveal a pericardial effusion. An ANA, BUN and tuberculin skin test are indicated when the cause of pericariditis is not readily evident.

OTHER CONDITIONS. Only a few musculoskeletal disorders require chest x-ray: suspected rib fractures and cervical or thoracic spine disease. If a gastrointestinal etiology is suspected, a contrast study may be in order. The ECG may show T-wave depression in cholecystitis and pancreatitis and may mistakenly be interpreted as evidence of coronary disease.

The anxious patient with psychogenic pain may find a chest x-ray and/or electrocardiogram reassuring. In most instances, however, a thorough history and careful physical examination combined with a detailed explanation should suffice. Repeating tests "just to be sure" may begin to undermine the patient's confidence in the physician's explanation and even heighten anxiety, especially if there are repeat studies.

It is important to realize that as many as 10 to 15 per cent of cases remain undiagnosed, even after careful and thorough evaluation. Nevertheless still, in such instances it is possible to rule out the presence of an acutely serious etiology. Most patients with chest pain that initially eludes diagnosis can be followed expectantly for the time being.

SYMPTOMATIC RELIEF

Relief of pain must be based on an etiologic diagnosis. To simply suppress the pain with analgesics or sedatives before a diagnosis is made may hide important clues. However, musculoskeletal forms of chest pain may require analgesia. When the diagnosis of costochondritis is certain, local injection with lidocaine into the point of maximal tenderness (Xylocaine) can provide dramatic relief.

PATIENT EDUCATION

A careful and thorough explanation is essential to avoid precipitating a cardiac neurosis or unnecessary visits to multiple physicians for evaluation of chest pain. Patients making many visits usually harbor unexplored concerns that have not been adequately addressed in an open and detailed explanation. Discussion of concerns can be extremely reassuring and comforting to the patient and family; this must not be overlooked when workup reveals a benign etiology.

ANNOTATED BIBLIOGRAPHY

Diamond, G.A., and Forrester, J.S.: Analysis of probability as an aid in the clinical diagnosis of coronary artery disease. N. Engl. J. Med., *300*:1350, 1979. *(Provides data on probability of coronary disease by history and lab studies.)*

Kayser, H.L.: Tietze's syndrome—A literature review. Am. J. Med., *21*:982, 1956. *(Points out the often epidemic nature of the illness; best review.)*

McElroy, J.B.: Angina pectoris with coexisting skeletal chest pain. Am. Heart J., *66*:296, 1963. *(Makes the important point that more than one etiology of chest pain can be present at the same time, and that skeletal pain is often found in patients with coronary disease.)*

McNeil, B.J., Hessel, S.J., Branch, W.T., et al.: The value of the lung scan in the evaluation of young patients with pleuritic chest pain. J. Nucl. Med., *17*:163, 1976. *(History, physical and chest x-ray detected 95 per cent of cases of embolism, but the false-positive rate was 39 per cent. The lung scan had only a marginal impact on sensitivity in case detection [increased detection rate to 100 per cent], but it did improve specificity by substantially reducing the false-positive rate to 16 per cent.)*

Robin, E.D.: Overdiagnosis and overtreatment of pulmonary embolism. Ann. Intern. Med., *87*:775, 1977. *(A critical discussion of the shortcomings of methods of diagnosis of pulmonary embolism; argues that lung scan should be limited to ruling out embolism in young patients and that arterial blood gases are of no help.)*

Spodnick, D.H.: Differential characteristics of the electrocardiogram in early repolarization and acute pericarditis. N. Engl. J. Med., *295*:523, 1976. *(Presents data suggesting that one can differentiate the two based on location and occurrence of ST and PR segment changes.)*

15
Evaluation of Systolic Ejection Murmur

Systolic ejection (crescendo–decrescendo) murmurs are frequently noted in otherwise asymptomatic patients. Most are harmless, but it is important to identify those that may represent hemodynamically significant lesions and thus require more extensive evaluation such as cardiac ultrasound, fluoroscopy, and catheterization. In most cases, one should be able to make the initial assessment in the office by a careful history and cardiac examination supplemented by chest x-ray and ECG.

PATHOPHYSIOLOGY AND CLINICAL PRESENTATION

"Physiologic" murmurs occur when there is increased ejection velocity across a normal valve creating turbulence. Causes of increased velocity include fever, anemia, pregnancy, hyperthyroidism, exercise, and conditions associated with a large stroke volume (e.g., aortic regurgitation, bradycardia, atrial septal defect). Dilation of the aorta, as in hypertension or aging, may also produce a flow murmur by causing turbulent flow in the dilated segment.

"Innocent" murmurs occur in normal hearts under resting conditions. The origin of such murmurs is a subject of debate, with recent evidence pointing to the aortic root. Since there is no obstruction in the outflow tract, the murmur reflects the normal ejection pattern of blood from the ventricles and is early systolic and crescendo-decrescendo. Since chamber pressures are normal, there is normal splitting of heart sounds. Valves are normal; there are no adventitious sounds or other murmurs.

Early *aortic* and *pulmonic valve disease* may produce murmurs identical to physiologic ones, except that the former are often accompanied by ejection clicks. If outflow tract obstruction increases, the murmur will usually become louder and more prolonged and, peak intensity will occur later in systole. In pulmonic stenosis, the murmur increases with inspiration, and the pulmonic component of the second sound is delayed as disease progresses.

Atrial septal defects (*ASD*) produce physiologic murmurs due to increased right ventricular stroke volume. However, unlike other physiologic murmurs, there is often wide and fixed splitting of the second sound due to left-to-right shunting of blood and a delay in right ventricular ejection.

Asymmetric septal hypertrophy (*ASH*) produces an ejection quality murmur that is affected by the size of the left ventricular cavity. Any maneuver that decreases blood flow to the left ventricle (e.g., Valsalva) will increase the degree of obstruction and make the murmur louder. When there is marked obstruction, the murmur lasts through most of systole and its peak is delayed beyond midsystole.

Patients with physiologic or innocent murmurs are generally asymptomatic from a cardiac standpoint and usually have no previous history of heart disease. Patients with mild varieties of aortic or pulmonic stenosis, ASH, or a small ASD may be asymptomatic as well. Only in later stages of these illnesses do patients begin to complain of dyspnea on exertion, fatigue, etc. Symptoms may not develop until the problem is far advanced, as in aortic stenosis (see Chapter 28).

DIFFERENTIAL DIAGNOSIS

The differential diagnosis can be listed according to the underlying pathophysiology. Thus, systolic ejection murmurs can be classified as innocent, physiologic, aortic and pulmonic (Table 15–1).

WORKUP

The primary physician needs to separate cases which require extensive investigation from those which do not, on the basis of a careful history, physical examination, ECG, and chest x-ray. Patients suspected of having correctable, hemodynamically significant lesions often require further noninvasive study and cardiac consultation. In an occasional case, cardiac catheterization is indicated, for example, the asymptomatic athlete with marked aortic stenosis.

The first step in evaluation is to distinguish the systolic ejection murmur from other systolic mur-

Table 15–1. Differential Diagnosis of
Systolic Ejection Murmur

1. Innocent Murmurs
2. Physiologic Murmurs
   a. Exercise or emotion
   b. Fever
   c. Anemia
   d. Hyperthyroidism
   e. Conditions with large stroke volumes: atrial septal defect, aortic regurgitation, bradycardia
   f. Pregnancy
3. Aortic Murmurs
   a. Aortic stenosis
   b. Asymmetric septal hypertrophy
   c. Sub- and supravalvular fixed stenoses
4. Pulmonic Murmurs
   a. Pulmonic stenosis

murs. Timing, quality, and location are the most helpful features. Ejection quality murmurs are crescendo-decrescendo, harsh, best heard with the bell, usually loudest at the base and radiate into the neck and down to the apex. In some patients, the murmur may be higher-pitched and maximal at the apex, as in elderly people with aortic stenosis. The systolic murmurs of mitral and tricuspid regurgitation are characteristically high-pitched, well localized to the apex or left sternal border (unless very loud) and pansystolic or late systolic. A mid-systolic click may precede the regurgitant murmur of mitral valve prolapse.

Next, one must separate innocent and physiologic ejection murmurs from those due to significant aortic and pulmonic outflow tract obstructions and atrial septal defects. The former are usually midrange in frequency, less than 3/6 in intensity, peak in early systole, stop long before S_2, are heard best at the base and can radiate to neck and apex. Valsalva maneuvers and standing decrease their intensity. The second sound is normally split; there are no clicks, heaves, $S_3 S_4$, or other murmurs. The ECG and chest x-ray are normal. Signs of anemia, fever, hyperthyroidism and anxiety should be sought.

The murmurs due to atrial septal defect and hemodynamically insignificant aortic and pulmonic stenoses may resemble physiologic murmurs. However, in most cases of ASD, there is widened and fixed splitting of S_2, and in over 90 per cent, there is a conduction defect of the right bundle branch type producing a QRS and lead V_1 with an RSR′ configuration. A normal ECG and normal splitting of S_2 make an ASD unlikely. When one is in doubt, an echocardiogram can be used to look for abnormal septal motion and right ventricular enlargement; a normal study rules out the diagnosis.

Mild aortic stenosis in the young patient may be

impossible to distinguish from a physiologic murmur; the presence of an ejection click is an important clue to the former. As severity progresses, the murmur gets louder, a thrill becomes palpable, and the carotid upstroke becomes delayed. (In the elderly, the upstroke may be normal due to a loss of vessel compliance.) As stenosis progresses, the murmur tends to peak later in systole; however; this does not always occur. Left ventricular enlargement may begin to develop on chest film, and signs of hypertrophy appear on ECG. The absence of these findings does not rule out serious aortic stenosis (see Chapter 28). In older patients, the degree of valve calcification corresponds roughly to the severity of stenosis. Cardiac fluoroscopy and echocardiogram are useful for detection of valve calcification.

In asymmetric septal hypertrophy, the systolic ejection murmur peaks around midsystole, which helps distinguish it from an innocent murmur. Moreover, it is usually heard most clearly along the left sternal border, often increases with Valsalva maneuvers and standing and decreases with squatting. The carotid upstroke is brisk and sometimes bisferiens in quality. The echocardiogram is diagnostic.

Hemodynamically significant pulmonic stenosis is suggested by wide splitting or absence of the pulmonic component of the second heart sound, an ejection click that decreases with inspiration, a prolonged and loud murmur (greater than 3/6) that may increase with inspiration, evidence of pulmonary artery dilation on chest film, and prominent R-wave in V_1 indicative of right ventricular hypertrophy. A normal ECG and an early systolic murmur rule out significant pulmonic stenosis. Mild hemodynamically insignificant pulmonic stenosis may be indistinguishable from an innocent murmur, but there is no therapy indicated (other than the need for dental prophylaxis), and therefore misdiagnosis is of little consequence.

In summary, the key components of the initial evaluation of the systolic ejection murmur in the asymptomatic patient include attention to carotid upstroke, second sound, clicks, quality, timing, intensity and location of the murmur effects of provocative maneuvers, ECG and chest x-ray.

PATIENT EDUCATION

If the murmur is determined to be innocent, it is essential to provide careful explanation and reassurance. Anxiety may be precipitated by repeated auscultation and laboratory work that focuses on the heart. Excessive workup, if left unexplained, can lead to unnecessary concern and self-restriction of activity. Reassurance should include a discussion of the cause of the murmur and emphasize that other forms of heart disease have been ruled out. The patient with a harmless murmur should be specifically told that there is no need to restrict activity or undergo further evaluation at the present time.

ANNOTATED BIBLIOGRAPHY

Burde, G.D., and DePasquale, N.P.: Electrocardiography in the Diagnosis of Congenital Heart Disease. Philadelphia: Lea and Febringer, 1967. *(Describes right bundle branch pattern in patients with ASD.)*

Epstein, S.E., *et al.*: Asymmetric septal hypertrophy. Ann. Intern. Med., *81*:650, 1974. *(A detailed discussion of ASH, including clinical findings; 67 refs.)*

Finegam, R.E., Gianelly, R.D., and Harrison, D.C.: Aortic stenosis in the elderly: Relevance of age to diagnosis and treatment. N.Engl. J. Med., *281*:1261, 1969. *(Physical findings such as carotid upstroke and quality and location of the murmur may be misleading in assessing aortic stenosis in the elderly.)*

Stein, P.D., and Sabbah, H.: Aortic origin of innocent murmur. Am. J. Cardiol., *39*:665, 1977. *(Presents extensive data for the aortic origin of innocent murmurs.)*

Tavel, M.E.: The systolic murmur—innocent or guilty. Am. J. Cardiol, *39*:757, 1977. *(An editorial arguing that evaluation of the systolic murmur can be done without resorting to invasive procedures.)*

16
Evaluation of Leg Edema

Leg swelling can be a bothersome problem as well as an initial symptom of important underlying disease. Many suffer from chronic venous insufficiency, but occasionally the cause of the swelling is acute deep vein thrombophlebitis, nephrotic syndrome, or another condition of similar seriousness. Accurate determination of etiology is essential to avoidance of such common mistakes as treating edema in elderly persons with digitalis when the actual cause is venous disease.

PATHOPHYSIOLOGY AND CLINICAL PRESENTATION

Edema is defined as an increase in extracellular volume. It develops if hydrostatic pressure exceeds colloid oncotic pressure, capillary permeability increases, or lymphatic drainage becomes impaired. Hydrostatic pressure is a function of intravascular volume, blood pressure, and venous outflow. Colloid oncotic pressure is dependent on the serum albumin concentration.

Decreased oncotic pressure is usually due to hypoalbuminemia, which can occur secondary to malnutrition, hepatocellular failure, or excess renal or gastrointestinal loss of albumin. The resultant fall in intravascular volume from excessive transudation of fluid stimulates salt retention. This compensatory effort to maintain adequate intravascular volume leads to further edema formation because the underlying oncotic deficit remains. Edema sets in when the serum albumin concentration falls below 2.5 gm. per 100 ml. Leg swelling due to hypoalbuminemia is typically bilateral, pitting, and sometimes accompanied by edema of the face and eyelids (especially upon awakening).

Increased hydrostatic pressure may result from excessive fluid retention (such as seen with congestive heart failure) or impairment of venous outflow. A localized increase in hydrostatic pressure develops in the legs during prolonged standing, especially if the valves in the leg veins are incompetent. Increased hydrostatic pressure due to fluid retention produces bilaterally symmetrical edema, whereas swelling due to venous insufficiency may be asymmetrical and accompanied by varicosities and other signs of venous disease (see Chapter 30). At times, the only sign of deep vein thrombophlebitis is an acutely swollen leg. A stroke that causes paresis in one leg may result in unilateral edema due to reductions in vascular tone and venous and lymphatic drainage; thrombophlebitis may ensue.

Increased capillary permeability can occur with immunologic injury, infection, inflammation or trauma. A permeability defect is also believed to be responsible for *idiopathic edema*, a poorly understood but common problem seen almost exclusively in women. Although some patients report a periodicity to the problem that seems to parallel the menstrual cycle, careful studies have failed to find sufficient evidence to warrant the label "cyclic edema." The condition is especially aggravated by hot weather and standing, more so than occurs with venous insufficiency. Transient abdominal distention is frequent, and weight may fluctuate several pounds over the course of the day. The disorder is not progressive, but it can cause considerable discomfort. It is often accompanied by headache, fatigue, anxiety and other functional symptoms. Some patients are bothered by nocturia.

Lymphatic obstruction hinders reabsorption of interstitial fluid. The swelling usually starts in the feet and progresses upward; often the problem is unilateral. The edema of lymphatic obstruction tends to have a brawny quality and evidences little pitting, except in its early stages. Recumbency provides only minor relief compared to edema from other causes.

DIFFERENTIAL DIAGNOSIS

The differential diagnosis of edema can be organized according to clinical presentations and pathophysiologic mechanisms (see Table 16–1). Certain infiltrative conditions may be mistaken for edema, such as pretibial myxedema and lipedema (a familial, bilateral deposition of excess fat).

Table 16–1. Important Causes of Leg Edema

I. Unilateral or Asymmetric Swelling
  A. Increased hydrostatic pressure
    1. Deep vein thrombophlebitis
    2. Venous insufficiency
  B. Increased capillary permeability
    1. Cellulitis
    2. Trauma
  C. Lymphatic obstruction (local)
II. Bilateral Swelling
  A. Decreased oncotic pressure
    1. Malnutrition
    2. Hepatocellular failure
    3. Nephrotic syndrome
    4. Protein-losing enteropathy
  B. Increased hydrostatic pressure
    1. Congestive heart failure
    2. Renal failure
    3. Use of salt-retaining drugs (e.g., corticosteroids, estrogens)
    4. Venous insufficiency
    5. Menstruation
    6. Pregnancy
  C. Increased capillary permeability
    1. Systemic vasculitis
    2. Idiopathic edema
    3. Allergic reactions
  D. Lymphatic obstruction (retroperitoneal or generalized)

WORKUP

History. The distribution of the swelling should be ascertained from the patient. If edema is predominantly unilateral, the patient ought to be questioned about risk factors for thrombophlebitis such as use of oral contraceptives, recent surgery, previous phlebitis and prolonged inactivity. Inquiry into recent injury, redness, tenderness or fever may prove productive. If the edema is bilateral, it is important to check for a history of dyspnea on exertion, orthopnea, ascites, jaundice, proteinuria, chronic kidney disease, malnutrition, varicose veins, chronic diarrhea, rash and use of salt-retaining drugs such as corticosteroids and estrogens. A report of acute facial swelling suggests an allergic reaction or hypoalbuminemia if the swelling is more chronic.

Physical examination should be used to detail the extent of the edema. Careful measurements of calf and thigh diameters can be very helpful. If the swelling is predominantly limited to one leg, the limb ought to be examined for tenderness, redness, increased warmth, varicosities and a palpable thrombosed vein. Unfortunately, the utility of the physical examination for detection of deep vein thrombophlebitis is limited. The often mentioned signs of deep venous thrombosis—calf tenderness, palpable cord, positive Homan's sign—have not proved to be very sensitive or specific; unilateral edema may be the only clue aside from a suggestive history. It is important to check for pitting; if edema is prominent but pitting is only minimal, it suggests that lymphatic obstruction might be the cause.

The patient with bilateral leg edema should have the blood pressure measured for elevation, especially if there is a history of kidney problems; new onset of hypertension may be a sign of renal failure. The skin is checked for signs of hepatocellular failure (jaundice, spider angiomata, ecchymoses), the jugular veins for distention, the chest for rales and evidence of a pleural effusion, the heart for a third heart sound indicative of failure, the abdomen for masses, ascites, and other manifestations of portal hypertension, and the pelvis for masses. Any lymphadenopathy should be noted.

Laboratory studies. The patient with unilateral edema requires a venogram if there is any possibility of deep vein thrombosis. The venogram remains the definitive test for detection of deep venous occlusion, in spite of the advent of numerous noninvasive diagnostic procedures. The noninvasive methods have not yet achieved the sensitivity or the specificity of the venogram (see Chapter 30). A venogram may also detect the cause of lymphatic obstruction and should be obtained before lymphangiography is attempted. Severe lymphatic obstruction may interfere with attaining a satisfactory lymphangiogram.

The patient with more generalized edema involving both legs should have a chest film in search of heart failure and pleural fluid, a urinalysis for detection of albuminuria, determinations of the serum creatinine and the BUN for evidence of renal insufficiency, and measurements of the prothrombin time and bilirubin for further documentation of hepatocellular failure. If the serum albumin is low and protein is detected in the urine, a 24-hour urine collection for albumin and creatinine is indicated (see Chapter 124).

PATIENT EDUCATION AND SYMPTOMATIC THERAPY

When edema is due to increased hydrostatic pressure or decreased oncotic pressure, a number of simple measures can provide the patient some symptomatic relief. The patient should be advised to restrict salt intake, avoid prolonged standing or prolonged sitting with the legs dependent, elevate the legs whenever possible and avoid wearing garments which might restrict venous return (e.g., garters and girdles). Proper support stockings might provide some added benefit (see Chapter 30). If possible, use of salt-retaining drugs should be discontinued or minimized. Severe edema may require diuretic therapy (see Chapters 27, 30, 71, 124 and 135). Lymphatic obstruction and increased capillary permeability do not respond well to these measures.

Patients with idiopathic edema are sometimes helped by salt restriction, support hose, elevation and diuretic use in the early evening. There are reports that propranolol may have beneficial effects. It is important to reassure the patient with this condition that the edema poses no threat to health.

Patients with chronic leg edema should be instructed to call the physician at the first sign of inflammation or unilateral increase in swelling.

ANNOTATED BIBLIOGRAPHY

Coggins, C.P.: Edema. In R.S. Blackow (ed.): Signs and Symptoms, Philadelphia: J.B. Lippincott, 1977. *(Excellent review of pathophysiology of edema.)*

Cranley, J.J., Canos, A.J., and Sull, W.J.: The diagnosis of deep vein thrombosis, fallibility of clinical symptoms and signs. Arch. Surg., *111*:34, 1976. *(Classic signs of deep vein thrombosis, muscle pain, tenderness, swelling and the presence of Homans' sign occurred with approximately equal frequency in people with and without deep vein thrombosis.)*

Galloway, J.M.D.: The swollen leg. Practitioner, *218*:676, 1977. *(A clinically useful review that concentrates on the swollen limb resulting from local vascular problems.)*

Haeger, K.: Venous and Lymphatic Disorders of the Leg. Philadelphia: J.B. Lippincott, 1966. *(Detailed discussion of lymphatic obstruction.)*

Streeten, D.H.P.: Idiopathic edema: Pathogenesis, clinical futures and treatment. Metabolism, *27*:353, 1978. *(Absolutely comprehensive review of the syndrome of idiopathic edema. All of the etiologic theories are studied with the conclusion that upright posture is an important contributor to excess transudation of fluid in over 30 per cent of the patients studied. Treatment is suggested, including reducing salt intake, reducing the duration of standing and sitting, and administration of diuretic if done at 7 or 8 p.m. followed by recumbency for several hours. 84 refs.)*

17
Evaluation of Arterial Insufficiency of the Lower Extremities

DAVID C. BREWSTER, M.D.

Vascular occlusive disease of the lower extremities is seen with greater frequency as atherosclerosis becomes more prevalent and as people continue to live longer. Proper management requires the physician to first recognize the manifestations of ischemic disease and to carefully evaluate its severity. Many patients with mild to moderate vascular insufficiency may be managed conservatively, while others with acute ischemia or more severe chronic ischemia that threatens to cause tissue necrosis require more intensive investigation and often surgery.

Intermittent claudication is the hallmark of arterial insufficiency. It is defined as pain brought on by using the limb and relieved by rest. It is a common complaint; prevalence is higher in males and increases sharply with age. The primary physician must be able to differentiate patients with arterial insufficiency from those with exertional pain due to other causes. Moreover, one needs to know the indications for and limitations of the newer noninvasive techniques for determining arterial insufficiency as well as when to employ angiography.

PATHOPHYSIOLOGY AND CLINICAL PRESENTATION

The pathophysiology of claudication is ischemic. The pain is analogous to angina pectoris, occurring when the oxygen requirements of the functioning muscle cannot be met because blood flow is inadequate. The major cause of reduced blood flow is atherosclerotic disease in the aorta or its branches supplying the lower extremity. The exact etiology of atherosclerosis is still unsettled.

Atherosclerotic plaques producing stenosis or occlusion of the arterial lumen are often segmentally distributed with a predilection for arterial bifurcations. The infrarenal abdominal aorta and aortic bifurcation are frequent sites of disease, as are the iliac and femoral artery bifurcations. As stenotic lesions progress, they may remain asymptomatic; pressure and flow may not be impaired until the cross-sectional area of the vessel lumen is reduced by approximatley 75 per cent (50 per cent diameter reduction). More severe stenoses or even total occlusions may remain essentially asymptomatic as long as collateral circulation maintains sufficient blood flow around the lesion to satisfy the metabolic demands of the distal limb at rest and during exercise. Development of ischemic symptoms in the leg implies either inadequate collateral circulation or additional occlusive disease distal to the particular collateral bed. Thus, lesions in the aortoiliac segment may cause little difficulty unless, as is commonly the case, there is associated disease in the femoropopliteal segments.

The earliest manifestation of impaired arterial circulation is usually intermittent claudication, brought on regularly by a given amount of exercise and relieved within 10 minutes by rest. Blood flow, while adequate for local metabolic demands at rest, is insufficient when the oxygen demands of the muscle mass are increased with exercise. The relatively high resistance across collateral vessel beds limits the amount of blood available, while the demand in the normal limb may be increased three- to fourfold with vigorous activity.

As the occlusive process becomes more severe, blood flow becomes inadequate for tissue needs even at rest, resulting in manifestations of more severe arterial insufficiency: ischemic "rest" pain and tissue necrosis (gangrene or ischemic ulceration).

DIFFERENTIAL DIAGNOSIS

Lower extremity ischemia may also be caused by embolism, arterial dissection, trauma, thrombosis of an aneurysm or thromboangiitis obliterans. Symptoms of other nonvascular conditions may mimic those of claudication, ischemic rest pain or tissue necrosis. Pain in the hip, thigh or knee region with walking is not infrequently due to degenerative disc disease, osteoarthritis of the hip or knee, or Paget's disease. Sciatic or other radicular pain may be involved. Various other neurologic or musculoskeletal disorders may be at fault. Cauda equina compression by disc or tumor produces a well-known pseudoclaudication syndrome. Most of these conditions are suspected when pain is not clearly related to a predictable amount of exercise and not promptly relieved by rest. The presence of paresthesias in addition to pain suggests a neurologic etiology. Diabetic neuropathy can frequently cause a burning discomfort in the foot and toes, and may be difficult to differentiate from pain due to ischemia, particularly in a patient with absent pulses.

WORKUP

The diagnosis of peripheral vascular disease and an accurate assessment of its level and severity may be made by a careful history and physical examination to an extent not possible in many other disease states. The availability of effective treatment for vascular disease makes it mandatory that earlier and more accurate diagnosis be established prior to progression to end-stage problems resulting in inevitable limb loss.

History. The most common manifestation of hemodynamically significant arterial insufficiency is claudication, and a reliable history can be diagnostic. The pain of claudication is usually described as a cramp or ache in the calf or thigh muscles after walking a predictable distance. The location of pain in either calf or thigh and hip region may help to localize the occlusive process to the femoropopliteal or aortoiliac level, respectively, but is often misleading in this regard. The pain should be reproducible by walking a certain distance and should be relieved within minutes of stopping. If the walking distance required to produce the pain varies considerably from day to day, or if the pain requires the patient to sit down or lie down for more than several minutes for relief, the physician should suspect other etiologies. Similarly, the pain should involve the same areas consistently, and not different portions of the leg from one day to the next. Crampy pain in the calf region at rest only or at night rarely signifies a vascular problem.

Complaints of pain at rest as well as with exertion suggests advanced ischemia. A history of claudication should be present in almost all such patients unless the distribution of the occlusive process is quite distal or in small vessels only. Ischemic rest pain typically involves the toes or forefoot, not the calf or thigh. It is usually improved with dependency

of the limb and, therefore, worse at night. Pain not confined to the distal foot, better with elevation, or occurring in a patient without intermittent claudication should alert the physician to look for other possible causes, such as diabetic neuropathy or other neuro-orthopedic problems.

Patients with advanced ischemia will almost always give a long history of progressively severe claudication leading to ischemic pain at rest. Symptoms of tissue necrosis will usually be quite apparent. Peripheral gangrene without such prior symptoms should raise the possibility of embolic disease or small vessel occlusions due to conditions other than chronic arteriosclerosis. In patients with extremity ulceration, historical clues suggesting a traumatic, dermatologic or venous etiology should also be looked for, as many leg or foot ulcers are not ischemic in origin.

A complete history should include questioning for sexual difficulties; erectile impotence has long been associated with severe aortoiliac occlusive disease and termed the Leriche syndrome after the French surgeon who first reported its significance in 1923. Finally, it is of utmost importance to note the existence of known risk factors for arteriosclerosis (family history, smoking, diabetes mellitus, hypertension, lipid disorders) as well as similar diseases (coronary or cerebrovascular symptoms) indicative of the systemic nature of arteriosclerosis. There is a high prevalence of coronary disease, stroke and congestive failure in these patients.

Physical examination can help confirm, localize and establish the severity of the arterial lesion. Palpation of peripheral pulses is the keystone of the examination. Femoral, popliteal, posterior tibial and dorsalis pedis pulses should all be examined carefully. Absence of a dorsalis pedis pulse may occasionally be found in a normal individual, but the finding of an absent or markedly diminished pulse in the area of complaint is virtually diagnostic. Local factors such as edema or marked obesity may hinder palpation. Abnormally prominent pulsation suggests aneurysmal disease. Auscultation of the aortic and groin regions should also be performed, with the finding of bruits further indicating the existence of arterial disease. The absence of bruits has little meaning, since marked reduction of flow in a severely stenotic or occluded vessel will not produce a bruit.

Other useful findings are abnormal pallor on elevation of the legs, rubor on dependency and prolonged capillary filling time (especially when one leg is compared to the other). Temperature differences and atrophic skin changes are less reliable indicators of chronic arterial insufficiency.

Careful spine, hip, knee and neurologic examinations are needed to rule out nonvascular causes of exertional lower extremity pain. Atheroembolism is suggested by the sudden onset of distal cyanosis in one or more digits in a patient with an abdominal aortic aneurysm. Evidence of embolic involvement of the kidneys (new onset of hypertension and renal insufficiency) and other viscera is often present. Diagnosis is confirmed by the finding on biopsy of cholesterol clefts in small arteries of involved skin or muscle.

History and physical are usually sufficient to establish the diagnosis and provide a rough estimate of severity. In patients with mild to moderate disease who are not unacceptably hindered, no further investigation is necessary other than to check for treatable, potential risk factors such as hypertension, hyperlipidemia and smoking. A blood sugar determination may detect a previously undiagnosed diabetic, but there is no firm evidence that tight control of the serum glucose level prevents or ameliorates vascular disease.

Noninvasive vascular laboratory studies are indicated when the diagnosis or degree of impairment is uncertain, or when the disease is severe enough to warrant consideration of surgery. Doppler ultrasound segmental limb pressures combined with pulse-volume recordings provide simple, safe, reliable and sensitive measures of blood supply. Sensitivity is improved upon when treadmill exercise is added to the evaluation. Noninvasive methods can also provide anatomic information as to the site of occlusion and can be used repetitively to follow the course or results of therapy.

In summary, while not required in most instances, noninvasive testing can clearly confirm the diagnosis, clarify severity of disease, and serve as a baseline for follow-up care. Angiography has little place in the diagnosis or evaluation of peripheral vascular disease. It is reserved for those patients who have been selected as operative candidates and is intended for planned surgery.

SYMPTOMATIC MANAGEMENT

See Chapter 29 on management of peripheral arterial disease.

ANNOTATED BIBLIOGRAPHY

Carter, S.A.: Response of ankle systolic pressure to leg exercise in mild or questionable arterial disease. N. Engl. J. Med., *287*:578, 1972. *(A paper demonstrating that measuring ankle pressure after exercise increases the sensitivity of detecting arterial disease.)*

Dean, R.H., and Yao, J.S.T.: Hemodynamic measurement in peripheral vascular disease. In *Current Problems in Surgery.* Chicago: Year Book Medical Publishers, August, 1976. *(Excellent monograph describing methodology and advantages of various noninvasive techniques and their application to diagnosis and management.)*

Gilfillan, R.S., Jones, O.W., Roland, S.I., and Wylie, E.J.: Arterial occlusion simulating neurologic disorders of the lower limbs. JAMA, *154*:1149, 1954. *(Discussion of possible confusion in differential diagnosis of limb ischemia.)*

Raines, J.K., Darling, R.C., Buth, J., Brewster, D.C., et al.: Vascular laboratory criteria for the management of peripheral vascular disease of the lower extremities. Surgery, *79*:21, 1976. *(Description of noninvasive methods and criteria for evaluation of peripheral vascular disease.)*

18
Evaluation of Syncope

When confronted with a report of loss of consciousness, the primary physician needs to determine whether the patient has an underlying cardiovascular or seizure disorder that requires prompt attention or a less threatening condition which can be approached in a more leisurely fashion.

PATHOPHYSIOLOGY AND CLINICAL PRESENTATIONS

The pathophysiological common denominator of circulatory syncope is inadequate cerebral perfusion that does not meet the brain's metabolic demands.

Mechanisms that may be responsible include sudden decrease in peripheral vascular resistance, inadequate cardiac output, failure of vasoconstrictive reflexes, and functional or anatomic cerebral vascular occlusion; any number of these may be operative in a given case. Psychoneurologic mechanisms of syncope include hysteria and seizure activity. Metabolic disturbances usually do not result in syncope, though they may alter consciousness.

Vasodepressor syncope (the common faint) accounts for most episodes. Although vagal activity plays some role, and the episode is often labeled "vasovagal," the condition can be induced even when vagal activity is blocked by atropine. In response to an emotionally uncomfortable situation, fight or flight reactions are only partially mobilized. Marked peripheral arterial dilatation takes place, particularly in the muscular bed, resulting in reduced total peripheral vascular resistance. The fall in resistance is not accompanied by a compensatory increase in cardiac output. The failure of the heart to respond is believed to be a function of inadequate filling volume due to a shift of blood to the vascular bed in the muscles which is outside the central venous reservoir. Perfusion pressure drops over the course of minutes, and lightheadedness syncope ensues.

The patient experiences premonitory symptoms of sweating, epigastric queasiness, lightheadedness and pallor. Dilation of the pupils, blurring of vision, yawning and sighing or hyperventilation occur; the patient feels restless and unable to concentrate. The heart rate is rapid prior to loss of consciousness. By the onset of syncope, the pulse slows due to vagal influence. Shortly afterward, the person regains consciousness but feels weak, sweaty and nauseated. Control of bladder and bowels is never lost.

Orthostatic hypotension is another cause of reduced cerebral perfusion pressure. Upon standing, reflex vasoconstriction and increase in heart rate fail to occur because of autonomic insufficiency. Hypotension progresses over seconds to a few minutes, until perfusion is inadequate for maintainence of consciousness. During the presyncopal period, there is no change in heart rate, nor do other signs of autonomic response, such as pallor, nausea or sweating, occur. The period of syncope is brief, and consciousness returns promptly. Near syncope is common among these patients, as are impotence and bladder and bowel disturbances.

Carotid sinus hypersensitivity can cause marked reflex bradycardia and a fall in arterial resistance. Most patients with this condition are elderly and have underlying atherosclerotic heart disease manifested by ischemic changes on electrocardiogram.

Massage of the carotid sinus often results in long asystolic pauses. Digitalis administration seems to aggravate the condition. Carotid sinus syncope may also cause a vasodepressor form of syncope in which heart rate remains unchanged. Minor events can trigger symptoms; wearing a tight collar, turning the head or shaving may cause light-headedness, sweating, pallor and nausea, followed by fainting. When the predominant mechanism is asystole, the loss of consciousness can be precipitous.

Post-tussive syncope is characterized by loss of consciousness which follows a prolonged bout of forceful coughing. Men with chronic bronchitis are most often affected. The mechanism is believed to involve decreased cardiac output due to decreased venous return, increased cerebral vascular resistance secondary to hypocapnia, and compression of cerebral vessels by an increase in cerebrospinal fluid pressure. Prolonged Valsalva maneuvers have a similar effect; the increase in intrathoracic pressure impedes venous return and decreases cardiac output.

Postmicturition syncope takes place in the context of emptying a distended bladder. The typical setting involves a male who has gotten up at night to urinate after consuming considerable amounts of alcohol. Consciousness is lost without much warning. Drainage of ascitic fluid or a distended bladder may produce a similar effect. The mechanism is unknown. Valsalva maneuver and reflex vasodilatation have been implicated.

Cerebral vascular disease leads to syncope only when there is total or near total occlusion of most major vessels supplying the brain. Lesser degrees of obstruction may contribute to minor lightheadedness upon standing. Patients with substantial cerebrovascular disease often have evidence of previous strokes manifested by focal neurologic deficits.

The subclavian steal syndrome results from occlusion of the proximal subclavian artery, leading to reversal of flow in the adjacent vertebral artery. When vascular resistance in the arm falls, e.g., during exercise, flow is redirected away from the brain, and ischemic symptoms may ensue.

Effort syncope suggests underlying cardiac disease. Exercise induces peripheral vasodilatation, but cardiac output cannot adequately be increased, and syncope results. Severe aortic stenosis and marked asymmetric septal hypertrophy (ASH) obstruct the ventricular outflow tract to a degree sufficient to limit cardiac response to exercise. Total blockade of the mitral orifice from an atrial myxoma and pulmonary hypertension can have similar consequences. Loss of consciousness comes with little warning.

Cardiac arrhythmias and *heart block* may precipitate drop attacks that have none of the premonitory manifestations of vasodepressor syncope. Fewer than 5 seconds of consciousness remain once effective systoles have ceased. Palpitations are sometimes reported, and loss of consciousness can occur while the person is supine. Important conditions associated with heart block and/or dysrhythmias include acute ischemia, sick sinus and preexcitation syndromes, prolapsed mitral valve and digitalis toxicity. It seems that patients with chronic bifascicular and trifascicular block are more likely to have syncopal attacks, but those with syncope have not been found to have an increased risk of sudden death.

Vasovagal syncope refers specifically to instances where the entire reflex is vagally mediated. Distention of a viscus (as occurs in esophagoscopy) is an example of a vasovagal etiology. Vagal influences also play roles in vasodepressor syncope and carotid sinus hypersensitivity by contributing to bradycardia and suppressing AV node conduction.

Metabolic factors (hypoxia, hyperventilation, hypoglycemia) are more likely to alter consciousness than to cause actual syncope. Restlessness, confusion and anxiety are prominent and precede loss of consciousness. When hyperventiliation is responsible, the patient first complains of a smothering or suffocating feeling in conjunction with paresthesias in the limbs and circumorally (see Chapter 214). Syncope may take place while the patient is sitting or lying down. Hypoglycemia rarely causes loss of consciousness (see Chapter 95).

Hysteria produces syncope characterized by graceful fainting to the floor or couch, frequent presence of an audience, normal pulse, skin color and blood pressure, and an emotionally detached description of the episode.

Seizures differ from other causes of syncope in that aura, postictal symptoms, incontinence and tonic-clonic movements often dominate the clinical picture. However, akinetic petit mal attacks have few of these features, though normal blood pressure and pulse help distinguish them from seizures having cardiovascular etiologies (see Chapter 158).

DIFFERENTIAL DIAGNOSIS

Important causes of syncope are listed in Table 18–1. Vasodepressor syncope (the common faint) secondary to emotional upset is the most frequent and least worrisome type. Syncope having a cardiac etiology is of great concern, because it may be a manifestation of a serious lesion. Most vascular or reflex causes are annoying but certainly not life-

Table 18–1. Important Causes of Syncope

1. Cardiac
   a. Arrhythmias (sick sinus syndrome, ventricular tachycardia, very rapid supraventricular tachycardia)
   b. Heart block (Stokes-Adams attacks)
   c. Aortic stenosis, severe
   d. Asymmetric septal hypertrophy, severe
   e. Primary pulmonary hypertension
   f. Atrial myxoma
   g. Prolapsed mitral valve
2. Vascular-Reflex
   a. Vasodepressor syncope (emotional upset)
   b. Orthostatic hypotension (ganglionic blocking agents, diabetes, old age, prolonged bed rest)
   c. Carotid sinus hypersensitivity
   d. Cerebral vascular disease, severe
   e. Subclavian steal syndrome
   f. Post-tussive syncope
   g. Valsalva syncope
   h. Post-micturition syncope (emptying distended bladder)
   i. Vasovagal syncope (distention of a viscus)
3. Psychological-Neurologic
   a. Seizures
   b. Hysteria
4. Metabolic
   a. Hyperventilation
   b. Hypoxia
   c. Hypoglycemia (rarely)

threatening. Seizures, hysteria, metabolic disturbances and vertigo must be distinguished from true syncope of a circulatory nature.

WORKUP

History. One immediate objective is to determine whether a cardiac problem is responsible for the loss of consciousness. The absence of premonitory symptoms in the presyncopal period suggests a sudden fall in cardiac output, whereas nausea, diaphoresis, pallor, and lightheadedness are more typical of reflex and vascular etiologies. Identification of precipitants requires asking about emotional upsets, crowded hot surroundings, sudden standing, prolonged and forceful coughing, Valsalva maneuvers, micturition, and vigorous exercise. Effort syncope is characteristic of hemodynamically significant obstruction in the ventricular outflow tract. Position just prior to syncope is worth noting because loss of consciousness while recumbent argues against a reflex or vascular mechanism. In considering heart disease, one needs to ask about a history of infarction, palpitations, chest pain, heart murmur, dyspnea on exertion and use of digitalis and antiarrhythmic drugs, especially quinidine. History of diabetes, stroke, use of antihypertensive agents, prolonged bed rest, impotence and bladder and bowel incontinence should be checked for when the patient reports lightheadedness or syncope on standing.

It is important not to mistake other conditions for true loss of consciousness. Vertigo (see Chapter 154), neuroglycopenic symptoms (see Chapter 95) and the lightheadedness associated with an anxiety attack are sometimes confused with syncope.

A seizure disorder is usually not difficult to distinguish from circulatory syncope because of the preceding aura, motor activity, incontinence and postictal symptoms of confusion, drowsiness and paresis. However, when there are no motor manifestations, as in akinetic petit mal seizures, the differentiation may be impossible to make by history alone.

Reports from witnesses should be sought whenever possible. Activity, position, complaints, and appearance prior to syncope as well as duration of the episode, associated motor activity and behavior upon regaining consciousness deserve attention. Some observers will even be able to report pulse and respirations.

Physical examination concentrates on the cardiovascular system. Blood pressure and pulse should be measured supine and standing and in both arms in order to detect postural effects and any occlusion of the subclavian artery. It may be necessary on occasion to wait as long as 5 minutes to obtain a postural fall. Head and torso require scrutiny for signs of trauma sustained during a motor seizure. Carotid pulses are auscultated for bruits and gently palpated for volume and carotid upstroke (see Chapter 15). If there is no evidence of carotid artery disease, one can massage the carotid and observe for reflex bradycardia and hypotension. The maneuver is indicated when a hypersensitive carotid sinus reflex is suspected. However, because it may also cut off blood supply and cause syncope when there is severe cerebral occlusive disease, it should not be attempted. The neck veins are noted for distention and the chest for rales and rhonchi. The heart is palpated for heaves and thrills and is auscultated for clicks and murmurs with the patient in the supine, decubitus and sitting positions. Systolic murmurs should be evaluated for evidence of aortic stenosis, ASH and mitral valve prolapse (see Chapter 15). A variable diastolic murmur raises the question of atrial myxoma. Neurologic assessment includes searching for focal deficits indicative of prior stroke.

Provocative maneuvers are particularly helpful in identifying conditions which alter consciousness but do not cause syncope. Asking the patient to voluntarily hyperventilate or spin around may reproduce symptoms and confirm a clinical suspicion. Exercising the arm is worthwhile if subclavian steal syndrome is suspected.

Laboratory studies. When the history suggests a common faint and the physical examination is normal, no laboratory studies are needed. Sudden loss of consciousness without warning is an indication for an electrocardiogram (ECG), looking not only for heart block and arrhythmias, but also for subtle clues such as a short PR interval, delta waves, or new onset of bundle branch block. If the ECG is unrevealing and if transient heart block or arrhythmias are strongly suspected, a Holter monitor can be worn for 24 hours. An electroencephalogram is best reserved for patients who have sudden drop attacks that occur without premonition and are devoid of clinical evidence for heart disease, as well as those suspected of having a seizure disorder (see Chapter 158). A person with a systolic heart murmur and effort syncope requires an echocardiogram for detection of ASH or aortic stenosis. The same test might identify a prolapsed mitral valve or an atrial myxoma. Random blood sugar determinations are of little use in documenting hypoglycemia; a blood sugar at the time of symptoms is the best test (see Chapter 95).

SYMPTOMATIC THERAPY AND PATIENT EDUCATION

Vasodepressor syncope can be prevented by instructing the patient to lie down or at least put his head below his knees during the presyncopal period. The patient bothered by orthostatic hypotension needs to avoid abrupt postural changes by sitting on the edge of the bed in the morning before getting up. Girdles, garters and other constricting garments should not be worn, but elastic stockings may be helpful in increasing venous return. One can advise the patient to avoid prolonged standing and to contract the calf muscles when standing in order to increase venous blood flow. It may be necessary to discontinue or alter dosages of drugs that contribute to postural hypotension, particularly diuretics, antihypertensive agents and hypnotics. Loosening the collar is sometimes helpful for the person with a hypersensitive carotid sinus reflex. A demand pacemaker is indicated only when heart block or severe bradycardia has been proven responsible for syncope.

INDICATIONS FOR ADMISSION

Pending further study, it is probably safest to hospitalize patients with syncope suspected to be of cardiac origin or due to a seizure disorder of recent onset. If serious heart and neurologic diseases have been ruled out, further evaluation can safely proceed on an outpatient basis even though the etiology may remain undetermined. Family members should be instructed to make careful note of all events surrounding the syncopal period, including appearance, position, activity, complaints, and behavior. They might be taught to palpate the radial or femoral pulse in order to provide data on heart rate and rhythm during the episode. Admission to the hospital for observation of the obscure case is a difficult decision, but is most useful when episodes are frequent.

ANNOTATED BIBLIOGRAPHY

Dhingra, R.C., Denes, P., Wu, D., *et al.*: Syncope in patients with chronic bifascicular block. Ann. Intern. Med., *81*:302, 1974. *(An analysis of 186 patients with bifascicular block. Syncope in 27 was fully evaluated, revealing a variety of causes with a tendency not to recur. The incidence of sudden death was the same in patients with and without syncope.)*

Ibrahim, M.M., Tarazi, R.C., and Dustan, H.P.: Orthostatic hypotension: Mechanisms and management. Am. Heart J., *90*:513, 1975. *(Good discussion of the mechanisms by which blood pressure is maintained as well as the failures resulting in orthostatic hypotension.)*

Noble, R.J.: The patient with syncope. JAMA, *237*:1372, 1977. *(An excellent discussion detailing approach to the patient.)*

O'Connor, P.J.: Syncope. Practitioner, *216*:276, 1976. *(A helpful review from the British litera-ture emphasizing the conditions from which syncope must be distinguished.)*

Weissler, A., Warren, J., Estes, E., *et al.*: Vaso-depressor syncope: Factors influencing cardiac output. Circulation, *15*:875, 1957. *(Vasodepressor syncope may occur even when vagal activity is blocked by atropine, thus arguing against a primary role for vagal effects in syncope associated with emotional upset.)*

Wright, W.E., Jr., and McIntosh, H.D.: Syncope: A review of pathophysiological mechanisms. Prog. Cardiovasc. Dis., *13*:580, 1971. *(A good discussion of pathophysiology.)*

The following references document the association of syncope with various conditions and precipitants:

Engel, G.L.: Psychologic stress, vasodepressor (vasovagal) syncope, and sudden death. Ann Inter. Med., *89*:403, 1978.

Ferrer, M.: "Sick sinus syndrome." Circulation, *47*:635, 1973.

Klotz, P.G.: Syncope during prostatic examination. N. Engl. J. Med., *282*:1046, 1970.

Levin, B., and Posner, J.B.: Swallow syncope: Report of a case and review of the literature. Neurology, *22*:1086, 1972.

Mannick, J., Suter, C., and Hume, D.: The subclavian steal syndrome: A further documentation. JAMA, *182*:254, 1962.

McIntosh, H., Estes, E., and Warren, J.V.: Mechanisms of cough syncope. Am. Heart J., *52*:70, 1956.

Peters, M., Hall, R., Cooley, D., *et al.*: Clinical syndrome of atrial myxoma. JAMA, *230*:695, 1974.

Proudfit, W.L., and Forteza, M.E.: Micturition syncope. N. Engl. J. Med., *260*:328, 1959.

Thomas, J.E.: Hyperactive carotid sinus reflex and carotid sinus syncope. Mayo Clin. Proc., *44*:127, 1969.

19

Evaluation of Atrial Fibrillation in the Ambulatory Setting

Not infrequently, atrial fibrillation (AF) is discovered incidentally during a routine office examination. Unless cardiac output falls precipitously, few symptoms may be noted by the patient. The primary physician's initial tasks are to: (1) assess the need for hospitalization, (2) control the ventricular response rate (see Chapter 23), (3) establish the etiology of AF by noninvasive means, and (4) consider the need for prophylaxis of an embolic complication (see Chapter 23).

PATHOPHYSIOLOGY

Most investigators support the unifocal theory of atrial fibrillation, which postulates that a single ectopic atrial focus is responsible for the dysrhythmia. By depolarizing at over 400 times per minute, the focus puts the atrium into fibrillation; a coordinated atrial contraction cannot occur at such rates because repolarization time is inadequate. Factors which may precipitate and/or perpetuate fibrillation include increased atrial size, increased vagal tone, varying repolarization times of neighboring areas of atrial myocardium, and occurrence of an atrial premature beat during the vulnerable period of an atrial cycle. Increase in catecholamines may precipitate atrial premature beats, which in turn may lead to atrial fibrillation. Ischemia or disease of the sinoatrial node also predisposes to atrial dysrhythmias by suppressing this pacemaker and allowing other foci to fire.

CLINICAL PRESENTATION

The majority of patients with incidentally discovered atrial fibrillation are asymptomatic. If the AF is paroxysmal or the ventricular rate very rapid, palpitations may be reported. If cardiac output falls precipitously, symptoms of heart failure may occur. Systemic embolization may be the first evidence of AF and present as an acute neurologic or peripheral vascular deficit.

Some of the causes of AF have characteristic clinical presentations. *Lone atrial fibrillation* was found in about 1 in 10,000 military recruits. It is a harmless condition of young people, in which the episodes are precipitated by emotional stress, alcohol or smoking. There is no underlying heart disease, and prognosis is excellent. *Hyperthyroidism of the elderly* may be manifested by marked apathy and weight loss in conjunction with AF. Often, AF may be the only sign of the thyroid disease; it reverts to sinus rhythm with treatment.

Paroxysmal atrial fibrillation may be the presenting sign of underlying heart disease (as in mitral stenosis, Wolff-Parkinson-White syndrome or sick sinus syndrome). It may also occur in the context of an acute cardiac event such as the onset of congestive

Table 19-1. Important Causes of Atrial Fibrillation

1. Chronic Atrial Fibrillation
   a. Mitral valve disease
   b. Coronary artery disease
   c. Congestive cardiomyopathy
   d. Hyperthyroidism
   e. Chronic lung disease
   f. Atrial septal defect
   g. Chronic pericarditis
   h. Late stages of aortic valve disease
2. Paroxysmal Atrial Fibrillation
   a. Acute ischemia
   b. Acute congestive failure
   c. Sick sinus syndrome
   d. WPW syndrome
   e. Pulmonary embolization
   f. Rheumatic fever
   g. Normal young people
   h. Alcohol excess
   i. All of the causes of chronic AF

failure, acute pericarditis, ischemia, rheumatic fever or pulmonary embolization.

Many patients with chronic AF have other symptoms and signs of underlying heart disease. In fact, the AF may be a manifestation of advanced disease that has resulted in marked atrial enlargement and/or elevated atrial pressure. For example, the late stages of aortic stenosis and asymmetric septal hypertrophy are at times complicated by AF. AF is seen in less advanced stages of mitral stenosis and regurgitation, because left atrial enlargement is apt to occur sooner.

DIFFERENTIAL DIAGNOSIS
(Table 19-1)

Atrial fibrillation is only one of a number of dysrhythmias that present as an irregularly irregular pulse. Frequent atrial premature beats, multifocal atrial tachycardia, atrial flutter with variable block, sinus arrhythmia, and frequent ventricular premature beats may give a similar pattern to the pulse.

WORKUP

The etiology of AF can usually be determined by noninvasive means. The identification of AF is based on the characteristic ECG findings of an irregularly irregular ventricular response and atrial fibrillatory waves. In some instances, the routine 12-lead ECG may show no atrial activity, yet the ventricular response is irregularly irregular, and the QRS is normal in duration. Leads V_1 and V_3R are the best leads in which to look for atrial activity, followed by leads II, III and AVF. Multifocal atrial tachycardia, atrial flutter with variable block, frequent atrial premature beats, frequent ventricular premature beats and sinus arrhythmia may at times be confused clinically with atrial fibrillation. However, they are easily distinguished on ECG from atrial fibrillation if there are discrete P waves present.

After the electrocardiographic diagnosis of atrial fibrillation is established, one needs to determine whether hospitalization is necessary. Criteria for admission include evidence of marked congestive heart failure, ischemia, embolization, hypotension or very rapid ventricular response (>150). If the rhythm is well tolerated, an outpatient workup can commence.

History. The patient with paroxysmal atrial fibrillation should be questioned about alcohol, coffee, and tea intake, emotional stress, pleuritic chest pain, prior paroxysms of AF and symptoms of rheumatic fever, congestive heart failure and angina. Patients with chronic atrial fibrillation need to be asked about previous rheumatic fever, heart murmur, weight loss and apathy (especially if they are elderly), hypertension, ischemic heart disease, and congestive heart failure.

Physical examination. Particular note should be made of apathetic general appearance, rapid heart and respiratory rates, hypertension, elevated jugular venous pressure, goiter, rales, wheezes, rubs, opening snaps, diastolic and systolic murmurs, calf tenderness and asymmetry, and tremor. In evaluating heart rate, the apical pulse should be determined at rest and after mild exertion (e.g., 10 situps). An acceptable rate at rest may rise markedly with only modest exertion.

Laboratory evaluation should begin with a full 12-lead electrocardiogram; the configuration of the fibrillatory waves can be of help diagnostically. Coarse fibrillatory waves are characteristic of atrial fibrillation due to rheumatic, thyrotoxic, congenital and functional causes, whereas fine fibrillatory waves are more common in atherosclerotic and hypertensive heart disease. Moreover, cardioversion is more likely to be successful in patients with coarse fibrillatory waves. The ventricular rate provides a means to judge the need for and adequacy of therapy. ST segments and T-waves should be observed for signs of pericarditis (see Chapter 14) and ischemia. Prominent septal Q-waves in leads II, III and F, V_5 and V_6

point to asymmetric septal hypertrophy. Between episodes of AF, short PR intervals and delta waves suggest Wolff-Parkinson-White syndrome.

Determination of left atrial size is helpful since size correlates inversely with the probability of successful cardioversion. This determination can best be done by ultrasound, because there is no correlation between the size of the fibrillatory wave and the size of the left atrium, and because chest x-ray and ECG do not give reliable estimates of the left atrial size. When the left atrial dimension exceeds 45 mm., cardioversion is unlikely to produce a sinus rhythm that can be maintained longer than 6 months.

The echocardiogram is also important for further definition of conditions that may be responsible for AF such as valvular disease, pericarditis, atrial septal defect and asymmetric septal hypertrophy. Chest x-ray is the best simple test for congestive heart failure. Measurement of thyroid indices, in particular the free T_4 and the total T_3, can help in assessing the elderly patient with atrial fibrillation for apathetic hyperthyroidism. A recent report suggests that a TRH stimulation test may be more sensitive for diagnosis in some cases. A digitalis level may at times be helpful in detecting the rare instance in which atrial fibrillation is due to digitalis intoxication.

In summary, the evaluation can be performed on an outpatient basis if the patient is tolerating the rhythm well and there is no evidence of failure, ischemia or embolization. Careful history and physical examination supplemented by electrocardiogram, chest x-ray and echocardiogram complete the evaluation in most patients. In the elderly, thyroid indices can be helpful, and in rare instances a digitalis level is indicated.

ANNOTATED BIBLIOGRAPHY

Culler, M.R., Boone, J.A., and Gazes, P.C.: Fibrillatory wave size as a clue to etiologic diagnosis. Am. Heart J., *66*:425, 1963. *(Coarse atrial fibrillation found most frequently in mitral valve disease, thyrotoxicosis, and lone atrial fibrillation.)*

Forfar, J.C., Miller, H.C., and Toft, A.D.: Occult thyrotoxicosis: A correctable cause of "idiopathic" atrial fibrillation. Am. J. Cardiol., *44*:9, 1979. *(Ten of 75 patients presenting with AF of unknown etiology were hyperthyroid by TRH stimulation testing. In a number of cases, the T_4 and total T_3 were normal.)*

Garber, E.B., Morgan, M.G., and Glasser, S.P.: Left atrial size in patients with atrial fibrillation. Am.

J. Med. Sci., *272*:57, 1976. *(An echocardiographic study showing no significant correlation between F-wave size and left atrial dimension.)*

Hanson, H.H., *et al.*: Auricular fibrillation in normal hearts. N. Engl. J. Med., *240*:947, 1949. *(Discusses and documents the entity of lone fibrillation.)*

Hurst, J.W., Paul, K., Proctor, H.D., *et al.*: Management of patients with atrial fibrillation. Am. J.

Med., *37*:728, 1964. *(Excellent, though slightly, dated review.)*

Thomas, F.B., Mazzaferri, E.L., and Skillman, T.G.: Apathetic thyrotoxicosis: A distinctive clinical and laboratory entity. Ann. Intern. Med., *72*:679, 1970. *(Describes the presentation of hyperthyroidism in the elderly; it may present with apathy, atrial fibrillation, and marked weight loss.)*

20
Evaluation of Palpitations

Palpitations are disconcerting and often incite fear of serious heart disease, although the majority of cases seen in the office occur among the worried well. The patient with palpitations reports a disquieting awareness of his heartbeat, which may be described as a pounding, racing, skipping, flopping or fluttering sensation. The primary physician must be able to diagnose and treat important dysrhythmias and provide convincing reassurance to the anxious persons with no underlying heart disease. The development of ambulatory monitoring (Holter monitoring) has improved detection of arrhythmias; its indications and limitations need to be understood.

PATHOPHYSIOLOGY AND
CLINICAL PRESENTATION

Most healthy individuals are unaware of their resting heartbeat. Increase in stroke volume or contractility, sudden change in rate or rhythm, or unusual cardiac movement within the thorax may cause a perceptible beat. Isolated palpitations are noted when premature atrial or ventricular contractions are followed by a long pause; the prolonged filling time leads to an increase in stroke volume and the vigorous ejection of a large volume of blood on the next beat. A constant pounding is felt at rest by patients with hyperkinetic states (e.g., fever, severe anemia, hyperthyroidism); the rate is rapid and the rhythm is regular. A regular rhythm is also noted in those with large stroke volumes due to aortic regurgitation and other forms of valvular heart disease.

Excess adrenergic stimulation results in increased contractility and sinus tachycardia which may present as palpitations. Anxiety is a common cause of such catecholamine-induced palpitations. A heightened awareness of bodily sensations often compounds the problem. The normally perceptible heartbeat that occurs with exercise is not unpleasant unless one is preoccupied with worries about health. Hyperthyroidism may have a presentation similar to anxiety (see Chapter 99).

In rare instances, the source of adrenergic outpouring is a pheochromocytoma. Its incidence is less than 0.1 per cent, with about half of cases presenting as paroxysms of palpitations, hypertension, perspiration, tremor, nervousness and other signs of adrenergic stimulation. Episodes are often spontaneous in origin, but may be triggered by emotion and thus mimic an anxiety attack. An insulin reaction can produce a similar clinical picture (see Chapter 95). Onset of palpitations from adrenergic stimulation can be abrupt; resolution is usually more gradual.

Any sudden change in rate or rhythm may be perceptible. Attacks of palpitations which are regular in rhythm and rapid in rate are not unique to catecholamine excess; paroxysms of supraventricular tachycardia (SVT), often referred to as paroxysmal atrial tachycardia (PAT), are an important cause. SVT occurs in a wide variety of patients, including those with normal hearts, sick sinus syndrome, mitral valve prolapse and other forms of valvular disease, coronary artery disease, cardiomyopathy, and the pre-excitation syndromes (e.g., Wolff-Parkinson-White syndrome). Onset of SVT is characteristically sudden and may be precipitated by excess coffee, alcohol consumption, emotional upset or strenuous exertion. Often there is no obvious precipitant. Resolution is typically abrupt. A reentrant mechanism is postulated to account for SVT. Pathways which have been implicated involve the AV node, atria, and accessory conduction fibers. The dysrhythmia seems to be initiated by the occurrence of premature beats which alter conduction in the normal pathway. Paroxysms cease when the conducting properties of the reentrant circuit are disturbed by changes in vagal tone.

Some of the conditions associated with SVT are responsible for other dysrhythmias as well. For example, almost half of patients with sick sinus syndrome experience heart block or marked bradycardia in addition to bouts of SVT.

Sudden onset of palpitations with an irregular rhythm and rapid rate typifies paroxysmal atrial fibrillation (PAF) and may also be seen if there are runs of multifocal atrial tachycardia (MAT). PAF occurs in a host of settings (see Chapter 19) including alcohol excess, infection, and acute worsening of congestive heart failure; the condition is also found among otherwise healthy young people. MAT takes place in the context of severe pulmonary disease, particularly when there is an acute fall in PO_2 or pH. Frequent atrial or ventricular premature contractions can lead to a similarly irregular rhythm and rapid rate. Most chronic tachyarrhythmias do not produce palpitations.

Abnormal motion of the heart may be felt as a "turning over" or "flopping." The sensations are isolated and can occur with premature beats, the beat after a compensatory pause, or the beat after a blocked beat.

When there is serious underlying heart disease, palpitations are usually not the major or sole symptom. Syncope, near syncope, chest pain, or dyspnea suggests the presence of a significant cardiopulmonary illness.

DIFFERENTIAL DIAGNOSIS

The causes of palpitations can be listed in terms of their clinical presentation (Table 20–1).

WORKUP

History. The first priority is the detection of underlying heart disease. Inquiries into dyspnea, chest pain, and syncopal or near syncopal episodes are essential, as are questions about risk factors for coronary disease (see Chapters 8, 9, 10) and prior history of a heart murmur, rheumatic fever, myocardial infarction and other forms of cardiac illness. A costly error is to mistake symptoms of anxiety, such as chest tightness and air hunger at rest, for evidence of

Table 20–1. Important Causes of Palpitations

1. Isolated Single Palpitations
   a. Premature atrial or ventricular beats
   b. The beat following a blocked beat
   c. The beat after a compensatory pause
2. Paroxysmal Episodes with Abrupt Onset and Resolution (Rate Usually Rapid)
   a. Rhythm irregular
      1) Paroxysmal atrial fibrillation
      2) Paroxysmal atrial tachycardia with variable block
      3) Frequent atrial or ventricular premature beats
      4) Multifocal atrial tachycardia
   b. Rhythm regular
      1) Supraventricular tachycardias with constant block or 1:1 conduction
3. Paroxysmal Episodes with Less Abrupt Onset or Resolution (Rhythm Usually Regular, Rate Rapid)
   a. Exertion
   b. Emotion
   c. Drug side effect (e.g. sympathomimetics, theophylline compounds)
   d. Stimulant use (coffee, tea, tobacco)
   e. Insulin reaction
   f. Pheochromocytoma
4. Persistent Palpitations at Rest with Regular Rhythm (Rate Normal, Slow, or Rapid)
   a. Aortic or mitral regurgitation
   b. Large ventricular septal defect
   c. Bradycardia
   d. Severe anemia
   e. Hyperthyroidism (may also cause atrial fibrillation)
   f. Pregnancy
   g. Fever
   h. Marked volume depletion
   i. Anxiety neurosis

organic heart disease. Use of all cardiotonic drugs should be detailed, including digitalis preparations, theophylline compounds, sympathomimetics, and anticholinergics. Use of tricyclic antidepressants is frequently associated with palpitations (see Chapter 215). Many over-the-counter cold remedies contain catecholamines or theophylline derivatives; their abuse may be responsible for symptoms.

A careful description of the palpitations in terms of onset, frequency, rate, rhythm, and pattern of resolution can sometimes be of help in diagnosis (see Table 20–1). Unfortunately, many patients are unable to give accurate or a detailed account of their symptoms. The relationship of the onset of symptoms to exertion can aid in separating the anxious individual, whose symptoms may occur at rest, and are usually not worsened by exertion from the patient with heart disease and impaired exercise tolerance. Identification of precipitants such as emotional upset, stimulant intake, fever, pregnancy, volume depletion, and severe anemia is essential, for their recognition can contribute to design of proper therapy. Inquiry into symptoms of an insulin reaction (see Chapter 95) and hyperthyroidism may also prove productive.

Physical examination. At the beginning of the physical examination, one should look for evidence of excessive anxiety, such as tremor, sighing, and nervous mannerisms. Other important observations include determination of the blood pressure for elevation, marked postural change and widened pulse pressure. The apical pulse is noted for rate and rhythm disturbances; relying on the peripheral pulse may be misleading when there is a pulse deficit, as occurs in atrial fibrillation or premature beats. The temperature should be recorded. The skin is examined for pallor and signs of hyperthyroidism, eyes for exophathalmos, neck for goiter, carotid pulse for upstroke, jugular venous pulse for distention and cannon waves, chest for rales, rhonchi, wheezes and dullness, heart for heaves, thrills, clicks, murmurs, rubs, and S_3, and extremities for edema and calf tenderness. In addition to possibly providing important diagnostic information, the careful, unhurried physical examination can be of considerable use in reassuring the worried patient.

Laboratory studies. Most patients with palpitations should have a resting 12-lead ECG. Even if physical examination is completely normal and no disturbances of rate or rhythm are noted, one might detect evidence of conduction system disease (e.g., bundle branch block or preexcitation) or signs of ischemia. In particular, the ECG needs to be studied for axis shifts, QRS widening, short PR intervals, and delta waves. If a dysrhythmia is noted on examination, it is worth obtaining a 2-minute rhythm strip to better characterize the problem. The anxiety-laden person often insists on having an ECG and finds comfort in a normal result; unfortunately in many cases the reassurance is only transient.

The development of continuous ambulatory electrocardiographic monitoring has proved to be an important addition to the diagnosis and understanding of dysrhythmias. When history, physical examination and resting ECG have not provided a definitive diagnosis, it may be helpful to utilize ambulatory monitoring, particularly true if the patient reports syncope or near syncope that seems to be cardiac in origin (see Chapter 18). Even when there is no syncopal history, patients with a preexcitation syndrome or bundle branch block on ECG, or evidence of mitral valve prolapse, cardiomyopathy, or coronary disease are candidates for monitoring, because they are at increased risk of having a clinically significant arrhythmia that requires treatment. The utility of the test in otherwise healthy patients who complain of palpitations is unclear at the present time, for it is known that healthy asymptomatic patients subjected to monitoring demonstrate a variety of dysrhythmias ranging from premature ventricular beats to very slow rhythms. Since the range for normals has not been established, interpretation is difficult. However, interpretation of results is facilitated by having the patient keep a log of his activities and symptoms during the course of the monitoring. When ECG findings can be correlated with symptoms, interpretation is improved and their significance becomes clearer. The optimal duration of monitoring is thought to be 24 hours, which seems to maximize arrhythmia detection and allows for observation of the patient through a full range of daily activities.

When palpitations are precipitated by exertion, exercise stress testing can contribute to assessment, especially in the patient with known or suspected coronary disease (see Chapter 31). In a study comparing the stress test to ambulatory monitoring, monitoring was found to be the more sensitive test for detecting most types of ventricular irritability in patients with coronary disease; however, there were instances in which ventricular tachycardia occurred on stress testing but did not appear on monitoring. Thus the tests could be considered complementary.

Routine screening for endocrinologic causes of palpitations in the absence of clinical findings is of low yield. Patients with paroxysms of palpitations in conjunction with labile hypertension probably deserve to be screened for pheochromocytoma, though the condition is rare and screening tests have lacked the specificity and sensitivity required to minimize the rather high frequency of false-positive and false-negative results. Recent study of the plasma catecholamine determination suggests that it is a more sensitive and specific test than the urinary VMA or metanephrines and better suited for screening for pheochromocytoma. The test requires only a single venipuncture, rather than the 24-hour urine collection needed for VMA and metanephrine determinations; the patient needs to be supine for 30 minutes prior to the venipuncture. Metanephrines provide a more reliable index of pheochromocytoma than does the VMA.

SYMPTOMATIC RELIEF

When palpitations are a manifestation of neurotic concern, efforts should be addressed toward providing reassurance. Hasty words of comfort are worthless. Careful history and physical examination, combined with eliciting and responding to patient concerns, views, and requests, must take place before the patient can be told the palpitations are harmless. Such reassurance may be all that is needed, especially when combined with advice to increase physical activity and cut down on alcohol, coffee, smoking and stress. Exercise stress testing may have a role in helping to reassure the anxious patient. If the palpitations persist and are bothersome, a trial of propranolol therapy may be beneficial. Often as little as 80 mg. per day decreases the frequency of symptoms to the point where they are tolerable. Use of minor tranquilizers is also worth incorporating into the program, but only in an episodic manner (see Chapter 214). All nonessential drugs capable of causing palpitations should be stopped.

Vagal maneuvers are often effective in halting SVT. Valsalva and carotid sinus massage (in the absence of carotid disease) can be taught to the patient and suggested as the first line of therapy after the onset of an attack. Digitalis and propranolol are effective in terminating SVT, but when SVT is due to a preexcitation syndrome, e.g., Wolff-Parkinson-White syndrome, propranolol is preferred, since digitalis may only prolong the problem by enhancing conduction in the accessory pathway. Prophylaxis of SVT attacks can be accomplished by avoidance of known precipitants, such as alcohol and stimulants, and by use of digitalis or propranolol; sometimes quinidine proves helpful by reducing the frequency of premature beats (the agent should usually be used in conjunction with digitalis, because of its vagolytic effects). Digitalis is the drug of choice for PAF. If SVT or PAF is accompanied by ischemia or failure, admission is urgent.

Treatment of MAT requires correction of the underlying pulmonary problem, rather than use of antiarrhythmic drugs. Improvement in oxygenation and pH status is essential. The approach to ventricular irritability depends on the setting in which it occurs (see Chapter 24). Correction of severe anemia, volume depletion, hyperthyroidism (see Chapter 99), fever (see Chapter 6) or congestive failure (see Chapter 27) is of prime importance to attaining symptomatic relief.

ANNOTATED BIBLIOGRAPHY

Bravo, E.L., Tarazi, R.C., Gifford, R.W., and Stewart, B.H.: Circulating and urinary catecholamines in pheochromocytoma. N. Engl. J. Med., 301:682, 1979. (*The serum catecholamine concentration proved to be the most sensitive and specific test for diagnosis, followed by the urinary metanephrines; the VMA determination was the least reliable.*)

Giffort, R.W., Jr., Kvale, W.F., Maher, F.T., et al.: Clinical features, diagnosis and treatment of pheochromocytoma: A review of 76 cases. Mayo Clin. Proc., 39:281, 1964. (*A classic article on the condition, emphasizing that it may mimic various common problems and requires biochemical confirmation for diagnosis.*)

Harrison, D.C., Fitzgerald, M.D., and Winkle, R.A.: Ambulatory electrocardiography for diagnosis and treatment of cardiac arrhythmias. N. Engl. J. Med., 294:373, 1976. (*Thorough review of the subject; 53 refs.*)

Josephson, M.E., and Kastor, J.A.: Supraventricular tachycardia: Mechanisms and management. Ann. Intern. Med., 87:346, 1977. (*Excellent discussion of pathophysiology and rational basis for therapy; 78 refs.*)

Narula, O.S.: Wolff-Parkinson-White syndrome: A review. Circulation, 47:872, 1973. (*A detailed description of the syndrome; 38 refs.*)

Peters, R.W., Scheinman, M.M., Mondin, G., et al.: Prophylactic permanent pacemakers for patients with chronic bundle branch block. Am. J. Med., 66:978, 1979. (*Prophylactic permanent pacemaker insertion in 40 symptomatic patients with chronic bundle branch block and prolonged infranodal conduction times did not protect against sudden death. The incidence of sudden death appears to be related to the type and severity of underlying heart disease.*)

Rubenstein, J.J., Schulman, C.L., Yurchak, P.M., and DeSanctis, R.W.: Clinical spectrum of the sick sinus syndrome. Circulation, 46:5, 1972. (*Classic article reporting on a series of 56 patients; over 60 per cent of patients had bradycardia and SVT.*)

Ryan, M., Lown, B., and Horn, H.: Comparison of ventricular ectopic activity during 24-hour monitoring and exercise testing in patients with coronary heart disease. N. Engl. J. Med., 292:224, 1975. (*Monitoring proved better in exposing ventricular irritability, but there were instances when ectopic activity was detected only by stress testing.*)

Shand, D.G.: Propranolol. N. Engl. J. Med., 293:280, 1975. (*A terse review of the drug; includes discussion of its use in anxiety to control palpitations; 20 refs.*)

21
Management of Hypertension
EVE E. SLATER, M.D.

Few conditions in medicine can be readily detected and effectively treated in the asymptomatic period before irreparable harm is done. Fortunately, hypertension is one such condition. The frequency and importance of the problem demand that the primary physician be expert in its management.

PRINCIPLES OF THERAPY

No study to date has successfully determined exact guidelines for antihypertensive treatment in the general population. Nevertheless, data from the Veterans' Administration and Framingham studies appear to be the most generally applicable. The former report provides strong support for the treatment of patients with *diastolic blood pressure ≥ 105 mm. Hg,* since treatment was shown to reduce morbidity and mortality related to congestive heart failure, renal failure and stroke. Reduction in the number of myocardial infarctions was shown to accompany the treatment of diastolic blood pressure ≥ 115 mm. Hg; at lower pressure levels, the efficacy of treatment in preventing this complication has not been demonstrated, owing to the lack of a long-term study employing early intervention.

The decision to treat *diastolic blood pressure of 100-104 mm. Hg* has been the subject of controversy, but evidence now weighs in favor of early therapeutic intervention if patients have other cardiovascular risk factors (from the Framingham data). Thus, we agree with the current recommendations of the Joint National Committee on Detection, Evaluation and Treatment of High Blood Pressure, which are summarized in Table 21–1. Goal of therapy is reduction of diastolic blood pressure to below 95 mm. Hg with a minimum of adverse side effects.

Recently released reports showing a significant reduction in deaths from cardiovascular complications attributes awareness and more effective control of blood pressure as primary factors.

Definition and indications for treatment of isolated *systolic hypertension* are less clear. While epidemiologic data shows an increased risk from systolic hypertension, benefits of treatment have not been

Table 21–1. Algorithm for the Identification of High Blood Pressure

DIASTOLIC BP	ACTION
1. ≥ 120 mm. Hg	Immediate evaluation and treatment
2. 105-119 mm. Hg	Evaluation and treatment
3. 90-104 mm. Hg in males 95-104 mm. Hg in females	Confirm elevation on one separate occasion; decision to treat based upon age and presence of other cardiovascular risk factors
4. Below 90 mm. Hg in males Below 95 mm. HG in females	Remeasure blood pressure at yearly intervals (or more frequently in patients with prior hypertension or a familial tendency to hypertension)

demonstrated. Moreover, systolic hypertension is often very difficult to control. Therefore, treatment recommendations are conservative; reduce systolic blood pressure by 10 per cent in individuals under 35 years of age with systolic pressure greater than 140 mm. Hg; in those 35-59 with systolic pressure greater than 150 mm. Hg; and in those 60 or older with systolic pressure greater than 160 mm. Hg. Systolic hypertension due to high output states such as aortic regurgitation or anemia should not be treated with antihypertensive medications.

It has been argued that the therapy of hypertension is largely empirical; individualization is dictated by factors such as severity of disease and drug side effects. The hypertensive patient should first be instructed in a no-added-salt diet and in weight reduction when indicated. If these modifications alone are insufficient to reduce blood pressure, drug therapy should be initiated. Agents used in the treatment of hypertension can be classified as diuretics, sympatholytics or vasodilators. Some combination therapy is based on the observation that efficacy of any single agent is usually offset by homeostatic compensation. Sympatholytic and vasodilator agents induce a secondary increase in intravascular volume; conversely, diuretics, by virtue of volume depletion, cause a compensatory increase in PRA, leading to increased vascular resistance. Table 21–2 presents agents valuable in the treatment of hypertension, their dosages, and their side effects.

Table 21-2. Antihypertensive Drugs

CLASS	DRUG	TRADE NAME	INITIAL/MAXIMUM DOSE (MG./DAY)	FREQUENCY OF DOSAGE	RELATIVE COST (DOSE IN MG.)
	Thiazides				
	Chlorothiazide	Diuril Esidrix	500/1,500	b.i.d.	1.08 (1,000)
	Hydrochlorothiazide	HydroDiuril Oretic Thiuretic	50/150	b.i.d.	1.00* (100)
	Hydroflumethiazide	Saluron	100/150	b.i.d.	2.38 (100)
	Bendroflumethiazide	Naturetin	10/15	q.d.	2.93 (10)
	Trichlormethiazide	Naqua Metahydrin	4/8	q.d.	0.97 (4)
	Methyclothiazide	Enduron	10/15	q.d.	1.77 (10)
	Benzthiazide	Exna Aquatag	100/150	b.i.d.	2.36 (100)
	Polythiazide	Renese	2/8	q.d.	3.04 (4)
	Cyclothiazide	Anhydron	2/6	q.d.	2.39 (4)
	Phthalimidine derivatives				
	Chlorthalidone	Hygroton	50/100	q.d.	0.81 (50)
	Metolazone	Zaroxolyn	2.5/5	q.d.	1.39 (5)
	Loop diuretics				
	Furosemide	Lasix	40/160	b.i.d.	1.69 (80)
	Ethacrynic acid	Edecrin	50/200	b.i.d.	2.84 (100)

Diuretics

SIDE EFFECTS: *Chemical:* $\downarrow$K+, alkalosis, $\uparrow$uric acid, $\uparrow$blood sugar, $\uparrow$Ca++, ?$\uparrow$lipids
Dermatologic: dermatitis, photosensitivity
Hematologic: $\downarrow$platelets, $\downarrow$WBC, $\downarrow$RBC
Renal: $\uparrow$PRA, may $\downarrow$glomerular filtration rate (GFR)
GI: GI or hepatic toxicity, pancreatitis
GU: impotence

	Distal tubular diuretics				
	Spironolactone	Aldactone	25/100	t.i.d.	4.87 (100)
	Triamterene	Dyrenium	100/300	q.d.	1.29 (100)

SIDE EFFECTS: *Chemical:* $\uparrow$K+
Dermatologic: rash, hyperpigmentation
Hematologic: megaloblastic anemia (triamterene)
Renal: $\uparrow$PRA, $\downarrow$GFR
GI: nausea, vomiting, diarrhea
GYN/GU: menstrual irregularities and gynecomastia (spironolactone), impotence
Neurologic: drowsiness, ataxia

	Combination drugs				
	Spironolactone and hydrochlorothiazide	Aldactazide	1-4 tablets	b.i.d.	2.23 (2 tablets)
	Triamterene and hydrochlorothiazide	Dyazide	1-2 tablets	b.i.d.	1.60 (2 tablets)
	Methyldopa	Aldomet	250/3,000	t.i.d. or q.d.	6.11 (2,000)

SIDE EFFECTS: Orthostatic hypotension, drowsiness (usually transient), depression, dry mouth, flulike syndrome, drug fever, positive direct Coombs' test (usually without clinical hemolysis), impotence, hepatotoxicity, myocarditis, $\downarrow$PRA, $-$GFR

	Clonidine	Catapres	0.1/2.4	b.i.d. or q.d.	4.57 (0.6)

SIDE EFFECTS: Drowsiness (usually transient), depression, dry mouth, constipation, weakly positive Coombs' test (usually without clinical hemolysis), impotence, sudden rebound hypertension with abrupt discontinuation of drug, bradycardia or heart block, impaired glucose tolerance, $\downarrow$PRA, $-$GFR

	Propranolol	Inderal	40/2,000	q.i.d. or b.i.d.	2.76 (160)

SIDE EFFECTS: Nausea, vomiting, diarrhea, constipation, bradycardia, weight gain, congestive heart failure, bronchospasm, insomnia, depression, paresthesias, claudication, masking of hypoglycemia, impotence (rare), sedation (rare), possible precipitation of angina with abrupt discontinuation of drug, $\downarrow$PRA, $\downarrow$GFR, $\uparrow$K+

(Continued)

Table 21-2.   Antihypertensive Drugs

CLASS	DRUG	TRADE NAME	INITIAL/MAXIMUM DOSE (MG./DAY)	FREQUENCY OF DOSAGE	RELATIVE COST (DOSE IN MG.)
Sympatholytics	Metoprolol	Lopressor	100/400	b.i.d.	5.79 (300)
	SIDE EFFECTS: Reported similar to propranolol with the exception of absence or reduction in bronchospasm. Experience limited.				
	Nadolol	Corgard	40/320	q.d.	0.57 (120)
	SIDE EFFECTS: Similar to Propranolol, experience limited.				
	Guanethidine	Ismelin	10/300	q.d.	1.78 (25)
	SIDE EFFECTS: Orthostatic hypotension (A.M.), weakness, bradycardia, diarrhea (dose related), nasal congestion, sedation (rare), impotence (retrograde ejaculation), ↑PRA				
	Reserpine	Raudixin	100/300	q.d.	0.59 (0.25)
		Serpasil Sandril	0.1/0.5		
	SIDE EFFECTS: Drowsiness, nasal congestion, increased appetite, bradycardia, depression (can be severe), nightmares, ↑gastric acidity (may be ulcerogenic), parkinsonian rigidity, galactorrhea, postural hypotension (rare), impotence (rare), ?breast cancer (may promote development of preexisting disease)				
	Prazosin	Minipress	3.0/20	t.i.d.	3.96 (6)
	SIDE EFFECTS: Dizziness, drowsiness, headache, weakness, depression, palpitations, tachycardia, orthostatic hypotension, syncope (may occur suddenly after first dose), nausea, diarrhea, constipation, edema, dyspnea, rash, pruritus, dry mouth, blurred vision, impotence, urinary frequency, hallucinosis, ↓PRA				
Vasodilators	Hydralazine	Apresoline	40/400	q.i.d. or b.i.d.	1.22 (200)
	SIDE EFFECTS: Headache, tachycardia, palpitations, fever, weight gain, edema, lupus erythematosus-like syndrome (rare if dosage <200 mg./day), exacerbation of coronary insufficiency, ↑PRA, ↑ or −GFR				
	Minoxidil	Loniten	5/40	q.d.-q.i.d.	0.23 (20)
	SIDE EFFECTS: Sodium retention, peripheral edema, ?pulmonary hypertension, hirsutism, ?atrial lesions, pericardial effusion				
Renin-blocking agent	SQ14225†	Captopril	100/400	t.i.d.	
	SIDE EFFECTS: Fever, rash, proteinuria, ?glomerulonephritis, stomatitis, taste alteration, agranulocytosis				

Note: Lists of side effects may be incomplete. Consult package insert before prescribing.

*Approximately $36 per year. Calculations are based on lowest available price and estimated for mean doses indicated in parentheses. Considerable regional variations in price may exist.

From Slater, E. E., and Haber, E.: High blood pressure. *In* Principles and Progress for Practicing Physicians. New York: Scientific American, 1978.

Diuretics

Diuretics are the most commonly used drugs in both initiation and maintenance of therapy. Regardless of severity of hypertension, diuretics are usually necessitated throughout treatment to offset the volume-retaining effects of sympatholytic or vasodilator agents. *Thiazides* are the most commonly used diuretics. Certain thiazides are taken only once daily, which often augments patient compliance. Cost should also enter into the choice of a thiazide (see Table 21-2).

Significant diuretic-induced hypokalemia is a side effect which most commonly involves excessive salt intake, or, rarely, mineralocorticoid hypertension. Serum potassium should be checked routinely in patients receiving diuretics. If hypokalemia develops, supplementary potassium or a potassium-sparing distal tubular diuretic may have to be added to the regimen. Any degree of hypokalemia must be avoided in patients simultaneously receiving digitalis or in patients with coronary artery disease or ventricular irritability. In the hypertensive patient without concomitant cardiac failure, the weakness associated with even mild degrees of hypokalemia often limits compliance. Thus, careful correction of even mild hypokalemia is necessary.

A recently reported increase both in cholesterol

and triglyceride levels observed during short-term diuretic administration and in possible deterioration of glucose tolerance after long-term diuretic therapy warrant further investigation. Hypersensitivity reactions mandate immediate discontinuation of the thiazides and substitution of a loop, distal tubular, or phthalimidine derivative, although similar reactions may occur with each of these.

The *more potent loop diuretics,* furosemide and ethacrynic acid, should be reserved for patients with evidence of renal insufficiency (creatinine clearance less than 30 per cent of normal) or with allergy to the thiazides.

The *distal tubular diuretics,* spironolactone and triamterene, provide no special advantage in initial management. Side effects—for example, gynecomastia with spironolactone—often limit compliance. We use these drugs in patients with mineralocorticoid hypertension, thiazide hypersensitivity, or gout. In patients simultaneously receiving digitalis preparations or with ventricular irritability, in whom hypokalemia is a special risk, the potassium-retaining properties of these agents are advantageous whether used alone or in combination with thiazides. These drugs must be used with extreme caution in patients with a tendency to develop hyperkalemia—for example, patients with renal insufficiency, or insulin-requiring diabetics with renin deficiency. It is well to avoid starting with a preparation that has a fixed combination of a thiazide and a distal tubular diuretic, until the necessary dose of each is established. Fixed combinations may not provide proper doses and are usually more expensive.

Sympatholytics

Either propranolol or methyldopa is commonly begun when diuretic therapy fails to control the hypertension. Some physicians are initiating antihypertensive therapy with *propranolol.* This practice may offer a relative advantage in patients with concomitant angina pectoris or arrhythmias, lipid disorders, autonomic nervous system overactivity (for example, borderline hypertensives) and high plasma renin activity. In addition, we currently favor propranolol as initial therapy in the very young patient because of its efficacy, ease of administration, and low incidence of side effects. A long-term prospective study comparing propranolol *vs* diuretics as initial therapy in young patients is very much needed. If therapy is initiated with propranolol, the physician should be aware of a possible paradoxical increase in blood pressure in certain patients with low plasma renin levels, and poor responsiveness often observed in elderly patients. It should be noted that although propranolol is recommended as a more appropriate initial agent for therapy of patients with high levels of plasma renin activity, studies to date do not confirm the postulated unique responsiveness of this group to beta-adrenergic blockade. The efficacy of propranolol alone is often blunted by fluid retention, which necessitates concomitant diuretic administration. Propranolol is remarkably free of unpleasant side effects, although patients with heart failure, bradycardia, or asthma will probably be unable to tolerate the drug. Diabetic patients should be given propranolol with caution, for it can mask hypoglycemic symptoms and signs. It is best to begin treatment with modest dosages (10-20 mg. q.i.d.) and gradually increase dosages until the desired fall in blood pressure is obtained. Up to 1 to 2 gm. of propranolol per day has been used with good effect. In most patients with mild or moderate hypertension, propranolol is effective on a twice-daily schedule, which often improves compliance.

Metoprolol is a selective beta-1 antagonist. Its properties are similar to those of propranolol; however, it is less likely to cause bronchospasm in susceptible patients. This drug may also be safer than propranolol in insulin-requiring diabetics who also require a beta-blocking agent. Metoprolol is more costly than propranolol.

Methyldopa has been used safely and reliably for a long time. Compared to propranolol, side effects occur with greater frequency. Orthostatic hypotension, drowsiness, and impotence are common. Drowsiness can sometimes be offset by nighttime administration of the complete dose, since methyldopa is often effective on a once daily schedule. Increased therapeutic efficacy is rarely observed above a dosage of 2 gm./day. Like propranolol, methyldopa's efficacy is usually potentiated by concomitant diuretic therapy.

Reserpine and *guanethidine* are still used by many physicians, but their popularity has waned owing to bothersome side effects that are especially apparent with higher dosages. Reserpine may be associated with severe depression and with an increased frequency of peptic ulcer disease.

Guanethidine is effective in severe hypertension. Patients can be taught to compensate for the orthostatic hypotension it causes. Diarrhea is almost invariable but can be treated symptomatically. Impotence is common and takes the form of retrograde ejaculation. Despite the relatively high incidence of side effects, the drug is used because it is inexpensive and can be given in a single daily dose, has a wide dose-response range, and produces little sedation.

Clonidine is rapidly replacing guanethidine as the drug of choice in severe hypertension, especially if PRA is high. Clonidine acts upon the central nervous system to decrease sympathetic output. Side effects are similar to methyldopa, although orthostatic hypotension and impotence are said to be less frequent. Sedation can be severe initially but usually resolves to a tolerable level after 4 to 8 weeks. Rebound hypertension may occur following rapid discontinuation of clonidine, but is rare. Because of the potential for rebound, the drug should not be used in unreliable patients, and dosage must be tapered when the drug is discontinued. Treatment for clonidine rebound is identical to that for pheochromocytoma crisis.

Though initially classified as a vasodilator, *prazosin* is now thought to have a mechanism of action that is predominately mediated by alpha-adrenergic inhibition. When administered as a single agent in mild to moderate disease, prazosin is less effective and more costly than a thiazide diuretic. Nevertheless, it is a useful supplement as a third agent in the therapy of moderate to severe disease. Sudden syncope, presumably resulting from mesenteric pooling of blood, requires that therapy be initiated with a low dose and first administered in the office to observe response and to minimize risk. The drug is easily tolerated and side effects are few.

Vasodilators

Hydralazine is most commonly used as a third agent in combination with propranolol and a diuretic. When administered in this manner, its efficacy is impressive, and side effects such as tachycardia and headache are minimized. Hydralazine should be used with caution in patients with ischemic heart disease because it augments cardiac output. Hydralazine may produce a lupus-erythematosuslike syndrome, which, however, is extremely rare when the daily dose does not exceed 200 mg.

Captopril (SQ 14225) is a soon to be released, orally administered dipeptide with potent hypotensive properties either alone or in combination with a diuretic or another antihypertensive agent. Its primary mechanism of action is inhibition of the conversion of angiotensin I and II; however, other hypotensive effects are likely, given the lack of direct correlation between efficacy and level of plasma renin activity. Side effects include rash, which occurs in approximately 10 per cent of patients and is usually dose-related, possible renal involvement with proteinuria, and agranulocytosis.

Other Approaches

The *relaxation response,* a form of medication, has been publicized as a means of controlling high blood pressure. While any form of regular relaxation can be helpful in treatment, objective studies show that, at best, such approaches have only a minimal effect in ameliorating established hypertension and rarely obviate the need for pharmacologic intervention.

THERAPEUTIC RECOMMENDATIONS

Confronted with a bewildering array of drugs and drug combinations, the physician should be reassured that it is possible to proceed in a logical manner to treat the hypertensive patient. A thiazide diuretic is almost always the first drug to be used. Many patients with mild or moderate hypertension are controlled with this agent alone. Propranolol or methyldopa is then added if needed. When hypertension persists, hydralazine or prazosin is given as a third agent. This program will control 80 to 85 percent of all hypertensive patients, with minimal side effects. As an alternative to this three-drug approach, another sympatholytic agent, such as clonidine, guanethidine or reserpine may be used in combination with a diuretic for moderate or severe hypertension. For the few patients who cannot be controlled by either of these combinations, one might employ two sympatholytic agents that act by different mechanisms, such as clonidine and propranolol, together with a diuretic (Figure 21–1).

COMPLIANCE

Unfortunately, most antihypertensive agents cause some uncomfortable side effects. These factors naturally favor noncompliance with therapy. Attrition from treatment programs is high, and even when patients do keep their appointments faithfully, they may not be taking medications as prescribed. Nevertheless, recent evidence suggests that behavioral and educational efforts directed toward better compliance can be effective.

INITIAL

Thiazide diuretic or *Propranolol*

Favor if: Favor if:

1. Elderly patients
2. Patient with low plasma renin level

1. Young patient
2. Patient with evidence of autonomic overactivity
3. Patient with high plasma renin level

NEXT

Combine diuretic with propranolol or another sympatholytic agent such as methyldopa or clonidine (in specific cases reserpine or prazosin).

In Severe Diseases

Add hydralazine to combined diuretic and sympatholytic

Substitute guanethidine in combination with diuretic.

Combine two sympatholytic agents that act by different mechanisms (for example, propranolol and clonidine or prazosin) together with diuretic

Fig. 21–1. Algorithm for treating high blood pressure.

Home blood pressure determinations can successfully and inexpensively foster compliance. Provided the patient does not become obsessed or excessively alarmed, such determinations can provide useful information regarding blood pressure and its fluctuations in the home environment. Office visits can be minimized or promptly instituted if control is lost.

The increasing number of effective antihypertensive agents is allowing a greater degree of flexibility in treatment. Thus, unpleasant side effects can be circumvented by alternate therapeutic regimens. It is worthwhile mentioning in this regard the problem of impotence, which has been reported with the use of every available antihypertensive agent (although with particular frequency with certain sympatholytic

agents). Both men and women should be questioned about sexual dysfunction shortly after initiation of antihypertensive therapy. Often the substitution of another drug or alteration in dosage will eliminate this problem.

SPECIAL TOPICS

Hypertension Associated with Estrogen-Containing Contraceptives

Elevation of systolic and diastolic blood pressure occurs in most patients receiving estrogen therapy over prolonged periods. Five per cent of patients become hypertensive, and approximately one-half of these remain hypertensive after hormonal therapy has been discontinued. Factors which predispose to the development of hypertension include family history or past history of high blood pressure, chronic renal disease, and hypertension with a previous pregnancy. A patient should be started on oral contraceptive or estrogen therapy only after a careful history has excluded these predisposing factors; once therapy is begun, continued blood pressure monitoring is required for the duration of treatment. The development of hypertension should prompt immediate cessation of therapy.

Hypertension Associated with Pregnancy

Hypertension that develops during pregnancy may represent either preeclampsia or exacerbation of preexisting hypertension. In the latter case, hypertension appears before 20 weeks of gestation, blood pressure is often quite high, and end-organ damage may already be evident. Patients with chronic hypertension are usually multigravidas. These patients are best managed by standard antihypertensive therapy as indicated. Each of the commonly used agents appears safe and without adverse effects upon the fetus, although widest experience has been gained with thiazide diuretics, hydralazine, and methyldopa.

Preeclampsia is characterized by a blood pressure of 140/90 mm. Hg or higher, edema, and proteinuria; all of which appear in the third trimester. The typical patient is a very young primagravida. Multiple births, diabetes, or hydatidiform mole are frequent associated factors. It is now recognized that in early pregnancy blood pressure of normal women is low. This observation has led to clinical tests aimed at identifying patients at risk of the development of preeclampsia. Thus, a resting blood pressure above 110/75 mm. Hg while the patient is sitting, or above 100/65 mm. Hg while the patient is in the left lateral decubitus position, at 17 to 20 weeks of gestation, should alert one to the possibility of preeclampsia. Once diastolic blood pressure rises above 90 mm. Hg, bed rest and, if necessary, hospitalization are indicated. Salt restriction and diuretic administration as therapies for preeclampsia are controversial; it is currently thought that they have the potential to aggravate this syndrome by stimulating the renin-angiotensin-aldosterone system.

Borderline Essential Hypertension

Borderline essential hypertension has become the focus of recent investigative interest. A subgroup of borderline hypertensive patients has been identified in whom excessive central nervous system sympathetic overactivity and parasympathetic underactivity result in a hyperdynamic, hyperkinetic state. These patients are characterized by increased cardiac output and heart rate. While such patients respond well to therapeutic intervention with propranolol, the impact of treatment upon disease progression and ultimate outcome has yet to be determined.

ANNOTATED BIBLIOGRAPHY

Alderman, M.H., and Schoenbaum, E.E.: Detection and treatment of hypertension at the work site. N. Engl. J. Med., 293:65, 1975. *(One of the few studies to demonstrate improved patient compliance based upon patient education and follow-up.)*

Benson, H., Rosner, B.A., Marzetta, B.R., and Klemchuck, H.M.: Decreased blood pressure in pharmacologically treated hypertensive patients who regularly elicited relaxation response. Lancet, 1:289, 1974. *(Presents the concept of relaxation response in treatment of hypertension.)*

Fries, E.D., et al.: Veterans Administration cooperative study group on antihypertensive agents. 1. Effects of treatment on morbidity in hypertension: Results inpatients with diastolic blood pressures averaging 115 through 129 mm. Hg. JAMA, 202:1028, 1967. II. Results in patients with diastolic blood pressure averaging 90 through 114 mm. Hg. JAMA, 213:1143, 1970. *(The classic studies demonstrating that treatment of hypertension reduced morbidity and mortality from heart failure, renal failure and stroke.)*

Gavras, H., et al.: Antihypertensive effect of the oral angiotensin converting enzyme inhibitor SQ 14225 in man. N. Engl. J. Med. 298:991, 1978. *(Preliminary data on this new drug.)*

Hypertension Detection and Follow-up Program: 5-year findings of the Hypertension Detection and Follow-up Program. JAMA, 242:2562;2572, 1979.

Levy, R.I.: Stroke decline: Implications and prospects. (Editorial.) N. Engl. J. Med., 300:490, 1979. *(Analyzes the exciting recent decline in stroke deaths.)*

Moser, M., et al.: Report of the Joint National Committee on Detection, Evaluation and Treatment of High Blood Pressure, A Cooperative Study.

JAMA, *237*:255, 1977. *(This report summarizes the consensus on whom to call hypertensive and whom to treat.)*

Slater, E.E., and Haber, E.: High blood pressure. *In* Scientific American's Medicine—Principles and Progress for Practicing Physicians, New York: Scientific American, 1978. *(This chapter presents a detailed review of the pathophysiology, approach to diagnosis, and management of high blood pressure.)*

Taguchi, J., and Fries, E.D.: Partial reduction of blood pressure and prevention of complications in hypertension. N. Engl. J. Med., *291*:329, 1974. *(This article makes the important point that even partial reduction of blood pressure reduces significantly the complications of hypertension.)*

Weinberger, M.H.: Oral contraceptives and hypertension. Hosp. Pract., *10*:65, 1975. *(This review summarizes current knowledge on oral contraceptives and hypertension.)*

Woods, J.W., *et al.*: Renin profiling in hypertension and its treatment with propranolol and chlorthalidone. N. Engl. J. Med., *294*:1137, 1976. *(This article presents strong evidence that patients can be treated effectively without knowledge of their renin status.)*

Zacest, R., Gilmore, E., and Koch-Weser, J.: Treatment of essential hypertension with combined vasodilation and beta-adrenergic blockade. N. Engl. J. Med., *286*:617, 1972. *(This paper presents evidence for the efficacy of combined diuretic-vasodilator-beta blocking therapy.)*

22
Management of Hyperlipidemia

Hyperlipidemia is a major risk factor for atherosclerotic cardiovascular disease (see Chapter 9). Elevated levels of cholesterol and/or triglyceride may be due to a primary, inherited disorder of lipid metabolism, to an underlying disease which causes secondary elevation of lipid levels, or to dietary habits. The heterogeneity of hyperlipidemia can be a source of confusion in the management of patients with elevated lipid levels. An understanding of the still-evolving taxonomy is necessary to avoid confusion and to follow new developments that may affect management.

LIPOPROTEIN AND GENETIC
CLASSIFICATIONS OF HYPERLIPIDEMIA

Plasma lipids circulate in the form of lipoprotein complexes. Properties of these complexes—chylomicrons, very low-density lipoproteins (VLDL), low-density lipoproteins (LDL), and high-density lipoproteins (HDL)—are summarized in Table 22–1. Hypercholesterolemia can result from sufficient elevation of any of the lipoprotein types, alone or in combination. Elevation of chylomicrons or VLDL, alone or together, results in hypertriglyceridemia.

The most commonly used classification of lipid disorders is based on the distinction between *hyperlipidemia* and the underlying *hyperlipoproteinemia*. Six patterns of lipoprotein elevation have been identified. The lipid abnormalities associated with each of these phenotypes are summarized in Table 22–2.

Genetic typing of hyperlipoproteinemia provides a preferable classification scheme for primary lipid disorders. Five disorders, each apparently inherited by a single gene mechanism, have been described. *Familial hypercholesterolemia, familial combined hyperlipidemia* and *broad-beta disease* are of particular interest because of strong associations with premature cardiovascular disease. *Familial lipoprotein lipase deficiency* does not increase coronary risk. Risk associated with *familial hypertriglyceridemia* has been suggested by some authors but remains unproven. (A severe form of familial hypertriglyceridemia has been called familial Type 5 disease and is considered a sixth monogenic disorder by some.)

It should be kept in mind that all patients with monogenic disorders constitute a minority—probably less than 20 per cent—of patients with hyperlipidemia. Polygenic hypercholesterolemia is far more common, affecting 5 per cent of the general popula-

Table 22-1.   Properties of Plasma Lipoproteins

	ELECTROPHORETIC MOBILITY	PERCENT PROTEIN	PERCENT LIPID		
			CHOLESTEROL	TRIGLYCERIDE	PHOSPHOLIPID
Chylomicrons	Remains at origin	1-2	2-12	80-95	3-15
Very low-density lipoproteins (VLDL)	Prebeta	10	9-24	50-80	10-25
Low-density lipoproteins (LDL)	Beta	25	57	13	30
High-density lipoproteins (HDL)	Alpha	50	30	10	60

Table 22-2.   Characteristics of Hyperlipoproteinemic Phenotypes

PHENOTYPE	LIPOPROTEINS	PLASMA CHOLESTEROL	PLASMA TRIGLYCERIDES	PLASMA APPEARANCE AFTER OVERNIGHT REFRIGERATION
Type I	Chylomicrons	Normal or increased	Increased	Creamy layer with clear infranatant
Type IIA	LDL increased	Increased	Normal	Clear
Type IIB	LDL increased VLDL increased	Increased	Increased	Uniform turbidity
Type III	Abnormal floating beta lipoprotein	Increased	Increased	Uniform turbidity (rarely, a creamy layer is also present)
Type IV	VLDL increased	Normal or increased	Increased	Uniform turbidity
Type V	Clylomicrons LDL increased	Normal or increased	Increased	Creamy layer with turbid infranatant

Table 22-3.   Genetic Classification of Hyperlipidemia

TYPE	LIPOPROTEIN PHENOTYPE	GENETIC MECHANISM	PREVALENCE	PREVALENCE AMONG PATIENTS WITH MYOCARDIAL INFARCTION BEFORE AGE 50	PRESUMED CONTRIBUTION TO CORONARY RISK
Polygenic hypercholesterolemia	IIA or IIB	Polygenic	5%	Increased	2+
Familial combined hyperlipidemia	IIA, IIB, or IV (rarely V)	Autosomal dominant	1.5%	10-20%	3+
Familial hypertriglyceridemia	IV (rarely V)	Autosomal dominant	1%	5%	1+
Familial hypercholesterolemia	IIA (rarely IIB)	Autosomal dominant	0.1-0.5%	3-6%	4+
Broad-beta disease	III	Autosomal dominant	Rare	1%	4+
Familial lipoprotein lipase deficiency	I	Autosomal recessive	Very rare	—	0

Modified from Motulsky, A. G., N. Engl. J. Med., *294*:823, 1976.

tion. The phenotypic expression by lipoprotein type for each of the genetic disorders, their relative frequencies, and apparent association with premature coronary disease are summarized in Table 22-3.

DIAGNOSTIC PRINCIPLES

A number of diagnostic steps should be taken when hyperlipidemia is identified in an individual.

1. Underlying disease should be excluded. Secondary hyperlipidemia is most often due to diabetes, hypothyroidism, obstructive liver disease, dysproteinemias or the nephrotic syndrome. Fasting blood sugar, thyroid function tests, liver function tests, and screening tests for urine protein are indicated.

2. Hyperlipidemia should be further characterized. Cholesterol and triglyceride should be measured after an overnight fast. Variables that may acutely affect levels (see Chapter 9) should be controlled. Lipoprotein electrophoresis is not necessary for classifying patients by type of lipoprotein elevation; cholesterol and triglyceride levels and examination of plasma after overnight refrigeration will suffice. For example, the patient with elevated cholesterol and normal triglyceride levels is almost certainly Type IIA. Elevated cholesterol and moderately elevated triglycerides (less than 400 mg. per 100 ml.) suggest either Type IIB, IV or, less often, III. Triglyceride levels of 400 to 1000 mg. per 100 ml. are found in Types IV or V, and levels greater than 1000 mg. per 100 ml. indicate Type I or V. The presence of a cream layer over a clear or turbid infranate after serum has been refrigerated overnight distinguishes Types I and V respectively. Distinguishing between Types IV and III (or sometimes IIB) can be difficult without electrophoresis, but the distinction rarely has therapeutic significance. The occasional clue provided by physical findings should not be missed. Abdominal pain or hepatosplenomegaly may occur in patients with the Type I disorder. Eruptive xanthomas should suggest either Type I, IV, or V. Xanthelasma and the corneal arcus can be seen in normals, but are frequently found with Type II disease. Tendon xanthomas are more specific indicators of Type II.

3. Family history should be explored and, when appropriate, first-degree relatives should be screened for elevated cholesterol. This step is necessary to assess the likelihood of primary genetic disease. Potential benefits of identifying lipid disorders in young first-degree relatives is another reason for screening.

PRINCIPLES OF MANAGEMENT

It has yet to be demonstrated that lowering serum lipids reduces risk of atherosclerotic disease. Nevertheless, the epidemiologic association of hyperlipidemia with coronary disease and the effectiveness of dietary and drug therapies lead most clinicians to the conclusion that treatment is worthwhile. However, the vast majority of patients can and should be treated with diet alone.

Calorie restriction with weight reduction is the most important intervention in obese patients with hypercholesterolemia. These patients most often have moderate or marked elevations of triglyceride levels as well (Type IV). Reduction of saturated fat consumption and increase in polyunsaturated fat consumption is the objective in patients with hypercholesterolemia and normal or moderately increased triglyceride levels (Type II). In addition to restriction of red meat and dairy products and replacement of saturated fat with vegetable oil, dietary cholesterol should also be limited.

Drug therapy should be added only after vigorous attempts to modify the patients' diet have failed to reduce serum cholesterol to acceptable levels. All drugs currently used to lower lipids have significant side effects. The European primary prevention trial has raised concerns about long-term ill effects of lipid lowering drugs (see Chapter 9). The side effects of therapy must be judiciously balanced against potential benefits.

What level of cholesterol elevation should be considered an indication for therapy? Since cholesterol level is of greater prognostic significance at earlier ages and treatment is likely to be of more value if initiated before atheromatous disease has reached an advanced stage, lower cholesterol levels should prompt treatment in younger individuals. Since coronary risk rises continuously with cholesterol level within age groups, the choice of cutoff levels is necessarily arbitrary. Treatment should be considered if the cholesterol level is greater than 220 mg. per 100 ml. in a young adult (roughly, those 20 to 45 years old). Lower levels are of concern in those under 20. While higher levels should be tolerated in older adults, simple dietary instruction may be of benefit and is recommended for all patients with "normal" high cholesterol levels.

THERAPEUTIC RECOMMENDATIONS

Simple treatment approaches are sufficient for management of the vast majority of patients with hyperlipidemia.

Isolated Hypercholesterolemia

Elevation of low-density lipoprotein is the underlying abnormality in most patients with isolated hypercholesterolemia (Type IIA). Dietary manipulation is directed at lowering cholesterol. Cholesterol intake should be restricted to less than 300 mg. per day. The ratio of polyunsaturated to saturated fats should be increased from the usual 1:5 to 2:1 or more. Reduction of total calorie intake is not necessary in Type IIA patients. When there is accompanying mild or moderate elevation of triglyceride level (Type IIB), calorie restriction to achieve ideal body weight should be advised.

In familial Type II disease, diet is often not sufficient. Bile acid sequestration with cholestyramine has emerged as the drug treatment of choice. The initial dose of the resin is 16 gm per day in four divided doses. Constipation, nausea, abdominal distention or cramps may prove to be limiting side effects. In the patient with hypertension or heart disease, it must be remembered that cholestyramine decreases absorption of a number of drugs, including thiazides, digitalis, antiarrhythmics and warfarin. Nicotinic acid, D-thyroxine and sitosterol have also been used in patients with Type II hyperlipidemia and may have an adjunctive role.

Elevation of Cholesterol and Triglyceride Levels

High cholesterol and moderately or markedly elevated triglyceride levels most often reflect elevation of very low-density lipoproteins (Type IV). Most patients with Type IV disease are obese; even in the patient who is only slightly overweight, calorie restriction with reduction to ideal body weight is the key therapeutic step. Polyunsaturated fats should be recommended, and cholesterol intake moderately restricted to less than 500 mg. per day. Alcohol intake must be strictly limited.

As discussed in Chapter 9, an independent association between cardiovascular risk and increased triglycerides has not been demonstrated conclusively. For this reason, drug therapy of Type IV disease is recommended only when effective dietary therapy fails to reduce serum *cholesterol* to acceptable levels.

Clofibrate is considered the drug of choice for Type IV disease. It has a variable effect and rarely reduces lipid levels to normal. Clofibrate doses range between 1 and 2 gm per day in two divided doses. Infrequent side effects include nausea, diarrhea, weight gain and decreased libido. Most serious complications include ventricular ectopy and myositis. Increased risk of cholelithiasis has been suggested by large-scale clofibrate trials. The increase in noncardiovascular mortality in clofibrate-treated patients in the European cooperative study has been noted. The effect of oral anticoagulants is usually potentiated by clofibrate administration.

Nicotinic acid has also been used. An initial dose of 100 mg. three times per day is increased by 300 mg. per day each week until a maintenance dose of 3 to 9 gm per day is reached. The initial symptoms of cutaneous flushing and itching usually diminish after the first several weeks of therapy. Abnormal liver function tests, decreased glucose tolerance and increased uric acid are more troublesome side effects that usually disappear when the drug is discontinued.

The reader is referred to recent reviews cited in the bibliography for further discussion of therapy and approaches to the less common lipid disorders.

PATIENT EDUCATION

The importance of patient education in the management of hyperlipidemia, as with other cardiovascular risk factors, cannot be overemphasized. The first step in therapy should be a careful review by the physician of the indications for attempts to lower lipid levels. Detailed dietary instruction will often require several visits with a dietitian. Careful attention to weight at each visit and periodic measurement of serum cholesterol and triglyceride should provide reinforcement.

ANNOTATED BIBLIOGRAPHY

Fisher, W.R., and Truitt, D.H.: The common hyperlipoproteinemias: An understanding of disease mechanisms and their control. Ann. Intern. Med., *85*:497, 1976. (*A good update focusing on pathophysiology of increased LDL and VLDL.*)

Fredrickson, D.S., Goldstein, J.L., and Brown, M.S: The familial hyperlipoproteinemias. *In* J.B. Stanbury *et al.* (eds.): The Metabolic Basis of Inherited Disease, ed. 4. New York: McGraw-Hill, 1978. (*A description of hereditary forms.*)

Levy, R.I., Fredrickson, D.S., *et al.*: Dietary and drug therapy of primary hyperlipoproteinemia. Ann. Intern. Med., 77:267, 1972. (*A good roundtable review of the relationship of hyperlipidemia to hyperlipoproteinemia as well as dietary and drug therapy.*)

Levy, R.I., Fredrickson, D.S., *et al*: Cholestyramine in type II hyperlipoproteinemia. Ann. Intern. Med., *79*:51, 1973. (*Cholestyramine lowered cho-*

lesterol levels more than 20 per cent among patients already treated with diet.)

Levy, R.I., Morganroth, J., and Rifkind, B.M.: Treatment of hyperlipidemia. N. Engl. J. Med., 290:1295, 1974. (A succinct review of classification by lipoprotein type and therapy.)

Motulsky, A.G.: The genetic hyperlipidemias. N. Engl. J. Med., 294:823, 1976. (A clear, succinct review of the confusing genetics of increased lipids with its own annotated bibliography.)

Smith, L.K., Leupker, R.V., et al.: Management of type IV hyperlipoproteinemia. Evaluation of practical clinical approaches. Ann. Intern. Med., 84:22, 1976. (Successful outpatient management of Type IV patients with triglyceride reduction of more than 50 per cent with dietary therapy.)

Yeshurun, D., and Gotto, A.M.: Drug treatment of hyperlipidemia. Am. J. Med., 60:379, 1976. (A more detailed review of drug therapy with specific recommendations.)

23
Management of Atrial Fibrillation in the Office Setting

Atrial fibrillation (AF) that is discovered incidentally in the office can usually be well managed on an outpatient basis as long as there is no evidence of failure, ischemia, or embolization. Although the number of causes of AF is large, the first therapeutic task, regardless of etiology, is control of the ventricular response rate. In addition, patients who are candidates for anticoagulant therapy and/or cardioversion need to be identified and treated. Then attention can be directed to correcting the underlying etiology (see Chapter 19). On occasion, atrial fibrillation may be refractory to standard methods of rate control, necessitating a more aggressive approach to the cause of the dysrhythmia.

CLINICAL COURSE AND NATURAL HISTORY

Atrial fibrillation may be intermittent or chronic. Paroxysmal AF resolves spontaneously when it occurs in the absence of underlying heart disease. When the episode is precipitated by infection, alcohol excess or congestive failure, correction of the inciting event is necessary for return to sinus rhythm. Most cases of AF due to valvular heart disease (e.g., mitral stenosis) or cardiomyopathy begin as paroxysms of AF, but as left atrial pressure rises and left atrial size increases, the episodes last longer, until chronic AF ensues. In the early stages of chronic AF, cardioversion may be successful in reverting the rhythm to sinus, but unless the underlying pathophysiology is corrected, the AF returns within days to months.

Systemic embolization is among the most serious complications of AF. Both prospective and retrospective studies have documented increased risk of embolization in patients with AF. It used to be felt that such risk was present only in patients who had mitral stenosis and atrial fibrillation, but data from the Framingham study and elsewhere demonstrate that underlying coronary artery disease and other forms of nonvalvular heart disease are associated with increased rates of embolization that approach those reported for mitral stenosis. No definite correlation has been found between duration of AF and risk of embolization, but there was a trend for risk to increase with duration of AF in the Framingham population.

AF may precipitate acute congestive failure as well as result from it. Heart failure that ensues in cases of AF is a sign of limited myocardial reserve due to severe underlying heart disease. The patient who develops heart failure from the onset of AF is so tenuously compensated that the rapid rate and loss of atrial pump function are sufficient to reduce cardiac output to inadequate levels. At times, the compromised state of the myocardium is transient, as occurs in cases of acute ischemia triggered by rapid ventricular response rates.

PRINCIPLES OF MANAGEMENT

Regardless of cause, the first priority is of *control rate*, i.e., to slow the ventricular response to less than 85 at rest and less than 110 after mild exercise (e.g., 10 sit-ups or 10 stand-ups from a chair). Heart rate may be well controlled at rest, but rise markedly with mild effort, making evaluation of rate control necessary both at rest and on exertion. *Digoxin* is the drug of choice for achieving a slowing of the ventricular rate. The only exception to the use of digoxin in AF is in cases of AF due to Wolff-Parkinson-White syndrome, where the drug may only aggravate the situation by decreasing conduction in the AV node and favoring conduction through the bypass tract; moreover, digoxin shortens the refractory period of the bypass tract, which can further accelerate the ventricular response. However, in the vast majority of cases, the AF is not from a preexcitation syndrome and responds well to digoxin, which impedes conduction of the flurry of atrial impulses arriving at the AV node. At times, AF converts to sinus rhythm upon initiation of digitalis therapy.

If the patient is tolerating the ventricular rate without showing signs of ischemia or failure and the rate is not dangerously rapid (i.e., over 150), the patient can be treated in the outpatient setting, starting with the oral administration of a rapid-acting cardiac glycoside such as digoxin. Initiating therapy with maintenance doses of digoxin is reasonable if the ventricular rate is less than about 120 and well tolerated. About 5 days are required to achieve standard therapeutic serum levels. If the ventricular rate is between 120 and 150 and the patient appears uncompromised, outpatient management is still reasonable as long as the patient is reliable and the home situation supportive. In such circumstances, more rapid digitalization is preferable in order to attain rate control more promptly. A loading dose of digoxin is given orally over the first 24 hours and rate monitored to assess need for further doses in the acute phase and to establish a maintenance dose. At the first sign of congestive failure or ischemia, the patient requires hospital admission.

At times, it is difficult to slow the ventricular response. Occult hyperthyroidism (see Chapter 99), refractory heart failure, pulmonary embolization, poor compliance, and preexcitation syndrome are important causes of the problem. Treatment needs to be directed at the underlying condition rather than at increasing cardiac glycoside therapy to the point of toxicity. Hospitalization should be considered in such instances.

In the patient with AF and a slow ventricular response due to the presence of preexisting conduction system disease, there is no need to intervene pharmacologically with digoxin unless there is coexisting heart failure.

In addition to rate control, it is important to assess the risk of embolization and the indications for *anticoagulant therapy*. Although the risk of embolization is the greatest in AF patients with mitral stenosis (17 times greater than the population at large in the Framingham study), it is also considerable in those with AF of nonrheumatic origin (fivefold increase in risk). Other factors reported to increase the chances of embolic stroke include evidence of previous embolization, presence of coronary artery disease, and chronicity of atrial fibrillation. Because the consequences of cerebral embolization are often devastating and occur in patients who were functioning independently prior to the episode, some clinicians have argued that all patients with AF should receive anticoagulant therapy prophylactically. Others have taken a more cautious stance in view of the potential complications of anticoagulant use in an elderly population, and suggested that controlled trials be conducted. Most agree that the patient with AF and mitral stenosis is a candidate for anticoagulant therapy as well as the patient with previous embolization.

Another major management decision in cases of atrial fibrillation regards the indications for pharmacologic or electrical conversion to sinus rhythm, i.e., *cardioversion.* Cardioversion is the treatment of choice in acute situations for patients who manifest hemodynamic deterioration with the onset of AF, increase in angina pectoris, or an extremely rapid ventricular response. Less urgent indications include symptomatic palpitations, persistence of AF after successful treatment of hyperthyroidism, and systemic embolization thought to arise from the left atrium. Maintenance of sinus rhythm for more than 6 months after cardioversion is most likely to be attained in patients with recent onset of AF, coarse fibrillatory waves on ECG, and a normal-sized left atrium. Conversely, those with chronic AF, large left atria, advanced mitral stenosis or chronic congestive failure are the worst candidates for attempting restoration of sinus rhythm, since AF almost always returns quickly.

Electrical cardioversion is the procedure of choice for converting AF to sinus rhythm. When preceded by treatment with *quinidine* to prevent reversion to AF, electrical cardioversion is safer than purely pharmacologic cardioversion, which requires near toxic doses of quinidine, and is more effective than electrical cardioversion alone without use of quinidine. Quinidine must never be given to the undigitalized patient with AF, because the drug enhances conduction through the AV node and may result in development of very rapid ventricular response rates.

Most cardiologists administer anticoagulant therapy prior to cardioversion in those people in the high-risk group for embolization, because there is a small risk of embolization associated with the procedure. Usually, oral anticoagulants are prescribed for 3 to 4 weeks to allow organization of clots which may be present in the left atrium and to prevent the formation of a new thrombus. Digoxin is withheld for 2 days before cardioversion, because there is an increased risk of ventricular dysrhythmias when the heart is countershocked in the presence of high digitalis levels.

Once rate has been controlled and the need for cardioversion, anticoagulant therapy, and hospitalization assessed, treatment can be directed at the underlying cause of the AF. For example, definitive management of valvular disease may require commissurotomy or valve replacement (see Chapter 28). AF due to hyperthyroidism often responds to antithyroid treatment; in many instances propranolol is effective in helping to control the ventricular response rate when digoxin alone does not suffice.

PATIENT EDUCATION

The patient with lone fibrillation (see Chapter 19), free of underlying heart disease, needs to be carefully reassured. The physician should try to prevent fostering cardiac neurosis and the unnecessary restriction of activity. Teaching relaxation techniques or providing the patient with small amounts of a mild sedative can help lessen the frequency of episodes precipitated by emotional stress. The patient should be instructed to avoid sleep deprivation and excessive use of alcohol or stimulants, and to stop smoking.

Regardless of etiology, it is important to teach the patient and his family how to detect signs of congestive failure and rapid ventricular rate. The person with AF should be advised to regularly check his pulse and weight and call the physician when there is a rapid and unexplained increase, especially if it occurs in the context of increasing dyspnea on exertion, orthopnea, or chest discomfort. Patients appreciate knowing that proper daily use of digitalis is not habit-forming or injurious to the heart, concerns harbored by a surprising number. However, they need to be aware of the symptoms of digitalis toxicity so that correction of excess dose is not unnecessarily delayed

(see Chapter 27). Teaching the patient and family to check the radial pulse can facilitate detection of digitalis toxicity, for slow rates or regular rhythms could well be manifestations of excessive drug levels.

THERAPEUTIC RECOMMENDATIONS

- If the ventricular response rate is less than 150 and the patient shows no signs of congestive failure or ischemia, outpatient management can be undertaken, provided the patient is reliable and there is a supportive home environment.
- The first priority is slowing the ventricular rate. Digoxin is the drug of choice. If the initial rate is less than 110 to 120 and the AF is being well tolerated, digoxin therapy can begin with maintenance level oral doses of 0.25 to 0.375 mg. per day and adjusted according to ventricular response rate. Optimal control should be achieved within 5 days, the time it takes to reach maximal therapeutic serum levels.
- If the initial rate is between 120 and 150 per minute and there are no signs of hemodynamic compromise, the patient might be given a loading dose of digoxin to achieve rate control more rapidly. If there are any signs of ischemia or failure, hospitalization is urgent and electrical cardioversion indicated. When outpatient management is deemed safe, the oral loading dose of digoxin is 1.0 to 1.25 mg. given over 24 hours in divided doses. Ventricular rate is monitored to adjust dose.
- If the rate cannot be controlled by use of moderate doses of digoxin, it is necessary to search for a cause of refractory rapid AF such as pulmonary embolization or hyperthroidism. Further increases in digoxin dose should be approached with caution and hospitalization considered.
- The goal of rate control should be a heart rate of less than 85 at rest and less than 100 to 110 after mild exercise (e.g., 10 stand-ups). The rate must be checked after exercise because it may rise markedly, even though it appears well controlled at rest.
- Digoxin is contraindicated in AF due to preexcitation syndromes such as Wolff-Parkinson-White syndrome. Quinidine or cardioversion is often necessary.
- Anticoagulation to prevent systemic embolization is indicated in patients with mitral stenosis or a prior history of embolization. Oral anticoagulant therapy can be initiated safely in the outpatient setting

(see Chapter 84). There seems to be increased risk of embolic stroke in AF patients with nonrheumatic heart disease; such patients should also be considered for prophylaxis, as long as there are no major contraindications to therapy.

- Elective cardioversion is indicated for treatment of symptomatic palpitations, persistence of AF after successful treatment of hyperthroidism, systemic embolization thought to arise from the left atrium, and difficulty in controlling ventricular rate. Urgent, nonelective cardioversion is needed for hemodynamic deterioration, increase in angina or other signs of ischemia, and extremely rapid rates (e.g., 200 or more).

- Electrical cardioversion, preceded by a brief course of quinidine, is the preferred method of elective cardioversion. Because of a small risk of embolization associated with cardioversion, patients at high risk for embolization should receive oral anticoagulant therapy for 3 to 4 weeks prior to elective cardioversion. Two days before cardioversion, digoxin is omitted and quinidine sulfate, 200 mg. every 6 hours, is given orally. The quinidine is continued indefinitely at the same level after restoration of sinus rhythm to prevent relapse to AF. The patients most likely to remain in sinus rhythm beyond 6 months after cardioversion are those with recent onset of AF, normal left atrial size, and coarse fibrillatory waves on electrocardiogram. Chronic AF, advanced mitral stenosis, and chronic congestive failure are poor prognostic signs for successful cardioversion.

- Once rate control has been achieved, therapy should be directed at the underlying etiology.

ANNOTATED BIBLIOGRAPHY

Freeman, I., and Wexler, J.: Anticoagulants for treatment of atrial fibrillation. JAMA, *184*:1007, 1963. *(Classic study documenting the reduction in mortality and morbidity from embolization in patients treated with anticoagulants.)*

Goldman, S., Probst, J., Selzer, A., *et al.*: Inefficacy of "therapeutic" serum levels of digoxin in controlling the ventricular rate in atrial fibrillation. Am. J. Cardiol, *35*:651, 1975. *(Amounts of digoxin sufficient to achieve "therapeutic" serum concentrations may fail to lower the ventricular rate below 100 beats a minute when serious complicating illness coexists. Patients who are clinically stable usually require no more than "therapeutic" levels to maintain rate control.)*

Henry, W.L., Pearlman, A.S., and Clark, G.E.: Relation between echocardiographically determined left atrial size and atrial fibrillation. Circulation, *53*(2):273, 1976. *(A carefully performed study showing that atrial fibrillation is rare when the left atrial dimension was below 40 mm. and common when the dimension exceeded 40 mm. In addition, when left atrial dimension exceeded 45 mm; cardioversion was unlikely to produce sinus rhythm maintained at least 6 months. This study also documented a high incidence of embolization in patients with atrial fibrillation and asymmetric septal hypertrophy.)*

Hinton, R.D., Kistler, P., Fallon, J.T., *et al.*: Influence of etiology of atrial fibrillation on incidence of systemic embolization. Am.J.Cardiol., *40*:509, 1977. *(An autopsy study of patients with AF demonstrating that the incidence of embolization was increased almost as much for AF due to other forms of heart disease as for AF due to mitral stenosis.)*

Sodermark, T., Jonsson, A., Olsson, L., *et al.*: Effect of quinidine on maintaining sinus rhythm after cardioversion of atrial fibrillation or flutter. Br. Heart J., *37*:486, 1975. *(A multicenter controlled study showing significant reduction in reoccurence of atrial fibrillation after electrical cardioversion in patients pretreated with quinidine.)*

Wolf, P.A., Dawber, T.R., Emerson, H., Jr., *et al.*: Epidemiologic assessment of chronic atrial fibrillation and risk of stroke: The Framingham study. Neurology, *28*:973, 1978. *(Chronic AF due to mitral stenosis was associated with a seventeen fold increase in stroke incidence, but nonrheumatic causes of AF also showed an increased incidence.)*

24

Management of
Premature Ventricular Contractions
in the Ambulatory Setting

LEE GOLDMAN, M.D.

Decisions regarding treatment of premature ventricular contractions (PVCs) discovered on an office visit are among the most difficult in outpatient medicine. At issue is whether the PVCs represent increased risk of sudden death or are merely an incidental, harmless finding. Treatment is not without its own risks and is fraught with considerable expense and morbidity. The tasks are to determine which PVCs signify a poor prognosis, how best to detect them, and which therapy, if any, to institute.

CLINICAL PRESENTATION AND COURSE

In studies of the general population, at least one PVC in a single routine electrocardiogram (ECG) was found in 1 per cent of Air-Force recruits, 4 per cent of life insurance applicants, 7 per cent of men over the age of 34, and up to 15 per cent of men over the age of 60. If ECGs are continuously recorded for 6 to 24 hours by telemetry or ambulatory Holter monitoring, these percentages increase about fivefold.

In the ambulatory setting, PVCs usually present in one of several ways: (1) as an incidental finding on routine examination or ECG; (2) as an ECG finding in a patient being evaluated for palpitations, dizziness or syncope; (3) as a complication of coronary artery disease noted on resting ECG, exercise stress test or ambulatory ECG monitoring. In terms of assessing the prognostic and therapeutic importance of the PVCs, the crucial criterion seems to be the presence or absence of underlying heart disease.

Prospective studies of large populations of ambulatory men have shown a correlation between PVCs on routine ECG and subsequent sudden death. When controlled for other cardiac risk factors, these surveys found that PVCs were not an independent predictor of cardiac death in the general population. Other natural history surveys have also emphasized that in the absence of hypertension, angina, history of myocardial infarction, cardiomegaly on chest x-ray, or ECG signs of ischemia, left ventricular hypertrophy or bundle branch block, people with PVCs are at no greater risk for myocardial infarction or sudden death than are those without PVCs.

PVCs are frequent in patients who survive for more than two weeks after a myocardial infarction; they occur in about 12 per cent on routine ECG and in 60 to 80 per cent of those studied by 6- to 24-hour ECG monitoring or supervised stress testing. In the Coronary Drug Project study of over 2000 survivors of myocardial infarction, the occurrence of even a single PVC on an ECG taken three months or more after the infarct was associated with a doubled (21 per cent versus 12 per cent) mortality during a three-year follow-up period. Among those with PVCs, the number or configuration of PVCs on the single ECG did not significantly affect the prognosis. Two recent multifactorial studies have confirmed that in the postinfarct patient, even one PVC per hour is an independent prognostic factor, but also found that more complex PVCs seem to carry even higher risk. However, it has also been shown that postinfarction PVCs increase in direct proportion to the degree of cardiac muscle dysfunction and coronary artery stenosis. Thus, the higher mortality of patients with PVCs is related at least in part to reinfarction and congestive heart failure.

PRINCIPLES OF MANAGEMENT

At present, there are absolutely no data documenting that treatment specifically aimed at chronic PVCs will in any way influence the chances of recurrent infarction or sudden death, even in the postinfarct patient. Of patients studied while on therapy with quinidine or procainamide, only about 20 to 35 per cent have a significant reduction in PVC frequency, even when blood concentrations of the drug used can be shown to be in the high therapeutic range. In addition, troublesome side effects of the medications develop in 25 to 40 per cent of patients.

Recently, a multicenter international study of practolol, a beta-adrenergic blocking agent related to propranolol, has been shown to reduce the incidence of sudden death and overall cardiac death in post-infarction patients. It is suspected that the mechanisms responsible for the effect involve reduction of myocardial oxygen demand as well as direct suppression of PVCs. Unfortunately, practolol has been found to have unacceptable noncardiac toxicities and has been removed from the market. The literature should be followed closely for further data on the use of other beta-blocking agents for prevention of sudden death.

THERAPEUTIC RECOMMENDATIONS

Based on the knowledge at hand, the following recommendations can be forwarded:

- The patient should be assessed for (a) symptoms (dizziness or syncope) related to ventricular irritability and documented by ECG monitoring; (b) evidence of ischemic heart disease (angina, ischemic changes on ECG), congestive heart failure, cardiomegaly, left ventricular hypertrophy, bundle branch block or hypertension; (c) history of a myocardial infarction more than 2 weeks previously. (PVCs early in the post-MI period do not signify increased long-term risk.)
- In the presence of dizziness or syncope related to recurrent ventricular arrhythmias (usually bursts of ventricular tachycardia), the patient should be hospitalized and treated in the routine manner for malignant ventricular irritability as outlined in standard texts.
- In the asymptomatic patient with PVCs but no other evidence of heart disease, there is no association between PVCs and prognosis and no reason to treat the PVCs. Some authors suggest that such patients be studied with exercise electrocardiography and that patients who develop (a) ST-segment depression or (b) a worrisome increase in PVCs be treated. There are no data to document that such totally asymptomatic patients will benefit from therapy.
- The patient with heart disease and PVCs who has no dizziness or syncope should be studied with exercise testing and Holter monitoring. If complex forms of ventricular irritability develop (i.e., two or more PVCs in a row, multifocal PVCs, prolonged periods of bigeminy, or PVCs which occur on the T-wave of the preceding normal beat), outpatient antiarrhythmic therapy should probably be attempted.
- In the patient with heart disease but no history of myocardial infarction and no serious PVCs, specific antiarrhythmic therapy with presently available drugs does not seem worthwhile. If such patients have angina, propranolol should already be part of the regimen; for the other presently available drugs, side effects of medication are more likely than therapeutic response. Alternatively, if treatment is undertaken, it would seem incumbent upon the physician to demonstrate the efficacy of therapy by repeat monitoring or stress testing before subjecting the patient to a lifetime of medications. Because of the known variability of PVCs from day to day in an individual patient, PVCs must be decreased by about 80 per cent for the change to be specifically attributable to the therapeutic intervention.
- Evidence currently at hand suggests that propranolol is the only medication presently available which might prolong life in the patient with a documented history of infarction. If there are no contraindications, the drug should be given to postinfarct patients with complex ventricular arrhythmias; based on the practolol study, some would suggest it be given to all survivors of anterior infarctions as well. Quinidine, disopyramide, or procainamide should be added to propranolol therapy if potentially lethal arrhythmias are still observed on monitoring 2 weeks or more after an infarction. Routine 6- to 24-hour monitoring just prior to hospital discharge is recommended as an aid to planning rational management.
- Before using propranolol, check for contraindications to beta-blockade (insulin use, heart failure, asthma, severe obstructive lung disease, bradycardia, hypotension, heart block). Begin with 10 mg. every 6 hours and increase gradually until complex irritability is suppressed as documented by Holter monitoring and, in cases of persons accustomed to regular physical exercise, by stress testing. The major cardiac side effects of propranolol are postural hypotension and bradycardia, but resting bradycardia (below about 65 beats per minute) is mandatory if beta-blockade is to be achieved. Propranolol dosage is adequate if there is a less than 10-beat-per-minute pulse rise after moderate (one to two flights of stairs) exertion. The direct antiarrhyth-

mic action of propranolol may occur at subblockade doses.

- Quinidine preparations can be used as long as "therapeutic" blood levels are maintained. The most common dosages range from 200 to 400 mg. of quinidine sulfate every 6 hours. A steady-state blood concentration will not be reached for about 3 days. Loading dose regimens are not recommended in the outpatient setting. Disopyramide (Norpace), a new medication with antiarrhythmic properties similar to those of quinidine, is usually given in a dose of 150 to 200 mg. every 6 hours; the drug is often used for patients who develop gastrointestinal problems with quinidine, but disopyramide's own side effects include dry mouth, urinary retention, and myocardial depression. This myocardial depression is more marked than that found with quinidine and may lead to a clinically important decompensation in ambulatory patients with preexisting heart failure.

- If propranolol, quinidine, and disopyramide (singly and in combination) fail to suppress complex forms of ventricular irritability, procainamide (250 to 500 mg. every 3 to 4 hours) can be tried. Side effects are especially common with procainamide. Because development of a lupuslike syndrome is a risk, a pretreatment antinuclear antigen titer should be obtained; if the titer is elevated, procainamide should be avoided if possible.

- Patients with complex PVCs unresponsive to conventional medical therapy should be referred to a cardiologist for consideration of newer medications, cardiac catheterization, or overdrive pacemaker therapy.

ANNOTATED BIBLIOGRAPHY

Coronary Drug Project Research Group: Prognostic importance of premature beats following myocardial infarction. JAMA, 223:1116, 1973. (The classic article with univariate analysis showing a poorer prognosis in postinfarct patients with PVCs on routine ECG, but no difference based on the "malignancy" of the PVCs.)

Fisher, F.D., Tyroler, H.A.: Relationship between ventricular premature contractions on routine electrocardiography and subsequent death from coronary heart disease. Circulation, 47:217, 1973. (Patients with PVCs but no other evidence of heart disease do well, while those with evident heart disease have increased mortality.)

Jelinek, M.V., Lohrbauer, L., and Lown, B.: Antirhythmic drug therapy for sporadic ventricular ectopic arrhythmias. Circulation, 49:649, 1974. (The success rate of quinidine or procainamide against PVCs is less than 40 per cent; increasing either drug to its maximum dose causes as much toxicity as therapeutic benefit.)

Koch-Weser, J.: Disopyramide. N. Engl. J. Med., 300:957, 1979. (Terse and critical review of the use of this new antiarrhythmic agent; 59 refs.)

Luria, M.H., Knoke, J.D., Margolis, R.M., Henricks, F.H., and Kuplic, J.B.: Acute myocardial infarction, prognosis after recovery. Ann. Intern. Med., 85:561, 1976. (This study's multivariate analysis supports the prognostic importance of even one PVC per hour in the post-infarct patient.)

Moss, A.J., DeCamilla, J., Davis, H., and Bayer, L.: The early post-hospital phase of myocardial infarction: Prognostic stratification. Circulation, 54:58, 1976. (This article indicates that frequency or coupling [two or more in a row] of PVCs is even more ominous than infrequent PVCs as a prognostic sign after an infarction.)

Multicentre International Study: Improvement in prognosis of myocardial infarction by longterm beta-adrenoreceptor blockade using practolol. Br. Med. J., 3:735, 1975. (Practolol [related to propranolol], when given to postinfarct patients, reduced the rate of development of angina, reinfarction, and sudden death without increasing the rate of heart failure in those without contraindications to its use. Benefit was especially significant in those with prior anterior or lateral infarctions; in those after an inferior infarct, incidence of sudden death was reduced but overall mortality was not.)

Rodstein, M., Wolloch, L., and Gubner, R.: Mortality study of the significance of extrasystoles in an insured population. Circulation, 44:617, 1971. (Supports data of Fisher, et al.)

Ruberman, W., Weinblatt, E., Goldberg, J.D., et al.: Ventricular premature beats and mortality after myocardial infarction. N. Engl. J. Med., 297:750, 1977. (Patients with complex forms of PVCs detected by 1 hour of ECG monitoring had a threefold increase in mortality.)

Ryan, R., Lown, B., and Horn, H.: Comparison of ventricular ectopic activity during 24-hour monitoring and exercise testing in patients with coronary disease. N. Engl. J. Med., *292*:224, 1975.

(In some patients, exercise stress-testing brought out more worrisome forms of ventricular ectopy, but Holter monitoring detected ventricular arrhythmias with greater frequency.)

25

Management of Chronic Stable Angina

The advent of beta-adrenergic blocking agents, long-acting nitrates, coronary artery bypass surgery and exercise programs has provided new options for the management of chronic stable angina. Although the ultimate goal is to improve life expectancy, this is not yet possible in most instances. Consequently a more attainable objective is to help the patient achieve a personally satisfactory level of daily activity. The primary physician needs to know the indications and limitations of the available treatment modalities and the life-style of the patient in order to design an optimal program for management of chronic angina.

PATHOPHYSIOLOGY

Angina is a manifestation of myocardial ischemia; it occurs when oxygen demand exceeds supply. Coronary artery occlusion due to atherosclerotic disease is by far the most common etiology. Coronary vasospasm that involves otherwise normal vessels has also been documented, especially in some patients with Prinzmetal's angina. Hemodynamically significant aortic stenosis can limit flow to the coronary circulation and produce angina. In addition, conditions that increase myocardial oxygen demand (e.g., hyperthyroidism) or decrease oxygen supply (e.g., severe anemia) can aggravate or precipitate angina when there is preexisting coronary disease.

NATURAL HISTORY

Coronary angiographic studies have shown that prognosis is a function of the severity and site of stenosis. Combined data reveal that patients with significant disease in one vessel have a mean annual mortality rate of 2.2 percent; this figure increases to 4.5 to 7 percent when the single obstruction involves the left main coronary artery. With stenosis of two vessels, the mean annual mortality rate is 6.8 per-

cent; the rate increases to 11.4 percent for three vessel disease. Other correlates of increased risk include cardiomegaly, symptoms of congestive failure, and resting tachycardia.

Studies of work status in patients with angina have found that 50 to 75 percent maintain full-time employment. Data from a community-wide surveillance in Seattle identified several factors which affected the chances of staying on the job. Age greater than 55, less than 12 years of formal education, involvement of more than one vessel on angiogram, and functional Class III or IV were among the variables that reduced the likelihood of remaining in full-time work over the 1-year period of the study. Ejection fraction and amount of activity required by the job did not affect employment status in patients treated medically, but did in the surgical group.

PRINCIPLES OF MANAGEMENT

Most medical therapies are designed to decrease myocardial oxygen demand; surgical treatment aims at improving blood supply to the myocardium. Oxygen needs can be lessened for a particular level of activity by reducing heart rate, contractility, or heart size. Other means of improving exercise tolerance include redistribution of myocardial blood flow, improvement in peripheral oxygen extraction, and promotion of psychological well-being. Therapeutic methods of decreasing oxygen demand include nitrate administration, beta blockade, exercise restriction, exercise training, modification of life-style to limit stress, and cessation of smoking. Correction of any preexisting hypertension (see Chapter 21), congestive heart failure (see Chapter 27), severe anemia (see Chapter 77), hyperthyroidism (see Chapter 99) or pulmonary disease is also essential to an optimal outcome.

Nitrates are a mainstay of therapy for angina. Their mechanism of action in relieving anginal pain is still not fully understood. These agents are smooth muscle relaxants that cause vascular dilatation, predominantly of capacitance vessels, though they also have a lesser effect on the arterial bed. Nitrates have no proven direct action on heart rate or contractility, but are believed to decrease myocardial oxygen demand by reducing heart size (a consequence of lowering left ventricular filling pressure) and blood pressure. There is some suggestion that regional myocardial perfusion may also be improved, but total coronary blood flow is not. Nitrates may lessen coronary vasospasm.

Sublingual nitroglycerin (TNG) is effective for relief of anginal pain and can provide short-term (up to 30 minutes) improvement in exercise tolerance when taken prophylactically. Its advantages are low cost, rapid onset of action (30 seconds to 3 minutes), safety and proven efficacy in providing symptomatic relief. Its main drawback is its short duration of action. TNG must be taken sublingually because oral doses are denitrified and inactivated on the first pass through the portal circulation. Since the drug is volatile, it must be kept in a stoppered, amber vial and stored in a cool place. Once a bottle of TNG is opened, the contents remain maximally effective for up to 6 months; after that it is best to assume that the TNG has lost some of its potency, and a fresh supply should be prescribed. Often the patient using old TNG will note that the side effects of the drug, such as headache, are less pronounced, and there is less relief from angina.

Isosorbide dinitrate is the best studied of the oral nitrates that have been developed in efforts to improve upon the short duration of action characteristic of TNG. Early studies failed to demonstrate any prolonged action for these so-called long-acting nitrates when they were compared with TNG. It was not until larger single doses of isosorbide were utilized (20 to 40 mg.) that controlled studies showed statistically significant improvements in hemodynamic parameters and exercise tolerance that persisted for up to 4 hours after a dose.

The onset of action of isosorbide is 15 to 30 minutes when taken orally. A sublingual form has also been developed that has a more rapid onset of action, 5 to 15 minutes; its duration of action is about 2 hours. In addition, a chewable isosorbide preparation is marketed; its characteristics are similar to those of sublingual isosorbide. It remains unsettled whether the faster but shorter acting forms of isosorbide are so superior to TNG for prophylaxis that they are worth the much greater cost. Long-acting prophylaxis appears to be best achieved by use of oral isosorbide or nitroglycerin ointment.

Nitroglycerin ointment has been rediscovered in recent years as an effective method for providing long-acting prophylaxis. Improved exercise tolerance and hemodynamic effects have been found to persist for 3 to 6 hours after application. Because the ointment is messy and becomes irritating to the skin of some patients if applied to the same area around-the-clock, it is best suited for nocturnal use.

Selection of the proper dose of isosorbide or nitropaste can be achieved by monitoring the effect of the agent on heart rate, blood pressure, and exercise tolerance. Dose can be increased until (1) customary activity can be undertaken without pain, (2) the heart rate at rest rises by 10 to 15 beats per minute, or (3) the blood pressure falls to the point of causing postural light-headedness. The development of headache is not a reliable therapeutic end point, because it usually disappears with continuation of therapy.

The role of nitroglycerin in the symptomatic management of stable angina is well established; its effect on survival is undetermined. There is still some uncertainty concerning the place of long-acting nitrates in the treatment of ischemic heart disease. For example, the questions of nitrate tolerance and dependence are unsettled. Anginal symptoms have developed in previously healthy munitions plant workers (who are chronically exposed to nitrates) when they are away from the factory. Some patients taking large doses of long-acting nitrates have reported an attenuated response to nitroglycerin, suggesting the development of tolerance. Thus, enthusiasm for long-acting nitrate therapy should be tempered a bit, pending further study. Nevertheless, it is quite reasonable to employ long-acting nitrate therapy for prophylactic management of patients with angina who cannot be controlled by TNG alone. Some authorities advocate a trial prophylactic dose of TNG, because benefit from TNG predicts a strong likelihood of benefit from isosorbide.

Propranolol. Many clinicians add propranolol to the patient's program at the time that isosorbide is begun; there is evidence that the two agents might be complementary in effect. Propranolol slows the heart rate, lowers systolic blood pressure, and decreases contractility; these actions diminish myocardial oxygen demands. Propranolol can counter the tachycardia induced by nitrates, and nitrates can help minimize any increase in left ventricular end diastolic pressure that may result from propranolol's negative inotropic effect. Thus their combined use is potentially advantageous.

Data are becoming available on the effects of

long-term propranolol use. Results from a study of anginal patients with New York Heart Association functional Class III or IV disease (symptoms on minimal activity or at rest) who took the drug for 5 to 8 years showed that 84 per cent had at least a 50 per cent reduction in anginal episodes. There was no evidence of tachyphylaxis. Heart failure was seen in 25 per cent, but two thirds of these patients had a history of heart failure prior to propranolol therapy. All patients with a cardiothoracic ratio greater than 1:2 developed some degree of heart failure on propranolol. The only adverse long-term effect seemed to be a slight increase in risk of cardiogenic shock with acute myocardial infarction. The incidence of asthma was 4 per cent, was dose-related, and did not require complete discontinuation of the drug. The overall annual mortality rate for patients in the study was only 3.8 per cent, but 50 per cent of patients dropped out of the study, rendering mortality figures uninterpretable. However, data on patient survival from a controlled, multicenter, English study of patients with prior myocardial infarction treated chronically with a beta-blocking agent or placebo demonstrated improved life expectancy for those with anterior infarction treated with beta-blocking therapy. Other studies on survival are in progress.

Propranolol has a negative chronotropic effect and is relatively contraindicated in patients with heart block. The drug interferes with epinephrine response to hypoglycemia and therefore must be used with caution in diabetics who require insulin therapy. Reports of the development of angina after immediate cessation of propranolol therapy have led to the recommendation that propranolol be tapered over several days before discontinuation or that activity be limited when tapering is impossible.

The study of long-term propranolol use revealed a subgroup of patients who did not respond to the agent; they had a fourfold increase in mortality compared to responders. The same study revealed that the heart rate could be lowered to 40 beats per minute in most patients without adverse effect. The mean dose necessary to reduce anginal pain was 250 mg. per day, but some patients required two to three times that amount.

There are two important contraindications to use of propranolol in angina: (1) patients with critical aortic stenosis need a maximal amount of inotropy to maintain cardiac output; they may be jeopardized by the loss of contractility from propranolol (see Chapter 28); (2) patients with documented coronary vasospasm may have their condition aggravated by use of a beta-blocking agent.

Digitalis. When heart failure complicates angina, digitalis and/or a diuretic can provide some symptomatic relief (see Chapter 27). Digitalis may be needed to counter failure associated with the use of propranolol; nitrates cannot prevent the development of clinically significant congestive failure induced by beta blockade. Although the positive inotropic effect of digitalis may increase myocardial oxygen demand, this increase can be offset by a reduction in heart size; a net decrease in oxygen requirements often results. Nocturnal episodes of angina that are triggered by failure will respond to treatment of the congestive failure. Sometimes symptoms of failure that occur at night are due to ischemia and labeled an "anginal equivalent"; reducing myocardial oxygen demands may alleviate the symptoms.

Minor tranquilizers have a limited, specific role in management of angina. When acute anxiety or situational stress precipitates chest pain, use of a benzodiazepine, such as chlordiazepoxide, may be helpful. Constant use may result in some loss of effect; the agent should be reserved for the occasion when other anxiety-reducing efforts do not suffice (see Chapter 214).

Smoking is a major aggravating factor for angina, not only because it contributes to the development of coronary disease, but also because the absorbed nicotine increases blood pressure and heart rate, thus increasing myocardial oxygen demands. Moreover, the rise in carboxyhemoglobin levels in the blood cuts down on oxygen supply to the heart. Even passive smoking, i.e., breathing the air in a smoke-filled room, has been shown to significantly reduce exercise tolerance in patients with chronic stable angina. Cessation of smoking is certainly not easy to achieve and may even produce some additional stress; nevertheless, the benefits in terms of symptomatic improvement may be impressive and may obviate the need to consider more aggressive antianginal therapy. Working with the patient to quit smoking is certainly worth a serious attempt and often succeeds when the physician takes a strong interest (see Chapter 49).

Weight reduction should be advised in the obese patient in an effort to reduce work load and oxygen requirements. The psychological benefits are often substantial as well. It is hoped that adherence to a *low cholesterol, low saturated fat diet* will prove effective in reduction of morbidity and mortality from coronary disease, though this remains unproven (see

Chapters 9 and 22). Other dietary factors, such as coffee and alcohol, do not appear to be of major significance, though there is one report suggesting reduced exercise tolerance with intake of alcohol.

The impact of life-style and environmental stress on the patient should not be overlooked, though it is probably imprudent to force the patient to radically alter his life-style or avoid pleasurable activities; any such attempts may be counterproductive. The simplest advice is to guide the patient away from unnecessary physical stress (e.g., heavy exertion during extremes of heat and cold) and excessive emotional upset.

An exercise program can improve exercise tolerance. Uncontrolled data suggest that survival may be prolonged by exercise training; the issue remains controversial (see Chapter 26). Exercise programs may improve exercise tolerance by reducing peripheral oxygen demands (skeletal muscle efficiency improves), by decreasing the increment in heart rate and blood pressure that occurs with exercise, and by promoting a sense of psychological well-being.

Careful screening of patients who are potential candidates for exercise training is necessary to ensure safety. Patients should *not* take part in an exercise program if they have congestive heart failure, unstable angina, severe systemic hypertension, brittle insulin-dependent diabetes, severe lung disease, hemodynamically significant valvular heart disease, heart block, exertional hypotension, or poor motivation. Patients using ganglionic blocking agents are also advised against participating.

All patients who are enrolled should have an exercise stress test to determine the maximum heart rate at which they can safely exercise (see Chapter 26). Once this rate is established, the patient should be taught to measure his own pulse and instructed not to exceed the target rate. The optimal rate for achieving training benefit is 75 to 85 per cent of the maximum for the patient's age, but the level may have to be set lower if angina, ischemic ST and T-wave changes, or arrhythmias occur at such rates.

The best exercises are isotonic ones that utilize the large muscles of the body (e.g., walking, swimming, jogging, and cycling). Isometrics are to be avoided, because they are capable of inducing marked elevations in blood pressure and precipitating ventricular irritability. A 10- to 15-minute warm-up period should start the session, followed by 20 to 30 minutes of more strenuous activity. In order to attain the optimal training benefit from exercise, there should be two to three periods of about 5 minutes each, during which the target heart rate is achieved. The session ends with time for cooling down. Conditioning requires at least three sessions per week.

Training should begin slowly, advance gradually, and not involve competitive activities until a full 3 months of activity at the target heart rate has been achieved and is well tolerated. Many patients report a new sense of confidence and well-being and a return to productive work; they avoid unnecessary restrictions of lifestyle, and depression often resolves.

Coronary artery bypass surgery is the most radical therapeutic modality available. At present, the major indication for surgery in the patient with chronic stable angina is persistence of intolerable angina in spite of a maximal medical regimen. There is no evidence that surgery prolongs survival or prevents infarction, except in the case of significant occlusion of the main left coronary artery. Randomized studies indicate that surgery for other than main left disease is no better than medical therapy with regard to improvement in life expectancy or return to full-time employment. However, symptomatic improvement is more likely to be achieved in patients subjected to surgery. Unfortunately, there is no clinical or noninvasive means of identifying patients with main left coronary disease. The decision to refer the patient for angiography and consideration of surgery needs to be carefully individualized. At present, only those who have failed a full trial of medical therapy and could tolerate surgery if a bypassable lesion were found should be referred for angiography.

PATIENT EDUCATION

Patient education is pivotal in the management of the person with angina, because the success of a medical regimen requires the intelligent use of drugs by the patient. If the patient lacks an understanding of the rationale behind therapy, he is apt to misuse the agents prescribed or to comply poorly. Counseling can prevent unnecessary restrictions in activity, excessive fear, and decline in life-style. Of particular concern to many patients is the safety of engaging in sexual intercourse. The issue should be addressed openly and directly, even if the patient does not raise the subject, for the worry and interference with marital life can worsen emotional stress and aggravate symptoms. Guidelines for engaging in sexual activity are similar to those for any other form of physical exertion. The oxygen demands of intercourse among married, middle-aged partners are about the same as those for climbing a flight of stairs. If intercourse takes place among unaccustomed partners, the physical and emotional stress may be greater and the oxygen requirements increased. When there is a question of how much activity the patient can safely tolerate, an exercise stress test can be of help; moreover, the test may have a reassuring effect on the overly cautious patient who has been needlessly limiting his activity.

The patient has an important role in helping the physician to gauge the effectiveness of therapy. Subjective reports of exercise tolerance have been found to correlate with objective ergometric findings. Thus a careful history that reveals how well the patient is managing can provide a very practical means of judging the adequacy of the therapeutic program.

INDICATIONS FOR ADMISSION AND REFERRAL

Admission is required when the anginal pattern is increasing in frequency and/or severity and is becoming harder to control. Episodes that last more than 15 minutes suggest the development of acute coronary insufficiency, especially when associated with new ST and T-wave changes on ECG. Hospitalization may also be of benefit to judge the adequacy of a medical regimen when a patient reports insufficient relief, and poor compliance is suspected. Referral to a cardiologist can be helpful when angina is stable but difficult to control and surgery is being entertained. Angina in the setting of aortic stenosis also deserves a review by the cardiologist. The same is true for cases of Prinzmetal's angina that are proving difficult to treat by nitrates alone.

THERAPEUTIC RECOMMENDATIONS

- Advise the patient to eliminate or reduce aggravating factors such as smoking, marked obesity or excessive emotional stress.
- Treat any preexisting hypertension, heart failure, severe anemia, hyperthyroidism, or hypoxia.
- Employ nitroglycerin, 0.3 or 0.4 mg. sublingually, for treatment of anginal pain; instruct the patient to rest at the time of pain and to repeat the nitroglycerin if the pain does not resolve within 5 minutes.

- Have the patient use nitroglycerin sublingually before engaging in any activity which usually causes angina.
- Add oral isosorbide dinitrate for prophylaxis of angina if nitroglycerin alone is inadequate for prevention of pain; begin with 10 mg. every 6 hours and increase dose in 5-mg. increments. If anginal pain is occurring toward the end of the 6-hour period, reduce the interval between doses to 4 hours. Increase dose until angina is adequately controlled, postural light-headedness develops, or resting heart rate increases by 10 to 15 beats per minute.
- Use nitroglycerin paste as an adjunct to isosorbide therapy for nocturnal pain. Instruct the patient to apply the ointment to the precordium or another area on the body before bed. Begin with 1 inch of paste and increase dose by half inches until therapeutic end point is reached.
- Add propranolol to the regimen at the time isosorbide is begun or after nitrates have been tried alone and proven inadequate. Begin with 10 to 20 mg. of propranolol every 6 hours and increase by 40 mg per day every few days until control is achieved, heart rate falls below 40 beats per minute, or heart failure ensues. If propranolol is to be stopped, taper for 2 to 7 days or have the patient markedly reduce activity. Add digoxin to the propranolol program if mild heart failure is a problem.
- Begin an exercise program for the motivated patient; obtain stress test first.
- Refer for angiography only those patients whose angina remains uncontrolled after a maximal medical program has been tried.

ANNOTATED BIBLIOGRAPHY

Natural History

Kannel, W. G., and Feinleib, M.: Natural history of angina pectoris in the Framingham study. Prognosis and survival. Am. J. Cardiol., 29:154, 1972. *(A community-based study showing an overall annual mortality rate of 4 per cent.)*

Reeves, R.J., Oberman, A., Jones, U.B., et al.: Natural history of angina pectoris. Am. J. Cardiol., 33:434, 1974. *(A terse review of natural history studies and prognostic indicators. Concludes that extent of coronary disease and performance of left ventricle are best determinants of prognosis.)*

Nitrates

Battoch, D.J., Levitt, P.W., and Steele, P.P.: Effects of isosorbide dinitrate and nitroglycerin on central circulatory dynamics in coronary artery disease. Am. Heart J., *92*:455, 1976. *(Compared effects of long-acting nitrates with nitroglycerin. Finds that all nitrates have a significant effect on both preload and afterload, but that duration of action of oral isosorbide is 4 hours, compared to 15 to 30 minutes for sublingual TNG.)*

Danahy, D.T., Burwell, D.T., Aronow, W.S., et al.: Sustained hemodynamic and antianginal effect of high dose oral isosorbide dinitrate. Circulation, *55*:381, 1977. *(A double-blind, crossover study demonstrating long-acting effect of oral isosorbide on blood pressure, heart rate, and exercise tolerance in patients with known stable angina. Average dose was 29 mg.)*

Koch, J.C.: Nonocclusive coronary disease after chronic exposure to nitrates. Am. Heart J., *89*:510, 1975. *(Case report of documented coronary artery spasm on withdrawal from chronic nitrate exposure. Also brief literature review; 14 refs.)*

Meister, S.G., Furr, C., Feitosa, G., et al.: Sustained hemodynamic effects of nitroglycerin ointment. Am. J. Cardiol. *37*:155, 1976. *(Reports significant effects noted 4 hours after ointment is applied.)*

Warren, S.E., and Francis G.S.: Nitroglycerin and nitrate esters. Am. J. Med., *65*:53, 1978. *(A terse and well-documented review; 127 refs.)*

Propranolol

Alderman, E.L., Coltart, J., Wettach, G.E., et al.: Coronary artery syndromes after sudden propranolol withdrawal. Ann. Intern. Med., *31*:625, 1974. *(Original report of unstable angina occurring on sudden cessation of therapy.)*

Crawford, M.H., Lewinter, M.M., O'Rourke, P.A. et al.: Combined propranolol and digoxin therapy in angina pectoris. Ann. Intern. Med., *83*:449, 1975. *(Digoxin helped avoid exercise limitation due to propranolol-induced heart failure.)*

Multicenter International Study: Improvement in prognosis of myocardial infarction by long-term beta-adrenoreceptor blockade using practolol. Br. Med. J., *3*:735, 1975. *(Demonstrates reduction in mortality compared to control group.)*

Warren, S.G., Brewer, D.L., and Orgain, E.S.: Long-term propranolol therapy for angina pectoris. Am. J. Cardiol., *37*:418, 1976. *(An 8-year study of patients on long-term therapy. Eighty-four percent had over 50 per cent reduction in frequency and severity of angina. Congestive failure occurred in 25 per cent, but most had failure previously. No tachyphylaxis was noted. Mortality 3.8 per cent but many dropouts from the study make this figure uninterpretable.)*

Other Aspects

Aronow, W.S.: Effects of passive smoking on angina pectoris. N. Engl. J. Med., *299*:21, 1978. *(Exercise tolerance was significantly reduced.)*

Hammermeister, K.E., DeRouen, T.A., English, M.T., and Dodge, H.T.: Effect of surgical versus medical therapy on return to work in patients with coronary artery disease. Am. J. Cardiol., *44*:105, 1979. *(Neither therapy proved superior to the other in regard to work; in both groups, 62 per cent were engaged in full-time work 1 year after surgery or angiography.)*

Murphy, M.L., Hultgren, H.N., Detre, K., et al.: Treatment of chronic stable angina. N. Engl. J. Med., *297*:621, 1977. *(Multicenter randomized study showing no difference in survival between surgically and medically treated groups. [Patients with left main lesions not included in the study.])*

Orlando, J., Aronow, W.S., Cassidy, J., et al.: Effect of ethanol on angina pectoris. Ann. Intern Med., *84*:652, 1976. *(Ethanol decreased exercise tolerance.)*

Peduzzi, P., and Hultgren, H.N.: Effect of medical vs. surgical treatment on symptoms in stable angina pectoris. Circulation, *60*:888, 1979. *(A randomized multicenter VA study of over 300 patients. At 1 year, 60 per cent of surgical patients were improved, compared to 16 per cent of medical patients.)*

Redwood, D.R., Rosing, D.R., and Epstein, S.E.: Circulatory and symptomatic effects of physical training in patients with coronary-artery disease and angina pectoris. N. Engl. J. Med., *286*:959,

1972. *(Physical training improves exercise performance by reducing responses of heart rate and arterial pressure to exercise.)*

Takaro, T., Hultgren, H.N., Lipton, M.J., *et al.*: VA cooperative study of surgery for coronary arterial occlusive disease: Subgroup with significant left main lesions. Circulation, *53 (Suppl. III)*:107, 1976. *(Patients treated surgically had one-quarter the mortality of the medical group.)*

Wilmore, J.H.: Individual exercise prescription. Am. J. Cardiol., *33*:757, 1974. *(An essay on constructing a workable exercise program.)*

26
Postmyocardial Infarction Rehabilitation

Each year over 400,000 individuals who have survived a myocardial infarction are discharged from hospitals. At least half of the patients have uncomplicated, mild infarctions. Over 85 per cent of previously employed patients under age 65 return to work within 2 to 4 months of sustaining a heart attack, but one quarter of these people do not return to prior levels of activity. A considerable number of survivors remain on the disabled list for physical and/or emotional reasons.

The goals of postmyocardial infarction rehabilitation are to help the patient regain function, return to self-sufficiency as quickly as possible, and avoid future disability. The primary physician has a pivotal role in this effort, which begins in the hospital and continues throughout the recovery period at home. Individualized, coordinated, continuous care is essential if psychological invalidism that retards resumption of activity is to be avoided. With growing emphasis on early discharge and home care, the role of the primary physician and the importance of a rehabilitation program grow.

PRINCIPLES OF REHABILITATION

A successful program requires a combination of health education, psychosocial and job counseling, reduction of risk factors, careful medical follow-up and a well-developed activity prescription. The effort needs to include the patient's family as well as the individual himself. Community rehabilitation and mental health personnel can often play an important role when their skills are enlisted and coordinated by the primary physician.

Health education is the first step in rehabilitation. Patient and family are apt to be depressed and frightened by the diagnosis of "heart attack," believing the prognosis to be grim and invalidism likely. They need to be informed that in the vast majority of uncomplicated cases, a return to former job and activity is possible.

Long-term prognosis after recovery has been the subject of recent prospective epidemiologic studies. Average annual mortality in the Framingham study was 5 per cent for men, 7 per cent for women. Patients at greatest risk for late cardiac death were found to have "malignant" ventricular irritability beyond the acute phase of illness, azotemia, previous infarction, persistent congestive failure, angina or advanced age; once congestive failure ensued, 50 per cent were dead by 5 years. Many of the complications of infarction are a function of the degree of myocardial damage; this is consistent with the observation that prognosis correlates with extensiveness of disease, a finding also supported by angiographic studies (see Chapter 25). Risk of postinfarction angina was 5.2 per cent per annum; risk of a second infarction was 2.9 per cent for men, 9.6 per cent for women; risk of failure was 2.3 per cent. Specific statements to the patient and family concerning exercise capacity can be based on graded treadmill stress testing during the recovery period. There are some data suggesting that 1-year survival can also be estimated from a limited, treadmill exercise test done prior to discharge.

Discussions with patient and family about the schedule for recovery period and return to work, resumption of sexual activity and social responsibilities, and modification of risk factors for coronary disease should begin while the patient is still in the hospital. Providing information and an opportunity to voice concerns may be of considerable help toward improving morale, lessening anxiety and obtaining cooperation. Much invalidism is due to fear and ignorance; it should be preventable. Further discussion will be needed during the posthospital period to reinforce the teaching begun prior to discharge.

Medical follow-up is useful for assessments of myocardial status and progress in resumption of daily activity. History, physical and ECG should be checked for evidence of recurrent angina, congestive failure, ventricular irritability, heart block and exercise capacity. Any suggestion of congestive failure should be evaluated by chest x-ray. A walk down the hall or up a flight of stairs can provide a rough estimate of exercise capacity. Assessment of any unexpected limitation may be aided by a graded exercise stress test evaluation under continuous ECG and blood pressure monitoring.

It is important not only to assess myocardial status, but to evaluate the patient's total functioning in regard to resumption of daily activities. Encouraging discussion of fears and family and job responsibilities, and answering any further questions regarding allowable activity and prognosis are integral to the rehabilitation effort. Frequency of visits obviously depends on the severity of the patient's condition. In uncomplicated cases, visits at 2, 6 and 12 weeks postdischarge should suffice. However, some patients remain quite anxious and dependent. In such instances, visits every 2 weeks for the first 2 months may be helpful. Return visits that are too frequent may foster excessive concern and preoccupation with one's heart.

Exercise programs are an exciting development in postinfarction rehabilitation. Numerous small-scale pilot studies in selected populations have shown that patients undergoing early mobilization and exercise programs have reduced morbidity, improved exercise capacity, earlier return to work, better psychological adjustment, and, in some instances, decreased rates of reinfarction and death. It must be emphasized that there are still no well-controlled randomized studies on the effects of exercise in postinfarction patients. The benefits noted above may be due more to patient selection than to exercise itself. Nevertheless, many experts in postinfarction rehabilitation feel that the evidence currently available indicates that inclusion of exercise in the total rehabilitation program is warranted.

The exercise program can be divided into three phases: early in-hospital mobilization, postdischarge convalescence and late convalescence-physical training. The first covers the inpatient period. *Early mobilization* and discharge by the end of the first week

have been carried out in patients with uncomplicated mild cases; this resulted in fewer medical complications, greater emotional recovery, and a substantial economic saving when compared to data from patients subjected to the traditional 10- to 14-day hospital stay.

The *convalescence phase* lasts about 8 to 12 weeks, depending on severity of disease. The goal is to achieve (by gradual increase in daily activity) an activity level sufficient for independent functioning. Return to work usually can occur by 8 to 12 weeks. If work is strenuous (requiring 6 to 8 multiples of resting oxygen consumption) then more time may be needed for reconditioning.

Activity in the convalescence period begins with walking around the house and doing light housework; it progresses to daily walks, stair climbing and sexual intercourse by the end of the month. To assure reconditioning, a given amount of daily exercise is specified and raised by small, well-tolerated increments. Isometric exertion, such as lifting, is to be avoided since it inordinately raises blood pressure and precipitates arrhythmias. Leisurely walks of 5 to 10 minutes are begun by the third or fourth week, then built to 30 minutes of brisk walking by the tenth week. Contraindications to progression are onset of angina, dyspnea on exertion, marked fatigue, or arrhythmias. Stress testing can always be carried out whenever the patient or physician questions the safety of a given level of activity and desires objective assessment.

Studies have shown the energy cost of sexual activity in unconditioned middle-aged men having intercourse with their long-time spouses to be approximately 6 calories per minute at maximal activity (which lasted less than 30 seconds) and 4 calories per minute during pre- and post-orgasmic periods. This level is the equivalent of walking briskly on the street or climbing one flight of stairs. In other words, once the patient is able to climb a flight of stairs, intercourse can be permitted.

Modern industrial jobs and white collar work do not require more than the same 4 to 6 calories/minute expense of energy. *Return to work* can be initiated when this degree of physical activity becomes comfortable. The limits to resumption of normal activity in patients with uncomplicated infarctions are most often psychological and usually are not due to reduction in myocardial reserve or persistent angina. It cannot be overemphasized that the design of a rehabilitation program must be individualized and take into account the patient's personality style, attitudes toward heart disease, job, social situation and family response, as well as the status of the myocardium and its blood supply.

The *late convalescence-physical training phase* is characterized by return to work for most patients and the initiation of a formal training program for highly motivated individuals interested in further improving their exercise capacity. At present, no definite statement can be made that the chances of future infarction and death are reduced by such programs. The effect of training is, however, clearly measureable in terms of increased exercise capacity. Only those patients who have made uncomplicated recoveries and are willing to invest the time and effort should be considered.

Exercise raises the amount of activity that can be performed prior to the onset of angina by lowering the increments in blood pressure and heart rate that occur with exercise. The psychological effect is often impressive, helping to dispel the fear that one's heart disease is permanently disabling. Recent evidence indicates that the intensity of training plays a key role in achieving benefit from exercise.

Exercise training programs must be preceded by treadmill testing to determine the level of activity allowable for the patient (see Chapter 31). The exercise prescription provides for activity which achieves a maximum of 70 to 85 per cent of the maximum predicted heart rate. Endurance exercises of the isotonic variety are used (walking, running, jogging, swimming, cycling) (see Chapter 10). Isometric exercises are avoided.

Group training programs are available on a community basis, and are usually conducted under the supervision of an individual skilled in training and resuscitation. Equipment for resuscitation, including a defibrillator, should be at the training site. To be beneficial, sessions must be scheduled at least two to three times per week. A typical session begins with a 5- to 10-minute warm-up period of walking or gentle jogging, followed by 15 to 20 minutes of exercise (e.g., jogging or cycling) designed to maintain the heart rate at 60 to 75 per cent of maximum. Patients are taught to monitor their rates. A 5-minute cooling down period of stretching or walking completes the session. Many groups begin or end their session with discussion.

Long-term activity programs should be considered after physical conditioning has been achieved. Since the patient will be exercising on his own without direct supervision, he should again undergo an exercise stress test. If he achieves a performance of 10 to 12 mets, jogging, cycling and similar activities are probably safe. Again, isometric exercises should be avoided, as well as major competitive sports activities. Exercise must be maintained on a regular basis. Weekend bursts of unaccustomed activity are dangerous.

Alleviation of risk factors for coronary disease deserves attention. Cessation of smoking and lowering of blood pressure are essential and can often be accomplished for the first time now that motivation is high. The ability of such efforts to change prognosis is as yet unproven, but most feel they are worthy of implementation based on the strong epidemiologic evidence available implicating them in causation of coronary artery disease. Whether weight reduction and dietary change to a low-cholesterol, low-saturated fat intake can improve prognosis is unknown at present (see Chapters 9 and 22). *Job counseling* is indicated if the patient's job is too stressful or his heart disease is too severe to allow return to his former occupation. Short-term *psychotherapy* may be considered if the patient's adjustment to his illness has been poor and is adversely affecting resumption of activity and responsibilities.

ANNOTATED BIBLIOGRAPHY

Haskell, W. L.: Physical activity after myocardial infarction. Am. J. Cardiol., *33*:776,1974. *(Physical activity reduces psychological maladjustment and improves success of return to gainful employment. Also provides good review of the literature; 66 refs.)*

Kannel, U. B., Sorlie, P., and McNamara, P. M.: Prognosis after initial myocardial infarction: The Framingham study. Am. J. Cardiol., *44*:53, 1979 *(A prospective epidemiologic study detailing rates of reinfarction, angina, congestive failure and death.)*

Luria, M. H., Knoke, J. D., Margolis, R. M., et al: Acute myocardial infarction: Prognosis after recovery. Ann. Intern. Med., *85*:561, 1976. *(Discriminant analysis showed in this study that persistent angina, previous infarction and more than one ventricular ectopic beat per hour were among the variables that correlated with increased risk of mortality.)*

McHenry, M. M.: Medical screening of patients with coronary artery disease. Am. J. Cardiol., *33*:752, 1974. *(Presents criteria for entry into and exclusion from exercise programs.)*

McNeer, J. F., Wagner, G. S., Ginsberg, P. B., et al: Hospital discharge one week after acute myocardial infarction. N. Engl. J. Med., *28*:229, 1978. *(A controlled study of early discharge in patients with uncomplicated acute infarctions. There was no difference between groups in mortality, com-*

plications, or functional status at 6 months post-infarction.)

Rechnitzer, P. A., Pickart, H. A., Paivio, A. U., et al: Long-term follow-up study of survival and recurrence rates following myocardial infarction in exercising and control subjects. Circulation, 45:853, 1972. (A loosely controlled study showing that an exercise program improved chances of survival and reduced rate of reinfarction. Unfortunately the study did not control for selection bias, blood pressure, or recurrent angina, which could have affected results.)

Redwood, D. R., Rosing, D. R., and Epstein, S. E.: Circulatory and symptomatic effects of physical training in patients with coronary artery disease and angina pectoris. N. Engl. J. Med., 286:956, 1972. (Exercise training raised the amount of activity that could be performed prior to the onset of angina and seemed to do so by lowering the increments in blood pressure and heart rate that occur with exercise.)

Théroux, P., Waters, D. D., Halphen, C., et al: Prognostic value of exercise testing soon after myocardial infarction. N. Engl. J. Med., 301:341, 1979. (When there was angina or ST segment depression on a limited treadmill test done 1 day before hospital discharge, the risks of developing angina subsequently and dying within 1 year were greatly increased.)

27
Management of Chronic Congestive Heart Failure

Chronic congestive heart failure (CHF) ranks among the most frequently encountered cardiac problems in office practice. Because of the high prevalence of CHF, the primary care physician must be skilled in its management. A well-conceived outpatient treatment program that includes thorough instruction of patient and family should help to minimize the rate of complications and hospitalizations. Digitalis and diuretics remain cornerstones of therapy, but widespread misuse of cardiac glycosides has led to many instances of excess morbidity and mortality. The use of vasodilators for CHF is a recent development derived from research on the effects of altering preload and afterload; the approach appears to have some promise in patients refractory to conventional therapy.

Successful management of CHF in the outpatient setting requires identification and correction of treatable underlying causes, elimination of precipitating factors, well-reasoned application of digitalis, diuretics, and vasodilators, and much effort at educating the patient and family.

CLINICAL PRESENTATION AND COURSE

Regardless of etiology, the clinical manifestations of CHF are quite stereotyped and reflect the magnitude of the fall in cardiac output and the rise in pulmonary and systemic venous pressures. Initially and in mild cases, the patient may complain of fatigability, dyspnea on exertion or unexplained weight gain; there may be few overt physical signs of failure, but chest x-ray often shows redistribution of pulmonary venous flow to the upper lung fields and/or an enlarged heart. Fatigue becomes increasingly prominent as cardiac output falls. As pulmonary congestion increases, dyspnea worsens, orthopnea is noted and paroxysmal nocturnal dyspnea may be reported. At this stage, rales are frequently found on physical examination, but their absence does not rule out the presence of CHF. Sometimes failure-induced bronchospasm dominates the pulmonary examination. In severe cases, the chest film will show interstitial pulmonary edema. In chronic CHF, right-sided or bilateral pleural effusions are common. Ankle edema, jugular venous distention and hepatojugular reflux are indicative of elevated systemic venous pressure; if CHF is predominantly left-sided, these findings may not be present. An S3 gallop is among the most specific physical signs of failure, but it is often difficult to hear. If left ventricular dilatation becomes very marked, a mitral regurgitant murmur may become evident. Pedal edema is one of the least specific signs of CHF; in the elderly, isolated pedal edema is more likely to be a result of venous insufficiency (see Chapter 16).

Since congestive failure is not a single disease, it does not have a uniform natural history. Clinical course and response to therapy depend on the nature of the underlying etiology and the state of the myocardium at the time of presentation. For example, the appearance of CHF in a patient with aortic stenosis is an ominous prognostic sign associated with a mean survival of no more than 2 to 3 years. However, if the valve is replaced before irreversible myocardial decompensation has occurred, the prognosis is altered dramatically (see Chapter 28). Cases of CHF due to alcoholic cardiomyopathy, thiamine deficiency, hypertensive heart disease, and hyperthyroidism also have favorable outcomes if detected and treated early.

The Framingham study has provided interesting epidemiologic data concerning CHF in the community setting. The annual incidence rate for development of failure was 2.3 per 1000 for men and 1.4 per 1000 for women. The major causes were hypertension in one third of the patients, hypertension in combination with coronary disease in another one third, isolated coronary disease in about 10 per cent, and valvular disease in another 10 per cent. Sixty per cent of patients had a serious noncardiac illness along with CHF. Five-year survival rates, regardless of cause, were only 50 percent.

PRINCIPLES OF MANAGEMENT

The first task is to search for and treat a reversible underlying etiology. All too often, many cases are encountered at the time irreversible myocardial damage has occurred, but when a treatable cause is present and detected early, there is an opportunity for definitive measures to bring about a successful outcome. Valvular disease (see Chapter 28), alcohol excess (see Chapter 216), hypertension (see Chapters 13 and 21), hyperthyroidism (see Chapter 99) and myxedema (see Chapter 100) are examples of conditions requiring etiologic therapy. A stereotyped approach with digitalis and diuretics that ignores etiology may lead to omission or delay of proper measures and result in loss of a unique therapeutic opportunity.

Correct selection and application of supportive treatment also requires identification of etiology. For example, digitalis usually proves helpful when there is an excess pressure load on the left ventricle, but if the specific cause of the pressure work is hypertrophic subaortic stenosis, addition of digitalis can increase contractility to the point of worsening outflow tract obstruction. The decision regarding initiation of therapy with digitalis or a diuretic is dependent on a clear formulation of the underlying pathophysiology.

Attention must be directed to the presence of precipitating factors. Severe anemia (see Chapter 77),

high fever (see Chapter 6), tachycardia (see Chapters 19, 20 and 23), pulmonary infection (see Chapter 43), pulmonary embolization (see Chapter 14), excess salt intake, marked obesity (see Chapter 221) and excess exertion or emotional stress may worsen or precipitate failure in patients with decreased myocardial reserve. Use of propranolol (see Chapter 25) or other negatively inotropic agents may also bring on CHF. A careful search for these factors is essential.

The mainstay of supportive, symptomatic management is drug therapy. Digitalis, diuretics and vasodilators each have specific roles determined by their different hemodynamic effects. Digitalis is used mainly for its positive inotropic action, diuretics for their ability to reduce volume, and vasodilators to lessen preload and afterload.

Digitalis works best to improve cardiac output when there is an increase in the volume or pressure load on the ventricle, yet some myocardial reserve remains. Cardiac glycosides may not provide much benefit when the heart has reached an irreversible congestive cardiomyopathic state characterized by marked chamber enlargement and low ejection fraction. However, regardless of the state of the myocardium, digitalis is the drug of choice for failure induced by rapid atrial fibrillation, since the vagal effects of the drug can slow the ventricular response rate (see Chapter 23).

Digitalis is of no proven benefit in cases of mitral stenosis not complicated by atrial fibrillation. The drug is contraindicated in hypertrophic subaortic stenosis and in second degree or unstable heart block. There is no evidence that digitalis given for treatment of acute congestive failure precipitated by an acute ischemic event needs to be given indefinitely in the absence of failure. The efficacy of digitalis in cor pulmonale is in question; the drug is occasionally beneficial, but the results are usually not impressive and the risks of toxicity are increased in severe pulmonary disease.

If digitalis is to be used, it should probably be started at the earliest signs of failure to minimize the consequences of unchecked progressive CHF. As long as the underlying disorder responsible for failure persists, the drug should be continued. However, many patients are placed on digitalis for unclear reasons and never taken off of the glycoside. When such a patient is encountered and no evidence of failure or its cause is found, a cautious attempt to discontinue the agent is warranted.

Patients who are relatively stable can be started

on a maintenance oral dose without resorting to a loading dose. Full therapeutic serum levels can be achieved in 5 to 7 days with digoxin (see Digitalis Supplementation, below). If the patient is less stable, but not so compromised as to require hospitalization, an oral loading dose can be given in divided amounts over 24 hours.

The decision to initiate digitalis therapy should not be made casually. The incidence of digitalis toxicity was found to be 23 per cent in a prospective study of 900 consecutive admissions to the Boston City Hospital general medical service. Mortality from digitalis intoxication has averaged 22 per cent in published series. Use of serum concentration measurements seems to have helped limit the incidence of toxicity. However, one cannot depend on serum levels alone for the diagnosis of digitalis toxicity, because there is considerable overlap in serum concentrations among those with and without evidence of toxicity (see Appendix).

Diuretics are indicated when there is excessive fluid retention. Most patients with failure begin to retain sodium as cardiac output falls and renal perfusion diminishes. Initially, the increase in volume helps to produce a rise in diastolic filling pressure and maintain cardiac output by the Frank-Starling mechanism. However, the degree of fluid retention is often excessive, resulting in pulmonary congestion and/or peripheral edema.

Therapy of CHF can be initiated with a diuretic when digitalis is not the drug of choice. If treatment has begun with digitalis, but volume overload persists, a diuretic can be added to the program; however, overzealous use of diuretics may worsen the situation by producing prerenal azotemia or a dangerous fall in filling pressure (as in critical aortic stenosis, see Chapter 28). Moreover, escalating diuretic therapy in mitral or aortic valve disease may inappropriately delay the timing of surgical therapy (see Chapter 28).

Diuretic therapy can be initiated with a *thiazide* when the symptoms of failure are mild or when the patient is asymptomatic but showing weight gain or x-ray findings indicative of early CHF. The degree of dyspnea on exertion and weight changes are the simplest clinical parameters to follow for gauging response to therapy in mild cases. Patients with dyspnea at rest, orthopnea, or paroxysmal nocturnal dyspnea represent the other end of the spectrum; if it is judged reasonable to attempt outpatient management, a *loop diuretic,* i.e., furosemide or ethacrynic acid, is necessary. Small doses of loop diuretics may also benefit patients with mild to moderate failure that cannot be adequately controlled by thiazides. Caution is warranted when treating a patient for the first time with a loop diuretic, because a marked diuresis may be evoked, even from a small dose. If a thiazide had been used previously, it should be stopped rather than continued in conjunction with the loop diuretic, because the two agents are very potent when used together. The combination of a thiazide and loop diuretic is indicated in cases of failure refractory to large doses of the loop diuretic alone. The maximal effect of a loop duretic can be achieved by using a single daily dose. Monitoring postural signs, BUN and creatinine is essential to avoid excess volume depletion and severe prerenal azotemia (see Appendix).

The *potassium-sparing diuretics* are weak agents used mainly in conjunction with other diuretics to avoid the need to prescribe potassium preparations and to augment diuresis. Their onset of action is slow; full effect may take up to a week to become evident. The *mercurials* have dropped from use because of the need to administer them parenterally, but they are more potent than the thiazides and can sometimes be used intramuscularly on an intermittent basis, e.g., by the visiting nurse, to supplement oral diuretic therapy. At times, intravenous administration of a loop diuretic in the office is needed to counter worsening failure refractory to oral therapy.

When a potassium-wasting diuretic is being used in conjunction with digitalis therapy, it is critical to carefully monitor the serum potassium and supplement potassium intake or add a potassium-sparing diuretic (see Appendix). The incidence of digitalis toxicity rises appreciably in the setting of hypokalemia.

Vasodilators. Advances in understanding the effects on cardiac output and pulmonary congestion of reducing preload and afterload in the failing heart have led to small-scale trials of oral vasodilators in patients with chronic CHF refractory to digitalis and diuretics. Agents which act predominantly on the arterial bed have been used to lower systemic resistance and reduce impedance to the ejection of blood from the left ventricle, thus augmenting cardiac output. Hydralazine has been the most widely studied of the oral arterial vasodilators and appears to have a sustained beneficial effect on cardiac output in patients with severe failure. Prazosin, a recently developed antihypertensive drug which produces both arterial and venous dilatation, is also capable of increasing cardiac output by lowering systemic vascular resistance, but there is evidence suggesting its effect on cardiac output is short-lived.

Best results with oral arterial vasodilators have been obtained in CHF patients with normal or elevated blood pressures. Often the blood pressure does not change much in response to therapy, because the fall in systemic resistance is offset by the rise in cardiac output. Successful use of these agents in patients with low blood pressure has also been achieved, but requires very careful titration of dose and close monitoring to avoid a precipitous fall in pressure. CHF due to severe mitral insufficiency has responded well to arterial vasodilators; the regurgitant fraction decreases substantially with reduction in afterload.

Vasodilators which act predominantly on the venous bed decrease preload, but their effect on cardiac output is less pronounced. The long-acting oral nitrates are among the best studied of these agents. Their major hemodynamic effect is to increase venous capacitance and reduce pulmonary venous and end diastolic pressures. Nitrates also cause some arterial dilatation, but the effect on the venous side is greater. Changes in cardiac output have been variable; output seems to increase most in patients with high systemic vascular resistance. The main benefits of nitrates appear to be related to alleviation of pulmonary venous hypertension, with reduction of dyspnea and improvement in exercise tolerance being reported.

Combined use of oral nitrates and hydralazine has been advocated, since most cases of severe CHF are characterized by low cardiac output *and* pulmonary venous congestion. Reductions in both preload and afterload have been measured, and improvements in cardiac output and pulmonary congestion have been achieved by combining oral isosorbide dinitrate with hydralazine. The hope that prazosin would accomplish the same thing has been dimmed by recent reports of its inability to sustain improvement in cardiac output.

Patients who are refractory to conventional treatment might be considered candidates for vasodilators, but such therapy for CHF is still in the investigational stage; it is too early to draw definitive conclusions or make specific recommendations concerning vasodilators for routine use in outpatient management of chronic failure. As yet, there are no long-term, large-scale studies of these agents in CHF. Available data derive from carefully selected, refractory cases that have been subjected to very close supervision and monitoring; observations have been limited to a few hours in the catheterization laboratory or several weeks outside the hospital. Data on prolonged use and patient selection are not complete; the literature should be followed closely for developments in this promising area.

Salt restriction has traditionally occupied an important place in supportive therapy. It is probably most helpful in preventing unnecessary exacerbations of failure. Patients are placed on a no-added-salt diet, which provides about 4 gm. of sodium per day. The patient and family are instructed to prepare and serve meals without addition of salt and to avoid foods with large salt content, including canned ham (which is packed in salt water), bacon, catsup, etc. Rarely is extreme salt restriction (e.g., 1 to 2 gm. sodium diet) urged on the patient since it is often unrealistic and unpalatable, leading to poor caloric intake and depression. Fluid restriction is reserved for severe cases which are complicated by hyponatremia.

The activity prescription has an important function in minimizing myocardial work demands while maintaining the patient's ability to live as fully as possible. The level of allowable activity needs to be tailored to the patient's medical status, life-style and responsibilities. Patients with symptoms of failure on moderate exertion (New York Heart Association Class II disease) can continue to work as long as reasonable limits are placed on emotional and physical demands. It may be more stressful psychologically (and consequently physically) to have to quit one's job than to continue working in a somewhat more limited capacity. In most instances, the amount of allowable activity can be determined from an office visit by a careful story that elicits the degree of exertion that precipitates symptoms. At times, symptoms may be out of proportion to physical findings; taking a walk up a flight of stairs with the patient can provide helpful data regarding exercise tolerance. Treadmill testing is sometimes necessary to gauge exercise capacity, especially if the patient has coronary disease and it is unclear whether it is failure or ischemia that is limiting the patient. Regardless of etiology, a daily rest period and reduction of psychological stress are key means of lessening myocardial work in the patient with failure.

If weight is increasing, orthopnea worsening, and dyspnea on exertion more severe and brought on by less exertion, activity should be further restricted. A few days of bed rest are often beneficial and may obviate the need for hospitalization. The patient with failure who is put to bed should use a footboard or get out of bed periodically to avoid prolonged venous stasis and thrombus formation.

Anticoagulant therapy in management of CHF depends on the nature of the underlying heart disease and the presence of additional risk factors for thrombophlebitis or systemic embolization, such as prolonged bed rest or atrial fibrillation. Although CHF *per se* may not be an absolute indication for anticoagulants, its occurrence in a condition that predisposes one to clot formation may substantially increase the risk of embolization (see Chapters 23, 28, and 84).

PATIENT EDUCATION

Because the medical program is often complex and the need for compliance is great, the physician must take the time to discuss with patient and family the rationale behind therapy and to set with them the guidlines for activity, diet, and use of medication. In this way they can become valuable partners in the treatment effort.

Patients should be instructed to weigh themselves each morning before breakfast and to keep a *weight record*. If their clinical status, weight and medication program are stable, less frequent recordings are necessary. Patients are advised to call their physician when weight increases suddenly by more than 2 or 3 pounds, because this may be the earliest sign of increasing CHF and a forerunner of more severe symptoms. Reliable, intelligent patients may be instructed to adjust their diuretic doses according to weight. Debilitated or uncooperative individuals should have a family member or visiting nurse obtain weight recordings. Weight is among the most helpful parameters to follow in outpatient management of failure.

Patients and their families must know the identity of the medication being used. It is easy for the patient to become confused because multiple-drug regimens are common and many of the pills are similar in appearance. Medication booklets are invaluable. Each tablet is taped to the page alongside its generic and brand names, dose schedule, indication for use and warning signs of toxicity. For patients with poor eyesight, a family member or visiting nurse should put out and set aside the pills to be taken each day.

INDICATIONS FOR REFERRAL AND ADMISSION

Patients with refractory failure should be considered for hospital admission, because valuable observations can be made under controlled conditions which assure compliance with the medical regimen.

Moreover, it may provide an opportunity to search for a treatable underlying etiology which may not have been appreciated initially. If the patient is still refractory to therapy while in the hospital, it may be helpful to obtain a cardiac consultation regarding the use of oral vasodilator therapy. Starting such therapy in the hospital is the safest way to initiate a vasodilator program and allows close monitoring of response. Other indications for admission include worsening failure, evidence of digitalis toxicity (see Appendix) and inadequate support and supervision at home.

THERAPEUTIC RECOMMENDATIONS

- Identify the etiology of the CHF and any precipitating factors; treat these specifically if they are amenable to therapy rather than relying solely on symptomatic measures.
- Help the patient reduce emotional stresses and set aside time for a daily period of rest; advise against heavy physical exertion.
- Initiate a no-added-salt diet, but do not restrict water intake unless dilutional hyponatremia has set in.
- Begin digitalis if the predominant pathophysiology is ventricular overload, either from a pressure load or a large regurgitant volume. Also start with digitalis if atrial fibrillation has precipitated the CHF. Contraindications to use of digitalis are hypertrophic subaortic stenosis, unstable or second degree heart block, and dysrhythmias indicative of digitalis toxicity.
- Digitalis may benefit ischemia-induced failure if heart size can be reduced. Obtain chest films before and after onset of therapy.
- When CHF is mild, one can begin digitalis therapy with 0.25 mg. per day of digoxin given orally; check serum level in 1 week and make any further dose adjustment on the basis of clinical response, serum level, BUN and creatinine.
- If there is no evidence of improvement with digitalis after a therapeutic serum level has been achieved (around 1.5 ng. per ml. for digoxin), do not increase dose further; consider discontinuing cardiac glycoside therapy.
- If the patient shows response to therapy, but the underlying etiology of the failure persists, do not stop digitalis.
- If CHF is marked, but the patient does not require immediate hospitalization, one can start digitalis therapy with a loading dose of 1 to 1.25 mg. of di-

goxin orally, given in divided doses over the first 24 hours. Then adjust dose as noted above.

- If a change in rate or rhythm is noted of if the serum level goes above 2.0 ng. per ml., hold digoxin if CHF is mild and check ECG and serum potassium. Admit to the hospital if there is a disturbance of rate or rhythm.
- Initiate a thiazide diuretic when there is evidence of excessive fluid retention that is mild to moderate in severity; a reasonable starting program is 100 mg. per day of hydrochlorothiazide or 1 gm. of chlorothiazide. Other thiazides offer little advantage and are much more expensive because they are usually not available as generic preparations.
- Switch to or begin with a loop diuretic if fluid retention is severe. Beware of the possibility of severe volume depletion and marked response to even a modest initial dose. A typical oral starting dose is 20 to 40 mg. per day of furosemide. Exert particular caution in cases requiring high filling pressures (e.g., aortic stenosis).
- Divide daily dose of loop diuretic to minimize single large diuresis; avoid evening dose if sleep is being interrupted by need to urinate frequently.
- If patient appears refractory to a loop diuretic that is being given in divided aliquots, try giving the entire daily dose at one time rather than escalating dose; an occasional intravenous dose of a loop diuretic in the office may also help.
- If the patient still does not respond adequately to a loop diuretic, add a thiazide or a potassium-sparing agent to the program (e.g., 100 mg. per day of hydrochlorothiazide or 100 to 200 mg. per day of triamterene).
- In all forms of diuretic therapy, monitor postural signs, potassium, BUN and creatinine; reduce dose if postural hypotension or severe prerenal azotemia is noted.
- Prevent potassium depletion with a dietary supplement (usually sufficient in thiazide therapy), an oral potassium preparation (usually needed when loop diuretics are used), or a potassium-sparing diuretic. If a potassium-sparing agent is prescribed, halt all other forms of potassium supplementation and monitor serum level.
- If an oral potassium preparation is employed, begin with an agent that provides chloride as well as potassium in order to avoid diuretic-induced alkalosis; however, do not utilize enteric-coated or sustained release KCl preparations because of their risk of mucosal injury.
- Consider oral anticoagulant therapy if prolonged

bed rest, atrial fibrillation, or congestive cardiomyopathy is encountered.
- Consider vasodilator therapy in patients refractory to digitalis and diuretics, provided that all precipitating factors and correctable etiologies have been attended to.

APPENDIX: DIGITALIS, DIURETICS, AND POTASSIUM SUPPLEMENTATION

Digitalis

Numerous digitalis preparations are available; the physician should become familiar with one or two, learn their pharmacokinetics and use them predominantly. *Digoxin* is the most widely used. In the past, some variations in bioavailability had been noted among different brands; this seems to have been corrected. Half-life of digoxin is 36 hours; onset of action is 1 to 2 hours when taken orally; absorption from the GI tract ranges from 50 to 75 per cent complete. Excretion is renal and decreases significantly with reduction in creatinine clearance. Therapeutic serum levels can be achieved in 5 to 7 days by prescribing a daily maintenance dose of 0.25 mg. When more rapid oral digitalization is desired, a loading dose of 1 to 1.25 mg. can be given in divided doses over 24 hours.

If a patient presents taking a digitalis preparation other than digoxin, it is best to leave him on the drug he is used to. The exception to this generalization concerns patients taking *digitalis leaf.* Because of its variable and unpredictable composition of digoxin and digitoxin, digitalis leaf should be discontinued and one of the preparations containing only a single active ingredient used instead. *Digitoxin* may be beneficial when digitalis must be given to a patient with renal failure, because elimination of digitoxin is not dependent on renal function. However, a major disadvantage with digitoxin is its long half-life of 4 to 6 days, making for serious problems if toxic levels occur. Digoxin can be used safely in renal failure as long as renal function and serum levels are frequently checked and necessary dosage adjustments made.

Digitalis therapy requires careful monitoring. *Serum levels* should be measured at least three or four times per year, more frequently if there are changes in the patient's clinical status. It is hoped that this will help reduce the incidence of digitalis toxicity. A sample should be drawn at least 6 hours after the last dose, since there is a 4 to 6 hour rise in serum level after an oral dose. In most instances it is best to have the patient omit the day's dose when he comes to the office for a serum determination.

A number of factors can affect serum concentration, including renal function when digoxin is being used and hepatic function in digitoxin therapy. Absorption of digitalis from the gut remains adequate in CHF, but may fall in severe cases of malabsorption. Thyroid status can affect digitalis metabolism; hypothyroidism prolongs the half-life and hyperthyroidism shortens it. Treatment of thyroid disease needs to be accompanied by an adjustment of dose.

The serum level of digitalis is not in itself diagnostic of toxicity, because there is considerable overlap in serum concentrations among those with and without evidence of toxicity; but if the digoxin level is above 2.0 ng. per ml., the probability of encountering toxicity increases considerably. In one series, 80 per cent of patients without evidence of toxicity had a digoxin level below 2.0 ng. per ml.; in 87 per cent with toxicity, the level was above 2.0.

To avoid *digitalis toxicity,* even when dose is closely followed, the physician needs to monitor factors that increase the "sensitivity" of the myocardium to the toxic effects of the drug. These include hypokalemia, elevations in serum calcium and magnesium, acute hypoxia, organic heart disease and pulmonary disease with acute hypoxia.

Symptoms of digitalis toxicity can be divided into noncardiac and cardiac manifestations. Anorexia, nausea, vomiting, diarrhea, visual disturbances including yellow halos around lights, and, in rare instances, delirium have been described since Withering's time. Arrhythmias are the predominant cardiac manifestation of toxicity. Digitalis can cause any type of rhythm and/or conduction disturbance since it affects automaticity of myocardial tissues as well as the conduction system. Ventricular irritability (especially bigeminy), paroxysmal atrial tachycardia with block and junctional tachycardia are particularly characteristic of digitalis excess.

The unexplained onset of an arrhythmia in a patient on digitalis raises the possibility of drug-related toxicity. The drug should be withheld, a serum level obtained, a stat potassium level checked and serious consideration given to immediate hospitalization for monitoring and parenteral antiarrhythmic therapy. The high incidence and mortality rate of this preventable and often treatable condition call for vigilance.

A few pitfalls in use of digitalis must be pointed out: (1) digitalis should not be used unless there is genuine evidence of heart failure or atrial fibrillation.

A most common error is to assume that ankle edema in the elderly is related to CHF and to begin digitalis for this reason. Most of the time the ankle edema is due to venous insufficiency. (2) Unless failure has a reversible cause that has been corrected, digitalis should not be discontinued. Patients who respond to digitalis need the drug chronically; they have been shown to deteriorate clinically and hemodynamically when the drug is withdrawn in experimental circumstances. (3) The ST-T wave changes on the ECG have no correlation with optimal or toxic dose levels and cannot be used for such determinations.

Diuretics

Thiazides are believed to inhibit sodium reabsorption in the cortical tubule. Although the number of thiazides is large, they differ only in cost and duration of action. Chlorothiazide and hydrochlorothiazide are the least expensive. Thiazides cause potassium depletion, and their use requires potassium supplementation and monitoring of the serum potassium level, especially when digitalis is being taken. Sometimes a potassium-sparing diuretic may be used instead of KCl supplement (see below). Hyperglycemia and hyperuricemia are commonly encountered when thiazides are used. Glucose intolerance is not usually of major significance and is not a contraindication to the drug's use in diabetics; it may be lessened to some extent by careful potassium replacement. Severe hyperuricemia can sometimes lead to gout and may force the use of allopurinol concomitantly (see Chapter 146). During the first 7 to 10 days of therapy, the serum calcium may rise, but it will stay elevated indefinitely only in patients with underlying hyperparathyroidism. Absorption from the gastrointestinal tract is rapid; onset of action is 1 hour, and half-life 12 to 24 hours.

The potent diuretics which act at the loop of Henle are *furosemide* and *ethacrynic acid.* Their absorption is rapid, and onset of diuretic action occurs within 30 to 60 minutes and lasts 6 to 8 hours. Caution must be exercised, since serious volume depletion may occur with their use. Prerenal azotemia (manifested by BUN-creatinine ratio of more than 20:1), postural hypotension, lightheadedness and fatigue are clues to marked hypovolemia. Hypokalemia, hyperglycemia and hyperuricemia may occur. Ethacrynic acid is potentially ototoxic, especially when used in combination with an aminoglycoside antibiotic such as kanamycin. Audiograms should be obtained if ethacrynic acid is to be given for a prolonged period.

Frequent urination is a common complaint in patients using these potent diuretics; evening doses should be avoided if possible. Starting dose of furosemide is 20 to 40 mg. per day. If this amount does not produce the desired effect, the single dose should be increased rather than the frequency of doses. In many instances, one daily dose is sufficient, maximally effective and well tolerated by the patient. Potassium loss can be countered by prescribing potassium supplements or adding a potassium-sparing diuretic (see below).

Spironolactone and *triamterene* are the commonly used potassium-sparing diuretics. The former is an antagonist of aldosterone, the latter is not, but clinically it behaves in a manner similar to spironolactone. Both are weak diuretics when used alone and should never be used initially in CHF. Their role is to help preserve potassium and supplement diuresis. Serious hyperkalemia may occur, necessitating frequent serum potassium determinations and discontinuation of potassium supplements. Neither drug should be used in renal failure, since life-threatening hyperkalemia may ensue. Spironolactone has been known to cause gynecomastia; there is also a question of increased risk of carcinogenesis based on experiments in which high doses were given to rats.

Fixed combinations containing a potassium-sparing diuretic and a thiazide are heavily promoted. Not only are these more expensive than if each drug is prescribed separately, but the doses of the diuretics in the combination tablet are usually half the usual minimum doses. When a fixed combination is used, any increase in the dose of one component forces an increase in the other, which may not be desired or needed. At times, the use of a fixed combination may lead to inadvertent administration of a toxic dose of one ingredient in attempting to give enough of the other. The doses of each agent should be determined separately. The combination preparation is reasonable to use only if it can provide the exact dosages desired.

Potassium Supplementation

Potassium supplementation needs close attention because diuretic-induced hypokalemia is frequent and potentially dangerous, especially in patients with underlying cardiac disease who are taking digitalis. Hypokalemia may precipitate "dig-toxic" arrhyth-mias or cause weakness. Individual requirements for potassium replacement vary widely, necessitating regular checks of the serum potassium level, which is not an exact measure of body potassium levels, but rather, a rough guide to potassium requirements.

Supplements may be taken in the form of dietary additions or potassium-containing preparations. Amount needed is usually determined empirically, ranging from 0 to 60 mEq of supplement per day over and above normal dietary potassium intake. For patients on thiazides, dietary replacement often suffices. When furosemide or ethacrynic acid is used, a potassium preparation is usually a must (unless a potassium-sparing diuretic is used). Dietary supplements are the most palatable way to provide potassium. There are 15 mEq in a 10-oz. glass of orange, pineapple or grapefruit juice, a medium-sized banana, a baked potato or two oranges. Tomato juice has almost twice the potassium content of orange juice but is high in sodium.

Oral potassium supplements combine potassium with a number of different anions. Only the potassium chloride form is effective in correcting the hypokalemic alkalosis that results from diuretic use. However, any form will prevent potassium depletion unless sodium depletion is very severe. Potassium chloride elixir is probably the cheapest form; 15 cc. contains 20 mEq. It is most palatable when given in orange juice. Patients may refuse it because of its taste. Salt substitutes contain KCl, but some also contain 50 percent NaCl. They provide some KCl but are not sufficient in themselves. Slow-release and enteric-coated KCl tablets should not be used because they are associated with mucosal irritation, ulceration and stricture formation. Potassium gluconate and bicarbonate forms are palatable, but more expensive and lacking in chloride. They should be used in the patient who requires an oral preparation but refuses KCl elixir. If all attempts at potassium supplementation fail, then a potassium-sparing diuretic is indicated. These agents are expensive and not without risk (e.g., hyperkalemia). Therefore, they should not be used until other methods of potassium management have been tried.

ANNOTATED BIBLIOGRAPHY

Arnold, S.B., Williams, R.L., Ports. T.A., *et al.*: Attenuation of prazosin effect on cardiac output in chronic heart failure. Ann. Intern. Med., *91*:345, 1979. *(A study of 12 patients with severe conges-*

tive failure demonstrating only a transient improvement in cardiac output with prazosin.)

Beller, G.A., *et al.*: Digitalis intoxication. N. Engl. J. Med., *284*:989, 1971. *(A prospective study showing a 23 percent incidence of digitalis intoxication among unselected patients on digitalis admitted to a general hospital.)*

Chatterjee, K., Massie, B., Gelberg, H., *et al.*: Long-term outpatient vasodilator therapy of congestive heart failure. Am. J. Med., *65*:134, 1978. *(Presents evidence of reduction in left ventricular filling pressure and improvement in cardiac output with combined use of nitrates and hydralazine. Improvement in exercise tolerance also occurred. Sample sizes were small and duration of studies was short.)*

Cohn, K., *et al.*: Variability of hemodynamic responses to acute digitalization in chronic cardiac failure due to cardiomyopathy and coronary disease. Am. J. Cardiol., *35*:461, 1975. *(A careful catheterization study in a small series of patients with congestive cardiomyopathies showing that acute digitalization did not produce significant or lasting hemodynamic improvement.)*

Dall, J.L.C.: Maintenance digoxin in elderly patients. Br. Med. J., *2*:705, 1970. *(When Digoxin was stopped in 80 elderly patients on chronic therapy, only one quarter showed signs of increasing failure. Most who had no change had little indication for being on the drug in the first place.)*

Dobbs, S.N., *et al.*: Maintenance digoxin after an episode of heart failure. Br. Med. J., *1*:749, 1977.

(Demonstrated persistent hemodynamic effect of digoxin; CHF returned if drug was stopped in patients on long-term therapy for heart failure. Points out justification for chronic therapy in properly selected patients.)

Green, L.H., and Smith, T.W.: Use of digitalis in patients with pulmonary disease. Ann. Intern. Med., *87*:459, 1977. *(A literature review which concludes that the efficacy of digitalis in cor pulmonale is in question; there may be an associated increase in risk of digitalis toxicity.)*

McKee, P.A., *et al.*: Natural history of congestive heart failure: The Framingham study. N. Engl. J. Med., *285*:1444, 1971. *(A community-based study of the epidemiology of CHF. Over two thirds of patients with CHF had hypertension alone or in combination with coronary artery disease.)*

Slow-release potassium. Medical Letter, *20*:29, 1978. *(Reviews use of slow-release potassium tablets and concludes that small bowel ulceration continues to be reported in patients using these preparations.)*

Smith, T.W.: Digitalis toxicity: Epidemiology and clinical use of serum concentration measurements. Am. J. Med., *58*:470, 1975. *(A review of the appropriate use of serum digitalis levels, arguing for cautious interpretation and use of results, since there is overlap between normals and those with evidence of toxicity.)*

28

Management of Acquired Valvular Heart Disease

As a result of increased physician awareness and improvements in noninvasive diagnostic techniques, the diagnosis of acquired valvular heart disease is being made earlier in the course of illness. Outpatient management has become commonplace because symptoms are frequently absent or mild at the time the condition is discovered. Although consultation with a cardiologist is often obtained, the responsibility for long-term care usually falls on the primary physician.

In order to properly manage the patient with valvular heart disease, the primary physician must be familiar with the condition's natural history, early warning signs of hemodynamic deterioration, and indications for and types of medical and surgical therapies. Of major importance is the proper timing of surgery.

NATURAL HISTORY

Mitral Stenosis (MS)

Most cases of mitral stenosis are rheumatic in origin, even though as many as 50 per cent of patients cannot give a history of rheumatic fever. The symptom-free interval averages about 10 years (range is 3 to 25 years). In most instances, symptoms develop gradually over a decade, roughly paralleling the progression of stenosis; however, some people remain relatively free of complaints until stenosis becomes severe. Increases in left atrial and pulmonary venous pressures often become substantial as valve area falls below 1.5 cm²; at this point, many patients begin to experience dyspnea on exertion. Any stimulus which rapidly increases blood flow or decreases the time available for diastolic filling can precipitate a sudden increase in pulmonary congestion and result in acute shortness of breath; in addition to strenuous activity, fever, emotion, and atrial fibrillation are often responsible.

Progressive narrowing of the valve orifice is accompanied by worsening exercise tolerance and increasing dyspnea. In patients with tight stenosis (valve area less than 1.0 cm²) the period from onset of symptoms to incapacity averages 7 years, but the decline can be precipitous with the onset of atrial fibrillation or pneumonia. Persistence of chronic pulmonary congestion is followed by development of pulmonary hypertension, in which pulmonary vascular resistance rises out of proportion to the increase in wedge pressure. Cardiac output usually falls with onset of pulmonary hypertension, and fatigue may become a prominent symptom. The right ventricle hypertrophies in response to the rise in pulmonary artery pressure, but eventually right heart failure and death ensue unless intervention occurs; deterioration may be rapid at this stage.

Atrial fibrillation complicates 40 to 50 per cent of cases of symptomatic mitral stenosis. The correlation between development of atrial fibrillation and the severity of stenosis is only slight and not due solely to the degree of left atrial enlargement. The loss of atrial systole and the increase in heart rate that characterize atrial fibrillation markedly reduce flow across the mitral valve and boost left atrial pressure. Premature atrial contractions and paroxysmal atrial fibrillation often precede sustained atrial fibrillation due to mitral stenosis.

Systemic embolization occurs in 10 to 20 per cent of patients with MS. Age and presence of atrial fibrillation are the major determinants of risk; severity of stenosis is not a determinant, and, in fact, embolization may be a presenting symptom of MS.

In sum, there is typically a symptom-free period of about 10 years. Patients then begin to note dyspnea on exertion over the next 10 years, which progresses in many instances in the following decade. Once symptoms are present on minimal exertion, survival becomes markedly reduced. Patients with New York Heart Association Class IV disease (symptoms at rest) have been found to have a 5-year mortality rate of 85 per cent. Some patients have disease that does not progress and may remain stable indefinitely. In another subset of patients, symptoms do not develop until late in the illness.

Mitral Regurgitation (MR)

Patients with rheumatic MR can remain asymptomatic for many years, because the left ventricle dilates and adjusts well to the increase in volume load. Onset of dyspnea and fatigue may not occur for decades, and symptoms take an average of 10 years to progress to the point of disability and need for surgery. It is not until very late in the disease that myocardial reserve falters. Once this occurs, the patient progresses to worsening dyspnea and much fatigue; symptoms are present at rest (functional Class IV disease), and there may be signs of right heart failure as well, especially if pulmonary hypertension has set in. Prognosis is poor at this stage.

Atrial fibrillation is found in upwards of 75 per cent of cases, but the abrupt episodes of pulmonary congestion that typify mitral stenosis do not happen as frequently in MR; however, rupture of one of the chordae tendineae can result in sudden deterioration.

Nonrheumatic forms of chronic mitral regurgitation encountered in ambulatory patients probably account for the majority of MR that occurs. Etiologies include papillary muscle dysfunction, mitral valve prolapse, and calcified valve annulus.

Papillary muscle dysfunction is responsible for as much as 10 per cent of MR found clinically. It may result from ischemia, left ventricular dilatation, or cardiomyopathy, among other causes. Coronary disease is the most frequent etiology, with 40 per cent of posterior infarcts and 20 per cent of anterior infarcts accompanied by the development of MR. The amount of regurgitant flow produced is highly variable from case to case. Severe MR and marked pulmonary congestion can occur, even in the context of only a minimal reduction in left ventricular ejection fraction. Prognosis, on the other hand, does depend on left ventricular systolic performance.

Mitral valve prolapse usually does not produce hemodynamically significant regurgitation. Consequently, patients are rarely bothered by dyspnea. Palpitations and atypical chest pain are the most frequent complaints. With the exception of a subset of patients who are bothered by ventricular irritability, prognosis is excellent. The amount of regurgitant flow has not been found to increase with time; however, there is an increased incidence of bacterial endocarditis in patients with mitral valve prolapse.

Calcification of the mitral annulus occurs in older people, often in conjection with calcification of the aortic valve. The mitral lesion is usually not of hemodynamic significance, but heart block can develop if calcification extends into the ventricular septum.

Mixed mitral disease. Mortality is increased when signigicant stenosis and regurgitation occur simultaneously. In one large series of patients managed medically, the 10-year survival rate from the time of diagnosis was 33 per cent.

Aortic Stenosis (AS)

Because of the marked ability of the left ventricle to hypertrophy and compensate for the pressure load, patients can remain symptom-free for many years, even with tight stenosis (valve area less than 0.7 cm²). This is especially true in young patients; however, it must be remembered that sudden death can occur in asymptomatic individuals with critical AS. Onset of angina and effort syncope suggest a hemodynamically critical lesion that is limiting cardiac output, although in as many as 30 to 60 per cent of AS patients with angina, there coexists significant occlusion of a coronary vessel. Survival averages about 3 years from the onset of angina or effort syncope. The development of congestive failure is an ominous sign, for it signals the inability of the myocardium to continue tolerating the enormous pressure load; survival averages about 2 years from the time failure is first noted. Over half of patients with AS die of congestive failure. Sudden death accounts for another 20 per cent. The mean age of patients dying suddenly is 60; the mechanism of death in these cases is believed to be a dysrhythmia triggered by myocardial ischemia. The rate of stenosis is unpredictable and can progress rapidly over a few years, especially as the patient enters his 60s. Figures for survival are only averages; the range is wide, and many patients die soon after the onset of symptoms.

Age at clinical onset of AS is dependent in part on the underlying etiology. Significant AS appearing in a patient under the age of 30 is congenital in origin, due to a *unicuspid valve*. Patients presenting between 30 and 70 have either a *bicuspid valve* or a valve damaged by *rheumatic fever*. Those who present with significant AS due to rheumatic fever are about 10 to 15 years older than patients who present with mitral stenosis, due to the more gradual progression of the illness associated with AS; nevertheless, the course can be one of rapid deterioration. Many patients over 60 often develop a systolic ejection murmur; by age 80, half of the population has such a murmur. In a small percentage of these *elderly patients,* hemodynamically significant stenosis develops due to heavy calcification of a tricuspid aortic valve.

Aortic Regurgitation (AR)

Rheumatic fever accounts for the largest number of cases. Most patients can live for decades with little incapacity, as the left ventricle dilates and eccentrically hypertrophies to accommodate the extra volume load. The latent period from occurrence of rheumatic fever to onset of clinical manifestations is about 10 years. During the following decade, symptoms appear and progress. The onset of symptoms is typically gradual, with palpitations being among the earliest changes noted by the patient, followed by dyspnea on exertion and fatigability. Appearance of LVH with strain and worsening cardiomegaly are associated with a markedly increased risk of heart failure and death within 5 years. If exertional dyspnea worsens, other manifestations of congestive failure are likely to follow and signal the beginning of a rapidly declining phase of the disease due to left ventricular decompensation. At this stage, deterioration is rapid, with death occurring within 1 to 2 years of the onset of congestive failure. Angina is common, reported by almost 30 per cent of patients; unlike the angina of aortic stenosis, it typically takes place at rest rather than upon exertion. Angina becomes more frequent when there is worsening heart failure.

Nonrheumatic causes of chronic AR include syphilis, myxomatous degeneration, and connective tissue disease. Aortic regurgitation secondary to untreated *syphilis* appears about 15 to 25 years after the initial infection and often has a more rapidly downhill course than AR due to rheumatic fever. It accounts for an average of 10 per cent of AR cases seen in hospital populations. *Myxomatous transformation* has been found in 10 to 15 per cent of cases of AR studied pathologically. The process is progressive and becomes clinically evident between the ages of 30 and 60. *Ankylosing spondylitis* is complicated by AR in about 3 per cent of cases. The severity of the lesion is highly variable, and conduction defects are frequent. AR may appear before the onset of other symptoms, but in most instances it follows the appearance of arthritic symptoms by 10 to 20 years. The presence of severe AR shortens the otherwise normal life expectancy of patients with anklyosing spondylitis. *Reiter's syndrome* is associated with the development of AR in 5 per cent of cases, typically in those with florid manifestations of the disease such as iritis, mucocutaneous changes and extensive sacroiliac inflammation. Onset of AR occurs on an average of 15 years after the disease is first noted, often preceded by conduction disturbances. The severity and course of the AR are highly variable.

Mixed aortic valve disease. Many patients with AS have some degree of AR, and vice versa. Whenever the gradient across the aortic valve is greater than 25 mm. Hg in the context of significant regurgitation, there begins to develop a substantial pressure load as well as an increased volume load on the left ventricle. The clinical course is similar to that for isolated aortic stenosis of the same degree, although some clinicians believe there is an earlier onset of symptoms.

Combined aortic and mitral disease. The etiology is mostly rheumatic; in fact, most cases of rheumatic fever produce some degree of multiple valve damage, though disease of one valve often dominates the clinical picture. The most common combination is aortic regurgitation in conjunction with mitral disease. Atrial fibrillation and systemic embolization are more frequent than in isolated AR, as is the severity of pulmonary symptoms. Less common is the coexistence of AS and MS. Symptoms and signs of AS are blunted by significant MS, such that pulmonary symptoms, atrial fibrilltation and systemic embolization may dominate the presentation, but there may be more angina and syncope than expected from isolated MS. Course is dictated by the severity of the individual lesions, but MS can delay the appearance of some of the manifestations of advanced AS.

ESTIMATING SEVERITY OF DISEASE

Mitral Stenosis

Symptoms provide crude indications of the severity of stenosis. Dyspnea correlates with increase in left atrial pressure and development of pulmonary venous congestion, but the relationship between degree of stenosis and elevation of left atrial pressure is variable. Fatigue occurs most often in the context of pulmonary hypertension, but the nonspecific nature of the symptom lessens its utility in estimating severity. Hemoptysis is related to pulmonary venous hypertension, but does not necessarily imply severe stenosis. Thus, history alone may fail to detect severe stenosis that is unaccompanied by marked pulmonary congestion; however, a worsening of dyspnea and a decline in exercise tolerance suggest hemodynamic deterioration and require further investigation.

On physical examination, the interval between the second heart sound and the opening snap, referred to as the S_2-OS interval, and the duration and timing of the diastolic murmur provide additional clues of severity. The S_2-OS interval is a function of the elevation in left atrial pressure. The greater the pressure, the shorter the interval. Unfortunately, the degree of MS is not the only determinant of left atrial pressure; the interval can be affected by factors other than valve area, such as heart rate and left ventricular pressure. Moreover, the valve must be mobile to snap; in advanced disease, the valve may calcify and the snap becomes inaudible. Nevertheless, the S_2-OS interval is useful because it can be determined at the bedside and does provide data which may help in judging severity when considered in the context of other findings. Perhaps the most precise uses of the interval is in separating hemodynamically insignificant disease from moderate and severe MS. An interval of greater than 0.11 second at rest with a heart rate of 70 to 80 argues against a significant lesion (though there are exceptions). Patients with moderate to tight stenosis usually demonstrate intervals less than 0.08 second, which shorten with exercise. Proper estimation of the S_2-OS interval takes considerable practice, but can be achieved in many instances.

The intensity of the *diastolic murmur* does not correlate with severity of stenosis, but its duration through diastole does. However, development of pulmonary hypertension may decrease cardiac output from the right side of the heart, result in a diminution of flow across the mitral valve, and consequently shorten the duration of the murmur.

Chest x-ray provides important evidence of severity. The earliest radiologic sign of MS is dilatation of the left atrium, which is best seen on a lateral view in conjunction with a barium swallow to outline the esophagus. The finding is not a very reliable manifestation of severity. A better sign is redistribution of pulmonary venous blood flow, producing dilatation of the upper zone pulmonary veins. Upper zone redistribution becomes prominent at a left atrial pressure of 25 mm. Hg and parallels severity of stenosis. This change in pulmonary venous flow is very sensitive to changes in left atrial pressure, but not unique to mitral stenosis. Radiologic evidence of pulmonary hypertension (dilatation of the right pulmonary artery to 15 to 18 mm., rapid tapering of vessels, and right ventricular enlargement) strongly suggests advanced mitral stenosis, though again the findings are not specific for MS. Presence of Kerley B lines, perihilar haze and other manifestations of interstitial edema are seen in patients with severe dyspnea due to MS; the absence of interstitial edema on chest film does not rule out tight MS, but a patient with dyspnea at rest should always show these changes on x-ray; otherwise, one must question the meaning of the shortness of breath. In sum, no single radiologic finding is specific for severe MS, but x-ray data can provide important supporting evidence.

The electrocardiogram is of limited utility for estimation of severity. The best ECG sign appears to be the QRS axis; a rightward shift to greater than +60° is associated with a valve area of less than 1.3 cm² in over 85 per cent of cases. Like most clinical data, the absence of the rightward shift in axis means little. The greater the pulmonary artery pressure, the more likely right ventricular hypertrophy will appear on ECG.

Echocardiography has proven to be extremely sensitive for detection of MS and useful for estimation of valve mobility and degree of calcification. It is expected that development of two-dimensional echocardiography will provide a reliable noninvasive means of determining valve area.

Cardiac catheterization is resorted to when clinical data are contradictory, mixed or multiple valve lesions are suspected, or the coexistence of other types of heart disease is of concern.

Mitral Regurgitation

A reasonable estimate of the severity of mitral insufficiency can be obtained by history and physical examination. Dyspnea on exertion and fatigability are early symptoms of hemodynamically significant regurgitation, though the absence of such symptoms does not rule out severe disease. On physical examination, severe MR produces left ventricular enlargement with a hyperdynamic, slightly diffuse, apical impulse displaced to the left but of normal timing and duration. In addition, there is a pansystolic murmur (its loudness does not correlate directly with severity), a loud S_3, often a mid-diastolic rumble from increased flow across the mitral valve, and at times wide splitting of the second sound due to shortening of left ventricular systole and early aortic valve closure. Cardiomegaly and left atrial enlargement are pronounced on chest film. A normal heart on chest x-ray and absence of an apical pansystolic murmur rule out significant mitral regurgitation. The ECG and echocardiogram are of little specific help in evaluation of severity.

Cardiac catheterization is indicated in patients who are being considered for surgery, in order to quantitate the amount of regurgitation and assess ventricular function.

Aortic Stenosis

There are numerous pitfalls in the clinical estimation of severity, especially in the elderly. Nevertheless, careful history and physical examination can provide important clues. Effort syncope, angina, and symptoms of congestive heart failure point to advanced disease with markedly reduced chances of 5-year survival. At times, it is impossible to tell clinically if these worrisome symptoms are due to AS. Because of the high prevalence of coexisting coronary disease, the presence of angina must be interpreted cautiously; cardiac catheterization and coronary angiography may be necessary.

Delay in carotid artery upstroke is one of the most helpful physical signs of significant AS. A normal upstroke in a patient under age 60 is strong evidence against important stenosis; however, upstroke may be normal in the elderly patient with severe stenosis and a stiff, noncompliant carotid artery. When coincidental aortic regurgitation is present, the upstroke may also be normalized in the presence of marked stenosis. A misleading delay in carotid upstroke can occur from the combination of systemic hypertension and congestive heart failure. Elevation of systolic blood pressure does not rule out hemodynamically significant disease, though a pressure greater than 200 and a pulse pressure in excess of 80 mm. Hg are unusual when stenosis is marked.

In young patients, the intensity of the murmur

correlates with severity. A patient with less than a 3/6 murmur is unlikely to have significant AS. In patients with far advanced disease and a failing left ventricle, the murmur may decrease in intensity and appear rather insignificant as flow across the valve diminishes. In general, the longer the murmur takes to reach peak intensity, the greater the stenosis. Unfortunately, the timing of maximal intensity may not be delayed in some cases of severe stenosis, but if the murmur does peak after midsystole, the stenosis is usually significant. Because the murmur of AS in the elderly may lose its characteristic qualities, it is best to judge severity on the basis of symptoms and other findings.

A delay in the aortic component of the second heart sound is another sign of significant AS. It is manifested as a single second sound or a paradoxically split second sound. Calcification and increased rigidity of the valve will often diminish the aortic closing sound and can be mistaken for a delay. A prolonged left ventricular impulse on physical examination can be a helpful sign of important long-standing obstruction to flow.

The ECG can provide extremely valuable noninvasive data. In most cases of severe stenosis, there is evidence of left ventricular hypertrophy and a strain pattern, i.e., ST and T-wave depression in the lateral precordial leads. The likelihood of finding a strain pattern increases with the increase in gradient across the aortic valve. These ECG changes also identify patients at increased risk of sudden death, for less than 10 per cent of patients succumbing to sudden death demonstrate normal ECGs.

In the elderly, the degree of valve calcification on chest fluoroscopy correlates with severity of stenosis. The absence of significant calcification in a patient over 60 greatly reduces the probability of important valvular stenosis. Poststenotic dilatation of the aorta suggests aortic stenosis, but does not have quantitative meaning.

Echocardiography can sometimes help in assessment of AS by identifying calcification, thickening and decreased mobility of the aortic valve leaflets, findings which occur as AS progresses. Study is underway to try to determine the gradient across the valve by ultrasound techniques. Cardiac catheterization is indicated in the young asymptomatic patient with evidence of severe stenosis, as well as in the patient with known aortic stenosis who begins to develop clinical symptoms of angina, failure, or syncope. Elderly patients who would not be candidates for valve replacement under any circumstances need not be subjected to catheterization, but those who are should also have coronary angiography to identify significant occlusive disease that may be the source of symptoms and/or require correction to insure the best chances of surviving surgery.

Aortic Regurgitation

Severity of AR can usually be well assessed clinically in cases of isolated valvular insufficiency. Marked regurgitation that is long-standing produces dyspnea, a loud diastolic blow that extends beyond mid-diastole, an S_3, a bounding pulse, and a widened pulse pressure. The absence of a wide pulse pressure does not rule out hemodynamically significant AR, nor does the degree of widening correlate quantitatively with severity; changes in peripheral resistance alone can cause large variations in pulse pressure. ECG and x-ray evidence of left ventricular hypertrophy and enlargement are indicative of long-standing significant regurgitation and suggest worsening left ventricular function if they progress.

When aortic regurgitation occurs in the presence of mitral stenosis, compound aortic valve disease or heart failure, the estimation of severity can be very difficult to judge on clinical grounds alone. Consultation with a cardiologist and catheterization are often needed.

PRINCIPLES OF MANAGEMENT

The major therapeutic objectives are to preserve exercise capacity, life-style, and life expectancy. Minimizing the chances of endocarditis and systemic embolization are also of importance. Proper timing of surgical intervention is essential to successful treatment. A common management error is to inappropriately delay surgery, allowing irreversible myocardial decompensation to develop; this greatly increases the risk of operation and reduces the chances of survival. A physician can be lulled into a false sense of security by continuing to control symptoms through repetitive escalations of medical therapy. The need for progressive increases in medication suggests worsening myocardial function and the need for surgery. By ignoring the significance of such developments, the physician may miss the optimal opportunity for the best possible surgical outcome and long-term survival.

Early in the course of illness, symptoms of pulmonary congestion can be treated with digitalis and/or a mild diuretic regimen (see Chapter 27), but more advanced stages of disease require surgical intervention. Life expectancy and quality of life are clearly improved by properly timed valve surgery. Advances in design of prosthetic valves and improvements in operative technique have produced substantial reductions in surgical mortality. At present, hospital rates for patients undergoing valve surgery in major centers average less than 1 per cent for mitral valvulotomy and less than 5 per cent for mitral or aortic valve replacement. Operative mortality increases sharply when patients with advanced disease (e.g., functional Class IV) undergo surgery; nevertheless, imminent death is frequently inevitable unless surgery is undertaken. Consequently, patients with severe disease should not be denied an operation if there is any evidence of some myocardial reserve and the slightest chance of surviving surgery. The 5-year life expectancy rate for patients with Class IV disease who live through valve replacement is usually less than 50 per cent, but this figure is much better than the less than 5 per cent rate for similar patients managed medically. Thus, even when surgery is inordinately delayed, it may still offer the patient some opportunity for prolonging survival.

Contraindications to valve surgery include serious coexisting noncardiac illness that would compromise survival and existence of end-stage myocardial decompensation that would make surgery for naught.

Prior to surgery, medical therapy should be directed at control of failure (see Chapter 27) and atrial fibillation (see Chapter 23) and prevention of bacterial endocarditis (see Chapter 11) and embolization (see Chapter 84). Most people can be well managed on a outpatient basis for many years prior to the need for valve surgery.

THERAPEUTIC RECOMMENDATIONS AND INDICATIONS FOR REFERRAL AND ADMISSION

- All patients with any form of valvular heart disease should receive prophylaxis for bacterial endocarditis (see Chapter 11).
- Patients under the age of 35 with previous rheumatic fever should be considered for rheumatic fever prophylaxis (see Chapter12).
- Onset of rapid atrial fibrillation accompanied by acute hemodynamic deterioration is an indication for immediate hospital admission and cardioversion. Patients who tolerate the atrial fibrillation can be digitalized on an outpatient basis and need not be admitted (see Chapter 23).
- Occurrence of systemic embolization is an indication for urgent admission and intravenous anticoagulant therapy followed by long-term oral anticoagulant treatment (see Chapter 84). Some clinicians argue that valve surgery should be considered if embolization occurs; this is controversial.

Mitral Stenosis

- Asymptomatic patients with mild to moderate stenosis need no restriction of activity. Those with evidence of tight stenosis and relatively few symptoms should be advised of the risk of precipitating symptoms by extreme exertion or pregnancy.
- Patients with mild dyspnea which occurs only on exertion can be started on a mild diuretic program (e.g., 50 to 100 mg. hydrochlorothiazide per day) and advised to follow a no-added-salt diet. Digitalis is of no benefit in isolated mitral stenosis unless there is atrial fibrillation. Extremely vigorous exertion and emotional upset should be avoided to prevent precipitating symptoms.
- Development of signs of tight stenosis (see above), even if few symptoms are reported, is an indication for referral to a cardiologist for consideration of surgery. The same is true for worsening dyspnea that is inadequately controlled by a mild diuretic program and salt restriction.
- Young patients with evidence of isolated, tight MS with a pliable valve should be considered for surgery early in the course of their illness, even before symptoms are disabling, because valvulotomy can be performed. The procedure provides symptomatic improvement that may last for 10 to 20 years, is less risky than valve replacement, and does not require permanent oral anticoagulant therapy.
- Older patients with stiff valves (absent opening snap, heavy valve calcification, and limited motion as seen on echocardiogram) must undergo valve replacement if surgery is needed. Since surgical mortality and complications are greater for valve replacement than for valvulotomy, surgery need not be advised until symptoms are more disabling. However, surgery should not be delayed until symptoms occur at rest or upon minimal exertion, because operative risk and long-term mortality increase substantially.

- Cardiac consultation for consideration of catheterization is indicated in the patient being considered for surgery when there is a question of mixed mitral disease or involvement of multiple valves, or when symptoms are out of proportion to objective evidence of disease.

Mitral Regurgitation

- Asymptomatic young patients need no restriction of activity.
- Onset of fatigue and dyspnea can be treated with initiation of digitalis and diuretics, in conjunction with a no-added-salt diet. A modest diuretic program, such as 100 mg. of hydrochlorothiazide, that adequately controls symptoms may suffice for years in patients with mild to moderate MR and is not an indication for surgical consideration.
- The development of any increase in dyspnea that requires escalation of diuretic therapy is an indication for cardiac consultation concerning valve replacement. Progressive deterioration in clinical status and increasing heart size suggest presence of myocardial decompensation; prompt referral is indicated; medical therapy is no substitute for valve surgery.
- Refractory congestive failure due to MR is not a contraindication to surgery, though risk is increased. Prior to surgery, symptoms may be lessened by vasodilator therapy, which can diminish the proportion of regurgitant flow by decreasing afterload (see Chapter 27). Use of vasodilators can also benefit the inoperable patient.
- Patients with incapacitating dyspnea and pulmonary congestion felt to be due to *papillary muscle dysfunction* should be referred to the cardiologist for catheterization to determine if valve replacement will be of benefit. In one series, those with ejection fractions above 0.35 had the best surgical survival. If there is coexisting coronary disease, it should be treated (see Chapter 25).
- Patients with a *prolapsed mitral valve* may require treatment with propranolol for ventricular irritability if they are symptomatic or found to have runs of ventricular tachycardia (see Chapter 24). Dyspnea is uncommon and digitalis, diuretics and salt restriction are rarely necessary, since the degree of regurgitation is usually hemodynamically insignificant and not progressive. Occurrence of chest pain demands careful evaluation so that other etiologies are not mistakenly attributed to the valve disease (see Chapter 14).

- Patients with *calcification of the mitral valve annulus* should be followed for development of heart block. Regurgitant flow is usually small; consequently, dyspnea and pulmonary congestion are not major problems.

Aortic Stenosis

- Asymptomatic patients with mild to moderate AS do not require restriction of activity. However, young, asymptomatic patients with evidence of tight stenosis should be advised against extreme physical exertion (e.g., competitive sports) and referred to a cardiologist for further evaluation and consideration of valve replacement. Catheterization may be needed.
- Onset of angina, effort syncope or congestive heart failure dictates serious consideration of valve surgery, because these are signs of critical stenosis and predict a poor prognosis unless definitive therapy is undertaken. Patients with these symptoms are at risk for sudden death. Medical therapy is no substitute.
- Congestive failure can be treated symptomatically on a temporary basis by prescribing digitalis and a diuretic program (see Chapter 27). Cautious use of furosemide (20 to 40 mg. per day) may help reduce pulmonary congestion when fluid retention is marked, but the need for a high diastolic filling pressure must be kept in mind; overzealous diuretic therapy can cause a precipitous fall in cardiac output.
- Angina can be treated symptomatically with nitroglycerin pending surgery (see Chapter 25). Propranolol is contraindicated due to its negative inotropic effects. Coronary angiography is required at the time of cardiac catheterization to determine if there is coexisting significant coronary artery disease and the need for a bypass procedure at the time of valve replacement.
- Advancing age is not an absolute contraindication to valve replacement. Survival from surgery is predominantly a function of the patient's myocardial reserve. Consequently, patients in their 60s and 70s need not be denied surgery if they demonstrate good ejection fractions in the setting of severe AS.
- Because the lesion can progress rapidly over a few years, patients with AS should have careful longitudinal care and regular follow-up, even when disease appears hemodynamically insignificant and the patient is asymptomatic.

Aortic Regurgitation

- No activity restrictions are necessary in young asymptomatic patients.
- Patients with evidence of worsening left ventricular status (LVH with a strain pattern on ECG, increasing cardiomegaly on chest film) should be referred to a cardiologist for evaluation of surgery, even in the absence of disabling symptoms. Patients with these findings have been noted to have an increased 5-year mortality rate. Early identification of high-risk patients is suggested in the hope of correcting AR prior to the development of irreversible myocardial decompensation, which may occur rapidly at the time that symptoms of failure just begin to appear.
- Onset of early symptoms of pulmonary congestion (dyspnea on climbing more than one flight of stairs) in the absence of LVH with strain on ECG or marked cardiomegaly can be treated medically with digitalization and a mild diuretic (50 to 100 mg. hydrochlorothiazide). Progression of dyspnea to onset after climbing less than one flight of stairs or the appearance of LVH, strain, and an enlarging heart indicates the need for cardiac consultation and consideration of surgery.
- Patients with dyspnea prompted by minimal exertion, orthopnea or paroxysmal nocturnal dyspnea require prompt referral for surgery, because life expectancy is less than 1 year without surgery. Medical therapy with digitalis and diuretics may provide some symptomatic relief temporarily, but must not be used in place of valve surgery at this stage of illness.

PATIENT EDUCATION

By far, the most essential element of patient education is teaching the importance of endocarditis prophylaxis. The chances of compliance are certain to improve if time is taken to explain the rationale for prophylaxis and to inform the patient of the risks incurred if it is ignored. Proper procedure and situations requiring prophylaxis need thorough review (see Chapter 11). Patients who have had rheumatic fever require instruction prophylaxis against streptococcal infection (see Chapter 12).

Patients *and* their families should be fully briefed on allowable activity to avoid unnecessary restriction as well as the risk of sudden death (e.g., the young asymptomatic patient with critical AS). If the safety of unlimited activity is in doubt, the patient should have a cardiac consultation. Patient confidence can be maintained by regular follow-up by the primary physician in conjunction with a consulting cardiologist when needed. It is helpful to inform the patient of the treatability of his condition and its excellent prognosis when therapy is properly timed and applied. Teaching the early warning signs of worsening disease to the patient who is mature and intelligent can help to enlist him in the monitoring effort. If the patient cannot be depended upon to relate symptoms accurately, perhaps a family member might be recruited to watch for early manifestations of progressive disease. Reviewing the proper use of digitalis and diuretics (see Chapter 27) is important for prevention of inappropriate and unauthorized escalation of the medical program when symptoms worsen. Instruction in anticoagulant therapy is also essential if it is to be used on a long-term basis (see Chapter 84).

ANNOTATED BIBLIOGRAPHY

Barnhorst, D.A., Oxman, H.A., Connolly, D.C., *et al.*: Long-term follow-up of isolated replacement of aortic or mitral valve with Starr-Edwards prosthesis. Am. J. Cardiol., *35*:228, 1975. *(Valve replacement improves life expectancy and symptoms.)*

Brunnen, P.L., Finlayson, J.D., and Short, D.: Serious mitral stenosis with slight symptoms. Br. Med. J., *1*:1958, 1964. *(Symptoms may be slight but young patients with tight stenosis are at risk for sudden deterioration; pregnancy was a major precipitant in this series of 20 patients.)*

Chen, J.T.T., Beliar, V.S., Morris, J.J., *et al.*: Correlation of roentgen findings with hemodynamic data in pure mitral stenosis. Am. J. Roentgenol., *102*:280, 1968. *(When there is a prominent upper zone venous pattern and pulmonary artery dilation on chest film, the mitral stenosis is severe.)*

Fowler, N.O., and Van Der Bel-Kahn, J.M.: Indications for surgical replacement of the mitral valve. Am. J. Cardiol., *44*:148, 1979. *(A review which emphasizes timing of surgical therapy; 41 refs.)*

Frank, S., Johnson, A., and Ross, J., Jr.: Natural history of valvular aortic stenosis. Br. Heart J., *35*:41, 1973. *(In medically treated cases with significant stenosis, 50 per cent were dead within 5 years and 90 per cent within 10 years of diagnosis.)*

Friedman, W.F., and Braunwald, E.: Accurate estimation of left atrial pressure without cardiac catheterization in mitral valve disease. Am. J. Cardiol., *17*:123, 1966. *(Dilatation of upper zone pulmonary veins is prominent when left atrial pressure reaches 25 mm. Hg.)*

Goldschlager, N., Pfeifer, J., Cohn, K., *et al.*: Natural history of aortic regurgitation. Am. J. Med., *54*:577, 1973. *(Long asymptomatic period, but once symptoms occur, irreversible myocardial changes may have already taken place.)*

Graboys, T.B., and Cohn, P.F.: Prevalence of angina and abnormal coronary arteriograms in severe aortic stenosis. Am. Heart J., *93*:683, 1977. *(Twenty per cent of patients had >75 per cent luminal stenosis.)*

Kirklin, J.W., and Pacifico, A.D.: Surgery for acquired valvular heart disease. N. Engl. J. Med., *288*:133, 194, 1973. *(A slightly dated but thorough review of the subject; 58 refs.)*

Olsen, K.H., and Biden, H.: Natural history of mitral stenosis. Br. Heart J., *24*:349, 1962. *(Mortality for NYHA Class III patients managed medically was 6 per cent per annum and for Class IV, 17 per cent per annum.)*

Radford, M., Johnson, R.A., Buckley, M.J., *et al.*: Survival following initial valve replacement for mitral regurgitation due to coronary artery disease. Circulation, *60*: Suppl. II, 39, 1979. *(Survival was a function of preoperative ejection fraction. Long-term survivors experienced reductions in heart failure.)*

Rappaport, E.: Natural history of aortic and mitral valve disease. Am. J. Cardiol., *35*:221, 1975. *(In large series of medically treated patients with mitral regurgitation, the 10-year survival was 60 per cent.)*

Rothenberg, A.J., Clark, J.A., Carleton, R.A., *et al.*: Natural course of mitral stenosis. Clin. Res., *16*:246, 1968. *(Symptoms correlated roughly with reduction in valve area. Few symptoms occurred when valve area was greater than 1.5 cm².)*

Spagnuolo, M., Kloth, H., Tranta, A., *et al.*: Natural history of rheumatic aortic regurgitation. Circulation, *44*:368, 1971. *(Young patients with marked LV enlargement, LVH on ECG and wide pulse pressure with diastolic less than 40 mm. Hg are at high risk for failure or death.)*

Wood, P.: An appreciation of mitral stenosis. Br. Med. J., *1*:1051, 1954. *(Symptom-free interval from onset of rheumatic heart disease to onset of symptoms was 3 to 25 years with mean of 12 years. A classic study of mitral stenosis.)*

29

Management of Intermittent Claudication*

DAVID C. BREWSTER, M.D.

Although specific therapy for alleviation of atherosclerosis does not yet exist, there are a number of measures which can provide symptomatic improvement in patients with claudication. Both medical and reconstructive surgical approaches are available. The primary physician needs to know the indications for and effectiveness of each as well as the natural history of the disease.

NATURAL HISTORY OF CLAUDICATION

A number of studies have examined the clinical course and prognosis of patients with claudication. In a series of 520 nondiabetic patients from the Mayo Clinic followed over 5 years prior to the advent of surgical reconstruction, only 3 per cent came to amputation within 5 years if the only manifestation of their disease was claudication. Of the smokers who ceased smoking, none required amputation, but 11.4 per cent who continued to smoke lost a limb.

A more recent study of 104 patients with claudication who underwent angiography also noted a relatively benign prognosis. Over a 6-month to 8-year follow-up (average 2.5 years), 79 per cent remained stable or improved, and only 5.8 per cent came to amputation. When patients were divided into mild, moderate and severe disease groups on the basis of distance walked before onset of claudication, it was found that severity paralleled prognosis; the group with most severe disease accounted for 5 of the 6 amputations. Nevertheless, even in the most severe cases 69.4 per cent stayed the same or improved, and only 15.1 per cent came to amputation, underscoring the fact that progression to loss of limb is hardly inevitable. Angiographic finding showed that prognosis was also related to extent and degree of occlusion in vessels below the knee, regardless of involvement of more proximal vessels.

In the Mayo Clinic series, the 5-year survival rate was 77.2 per cent for patients with claudication, compared to 92.8 per cent for a normal population matched for age and sex. The cause of death in over 75 per cent of patients with claudication was believed to be coronary artery disease, underscoring the often systemic nature of the atherosclerosis and its adverse effect on prognosis.

PRINCIPLES OF MANAGEMENT

The basic tenet of nonoperative care is to control progression of the disease and stimulate collateral circulation. As long as improvement in collateral flow outpaces the development of existing or new occlusive lesions, blood flow will be maintained and symptoms will remain stable or actually improve. Perhaps the two most important methods of achieving these objectives are the cessation of smoking and daily exercise. Smoking appears to hasten progression of atherosclerosis and may also impair collateral flow by a vasoconstrictive effect. Significant occlusive disease is rare in nonsmokers. A possible stimulus for development of collateral circulation appears to be the demand created by daily exercise, though this is still unproven.

The best way to prevent limb loss is careful attention to foot care. It has been estimated that up to 80 per cent of amputations required in diabetics are attributable to poor foot care. Feet need to be inspected daily, especially when there is a coexistent peripheral neuropathy limiting sensation. Washing, moisturizing and padding friction points maximize skin protection. Properly fitting shoes and regular, careful nail-cutting are also essential.

Weight reduction can help by lessening work load and reducing metabolic demands of the extremities. It may also help lower lipid levels. Treatment of hypertension and hyperlipidemia is probably advisable since it may be of value in controlling progression of arteriosclerosis, although this has not been clearly documented (see Chapter 22). Tight control of diabetes does not seem to help (See Chapter 98).

Vasodilators are the most controversial and wide-

* See Chapter 17 for evaluation of arterial insufficiency.

ly used class of drugs in the treatment of symptomatic peripheral vascular disease. A wide variety of agents with different mechanisms of action is available. Little convincing evidence exists to support their use in obstructive vascular disease, either for claudication or ischemic problems at rest. Not only are they of no proven benefit and an unnecessary expense, but they dilate skin vessels and may divert blood away from muscles. Beta blockers have no role; some reports suggest that propranolol may exacerbate symptoms of claudication. Anticoagulants have not been found to prevent occlusion, but there is some suggestion that antiplatelet agents may be helpful. The literature should be followed for developments in this area.

Surgical referral is clearly indicated in patients with advanced ischemia resulting in gangrene, non-healing ischemic ulceration or ischemic rest pain. Such limbs are at risk, and arterial reconstruction is indicated, if feasible, to maximize chances of limb salvage. Noninvasive testing and arteriography are needed to assess site and extent of occlusion (see Chapter 17). The morbidity and mortality of common revascularization procedures are now in many instances less than that associated with major amputation. For poor-risk patients, various "extraterritorial" reconstructions are also available which may be done with even more safety.

The most controversial issue remains the role of arterial reconstruction in patients with claudication only. In such instances, the physician must attempt to determine the significance of ischemic symptoms in each individual patient. The age of the patient, work requirements, social circumstances, and general state of health should all be considered, as well as the severity of claudication. Noninvasive studies may provide sensitive measures of blood supply (see Chapter 17). In general, most vascular surgeons do not consider claudication by itself as an indication for surgery. However, if symptoms compromise the livelihood of the patient, operation may be indicated. Similarly, if a good-risk patient feels that ischemic symptoms seriously impair his life-style and are therefore intolerable, arterial reconstruction may be indicated. Referral for a surgical opinion is often useful in such instances.

Vascular reconstructive procedures require specialized training and judgment and are, therefore, best carried out by surgeons properly experienced in this field. In experienced hands, with good anesthetic and postoperative management, elective correction of aortoiliac occlusive disease should be associated with mortality of approximately 2 per cent, and with ex-

cellent long-term patency of approximately 85-90 per cent at 5 years. Femoropopliteal reconstruction may be done with even greater safety. Long-term patency is somewhat less, with approximately 70-75 per cent of saphenous vein grafts patent at 5 years. With improvement of direct reconstructive methods, lumbar sympathectomy is rarely considered a primary mode of treatment.

THERAPEUTIC RECOMMENDATIONS

- *Cessation of smoking.* The patient should be firmly told that he *must* stop smoking. The physician must be unequivocal about this, as patients often interpret half-hearted advice as only a suggestion (see Chapter 49).
- *Continued exercise.* In the patient with claudication, this is probably best achieved by daily walking. Patients are advised to walk to the point of discomfort, stop briefly, and then resume walking. It is important to emphasize to the patient that pain does not indicate harm or damage to the muscle, and that such a program will help rather than aggravate his condition. Any tendency to restrict activity, sometimes to the point of invalidism or confinement to the home, should be avoided, unless severe ischemia is present.

  Patients with more advanced ischemia and rest pain at night will often benefit from raising the head of the bed on 6- to 8-inch blocks so that the feet and legs are made slightly dependent; gravity may aid blood flow enough to allow more comfortable sleep.
- *Foot care.* This aspect of preventive medicine is of extreme importance, particularly in the diabetic patient who often lacks protective sensation due to neuropathy and who may be more susceptible to infection. Because there is often a great deal of confusion about what is meant by "foot care," its components require elaboration:
  1. *Inspection.* The feet should be inspected daily for any scratches, cuts, fissures, blisters or other lesions, particularly around the nail beds, between the toes, and on the heels.
  2. *Washing.* The feet should be washed daily with mild soap and lukewarm water (never hot). Rinse thoroughly and dry gently but completely, particularly between the toes. Excessive soaking, leading to maceration, should be avoided.
  3. *Lanolin.* A moisturizing cream such as lanolin or Eucerin should be applied to the skin of the

foot and heel, but not between the toes. A light film, well rubbed in, will prevent drying and cracking of the skin, often the genesis of a lesion, particularly on the heel. This should not be applied thickly or allowed to "cake" on the foot.

4. *Lambswool.* A small amount of this or dry cotton or gauze may be placed between the toes to prevent lesions which may occur if toes are allowed to rub together, particularly if orthopedic deformities of the toes are present.

5. *Powder.* An antifungal powder, such as tolnaftate, may be used between the toes if excessive moisture or maceration is a problem.

6. *Proper footwear.* Properly fitting shoes, with ample space in the forefoot, are essential. Special shoes are not necessary.

7. *Podiatry.* Nails should be cut with extreme care, in good light, and only if vision is normal. They should be cut straight across and even with the end of the toe, never close to the skin or into the corner of the nail bed. Any abnormality of the nails, corns or calluses are better handled by a physician or podiatrist in the case of the ischemic foot.

8. *Avoidance of trauma.* Never use adhesive tape on the skin (paper tape is better), or any strong antiseptic solution. Avoid heating pads, hot packs or heat lamps. Never walk barefoot.

It is the physician's responsibility to educate his patients in these points, and to urge them to contact him at the first sign of difficulty.

- *Weight reduction* (see Chapters 221 and 222).
- *Control of other risk factors* (e.g., hypertension [see Chapter 21], hyperlipidemia [see Chapter 22]).
- *Surgical referral*
  1. *Patients with claudication alone.* An operation should be considered only in patients who are so significantly disabled by claudication that their livelihood or life-style is intolerably compromised by their inability to walk distances.
  2. *Patients with more severe disease.* People with rest pain, nonhealing ulcers or early gangrene who have a limb which is in jeopardy should be considered for operation with some urgency.

PATIENT EDUCATION

Patient education is vital, as implementation of many of the above measures requires that the patient understand the nature of the problem as well as the factors which may aggravate the severity of symptoms. Patient compliance is essential in most nonoperative recommendations. Many patients come to the physician with great fear of limb loss. The favorable prognosis and likelihood of improvement are usually of great comfort and reassurance to the patient and family. The psychological management of the patient is essential to prevention of depression and invalidism. Emphasis should be on the positive prognosis and the patient's ability to improve his physical condition. The patient with new claudication should be seen at 2- to 3-month intervals for assessment of exercise tolerance and inspection of the feet for potential pressure points and ulcers. The need for foot care and immediate attention to the most trivial injury or lesion must be emphasized.

ANNOTATED BIBLIOGRAPHY

Boyd, A.M.: The natural course of arteriosclerosis of the lower extremities. Angiology, *11*:10, 1960. *(A cohort of 1440 patients with claudication was followed for 5 to 15 years. Mortality was high, with 5-, 10- and 15-year survivals of 73 per cent, 38 per cent and 22 per cent, but the risk of a major amputation was low, 7.2 per cent and 10 per cent at 5 and 10 years.)*

Coffman, J.D.: Vasodilator drugs in peripheral vascular disease. N. Engl. J. Med., *300*:713, 1979. *(A critical review of the literature arguing that vasodilators are not effective in treatment of intermittent claudication or ischemic rest pain due to obstructive vascular disease; 32 refs.)*

Humphries, A.W.: Relation of the natural history of arteriosclerosis to surgical management. In W.A. Dale (ed.), *Management of Arterial Occlusive Disease.* Chicago: Year Book Medical Publishers, 1971. *(Excellent review of certain aspects of natural history and collateral circulation which enter into selection of patients for operation.)*

Imparato, A.M., Kim, G.E., Davidson, T., and Crowley, J.G.: Intermittent claudication: Its natural course. Surgery, *78*:795, 1975. *(Study of 104 claudicators with angiographic control. Over a 6-month to 8-year follow-up, 79 per cent remained stable or improved, and only 5.8 per cent came to amputation; 25 per cent eventually underwent arterial reconstruction.)*

Intermittent claudication (editorial): Brit. Med. J., *1*:1165, May 15, 1976. *(An appropriately con-*

servative review of the limited value of therapy available for claudication.)

Juergens, J.L., Barker, N.W., and Hines, E.A.: Arteriosclerosis obliterans: Review of 520 cases with special reference to pathogenic and prognostic factors. Circulation, *21*:188, 1960. *(General review of factors applying to natural history. Of patients who continued to smoke, 11.4 per cent required amputation during the 5-year period, while none who stopped smoking had an amputation.)*

Larsen, O.A., and Lassen, N.A.: Effects of daily muscular exercise in patients with intermittent claudication. Lancet, *1*:1093, 1966. *(Controlled study showing benefit of exercise. No measurable increase in blood flow could be documented, however.)*

McAllister, F.F.: The fate of patients with intermittent claudication managed nonoperatively. Am. J. Surg., *132*:593, 1976. *(A study of 100 patients with intermittent claudication followed for an average of 6 years; 78 per cent either improved or remained stable. The study argues for restraint in bypass grafting.)*

Peabody, C.N., Kannel, W.B., and McNamara, P.M.: Intermittent claudication: Surgical significance. Arch. Surg., *109*:693, 1974. *(Study of Framingham cohort with claudication followed an average of 8.3 years. Only 5 per cent progressed to amputation, and 81 per cent remained stable or improved. Effect of various risk factors on significant cardiovascular morbidity and mortality is emphasized.)*

Raines, J.K., Darling, R.C., Buth, J., Brewster, D.C., Austen, W.G.: Vascular laboratory criteria for the management of peripheral vascular disease of the lower extremities. Surgery, 79:21, 1976. *(Description of noninvasive methods and criteria useful for clinical management of vascular patients, from original work at Massachusetts General Hospital.)*

Siperstein, M.D., Foster, D.W., Knowles, H.C., et al.: Control of blood glucose and diabetic vascular disease. Editorial. N. Engl. J. Med., 296:1060, 1977. *(Presents the data arguing that tight control of blood sugar does not prevent occurrence of vascular complications.)*

30

Management of Venous Disease
DAVID C. BREWSTER, M.D.

Problems of the venous system (varicose veins, venous insufficiency and phlebitis) are extremely common and a cause of much misery. Many physicians do little for the more mundane complaints attributable to the venous system because they are poorly informed regarding pathophysiology and proper management. Such incomplete knowledge is unfortunate, because neglected venous problems can cause considerable disability and even become life-threatening. The primary management of venous diseases is still largely nonoperative, and great benefit is possible with well-conceived office care.

PATHOPHYSIOLOGY AND CLINICAL PRESENTATIONS

The high frequency of venous disorders of the lower extremities is unique to man and undoubtedly reflects the consequences of an upright posture and the effects of gravity. In order to return blood from the periphery to the right heart, the venous system in the legs must work against the forces of gravity without the aid of organs specifically designed for this purpose. A number of factors act to lessen venous pressure in the leg and propel blood toward the heart; these include the "muscular pump" effect of the exercising calf musculature, the negative intrathoracic pressure created by the "bellows effect" of the chest wall with respiration, and the presence of multiple valves in both superficial and deep venous systems. The valves prevent reflux of blood and serve to reduce pressure in the veins that would otherwise equal the weight of an uninterrupted column of blood from the heart to the foot (approximately 100 mm. Hg).

A knowledge of basic anatomy of the venous system is vital to evaluation and management of lower extremity venous problems. The existence of two venous systems, superficial and deep, is well known. A third system that links the superficial and deep systems, the communicating or perforating veins, is less well recognized but of great importance. Valves also exist in the communicating veins, permitting flow from the superficial to the deep system but preventing retrograde flow.

When they are functioning properly, these three systems operate in a coordinated manner. The deep system, comprised of paired anterior and posterior tibial and peroneal veins, popliteal veins, and superficial and deep femoral veins, accommodates approximately 80 to 90 per cent of venous return; the superficial network of greater and lesser saphenous systems is much less important in this respect.

Clinical disorders of the venous system usually stem from obstruction to venous return due to thrombosis of the vein lumen, or from incompetent venous valves which allow reflux of blood and persistent elevation of venous pressure in the leg and foot.

Varicose Veins

Because the superficial venous system is located in the subcutaneous tissue and lacks the support afforded by muscle and fascial compartments, it is most prone to difficulty. Varicose veins are extremely common and probably affect some 10 to 20 per cent of the adult population. They are more common in women, who also seem more likely to consult a physician for advice.

A family history of varicosities is present in the majority of patients with venous disease, which lends support to the concept of a hereditary or congenital etiology. It is unclear whether the primary problem is a congenital incompetence of valves or a weakness of the venous wall itself that causes dilatation of the vein lumen and subsequent valve inadequacy. In either case, a self-perpetuating cycle is established in which venous reflux leads to further vein dilatation and valve failure, which in turn causes still more reflux. In time, the poorly supported superficial veins widen, elongate, and become tortuous. In a small percentage of patients, the initial defect may be in the communicating veins, where poorly functioning valves allow abnormal flow toward the superficial system, causing eventual overdistension. In other patients, acquired factors such as previous trauma or venous thrombosis may play a role. Factors that raise intraluminal vein pressure, such as repeated pregnancies, obesity, or wearing tight garments that constrict the thigh, may be of importance. Nevertheless, the common element in all of these conditions remains valvular incompetence.

Varicosities most commonly involve the greater saphenous system or its tributaries thus producing symptoms and signs in the medial and anterior thigh and calf region and less frequently in the medial ankle or instep area of the foot. The lesser saphenous system may also be involved, producing varicosities of the posterior calf and lateral ankle region. The exact distribution of involved branches is of importance only when surgical correction is being considered.

The presenting symptoms of varicose veins are extremely variable, and often seem to bear little relationship to the apparent severity of the varicosities. It is well recognized that complaints are more frequent in women, particularly young women at the time of the menstrual period. Clearly, hormonal factors that favor fluid retention may aggravate venous distension. Concern over the cosmetic appearance of minor varicosities may also trigger a visit to the physician.

Typically, patients complain of local aching or burning pain in the area of the varicosities, particularly at the end of the day after having been on their feet at work. Tiredness, heaviness, or a bursting sensation are common. Itchiness due to a stasis dermatitis may occur in the region of a severe and chronic varix, especially in the region of an incompetent perforating vein. Mild swelling in the ankle region may occur; however, this is relatively unusual with uncomplicated varicose veins. Similarly, ulceration due to primary varicose veins is rare. Severe swelling or recurrent ulceration almost always implies problems with the deep venous system.

Large varices may be subject to trauma and bleeding. Much more commonly, however, a thrombus may form in a distended vein with sluggish blood flow and present as a superficial phlebitis.

Chronic Venous Insufficiency

Chronic venous insufficiency, also called the postphlebitic syndrome, is a common chronic disorder that is particularly disabling if stubborn venous ulcers develop. The principal defect lies in the deep venous system; varicose veins of the superficial venous system may develop secondarily.

Although a documented history of deep venous thrombosis can be obtained in less than one half of patients with chronic venous insufficiency, this is felt to be the etiology in most instances. Deep venous thrombosis may be clinically silent, as documented by prospective I^{125}-fibrinogen scanning studies in postoperative patients. Despite subsequent recanalization of deep venous occlusions, venous valves in the deep system become incompetent, leading to reflux and increased venous pressure. Similar valvular incompetence may also develop in communicating veins due to valvular damage or simply by exposure to chronically elevated pressure from the deep venous system. Some authorities feel congenital valvular incompetence may also play a role. Regardless of cause, high venous pressure generated by muscular contraction forces blood through damaged valves in communicating veins toward the superficial system, resulting in "ambulatory venous hypertension." Such venous hypertension results in edema, usually most prominent in the calf and ankle region. Swelling of the thigh may occur, denoting valvular incompetence at the ileofemoral level as well. This edema is usually less severe and less troublesome than that of the lower leg; it is one of the hallmarks of chronic venous insufficiency and clearly differentiates the problem from simple varicose veins.

Venous hypertension leads not only to interstitial fluid accumulation, but also to extravasation of plasma proteins and red blood cells into subcutaneous tissues. In time, this results in brawny induration of the skin and pigmentation of the thickened but fragile tissue. The presence of edema and continual high venous pressure results in reduced local capillary flow and relative hypoxia, and further increases the likelihood of tissue breakdown and subsequent healing difficulties. Eventually these processes and accompanying infection lead to damage of the lymphatics, aggravating swelling and local tissue breakdown.

The presenting complaints of patients with chronic venous insufficiency usually result from swelling or ulceration of the lower leg. Chronic recurrent swelling causes a sensation of tightness or bursting, as well as heaviness or aching of the limb. Naturally, this is often worst at the end of the day and may largely disappear overnight.

Thrombophlebitis

The cause of acute thrombus formation in the venous system is often unclear, but in most instances circumstances contributing to the three basic elements of Virchow's triad (intimal damage, stasis and hypercoagulability) can be identified. *Superficial thrombophlebitis* almost always occurs in varicose veins and is clearly a result of stasis in these channels. Trauma may occasionally be implicated. In the upper limbs, the cause is most often iatrogenic following intravenous cannulation. On examination, there will be pain and tenderness along the course of the vein,

which may also be palpated as a tender cord or knot. There is often a local inflammatory erythema.

Superficial thrombophlebitis that occurs in several locations over a short time span is sometimes called *migratory superficial phlebitis*. It can be an important clue to occult malignancy, especially adenocarcinoma of the pancreas. A hypercoagulable state seems to occur due to the tumor.

Deep venous thrombophlebitis is notoriously more variable in its clinical presentation than superficial thrombophlebitis. Although most authorities no longer emphasize the distinction between thrombophlebitis and phlebothrombosis, there may be considerable differences in presenting complaints and physical findings. In phlebothrombosis, extensive deep venous clot may be present in limbs with little or no pain, swelling, or tenderness. Thrombophlebitis often produces marked clinical symptoms and signs; classically, the patient complains of pain in the limb that is worse with motion, walking or dependency and better with rest or elevation. There is frequently some swelling below the level of venous occlusion and tenderness upon calf compression. Calf pain produced by dorsiflexion of the foot (Homans' sign), is a classic finding, but often it is lacking. With extensive deep venous thrombosis, there may be a dusky cyanosis. Engorged or prominent superficial veins may be apparent and are highly suggestive of deep venous obstruction.

EVALUATION

Varicose Veins

In the physical examination, the extent and location of the varicosities should be noted, and, more important, signs possibly indicating pathology in the deep venous system, such as stasis changes, ulceration, and swelling. Complaints of pain should be carefully evaluated to rule out other possible contributing causes in addition to the obvious varicosities, such as arterial insufficiency, orthopedic or joint disorders or neurologic problems. Severe varicosities that occur at a young age or follow trauma indicate the possibility of an arteriovenous fistula, which may be further suggested by auscultation of a bruit.

Venous Insufficiency

A prior history of deep vein thrombosis suggests chronic venous insufficiency. This condition needs to be distinguished from other causes of leg edema, such as obstruction to lymphatic drainage or hypoalbuminemia (see Chapter 16). Moreover, leg ulcerations may be due to chronic arterial disease, which also needs to be ruled out by inquiry into claudication that involves thigh or calf, rest pain that is relieved by dependency, and presence of numbness or paresthesias. On examination, arterial disease is manifested by absence of palpable pulses, dependent rubor, and atrophic changes as well as by ulceration. Bruits may be heard in the groin. If there remains a question of arterial disease, ultrasound flow and pressure studies should be obtained (see Chapter 17).

Thrombophlebitis

Superficial thrombophlebitis. Cellulitis and lymphangitis may resemble superficial thrombophlebitis. Both conditions can be distinguished from superficial thrombophlebitis by the absence of a palpable thrombosed vein, more widespread distribution of erythema and swelling not confined to the course of a vein, and identification of a possible focus of infection. Other musculoskeletal causes of pain and tenderness should be sought, as well as possible neurologic disorders such as neuritis or radicular pain which may cause confusion. Any generalized swelling in the extremity should also be carefully noted, because isolated superficial phlebitis does not contribute to generalized edema.

Deep vein thrombophlebitis. An accurate initial evaluation of patients with pain or swelling of one or both legs is of great importance, because deep venous thrombosis may lead to embolization. Differential diagnosis includes an extensive list of problems that may cause pain or swelling of the extremities. Truly unilateral swelling, particularly extending above the knee, indicates an increased likelihood of venous thrombosis, but cellulitis or lymphedema must be considered. Pain alone is a rather unreliable sign. The findings of calf tenderness and a Homans' sign are by no means conclusive. Numerous studies have now demonstrated the relative inaccuracy of diagnosis by clinical examination, which has been found to be incorrect in up to 50 per cent of cases.

The difficulty in evaluation of suspected deep venous thrombosis is the lack of reliable clinical findings. The use of recently developed, quite sensitive noninvasive screening techniques for deep venous thrombosis can be of help in selecting patients who should undergo venography. These methods include I^{125}-fibrinogen scanning, plethysmography and ultrasonic flow velocity detection (Doppler). A detailed evaluation of the advantages of each method is beyond the scope of this chapter, and obviously much will depend upon local availability of various techniques. One of the advantages of combined use of Doppler testing and venous outflow studies by cuff plethysmography is that the determination can be made immediately, whereas isotope must be given 24 hours in advance of I^{125} scanning.

If noninvasive testing strongly suggests a diagnosis of deep venous thrombosis, anticoagulant therapy may be initiated, but it is usually best to confirm the diagnosis by venography, which remains the definitive diagnostic method. If screening tests are negative and clinical suspicion is not high, the patient can be closely followed in the office and treated symptomatically. As noninvasive techniques improve, it is hoped that such methods will be of increasing use to the clinician in these difficult management decisions. The necessity of firmly establishing the diagnosis by methods other than history and physical examination cannot be overemphasized.

PRINCIPLES OF MANAGEMENT, THERAPEUTIC RECOMMENDATIONS, PATIENT EDUCATION AND INDICATIONS FOR REFERRAL

Varicose Veins

Management of varicose veins can very often be satisfactorily accomplished by nonoperative means, if attention is directed to the principal problems of valve incompetence and poor soft tissue support. Untreated, most varicose veins will slowly worsen, and may progress to causing discomfort and disability. Almost all patients will benefit from proper *elastic support* of medium weight, together with periodic *elevation* of the involved extremity during the day. Elastic support is best achieved by a properly fitted surgical stocking obtained from a hospital or commercial surgical company such as Jobst. The various stockings sold in department or drug stores are usually too light in weight and do not fit properly. Ace wraps are cumbersome and are often applied improperly, creating a "tourniquet" effect at the knee level. In almost all instances it is good practice to utilize only a below-the-knee stocking, because proper compression is difficult to achieve in the thigh, the stockings are difficult to keep up, and patient compliance is considerably lessened. Fortunately, varicosities in the thigh are much less often associated with symptoms or complications.

In addition, obese patients are urged to *lose weight*. Women are reminded to *avoid* the use of *tight garters* or panty girdles that will constrict superficial venous return at the thigh level. *Prolonged standing* should be avoided as much as is feasible.

Sclerotherapy has some advocates, but it is not currently in wide use. A sclerosing solution, such as 3 per cent Sotradecol is injected into the vein lumen and a pressure dressing applied and maintained for several weeks. An inflammatory reaction causing eventual fibrosis and obliteration of the vein lumen is hoped for. Although some occasionally employ this treatment for a small isolated varix, particularly a residual vein following surgical therapy, sclerotherapy is not indicated in the primary treatment of varicose veins.

Indications for *surgical referral* include persistently symptomatic varicose veins (particularly if a conservative program has failed), cosmetic dissatisfaction, or recurrent episodes of superficial thrombophlebitis. The option of surgery should probably be discussed before any treatment is initiated because some patients, particularly young women, will prefer surgery to chronic use of elastic support. In most instances of primary varicose veins, an excellent result can be expected from surgery. Operative morbidity is extremely low and only 2 to 3 days of hospitalization are required. In experienced hands, the "recurrence" rate of varicose veins is less than 10 per cent.

Venous Insufficiency

Treatment for venous insufficiency is best initiated prior to the occurrence of leg ulceration, which develops in many untreated cases. Again, elastic support and periodic elevation of the extremity are essential. Informing the patient of the rationale for therapy is likely to improve compliance. A *knee-length heavyweight elastic stocking* is prescribed and must be worn religiously from the moment the patient gets out of bed until he retires at night. The leg is best elevated on a pillow or by raising the foot of the bed. *Periodic elevation* during the day is essential for most patients; it must be emphasized to the patient that the leg should be above the level of the heart for elevation to be effective. Elevation must be done as often as necessary to prevent formation of edema. *Mild diuretic therapy* (e.g., 50 mg. of hydrochlorothiazide) may be of some help in lessening edema that still persists.

The chronic nature of venous insufficiency must be made clear to the patient, while reassurance is given that symptoms can be controlled and often prevented by careful adherence to the therapeutic program.

Progression of disease to the point of *ulcer formation* creates a much more troublesome problem. The ulcers may occur with even minor and unrecalled trauma due to the atrophic and vulnerable skin and subcutaneous tissues. Ulcers often develop in the lower medial leg just above the medial malleolus, usually overlying an incompetent communicating vein. These lesions will be refractory to all methods of care as long as the venous hypertension of the incompetent deep system continues to be transmitted to the superficial tissues. Secondary infection (bacterial or fungal) is common, further impairing any chance for local tissue repair.

Management at this stage is much more difficult, time-consuming, and often expensive. The preferred treatment is an extended period of bed rest with elevation of the involved extremity well above heart level at all times, combined with application of *wet to dry saline dressings* to the skin ulcer, three times daily. Such a program can usually be carried out at home by the family, perhaps with the help of a visiting nurse. Healing may take 2 to 4 weeks. Hospitalization is generally not necessary unless dictated by social circumstances or a failure of home treatment. Any skin infection should be cultured and treated with appropriate oral antibiotics. The patient should be urged to exercise the calf muscles repeatedly while in bed, ideally against a footboard, in order to minimize the possibility of acute deep venous thrombosis.

An alternative for patients who cannot afford extensive time off their feet is use of an *Unna paste venous boot*. Properly applied, this medicated bandage affords good compression, does not require much patient cooperation, and allows the patient to remain ambulatory. Such boot dressings are best changed every 7 to 10 days. Many venous ulcers may be successfully handled in this manner. Once the ulcer is healed, long-term use of a heavyweight elastic stocking is resumed.

Surgical referral is indicated for patients with recurrent or nonhealing ulcerations. Surgical interruption of incompetent communicating veins underlying the ulcer, together with stripping and ligation of associated superficial varicosities, may be indicated. Nevertheless, most cases of venous insufficiency may be adequately managed in the office by nonoperative means.

Thrombophlebitis

Superficial thrombophlebitis in the lower leg is best managed by a combination of local heat and compression with a good elastic stocking. Anti-inflammatory agents such as aspirin or indomethacin may be useful. Antibiotics have no role. Young women on birth control pills should discontinue their use. The patient is advised to avoid sitting or standing, but should remain ambulatory in order to minimize the chance of developing associated clot in the deep venous system. Pain and inflammation usually resolve within 1 to 2 weeks.

If superficial phlebitis extends above the knee, consideration of anticoagulant therapy or ligation of the saphenous vein at the level of the saphenofemoral junction in the groin may be indicated, and surgical consultation should be considered. This is particularly important if the process has ascended while under treatment and observation, because there is an increased risk of extension of the thrombus into the deep system.

Deep vein thrombophlebitis requires immediate hospitalization for heparinization and initiation of oral anticoagulant therapy. Warfarin is usually continued for about 6 months after hospital discharge (see Chapter 84).

ANNOTATED BIBLIOGRAPHY

Couch, N.P. (ed.): AMA Archives symposium on diagnostic techniques in phlebothrombosis. Arch. Surg., *104*:132, 1972. *(A good review by several experts of various techniques applicable to diagnosis of deep venous thrombosis.)*

Crombley, J.J., Canos, A.J., and Sull, W.J.: The diagnosis of deep venous thrombosis. Arch. Surg., *111*:34, 1976. *(Documentation of the inaccuracy of clinical diagnosis.)*

Dale, W.A.: The swollen leg. Curr. Probl. Surg., September 1973. *(Excellent monograph discussing differential diagnosis, pathophysiology, and treatment.)*

Hobb, J.J.: Surgery and sclerotherapy in the treatment of varicose veins. Arch. Surg., *109*:793, 1974. *(A good review of the advantages and proper indications for the use of each modality.)*

Linton, R.R.: Postthrombotic ulceration of the lower extermity: Its etiology and surgical management. Ann. Surg., *138*:415, 1953. *(Classic article on the etiology and management of venous ulcerations.)*

Lofgren, E.P., and Lofgren, K.A.: Alternatives in the management of varices. Geriatrics, *30*:111, 1975. *(Good summary of treatment options.)*

31

Exercise Stress Testing

The exercise stress test has become a widely employed method for detection of coronary artery disease. Assessments of exercise capacity, ventricular dysrhythmias, and severity of coronary disease can also be accomplished by stress testing. At present, the predominant method of stress testing is continuous ECG monitoring of the patient as he walks on a treadmill or pedals a bicycle. Thallium imaging techniques are being explored to improve upon ECG recording for detection of coronary disease. The primary physician needs to know the sensitivity, specificity, and predictive value of the ECG stress test and the factors that affect these parameters in order to appropriately order the study and properly interpret its results.

PHYSIOLOGICAL BASIS OF THE TEST

The exercise stress test provides an indication of the ability of the coronary circulation to supply the heart with sufficient blood to meet the increase in oxygen demand generated by exercise. Since myocardial oxygen extraction is relatively fixed, increased supply must be achieved by increased blood flow. When stenosis limits adequate blood supply, ischemia may result, often manifested by anginal pain and/or ECG changes. The demand made on the coronary circulation can be quantitated; the product of heart rate times systolic blood pressure closely parallels the measured oxygen consumption during isotonic exercise. Heart rate alone is almost as good an indicator of oxygen consumption. Since known quantities of work are being performed, the exercise stress test can provide a measure of exercise capacity as well as aid in detection of coronary disease.

STRESS TEST METHODOLOGIES

Exercise testing for detection of coronary disease utilizes dynamic (isotonic) rather than sustained-contraction (isometric) exercise, because isometric exercise produces lesser increases in heart rate, anginal pain and ST segment changes and greater increases in systolic blood pressure and frequency of ventricular dysrhythmias.

Isotonic testing protocols are divided into maximal and submaximal types, the difference being the criteria for termination of the test. *Submaximal* protocols usually require the patient to perform sufficient activity to achieve a target heart rate, in most instances 85 per cent of the age-predicted maximum. The *maximal* protocols have the patient continue exercising until onset of fatigue, dyspnea, chest pain, hypotension, arrhythmias or ischemic ECG changes. Submaximal testing is less commonly employed because it gives less accurate information regarding exercise capacity (the end point is artificial). It was believed by some that submaximal testing would be safer than maximal studies, but morbidity and mortality figures do not support this view. In fact, because the target heart rate for submaximal testing is a percentage of a theoretical maximum for *normal* persons, the level may actually be far in excess of what a patient with coronary disease is capable of; the designation "submaximal" may be a bit of a misnomer.

Most maximal and submaximal tests are multistage, i.e., graded amounts of work are performed, with the work load progressively increased. The objective of grading exercise is to obtain the greatest increase in heart rate that is possible before onset of musculoskeletal fatigue limits the amount of exercise that the patient can perform. The previously used Master's exercise test was a single stage test in which the intensity and amount of exercise were fixed; the test had a high rate of false-negative results because many patients did not sufficiently increase their heart rates during the performance of the test. Another disadvantage of Master's test was its inability to provide continuous ECG monitoring; cardiograms were taken before and after exercise only, often reducing the amount of information available from the test.

Currently the treadmill and bicycle are the most popular devices used for exercise testing. The bicycle has the advantage of producing less electrode interference, but the patient is able to vary the work load by changing the velocity of pedaling, thus potentially compromising the reproducibility of the test and reducing maximum oxygen consumption. The advantage of the treadmill test is that work load is observer-controlled and may provide more reproducible results. In both treadmill and bicycle tests, these is continuous ECG monitoring. A modified V_5 lead (CM_5) is the most commonly employed single lead. Test sensitivity can be increased by employing a three-lead system, since the CM_5 lead may not detect inferior ischemic changes. Because ischemic changes may not occur on ECG until after exercise, monitoring is continued for 5 to 7 minutes immediately following exercise.

SENSITIVITY, SPECIFICITY, AND PREDICTIVE VALUE[*]

Myocardial ischemia may be manifested during the stress test by ECG changes, abnormal blood pressure and heart rate responses, or chest pain. ECG changes, particularly the alterations in ST segments that occur on exercise in the context of ischemia, have received the most attention and study. Sensitivity and specificity of ST segment changes have been determined by correlating ECG findings with results obtained from subjecting the same patients to coronary angiography.

A number of factors affect sensitivity and specificity of the stress test, including severity of the underlying coronary disease and ECG criteria used for diagnosis of ischemia. For example, test sensitivity using the criterion of ST segment depression increased in one study from 40 to 76 per cent as the extent of disease went from one-vessel involvement to three-vessel stenosis. The magnitude of ST segment depression required for diagnosis affects sensitivity and specificity. One can achieve an increase in sensitivity by reducing the amount of ST depression necessary for the designation of ischemia, but at the cost of lowering specificity and obtaining more false-positive results. An analysis of pooled data showed that when the criterion for a diagnosis of ischemia was 1.0 to 1.5 mm. of ST depression, sensitivity was 23.3 per cent and specificity 89 per cent; when the amount of ST depression required was raised to 1.5

*For definitions of these terms, see Chapter 2.

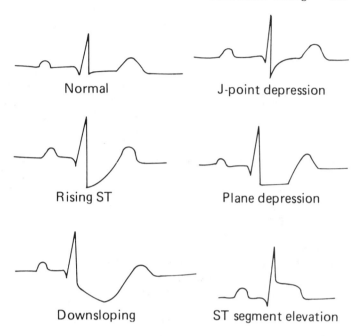

Normal   J-point depression

Rising ST   Plane depression

Downsloping   ST segment elevation

FIGURE 31–1 Exercise-induced ST-segment changes

to 2.0 mm. range, sensitivity fell to 8.8 per cent, but specificity rose to 97.8 per cent. This constant trade-off between sensitivity and specificity is characteristic of all tests having a quantitative standard for diagnosis (see Chapter 2).

Other aspects of ST segment change have been examined to improve sensitivity and specificity. Configuration of the ST segment has been subjected to careful study. A downsloping ST segment (see Fig. 31-1) was found to have a specificity of 99 per cent. Horizontal or plane depression of the ST had a specificity of 85 per cent, and a slowly upsloping ST (greater than or equal to 1.5 mm. ST depression at 0.08 sec. after the J point) had a specificity of 68 per cent. Simple J-point depression without a slowly upsloping ST is very nonspecific and not used as a diagnostic criterion. When the criterion for an ischemic response was at least 1 mm. of downsloping or horizontal ST segment depression, the stress test was found to have a sensitivity of 64 per cent and a specificity of 93 per cent. When a slowly upsloping ST was added to the list of acceptable criteria for ischemia, sensitivity increased to 76 per cent, but at the expense of specificity, which fell to 82 per cent.

A number of other factors alter the sensitivity and specificity of the ECG stress test, including the type of exercise protocol used (submaximal tests appear to be less sensitive) and the number of leads used (a three-lead system improves sensitivity by about 10 per cent over a single lead system). The specificity of ST changes is limited by the fact that ST depression is not unique to coronary disease. Patients with valvular, hypertensive, and nonischemic myocardial disease may demonstrate ST segment depression on exercise. In addition, recent glucose ingestion, hypokalemia, and sedatives may produce false-positive results. Digitalis is notorious for its ability to cause changes in ST segments.

Investigators have searched for other changes that occur during the ECG stress test which might help to better identify patients with coronary disease. The changes in ST segments which occur with exercise do not provide a definite answer, but rather a probability statement of the likelihood of the patient's having coronary disease. Among other variables studied have been timing and duration of ST changes, presence and severity of ventricular dysrhythmias, heart rate and blood pressure changes, and coexistence of exercise-induced chest pain. In a recent series of 302 patients undergoing stress testing and coronary angiography, the occurrence of typical angina during exercise had a sensitivity of 51 per cent and specificity of 90 per cent, compared with 76 per cent sensitivity and 76 per cent specificity for ECG changes alone. In essence, exercise-induced angina had about the same significance for diagnosis as did ST changes, especially when predictive values for these changes in the appropriate population were compared. A study that factored in all the possible exercise-induced variables that might help predict the presence of coronary disease (ST configuration, depth of ST depression, timing of onset and duration of ST changes, occurrence of hypotension or inappropriately slow heart rate, and presence of malignant ventricular irritability) found only a 10 to 15 per cent increase in test accuracy compared to that obtained by analyzing degree of ST segment depression alone. Some investigators are examining R wave changes to see if these might contribute meaningfully.

Knowledge of test sensitivity and specificity and attempts to improve them still do not provide the clinician with an estimate of the probability that coronary disease is present when a positive test result is encountered, i.e., the predictive accuracy or predictive value positive of the test. Figures for the predictive accuracy of the exercise stress test have varied greatly from series to series, and between men and women, because the prevalence of underlying coronary disease has probably differed widely in the populations studied. The predictive accuracy of any diagnostic test is directly related to the prevalence of the disease in the population examined (see Chapter 2). As a result, a test is going to have a low predictive accuracy when disease prevalence is low, regardless of how sensitive and specific the test is.

Asymptomatic patients who are subjected to stress testing and demonstrate "ischemic" changes are unlikely to have underlying coronary disease and much more likely to have a false-positive test. In asymptomatic populations, the incidence of coronary disease is about 6 percent, rising to 12 per cent by the sixth decade. Prevalence of coronary disease has been found to be 16 per cent in patients with nonanginal chest pain, 50 per cent in those with atypical pain and 89 per cent when typical angina is present. Consequently, the predictive value of a positive test can be expected to be greatest in patients with typical angina, but in such instances the history of angina is almost as good as the test's predictive value (about 90 per cent) in diagnosing coronary disease. The very high figures initially reported for the diagnostic utility and accuracy of the stress test resulted from studies conducted on a referred population that had a high probability of coronary disease in the opinion of their referring physicians; these were the people in whom angiography was deemed most appropriate.

In sum, the stress test is of little use for the diagnosis of coronary disease in patients with typical angina and cannot be used to rule out the diagnosis. Likewise, stress testing of asymptomatic patients will produce many more false-positives than true-positives and cause much needless concern; a negative test result will contribute little to what is already known. The test may be of help in diagnosis of patients with atypical anginal pain as long as the criteria for atypical pain are rather rigid (e.g., two or three characteristics of classic angina are present) though other features may be absent. In such settings, the predictive accuracy has been in the order to 40 to 50 per cent.

Further attempts to improve upon the stress test have led to development of imaging techniques, such as use of thallium, which behaves like potassium. Ischemic areas of myocardium are slow to take up the radionuclide; scans of such regions show decreased uptake that gradually normalizes, reflecting the decrease in blood supply but viability of the myocardium. Initial results regarding sensitivity and specificity are encouraging, but again the key issue is proper patient selection. It is too early in the development of this technique to make firm statements regarding its use; it has proven helpful in patients with resting ST abnormalities that render results of ECG stress testing difficult to interpret and in patients with suspected false-positive ECG stress tests.

OTHER APPLICATIONS OF EXERCISE TESTING

1. Severity of known coronary disease can be assessed by exercise stress testing. Factors correlating with severity and extensiveness of disease include depth of ST segment depression, early onset of ST changes, persistence of ST segment depression past 8 minutes into the recovery period, downward sloping ST configuration, hypotensive response at low work loads and impairment of heart rate response to exercise. In addition, occurrence of both angina and ischemic changes during exercise have been reported to predict an increased likelihood of multivessel disease. Recently, increase in R wave amplitude has been implicated as a sign of two- or three-vessel disease.

2. Assessment of prognosis of patients in the early postinfarction period may be aided by exercise testing. The greater the work load tolerated, the better the prognosis. Patients who developed angina on a limited stress test conducted just prior to hospital discharge had twice the rate of postinfarction angina. Those with no ST segment changes had a 2.1 per cent 1-year mortality, compared with a 27 per cent mortality for those who did develop ST segment depression during stress testing.

3. Determination of exercise capacity can be provided by the exercise stress test, since the patient is made to perform known quanities of work under direct observation and continuous ECG monitoring. This determination is essential for design of a safe cardiac rehabilitation program and may help to reassure the patient who is unnecessarily restricting his activity out of fear of sudden death or infarction. The work level achieved in the test can be used to define the degree of incapacity (when it is in question) as well as provide guidelines for establishing safe levels of activity which the patient can engage in on a daily basis.

4. Detection of ventricular dysrhythmias can sometimes be facilitated by stress testing, especially if the rhythm disturbance is felt to be exercise-induced. However, except in a few cases of ventricular tachycardia, Holter monitoring (ambulatory ECG monitoring) was found in a careful study to be better for detection of most types of ventricular irritability (see Chapters 20 and 24). Holter monitoring should be ordered in conjunction with an exercise test if the objective is optimal detection of dysrhythmias.

SAFETY AND CONTRAINDICATIONS

Reported mortality in a multicenter study involving 170,000 tests was 0.01 per cent. There was no relationship to type or severity of test. Morbidity requiring hospitalization was 0.2 per cent. Safety is enhanced by a preexamination history, a physical examination, and a resting ECG. Patients with unstable angina, recent infarction, congestive failure, severe anemia, high-grade heart block, severe aortic stenosis, cor pulmonale or severe hypertension should not undergo testing. A physician should be present throughout, and a defibrillator and other resuscitation equipment should be in the room. The test should be terminated if blood pressure or heart rate falls suddenly during exercise, or if exhaustion, angina, faintness, marked ST changes or serious arrhythmias occur (ventricular tachycardia, heart block, etc.).

ANNOTATED BIBLIOGRAPHY

Bartel, A.G., Behar, U.S., Peter, U.S., et al.: Graded exercise stress tests in angiographically documented coronary artery disease. Circulation, 49: 348, 1974. (The depth of ST-segment depression correlated with severity and extent of coronary disease.)

Bruce, R.A.: Methods of exercise testing. Am. J. Cardiol., 33:715, 1974. (A concise and thorough discussion of the differences in various methods of stress testing by one of the pioneers in the field.)

Cohn, K., Kamm, B., Feteih, N., et al.: Use of treadmill score to quantify ischemic response and predict extent of coronary disease. Circulation, 59: 286, 1979. (Test accuracy using a multifactorial analysis was improved by only 10 to 15 per cent over that achieved by use of ST criteria alone for evaluation of stress test results. Factors studied in the analysis included duration and onset of ST changes, blood pressure and heart rate responses, coexistence of exercise-induced chest pain, severity of ventricular irritability and magnitude and configuration of ST-segment changes.)

Ellestad, M.H., Cooke, B.M., and Greenberg, P.S.: Stress testing: Clinical application and predictive capacity. Prog. Cardiovasc. Dis., 21:431, 1979. (A worthwhile review with emphasis on specificity, sensitivity and predictive value of the stress test. Also discusses recent work on utility of R wave changes in test interpretation. 144 refs.)

Epstein, S.E.: Value and limitations of the electrocardiographic response to exercise in the assessment of patients with coronary artery disease. Am. J. Cardiol., 42:667, 1978. (Argues that the predictive value of the stress test is so low in asymptomatic patients that the test should not be used to screen for coronary disease. Agrees on its judicious use in symptomatic patients for providing information on prognosis and severity.)

Fortuin, N.J., and Weiss, J.A.: Exercise stress testing. Circulation, 56:699, 1977. (Excellent, detailed review with 126 references.)

Goldschlager, N., Selzer, A., and Cohn, K.: Treadmill tests as indicators of presence and severity of coronary artery disease. Ann. Intern. Med., 85:277, 1976. (A study of 269 patients with angiographically proven coronary disease. The configuration, time of onset, and duration of ST-segment depression correlated with presence and severity of coronary disease.)

Martin, C.M., and McConahay, D.R.: Maximum treadmill exercise electrocardiography. Circulation, 46:956, 1972. (Provides data on the changes in sensitivity and specificity associated with different diagnostic criteria. When 0.5 mm. ST de-

pression is used, false-positive rate equals 43 per cent and falls to 11 per cent with 1.0 mm. criteria.)

Rifkin, R.D., and Hood, W.B.: Bayesian analysis of electrocardiographic exercise stress testing. N. Engl. J. Med., *297*:681, 1977. *(Argues that the results of the stress test should be viewed as a probability statement, rather than as "positive" or "negative"; emphasizes the predictive value of various test results and the dependence of the predictive value on the prevalence of the disease in the population being studied.)*

Theroux, P.T., Waters, D.D., Halphen, C., *et al.*: Prognostic value of exercise testing soon after myocardial infarction. N. Engl. J. Med., *301*:341, 1979. *(Performance of a limited treadmill test just prior to hospital discharge provided useful prognostic information.)*

Weiner, D.A., Ryan, T.J., McCabe, C.H., *et al*:. Exercise stress testing. N. Engl. J. Med., *301*:230, 1979. *(A detailed study of data from the Coronary Artery Surgery Study examining the influence of the prevalence of coronary artery disease on the diagnostic accuracy of stress testing.)*

Weiner, D.A., McCabe, C., Heuter, D.C., *et al.*: The predictive value of anginal chest pain as an indicator of coronary disease during exercise testing. Am Heart J., *96*:458, 1978. *(The occurrence of anginal pain during exercise was found to be as predictive of coronary disease as ischemic ECG changes alone.)*

4

Respiratory Problems

32
Health Consequences of Smoking

Smoking has justifiably been called the most common self-inflicted injury. Epidemiologic and experimental information accumulated over the past 30 years has identified cigarette smoking as the primary cause of chronic obstructive pulmonary disease and lung cancer, and one of the most important risk factors for coronary disease. Despite efforts to inform the public of these dangers, millions continue to smoke. Because antismoking methods have been only moderately successful, some physicians have become somewhat nihilistic about their role. However, there is evidence indicating that personal health education from the primary care provider can be effective. Attempting to educate and change the behavior of smokers should be a high priority of the primary physician (see Chapter 49).

Epidemiology and Risk Factors

Between 30 and 35 per cent of American adults are smokers. Smoking has fallen off since 1955, when 68 per cent of the male population and 37 per cent of the female population over age 18 were smoking. Factors that influence the decision to smoke have not been well-characterized. Parental smoking habits have been shown to have a significant impact on the smoking status of young adults. Factors that influence the decision to quit smoking are discussed in Chapter 49.

Smoking as a Risk Factor for Premature Morbidity and Mortality

In 1964, the Surgeon General's report indicated that the death rate among male smokers was 68 per cent higher than that among nonsmoking males. Excess mortality was due to lung cancer, chronic obstructive pulmonary disease, coronary artery disease and cancers of the larynx, oral cavity and esophagus. Subsequent epidemiologic and experimental studies have confirmed the link between smoking and these common diseases.

Coronary artery disease. A strong relationship between cigarette smoking and coronary morbidity and mortality has been demonstrated by both retrospective and prospective epidemiologic studies. Male smokers are, in general, twice as likely to die of coronary disease than are male nonsmokers. Dose-response curves have been convincingly demonstrated. While dose-response curves for lung cancer show that risk progressively increases with the number of cigarettes smoked, curves for coronary disease level off somewhat—moderate smoking may confer maximal risk. Risks attributed to smoking are independent of other risk factors. Smoking may be the most important coronary risk factor for men under 50. More recent studies have demonstrated similar increases in risk for women who smoke. Autopsy studies documenting more frequent and severe atheromatous changes in smokers than in nonsmokers, and physiological studies documenting adverse effects of carbon monoxide and nicotine, support the epidemiologic evidence of increased risk.

Cerebrovascular disease and peripheral vascular disease. Data from the Framingham study indicate an association between smoking and atheromatous brain infarction and intermittent claudication, as well as coronary disease in men. Retrospective studies have demonstrated a strong association between smoking and peripheral vascular disease. The increased risk of stroke is less certain, particularly in postmenopausal women.

Lung cancer. The striking association between smoking and lung cancer has been demonstrated by prospective and retrospective epidemiologic studies as well as by autopsy results and experimental studies of carcinogenesis. These studies are reviewed in Chapter 33.

Other cancers. Studies indicate a significant increase in the risk of laryngeal cancer among smokers. Tobacco use, including pipe and cigar smoking and chewing as well as cigarette smoking, has been associated with an increased incidence of oral cancers. There seems to be synergism with alcohol use, the other most important risk factor. One study found a fifteenfold increase in incidence of oral cancers in smokers of more than 2 packs daily who consumed more than 1½ ounces of alcohol daily. The increased incidence was just over twofold for subjects who smoked at that rate but did not drink, or those who drank but did not smoke. Associations, with dose-response relationships, have been demonstrated between smoking and cancer of the esophagus and pancreas. No such relationship has been demonstrated for gastric cancer.

Chronic obstructive pulmonary disease. Cigarette smoking has been convincingly demonstrated by epidemiologic, autopsy and experimental data to be the primary cause of chronic bronchitis and emphysema. Marked increases in COPD mortality for male smokers have been repeatedly documented. There are dose-response curves for chronic bronchitis, with relative risks ranging from 4 to 21 times those of nonsmokers, and for emphysema, with risks increased 7 to 25 times. Studies of pulmonary function indicate that impairment exists in asymptomatic as well as symptomatic smokers. Experimental studies have indicated that smoking significantly compromises the defense mechanism of the lung.

Smoking during pregnancy. It has been known for more than 20 years that infants born to women who smoke during pregnancy are significantly smaller than infants born to nonsmokers. More recent data have convincingly linked smoking during pregnancy to increased rates of spontaneous abortion and perinatal mortality. The increased risk that can be attributed to smoking is particularly high for older mothers of higher parity. It has been estimated that approximately 5000 perinatal deaths occur each year in the United States as a result of maternal smoking.

Natural History of Smoking and Effectiveness of Cessation Methods

Most often, smokers begin their habit during late adolescence or early adulthood. There is a tendency to discontinue smoking—called natural discontinuance—that usually begins after age 30 and occurs at an increasing rate thereafter. The primary care provider can learn a great deal from the reasons people give for spontaneously discontinuing smoking. By far, the most common reason for quitting is, as documented by a British study, health. Most often the patient cites a minor ailment such as chronic cough or sore throat rather than fear of cancer, lung disease, or heart disease. Other reasons offered by patients who discontinued smoking are expense, social pressure, the example of physicians and other health workers, an attempt to test will power, and finally the feeling that smoking is a dirty or unpleasant habit.

No cessation method used by physicians or organized clinics has been very successful. However, evidence suggests that the primary physician has an advantage that he does not make the most of. The majority of exsmokers who stopped because of health reasons did so on their doctor's advice. It has been found in numerous studies, however, that only a minority of smokers are advised by their doctors to discontinue. Studies in the United States and Great Britain indicate that firm routine advice can lead to cessation for at least 3 to 6 months in 20 to 50 per cent of patients. These success rates compare well with those of programs using pharmacologic methods, behavioral techniques, group therapy or hypnosis (see Chapter 49).

CONCLUSIONS

- Conclusive evidence indicates that smoking is the single most important cause of currently preventable morbidity and mortality.
- No one cessation method is uniquely successful, but evidence indicates that primary care providers underestimate their potential influence on the behavior of smoking patients.
- It is recommended that the smoking status of all patients be carefully ascertained by the physician. All patients must be made aware of the multiple health effects of smoking and of how increases in risk and ill effects apply to them individually. This should be followed by firm advice to discontinue smoking. Pregnant patients or patients presenting with respiratory or coronary symptoms may be most responsive. Depending on local availability, other methods, including group therapy or hypnosis, should be tried if the physician's advice fails despite motivation on the patient's part to discontinue smoking (see Chapter 49).

ANNOTATED BIBLIOGRAPHY

Auerbach, O., et al.: Relation of smoking and age to emphysema. N. Engl. J. Med., 286:853, 1972. (Autopsy study demonstrating dose-response relationship between smoking and emphysema in men and women.)

Burt, A., Illingworth, D., Shaw, T.R.D., Thornley, P., White, P., and Turner, R.: Stopping smoking after myocardial infarction. Lancet, 1:304, 1974. (Infarction itself induced 28 per cent to stop smoking. Infarction plus an antismoking program persuaded 62 per cent to discontinue for 1 to 3 years.)

Doll, R., and Hill, A.B.: A study of the etiology of carcinoma of the lung. Br. Med. J., 2:1271, 1952. (Relative risk 13.8 times that of nonsmokers in this early retrospective study.)

———— The mortality of doctors in relation to their smoking habits; a preliminary report. Br. Med. J., 2:1071, 1956. (The first prospective report of historical interest—particularly for doctors.)

Friedman, G.D., Dales, L.G., and Ury, H.K.: Mortality in the middle-aged smokers and nonsmokers. N. Engl. J. Med., 300:213 1979. (Observations of over 4000 patients for 11 years suggesting a twofold increase in mortality during middle age among smokers.)

Gori, G.B.: Smoking and cancer: Research in etiology and prevention at the National Cancer Institute. Cancer, 30:1340, 1972. (Makes the case for the less hazardous cigarette.)

Kanzler, M., Jaffe, J.H., and Zeidenberg, P.: Long- and short-term effectiveness of a large-scale proprietary smoking cessation program—a 4-year follow-up of Smokenders participants. J. Clin. Psychol., 32:661, 1976. (70 per cent short-term success; 57 per cent long-term success among males, only 30 per cent among females.)

Russell, M.A.H.: Cigarette dependence. II Doctor's role in management. Br. Med. J., 2:393, 1971. (Good review of reasons for discontinuing, emphasizing the key role of the physician.)

U.S. Department of Health, Education and Welfare: Smoking and Health. Public Health Service Publication 1103, Washington, DC, 1964. (The "Surgeon General's Report" cataloging the ill effects of smoking.)

U.S. Department of Health, Education and Welfare: Smoking and Health: A Report of the Surgeon General. Washington, DC, 1979. (The first update of the case against smoking.)

Wald, N.J.: Mortality from lung cancer and coronary heart disease in relation to changes in smoking habits. Lancet, 1:136, 1976. (Hypothesizes that switching to filter cigarettes may explain leveling in lung cancer mortality rate that is not matched by change in coronary disease mortality rate.)

Wynder, E.L., Mabuchi, K., and Beattie, E.J.: The epidemiology of lung cancer. JAMA, 213:2221, 1970. (Retrospective study confirming high risk of smokers and decrease in risk after cessation. Also suggests decreased risk for smokers of filtered cigarettes.)

33

Screening for Lung Cancer

Lung cancer is the most common fatal malignancy among males. In recent years, it has claimed the lives of as many men as tumors of the colon and rectum, prostate, pancreas and stomach combined. The incidence of lung tumors in males has been rising dramatically since 1930. More recently, a dramatic increase among women, in whom it is already the third leading fatal malignancy, has been evident.

Most people are aware of the epidemic proportions of the lung cancer problem. Many have lost friends or relatives and know the grim prognosis of the disease. However, screening of asymptomatic individuals, whether or not it is restricted to those at high risk, can offer little reassurance. Efforts to improve the prognosis by early detection have been thwarted by the insensitivity of available tests, the characteristics of patients at high risk, and the aggressive natural history of most lung tumors. Without an understanding of these limitations, the primary care provider may expend resources that produce little more than exaggerated fear in some patients and inappropriate reassurance in others. Knowledge of the risk factors, the natural history, and the validity of available diagnostic tests provides a basis for the reasoned approach to many pulmonary symptoms (see Chapters 36 to 40).

EPIDEMIOLOGY AND RISK FACTORS

The epidemiology of lung cancer is dominated by its association with smoking. The dramatic increases in cancer death rates among men, and, more recently, among women are historically paralleled by increases in cigarette consumption. A dose-response relationship between duration of smoking and the number of cigarettes smoked per day and risk of lung cancer in men and women has been documented. When compared to nonsmokers, risks of lung cancer increase fivefold, tenfold and twentyfold for men who smoke less than ½ pack, ½ to 1 pack and 1 to 2 packs per day respectively. A decrease in risk has been demonstrated in smokers who are able to stop and in those who smoke filter-tipped cigarettes. Cigar and pipe smokers incur much less risk, but again a dose-response relationship has been documented.

The association between smoking and cancer is strongest for the epidermoid (squamous cell) and small cell undifferentiated (oat cell) tumors. The relationship is less certain for adenocarcinoma (alveolar cell) and large cell undifferentiated (anaplastic) histologic types.

The observation that lung cancer occurs in males far more often than in females can be explained for the most part by differences in smoking patterns. A slight apparent excess of lung cancer cases also occurs in urban areas and among low-income groups. The presence of polycyclic organic matter in urban pollution and in some occupational environments (see Chapter 35) may provide a partial explanation. On-the-job exposure to asbestos, chromate, nickel and uranium has also been associated with significantly increased rates of lung cancer.

NATURAL HISTORY OF LUNG CANCER AND EFFECTIVENESS OF THERAPY

Lung cancer's rapidly progressive and usually inexorable course frustrates screening efforts. The 5-year survival rate is between 5 and 10 per cent. At the time of symptomatic presentation, 75 per cent of patients have lesions that are clearly unresectable. Of the remainder, 60 per cent prove to be unresectable because of mediastinal involvement discovered by mediastinoscopy or thoracotomy. Five-year survival rates after resection in the relatively few remaining patients vary from about 9 per cent for patients with oat cell tumors to 28 per cent for patients with squamous cell tumors.

Reports of 5-year survival rates based on the symptoms present at the time of diagnosis are more relevant to the question of early detection. In a group of patients with overall 5-year survival of 7 per cent, the 6 per cent who were discovered while asymptomatic had an 18 per cent survival rate, compared with 10 to 15 per cent for patients with local symptoms and 6 per cent for those with systemic symptoms. Nearly one third of the patients had symptoms of metastatic disease; none was alive five years later.

There are reports of higher survival rates after resection of "in-situ" lung cancer diagnosed by means of chest x-ray or sputum cytology followed by bronchoscopy, but this may represent little more than selection of slow growing or otherwise benign lesions. Some highly speculative estimates of growth rate suggest that squamous cell carcinoma and adenocarcinoma take as long as 10 and 25 years respectively to reach a size likely to be detected by x-ray. If such estimates are accurate and if there is wide variability in natural history, overestimation of benefits of early detection are likely due to the problems of lead time and time-linked-bias sampling (see Chapter 3).

SCREENING AND DIAGNOSTIC TESTS

Chest X-ray

A controlled British study of 6-monthly chest x-rays in over 29,000 men detected 101 lung tumors over a 3-year period. Seventy-six were detected in a control population of 25,000. The overall 5-year survival rates among cancer patients from the screened and control groups were 15 per cent and 6 per cent respectively. Of the 101 cancers in the screened group, only 65 were detected by routine chest x-rays; the remainder presented symptomatically during screening intervals.

The most extensive American experience is that of the Philadelphia Pulmonary Neoplasm Project, which attempted to screen over 6000 male volunteers over age 45 with 6-monthly x-rays. Lung cancer developed in 121 patients during a 10-year period, with an ultimate mortality rate of 92 per cent at 5 years. The poor results were attributed to poor patient compliance with screening, patient and physician delay, advanced age or concomitant illness contraindicating surgical therapy, and inadequate sensitivity of the screening method.

While the specificity of radiographic screening has been shown to be 97 per cent, it is still too low to give an acceptable predictive value. A Veterans Administration study of lung cancer screens found 438 false-positive x-rays compared with 97 true-positive readings for suspected neoplasm.

Cytologic Screening

The sensitivity of cytologic screening varies with the cell type and location of the tumor and the methods of specimen collection. A single specimen will detect about 70 per cent of squamous cell lesions; three specimens may increase sensitivity to 90 per cent. Cytology is less sensitive in detecting tumors involving other cell types and is understandably less sensitive in detecting peripheral rather than hilar lesions.

The specificity of sputum cytologic examination is about 98 per cent, the same as that of chest x-rays.

It should be noted that, as diagnostic tests, x-ray and cytologic examination are complementary. In a Veterans Administration study, cytology alone had an overall screening sensitivity of 33 per cent and a specificity of 98 per cent. X-ray screening had a sensitivity of 42 per cent and specificity of 98 per cent. The sensitivity for combined x-ray and cytologic examination was 63 per cent.

SUMMARY AND CONCLUSIONS

- Lung cancer is a major cause of morbidity and mortality, especially among men. The incidence is increasing among women.
- Smoking is the overwhelming risk factor for lung cancer. Occupational exposures are also relevant.
- Little is known about the presymptomatic natural history of lung cancer. It is presumed to be very variable. The 5-year survival despite all forms of therapy is 5 to 10 per cent. Survival is slightly better when an asymptomatic lesion is detected.
- Cytologic examination of the sputum and chest x-ray are complementary diagnostic tests. Neither is sensitive or specific enough to serve as a screening test.
- Large-scale early detection programs have demonstrated little benefit. Such efforts to improve prognosis have been thwarted by the usually rapid course of lung cancer, the characteristics of the patients at risk and the relative insensitivity of available tests.

ANNOTATED BIBLIOGRAPHY

(Additional references concerning the relationship of lung cancer to smoking follow Chapter 32.)

Boucot, K.R., and Weiss, W.: Is curable lung cancer detected by semiannual screening? JAMA, *224*:1361, 1973. (Reviews the data of the Philadelphia Pulmonary Neoplasm Project, in which 5-year survival in men offered 6-monthly x-ray screening was only 8 per cent.)

Davies, D.F.: A review of detection methods for the early diagnosis of lung cancer. J. Chronic Dis., *19*:819, 1966. *(Somewhat dated but still useful review with 141 references.)*

Fontana, R.S.: Early diagnosis of lung cancer. Am. Rev. Respir. Dis., *116*:399, 1977. *(Editorial optimistically interpreting results of combined screening program at Mayo Clinic.)*

Lilienfeld, A., *et al.*: An evaluation of radiologic and cytologic screening for the early detection of lung cancer: A cooperative pilot study of the American Cancer Society and the Veterans Administration. Cancer Res., *26*:2083, 1966.

Schneiderman, M.A., and Levin, D.L.: Trends in lung cancer. Mortality, incidence, diagnosis, treatment, smoking and urbanization. Cancer, *30*:1320, 1972. *(Discusses increasing rates of smoking and lung cancer among women as well as cancer rates among urban dwellers and nonwhites.)*

Sterling, T.D.: A critical reassessment of the evidence bearing on smoking as the cause of lung cancer. Am. J. Public Health, *65*:939, 1975. *(Unconvincingly refutes the claim that cigarette smoking is a significant cause of lung cancer.)*

Weiss, W.: Smoking and cancer: A rebuttal. Am. J. Public Health, *65*:954. *(Refutes the Sterling argument.)*

———, *et al.*: The Philadelphia Pulmonary Neoplasm Project. Thwarting factors in periodic screening for lung cancer. Am. Rev. Respir. Dis., *111*:289, 1975. *(Describes lack of compliance with screening efforts, coexistent disease contraindicating surgery, and patient delay among patients at high risk.)*

Wynder, E.L.: Etiology of lung cancer. Cancer, *30*:1332, 1972. *(A brief review of the evidence incriminating cigarette smoking.)*

34
Screening for and Prophylaxis of Tuberculosis
HARVEY B. SIMON, M.D.

Active tuberculosis is now a relatively rare occurrence in ambulatory practice; however, the possibility of the diagnosis is often brought to mind by the patient presenting with hemoptysis, chronic cough, or severe weight loss. Tuberculin reactivity remains prevalent. On a daily basis, the primary physician faces the question of whether or not to test for reactivity and how to respond when it is present.

EPIDEMIOLOGY AND RISK FACTORS

The decline in prevalence of tuberculosis in the United States during this century has been dramatic. At the turn of the century, a majority of Americans were infected before they reached adulthood. Today, only 25 per cent of Americans over 50 and fewer than 5 per cent of young adults react positively to tuberculin skin testing. Overall, about 7 per cent of the population are positive reactors. Fewer than 5 per cent of these have a history of clinical tuberculosis. Approximately 90 per cent of new cases of clinical tuberculosis represent reactivation from the remaining pool of latent endogenous infection.

Not surprisingly, patients with tuberculosis tend to be clustered in certain population groups. The disease is more common in males, in the economically disadvantaged, in inner city residents, and in members of certain minority groups. The majority of patients with active disease are over 50 years of age, and the proportion of elderly patients appears to be increasing. Other population groups with a disproportionately high incidence of tuberculosis include immigrants, alcoholics, and patients with a history of gastrectomy, neoplasia and other debilitating diseases. Blacks, American Indians, and Eskimos seem to mount a less effective immune response and are likely to incur progressive disease if infected.

NATURAL HISTORY OF TUBERCULOSIS AND EFFECTIVENESS OF THERAPY

Mycobacterium tuberculosis is transmitted by way of fresh droplet nuclei expelled by an individual with cavitary tuberculosis. It cannot be spread by hands, utensils or other fomites, although organisms can be cultivated from room dust. While innoculation can occur via the gastrointestinal tract, the vast majority of infections in the United States begin in the lung (see Chapter 47). Rarely, primary infection results in early progressive disease; young children are at greatest risk for this complication. But in most cases, immunity develops over a period of several weeks and, hence the disease enters a latent stage.

Approximately 5 to 15 per cent of new tuberculous infections eventually progress to serious disease. Risk is greatest during the years immediately following infection. Only 3 to 5 per cent of patients without clinical disease 5 years after infection will suffer late reactivation.

Three strategies may be used in the prevention of clinical tuberculous infection. (1) biologic prophylaxis of uninfected individuals with BCG vaccine; (2) chemoprophylaxis of newly or recently infected individuals with isoniazid (INH); and (3) chemoprophylaxis of selected individuals with latent infections with INH.

Biologic prophylaxis in uninfected individuals is widely practiced in countries where tuberculosis is common. Bacillus Calmette-Guerin (BCG) vaccine is used for the prevention but not the therapy of tuberculosis. BCG vaccine is a live attenuated strain of *M. bovis* which has little virulence in man. BCG vaccine has been in clinical use since 1922 and has been shown to prevent tuberculosis in up to 80 per cent of vaccinated individuals. Current preparations of BCG are well tolerated. Despite its efficacy and safety, BCG is not recommended for routine use in the United States. The vaccine produces a positive tuberculin test in recipients, and because of the low prevalence rate of new tuberculous infections in the United States (estimated at 0.03 per cent), case-finding and INH prophylaxis are considered more effective. However, BCG vaccine may still have a place in certain high-risk populations, such as infants born to tuberculous mothers or tuberculin-negative members of groups with a high prevalence of tuberculosis and poor access to health care. BCG vaccine should not be administered to PPD-positive individuals.

Chemoprophylaxis of newly or recently infected individuals, as identified by recent conversion to tuberculin reactivity, is an important method of preventing clinical disease. In patients who have not received chemotherapy, a positive skin test implies the presence of a few dormant but viable tubercle bacilli, which have the potential for reactivation. In a sense then, patients with positive tuberculin skin tests serve as their own reservoir for future clinical disease. It has been demonstrated that the administration of INH daily for 1 year reduces the risk of reactivation by up to 80 per cent. Since the risk of progressive disease is greatest soon after infection, recent converters to tuberculin reactivity are most likely to benefit from such therapy. In general, individuals who have converted to tuberculin reactivity within 2 years should be considered for chemoprophylaxis. Close contacts of patients with active pulmonary tuberculosis deserve special attention. It has been recommended that children or adolescents who are exposed be treated with INH even if the tuberculin skin test is negative. If the test remains negative after 3 months of INH therapy, chemoprophylaxis can then be discontinued. Routine screening of all individuals below age 25 and INH treatment of positive reactors has also been recommended. Because the prevalence rate of positive reactions is less than 1 per cent among children and adolescents, a positive reaction in a young patient may indicate recent exposure.

The chemoprophylaxis of selected patients with latent infections and long-standing positive tuberculin reactivity has also been advised. Patients who have recovered from clinical tuberculosis without the benefit of adequate chemotherapy should be considered for prophylaxis. It also seems reasonable to administer INH to immunologically impaired hosts with positive tuberculin skin tests. Enthusiasm for INH prophylaxis must be tempered by the significant side effects of the drug. The major concern in the use of INH is its hepatotoxicity. This is quite rare in patients under age 20 and occurs in no more than 0.2 per cent of those between ages 20 and 34. On the other hand, among patients over 50, more than 2 per cent may develop INH-induced liver disease (see Chapter 47).

SCREENING AND DIAGNOSTIC TESTS

The tuberculin skin test, far more sensitive and specific than the chest x-ray, is the most useful test for the diagnosis of past or present tuberculous infection. The Mantoux test using the intradermal injection of Tween-80 stabilized purified protein derivative (PPD) is more reliable than multiple-puncture tests, such as the tine test. Three strengths of PPD are available: the first strength contains 1 tuberculin unit; the intermediate strength, 5 units; and the second strength, 250 units. Intermediate-strength PPD is the standard test material. The tuberculin skin test should be interpreted 48 to 72 hours after injection; the diameter of induration rather than erythema determines the interpretation: 0 to 4 mm. is a negative reaction; 5 to 9 mm. is doubtful; and 10 mm. or more is positive. First-strength PPD should be reserved for patients in whom a very strong reaction is anticipated. Second-strength PPD should be reserved for individuals with negative reactions to a lower strength. A positive second-strength test in the face of a negative or doubtful intermediate-strength test is suggestive of infection with atypical mycobacteria and resultant cross-sensitization to PPD. Obviously, a positive tuberculin test does not by itself prove active disease. Conversely, negative reactions have been documented in up to 20 per cent of patients with tuberculosis, particularly those individuals with overwhelming or advanced disease, malnutrition, or debility. Many of these patients are anergic, so that skin testing with *Candida* or streptokinase-streptodornase antigens can be useful in demonstrating overall immunologic impairment.

In addition to the immunologic incompetence of the host, false-negative skin tests may result from mishandling of the antigen or from faulty injection technique. Tuberculin should never be transferred from one container to another, and skin tests should be given as soon as possible after the syringe is filled. Subcutaneous rather than intradermal injection may result in false-negative reactions. Since tuberculin sensitivity develops 2 to 10 weeks after initial infection, early skin tests may be negative in newly infected individuals.

Tuberculin skin testing is highly specific; however, cross-reactivity with atypical mycobacterial antigens may cause intermediate skin test reactions to occur in people who have not been exposed to *M. tuberculosis*. More often, individuals infected with atypical mycobacteria will have positive second-strength PPD reactions and weak or negative intermediate PPDs.

RECOMMENDATIONS AND CONCLUSIONS

- While active tuberculous disease has become uncommon in the United States, the prevalence of latent infection remains approximately 7 per cent. Because the PPD test is useful in case-finding, BCG prophylaxis for PPD-negative patients is not recommended.
- For recent converters under age 35, or positive reactors under age 25, INH should be given for 1 year while the patient is monitored carefully for development of hepatitis. INH should also be given to close contacts of patients with active pulmonary disease, particularly if the contact is a child or an adolescent; treatment can be discontinued if the patient remains PPD-negative for a 3-month period. Older patients who have recovered from clinical tuberculosis, have no evidence of active disease, but have never received chemotherapy should be considered for INH therapy. The decision to treat asymptomatic older patients needs to be tempered by the increased risk of INH-induced hepatitis in this age group.
- The tuberculin skin test can be useful in apparently healthy individuals. Because of its prognostic value and the importance of recent conversion, the PPD status of children and young adults should be determined. Individuals with a high risk of exposure to tuberculosis, such as those in the health professions, should have tuberculin tests on an annual basis so long as they remain PPD negative.

ANNOTATED BIBLIOGRAPHY

Barlow, P.B., Black, M., Brummer, D.C. *et al.*: Preventive therapy of tuberculosis infection. Am. Rev. Respir. Dis., *110*:371, 1974. *(A good review with specific recommendations for INH prophylaxis.)*

Boyd, J.C., and Marr, J.J.: Decreasing reliability of acid-fast smear techniques for detection of tuberculosis. Ann. Intern. Med., *82*:849, 1975. *(Misleading title but very useful article pointing out high specificity [99 per cent] of smears but low predictive value [45 per cent] because of low prevalence. Sensitivity was 22 percent.)*

Comstock, G.W., Furculow, M.L., and Greenberg, R.A.: The tuberculin skin test. Am. Rev. Respir. Dis., *104*:769, 1971. *(Standards for the administration and interpretation of the tuberculin skin test.)*

Holden, M., Dubin, M.R., and Diamond, P.H.: Negative intermediate strength tuberculin sensitivity in active tuberculosis. N. Engl. J. Med., *285*:1506, 1971. *(Emphasizes loss of potency due to adsorption of antigen. Tween-80 stabilized antigen had a sensitivity of 83 per cent, superior to other preparations.)*

Hyde, L.: Clinical significance of the tuberculin test. Am. Rev. Respir. Dis., *105*:453, 1972. *(Skin tests on 100 patients with active pulmonary TB provoked reactions greater than 5 mm. in 90 per cent and greater than 10 mm. in 81 per cent.)*

Schacter, E.N.: Tuberculin negative tuberculosis. Am. Rev. Respir. Dis., *106*:587, 1972. *(Sixteen of 149 patients with clinical disease had negative tests. Ten with negative tests were infected with atypical organisms.)*

Smith, D.W.: Why not vaccinate against tuberculosis? Ann. Intern. Med., *72*:419, 1970. *(Reviews arguments against vaccination and concludes that BCG should be used for high-risk groups in the United States.)*

35
Screening for Occupational Respiratory Disease
JOHN D. STOECKLE, M.D.

"Occupational respiratory diseases" are cases of pulmonary inflammation, fibrosis, or neoplasia in which the etiologic agents are manmade, and which develop as a result of industrial or agricultural work. Estimates of the number of people exposed to such disease-producing agents include 250,000 workers involved in asbestos product manufacturing and insulation, 200,000 coal miners, 500,000 cotton and textile workers, and as many as one million workers exposed to silica. More than 20 per cent of urban industrial plants surveyed contain hazardous dusts. Smaller numbers of people are exposed to toxic metal compounds such as beryllium, cadmium oxide, tungsten carbide, and ferrous oxide. The list of toxic industrial agents is long, and new agents will certainly be identified in the future.

Despite recent factory and field surveys, a great deal remains to be learned about the epidemiology of occupational respiratory diseases, their natural histories, dose-response relationships, and reversibility at early stages.

Patients and physicians often fail to recognize the relationship between a toxic agent and the nonspecific acute respiratory symptoms it produces or the chronic pulmonary disease that develops long after exposure. For these reasons, disease incidence among exposed individuals is at best a rough estimate. Because some agents such as asbestos and detergent enzymes are ubiquitous, the size of exposed populations is also uncertain. As a result, only general estimates of populations at risk and disease prevalence can be made. Similarly, host factors (genetic, immune, economic, social, psychological) that predispose certain individuals rather than others to the development of debilitating disease are not often identified.

Despite these gaps in knowledge, it is critical that the primary physician be familiar with what is known about occupational lung disease if unnecessary morbidity is to be avoided. Since acute respiratory symptoms due to toxic exposure are nonspecific, recognition of their relationship to the toxic agent is essential; continued exposure may result in needless, irreversible functional abnormalities. The diagnosis of established chronic occupational respiratory disease is also important. In such instances, the rate of functional deterioration or the risk of secondary disease such as neoplasia may be reduced by removal from the exposure, control of infection and elimination of smoking.

CLINICAL DISORDERS

Occupational respiratory diseases may be caused by inert nonfibrogenic and fibrogenic mineral dusts such as coal and asbestos, by toxic chemicals such as isocyanates, or by organic dusts.

Mineral dusts. Coal worker's pneumoconiosis (CWP) results from the deposition of coal dust in peribronchial tissues and the distention of terminal bronchioles. Prevalence studies suggest that CWP among 140,000 active and 200,000 retired miners depends not only on the dustiness of the mine but on the rank of the coal. For example, anthracite miners have a higher prevalence of CWP than do bituminous miners. The hard coal anthracite is of the highest rank, having the most carbon and the least volatile matter compared to the bituminous soft coal and to lignite, a still softer coal. Such factors appear to explain regional differences in CWP prevalence. Results of the 1969 ongoing national coal study indicate a prevalence of 30 per cent of CWP among active miners in Appalachia. Because retired miners are not included in this study and because there is a latent period prior to development of clinical CWP, this figure probably underestimates the actual prevalence of the disease.

Asbestos and *silica* are among the mineral dusts that are fibrogenic. Obvious exposures occur in asbestos mining and insulation work. The fibers are also used in the manufacture of such diverse products as textiles, cement, rubber tires, vinyl plastics, graphite and resins. The widespread use of asbestos in the construction industry has raised concerns about general exposure among urban and school populations. It has been estimated that 3.5 million workers have been exposed to asbestos, but the number of resulting cases of pulmonary disease is not known.

Asbestos exposure most commonly causes pulmonary fibrosis with or without pleural fibrosis and calcification, occasionally produces benign pleural effusions, and is a major risk factor for bronchogenic carcinoma and mesothelioma. In the case of pulmonary fibrosis, severity and latency in development are related to the level and duration of exposure. Even at low levels of exposures, some 40 per cent of workers exposed for 10 to 20 years will develop fibrosing disease. Low-level exposure continued up to 30 years will produce detectable disease in 70 per cent. Their risk of lung cancer, a common cause of death among asbestos workers, is estimated to be 7 times that of the general population. Among workers who smoke, the risk is 90 times greater than that of nonsmoking, nonexposed individuals. In the case of mesothelioma, two thirds of reported cases have involved exposure to asbestos. In such cases, exposure usually antedates the development of the tumor by 30 to 35 years; neither level of exposure nor smoking appears to be a predictor of risk.

Toxic chemicals. Toluene diisocyanate (TDI) is one of a wide variety of chemicals that are bronchopulmonary irritants or injurious sensitizing agents. A highly volatile liquid polymerizing agent, TDI reacts with resins to produce polyurethanes which, on exposure, often produce acute but reversible symptoms of conjunctivitis, upper respiratory irritation, and bronchospasm. Continued low-level exposure may result

in chronic obstructive disease. It is estimated that as many as 100,000 workers are exposed to isocyanates.

Organic dusts. Farmer's lung and *byssinosis* are examples of occupational disease due to organic dusts. Farmer's lung is acute or chronic bronchitis-pneumonitis related to exposure to the dust of moldy hay or grain. Thermophilic actinomycetes have been incriminated as sensitizing agents. Byssinosis, characterized by bronchospasm, cough and sometimes dyspnea, results from exposure to textile dusts of cotton, flax or hemp. Although the mechanism of the disease is incompletely understood, these textile dusts release histamine *in vitro* and may act similarly *in vivo*, thereby producing bronchospasm. It has been estimated that 25 per cent of over 500,000 cotton and textile workers are affected by byssinosis.

It should be kept in mind that exposures to these agents also occur away from the work place. Toxic dusts can be brought home by the worker; in this way, family members may be exposed to an "occupational" respiratory disease, e.g., asbestosis. Exposure to these mineral dusts may occur in neighborhoods located near mines, construction sites or factories; likewise, chemical toxins, e.g., beryllium, may be present in the vicinity of manufacturing plants in concentrations sufficient to cause disease. Because thermophilic actinomycetes commonly contaminate home humidifiers, typical farmer's lung can result from home exposure.

NATURAL HISTORY OF DISEASE AND EFFECTIVENESS OF CONTROL

Although much remains to be learned about the natural history of most occupational lung diseases, practical control steps can be taken. It is worth distinguishing agents that commonly cause acute symptoms and, with repeated exposures, may produce irreversible disease from other agents that produce disease evident only after a long asymptomatic latent period.

Byssinosis and bronchitis-pneumonia due to diisocyanate exposure are examples of acute reversible diseases that can progress to chronic, irreversible diseases with repeated exposure. Both are characterized by acute symptoms of coughing and wheezing that occur when the worker is reexposed after a brief absence from work. Chronic obstructive changes can develop in those whose exposure continues despite symptoms. Some workers exposed to enzyme detergents have similar acute symptoms; progressive loss of elastic recoil is possible if exposure continues. Disorders due to organic dusts (farmer's lung) and toxic chemicals (beryllium) also produce both acute and chronic syndromes that are related to level and duration of exposure.

In contrast, diseases due to mineral dusts, such as coal worker's pneumoconiosis and asbestosis, become clinically manifest only after a long latent asymptomatic period. The clinical findings of coal worker's pneumoconiosis usually follow 10 years of exposure. Similarly, 10 to 20 years of low-level exposure is usually required to produce detectable pulmonary asbestosis. In the case of pleural asbestosis, exposure usually precedes the development of disease by 20 to 30 years. Silicosis also has a long latent period unless exposure is extremely intense. Despite improved dust control, termination of exposure has been advised for people with identifiable pulmonary disease. However, the extent to which progression of the disease can be influenced by cessation of exposure after the appearance of detectable abnormalities is not known.

SCREENING AND DIAGNOSTIC TESTS

Eliciting the occupational history is the most important step in preventing occupational lung disease. Four specific facts must be obtained: (1) the presence of symptoms and their relation to work, past or present, (2) the type of hazardous exposure, (3) the level and the duration of exposure, and (4) the presence of a similar illness in co-workers with similar jobs.

Besides periodic chest x-rays, the standard pulmonary function tests (including forced vital capacity, forced expiratory volume in 1 second, and the ratio of forced vital capacity to forced expiratory volume in 1 second) are adequate for assessing symptomatic disease but too insensitive for detecting mild abnormalities. Measurements obtained before and after a work shift may identify episodes of acute intermittent airflow obstruction. In general, obstruction in peripheral airways may be relatively advanced in the absence of spirographic abnormalities. Based on studies of lung function in smokers, some have advised the use of more sensitive tests in occupationally exposed individuals. Estimates of closing volume derived from single breath nitrogen tests have been used in occupational groups with varying levels of acceptability and reproducibility. The use of low-density gases to increase the sensitivity of maximum expiratory flow maneuvers has been proposed for field studies. Response to aerosolized histamine may provide an index of host factors that determine suscepti-

bility. While each of these new technologies for measuring respiratory impairment offers promise and deserves the attention of those dealing with groups who are occupationally exposed, their value must be further defined before their use as routine screening tests in exposed individuals can be recommended.

CONCLUSIONS AND RECOMMENDATIONS

- Occupational respiratory diseases are a heterogeneous mixture of allergic, inflammatory, and fibrotic pulmonary reactions, both acute and chronic, which occur in response to toxic agents usually encountered in the work place.
- Exposure to mineral dusts such as coal and asbestos causes pulmonary abnormalities that are evident after a variable, but usually long, latent period. Morbidity and mortality due to such exposures is increased by smoking and chronic infection. Cessation of exposure is recommended after disease is detected, but the effect of cessation on disease progression is not known. Environmental controls are essential.
- Exposure to toxic chemicals and organic dusts can cause either acute reversible or chronic irreversible disease. For patients with recurrent symptoms, rigid environmental controls, if possible, or removal from the work place is recommended.
- Spirometry, when performed before and after exposure, may be useful in documenting acute obstructive responses to toxic or sensitizing agents. Routine tests, however, are too insensitive to detect chronic disease at an early stage. While more sensitive methods offer promise to the epidemiologist and industrial physician, they cannot as yet be recommended for use by the primary physician to screen exposed individuals.
- It is important for primary physicians to consider occupational etiologies of acute respiratory disease; continued exposure in such situations must be prohibited in order to prevent irreversible disease.
- Asymptomatic patients with significant exposure history should be identified. Discussion of individual risk, firm advice to avoid smoking, and surveillance for subsequent pulmonary disease are indicated.

ANNOTATED BIBLIOGRAPHY

Barbee, R.A., Callies, O., and Dickie, H.A.: The long-term prognosis in farmer's lung. Am. Rev. Respir. Dis., *97*:223, 1968. *(Fifty patients fol-*

lowed for an average of 6 years. Chronic disease occurred most commonly in those with a history of mild recurrent episodes each winter.)

Bouhuys, A., Heapty, L.J., Schilling, R.S.F., and Welborn, L.W.: Byssinosis in U.S. N. Engl. J. Med., *277*:170, 1967. *(Chronic irreversible disease occurs mainly in reactors, those with acute reversible symptoms, often on a weekly basis with exposure after a weekend away.)*

Bouhuys, A., and Zuskin, E.: Chronic respiratory disease in hemp workers. A follow-up study, 1967. Ann. Intern. Med., *84*:398, 1976. *(Argues that disease is likely to progress even if exposure is discontinued.)*

doPico, G.A., Rankin, J., Chosy, L.W., Reddan, W.G., Barbee, R.A., Gee, B., and Dickie, H.A.: Respiratory tract disease from thermosetting resins. Study of an outbreak in rubber tire workers. Ann. Intern. Med., *83*:117, 1975. *(Example of a newly recognized toxic agent capable of producing both acute and chronic disease.)*

Dosman, J.A., and Cotton, D.J.: Grain dust and health. II. Early diagnosis in occupational pulmonary disease. Ann. Intern. Med., *89*:134, 1978. *(Describes newer more sensitive screening tests but points out need for validation and clearer understanding of natural history with population studies.)*

Murphy, R.L.H., Ferris, B.G., Burgess, W.A., Worcester, J., and Gaensler, E.A.: Effects of low concentration of asbestos. N. Engl. J. Med., *285*:1271, 1971. *(Documents risk among shipyard workers exposed to asbestos levels previously considered safe.)*

Selikoff, I.J., Hammond, E.C., and Churg, J.: Asbestos exposure, smoking and neoplasms. JAMA, *204*:106, 1968. *(Estimates sevenfold increase risk for asbestos-exposed nonsmoking workers and ninetyfold increase for asbestos workers who smoke.)*

Stoeckle, J.D., Hardy, H.L., King, W.B., and Nemiah, J.C.: Respiratory disease in U.S. soft coal miners: Clinical and etiologic considerations. J. Chronic Dis., *15*:887, 1962. *(Detailed study of 30 patients suggesting that coincident infection and smoking are important determinants of respiratory compromise.)*

Stoeckle, J.D., Hardy, H.L., and Weber, A.L.: Chronic beryllium disease, a report of 60 cases and selective review of the literature. Am. J. Med., *46*:545, 1969. *(Most patients were exposed during the manufacture of fluorescent lamps. Cor pulmonale was the usual cause of death.)*

Weiss, W.: Cigarette smoking, asbestos, and pulmonary fibrosis. Am. Rev. Respir. Dis., *104*:223, 1971. *(Documents higher prevalence of pulmonary fibrosis in asbestos workers who smoke compared to those who do not.)*

36

Evaluation of Chronic Dyspnea

Dyspnea is the subjective sensation of difficult or uncomfortable respirations; patients commonly use the term "short of breath" to describe their difficulty. Acute severe dyspnea is very often a manifestation of a serious cardiopulmonary problem and necessitates prompt hospitalization for evaluation. Chronic dyspnea, even when severe, can be evaluated on a outpatient basis as long as the patient's condition is relatively stable. The major causes of chronic dyspnea encountered in the office setting are chronic obstructive pulmonary disease (COPD) and chronic congestive heart failure (CHF). Many times these etiologies coexist; in such instances the diagnostic task requires a determination of which etiology is the predominant factor. Evaluation of chronic dyspnea should also include an assessment of prognosis and severity as well as a determination of etiology. In addition, one needs to identify precipitants and reversible components of the patient's illness.

PATHOPHYSIOLOGY AND CLINICAL PRESENTATION

The pathophysiology of dyspnea involves disturbances of ventilation. The work of breathing is often increased; this may result from decreased lung compliance, disturbances in the chest bellows system, airway obstruction, or exogenous factors such as obesity. Shortness of breath is experienced when ventilatory demands exceed the actual or perceived capacity of the lungs to respond. Operationally, greater respiratory effort is needed when airway resistance is increased and when the lungs are stiffer than normal. The location and workings of the system for detection of respiratory work are incompletely understood, but it has been hypothesized that an inappropriate relationship between length and tension in the respiratory muscles may be one triggering factor. The unmyelinated vagal nerve endings located between pulmonary capillaries and alveoli are believed to mediate the sensation of dyspnea experienced in interstitial pulmonary edema.

Congestive heart failure results in dyspnea as pulmonary compliance falls due to increase in pulmonary capillary pressure and fluid buildup in the interstitium. In mild CHF, the earliest symptom is dyspnea on exertion. More severe failure is manifested by orthopnea and paroxysmal nocturnal dyspnea (see Chapter 27). Crackles (rales), a third heart sound, distended neck veins and peripheral edema may be found on examination. Fever, ischemia, dysrhythmias, fluid overload, and poor compliance with a therapeutic regimen may precipitate or worsen failure. Other causes of increased pulmonary capillary pressure are also important sources of dyspnea; *mitral stenosis* is prominent among the chronic etiologies (see Chapter 28).

Airway obstruction at any level of the respiratory tract can produce chronic dyspnea. *Tracheal stenosis* from intrinsic disease or extrinsic compression is characterized by dyspnea in conjunction with stridor and inspiratory retraction of the supraclavicular space. Chronic obstructive pulmonary disease is the leading etiology of obstruction. *Chronic bronchitis* is the form of COPD defined as cough and sputum production that lasts for at least three months, two years in a row. Commonly there is a long-standing history of smoking, productive cough, and slowly progressive worsening of exercise capacity. In later stages, the patient appears plethoric, coughs incessantly, and may become cyanotic (the so-called blue bloater). Tobacco-stained fingers, wheezes, coarse rales, rhonchi and prolonged expiratory phase of respiration are often present on examination. *Bronchiectasis* is somewhat similar in presentation, except that the physical findings may be more localized and recurrent episodes of pneumonia and purulent sputum production may be more prominent in the history. Patients with COPD that is predominantly *emphysematous* are also bothered by airway obstruction, but sputum production is less prominent than in bronchi-

tis and there is less mismatching of ventilation and perfusion; consequently, hypoxia is milder, cyanosis is uncommon and cough is less of a problem. Gradual deterioration in exercise capacity takes place over many years. Patients with significant disease appear thin and barrel-chested. They may purse the lips during expiration to keep airways open. The chest is hyperresonant, breath sounds are distant, and a few end-expiratory wheezes may be noted; expiration is prolonged. In severe cases of COPD, accessory respiratory muscles are utilized along with pursed-lip breathing. Acute respiratory infection, CHF, and dehydration with inspissation of secretions can lead to acute deterioration (see Chapter 44).

Asthma is usually responsible for acute dyspnea, but airway obstruction may persist for a prolonged period after an acute attack and result in more chronic symptoms, including dyspnea, cough and wheezing; at times, cough may be the predominant symptom (see Chapter 45). Exercise-induced asthma may contribute to recurrent dyspneic episodes.

Diffuse *interstitial lung disease* alters pulmonary compliance and may lead to a disturbance in the balance between ventilation and perfusion. The process is usually very gradual, and often patients have few symptoms when pulmonary involvement is mild; however, tachypnea and cyanosis can occur in severe cases. Diffuse crackles are often heard on auscultation of the lungs. As the process progresses, dyspnea worsens and exercise tolerance deteriorates.

Kyphoscoliosis is the one type of chest wall deformity that is capable of producing major impairment of mechanical function and causing substantial respiratory difficulty; advanced cases can even terminate in cor pulmonale and respiratory failure. Extrinsic mechanical factors that can hinder lung mechanics include massive obesity, ascites and large pleural effusions. Dyspnea is often the chief complaint.

Pulmonary vascular disease due to recurrent embolization or primary pulmonary hypertension can be the source of severe dyspnea; mortality is high. Patients with *recurrent emboli* often have a history of long-standing venous disease and episodes of deep-vein thrombophlebitis, though at times the source of emboli is hard to uncover. *Primary pulmonary hypertension* is a diagnosis of exclusion, found most commonly among women between ages 20 and 40. In both conditions, there is often a history of recurrent chest pain (see Chapter 14), dyspnea on exertion, and fatigue. Hyperventilation may result and be mistakenly attributed to anxiety. A history of Raynaud's phenomenon can be obtained in a substantial percentage of patients with primary pulmonary hypertension. Secondary pulmonary hypertension may also cause dyspnea; it results from long-standing pulmonary congestion, as seen in mitral stenosis (see Chapter 28). Regardless of etiology, signs of right heart failure develop over time (see Chapter 27).

Anxiety attacks are often confused with more serious etiologies, because the patient may appear to be in severe respiratory distress. The patient often reports chest tightness or claims that he cannot get in enough air. The florid, acute case is represented by the hyperventilation syndrome (see Chapter 214), but commonly there is a less dramatic, chronic feeling of dyspnea and fatigue that is affected little by exertion. Frequent sighing, multiple bodily complaints, nervousness and a normal physical examination are typical of such patients.

DIFFERENTIAL DIAGNOSIS

The causes of chronic dyspnea encountered in the office setting are listed in Table 36–1.

Table 36–1.   Common Causes of
Chronic Dyspnea

Cardiac
1. Congestive heart failure
2. Other causes of pulmonary venous congestion (mitral stenosis, mitral regurgitation)

Pulmonary
1. Chronic obstructive pulmonary disease
2. Pulmonary parenchymal disease (including interstitial diseases)
3. Pulmonary hypertension
4. Severe kyphoscoliosis
5. Exogenous mechanical factors (ascites, massive obesity, large pleural effusion)

Psychological
1. Anxiety

WORKUP

History. The most difficult tasks in the evaluation of dyspnea are differentiating dyspnea due to cardiac disease from that resulting from pulmonary pathology and establishing the degree of functional impairment. With both cardiac and pulmonary etiologies, dyspnea is worsened by exertion. The occurrence of exacerbations at night are often thought to be more suggestive of heart failure than of respiratory disease, but excessive collections of sputum may occur at night, produce obstruction and force the patient to sit up and cough to clear his airways; this may be mistaken for a history of paroxysmal nocturnal dyspnea, unless the physician takes time to inquire about the details of the episode. In general, a past history dominated by chronic cough, sputum production, respiratory infections, and heavy smoking point more to lung disease than to a cardiac origin. The occurrence of wheezing may be a manifestation of heart-failure-induced bronchospasm, as well as a sign of airway obstruction from asthma or COPD. Thus, unless a strong history of prior lung disease or substantial sputum production is associated with exacerbations of dyspnea, it may be hard to distinguish a cardiac from a pulmonary source on the basis of history alone. Moreover, both may coexist in the same case with one responsible for an acute exacerbation; physical findings and laboratory observations are usually necessary for better differentiation.

Dyspnea that is a manifestation of a chronic anxiety state may superficially mimic cardiopulmonary disease and cause some confusion. Onset at rest in conjunction with a sense of chest tightness, suffocation, or inability to take in air are characteristic features of the history. Also, there is little evidence of significant heart or lung disease, though there may be much fear of it. Multiple bodily complaints, history of emotional difficulties, absence of activity limitations, and lack of exacerbation upon exercising argue for a psychogenic cause. Unfortunately, patients with pulmonary hypertension may have episodes that can resemble anxiety-induced bouts of dyspnea; sometimes a young patient with primary pulmonary hypertension is incorrectly labeled "neurotic."

It is helpful to define as precisely as possible the degree of activity that precipitates the sensation of dyspnea, in order to estimate the severity of disease, determine the extent of disability, and detect changes over time. One means of achieving these objectives is to relate symptoms to the patient's daily activities and interpret the degree of restriction in terms of the expected endurance of a patient of similar age.

Factors that may contribute to the occurrence or worsening of dyspnea should be documented, including cigarette smoking, occupational exposure, excessive salt intake, weight gain, and increasing sputum production. The patient should be asked about hemoptysis; the symptom raises the possibilities of tumor, embolization with infarction, and pneumonia (see Chapter 38). Suspicion of embolization requires an inquiry into use of oral contraceptives, recent surgery, recurrent thrombophlebitis, and pregnancy (see Chapter 14).

Physical examination should begin with a check for tachycardia, tachypnea, fever, and hypertension. Weight must not be forgotten, for it may be an early sign of worsening congestive failure (see Chapter 27). The patient's respiratory efforts need to be observed carefully to obtain an estimate of the amount of work expended in breathing; contractions of the accessory muscles of respiration suggest severe difficulty. Retraction of the supraclavicular fossa implies tracheal stenosis that has become critical. Pursed-lip breathing and a prolonged expiratory phase are signs of significant outflow obstruction; the best way to observe airflow obstruction is to have the patient take a deep breath and blow out as hard and fast as he can. The chest is examined for increased A-P diameter (suggestive of COPD) and deformity resulting from kyphoscoliosis or ankylosing spondylitis. Retraction of the intercostal muscles upon inspiration is characteristic of emphysema.

The chest should be percussed for dullness and hyperresonance and auscultated for wheezes, crackles, and quality of breath sounds. Crackles often represent fluid in the airway, as occurs with pneumonitis and CHF. A normal pulmonary examination does not rule out respiratory pathology, but lessens its probability of being severe. Cardiac examination should focus on the presence of jugular venous distention, a third heart sound, murmurs of mitral and aortic valve disease, heaves and carotid pulse abnormalities (see Chapters 27 and 28). It is important to recognize that many of the signs of right heart failure may be a consequence of long-standing pulmonary disease and therefore are not specific for a cardiac etiology. The abdomen is examined for ascites and hepatojugular reflux; the legs are checked for edema and other signs of phlebitis (see Chapters 16 and 30).

Laboratory studies. The chest x-ray is essential to evaluation and should be studied for pulmonary venous redistribution, effusions, interstitial changes, hyperinflation, infiltrates, enlargement of the pulmonary arteries (indicative of pulmonary hypertension), cardiac chamber enlargement, and valve calcification. Upper zone redistribution of pulmonary blood flow is among the earliest x-ray findings of CHF (see Chapter 27); however, redistribution may also occur in COPD from destruction of vessels in the lower lung fields. The chest film is valuable for detection of interstitial lung disease, because physical findings may be minimal.

Simple pulmonary function tests can be reliably performed in the office on an inexpensive spirometer. The FEV_1 and vital capacity are the most informative measurements for the detection of obstructive and restrictive defects, and for the determination of severity. The ratio of FEV_1 to vital capacity is markedly reduced in clinically important obstructive disease. In restrictive disease, the ratio is close to 1.0 but the vital capacity is significantly reduced. An FEV_1 can also provide prognostic information; a reading of less than 1.0 liter per second is associated with a poor 5-year survival rate among patients with COPD (see Chapter 44). Patients suspected of having tracheal stenosis may require flow-volume studies in order to identify the lesion and determine its severity; referral is indicated.

Arterial blood gases (ABGs) are not routinely available in most office settings, but are worth obtaining when there is a question of deteriorating ventilation (e.g., patient is observed to be breathing with accessory muscles); hospitalization should be considered when the pCO_2 is inappropriately elevated for the respiratory rate and repeat determinations reveal further pCO_2 increases. Drawing ABGs before and after exercise is helpful in assessing the severity of diffuse interstitial disease; a fall in pO_2 is evidence of a significant degree of interstitial disease. When use of accessory muscles is noted and the patient appears to be worsening, prompt hospital admission should be carried out, rather than taking time to obtain ABGs in the office.

Sometimes the combination of history, physical examination, chest x-ray and pulmonary function tests is not sufficient to determine the relative contributions of CHF and COPD to the patient's dyspnea. When findings are equivocal, it may be helpful to perform a circulation time; in patients with CHF, the circulation time is prolonged by 4 or more seconds beyond the upper limit of normal (16 seconds). Increasing sputum production or change to more purulent sputum indicates a pulmonary cause of worsening dyspnea in the patient with both CHF and COPD; a Gram stain of the sputum is often informative, especially when the patient is febrile, coughing more than usual, or reports a change in sputum.

The neurotic patient with anxiety-induced dyspnea often benefits from having a chest film and simple pulmonary function tests, for the confirmation of a well-functioning respiratory system may provide some reassurance and lessening of concern over bodily symptoms. At times, a walk with the patient up and down a few flights of stairs is just as convincing for both physician and patient. Climbing stairs with the patient complaining of dyspnea is also useful in those with suspected cardiopulmonary disease, for exercise tolerance can be quantitated in terms of flights climbed and the heart and respiratory rates attained.

SYMPTOMATIC MANAGEMENT AND PATIENT EDUCATION

Acute exacerbations of CHF (see Chapter 27), respiratory tract infections (see Chapter 43), large pleural effusions (see Chapter 39) and environmental irritants (see Chapter 35) can and should be dealt with promptly. Treatment of COPD (see Chapter 44), asthma (see Chapter 45), pulmonary venous congestion due to valvular heart disease (see Chapter 28), and anxiety (see Chapter 214) can also provide symptomatic relief. Regardless of cause, all patients with dyspnea should be advised to stop smoking; often the onset of even mild dyspnea is sufficient stimulus to quit, especially when combined with the physician's urging (see Chapter 49). Many patients with chronic dyspnea request oxygen treatment at home. Such requests are reasonable if there is no evidence of carbon dioxide retention and the patient is bothered by hypoxia (e.g., severe interstitial disease); however, the majority of patients have COPD and should not be given oxygen therapy unless it is clear that they do not retain CO_2 (see Chapter 44).

The etiologies and precipitants of the patient's dyspnea should be discussed. Prognosis also requires elaboration, especially if it is different from the patient's perception. Some clinicians encourage selected patients with COPD or heart disease to engage in an exercise program; exercise tolerance is often improved, although the effect on survival remains unproven (see Chapters 10, 26 and 44). It is important that patients be reminded to note the level of activity that they can tolerate and report any decrease. Precipitants of worsening exercise tolerance should also be watched for. In this manner, patients can be enlisted in the diagnostic and monitoring efforts; their inter-est may help ensure compliance and facilitate management.

ANNOTATED BIBLIOGRAPHY

Buehler, J.H., and Gracey, D.R.: Laboratory differentiation of cardiac and primary pulmonary dyspnea. Mod. Concepts Cardiovasc Dis., *43*:113, 1974. *(An excellent discussion of pathophysiology and the usefulness of pulmonary function tests in the evaluation of dyspnea.)*

Ebert, R.V.: The lung and congestive heart failure. Arch. Intern. Med., *107*:450, 1961. *(A review of pulmonary function in congestive heart failure, emphasizing the relationship of vital capacity to dyspnea.)*

Jones, N.L.: Exercise testing in pulmonary evaluation: Clinical application. N. Engl. J. Med., *293*:647, 1975. *(Describes the use of exercise PFTs in evaluating dyspnea; preceded by article, N. Engl. J. Med., 293:341, 1975, detailing methods and physiology of exercise testing.)*

Macklem, P.T.: New tests to assess lung function. N. Engl. J. Med., *293*:339, 1975. *(First article in a series reviewing applications of pulmonary function tests other than the routine forced expiratory spirograms.)*

Staub, N.C.: State of the art review: Pathogenesis of pulmonary edema. Am. Rev. Respir. Dis., *109*:358, 1974. *(An excellent review of the pathophysiology of pulmonary edema.)*

Stewart-Harris, C.H.: Shortness of breath. Br. Med. J., *1*:1203, 1964 *(A good review.)*

37
Evaluation of Chronic Cough

A chronic cough poses a difficult evaluation problem because etiologies range from trivial conditions to life-threatening illnesses. Although many patients attribute their cough to cigarette-smoking, the primary physician must be aware of early signs suggesting a more worrisome cause (such as bronchogenic carcinoma) so that a prompt, efficient and thorough evaluation can be undertaken with a minimum of unnecessary testing or excessive delay.

PATHOPHYSIOLOGY AND CLINICAL PRESENTATION

The physiological function of cough is to remove foreign substances and mucus from the respiratory tract. It is a three-phased mechanical process that involves a deep inspiration, increasing lung volume, muscular contraction against a closed glottis, and sudden opening of the glottis. The maneuver produces and sustains a high linear air velocity to expel material from the respiratory tree.

Cough is a reflex response mediated by the medulla, but subject to voluntary control. The afferent limb may involve receptors in the larynx, respiratory tree, pleura, acoustic duct, nose, sinuses, pharynx, stomach or diaphragm. The receptors respond to mechanical, inflammatory or irritant stimuli. The trigeminal, glossopharyngeal, phrenic and vagus nerves can carry the afferent signal. The efferent limb of the cough reflex involves the recurrent laryngeal, phrenic and spinal motor nerves, which innervate the respiratory muscles.

The most common cause of recurrent cough is *cigarette smoking,* which may trigger the cough reflex by direct bronchial irritation or may induce inflammatory changes and mucus production, stimulating a self-propagating productive cough. Chronic cough and decreased flow rates have been observed in teenagers after only 3 to 5 years of smoking. Pipe and cigar smoking cause lesser degrees of difficulty.

Environmental irritants play a majror role in production of cough in patients living in industrialized urban areas. Pollutants that are frequently involved are heavy smog, sulphur dioxide, nitrous oxide and industrial gases such as ammonia. In Britain, the relationship between air quality and production of cough has been documented. The dusts and particulate matter which are capable of producing pneumoconioses can contribute to the problem. The excessive drying of normal airway moisture that takes place in centrally heated homes (humidity may fall below 10 per cent unless a humidifier is utilized) results in a persistent dry cough.

Carcinoma of the lung may present with cough in its early stages, particularly when an endobronchial lesion is present. Often the cigarette smoker notes a change in the pattern of his chronic "cigarette cough." Hemoptysis is noted in about 5 to 10 per cent of early cases. Other clues are localized wheezing and purulent sputum suggestive of obstruction. In later stages, cough is present in conjunction with weight loss, anorexia, dyspnea, vomiting, etc. In some instances, a systemic syndrome (e.g., inappropriate ADH secretion, hypertrophic pulmonary osteoarthropathy, dermatomyositis or peripheral neuropathy) may precede appearance of tumor.

Cough may be the predominant manifestation of *asthma.* Recent studies of asthmatics have emphasized that cough can occur in the absence of wheezing, but in the presence of demonstrable airway obstruction. Marked mucus production is in part responsible for the cough (see Chapter 45).

Inflammation anywhere along the upper or lower respiratory tract is capable of producing cough, for receptors capable of transmitting impulses that stimulate cough are believed to be distributed throughout the respiratory system. The greater the inflammatory stimulus, the larger the white cell response and the more purulent the sputum. (The green coloration of very purulent sputum is due to the degeneration of white cells.) *Chronic bronchitis* is among the most common causes of chronic cough and sputum production. The condition is defined clinically as the presence of a productive cough that persists for at least three months, two years in-a-row. A morning cough is often prominent, and bronchospasm a frequent accompaniment (see Chapter 44). *Bronchiectasis* is also characterized by cough and sputum production, but differs clinically from bronchitis in that there are more likely to be repeated bouts of hemoptysis and pneumonia. Copious amounts of purulent sputum are often produced. Chronic cough and sputum production commonly persist between episodes of pneumonia. Focal destruction of supporting lung tissue leads to dilatation of bronchi and focal findings of rhonci and wheezes on physical examination. A history of suppurative pneumonia in childhood is sometimes elicited.

Nasal and *otic problems* are often overlooked as sources of chronic cough, but allergic rhinitis (see Chapter 212), sinusitis (see Chapter 209), impacted cerumen or external otitis may be responsible. A persistent postnasal drip can be quite bothersome (see Chapter 212). Otic problems cause a dry cough; nasal disease can lead to sputum production.

Interstitial lung disease and *extraluminal compression* may stimulate mechanical receptors and result in a nonproductive cough. Fibrotic diseases of the interstitium and pulmonary edema are examples of intrapulmonary etiologies, and hilar adenopathy, aortic aneurysm and neoplasm are important extraluminal mass lesions. Chronic interstitial pulmonary edema produces nocturnal cough due to increased venous return at night which worsens heart failure (see Chapter 27). When failure is severe, frothy pink or blood-tinged sputum may be noted.

Psychogenic cough is more prevalent in children but may occur in adults; characteristically, it is nonproductive, occurs at times of emotional stress and ceases during the night.

DIFFERENTIAL DIAGNOSIS

The common causes of chronic cough are listed in Table 37–1. Rarer etiologies of cough include irritation of the pleura, diaphragm, pericardium or stomach. Case reports of truly rare causes of cough in-

Table 37-1. Important Causes of Chronic or Persistent Cough

Environmental Irritants
  1. Cigarette smoking (cigar and pipe smoking to a lesser degree)
  2. Pollutants (sulfur dioxide, nitrous oxide, particulate matter)
  3. Dusts (all agents capable of producing pneumoconioses)
  4. Lack of humidity
Lower Respiratory Tract Problems
  1. Lung cancer
  2. Asthma
  3. Chronic obstructive lung disease (especially bronchitis)
  4. Interstitial lung disease
  5. Congestive heart failure (chronic interstitial pulmonary edema)
  6. Pneumonitis
  7. Bronchiectasis
Upper Respiratory Tract Problems
  1. Chronic rhinitis
  2. Chronic sinusitis
  3. Disease of the external auditory canal
  4. Pharyngitis
Extrinsic Compressive Lesions
  1. Adenopathy
  2. Malignancy
  3. Aortic aneurysm
Psychogenic Factors

clude osteophytes of the cervical spine and pacemaker malfunction.

WORKUP

History. Since many etiologies of chronic cough are serious but potentially treatable illnesses, the prime objective of evaluation is to search for them; these include early lung cancer, heart failure, asthma and tuberculosis. Moreover, identification of environmental precipitants is essential to successful therapy. Nonproductive cough should be distinguished from one that produces sputum or mucus. The color and nature of sputum and the timing of its production may be helpful in the diagnosis. Cough productive of purulent sputum indicates significant inflammation, while a scanty or nonproductive cough is usually noninflammatory. A productive morning cough is suggestive of chronic bronchitis, obstruction, interstitial lung disease, tumor and bronchiectasis. A cough described as "throat clearing" may be a manifestation of postnasal drip. The history should also detail smoking habits, environmental and occupational exposures, previous allergies, asthma, sinusitis, chronic respiratory infections and tuberculosis exposure. As-

sociated symptoms of orthopnea, dyspnea on exertion and paroxysmal nocturnal dyspnea strongly indicate heart failure; dyspnea may also reflect pneumonia or asthma. Hemoptysis suggests bronchitis, bronchiectasis, tumor or tuberculosis, but also may be due to blood loss from the upper respiratory tract. Generalized wheezing is associated with obstruction from asthma or bronchitis, but localized wheezing may be a sign of tumor. Hoarseness is usually indicative of tracheobronchial disease with laryngeal involvement, but may represent a tumor impinging on the recurrent laryngeal nerve.

Physical examination should emphasize the upper and lower respiratory tracts, ears, neck and cardiovascular system. The physician needs to examine the skin for cyanosis, the pharynx for postnasal discharge and tonsillar enlargement, the nose for polyps, discharge and obstruction, and the ears for impacted cerumen or otitis. The trachea is palpated for position and the neck for masses and adenopathy. Auscultation and percussion of the lungs (including the apices) are done to detect wheezing, crackles, and signs of consolidation or effusion. During cardiac examination, the physician should evaluate the jugular venous pulse for distention and listen for an S_3 indicative of heart failure.

Laboratory studies. Expensive testing can very often be held to a minimum when careful history and physical examination are combined with a few, simple, well-chosen studies. The chest film may be helpful when there is historical and/or physical evidence which raises the question of carcinoma, tuberculosis, heart failure, interstitial pneumonitis, bronchitis, or bronchiectasis. However, the test is overutilized. For example, many young previously healthy nonsmokers with a cough that lingers during the winter for 3 to 4 weeks after a typical upper respiratory tract infection come to the office because they are afraid they have pneumonia. If the chest is clear to auscultation, the sputum Gram stain without organisms, and the white count and differential normal, no chest film need be obtained, for the probability of encountering a process that requires antibiotic treatment is very small. Obviously, the chest film may be used to provide reassurance, but a careful history, physical, Gram stain and white count should suffice for this purpose.

When a chest film is obtained and an infiltrate identified, an acid-fast stain for tubercle bacilli should be performed in addition to a Gram stain; this may provide not only a diagnosis but also a crude indication of how infectious the sputum is.

Patients who give a history of producing purulent

sputum in conjunction with cough but who cannot raise sputum at the time of examination should be instructed to drink a few glasses of water (which may facilitate sputum production), and be asked to remain awhile until sputum can be raised. A common error in evaluation of a productive cough is failure to obtain and examine the sputum. Culturing the sputum is also important, especially when tuberculosis is a possibility, because the acid-fast examination is not a very sensitive test and the diagnosis cannot be ruled out with certainty until three early morning sputum samples have failed to produce growth by 4 to 6 weeks. (see Chapters 34 and 47).

When tumor is suspected (e.g., heavy smoker with change in cough pattern) but the chest film is unremarkable, one should avoid hastily ordering expensive and/or invasive tests such as tomography and endoscopy. Cytologic testing of three early morning sputum samples can be a useful screening test for pulmonary neoplasm (see Chapter 38) and should be obtained when concern about carcinoma of the lung persists in spite of a normal chest film. Pulmonary histiocytes must by demonstrated on each specimen to prove that the sample of pulmonary secretions is adequate. A "negative" test in the absence of histiocytes is meaningless and is the source of many false-negative results. Only if cytology is positive or clinical suspicion of cancer is extremely strong (new onset of hemoptysis in conjunction with cough) should the more invasive and expensive procedures be resorted to (see Chapter 33).

Evaluation of cough accompanied by shortness of breath should include a chest x-ray for signs of congestive failure (see Chapter 27) and a check of simple pulmonary function tests such as the FEV_1 and vital capacity in order to detect any significant bronchospasm which might be subject to treatment. A few whiffs of a bronchodilator can be given to measure the response to bronchodilators (see Chapters 44 and 45).

Patients with chronic bronchitis need not be subjected to repeated diagnostic studies whenever there is an increase or change in sputum production, because the most likely cause is an intercurrent tracheobronchitis due to pneumocci or *H. influenzae*.

SYMPTOMATIC THERAPY

The most effective therapy is to alleviate the underlying cause, although this is not always possible. Symptomatic management is directed at suppressing the cough and preventing complications that may re-

sult from coughing. Potential complications include musculoskeletal pain, rib fractures, pneumothorax, exhaustion, pneumomediastinum, post-tussive syncope (see Chapter 18), and rupture of subconjunctival or nasal veins. The occurrence of any of these complications may be a reason for occasionally suppressing a cough that has not been completely diagnosed.

The first priority and simplest manipulation is to remove or reduce irritants. Of paramount importance is cessation of smoking; this eliminated cough in 77 per cent and reduced it in another 17 per cent within a month. Second, a properly humidified environment should be maintained by placing pails of water near radiators and windows (an inexpensive maneuver) or by employing humidifiers. If a humidifier is used, it should be kept clean because it can become colonized with bacteria or fungi and cause infection or hypersensitivity pneumonitis. Third, adequate internal hydration should be encouraged by advising the intake of at least 1500 cc. of fluid daily, particularly water. These simple measures alone may abolish cough in many patients.

The patient with a chronic cough secondary to established underlying lung disease requires careful education. The patient must be informed that expectorating sputum is preferable to its remaining in the tracheobronchial tree. Patients with chronic bronchitis or bronchiectasis may benefit from improved pulmonary toilet. They can be taught how to cough with quiet, forceful expirations and how to perform postural drainage to promote removal of mucus from the bronchioles. Postural drainage is best timed before meals, before bedtime and on awakening in the morning. The aid of a chest physiotherapist can be invaluable for teaching the patient at home (see Chapter 44).

Patients with chronic cough often request and need temporary cough suppression, such as at bedtime to allow uninterrupted sleep, or when complications of cough arise. A wide variety of agents have been used to treat cough. The most effective are the narcotic antitussives which act centrally to suppress the medullary cough center. Other preparations are expectorants or mucolytic agents which merely help to mobilize sputum; they can have a mild placebo effect as well, but it is not an impressive one. When cough significantly interferes with sleeping or eating, a narcotic cough suppressant should be used. Codeine is the drug of choice. It should be used in relatively small doses of 8 to 15 mg., at intervals of 2 to 4 hours, according to the patient's needs. Liquid and tablet preparations are equally effective. If a small dose does not suppress the cough, doses of up to 60 mg. every 3 to 4 hours may be tried. It is worth noting that many patients expect to use a syrup for cough suppression; prescribing the drug in syrup form may provide some psychological benefit. Patients for whom a narcotic antitussive is prescribed should be given small quantities and followed closely to ensure that the cough resolves and excessive use does not result. The obvious exception to this precaution is the patient with incurable lung cancer, who should receive the doses necessary to provide relief from the discomfort of persistent cough.

Nonnarcotic antitussives lack addiction potential but are not as effective as codeine. The most popular over-the-counter cough suppressant is dextromethorphan, which has a mild suppressant effect. Many over-the-counter preparations contain alcohol, sympathomimetics, and antihistamines. The mucolytic effects of alcohol are minimal; the sympathomimetics and antihistamines are of little use except in patients whose cough derives from chronic rhinitis (see Chapter 212). Some over-the-counter agents dull the peripheral sensory receptors; this is the rationale for putting mild topical anesthetics in sprays, syrups, and cough lozenges. They are of questionable utility.

Expectorants are heavily consumed. There are over 60 preparations containing guaifenesin; terpin hydrate is another popular expectorant. These agents are often combined with an effective cough suppressant and, as such, are associated with a beneficial effect, but by themselves they have no proven effect and represent an unnecessary expense. They are given when the patient insists on something for cough but lacks clear indications for cough suppression, or because the patient believes expectorants help him. Expectorants are available over-the-counter and frequently promoted to the public in advertising (e.g., Robitussin).

ANNOTATED BIBLIOGRAPHY

Bloustine, S., *et al.*: Ear cough (Arnold's reflex). Otol. Rhinol. Laryngol. *85*:406, 1976. *(A clinical survey of 688 patients that revealed an incidence of the ear cough reflex of 1.74 per cent, a reminder to examine the ear.)*

Bucher, K.: Cough and antitussives: Considerations and experiments. Agents Actions, *4*:377, 1974. *(A scholarly presentation of what is known about the pathophysiology of cough and its application to developing experimental models for therapeutic agents.)*

Cattel, McK. (moderator): Conference on therapy: Treatment of cough. Am. J. Med., *114*:87, 1953. *(This report is a somewhat dated but thoughtful clinical approach.)*

Corrao, W., Braman, S.S., and Irwin R.S.: Chronic cough as the sole presenting manifestation of bronchial asthma. N. Engl. J. Med., *300*:633, 1979. *(Six patients whose asthma presented as cough and had no prior history of wheezing.)*

Irwin, R.S., Rosen, M.J., and Broman, S. S.: Cough—A comprehensive review. Arch. Intern. Med., *137*:1186, 1977. *(A superb review; unfortunately the bibliography is available only by sale.)*

Kiernan, K.E.: Chronic cough in young adults in relation to smoking habits, childhood environment, and chest illness. Respiration, *33*:236, 1976. *(This is a second article in a series following a cohort of young adults who show a strong correlation between the prevalence of chronic cough and smoking, with cessation reducing cough even when childhood factors predisposed to chronic cough.)*

McFadden, F.R., Jr.: Exertional dyspnea and cough as preludes to acute attacks of asthma. N. Engl. J. Med., *292*:555, 1975. *(Wheezing may be absent as an early manifestation of an acute attack, and cough may dominate the clinical picture.)*

38
Evaluation of Hemoptysis

Because of its well known associations with cancer and tuberculosis, hemoptysis is an alarming symptom for both patient and physician. Hemoptysis refers to coughing up of both blood-tinged and grossly bloody sputum. In the office, the primary physician is usually confronted with a patient who has noted sputum streaked with blood. Most patients prove to have inconsequential lesions, but a thorough evaluation is necessary because the seriousness of the etiology does not correlate with the amount of blood coughed up.

PATHOPHYSIOLOGY AND CLINICAL PRESENTATION

Inflammation of the tracheobronchial mucosa accounts for many cases of hemoptysis. Minor mucosal erosions can result from *upper respiratory infections* and *bronchitis;* blood-streaked sputum is often noted, especially if coughing has been vigorous and prolonged. Patients with *bronchiectasis* are more subject to recurrent episodes of grossly bloody sputum, because necrosis of the bronchial mucosa can be quite severe. Up to 50 per cent of those with bronchiectasis experience hemoptysis. In the U.S., hemoptysis occurring with *tuberculosis* is usually due to mucosal ulceration, although potentially fatal bleeding can occur when a blood vessel adjacent to a cavitary lesion ruptures. About 10 to 15 per cent of patients with tuberculosis report some form of hemoptysis; most of these episodes are minor, involving sputum tinged with small amounts of blood. Endobronchial inflammatory injury from granuloma formation is the mechanism of hemoptysis associated with *sarcoidosis;* small amounts of blood-streaked sputum are occasionally noted.

Mucosal injury can also be a consequence of *bronchogenic carcinoma.* Disruption of endobronchial tissue may be minimal and cause little more than a trace of hemoptysis from time to time; hemorrhage is rare. Between 35 and 55 per cent of patients with proven bronchogenic carcinoma report at least one episode of hemoptysis during the course of their ill-

ness; it is the presenting symptom in about 10 per cent of cases. Carcinoma metastatic to the lung rarely results in hemoptysis. *Bronchial adenomas* are quite vascular, and commonly central and endobronchial in location; as a consequence, they frequently bleed, and recurrent episodes of hemoptysis are reported in about half of cases.

Injury to the pulmonary vasculature is an important source of hemoptysis. *Lung abscess* may result in damage to adjacent vessels and frequently presents with bloody as well as purulent sputum. *Necrotizing pneumonias,* such as those produced by *Klebsiella,* can cause substantial vascular disruption; 25 to 50 per cent of patients cough up tenacious, bloody sputum referred to as "current jelly." *Aspergillomas* are also capable of vascular injury; hemoptysis is the most common symptom of the condition. The patient with an aspergilloma is typically a compromised host with prior cavitary disease from tuberculosis, bronchiectasis, etc. *Pulmonary infarction* secondary to embolization is characterized by sudden onset of pleuritic pain in conjunction with hemoptysis; embolization without infarction does not cause hemoptysis. Pulmonary contusion from blunt *chest trauma* may present with hemoptysis following a nonpenetrating blow to the thorax.

Marked elevations in pulmonary capillary pressure can cause vascular injury and leakage of red cells. The pink, frothy sputum of *pulmonary edema* is a manifestation of this process. More grossly bloody sputum sometimes occurs in severe *mitral stenosis* when a dilated pulmonary-bronchial venous connection ruptures. Vasculitic injury is responsible for the hemoptysis found in *Wegener's granulomatosis* (see Chapter 212) and *Goodpasture's syndrome.* Hematuria often accompanies both conditions. Hereditary vascular malformations are subject to recurrent bleeding. *Arteriovenous malformations* may be accompanied by an audible bruit on auscultation of the lung. In *hereditary hemorrhagic telangiectasia,* there is often a family history of bleeding problems or prior episodes of bleeding from multiple sites; telangiectasias may be visible in the buccal cavity and on the skin. Bleeding into the interstitium characterizes *idiopathic pulmonary hemosiderosis.* This rare disease, uncommon in adults, is manifested by diffuse interstitial infiltrates, anemia and hemoptysis.

Hemoptysis may be the first sign of a *bleeding disorder* or *excessive anticoagulant therapy;* however, there is usually an underlying bronchopulmonary lesion as well.

DIFFERENTIAL DIAGNOSIS

The most commonly reported etiologies of hemoptysis are chronic bronchitis and bronchiectasis, accounting for 50 to 70 per cent of cases in many series. Bronchogenic carcinomas account for less than 5 per cent of cases. Tuberculosis, pneumonia, and vascular lesions make up the remainder. Most incidence figures are obtained from chest clinics and inpatient units serving preselected populations; therefore, they cannot be extrapolated to the primary care setting. The declining incidence of tuberculosis (see Chapter 34), more widespread use of fiberoptic bronchoscopy, and increases in cigarette smoking and lung cancer in women are likely to change incidence figures in the near future. The more common and important etiologies of hemoptysis are listed in Table 38–1. One must also consider gastrointestinal and nasopharyngeal sources.

Table 38–1.   Important Causes of Hemoptysis

Gross Hemoptysis
1. Tuberculosis (with cavitary disease)
2. Bronchiectasis
3. Bronchial adenoma
4. Bronchogenic carcinoma (uncommon)
5. Aspergilloma
6. Necrotizing pneumonia
7. Lung abscess
8. Plumonary contusion
9. A-V malformation
10. Hereditary hemorrhagic telangiectasia
11. Bleeding disorder or excessive anticoagulant therapy
12. Mitral stenosis (with rupture of a bronchial vessel)

Blood-streaked Sputum
1. Any of the causes of gross hemoptysis
2. Upper respiratory tract infection
3. Chronic bronchitis
4. Sarcoidosis
5. Bronchogenic carcinoma
6. Tuberculosis
7. Pulmonary infarction
8. Pulmonary edema
9. Mitral stenosis
10. Idiopathic pulmonary hemosiderosis

WORKUP

History. Evaluation of the patient with hemoptysis should begin with consideration of the epidemiology of the serious underlying causes. Concern about pulmonary neoplasm should be highest in the older male with a long history of heavy smoking and/or asbestos exposure. The elderly patient with evidence of old disease on chest x-ray should be presumed to have reactivated tuberculosis infection. The adolescent with hemoptysis may have a new infection due to recent tuberculosis exposure. The compromised host with previous cavitary disease is at risk for an aspergilloma.

The patient's description of the sputum associated with hemoptysis can be of some diagnostic help. Pink sputum is suggestive of pulmonary edema fluid; putrid sputum is indicative of a lung abscess; current-jellylike material points to a necrotizing pneumonia; copious amounts of purulent sputum mixed with blood are consistent with bronchiectasis. The commonly described blood-streaked sputum is nonspecific.

History should also be checked for previous bleeding episodes, family history of hemoptysis, hematuria, concurrent pleuritic chest pain, known heart murmur or history of rheumatic fever, lymph node enlargement, blunt chest trauma, symptoms of heart failure (see Chapter 27), and use of anticoagulant drugs. Determining the amount of blood produced is not particularly helpful for diagnostic purposes beyond establishing whether the hemoptysis was gross or scant. It is important to be certain that there is no history of a coexisting nasopharyngeal problem or source of gastrointestinal bleeding that the patient may be mistaking for true hemoptysis.

Physical examination is directed at detecting nonpulmonary sources of bleeding as well as evidence of chest pathology and systemic disease. The vital signs should be checked for fever and tachypnea, the skin for ecchymoses and telangiectasias, and the nails for clubbing. Clubbing is associated with neoplasm, bronchiectasis, lung abscess and other severe pulmonary disorders (see Chapter 41). Nodes are examined for enlargement, suggestive of sarcoidosis, tuberculosis and malignancy (see Chapters 48 and 80). The neck is noted for jugular venous distention, consistent with heart failure and severe mitral disease. Examination of the chest should include a search for bruits, signs of consolidation, wheezes, crackles, and chest wall contusion.

The history and physical findings can be used to determine the pace at which workup should proceed, as well as the selection and sequence of laboratory tests. The patient with minimal hemoptysis may be followed at home while evaluation takes place on an outpatient basis, as long as the patient is given explicit advice to return immediately if severe bleeding ensues. The patient with a suspected bleeding diathesis should not be sent home.

Laboratory studies. The chest x-ray is essential to the assessment of most cases, for it may reveal a mass, abscess, infiltrate, interstitial changes, hilar adenopathy, signs of congestive failure (see Chapter 27) or evidence of significant mitral stenosis (see Chapter 28). Less common radiologic findings include peribronchial cuffing indicative of bronchiectasis and a crescentic radiolucency surrounding a coin lesion characteristic of an aspergilloma. Often the chest film is normal.

The sputum needs to be Gram stained if it appears grossly purulent or the patient is febrile. An acid-fast stain for tubercle bacilli is also essential, not only for diagnosis but for making a crude assessment of infectivity (see Chapter 47). The sensitivity of the acid-fast smear depends on the diligence with which the search for pathogenic organisms is made. In one series, only 20 per cent of culture-positive samples were identified in advance by acid-fast smear. It should also be remembered that despite a very high specificity, the predictive value of a positive smear may be as low as 50 per cent when the sputum specimens of low-risk patients are examined. A tuberculin skin test should be performed if the patient's PPD reactivity status in not known. It must be remembered, however, that approximately 7 per cent of all adults (25 per cent of adults over age 50) will have positive reactions. (See Chapters 34 and 47).

Sputum cytologies should be obtained in all patients in whom there is no clear diagnosis. The sensitivity of a single sputum cytology examination has been shown to be about 70 per cent in the detection of squamous cell lesions, lower for other cell types. Three cytologic examinations increase sensitivity to 90 per cent.

Additional diagnostic tests may be indicated in specific clinical settings; for example, tomography may further define a suspicious lesion seen on chest x-ray, and ventilation-perfusion scanning or angiography of the lung is indicated when the presentation suggests pulmonary embolization with infarction (see Chapter 14). Bleeding studies, such as a PT, PTT platelet count, and bleeding time are needed if more than one site of bleeding is noted.

A difficult decision is when to refer the patient for bronchoscopy. The procedure oftens provides useful information when the diagnosis is still in doubt after chest x-ray and sputum examination. Moreover, the sensitivities of cytologic and bacteriologic studies are enhanced when specimens are obtained by bronchoscopy. Bronchoscopy is mandatory in all patients with massive hemoptysis who are being seriously considered for surgery, in order to localize the bleeding site. Rigid bronchoscopy is preferred in this situation.

The more common indication for bronchoscopy is to exclude the possibility of a tumor. It must be remembered, however, that the prevalence of cancer in an unselected population presenting with hemoptysis is low and that the risks of morbidity associated with bronchoscopy are not insignificant. Among patients presenting at a chest clinic complaining of hemoptysis, only 2 per cent were subsequently found to have cancers. One could expect the prevalence among patients without suggestive chest x-ray findings and with negative sputum cytologies to be significantly lower.

Serious complications are rare with fiberoptic bronchoscopy, but they do occur. In a review of 48,000 procedures, fewer than 100 life-threatening cardiovascular or respiratory complications were reported, most often in older individuals with COPD and coronary disease. Hypoxia occurs commonly following bronchoscopy. In the low-risk patient, fiberoptic bronchoscopy is indicated for unexplained, recurrent, mild hemoptysis and can be safely performed without hospitalization.

ANNOTATED BIBLIOGRAPHY

Barrett, R.J., and Tuttle, W.M.: A study of essential hemoptysis. J. Thorac. Cardiovasc. Surg., *40*:468, 1960. *(Observed 81 patients with unexplained hemoptysis for 1 to 10 years; source of hemoptysis later identified in only 3 cases.)*

Boucot, K.R., *et al.*: Hemoptysis in older men. Geriatrics, *14*:67, 1959. *(A comprehensive statistical review of patients with hemoptysis from the Philadelphia Pulmonary Neoplasm Research Project. It found neoplasm in 80 per cent, but hemoptysis was generally a late finding.)*

Chaves, A.D.: Hemoptysis in chest clinic patients. Am. Rev. of Tub. *63:194*, 1951. *(A report of 325 patients with hemoptysis in a population of 4,771 consecutive patients seen in the Kips Bay Health Center Free Chest Clinic. Lung cancer was present in only 7 of 325 patients, suggesting the low prevalence that might be expected in an unselected primary care practice, but study done prior to advent of modern diagnostic methods.)*

Johnston, R.N., Lockhart, W., *et al.*: Hemoptysis. Br. Med. J., *1*:592, 1960. *(A paper from a chest clinic that revealed 324 cases of hemoptysis representing 15 per cent of the clinical population. Demonstrated that upper respiratory infection, bronchitis and "no apparent diagnosis" were the leading causes of hemoptysis in an ambulatory population, again done prior to advent of modern diagnostic techniques.)*

Pursel, S.E., and Lindskog, G.E.: A clinical evaluation of 105 patients examined consecutively on a thoracic surgical service. Am. Rev. Respir. Dis., *84*:329, 1961. *(A series of 105 patients with hemoptysis evaluated in the days prior to fiberoptic endoscopy;· it revealed 44.6 per cent with bronchiectasis, 9.5 per cent with carcinoma, 19.2 per cent with tuberculosis, and very much smaller numbers with a variety of other conditions.*

The severity of hemoptysis did not help establish a diagnosis.)

Selecky, P.A.: Evaluation of hemoptysis through the bronchoscope. Chest, *73*:7415, 1978. *(A good review that states that all patients with hemoptysis unless they have malignant cells or acid-fast bacilli in the sputum need bronchoscopy.)*

Smiddy, J.F., and Eliot, R.C.: The evaluation of hemoptysis with fiberoptic bronchoscopy. Chest, *64*:158, 1973. *(An article that establishes the utility of transnasal fiberoptic bronchoscopy in a prospective study evaluating hemoptysis. The source of bleeding was located in 66 of 71 patients.)*

Surratt, P.M., Smiddy, J.F., and Gruber, B.: Deaths and complications associated with fiberoptic bronchoscopy. Chest, *69*:747, 1976. *(Fifty-two severe respiratory complications and 27 severe cardiovascular complications in nearly 50,000 procedures.)*

39

Evaluation of Pleural Effusions

Most pleural effusions encountered in the office are discovered as incidental findings and often pose a diagnostic challenge, for etiology is frequently unclear. Outpatient evaluation of a pleural effusion requires skill in performance of a diagnostic thoracentesis in the office and the differentiation of a transudate from an exudate. Of major concern are the possibilities of tumor and infection. The primary physician should be able to safely carry out the initial evaluation of a pleural effusion in the ambulatory setting, provided the patient's respiratory status is satisfactory and there is no evidence of serious acute illness.

PATHOPHYSIOLOGY AND CLINICAL PRESENTATION

The pleural cavity normally contains a small volume of serous fluid that serves a lubricant function. Fluid is formed by transudation from the parietal pleural surface and reabsorbed predominantly by the visceral pleura. Effusion results from excessive transudation of fluid or from an exudative process. Increased hydrostatic pressure and decreased colloid oncotic pressure produce transudates. Exudates result from inflammatory or infiltrative disease of the pleura and its adjacent structures; damage occurs to capillary membranes, and protein-rich material accumulates in the pleural space. Obstruction to lymphatic flow can also produce an exudative effusion.

Transudates

Since transudates are rarely associated with pleural inflammation, they are not usually accompanied by pleuritic pain, but may lead to shortness of breath if they are large enough to interfere with respiratory mechanics. They may be unilateral, but are often bilateral. Physical examination of the lung reveals dullness and diminished breath sounds. If the effusion has produced some atelectasis, there may be bronchial breath sounds and increased vocal fremitus above the effusion. Most transudates have a protein concentration of less than 3.0 gm. per 100 ml., but chronic transudates may show higher concentrations. In a study of patients with long-standing effusions due to chronic congestive heart failure, a large percentage had pleural fluid protein concentrations in excess of 3.0 gm. per 100 ml.

Congestive heart failure is among the most common causes of transudative effusions. Left heart failure increases pulmonary capillary pressure (see Chapter 27), which forces excess fluid into the interstitium. Right ventricular failure contributes by raising central venous pressure, which elevates the hydrostatic force in the capillaries of the parietal pleura and diminishes fluid reabsorption. Most effusions due to congestive failure are bilateral, but at times there can be an isolated right-sided effusion; isolated left-sided effusions due to congestive failure are rare. The reason for the right-sided preference is unknown. Symptoms and signs of congestive failure (see Chapter 27) are usually evident. Over 85 per cent of effusions resulting from heart failure have protein concentrations less than 3.0 gm. per 100 ml. The concentration may be greater if the effusion is chronic or the patient has recently been undergoing a brisk diuresis. The pleural fluid is usually clear, but it may be bloody and have red cell counts in excess of 5,000 per ml.

Patients with an overexpanded extracellular volume due to severe *hypoalbuminemia* or *salt retention* develop edema in parts of the body where hydrostatic pressures are greatest, before showing evidence of pleural effusion. Cardiomegaly may be in evidence, but overt signs of congestive failure are usually absent. Edema is rare before the serum albumin falls below 2.0 to 2.5 gm. per 100 ml.

Intra-abdominal diseases are occasionally responsible for transudative effusions. Between 5 and 10 per cent of patients with ascites due to cirrhosis develop a right-sided pleural effusion; the composition of the effusion resembles that of the ascitic fluid. In cases of pancreatitis or a subphrenic abscess, a "sympathetic effusion" with the characteristics of a transudate sometimes forms; it soon changes into an exudate.

Exudates

Since most exudates form as a consequence of pleural injury, they are often accompanied by pleuritic chest pain, especially in the acute phase when a friction rub may be heard before much fluid accumulates. The fluid is initially free-flowing, but may be-

come walled-off and loculated when there is a marked inflammatory response. The protein content is usually greater than 3.0 gm. per 100 ml. The fluid is typically deep yellow or cloudy in appearance. The leukocyte count is often greater than 1,000 cells per ml.; a count greater than 10,000 is suggestive of an empyema, particularly if most of the cells are neutrophiles.

Neoplasms are often responsible for the development of effusions. The majority of pleural fluid accumulations due to malignancies have the characteristics of exudates, though at times the protein concentration is less than 3.0 gm. per 100 ml. *Bronchogenic carcinoma* is the tumor most frequently associated with a pleural effusion. Fluid collects in most instances as a direct result of pleural invasion; unilateral effusions are the rule. Patients report dyspnea when the effusion is large and occasionally complain of pleuritic chest pain. The pleural fluid is usually clear and straw-colored, but it may be bloody and its glucose level may be very low. The white count is typically around 2,500 per ml., with most cells being lymphocytes. Malignant cells are found in about 60 per cent of instances. Unfortunately, the disease and its effusions are progressive; thoracentesis is followed by rapid reaccumulation.

Pleural effusions due to *metastatic carcinoma* are more likely to be bilateral than those due to bronchogenic carcinoma, for they occur as a consequence of lymphatic obstruction or diffuse seeding of the pleura. Carcinoma of the breast is the leading metastatic tumor producing pleural effusions. The characteristics of the pleural fluid are similar to those of effusions due to bronchogenic carcinoma. *Lymphoma* is another malignant cause of bilateral pleural effusions. The formation of a large effusion is a sign of advanced disease; there is often evidence of pleural, parenchymal and lymph node involvement by the time a significant effusion appears. The pleural fluid may be a transudate or an exudate; most of the cells are lymphocytes. Cough and dyspnea accompany parenchymal involvement, but pleuritic pain is rare.

Mesotheliomas have become an increasingly important source of effusion as the incidence of asbestos exposure has increased. Only malignant mesotheliomas produce important pleural fluid accumulations. The latent period for mesothelioma formation ranges from 20 to 40 years after asbestos exposure; the degree of exposure may appear inconsequential (see Chapter 35). Chest pain, cough, and shortness of breath result from extensive pleural disease and large effusions. The fluid may be bloody and often contains malignant cells which are sometimes hard to identify specifically as those of a mesothelioma. Since the tumor is only locally invasive, there are no signs of extrathoracic disease.

Impressive effusions can form as a consequence of *benign ovarian neoplasms (Meigs' syndrome)*. The tumor produces ascites, and fluid tracks across the diaphragm and into the thorax. The effusion is typically on the right, but may be left-sided or even bilateral; it is exudative in quality, free of malignant cells and similar in composition to the ascitic fluid from which it derives. Removal of the ovarian tumor results in prompt resolution of the effusion.

Infections are an important source of exudative pleural effusions. The effusion due to *postprimary tuberculosis* represents a delayed hypersensitivity reaction to spillage of organisms into the pleural space during early bacteremia or subclinical parenchymal disease (see Chapter 47). The effusion is almost always unilateral. The patient may be relatively free of symptoms or complain of lethargy, fever and weight loss; at times, the clinical picture is dominated by acute onset of pleuritic pain and fever. Cough and sputum are conspicuously absent. The chest x-ray may show little more than an isolated effusion, but the intermediate-strength tuberculin skin test is usually positive. The pleural fluid has the qualities of an exudate; the glucose concentration may be low. The white cell count averages 1,000 to 2,000 cells per ml.; lymphocytes predominate; mesothelial cells are scarce (less than 2 per cent). Neutrophils may be seen early in the course of the illness. Organisms are rarely found on acid-fast stain of the fluid and can be cultured from the fluid in only 25 per cent of cases. Most of these effusions resolve spontaneously within a few months and leave little or no residual; however, symptomatic pulmonary parenchymal involvement eventually develops in over half of such patients (see Chapter 47).

Acute bacterial pneumonia may lead to the formation of a pleural effusion, but among the bacterial pneumonias encountered in ambulatory patients, effusions are uncommon. About 5 per cent of patients with pneumococcal pneumonia develop an effusion; it is usually small and transient. Empyema is a rare but much more worrisome event, seen in less than 1 per cent; most cases occur when proper antibiotic therapy is delayed. Cough, sputum production, fever, chills, and pleuritic pain are often prominent. Early on, the pleural fluid may be serous, but it quickly turns purulent with empyema formation. The fluid may be sterile if empyema does not develop; organisms can be isolated from most empyemas. In some instances, the pleural fluid offers the only opportunity for recovery of the causative organism. Characteristics of the pleural empyema fluid include a white cell count in excess of 5,000 to 10,000 per ml., with neutrophils predominating. The concentration of glucose is typically less than 20 mg. per 100 ml. Pleural scarring may be substantial if the empyema fluid is allowed to remain.

Viral pneumonitis and *mycoplasmal pneumonia* are sometimes associated with small pleural effusions in the course of illness, but the effusions are small, transient and of little consequence (see Chapter 43).

Pulmonary embolization has been found to be accompanied by pleural effusion in up to 50 per cent of cases. The effusions are usually small and not dependent on occurrence of pulmonary infarction. There is considerable variation in cell count, differential, and protein concentration. The effusions that result from infarction are more likely to be bloody. Bilateral effusions can be seen when emboli affect both lungs.

Many patients with *systemic lupus erythematosus* experience transient pleuro-pericardial involvement during the course of their disease, usually after other signs of the disease have appeared. There may be a brief period of pleuritic pain. On occasion, pleural involvement may be the disease's initial clinical presentation. In most instances, the pleural fluid has the characteristics of an effusion and may demonstrate low serum complement levels.

Rheumatoid arthritis is much less likely to produce a pleural effusion than is lupus, but the fluid often persists. Less than 5 per cent of patients experience pleuropericardial involvement; these individuals usually have a history of extra-articular manifestations and joint symptoms. Once in a while, the effusion is the first manifestation of rheumatoid disease. The effusion is an exudate, with a predominance of lymphocytes and a very low (less than 20 mg. per 100 ml.) glucose concentration. Although the fluid may contain rheumatoid factor, its presence is not unique to this disease.

Intra-abdominal pathology occasionally results in the production of a pleural effusion. Patients with a recent history of abdominal surgery, intestinal perforation, or hepatobiliary disease are at risk for development of a *subdiaphragmatic abscess*. In addition to gastrointestinal symptoms, these patients may complain of pleuritic pain, fever, weight loss and malaise. Often symptoms are nonspecific, causing considerable delay in the decision to seek medical help. The diaphragm on the involved side (which is the right in two-thirds of cases) is elevated and moves poorly on fluoroscopy. A pathognomonic subdiaphragmatic air-fluid level may be present on chest film. The pleural fluid is usually sterile, though it may have a high leukocyte count. If the diaphragm has been perforated, an empyema can form. *Pancreatitis* may lead to a pleural effusion, particularly in the early phase of the disease. The effusions are most often on the left, but may be bilateral or right-sided. The fluid characteristically has a high amylase concentration and is blood-tinged in one third of cases.

DIFFERENTIAL DIAGNOSIS

The etiologies of pleural effusions can be conveniently divided into those conditions which produce transudates and those which result in exudates (Table 39–1); nevertheless, some conditions can cause both. Chronic congestive heart failure is the etiology most frequently encountered in the ambulatory population. Neoplasms account for the majority of cases seen in referral populations. In a series reported from the Mayo Clinic, bronchogenic carcinoma was the leading cause of malignant pleural effusions, followed by breast cancer and lymphoma. Infection is the third most common etiology of fluid in the pleural space, with tuberculosis still accounting for a substantial proportion of effusions subjected to full evaluation. Bloody effusions are most often due to neoplasms, but are also seen with congestive heart failure, pulmonary embolization with infarction, tuberculosis, and pancreatitis. About 15 percent of effusions remain unexplained; most idiopathic effusions are exudates.

WORKUP

History. Although definitive evaluation of a pleural effusion requires analysis of the pleural fluid, history can provide important clues and supporting evidence. The patient should be asked about the presence of fever, cough, sputum production, chest pain, dyspnea, edema, abdominal pain, prior history of malignant, hepatic or renal disease, exposure to tuberculosis or asbestos, and symptoms of rheumatoid arthritis and systemic lupus (see Chapters 139 and 147). Cough, fever and sputum production in conjunction with pleuritic chest pain suggests pneumonitis with pleural involvement. Pleuritic pain is also

Table 39–1   Important Causes of Pleural Effusions

TRANSUDATES
Congestive heart failure
Hypoalbuminemia
Salt-retention syndromes
Ascites due to cirrhosis
Early phases of a sympathetic effusion
Neoplasm (on occasion)
Peritoneal dialysis

EXUDATES
Neoplasms
Bronchogenic carcinoma
Breast cancer
Lymphoma
Mesothelioma
Meig's syndrome
Infections
Tuberculosis
Bacterial pneumonia (including empyema)
Viral pneumonitis
Mycoplasmal pneumonia
Pulmonary embolization
Connective tissue disease
Rheumatoid arthritis
Systemic lupus erythematosus
Intra-abdominal disease
Subphrenic abscess
Pancreatitis
Idiopathic

consistent with embolization (see Chapter 14), malignancy and pleural inflammation with adjacent pericarditis due to connective tissue disease. Dyspnea may be induced by the effusion alone, but the symptom is indicative of congestive heart failure when accompanied by orthopnea and paroxysmal nocturnal dyspnea. A history of peripheral edema raises the possibilities of hypoalbuminemia, volume overload, and congestive failure. A history of alcohol abuse, recent abdominal surgery, or abdominal pain or distention points to a source below the diaphragm.

Physical examination should determine the size of the effusion and the degree of respiratory compromise associated with it, as well as provide evidence for an underlying etiology. The vital signs should be checked for fever, tachypnea, tachycardia, and weight change. The integument requires inspection for petechiae, purpura, spider angiomas, jaundice, clubbing (see Chapter 41), rheumatoid nodules, and rashes. The neck is noted for jugular venous distention and tracheal deviation; the lymph nodes, for enlargement. Findings of the effusion on examination of the lung include dullness to percussion and diminished breath sounds. If there is compression of adjacent lung, egophony and bronchial breath sounds may be heard above the effusion. A pleural friction rub may be audible, but is usually lacking when there is a considerable accumulation of fluid. The heart should be checked for an S_3, indicative of failure, and evidence of pericariditis, such as a 3-component friction rub. The abdomen is examined for signs of ascites, organomegaly, and focal tenderness. The pelvic examination is done to rule out the presence of an ovarian mass, and the extremities are noted for edema, calf tenderness, and joint changes.

Laboratory evaluation centers on chest film (for confirmation of the effusion's size and location) and on analysis of the pleural fluid. The chest x-ray should also be studied for pleural-based densities, infiltrates, signs of congestive heart failure (see Chapter 27), hilar adenopathy, coin lesions and loculation of fluid (detection of which requires lateral decubitus views). Elevation of a hemidiaphragm and presence of a subdiaphragmatic air-fluid level are important radiologic signs of a subphrenic abscess.

Although sampling of the pleural fluid is usually necessary for diagnosis, there are instances when thoracentesis need not be done on the first visit; these include the afebrile patient with clinical evidence of congestive heart failure and the young patient with a small effusion in conjunction with a viral or mycoplasmal pneumonia. These individuals can be followed expectantly with repeat chest films; failure of the effusion to clear with resolution of the presumptive etiology is an indication for thoracentesis.

A diagnostic thoracentesis can be done safely and comfortably in the office on patients who have free-flowing effusions confirmed by lateral decubitus films. Thoracentesis for loculated effusions is more difficult and has a greater risk of pneumothorax; it is best not to tap such effusions in the office. There are a few pitfalls in thoracentesis technique that must be avoided. A common error is to go into the chest too far below the meniscus of the effusion, risking penetrating the diaphragm or entering the diaphragmatic sulcus, which is likely to be sealed off from the effusion by lung tissue. To define the proper entry point, the lung fields should be percussed and auscultated to determine the upper border of the effusion. Because pleural fluid rises in a meniscus where it comes in contact with the parietal pleura, the needle should be passed into the chest one interspace *higher* than the upper border of the effusion as determined by examination. A few millimeters of penetration into the pleural space at the level of the meniscus will allow full drainage without the complications of a low entry. Injury to the neurovascular bundle along the in-

ferior surface of the rib is avoided by aiming the needle just above the rib's *superior* margin, accomplished by "walking the needle" over the anesthetized surface of the rib. Pneumothorax is minimized by withdrawing or changing needle position as soon as air bubbles begin to appear or one feels the visceral pleura contacting the needle tip; the onset of coughing is common at this stage. The patient should be advised to resist the impulse to cough, for the act may impale the lung on the needle. Use of a large-bore Intracath (14 or 16 gauge) minimizes the risk of needle injury to the lung. A post-thoracentesis chest film should be obtained to be sure that a significant pneumothorax has not been produced.

When analyzing an effusion of unknown etiology, the gross appearance of the pleural fluid should be noted and samples sent for determination of protein and glucose concentrations, cell count and differential, Gram stain, culture (including cultures for anaerobes and mycobacteria) and cytology. Because one cannot always distinguish an exudate from a transudate on the basis of the protein concentration alone, obtaining simultaneous serum and fluid LDH determinations is recommended. Exudative etiologies have been found to have pleural fluid LDH concentrations in excess of 220 units per ml. and ratios of pleural-to-serum LDH concentrations of greater than 0.6. Currently the combination of protein concentration, LDH concentration and LDH ratio provides the best means of distinguishing an exudate from a transudate. The cell count and differential are of little use for this purpose, because there is so much overlap. A very low glucose concentration suggests tuberculosis, malignancy, empyema, and rheumatoid arthritis. When an intra-abdominal source is suspected, an amylase level may be of some help, though conditions other than pancreatitis can produce elevations. When there is clinical evidence suggestive of rheumatoid disease, complement levels (CH_{50}, C_3 and C_4) may help in identification of the effusion's etiology.

One group has advocated measurement of the carcinoembryonic antigen (CEA) levels in pleural effusions as a means of distinguishing benign effusions from malignant ones. When used alone, a CEA concentration greater than 12 ng. per ml. had a sensitivity of only 34 per cent; specificity was 98 per cent. Sensitivity is increased to 54 per cent when CEA is combined with cytological examination for diagnosis of malignant effusion. Thus the CEA may make a contribution to diagnosis, mostly when judged in the context of other clinical and laboratory evidence.

In about 15 per cent of cases, the etiology of the effusion remains elusive after thoracentesis. Pleural biopsy is indicated when suspicion of tuberculosis or a pleura-based malignancy persists. Pleural biopsy is positive in up to 65 per cent of patients with tuberculosis; diagnostic accuracy is further enhanced by culturing part of the specimen. Pleural biopsy is positive in about 60 per cent of patients with bronchogenic carcinoma that has spread to the pleura. Suspicion of mesothelioma often requires confirmation by biopsy.

INDICATIONS FOR ADMISSION AND REFERRAL

The acutely tachypneic patient in much discomfort obviously requires hospitalization, especially when embolization, severe congestive failure, or acute severe pneumonitis is likely. Few of these patients will present to the physician in the office, but the patient with a chronic and enlarging collection of pleural fluid is apt to be encountered. The person who appears to be tolerating the effusion without much discomfort can be evaluated and managed on an outpatient basis as long as there is no evidence suggestive of an empyema or a subphrenic abscess, conditions which require surgical attention. Referral is appropriate when malignancy or tuberculosis is suspected and pleural biopsy deemed necessary.

SYMPTOMATIC MANAGEMENT

The patient can be made comfortable prior to establishing a diagnosis. Pleuritic pain often responds to indomethacin; the drug has the advantage over narcotics in that it does not have any suppressive effect on respiration. Removal of fluid is indicated when the effusion is compromising respiratory efforts. Usually no more than a liter should be removed at one time, in order to avoid intravascular volume depletion upon reequilibration.

ANNOTATED BIBLIOGRAPHY

Black, L.E.: Pleural space and pleural fluid. Mayo Clin. Proc. 47:493, 1972. (An excellent article reviewing pathophysiology.)

Fine, N.L., Smith, L.R., and Sheedy, P.F.: Frequency of pleural effusions in mycoplasma and viral pneumonias. N. Engl. J. Med., 283:790, 1970. (Small transient effusions are common in these conditions, but large effusions are rare.)

Hunder, G.G.: Pleural fluid complement in systemic lupus erythematosus and rheumatoid arthritis. Ann. Intern. Med., 76:356, 1972. (Complement levels are low.)

Light, R.W., and Ball, W.C.: Glucose and amylase in pleural effusion. J.A.M.A., 225:259, 1973. (Tuberculosis and malignant effusions were not universally associated with low glucose values.)

Light, R.W., et al.: Cells and pleural fluid. Arch. Intern. Med. 132:854, 1973. (Reviews the diagnostic significance of cell counts; concludes that the finding of many mesothelial cells is incompatible with tuberculosis; red counts greater than 100,000 suggested neoplasm, infarction, or trauma: predominant lymphocytes were consistent with tuberculosis or neoplasm.)

Light, R.W., et al.: Pleural effusions: The diagnostic separation of transudate and exudate. Ann. Intern. Med., 77:507, 1972. (A classic article that details rigorous criteria for the separation of transudates from exudates.)

Rittgers, R.A., Lowenstein M.S., Feinerman, A.E., et al.: Carcinoembryonic antigen levels in benign and malignant pleural effusions. Ann. Intern. Med., 88:631, 1978. (The CEA may be helpful when used in conjunction with other findings, but not by itself.)

40
Evaluation of the Solitary Pulmonary Nodule

The discovery of a solitary pulmonary nodule on chest x-ray is a worrisome finding, for it raises the possibility of malignancy. The patient is usually asymptomatic and has the lesion detected on routine chest film. Solitary pulmonary nodules represent the subgroup of pulmonary malignancies with the greatest potential for cure; consequently, thorough assessment is of utmost importance. On the other hand, many of these lesions are not cancers, and to subject all patients to invasive studies can lead to unnecessary morbidity. The primary physician needs to determine the likelihood of malignancy on the basis of clinical and radiological findings in order to identify the patient who requires referrral for consideration of bronchoscopy and/or thoracotomy. Workup can be initiated on an outpatient basis under the direction of the primary physician, pending the decision regarding the risk of cancer and the need for invasive study.

PATHOPHYSIOLOGY AND CLINICAL PRESENTATION

Solitary pulmonary nodules characteristically appear in the middle or lateral lung fields, surrounded by normal lung and unaccompanied by satellite lesions. They have smooth contours and are usually round ("coin" lesions) or oval. Neoplastic, granulomatous, vascular and cystic processes are responsible for their formation. The nodule displaces normal aerated lung parenchyma and does not cause symptoms unless there is airway obstruction, pleural invasion, interference with respiratory mechanics, or involvement of blood vessels or nerves. Inflammatory lesions double in volume in less than 5 weeks; malignancies take between 1 and 18 months to double; benign nodules take longer. A solitary nodule that does not change in size over 2 years is benign. The older patient, the greater the chances that the nodule is malignant; the probability is less than 2 per cent below age 30 and increases by 10 to 15 per cent with each succeeding decade.

DIFFERENTIAL DIAGNOSIS

The major etiologies are tumor and granuloma. The percentage of cases that are due to cancer is a function of the age and other epidemiologic characteristics of the patient population studied. In most series, at least 50 per cent of cases are malignant. Primary lung cancers account for the vast majority of pulmonary coin lesions that prove to be malignant; less than 10 per cent are due to metastatic disease. Tumors of breast, bowel, and testicles are particularly prone to metastasize to lung. Granulomas account for a large percentage of the solitary nodules in many series; most are tuberculous, but in endemic areas, histoplasmosis and coccidomycosis are important diagnostic considerations. Benign pulmonary tumors such as hamartomas occur in about 5 to 7 per cent of cases. The remaining 5 per cent of solitary nodules are bronchogenic cysts, hydatid cysts, pseudolymphomas, arteriovenous malformations, and bronchopulmonary sequestrations. Extrapulmonary lesion, such as skin lesions, moles, nipples, chest wall and rib lesions and pleural plaques may be confused with solitary parenchymal lesions.

WORKUP

A most difficult diagnostic issue regards the need for resection of the unexplained solitary pulmonary nodule. Many surgeons argue that the risk of thoracotomy is small and potential benefit considerable, because resection of a nodule that proves to be an early primary lung cancer may provide the patient with a chance for cure. On the other hand, pulmonologists have argued that lesions that possess many of the criteria of benignity can be managed conservatively, and that definitive tissue diagnosis can be approached by bronchoscopy or needle biopsy without resorting to early thoracotomy (see Chapter 42). A review of the literature reveals passionate advocates on both sides; conclusive data taking into account morbidity and mortality of both approaches are lacking.

Identification of the patients most likely to have malignant lesions on the basis of noninvasive findings can help to select those who would be best suited to undergo a definitive, invasive diagnostic procedure. The patient's age, the doubling time of the lesion and its x-ray appearance are among the most useful data for determining the chances of malignancy. The probability of cancer is 50 per cent for patients in their sixties, but less than 2 per cent for those under 30. Assessment of the doubling time, i.e., the period during which the tumor doubles in volume, can be achieved efficaciously by review of previous chest films, if available. Before any further studies are undertaken, every effort should be made to locate old chest x-rays to determine the age and speed of growth of the nodule. A lesion that has been stable for 2 or more years is most likely to benign; a nodule that has doubled in volume within 1 to 18 months is malignant until proven otherwise. If no previous films are obtainable, useful data can still be derived from the x-rays at hand; of particular importance are the pattern of calcification and the character of the lesion's borders. Patterns of uniformly dense calcification, central calcification, or definite lamination are strongly suggestive of a benign lesion. Tomography of the nodule may be necessary to clearly define the presence and distributution of calcification as well as the presence of hilar adenopathy. Lesions with irregular, poorly defined borders are suggestive of a malignant process.

History is occasionally of help in elucidating the etiology of the nodule. Although symptoms are often absent, it is worth inquiring into a history of smoking, hemoptysis (see Chapter 38), known previous breast, bowel or testicular cancer, and systemic symptoms such as fever, night sweats, and weight loss. History of exposure to tuberculosis or residence in an area in which fungal disease is endemic raises the possibility of a granulomatous etiology.

Physical examination is generally unrevealing, but breast or testicular mass, occult blood in the stool, clubbing (see Chapter 41), cutaneous or mucosal telangiectasia, and an audible bruit over the chest wall (suggestive of a vascular etiology) should be noted. Perhaps the most important part of the physical examinaton is careful palpation of lymph nodes, particularly those in the supraclavicular and axillary regions. If enlarged, such nodes can be biopsied, which may eliminate the need for thoracotomy or other invasive procedures.

Laboratory studies. A number of other ancillary diagnostic studies may be of some help. An intermediate strength tuberculin test should be implanted (see Chapter 34); in endemic areas, fungal cultures and histoplasmin complement fixation titers may be of importance. Sputum cytologic examination is the least invasive means of confirming the presence of a malignancy. Three first morning samples should be obtained on consecutive days; yield is highest when the sample contains pulmonary histiocytes (a sign of a deep sample) and the lesion is in the upper lobes, centrally located, communicating with a bronchus, and large (see Chapter 33).

A conservative approach to further evaluation is reasonable in some circumstances. Criteria for withholding invasive study are (1) cytologic diagnosis of lung cancer with evidence of metastases, (2) lesions that have not enlarged in 5 years, and (3) in young patients, x-ray evidence that suggests benignity, such as solid or laminated calcium and sharp borders.

If the risk of malignancy is still not established after outpatient evaluation, one can progress to bronchoscopy and transbronchial biopsy for diagnosis of central lesions or needle aspiration biopsy under fluoroscopic control for diagnosis of peripheral lesions. Thoracotomy with resection is a third alternative (see Chapter 42). The choice of procedure depends in part on loction of the lesion and available expertise. It is also important, when weighing the wisdom of an invasive procedure, to decide whether the patient could tolerate a resection. Patients with severe obstructive or restrictive disease should first undergo formal pulmonary fuction testing.

In sum, the management of the patient with a solitary pulmonary nodule remains controversial. It appears at present that a conservative approach to evaluation is justified in patients judged to be at low risk for malignancy based on epidemiologic, historical, physical and x-ray criteria. Patients at high risk for malignancy require a tissue diagnosis. A patient who falls between these two groups poses a dilemma, which should be shared with the patient so that a satisfactory plan can be devised. It may be reasonable to follow the patient with serial x-ray studies at 3-month intervals.

INDICATIONS FOR REFERRAL

Patients suspected on clinical and radiologic grounds of having a malignancy should be referred for tissue diagnosis. In situations where the probability of malignancy is unclear, the patient needs to be informed about the lack of diagnostic confidence based on noninvasive study, as well as the nature of further testing that would be undertaken. Patients who cannot emotionally tolerate the uncertainty should be advised to undergo a definitive procedure in order to end the constant worry about the possibility of malignancy. The patient who can live with such uncertainty and is relutant to have a thoracotmy or biopsy could be followed at 3-month intervals with serial chest films for a period of 2 years.

ANNOTATED BIBLIOGRAPHY

Lillington, G.A.: The solitary pulmonary nodule/ 1974. Am. Rev. Respir. Dis., *110*:699, 1974. *(A classic review of the problem.)*

Lillington, G.A., and Stevens, G.M.: The solitary nodule: The other side of the coin. Chest, *70*:322, 1976. *(An editorial that argues by example that early thoracotomy for every nodule, particularly in young people, would be uneconomic. It is suggested that needle biopsy or watchful waiting has a legitimate role in patients with low probability of malignancy.)*

Nathan, M.H.: Management of solitary pulmonary nodules: An organized approach based on growth rates and statistics. JAMA, *227*:1141, 1974. *(A very conservative approach advocated: observation of the nodule with serial x-rays for calculation of doubling time.)*

Ray, J.F., Lawton, B.R., *et al.*: The coin lesion story: Update 1976. Twenty years experience with ear-

lier thoracotomy for 179 suspected malignant coin lesions. Chest, *70*:332, 1976. (*This argues that low operative mortality and potential curability of small coin lesions justifies early thoracotomy.*)

41
Evaluation of Clubbing

The term "clubbing" refers to enlargement and sponginess of the nail beds of the fingers and toes and reduction in the angle created by the nail and the dorsum of the distal phalanx. Clubbing is sometimes accompanied by a chronic subperiosteal osteitis, hypertrophic osteoarthropathy. Patients rarely complain of clubbed fingers; it is the physician who detects this abnormality as an incidental finding on physical examination. Since clubbing or hypertrophic osteoarthropathy may be the first clinical sign of a serious underlying condition, such as a pulmonary neoplasm, it is important for the primary physician to recognize these findings and investigate their possible causes.

PATHOPHYSIOLOGY AND CLINICAL PRESENTATION

Hypotheses explaining the pathogenesis of clubbing and osteoarthropathy implicate autonomic influences, AV shunting, and bloodborne substances. The precise pathophysiology remains uncertain, but it is known that intrathoracic vagotomy can abolish clubbing and ostroarthropathy, as can correction of an AV shunt or removal of a pulmonary tumor.

Pathologic examination of clubbed fingers reveals increased vascularity. In hypertrophic osteoarthropathy, the periosteum is found to be edematous, hyperemic, and infiltrated by mononuclear cells. There is periosteal elevation, new bone formation, and endosteal resorption in the distal ends of long bones, metacarpals and metatarsals. Soft tissue swelling in the distal ends of the fingers and toes may lead to clubbing.

Clubbing is usually asymptomatic. Patients with hypertrophic osteoarthropathy may complain of pain in the wrists, ankles, hands and feet; erythema and effusions are sometimes noted. Hypertrophic osteoarthropathy may precede clubbing or occur without it, but most often the two appear together. Clubbing often takes place in the absence of osteoarthropathy. Either finding may develop prior to the clinical presentation of one of the conditions associated with it.

DIFFERENTIAL DIAGNOSIS

Clubbing and hypertrophic osteoarthropathy occur in as many as 5 to 10 per cent of cases of bronchogenic carcinoma; metastatic lung tumors are rarely responsible for such changes. With the decline in the incidence of chronic pulmonary infectious diseases (such as tuberculosis, lung abscess, and bronchiectasis), carcinoma of the lung has emerged as the leading cause of hypertrophic osteoarthropathy. Clubbing and/or osteoarthropathy are seen in patients with cyanotic congenital heart disease with right-to-left shunts, subacute bacterial endocarditis, inflammatory bowel disease, and biliary cirrhosis. Clubbing is a classic sign of chronic hypoxemia in patients with chronic obstructive lung disease. There are hereditary forms of clubbing and hypertophic osteoarthropathy that have no clinical significance. Unilateral clubbing is associated with impairment of the vascular supply to the arm that occurs with aortic, subclavian or innominate artery lesions. Jackhammer operators may develop clubbing.

Clubbing must be differentiated from a number of other phalangeal conditions that resemble it. Many normal people, particularly blacks, have increased curvature of the nails. Infections of the terminal phalanges such as felons and chronic paronychia may be confused with clubbing, as may thyroid acropachy. Bilateral wrist and ankle complaints suggest a host of inflammatory joint diseases (see Chapter 139), in addition to hypertrophic osteoarthropathy.

WORKUP

The evaluation of clubbing should begin with confirmation of the characteristic physical findings: loss of the angle made by the nail and increase in the ballotability of the nail bed. Hypertrophic osteoarthropathy is identified by x-ray of the long bones; the typical changes are increase in periosteal thickness and new bone formation at distal ends. Once it is clear that clubbing and/or hypertrophic osteoarthropathy are present, an evaluation for an underlying etiology can commence.

History. Before an elaborate search for a serious illness is undertaken, it should be established whether clubbing has been lifelong and is present in other family members, indicative of the harmless familial variety. Symptoms such as cough, sputum production, hemoptysis, and dyspnea point to a respiratory problem and may have already triggered an evaluation of the lungs (see Chapters 36–38). The patient should be questioned about history of a heart murmur and exercise intolerance, as well as prior liver disease, crampy lower abdominal pain, diarrhea, bloody stools and joint complaints. Smoking and other risk factors related to development of lung cancer (see Chapter 33) should be assessed. Exposure to tuberculosis also needs to be ascertained.

Physical examination requires a check for fever, tachypnea, tachycardia, cyanosis, tobacco stains, jugular venous distention, barrel chest, wheezes, rhonchi, rales (crackles), signs of consolidation or effusion, heart murmur, skin lesions of hepatocellular disease and signs of cirrhosis (see Chapter 71). Lymph nodes should be palpated for enlargement and joints for hypertrophic changes.

Laboratory studies. The only mandatory laboratory study is a chest x-ray, because an early pleural, pulmonary or mediastinal neoplasm may be asymptomatic. A CBC and stool examination for occult blood may be of help. Further evaluation of the liver, thyroid, heart or bowel should be undertaken only if symptoms or physical findings suggest pathology in these areas. Patients with new onset clubbing and a long smoking history should be followed for the development of pulmonary neoplasm; periodic examinations including sputum cytology and chest x-ray are appropriate.

SYMPTOMATIC MANAGEMENT AND PATIENT EDUCATION

There is no symptomatic therapy for clubbing. It is an innocuous cosmetic disturbance. Discomfort in the bones and joints secondary to hypertrophic osteoarthropathy can be treated with aspirin. Rarely, there are disabling joint symptoms; these may require extreme therapies such as corticosteroids or intrathoracic vagotomy. Such therapeutic options should be undertaken in consultation with a rheumatologist familiar with the condition.

Patient education is important in any condition where the physician discovers a potential sign of disease that is not obvious to the patient. It is likely that patients will be disturbed by the investigation and by the possibility of serious disease. The physician must take time to inform the patient that clubbing can be a harmless finding as well as a helpful guide to the early diagnosis of disease. The patient who smokes should be strongly advised to quit (see Chapter 49).

ANNOTATED BIBLIOGRAPHY

Holling, H.E., and Brody, R.S.: Pulmonary hypertrophic osteoarthropathy. JAMA, *178*:977, 1961. *(A good review of the condition, distinguishing between clubbing and osteoarthropathy. The pathogenisis suggested is disease of the pleura with neural reflexes affecting the limbs.)*

Schumacher, H.R., Jr.: Articular manifestations of hypertrophic pulmonary osteoarthropathy in bronchogenic carcinoma—A clinical and pathologic study. Arthritis Rheum., *19*:629, 1976. *(A detailed study and discussion.)*

Stenseth, J.H., Clagett, O.T., and Woolner, L.B.: Hypertrophic pulmonary osteoarthropathy. Dis. Chest, *52*:62, 1967. *(A review of 888 pulmonary neoplasms revealing a 9.2 per cent incidence of hypertrophic osteoarthropathy.)*

Trever, R.W.: Hypertrophic pulmonary osteoarthropathy in association with congenital heart disease: report of two cases. Ann. intern. Medicine *48*:660, 1958. *(Two case reports in a series of 3,000 cases of cyanotic heart revealing an incidence of 0.1 per cent. Clubbing is far more frequent.)*

42

Approach to the Patient
with Lung Cancer

JACOB J. LOKICH, M.D.

Carcinoma of the lung accounts for the highest number of annual cancer-related deaths, and yet is among the most preventable of all cancers, in that a causative agent, smoking, has been identified. Once established, most forms of bronchogenic carcinoma are minimally responsive to therapy, though there are important exceptions, e.g., oat cell tumors. The inability of members of the American public to alter their smoking habits has perpetuated the continuing incidence and death rate of lung cancer, which, in fact, is rising as a consequence of increased smoking among women. The primary physician needs to be alert to early signs of the disease, capable of initiating the evaluation, and familiar with various evaluation and management strategies.

CLINICAL PRESENTATION AND COURSE

The primary determinants of prognosis in patients with lung cancer are stage at the time of diagnosis, histopathologic classification, and the presence and duration of symptoms (Table 42–1). Lung cancer is staged according to involvement of the pulmonary parenchyma only (Stage I), spread to the draining hilar lymph nodes (Stage II), and extension to the mediastinal lymph nodes (Stage III). About 25 per cent of patients present with operable disease (Stages I and II), but the majority present with Stage III disease. The dismal prognosis in patients with lung cancer is related in part to the advanced stage of disease at the time of diagnosis. In those patients fortunate enough to have their disease confined to the lung (Stage I), almost half may be cured by surgical approaches alone. With involvement of hilar lymph nodes, survival rates decrease dramatically, except for epidermoid carcinoma.

Oat cell carcinoma (undifferentiated small cell carcinoma) is unique in that prognosis appears to be independent of the anatomic distribution of the tumor at the time of diagnosis. The 2-year survival for patients with oat cell disease, regardless of stage, had been approximately 6 per cent, but application of combined modality therapy (that employs a multi-

Table 42–1 Prognostic Determinants in Bronchogenic Carcinoma

Stage	Prognosis (2 yrs. Disease-free; %)	
Confined to lung	40–45	
Hilar node involvement	15*	
Mediastinum or chest wall involvement	10	

Histopathology	Incidence (%)	Median Survival (mo.)
Epidermoid	50	6–9
Adenocarcinoma	25	6–8
Undifferentiated large	15	36
Undifferentiated small (oat†)	10	2

Symptoms and Duration	5-Year Survival (%)	
None	18	
Local symptoms less than 6 months	16	
Local symptoms greater than 6 months	9	
Systemic symptoms with metastasis	6	

* With epidermoid type, prognosis improves to 40 percent.

† With combination chemotherapy and radiation, the median survival is 10 to 12 months.

drug regimen and radiation administered to the primary tumor as well as prophylactically to common sites of metastasis) has resulted in improvement of median survival from 1 or 2 months to 10 or 12 months.

Survival data reemphasize the importance of early detection when possible. Unfortunately, local and regional disease is most often asymptomatic, and the sensitivity and specificity of available screening tests are limited (see Chapter 33). Clinical presentation is partially a function of the tumor's location; central endobronchial lesions may produce symptoms early in the course of illness. Hemoptysis, cough, sputum production and a localized wheeze are among complaints reported in early phases; however, the frequency with which these symptoms are noted in early disease is low. Hemoptysis occurs as a presenting symptom in only 7 to 10 per cent of patients with lung cancer. On occasion, a systemic syndrome, such as hypertrophic osteoarthropathy (see Chapter 41), peripheral neuropathy, or innappropriate ADH secretion, may precede other evidence of disease.

Symptoms of advanced disease include anorexia, weight loss, nausea and vomiting, hoarseness (recurrent laryngeal nerve involvement), pleuritic chest pain, bone pain, and neurologic deficits. The metastatic pattern of bronchogenic carcinoma involves spread to the lymph nodes (25 to 45 per cent), to the liver (30 to 45 per cent), to the bone and bone marrow (20 to 40 per cent), and to the central nervous system (20 to 35 per cent). Variations in incidence figures for metastases are a function of the stage of disease and tissue type; for example, oat cell carcinoma more commonly spreads to the lymph nodes, marrow and brain relative to other cell types.

WORKUP

The patient who presents with an unexplained pulmonary nodule provides a diagnostic challenge (see Chapter 40). However, in view of the frequency of lung cancer and the relative infrequency of opportunistic infections and granulomatous diseases of the lungs, an unexplained pulmonary lesion should be considered malignant until proven otherwise. The histopathologic diagnosis may be obtained with a variety of procedures (Table 42–2). The principal guideline in evaluating pulmonary lesions suspected of being malignant is to begin with the most innocuous procedures, such as cytologic evaluation of the sputum, and proceed to more invasive ones, as needed (see Chapter 40). Many patients have concurrent

Table 42–2 Diagnostic and Staging Approaches to Lung Cancer*

Sputum cytology
Scalene node biopsy
Mediastinoscopy
Bronchoscopy
Transbronchial biopsy
Transpulmonary biopsy
Thoracotomy (Chamberlain procedure)

* In order of increasing invasiveness.

chronic lung disease and may be seriously compromised by a complication, such as pneumothorax, that results from an invasive study.

The diagnostic and therapeutic approach to the pulmonary nodule likely to be cancerous is determined by a history of malignancy, the "doubling time" or growth of the nodule, and the location and number of nodules observed.

In patients with established malignancy, the nodule may represent either a synchronous or metachronous metastatic lesion or a new primary cancer. If the previous cancer was gastrointestinal and the interval from previous tumor is more than 2 years, the pulmonary lesion is a new primary cancer in approximately 50 per cent of patients. If the previous tumor was a breast carcinoma and the interval is more than 2 years, the pulmonary lesion is a primary carcinoma of the lung or a metastasis from another tumor site in more than 75 per cent of patients. If there is no history of cancer, the malignant nodule turns out to be a lung cancer in over 80 per cent of patients.

Serial chest films can be obtained over a period of at least 4 to 6 weeks. The doubling time of the nodule is determined by sequential observations of its diameter, which may be plotted against time and translated into doubling times on semilogarithmic graphs. Retrospective, as well as prospective, studies of patients with single or multiple pulmonary nodules have demonstrated that malignant nodules grow with doubling times of 10 to 400 days; benign tumors grow at rates above or below these limits. In addition, doubling times in malignant tumors of less than 40 days are associated with a poor prognosis, and those with doubling times beyond 40 days have been found to have a median survival rate of beyond 2 years in spite of the presence of metastasis. These prognostic determinants can be used not only to determine the therapeutic approach but also to guide diagnostic workup.

The sites and number of nodules are also important to planning assessment. Peripheral lesions may be approached either with percutaneous aspiration or by a "mini-thoracotomy" (Chamberlain procedure); central lesions may be biopsied by transbronchial bronchoscopy.

In patients with clinically curable lesions, according to radiographic and anatomic criteria, the diagnostic procedure of choice is a thoracotomy with resection. Surgical excision is particularly indicated for nodules with long doubling times or long disease-free intervals, especially if the nodules are solitary and unassociated with extrathoracic disease.

Many thoracic surgeons believe that all patients should undergo *mediastinoscopy* for evaluation of the mediastinum and hilum prior to thoracotomy, since the presence of tumor in the mediastinum is a contraindication to resection. However, early peripheral coin lesions are uncommonly associated with hilar or mediastinal extension, and tomographic evaluation alone is often sufficient.

Bronchoscopy is advocated by some as a routine procedure in the evaluation of a pulmonary lesion, but for peripheral pulmonary lesions, the accessibility by fiberoptic bronchoscopy may be limited. The utility of radiographic and fluoroscopically guided procedures, such as transbronchial biopsy or transpulmonary biopsy, is reduced by the inadequacy of the specimen sometimes obtained, which is often cytologic material rather than a solid core of tissue; the architectural relationships may be obscured or unavailable in cytologic specimens. For patients with limited pulmonary reserve in whom the hazard of pneumothorax may be great, a controlled thoracotomy may also be preferable to needle aspiration.

Assessment of the patient with lung cancer for metastatic disease is contingent upon the prognostic and therapeutic implications; nevertheless, many routinely search for metastases to all possible sites. If there is no clinical evidence of metastatic disease, it is wasteful to routinely employ radionuclide scanning of the brain, bones and liver (see Chapter 86). Routine searches are not warranted when the results would make no difference in treatment.

Similarly, although the use of tumor markers to identify and monitor occult sites of disease is under development, the current lack of effective systemic therapy precludes the usefulness of such measures for treatment decision.

PRINCIPLES OF MANAGEMENT

Surgery is the most effective mode of therapy for bronchogenic carcinoma and is associated with the lowest rate of morbidity. Unfortunately, only 45 per cent of the patients who present with lung cancer can be explored with the possibility of successful resection. Of that group, only 60 per cent (27 per cent of all patients) have successful resections. Of this final group who undergo resection either by pneumonectomy or lobectomy, the 5-year survival or cure rate is approximately 25 per cent. Thus, 7 per cent of patients who present with lung cancer may be cured.

Less radical surgical procedures have become accepted for treatment of primary lung cancer. Pneumonectomy used to be performed in more than 70 per cent of patients; it generally incorporated the hilar as well as mediastinal lymph nodes. A regional excision that employs wedge resection or lobectomy for peripheral lobe lesions is now being performed. The general surgical dictum is to employ the minimal degree of surgery necessay to remove all macroscopic evidence of tumor. The subsequent use of radiation therapy may augment local control, allowing for lesser surgery.

Radiation therapy for bronchogenic carcinoma has been used preoperatively to promote or convert inoperable tumors to technically resectable lesions (with curative intent following resection) and as definitive therapy for patients with Stage III inoperable tumors without extrathoracic extension. As a *postoperative* adjunctive measure in bronchogenic carcinoma, radiation therapy has not significantly improved survival; however, it may reduce the extensiveness of local recurrence and consequently lower the incidence of severe pulmonary complications, such as superior vena cava syndrome or lobar collapse. Although there are reports of small improvements in long-term survival (less than 5 per cent) associated with radiation doses up to 6,000 rads for tumors confined to the hemithorax, the reports of improved survival are mostly anecdotal and not necessarily attributable to the administration of the radiation therapy.

Preoperative radiation therapy may promote the resectability of tumors and possibly extend survival rates. The superior sulcus tumor is one instance in which preoperative radiation therapy has improved the likelihood of cure in spite of contiguous extension of the tumor to bone or chest wall. In general, when surgery is used in combination with prior radiation, the resection almost always needs to be a pneumonectomy; in principle, surgery must incorporate all sites that were diseased prior to the radiation therapy.

Management of *Stage III disease* deserves special comment. More than 70 per cent of patients with bronchogenic carcinoma present with inoperable dis-

Table 42–3   Treatment of Oat-Cell Carcinoma:
Selected Series of Radiation and
Chemotherapeutic Programs

Time of Radiation in Relation to CT	Drug Combination	Complete Response Rate	Median Survival (Mo.)
Concomitant*	ADR + CTX + VCR	20/21	5–7+
Following CT	ADR + CTX + VCR + BCG	17/29	12+
Variable	CCNU + CTX + VCR	9/19	10+
Following CT	MTX + CTX + VCR	13/18	
Following CT	BCNU + CTX + VCR + PCZ	8/24	8+

* Plus prophylactic CNS radiation.

CT, Chemotherapy; ADR, adriamycin; CTX, cyclophosphamide; VCR, vincristine; CCNU or BCNU, nitrosourea; MTX, methotrexate; PCZ, procarbazine; BCG, bacill Calmette-Guerin.

Table 42–4   Clinical Problems in Lung Cancer

Superior vena cava syndrome
Superior sulcus tumor
Pleural effusion
Pulmonary nodules
Stage III (limited) disease
Oat cell carcinoma and paraneoplastic syndromes

ease, either on the basis of extrathoracic extension of the tumor or intrathoracic extension to mediastinal lymph nodes, chest wall, or bone cage. This latter group, with tumor limited to the chest at the time of presentation, is the most critical therapeutic challenge in bronchogenic carcinoma today. For patients with the *superior sulcus variant*, therapy that combines preoperative radiation with surgical resection has contributed to cures. With this singular exception, however, the majority of patients with Stage III bronchogenic carcinoma develop distant metastases regardless of control of the primary tumor. Survival is a function of the rate and extent of systemic dissemination. The development of improved drugs or new combinations of chemotherapy must occur before hope can be offered to the patient with this stage of disease.

The *small cell carcinoma* (oat cell) is a relatively infrequent variant of bronchogenic carcinoma, but recent progress in the therapeutic approach to this tumor has resulted in improved survival rates and even provided long-term control in a small but significant proportion of patients. The regimen involves an interdigitation of radiation with multiple-drug therapy (Table 42–3). The tumor exhibits an exquisite initial responsiveness to the combination program. Patients with this tumor should not be subjected to major surgical procedures in the thorax, since the prognosis is determined by the effectiveness of

the chemotherapy. The tumor is always considered disseminated or Stage IV at the time of diagnosis, regardless of anatomic localization within the chest.

MANAGEMENT OF COMPLICATIONS
(Table 42–4)

Obstruction to the superior vena cava produces the classic clinical syndrome of facial edema, proptosis, suffusion of the conjunctiva, and dilatation of the veins of the upper thorax and neck. In addition, the patient complains of relentless headache. The syndrome is invariably caused by tumor extending to the right side of the mediastinum. There is extrinsic compression of the venous system adjacent to the mediastinal lymph nodes. The secondary effects of compression are thrombosis and tumor invasion; if untreated, neurologic function may become compromised.

Treatment is achieved with immediate and often emergency radiation therapy. Venography and radionuclide scanning are not indicated to identify the site of obstruction, since the clinical syndrome is characteristic, and chest radiograph almost invariably demonstrates a localized lesion. Bronchoscopy, esophagoscopy, and biopsy should not be performed because of the hazard of severe, uncontrollable hemorrhage or tracheal edema. Furthermore, sputum specimens for cytology should not be obtained because the increased intrathoracic pressure from coughing may markedly exacerbate venous and intracranial pressures.

Treatment with radiation therapy is successful in more than 70 per cent of cases. Although patients with superior vena cava syndrome secondary to lung cancer have an inoperable tumor, the prognosis is no worse than that for patients with Stage III lung cancer. The histopathologic types of lung cancer that lead to the superior vena cava syndrome are variable, but most commonly the small cell undifferentiated tumor is the culprit.

Malignant pleural effusion is another important complication. It occurs in 10 to 15 per cent of patients with carcinoma of the lung and may be secondary to direct pleural implantation or a consequence of mediastinal obstruction to lymphatic drainage of the pleural surface. Only 20 to 30 per cent of pleural effusions that develop as a consequence of bronchogenic carcinoma are cytologically confirmed and many are transudates. Pleural biopsy is often required for definitive diagnosis.

The median survival for patients who develop a malignant pleural effusion is less than 3 months; therefore, the effusion should be monitored and treated only when it causes significant respiratory discomfort. The use of intrapleural chemotherapeutic agents or chemical irritants, such as tetracycline, talcum powder, or quinacrine, may be effective in 50 to 60 per cent of patients. The specific choice of agent for sealing the pleura is determined by morbidity of the treatment. The chemotherapeutic agents such as bleomycin or 5-flurorouracil are relatively innocuous. On the other hand, nitrogen mustard and the "inert" irritants may result in a major secondary inflammatory response with reactive effusion and fever. Quinacrine (Atabrine) must be instilled repeatedly over a 5- to 7-day period to be maximally effective. Radiation therapy to the mediastinum or to the pleura has been of limited effectiveness. Surgical drainage with an intrathoracic tube for 2 to 3 days may result in a secondary inflammatory response adequate to seal the pleural space.

Tumor-humoral syndromes are associated with oat cell carcinomas. The tumor has been known to produce ACTH, ADH and even serotonin on occasion, resulting in Cushing's syndrome, inappropriate ADH syndrome, and carcinoid syndrome, respectively. Treatment is directed at the tumor.

PATIENT EDUCATION (see Chapter 90)

ANNOTATED BIBLIOGRAPHY

Greco, F.A., and Oldham, R.K.: Small cell lung cancer. N. Engl. J. Med., *301*:355, 1979. *(Up-to-date summary of recent developments in evaluation and therapy; 21 refs. Combination chemotherapy has improved prognosis.)*

Paulson, D.L.: Carcinomas in the superior sulcus. J. Thorac. Cardiovasc. Surg., *70*:1095, 1975. *(Update of original series applying preoperative radiation with extensive regional surgery to effect cure.)*

Straus, M.J., and Selawry, O.S.: Diagnosis and treatment of lung cancer. Semin. Oncol., *1*:161, 1974. *(A perspective of the approach to diagnosis and therapy by the authorities in the field.)*

Takita, H., Marabella, P.C., Edgerton, F., and Rizzo, D.: CPD, Adriamycin, cyclophosphamide, CCNU and vincristine in non-small cell lung carcinoma. Cancer Treatment Rep., *63*:29, 1979. *(Up to 80 per cent of patients may respond to chemotherapy, and responders have a longer survival. This singular report is balanced against many others in which survival is unaffected because of rapid induction of tumor resistance.)*

43

Approach to the Patient with Acute Bronchitis or Pneumonia in the Ambulatory Setting
HARVEY B. SIMON, M.D.

Respiratory tract infections are among the most common acute problems seen in office practice; the majority are limited to the upper airway (see Chapters 46, 208–210). The cough, fever, chest discomfort and dyspnea which may accompany lower respiratory infections provoke great concern in the patient, and the physician should respond with a careful evaluation designed to elucidate three basic issues: (1) Is the process limited to the trachea and bronchi, or is a frank pneumonia present? In general, patients with bronchitis respond well to ambulatory care, while patients with pneumonia should be considered for hospital admission. (2) Is the patient at increased risk for cardiopulmonary complications? The elderly patient with underlying cardiac or chronic lung disease may decompensate acutely from bronchitis alone, while otherwise healthy young individuals have a much greater tolerance for these infections. (3) What is the causative organism—is it bacterial or nonbacterial? Bacterial processes are usually more severe and require antibiotics, while viral infections are managed symptomatically.

PATHOPHYSIOLOGY AND CLINICAL PRESENTATION

The distinction between bronchitis and pneumonia is anatomic rather than etiologic; the same organisms can cause both syndromes, and patients may present with similar complaints, including fever, malaise, cough and sputum production. Muscular-type chest wall discomfort produced from coughing occurs in both conditions, but individuals with pneumonia are more likely to have pleurisy or dyspnea as well as higher temperatures, chills, hypoxia and a more "toxic" appearance. Similarly, although either type of infection can lead to sputum production, patients with bacterial pneumonia generally produce more sputum and are more likely to have hemoptysis. The clinical distinction between bronchitis and pneumonia is based predominently on physical examination and chest x-ray findings. Patients with bronchitis can have clear lungs or diffuse rhonchi and/or wheezes due to large airway secretions and bronchospasm, while individuals with pneumonia classically have rales, rhonchi, bronchial breath and dullness to percussion over the involved areas of lung. Pleural effusions may accompany pneumonia. The chest x-ray in acute bronchitis usually reveals no infiltrate or signs of consolidation in contradistinction to the x-ray of the patient with pneumonia. But even this most clear-cut distinction between bronchitis and pneumonia can be misleading, for changes of chronic lung disease can simulate new infiltrates in some patients with bronchitis, while dehydration can minimize x-ray abnormalities in patients with pneumonia. Patients with pneumonia are far more likely to experience complications such as hypoxia, cardiopulmonary failure, local suppuration (lung abscess or empyema), and spread of infection to other organs via the bloodstream. Clinical presentations are, in part, a function of the causative organism.

Gram-positive organisms. Streptococcus pneumoniae is still the most common cause of bacterial bronchitis and pneumonia, accounting for about 60 to 80 percent of all bacterial pneumonias. It is especially likely to be the agent infecting healthy young ambulatory patients, but it may affect all age groups. Classical clinical features include abrupt onset of fever with a single rigor, cough with rusty sputum, and pleuritic chest pain. Radiologic evidence of lobar consolidation is typical, but infiltrates can be patchy, especially in patients with chronic lung disease. The sputum Gram stain reveals abundant polymorphonuclear leukocytes and gram-positive diplococci (classically lancet-shaped) in pairs or short chains.

The most common complication of pneumococcal pneumonia is bacteremia, which occurs in about one-third of patients. Bloodborne distant sepsis (septic arthritis, peritonitis, meningitis, etc.) is much less common. Sterile pleural effusions are common, while empyema is less frequent, and lung abscess is a rare complication. Delayed resolution of radiographic abnormalities is a relatively common occurrence and may take up to 6 to 8 weeks.

Staphylococcus aureus is the etiologic agent in up to 10 percent of bacterial pneumonias. Except in infancy, when it can be a primary infection, staphylococcal pneumonia most commonly follows a viral respiratory tract infection, particularly influenza. It may also occur as a nosocomial infection or as a result of bacteremic seeding of the lungs, especially in patients with staphylococcal endocarditis and/or intravenous drug abuse. Patients with staphylococcal pneumonia of respiratory or bloodstream origin are usually extremely ill. *S. aureus* produces tissue necrosis, and the distinctive feature of staphylococcal pneumonia is the tendency to produce multiple small lung abscesses. Healing usually leaves some degree of residual fibrosis. Abundant polymorphonuclear leukocytes and gram-positive cocci in pairs, clumps and clusters are found on the sputum Gram stain. Local suppurative complications, including lung abscess, empyema and pneumothorax, are relatively common. Bacteremia with metastatic seeding of distant sites such as endocardium, bone, joints, liver and meninges may occur.

Pneumonia caused by *Group A streptococci* is a rather uncommon infection, but has occurred in epidemics, especially in closed groups such as military units. Occasionally streptococcal pneumonia can occur following primary influenza pneumonia. Streptococcal pneumonia usually begins abruptly with fever, cough and severe debility. Chest pain is prominent in most patients. The distinctive clinical and radiological feature is rapid spread in the lung with resultant early empyema formation. Initially, the empyema fluid may be quite thin, possibly due to the many enzymes elaborated by Group A streptococci, but later frank purulence occurs. Other complications such as lung abscess, bacteremia, metastatic infection and poststreptococcal glomerulonephritis are uncommon. In patients with streptococcal pneumonia, the sputum Gram stain reveals numerous polymorphonuclear leukocytes and gram-positive cocci in pairs and short to long chains.

Gram-negative organisms. While *H. influenzae* has long been recognized as a common cause of bronchitis in adults with chronic lung disease, there has recently been a greater recognition of frank pneumonias due to this organism, sometimes with bacteremia. Most cases of bronchitis are caused by untypeable strains of *H. influenzae*, but pneumonias are often caused by the more invasive encapsulated strains, especially Type b. Radiographically, a bronchopneumonia pattern is typical. Abundant polymorphonuclear leukocytes and small pleomorphic gram-negative coccobacillary organisms are the characteristic findings in the sputum of patients with pneumonia or bronchitis due to *H. influenzae*. Complications of *H. influenzae* pneumonia in adults are uncommon, but in patients with underlying chronic lung diease, hypoxia and respiratory failure may develop.

Klebsiella pneumoniae typically produces pulmonary infection in debilitated patients, especially alcoholics, and is one of the only gram-negative bacillary pneumonias to occur with any frequency in ambulatory patients. It usually presents as an acute illness; rarely it may cause chronic pneumonitis. The organism has a high propensity to produce tissue necrosis, which accounts for the hemoptysis, dense lobar consolidation, and high incidence of abscess formation seen in this illness. Abundant polymorphonuclear leukocytes and large gram-negative bacilli, occasionally with thick capsules, are characteristically seen on sputum Gram stain. Lung abscess is a common complication and is really part of the natural evolution of the disease. Empyema may occur.

Other gram-negative bacillary pneumonias were once rare, but have increased over the past 15 years and now account for up to 20 percent of bacterial pneumonias. They are principally hospital-acquired infections and remain quite rare in the ambulatory population. Patients with gram-negative bacillary pneumonia are typically debilitated from other illnesses and frequently have received antibiotic therapy which alters their respiratory flora, thus accounting for the presence of these otherwise unusual pathogens. These pneumonias may result either from

aspiration of gram-negative organisms present in the upper airway (often related to inhalation therapy), or from seeding of the lungs in the course of gram-negative bacteremia. Bacteremic pneumonias are characterized by multiple small areas of infection in both lungs. Abundant polymorphonuclear leukocytes and gram-negative bacilli are seen on sputum Gram stain. Complications including lung abscess, empyema and bacteremia with metastatic spread of infection may occur.

Legionnaire's disease is an uncommon form of pneumonia caused by a newly recognized, very fastidious, filamentous gram-negative bacillus. The disease may occur in epidemics (summer months, usually related to contaminated soil or air-conditioning systems) or sporadically (year-round). Middle-aged and elderly adults are most often affected. The onset is typically acute with high fever, nonproductive cough and dyspnea. Pleuritic chest pain, diarrhea, and mental confusion may be seen. Abnormalities of renal function sometimes occur. Although the typical patient is severely ill and the mortality rate is high, milder cases have been recognized. Laboratory diagnosis is difficult since physical findings are nonspecific, sputum examination fails to reveal pathogens, leukocyte count is only mildly elevated, and chest roentgenograms may reveal either nonspecific interstitial infiltrates or patchy consolidation. Special stains of lung tissue are often required to demonstrate the organism.

Mixed flora. *Aspiration pneumonias* result from aspiration of mouth secretions and bacteria into the lower respiratory tree. They are usually mixed infections caused by the aerobic and anaerobic streptococci, bacteroides, and fusobacteria, which are harmless normal flora of the upper airway, that cause pneumonia if they attain a foothold in lung parenchyma. Predisposing factors include alteration of consciousness (drugs, anesthesia, alcohol, head trauma) and diminution of gag reflex, permitting aspiration to occur. Patients usually are mildly to moderately ill, but can be quite toxic, especially if lung abscess or empyema occurs. It must be stressed that hospitalized patients and ambulatory patients receiving antibiotics may have altered respiratory flora. Aspiration of mouth organism in such individuals may result in staphylococcal or gram-negative bacillary pneumonia, as discussed previously, rather than the pulmonary infection due to normal upper respiratory flora, as considered here. The sputum from patients with aspiration pneumonia may be malodorous, and characteristically shows abundant polymorphonuclear leukocytes and mixed flora, including gram-positive cocci in pairs and chains and pleomorphic gram-negative rods on Gram stain. Lung abscess and empyema are fairly common complications of aspiration pneumonia, especially if therapy is delayed.

Nonbacterial organisms. *Mycoplasma pneumoniae* is one of the most common causes of nonbacterial pneumonia, and accounts for up to 20 per cent of all pneumonias in some urban populations. The organism spreads via respiratory droplets and appears to have a long incubation period, so that slow spread among family members or other closed groups over a period of many weeks is characteristic. Although all ages can be affected, the greatest incidence of mycoplasmal pneumonia is in older children and young adults. The disease usually begins gradually. In addition to a nonproductive cough with fever and malaise, headache is a rather constant symptom. Physical examination discloses fine rales which are typically less extensive than the patchy alveolar densities (usually confined to one of the lower lobes) seen on chest x-ray. Occasionally examination of the tympanic membrane will also show a bullous myringitis. Laboratory studies reveal a normal white blood cell count and differential in most cases. The sputum is scant, with a predominance of mononuclear cells. Mycoplasma organisms are very small and lack cell walls; hence, they cannot be visualized with conventional microscopy. Mycoplasmal pneumonia is usually a mild, self-limited illness, but can produce severe pneumonia in children with sickle cell anemia, in immunosuppressed hosts, and in the elderly. Uncommon complications include hemolytic anemia, encephalitis, Guillain-Barré syndrome, myopericarditis and Stevens-Johnson syndrome.

VIRAL PNEUMONIA. Many viruses are capable of producing upper and lower respiratory tract infections, including adenoviruses, respiratory syncytial virus and parainfluenza virus. These infections are clinically indistinguishable except when part of a distinctive systemic viral illness such as rubeola in children or varicella in adults. Cytomegalovirus is a common cause of viral pneumonia in the immunocompromised host. The most important cause of viral pneumonia is influenza, which can be recognized by its epidemic spread and marked systemic symptoms such as fever and myalgias. Influenza pneumonia may be a mild or fulminant illness capable of causing lethal respiratory failure. Bacterial pneumonia, especially of the pneumococcal, staphylococcal or streptococcal variety, is a frequent complication.

PSITTACOSIS. Psittacosis is caused by a member of the *Chlamydia* group of obligate intracellular parasites which are also responsible for lymphogran-

uloma venereum and trachoma. The disease is transmitted from parrots or other birds (including pigeons and turkeys) to man. The clinical features of psittacosis are indistinguishable from those of other nonbacterial pneumonias, with prominent headache, nonproductive cough and fever. Occasionally a faint macular rash or splenomegaly develops.

Q FEVER. Caused by *Coxiella burnetii,* Q fever is unique among rickettsial infections in that pneumonia is prominent, there is no rash, and spread is through inhalation of infected dust particles rather than via the bite of an insect vector. The organisms reside principally in animals; human contact with cattle, sheep, goats or with infected animal hides or hide products is the most important epidemiologic factor, and is often the only clue to diagnosis. The clinical features of Q fever are similar to those of the other nonbacterial pneumonias, except that hepatitis occurs in up to one third of patients.

MANY OTHER ORGANISMS ranging from the tubercle bacillus (particularly during *primary tuberculosis,* see Chapter 47) to fungi (particularly histoplasmosis and coccidioidomycosis) and parasites (*Pneumocystis carinii* in the immunosuppressed host) can cause illnesses resembling the atypical pneumonias.

DIFFERENTIAL DIAGNOSIS

In addition to the conditions listed in Table 43–1 and detailed above, noninfectious diseases can occa-

Table 43–1.   Differential Diagnosis of Pneumonia

I. Bacterial Pneumonias
  A. Gram-positive
    1. *Pneumococcus*
    2. *Streptococcus*
    3. *Staphylococcus aureus*
  B. Gram-negative
    1. *H. influenzae*
    2. *Klebsiella*
    3. *Proteus, E. coli, Pseudomonas* and others (usually in hospitalized patients)
    4. Legionnaire's disease
  C. Mixed
    1. Aspiration pneumonia
  D. Mycobacterial
    1. Tuberculosis
II. Nonbacterial Pneumonias
    1. *Mycoplasma*
    2. Viral
    3. Psittacosis
    4. Q fever
    5. *Pneumocystis carinii*
    6. Fungi

sionally mimic infectious processes. Bronchial asthma (see Chapter 45) and hypersensitivity pneumonitis are common examples. The radiologic findings associated with chronic pulmonary diseases, especially chronic bronchitis (see Chapter 44), and bronchiectasis (see Chapter 37), may be misleading if previous x-rays are not available. Atelectasis, pulmonary infarction, pulmonary edema (see Chapter 27) and lung tumors may also be confused with pneumonia.

WORKUP

History. A careful history should be taken, looking particularly for recent viral upper respiratory infection and any exposure to respiratory tract infection. Impaired cough and gag reflexes due to anesthesia, head trauma, intoxication and neurologic disorders increase the risk of aspiration pneumonia. A history of recent travel may raise the question of unusual bacterial or fungal processes; and occupational exposures or animal (Q fever) and bird (psittacosis) contacts further broaden the differential diagnosis. It is particularly important to learn if the patient is a smoker and has underlying chronic lung disease or asthma.

It is important to distinguish between bacterial and nonbacterial diseases. Although this distinction can be difficult in individual patients, certain broad generalizations can be offered. Patients with bacterial pneumonias are more likely to have the abrupt onset of illness and to be clinically sicker with higher temperatures, a higher incidence of chills, more copious sputum production, and a greater likelihood of developing significant pleural effusions. While both types of pneumonia can affect all ages, nonbacterial pneumonias are more common in older children and young adults. Such patients characteristically report a more gradual onset of symptoms with only moderate fever. Patients with viral and mycoplasmal pneumonias will often complain of a severe hacking cough, but substantial sputum production is unusual.

Physical examination. The patient with bacterial pneumonia generally looks sicker, and chest examination usually reveals signs of consolidation or at least localized rales and rhonchi. In contrast, the chest examination of patients with nonbacterial pneumonias typically shows only fine rales, and often the physical findings are less extensive than the radiologic abnormalities.

Physical examination is important not only to elicit signs of pneumonia itself, but to assess the overall status of the patient. High fever, marked tachycardia, hypotension, cyanosis, signs of hypercarbia (asterixis, confusion, papilledema), and alterations of mentation are indications for emergency hospitalization.

Laboratory studies. When the patient is only mildly ill and has clear lungs, laboratory studies can be limited to a sputum Gram stain, sputum culture and a white blood cell count and differential. When pneumonia is suspected, PA and lateral chest x-rays are mandatory, and blood cultures should be obtained. If a sufficient volume of pleural fluid is present, thoracentesis should be performed and the fluid sent for Gram stain, culture, and protein, glucose and LDH determinations (see Chapter 39).

Laboratory studies help distinguish between viral and bacterial causes. Patients with bacterial pneumonias are more likely to have a polymorphonuclear leukocytosis. If the chest x-ray reveals lobar or segmental consolidation, abscess formation or significant pleural effusions, bacterial pneumonia is more likely; a patchy infiltrate can occur in either type of process, but a true interstitial infiltrate suggests a nonbacterial etiology.

The key to diagnosis is examination of sputum. The sputum of the patient with bacterial pneumonia is typically thick and green to brownish in color. It may be blood-tinged. A good sputum specimen for microscopic examination and culture is crucial. If the patient cannot expectorate spontaneously, pulmonary physiotherapy, intermittent positive pressure breathing with humidified air, or nasotracheal suction may be used to obtain the specimen. If these fail, transtracheal aspiration should be considered. Gram stain of sputum from patients with bacterial pneumonia usually reveals abundant polymorphonuclear leukocytes and will often disclose the primary pathogen. Patients with nonbacterial pneumonias generally produce only scant quantities of thin sputum, though in the case of influenzal pneumonia it can be bloody; the Gram stain is noteworthy for an absence of bacteria and a scant cellular response. In patients with mycoplasmal pneumonia, mononuclear cells may predominate.

The sputum should be cultured promptly and blood cultures should be obtained prior to administration of antibiotics, since transient bacteremias are frequent, especially with pneumococcal disease, and the organism may be too fastidious to grow from sputum specimens in some instances.

Diagnosis of Legionnaire's disease can be made

by isolation of the organism from sputum, lung or pleural fluid with the use of special media, by lung biopsy with fluorescent antibody staining, or by serologic studies.

Most viral pneumonias can be diagnosed on clinical grounds and epidemiologic evidence. Specific diagnosis depends on either serologic studies (which are retrospective) or viral cultures (which are not widely available). Recognition of influenza is important because contacts can be protected by prophylactic use of amantadine; diagnostic confirmation is worth seeking when influenza is suspected.

Mycoplasma can be grown in the laboratory only on specialized media. An important clue to diagnosis is the presence of cold agglutinins in the serum. Low titers (below 1:32 or 1:64) can occur in other disorders such as adenoviral and influenza infections, but high or rising titers are strongly suggestive of *M. pneumoniae* infection. Cold agglutinins may be absent, particularly in patients with mild disease, and specific serologic tests are then required.

For psittacosis, a history of bird exposure is the key to diagnosis, and specific serologies are required for confirmation. The diagnosis of Q fever depends on specific serologies.

PRINCIPLES OF MANAGEMENT

Many patients with lower respiratory tract infections, especially those with acute bronchitis or mild pneumonia due to virus, *H. influenzae,* pneumococci, or mycoplasma, can be managed on an outpatient basis, provided that they are alert, reliable, have help available to them, and have no signs of serious compromise such as high fever, tachycardia, tachypnea, hypotension, cyanosis or alterations of mentation. Oral antibiotic regimens can achieve therapeutic serum antibiotic levels. However, those with staphylococcal and gram-negative pneumonias must be treated with parenteral antibiotics and thus require hospitalization. The elderly and individuals with poor home environments also deserve consideration for inpatient treatment.

There are certain general principles of management which apply, regardless of etiology. Adequate hydration is essential to help clear secretions; this can be achieved via attention to fluid intake and also through local airway humidification. Expectorants such as guaifenesin may be helpful to some patients in loosening the sputum. Pulmonary physical therapy can further help with secretions. (See Chapters 37, 44, 46.) In general, the cough reflex should not be suppressed in patients with bacterial infections, because coughing is an important mechanism for clearing secretions. However, if severe paroxysms of coughing produce respiratory fatigue or severe pain, temporary relief may be obtained with small doses of codeine (see Chapter 37). Chest pain should be treated with analgesics which do not suppress cough. Aspirin should be tried first, but for more severe pain, pentazocine or opiates may be needed; if these agents are used, the patient must be carefully monitored for respiratory depression and excessive cough suppression. Fever can be controlled with aspirin or acetaminophen (see Chapter 6). If oxygen is administered prior to hospitalization, only very low FIO_2's (24 to 28 per cent) should be utilized. Individuals with

Table 43–2.   Antibiotics of Choice for Outpatient Treatment of Lower Respiratory Tract Infections

ORGANISM*	DRUG OF CHOICE	ALTERNATE DRUGS
S. pneumoniae (pneumococcus)	Penicillin	Cephalosporins Erythromycin Lincomycin Clindamycin
Hemophilus influenzae	Ampicillin	Tetracycline Trimethoprim- sulfamethoxazole
Mycoplasma pneumoniae	Erythromycin or Tetracyline	
Q fever	Tetracycline	Chloramphenicol
Psittacosis	Tetracycline	

* Lower respiratory infections due to Group A streptococcus, *Staphylococcus aureus,* Legionnaire's disease bacillus *(Legionella pneumoniae), Klebsiella pneumoniae, Pseudomonas aeruginosa, E. coli, Proteus mirabilis,* and other gram-negative bacilli require hospitalization for parenteral antibiotic therapy; the same is true for aspiration pneumonia due to mixed "normal" mouth flora.

Table 43–3.   Antibiotic Dosage Regimens for Ambulatory
Therapy of Acute Bronchitis
and Mild Cases of Pneumonia in Adults

DRUG	DOSE*	MAJOR TOXICITY†
Penicillin‡	250-500 mg. every 6 hrs.	Hypersensitivity
Ampicillin‡	250-500 mg. every 6 hrs.	Hypersensitivity GI intolerance
Amoxicillin‡	250-500 mg. every 8 hrs.	Hypersensitivity GI intolerance
Erythromycin	250-500 mg. every 6 hrs.	GI intolerance Hypersensitivity
Trimethoprim-sulfamethoxazole	2 tablets every 12 hrs.	Hypersensitivity
Tetracycline	250-500 mg. every 6 hrs.	GI intolerance Hypersensitivity
Clindamycin	150-300 mg. every 6 hrs.	Enterocolitis Hypersensitivity
Cephalexin‡,§	250-500 mg. every 6-8 hrs.	Hypersensitivity

*All doses are for average-sized adults with normal renal and hepatic function. Consult manufacturer's recommendations for details.

†Only major toxicity is listed; see manufacturer's literature for additional adverse reactions. In addition, all antibiotics predispose to superinfection with resistant organisms and should be used with caution.

‡Cross-sensitivity is shared among all of the penicillins. In addition, patients who are allergic to penicillins may be allergic to cephalosporins.

§Other cephalosporins used orally include cephradine (similar to cephalexin), cefaclor (somewhat more active than cephalexin against H.influenzae), cefadoxril (not yet approved for respiratory tract infection) and cephaloglycin (poorly absorbed; should not be used).

chronic lung disease who retain CO_2 depend on their hypoxic drive; excessive oxygen therapy may precipitate respiratory depression (see Chapter 44).

Specific therapy depends on the etiologic agent involved. While culture and sensitivity testing will require at least 24 to 48 hours to provide definitive information, the clinical setting, chest x-ray and sputum Gram stain usually enable the physician to make a reasonable presumptive diagnosis and to initiate therapy promptly. Treatment can then be modified as necessary on the basis of culture results.

THERAPEUTIC RECOMMENDATIONS
(see Tables 43–2 and 43–3)

Pneumococcal Disease

Penicillin is the drug of choice. Therapy should be continued until the patient has been afebrile for 3 to 5 days or for a total course of 10 to 14 days. A healthy young patient with disease confined to one lobe and a supportive home environment can be given an initial dose of intramuscular procaine penicillin and continued on oral penicillin at home with close follow-up. Most other patients should be considered for hospitalization initially and treated parenterally

until substantial improvement occurs. Table 43–2 lists alternative antibiotics for the penicillin-allergic patient; tetracyclines should *not* be used because many pneumococci are now resistant to these agents.

An important new development is the availability of a *vaccine* to prevent pneumococcal pneumonia. Although there are 83 capsular types of pneumococci, each with its own type-specific immunity, a relatively small number of serotypes account for most human infections. The vaccine incorporates 14 capsular types which together account for about 80 per cent of pneumococcal pneumonias in the United States, and field trials suggest that it should be at least 80 per cent effective in preventing pneumonia due to these 14 types. All patients who have undergone splenectomy or who have sickle cell disease should be vaccinated, because of their unique susceptibility to fulminating pneumococcal sepsis. In addition, immunosuppressed patients, the elderly, and individuals with chronic cardiopulmonary disease would seem to be good candidates for vaccination. Mild local pain and erythema are the only common adverse reactions to the vaccine, which is administered in a single 0.5-cc. intramuscular or subcutaneous dose. Repeat doses of vaccine are not required for at least 3 years.

Staphylococcus aureus

A parenterally administered semisynthetic penicillin (or penicillin, if the organism is not a penicillinase producer) is the drug of choice, requiring hospitalization. Therapy should be continued until clinical and x-ray healing is apparent; this usually requires at least 2 to 4 weeks.

Streptococcus pyogenes

Parenteral penicillin is the treatment of choice, requiring hospitalization. Therapy should be continued until clinical resolution, usually at least 2 weeks.

H. influenzae

Until very recently, ampicillin was the drug of choice for *H. influenzae* infections. In the past few years, an increasing number of ampicillin-resistant strains of this organism have been recognized. While ampicillin-resistant organisms still constitute a minority of strains, chloramphenicol should be used for initial therapy in the very sick patient, with a return to ampicillin if the organism proves sensitive. Cefamandole is a new parenteral cephalosporin-like drug which is proving very effective against *H. influenzae,* including ampicillin-resistant strains. For patients with bronchitis, the oral tetracyclines and trimethoprim-sulfamethoxazole have been excellent alternatives to ampicillin. In general, patients with bronchitis should be treated for 7 to 10 days, and patients with pneumonia for 10 to 14 days.

Klebsiella and Other Enterobacteriaceae

Hospital admission for parenteral antibiotic therapy is required. Gentamicin is the drug of choice, pending results of susceptibility testing.

Legionnaire's Disease

Therapy during outbreaks is often initiated on clinical and epidemiologic grounds before the diagnosis is confirmed. Erythromycin is currently the drug of choice, 1.0 gm. intravenously four times daily. Treatment failures have been reported when seriously ill patients are given oral erythromycin; very mild cases may be managed on an outpatient basis with 500 mg. erythromycin four times daily for 7 to 10 days. Close follow-up is mandatory.

Aspiration Pneumonia

A patient who aspirates cannot protect his airway and must be admitted. Penicillin is the drug of choice, and clindamycin is an excellent alternative.

Mycoplasma

Oral erythromycin or tetracycline is effective. The penicillins are inactive because mycoplasmas lack cell walls. Treatment should be continued for 1 to 2 weeks.

Viruses

While there is no effective treatment for any viral pneumonia, recognition of influenza is important because contacts of patients can be protected by the prophylactic administration of amantadine. Vulnerable individuals, such as the elderly and those with cardiopulmonary disease and diabetes should be protected by annual administration of influenza vaccine before the winter flu season. Serious reactions are rare unless the patient is allergic to egg protein. Minor febrile responses and myalgias are sometimes noted.

Tuberculosis

See Chapter 47.

MONITORING THERAPY

Temperature, respiratory rate, chest examination and white cell count will provide a reasonable estimate of recovery. Repeating chest x-rays at frequent intervals is wasteful if the patient is progressing well clinically. It is important to recognize that clearing of radiologic findings often lags far behind clinical resolution; continued presence of a slowly resolving infiltrate is neither a sign of poor response to therapy nor indicative of serious prognosis. This is particularly true for pneumococcal disease, in which the patient feels much better while x-rays may still show an infiltrate up to 6 weeks later. However, x-ray examination is important for detection of complications such as lung abscess and empyema, and films should be obtained when the patient's condition is worsening or fever is not resolving.

INDICATIONS FOR ADMISSION

High fever, tachypnea, tachycardia, cyanosis, poor home environment, presence of an organism necessitating parenteral therapy, aspiration, lung abscess, empyema, and positive blood cultures (except when positive for pneumococci) mandate inpatient management. Elderly patients and those with pre-existing cardiopulmonary disease should usually be admitted unless illness is very mild and close supervision is available at home.

PATIENT EDUCATION

Patients treated on an ambulatory basis need to be instructed to maintain a good fluid intake (approximately 2000 cc. of liquid daily) in order to avoid inspissation of secretions and poor pulmonary toilet. Temperature should be taken and recorded each evening. Caution against overuse of any cough suppressant is important; emphasis should be on nighttime use only, allowing for sleep but permitting cough and mobilization of sputum during the day. Many individuals think all coughing is bad; they need to understand its role in clearing the airways so they do not abuse their medication. If the patient is a smoker, he will probably have ceased smoking temporarily. This is an excellent opportunity to encourage the patient to quit, and, in fact, many do at this time (see Chapter 49). Patient and family should be instructed to watch for evidence of worsening (unremitting fever, drowsiness, dyspnea, etc.) and to call at first sign of difficulty.

ANNOTATED BIBLIOGRAPHY

General Aspects

Fekety, F.R., Caldwell, J., Gump, D., et al.: Bacteria, viruses, and mycoplasmas in acute pneumonia in adults. Am. Rev. Resp. Dis., 104:499, 1971. (A microbiologic study of the etiologic agents responsible for 100 consecutive cases of pneumonia in hospitalized adults. Sixty-two per cent were pneumococcal. In about 30 per cent the cause was uncertain. Other bacteria, viruses, mycoplasma were rarely implicated.)

Huxley, E.J., Viroslav, J., Gray, W.R., et al.: Pharyngeal aspiration in normal adults and patients with depressed consciousness. Am. J. Med., 74:564, 1978. (An interesting study which demonstrates that 45 per cent of normal subjects and 70 per cent of patients with depressed consciousness aspirate oropharyngeal contents into the lower airway during sleep. The authors speculate that aspiration probably occurs in all normals during deep sleep, but aspirated volumes are small and intact mucociliary clearance protects against pneumonia.)

Mostow, S.R.: Pneumonias acquired outside the hospital. Med. Clin. N. Am., 58:555, 1974. (A clinical overview of pneumonias in ambulatory patients.)

Newhouse, M., Sanchis, J., and Bienenstock, J.: Lung defense mechanisms. N. Engl. J. Med., 295:990, 1045, 1976. (A scholarly review of pulmonary defense mechanisms.)

Shulman, J.A., Phillips, L.A., and Petersdorf, R.G.: Errors and hazards in the diagnosis and treatment of bacterial pneumonias. Ann. Intern. Med., 62:41, 1965. (A nice summary of common problems in the clinical management of pneumonia, with 22 illustrative case reports.)

Sullivan, R.J., Dowdle, W.R., Marine, W.M., et al.: Adult pneumonia in a general hospital. Arch. Intern. Med. 129:935, 1972. (A prospective study of 292 consecutive hospital admissions of adults with pneumonia. The most important etiologic agents were pneumococci [62 percent], gram-negative bacilli [20 percent], and staphylococci [10 percent]. Eighty percent of these patients had underlying diseases and the overal mortality was 24 percent. The predominance of indigent and elderly patients with multi-system disease probably accounts for the unusually high incidence of staph and gram-negative bacilli and for the high mortality rate.)

Tager, I., and Speizer, F.E.: Role of infection in chronic bronchitis. N. Engl. J. Med., 292:563, 1975. (Challenges the notion that infections are responsible for exacerbations.)

Pneumococcal Pneumonias

Advisory Committee on Immunization Practices: Pneumococcal polysaccharide vaccine. Morbidity and Mortality Weekly Report, 27:25, January 27, 1978. (Recommendations for the use of pneumococcal vaccine.)

Austrian, R., and Gold, J.: Pneumococcal bacteremia with especial reference to bacteremic pneumococcal pneumonia. Ann. Intern. 60:759, 1964. (A *classic study of clinical features and prognostic indicators in bacteremic pneumococcal pneumonia.)*

Jay, S.J., Johannson, W.G., and Pierce, A.K.: The radiographic resolution of *Streptococcus pneumoniae* pneumonia. N. Engl. Med, *293*:798, 1975. *(A very helpful paper showing that delayed resolution of radiographic abnormalities is common in pneumococcal pneumonia, and that these x-ray findings in themselves need not raise concern about bronchial obstruction, neoplasia, or persistant infection.)*

Streptococcal Pneumonias

Basiliere, J.L., Bistrong, H.W., and Spence, W.F.: Streptococcal pneumonia: Recent outbreaks in military recruit populations. Am. J. Med., *44*:580, 1968. *(Clinical features of group A streptococcal pneumonia; based on 95 cases in naval recruits.)*

Staphylococcal Pneumonias

Musher, D.M., and McKenzie, S.O.: Infections due to *Staphylococcus aureus*. Medicine, *56*:383, 1977. *(A recent review of staphylococcal infections, including aerogenous and bacteremic pneumonias.)*

Gram-Negative Pneumonias

Tillotson, J.R., and Lerner, A.M.: Pneumonias caused by gram-negative bacilli. Medicine, *45*:65, 1966. *(A study of 38 hospitalized patients with gram negative pneumonias. Twenty-seven were community acquired, 7 were nosocomial, and 4 represented superinfection following pneumonococcal pneumonia. In all, these cases represented less than 4 percent of the pneumonias seen during the study period.)*

Wallace, R.J., Musher, D.M., and Martin, R.R.: *Hemophilus influenzae* pneumonia in adults. Am. J. Med., *64*:87, 1978. *(One of several recent and timely reminders that this "childhood" pathologen can cause serious infection in adults, particularly those with chronic lung disease.)*

Aspiration Pneumonias

Lorber, G., and Swenson, R.M.: Bacteriology of aspiration pneumonia: A prospective study of community-and hospital-acquired cases. Ann. Intern. Med., *81*:329, 1974. *(Mixed anaerobic oropharyngeal flora accounted for 21 of 24 community-acquired aspiration pneumonias, but for only 8 of 23 hospital-acquired aspiration pneumonias. In contrast, gram-negative bacilli and staphylococci were important pathogens in the nosocomial pneumonias but not in the community cases.)*

Nonbacterial Pneumonias

Denny, F.W., Clyde, W.A., and Glezen, W.P.: *Mycoplasma pneumoniae* disease: Clinical spectrum, pathophysiology, epidemiology, and control. J. Infect. Dis., *123*:74, 1971.

Maletzky, A.J., Cooney, M.K., Luce, R., *et al.*: Epidemiology of viral and mycoplasmal agents associated with childhood lower respiratory illness in a civilian population. J. Pediatr., *78*:407, 1971.

Murray, H.W., Masur, H., Senterfit, L.B., *et al.*: The protein manifestations of *Mycoplasma pneumonia* infection in adults. Am. J. Med., *58*:229, 1975. *(Three papers dealing with the epidemiologic features and clinical spectrum of mycoplasmal and viral pneumonias.)*

Legionnaire's Disease

Center for Disease Control: Legionnaire's disease: Diagnosis and management. Ann. Intern. Med., *88*:363, 1978. *(An overview of the clinical presentation, diagnosis and management of Legionnaire's disease.)*

Fraser, D.W., Tsai, T.R., Orenstein, W., *et al.*: Legionnaire's disease: Description of an epidemic of pneumonia. N. Engl., *297*:1189, 1977. *(A detailed account of the 1976 epidemic in Philadelphia which led to the identification of the unusual pulmonary pathogen.)*

44
Management of Chronic Obstructive Pulmonary Disease (COPD)

The chronic obstructive pulmonary diseases (chronic bronchitis and emphysema) are major causes of total disability, second only to coronary artery disease. The prevalence of COPD has been estimated to be almost 30 per 1000. Since COPD is incurable and often irreversible, the goal of management is to help the patient maintain his independence. In many instances, functional impairment can be minimized and exercise tolerance improved.

CLINICAL PRESENTATION AND COURSE

The earliest manifestation of COPD appears to be an increase in small airway resistance. Prior to the onset of symptoms, one can often detect an increase in the closing volume and a decrease in the maximum midexpiratory flow rate; measures of large airway resistance are usually within normal limits during this phase of illness. It is hypothesized that the presymptomatic, small airway stage of COPD may represent a period of reversible disease; however, early fibrotic changes have been found in airways of such patients. It is unresolved whether intervention at the time that small airway abnormalities begin to appear will alter the course of disease and affect prognosis.

The COPD patient may present clinically with any combination of cough, sputum production, wheezing and shortness of breath. The presentation is in part a function of the severity of illness and the relative contributions of chronic bronchitis and emphysema to the clinical picture. The majority of patients have mixed disease, with features of both forms, though one often predominates.

The person with *chronic bronchitis* is often a smoker who presents with a history of chronic, productive cough. By definition, the cough must be present for at least 3 months, during 2 consecutive years. At first, the sputum production and cough occur just in the winter months, but soon the patient becomes symptomatic year round, with a history of frequent exacerbations. By the time dyspnea on exertion sets in, the disease is well advanced. Patients may report having to sit up at night to breathe; at times this may be a manifestation of congestive heart failure, which is not uncommon, but more careful questioning often reveals that the difficulty was precipitated by cough and relieved by raising sputum. Patients with severe chronic bronchitis are at increased risk of developing cor pulmonale, because they often become chronically hypoxic and develop an increase in pulmonary artery resistance that leads to right heart failure.

The chronic bronchitic is typically in his fifties at the time of presentation. He appears plethoric and cyanotic at the stage of severe disease, a time when many first come for help. Tobacco stains on the fingers and teeth are common, and there may be signs of cor pulmonale (distended neck veins, a right ventricular heave, a right ventricular gallop, and peripheral edema). The lungs sound noisy; crackles and wheezes are readily evident. The expiratory phase of respiration is prolonged. Because of the mismatching of ventilation with perfusion, hypoxia may be found on measurement of arterial blood gases. The pCO_2 rises as the patient's ability to effectively move air declines. Secondary polycythemia is common.

The patient with *emphysema* as the predominant lesion frequently complains of dyspnea, particularly on exertion. Cough is only a minor part of the clinical picture, and sputum production is scant. The patient with advanced disease is thin and tachypneic, often using accessory respiratory muscles and pursed-lip breathing. The neck veins may seem distended, but only on expiration. The anterior-posterior diameter of the chest is increased, the percussion note is hyperresonant, and the breath sounds are distant. There are usually no signs of cor pulmonale, though the right ventricular impulse may be prominent due to displacement by the hyperinflated lungs. Hypoxia is minimal, because there is only minor mismatching of ventilation and perfusion in comparison to the major degree of imbalance that occurs in chronic bronchitis. Carbon dioxide retention is minimal if present at all.

The clinical course of COPD is generally progressive, though there are some individuals who seem to reach a plateau. Longitudinal studies of groups of symptomatic patients have shown a steady deterioration in pulmonary function with time. Using the forced expiratory volume at 1 second (FEV_1) as the measure of obstruction, an annual average decrease in flow rate of 50 to 60 ml. per second has been noted. By the time the FEV_1 declines to 1.0 liter per second, the mean annual mortality rate approaches 10 per cent. The onset of resting tachycardia and signs of cor pulmonale are other indicators of a poor prognosis. However, it is very difficult to predict the course of illness in a particular patient. Individuals with severe disease can often survive for years.

PRINCIPLES OF MANAGEMENT

The goal of management is to improve the patient's ability to perform his daily activities. Subjective improvement can often be achieved, though it may not always be accompanied by parallel changes in objective parameters. There is no clear evidence that any particular treatment modality prolongs survival. Consequently, it is sometimes necessary to choose among therapies on the basis of subjective responses. The success of any therapeutic program is facilitated by the physician's interest and the cooperation of patient and family.

Although the selection of treatment modalities is often empiric, it is helpful to identify the major physiological deficits, assess their severity, and direct therapy toward them. History-taking should include ascertaining the types of symptoms and activity limitations experienced in daily life, as well as smoking habits and exposure to pulmonary irritants such as aerosol sprays. In the physical examination, tachypnea, tachycardia, degree of prolongation of expiratory phase, use of accessory respiratory muscles, cyanosis, wheezing, signs of consolidation and evidence of right heart failure are noted. Small airway disease can be detected during the asymptomatic phase of illness by ordering closing volume and maximal midexpiratory flow rate determinations. The degree of obstruction in larger airways can be assessed by measuring expiratory flow rates on an office spirometer; the most helpful measurement is the ratio of the forced expiratory volume at 1 second (FEV_1) to the vital capacity. Crude estimates of obstruction can be provided by the FEV_1 alone. Results are compared to predicted values. Patients with a 50 per cent reduction in FEV_1 are often dyspneic on exertion; by the time the FEV_1 falls to 25 per cent of predicted, they may complain of shortness of breath at rest. De-

termination of expiratory flow rates before and after inhalation of a bronchodilator (e.g., isoproterenol) can provide a quick estimate of the benefit a patient may derive from bronchodilator therapy. The failure to obtain an improvement in flow rate from a few inhalations of a bronchodilator does not rule out the possibility of benefit, but it suggests the likelihood is not great.

A chest x-ray is helpful to detect complications of COPD, such as right heart failure, pneumonia, or a pneumothorax. Arterial blood gases provide measures of oxygenation and ventilation. Hypoxemia and hypercarbia are manifestations of severe chronic bronchitis. Blood gases are particularly useful for documenting acute decompensation. In patients with severe chronic bronchitis, baseline studies of blood gases should be performed, so that gases obtained at times of marked subjective worsening can be compared to baseline determinations. Hematocrit and hemoglobin concentration provides a rough indication of the severity and chronicity of hypoxemia and the need for phlebotomy. The electrocardiographic abnormalities which appear in COPD generally reflect the severity of the lung disease and the presence of cor pulmonale. The ECG should be studied for sinus tachycardia, multifocal atrial tachycardia, peaked P waves (P pulmonale) and signs of right ventricular hypertrophy (e.g., tall R wave in V_1 and deep S in lead V_6). Examination of the sputum is mandatory when acute pneumonitis is suspected.

Regardless of severity of disease or the types of deficits present, *all* patients should be urged in the most emphatic of ways to *stop smoking*. Although the percentage of smokers who give up cigarettes as a result of the physician's exhortations is small, it has been shown that the physician's advice does make some difference, particularly in patients who are symptomatic (see Chapter 49). The major hope for arresting progression of COPD is to halt the continuous insult to the airways produced by smoking. Patients exposed to other pulmonary irritants should be advised to reduce their contact with them if feasible. Readily avoidable pulmonary irritants include aerosol deodorants, hairsprays, paint sprays, and insecticides. Change in job or residence should be urged only when it is clear that the relationship between exposure and disease is strong (see Chapter 35); otherwise, more harm than good might come of the advice.

Another essential prophylactic measure is immunization against respiratory pathogens. Trivalent *influenza vaccine* should be given to every COPD patient in the fall of each year, before the onset of the influenza season. *Pneumococcal vaccine* has now been developed and is effective in immunizing against 80 per cent of pneumococcal strains. In adults, the pneumococcal vaccine need be given only once every 3 years. It is recommended that both vaccines not be given simultaneously, because it would be difficult to determine the source of a hypersensitivity reaction, should it occur. However, if there is any doubt as to the patient's chances of returning for the second vaccination, both should be given at the same time.

Patients with evidence of bronchospasm should be given a trial of bronchodilator therapy, especially if they show an improvement in FEV_1 after a few inhalations of isoproterenol. Bronchodilators can be quite helpful, though there is no evidence that they alter prognosis. They must be used cautiously in hypoxic patients because of the risk of inducing serious dysrhythmias; even the so-called selective $beta_2$ agents have cardiotonic effects when used in large enough doses. *Theophylline preparations* are effective and relatively inexpensive. They are best taken orally, because rectal administration can result in erratic absorption. Fixed-combination preparations containing low doses of theophylline in conjunction with a sympathomimetic such as ephedrine should be avoided; the sympathomimetic may potentiate toxicity without improving therapeutic effect. Adverse side effects of theophylline include gastrointestinal upset, nervousness, mild tremor, and tachycardia. The relatively selective *$beta_2$ sympathomimetic bronchodilators* such as metaproterenol and terbutaline are also effective. Use of both a theophylline preparation (e.g., aminophylline) and a $beta_2$ agent (e.g., terbutaline) can sometimes enhance bronchodilation and allow reduction in doses of each, helping to minimize side effects. Some patients report severe tremor with use of terbutaline; the tremor often decreases as therapy is continued, but there are patients who find the tremor disabling and stop the drug. Metaproterenol and other sympathomimetic bronchodilators can be used in aerosol form. Expensive intermittent positive pressure breathing equipment (IPPB) offers no advantage over simple hand-held nebulizers for inhalation therapy. Many patients use an aerosol preparation for relief of an acute exacerbation of bronchospasm; the risk of tachyphylaxis needs to be kept in mind.

Corticosteroids may be tried when bronchospasm is severe and refractory to other measures. The significant morbidity associated with chronic daily use of systemic steroids may be reduced by rapidly tapering the dosage as soon as control of bronchospasm is attained and switching to an inhaled preparation such as beclomethasone (see Chapters 45 and 101). Patients who cannot be controlled on inhaled beclomethasone may need alternate day prednisone therapy. Only the patient with totally refractory bronchospasm should be considered for chronic daily steroid treatment.

Patients bothered by heavy, tenacious sputum may obtain benefit by maintaining good *fluid intake*, and assuring the adequate *humidification* of the indoor environment (particularly in centrally heated homes), and practicing *postural drainage* when clearance of secretions is difficult and cough is incapacitating. The simplest method of postural drainage is to have the patient lean over the side of the bed, rest the elbows on a pillow placed on the floor, and cough as a family member or visiting nurse gently pounds on the chest. For hydration, ultrasonic nebulizers are no better than the simple maintenance of good systemic hydration, though the moisture they deliver does reach deep into the tracheobronchial tree. Occasionally, bronchospasm can be triggered by a nebulizer, and its reservoir can become contaminated and serve as a source of airway infection. Nebulized detergents are of no proven use, but *mucolytic agents* such as acetylcysteine are capable of thinning secretions; they are usually reserved for patients on respirators and not commonly used in outpatient practice. Oral *expectorants* are very popular with some patients, but without proven clinical efficacy. These preparations need not be denied to the patient who feels that they are of benefit, but should not be the mainstay of the therapeutic program. Glyceryl guaiacolate and potassium iodide are the most frequently prescribed expectorants; many are available without a prescription.

Acute exacerbations characterized by increased cough and purulent sputum production are usually treated with *antibiotic therapy*, although one group of investigators has questioned the role of infection in exacerbations. Since pneumococci and *H. influenzae* are the predominant organisms infecting patients with COPD, most clinicians prescribe ampicillin or tetracycline for those who develop purulent sputum and increased cough. Several British studies have demonstrated that prophylactic use of antibiotics during the winter months can reduce the number of exacerbations and days lost from work. Attention to pulmonary toilet and hydration is probably as important to prevention and treatment of acute episodes.

Among the simplest and most effective measures for improving exercise tolerance is an *exercise training* program. Walking has proven to be the best form of exercise for increasing the duration and intensity of activity in COPD patients. Three of four sessions per day are prescribed, ranging from 5 to 15 minutes each. The pace and duration of activity are matched to the patient's capabilities; most begin the program walking at a half-maximal pace and build gradually over a period of several weeks. At the end of the training period, heart and respiratory rates for a given level of activity are decreased; oxygen consumption also falls. Tests of ventilatory function are not significantly changed, but increases of 25 per cent are attained in maximum duration and intensity of exercise. Many patients enjoy marked improvement in ability to carry out their daily activities.

Breathing exercises may have some beneficial effect, particularly in those patients who easily panic and hyperventilate when dyspneic. Teaching such individuals to take slow, deep, relaxed breaths and exhale against pursed lips can lessen the work of moving air and provide the patient who tends to panic with a sense of control over his breathing and a more relaxed respiratory pattern.

Patients who are severly incapacitated by hypoxia and require frequent phlebotomies for control of secondary erythrocytosis (see Chapter 78) are candidates for *chronic oxygen therapy*. Although prevention of cor pulmonale by oxygen therapy has not been proven, correction of severe hypoxia can lower pulmonary artery pressure and serve as a means of treating acute pulmonary hypertension. Oxygen therapy should never be attempted until it is established that the patient does not retain carbon dioxide when given oxygen, even at the low flow rates of oxygen available from portable units. Prior evaluation in the hospital is usually necessary before initiation of an outpatient program of oxygen administration. Patients being considered for this form of therapy should have arterial pO_2 levels of less than 50 to 55 mm. Hg. Oxygen is administered by a "low-flow" apparatus during sleep, when hypoxia is often greatest, and continued for up to a total of 18 hours per day. Patients who are known to become hypoxic during exercise may be helped by oxygen supplementation before exertion. Besides the risk of respiratory drive suppression, the drawbacks of this treatment modality are cost and the lack of proven effect on long-term survival. The literature should be followed for further developments in this area.

Patients with chronic cor pulmonale can often be made more comfortable by careful attention to their volume status, degree of hypoxemia, and hematocrit. Reduction of excess intravascular volume can reduce edema; diuretic therapy (see Chapter 27) is an effective means of volume control. Phlebotomy is indicated when secondary erythrocytosis is severe enough to significantly reduce blood viscosity and impair oxygen delivery; this occurs when the hematocrit rises above 55. Low-flow oxygen therapy can acutely lower pulmonary vascular resistance and provide some symptomatic relief during acute exacerbations; hospitalization is often necessary in this setting. Bronchodilators such as aminophylline can also reduce pulmonary vascular tone; in addition, they have a positive inotropic effect which may result in an increase in cardiac output. Use of digitalis in cor pulmonale is a subject of debate. The incidence of toxicity is increased, and the clinical responce is often equivocal. Patients who do appear to improve with digitalis therapy should be given a minimum maintenance dose and monitored closely for manifestations of digitalis toxicity (see Chapter 27).

Patients with severe COPD, especially those with known carbon dioxide retention, should not be given sedatives or tranquilizers. Anxiety and difficulty sleeping due to the symptoms of COPD should be treated by attending to the underlying disease.

PATIENT EDUCATION AND MONITORING

The first priority is to stress the importance of cessation of smoking; this should be followed by recommendations for ways of accomplishing the objective (see Chapter 49). Patients should be encouraged to maintain as much activity as possible and be provided with an exercise program if they can be motivated to comply. Patient, family and physician should be involved in setting reasonable and realistic goals of therapy. It is essential to warn against excessive use of oxygen therapy and intake of sedatives or tranquilizers. Advice regarding adequate hydration and pulmonary toilet should be given, as well as the importance of maintaining a well-humidified indoor environment in the winter. Careful instructions regarding the indications and adverse effects of therapy can help the patient to properly carry out the prescribed program. Complex regimens should be written down and reviewed with both patient and family. The interest and concern of the physician can have a considerable effect on the progress made by the COPD patient.

Part of the patient education process should include instructions on self-monitoring and on reporting symptoms to the physician. The number of stairs that can be climbed or the distance walked without stopping can be used to provide a crude estimate of clinical status. Serial determinations of arterial blood gases and expiratory flow rates can help in objectively following the course of disease and detecting acute deteriorations. Patients with known carbon dioxide retention should be checked for asterixis, an indication of worsening ventilatory status, further carbon dioxide retention and encephalopathy.

INDICATIONS FOR ADMISSION AND REFERRAL

The patient who develops asterixis should be promptly admitted to the hospital; no oxygen should be administered for fear of further suppressing respiration. The same holds for the lethargic patient. Patients with refractory bronchospasm, severe cor pulmonale or acute pneumonitis also require inpatient management. A hospital admission is needed to assess the safety and utility of low flow oxygen therapy for future outpatient use. A specialist in pulmonary medicine should be consulted when oxygen therapy is being considered for long-term management.

THERAPEUTIC RECOMMENDATIONS

- Insist on cessation of smoking.
- Advise the patient to remove environmental irritants and allergens and to maintain adequate humidity and hydration, particularly during the winter in cold climates.
- Be certain that influenza and pneumococcal vaccines are given.
- Employ a trial of bronchodilators, using aminophylline 200 mg. q.i.d. alone or in combination with a beta$_2$ agent such as terbutaline 5 mg. orally every 8 hours. The aerosolized beta$_2$ agent metaproterenol administered by hand nebulizer is helpful for acute use and as an alternative in patients who do not tolerate oral terbutaline, but there is no advantage to combined regular use of aerosol plus oral beta$_2$ agents. Reserve steroids for refractory cases.
- Teach slow, relaxed, deep breathing to the patient likely to panic and hyperventilate when dyspneic.
- Institute an exercise program in patients able to walk and motivated to carry out a daily activity program.
- Teach postural drainage techniques to patients bothered by difficulty raising sputum; a respiratory therapist may be of help in the teaching effort.
- Provide the reliable patient with a supply of ampicillin or tetracycline to be taken when the sputum turns purulent.
- Begin a diuretic program (e.g., 20 mg. furosemide per day) when edema formation begins to occur secondary to cor pulmonale; increase the program as needed to control fluid retention.
- Phlebotomize the patient with secondary erythrocytosis when the hematocrit reaches the 55 to 60 range.
- Consider chronic low-flow oxygen therapy when the patient is limited by severe hypoxia (pO$_2$ less than 50 mm. Hg), when recurrent phlebotomies are unable to control the erythrocytosis, or when cor pulmonale is difficult to control; obtain consultation.
- Use digitalis only in refractory cases of cor pulmonale, and only when an objective improvement can be demonstrated; monitor closely for signs of digitalis toxicity.

ANNOTATED BIBLIOGRAPHY

Cherniak, R.M., and Svanhill E.: Long-term use of intermittent positive pressure breathing (IPPB). Am. Rev. Respir. Dis., *113*:721, 1976. *(A summary of the evidence indicating the limited efficacy of expensive IPPB therapy.)*

Diener, C.F., and Burrows, B.: Further observations on the course and prognosis of chronic obstructive lung disease. Am. Rev. Respir. Dis., *111*:719, 1975. *(An important prospective study of prognosis in 200 patients with chronic airway obstruction. Reviews previous reports from this group.)*

Editorial: Domiciliary oxygen in advanced chronic bronchitis. Br. Med. J., *1*:484, 1976. *(A succinct review of the use of oxygen in the management of chronic obstructive pulmonary disease.)*

Foster, L.J., Corrigem, K., and Goldman, A.L.: Effectiveness of oxygen therapy in hypoxic polycythemic smokers. Chest, *73*:572, 1978. *(Low-flow oxygen is partially effective in decreasing polycythemia in nonsmokers. In smokers, high carboxyhemoglobin limits the benefit of correcting hypoxia.)*

Green, L.H., and Smith, T.W.: Use of digitalis in patients with pulmonary disease. Ann. Intern. Med., *87*:459, 1977. *(Digitalis is of questionable benefit, and risk of toxicity is increased.)*

Laforet, E.G.: Surgical management of chronic obstructive lung disease. N. Engl. J. Med., *287*:175,

1972. *(A review of extreme therapeutic measures.)*

Lefcoe, N.M., and Patterson, N.: Adjunct therapy in chronic obstructive pulmonary disease. Am. J. Med., *54*:343, 1973. *(A review of the use of exercise, IPPB and oxygen supplementation to ameliorate long-term complications of chronic pulmonary disease.)*

Lertzman, M.M., and Cherniack, R.M.: Rehabilitation of patients with chronic obstructive pulmonary disease. Am. Rev. Respir. Dis., *114*:1145, 1976. *(A superb review of therapeutic medalities in the management of chronic obstructive pulmonary disease.)*

Levy, D.: Therapy of obstructive bronchial diseases: The physicochemical approach. J. Asthma Res., *8*:161, 1971. *(A thorough review of physical therapeutic measures that produce subjective improvement without significant change in physiological parameters.)*

Petty, T.L., and Nett, L.N.: For those who live and breathe. A manual for patients with emphysema and chronic bronchitis. Springfield, IL: Charles C Thomas, 1972. *(A useful monograph emphasizing patient education in the management of COPD.)*

Pierson, D.J.: When to hospitalize the COPD patient. Chest, *73*:126, 1978. *(Little objective evidence exists to help make this decision, but this well-conceived editorial provides intelligent guidance on treating people without hospitalization.)*

Sackner, M.A.: Diaphragmatic breathing exercises. JAMA, *231*:295, 1975. *(A guide to applying this adjunctive therapy.)*

Sahn, S.A.: Corticosteroids in chronic bronchitis and pulmonary emphysema. Chest, *73*:389, 1978. *(A review of 17 published studies on the use of steroids concluding that benefit is restricted to individual patients; considers objectively monitored trials only.)*

Tager, I., and Speiser, F.E.: Role of infection in chronic bronchitis. N. Engl. J. Med., *292*:563, 1975. *(Argues that many exacerbations are not clearly due to infection.)*

Vandenbergh, E., Clement, J., and Vande Woestijne, K.P.: Course and prognosis of patients with advanced chronic obstructive pulmonary disease. Am. J. of Med., *55*:736, 1973. *(Increased pCO_2 and decreased pO_2 with exercise were among five indices predicting poor prognosis.)*

45

Management of Bronchial Asthma

Asthma affects about 2.5 per cent of the population and is a common outpatient problem. Bronchial asthma is characterized by reversible airway obstruction and manifested by cough, wheezing, sputum production and shortness of breath. The obstruction results from hyperreactivity of the airway causing excessive mucus production, smooth muscle contraction, and edema of the bronchial wall. Cases are sometimes classified as "extrinsic" (triggered by a known allergen and often associated with elevated levels of IgE) or "intrinsic" (adult onset, no specific allergen evident). Although there are no cures for asthma, there are effective means of treatment. The role of the primary physician is to minimize the frequency and severity of attacks and to treat them early and vigorously when they do occur.

PATHOPHYSIOLOGY, CLINICAL PRESENTATION AND COURSE

The increased reactivity of the bronchial airway is believed to be due in part to a reduction in the normal amount of cyclic AMP in the bronchial tissues. Cyclic AMP is a potent mediator of bronchodilatation. Beta-adrenergic stimulation increases adenyl cyclase activity, which results in increased production of cyclic AMP and, consequently, bronchodilatation. Alpha-adrenergic stimulation reduces cyclic AMP synthesis. A number of substances have been noted to produce bronchoconstriction. One of the major mediators of bronchoconstriction in asthma is slow reacting substance of anaphylaxis (SRS-A). Its release from mast cells can be triggered by infection, IgE, emotional factors and physical irritants. Cholinergic agents promote release of SRS-A. Excessive cholinergic activity in response to stress is thought to be responsible for emotion-induced bronchospasm. The exact role of prostaglandins in asthma is currently unsettled; they may prove to be quite important.

Patients with *extrinsic asthma* often experience the onset of symptoms before age 5. Prognosis is relatively good, with 70 per cent of patients found to be symptom-free after 20 years. Extrinsic asthma occurs in patients with an atopic history. It may be seasonal or year-round and is precipitated by an allergen, anxiety, or inhalation of irritants. The course of attacks is usually self-limited, though some patients can have severe bouts requiring hospitalization. IgE levels may be elevated in patients with extrinsic asthma.

Patients with *intrinsic asthma* typically begin having symptoms in the third or fourth decade. No identifiable allergen precipitates attacks in these patients. At times, there is much sputum production, making differentiation from chronic bronchitis difficult. The role of minor upper respiratory infection in the precipitation of attacks is often prominent. Some patients present with exertional dyspnea or cough and no demonstrable wheezing, though expiratory flow rates are clearly reduced. Patients with intrinsic asthma are sometimes more refractory to treatment than those with extrinsic disease.

Not all patients fall into the extrinsic or intrinsic categories. One group of asthmatics is notable for nasal polyps and hypersensitivity to aspirin. Some patients with no prior history of atopy or bronchospasm develop symptoms when air pollution is heavy.

Regardless of the type of asthma, subclinical but significant bronchospasm remains for days to weeks after the wheezing of an acute attack subsides. The continuing obstruction is believed to result from residual small airway bronchoconstriction that resolves more slowly than large airway bronchospasm. The clinical recurrences that often develop shortly after severe episodes are most often not new attacks, but rather the result of the previous one.

Overall mortality for all forms of asthma is 0.1 per cent per year; the rate increases markedly to 3.3 per cent for patients with episodes of status asthmaticus.

PRINCIPLES OF MANAGEMENT

The goals of therapy are to prevent exacerbations and control flares when they do occur. Before initiation of therapy, it is important to verify that non-asthmatic etiologies of bronchospasm are not involved (see Chapters 27, 36, and 44). Most patients with *acute asthmatic attacks* can be managed on an outpatient basis, provided that proper treatment is promptly instituted. Reliable individuals should be instructed to initiate a full bronchodilator program at the first signs of a flare, and to report quickly to the physician if treatment does not seem to be working.

Initiation of bronchodilator therapy at home can begin with a theophylline or beta-adrenergic preparation. Occasionally, the patient will be on a small maintenance dose of one of these medications at the time of an attack and require an increase in dose and/or addition of a second agent. The *theophylline preparations* are widely used, effective and relatively inexpensive bronchodilators. They inhibit phosphodiesterase (an enzyme that cleaves cyclic AMP); this action is believed to be the basis for their bronchodilating effect. *Aminophylline* is a salt of theophylline and is converted to the parent compound in vivo. It is the least expensive theophylline preparation. Theophylline elixirs are perhaps a bit more rapidly absorbed, but they are also more expensive and shorter acting. Suppositories are not to be used because they are erratically absorbed and result in unpredictable serum levels. Although the half-life of aminophylline averages 4 to 6 hours, there is wide individual variation; determination of the serum theophylline level is useful in adjusting dosage, especially when there is difficulty controlling symptoms. Therapeutic serum levels can be obtained by oral therapy, since 90 per cent of the drug is absorbed. Adverse effects include nausea, vomiting, nervousness and cardiac arrhythmias. Because there is a narrow margin between toxic and therapeutic effects, the drug should be started at moderate doses when used in the outpatient setting and cautiously increased as needed. The long-acting theophylline preparations with 12-hour duration of action (e.g., Slophyllin) are promising for nighttime use. These are not to be confused with enteric-coated forms, which offer no significant advantages and are expensive.

Beta-adrenergic agents may be used alone or in addition to theophylline compounds. They cause bronchodilatation by stimulating beta$_2$ receptors. Unfortunately, these agents usually possess some beta$_1$ activity and can have a prominent effect on the heart, especially when large doses are used. *Isoproterenol* is the time-honored sympathomimetic for asthma. It is usually administered by the aerosol route and can provide prompt relief, but its usefulness is limited by its short duration of action, considerable beta$_1$ activity, and strong potential for tachyphylaxis. The highly touted, relatively more *selective beta$_2$ sympathomimetics* are less cardiotonic, but they still have some beta$_1$ effect, particularly at higher doses. These agents have longer durations of action than isoproterenol and can be given orally. *Terbutaline* and *metaproterenol* are the two most commonly used beta$_2$ agents at the present time. Metaproterenol has the advantage of being available in inhalant form as well as in an oral preparation. Terbutaline can cause disturbing tremulousness in some patients; at times, this side effect lessens with continued use of the drug. Salbutamol, an even more selective beta$_2$ agent, is not presently available in the U.S. because of possible oncogenesis associated with its use. *Isoetharine* is a popular inhalation agent of the beta$_2$ variety. Combined use of a beta$_2$ agent and a theophylline derivative is often very effective and may allow reductions in the doses of each agent, thus minimizing side effects and maximizing bronchodilation. Use of more than one beta$_2$ preparation is probably unnecessary, though, at times, some patients are given oral terbutaline and a metaproterenol inhaler.

Epinephrine and ephedrine have been used for years; they are examples of less selective, but effective adrenergic bronchodilators. *Epinephrine* is the drug of choice for treatment of a severe acute asthmatic attack. Its disadvantages are the need for parenteral administration, short duration of action (less than 30 minutes), and a capacity to cause a significant rise in blood pressure. Patients who abuse sympathomimetics may become tachyphylactic to them and may not respond to epinephrine. *Ephedrine* has been replaced by the more selective beta$_2$ drugs, though it is still found in many fixed-combination preparations.

Fixed-combination preparations are expensive, offer few advantages, and have a greater risk of toxicity. Many such products contain theophylline and ephedrine. There is no evidence that a fixed combination is more effective than theophylline alone, and there are data showing that toxic amounts of ephedrine can accumulate when a fixed combination is given in sufficient dose to achieve therapeutic levels of theophylline.

Phenobarbital is also found in many combination preparations. It is added to offset the CNS-stimulating effects of ephedrine and theophylline. The dose of phenobarbital in each tablet is small, (8 to 15 mg.) but if 8 to 10 tablets are taken daily (which is not unusual during a flare-up), sufficient drug may be ingested to potentially compromise respiratory drive in the seriously affected patient. Phenobarbital and other sedatives have little place in the treatment of an asthmatic attack; the most effective treatment for alleviation of the anxiety caused by difficulty breathing is to ease the patient's respiratory distress. Sedatives, antianxiety agents and combination preparations which contain these drugs should be avoided.

Patients experiencing acute attacks that do not abate promptly at home with initiation of oral bronchodilator therapy require prompt physician evaluation. A telephone call to the patient can be very helpful in making triage decisions, for the patient who cannot complete a sentence on the telephone needs urgent hospital admission. The patient who arrives in the office breathing with the help of accessory respiratory muscles (i.e., shows sternocleidomastoid retraction) or demonstrates pulsus paradoxus or an FEV$_1$ of less than 1.0 liter per second should also be hospitalized. A subcutaneous injection of epinephrine may ease an acute attack and is worth giving at the outset of the office visit. If there is not an adequate response, the injection can be repeated every 20 minutes over the course of 1 hour. Patients who have been making heavy use of sympathomimetic inhalers may be refractory to epinephrine.

An attack that is not fully controlled by maximal doses of xanthines and sympathomimetics may necessitate a short course of oral corticosteroid therapy. A 7-to 10-day program of *prednisone* in a rapidly tapering schedule is often very effective in controlling an otherwise refractory episode and will not cause adrenal suppression. Switching to an inhaled steroid preparation that does not significantly suppress adrenal function can be done as prednisone is tapered; the changeover helps to maintain control without subjecting the patient to further systemic steroids.

Beclomethasone has proved useful in this regard. At times, prednisone cannot be tapered without inducing a recrudescence of symptoms; in such situations, it may be possible to utilize an alternate day prednisone program to control bronchospasm without risking the major side effects of long-term steroid use (see Chapter 101). Prolonged daily prednisone therapy should be reserved for truly refractory cases. Patients who can be brought under control by nonsteroidal agents, but have trouble tolerating the side effects from the large doses necessary, may be candidates for a trial of beclomethasone, which may allow reduction in oral bronchodilator doses. Clinically significant adrenal suppression does not occur with beclomethasone, as long as the total daily dose is less than 1000 mcg. (20 inhalations); usually 6 to 8 inhalations per day suffice to ease symptoms.

The adequacy of systemic steroid therapy can be determined by checking the *total eosinophil count,* as well as by monitoring clinical parameters. The count frequently provides a reliable measure of disease activity. When steroids are necessary, they should be prescribed in doses sufficient to reduce the eosinophil count to normal. Tapering can then be initiated while monitoring the count for elevation, a sign of inadequate therapy. A rise in the eosinophil count often occurs before the onset of symptoms; thus the count can be used to warn of impending flares.

Once an attack is terminated, the goal of management shifts to prevention of future episodes. Identification of the responsible allergen is sometimes helpful in patients with extrinsic asthma, but in most instances extensive skin testing reveals a large number of allergens to which the patient is sensitive. Consequently, *desensitization* is ineffective is such situations. Even in cases where a single known allergen has been identified, controlled studies have failed to demonstrate the efficacy of desensitization injections. Avoidance of the offending agents is good therapy, where practical (e.g., remaining indoors when air pollution is heavy); unfortunately this is not always feasible and other methods of prophylaxis have to be used.

The inadequacy of immunotherapy is not critical in view of the availability of effective pharmacologic agents for prophylaxis. It is felt that daily maintenance doses of bronchodilators can help curb the frequency and severity of attacks. Aminophylline, terbutaline and related agents are very commonly used for such purposes. Controlled studies demonstrating the superiority of maintenance therapy over intermittent use are lacking, but most authorities recommend

a maintenance program when attacks are frequent and severe. Cromolyn sodium and steroids are reserved for the more refractory cases.

Cromolyn sodium has been found to be most effective for prevention of asthmatic attacks in children and those with exercise-induced bronchospasm. The agent has no direct bronchodilating or anti-inflammatory actions; rather, it works by preventing degranulation of mast cells. Cromolyn has no role in treatment of established, acute asthmatic attacks; its place is in prevention. The drug is worthy of consideration in children and those with asthma brought on by exercise if maintenance bronchodilators have not proven adequate. The drug is administered as an inhaled powder. Unfortunately, some patients experience a hypersensitivity reaction to the agent, thus limiting its usefulness. Cromolyn is less likely to work in adults than it is in children, but should be considered before a patient is committed to chronic prednisone therapy. A 4- to 8-week trial is needed to assess efficacy.

Patients who do not achieve adequate prophylaxis from use of oral bronchodilators are candidates for *beclomethasone,* before one resorts to systemic corticosteroid therapy. This inhaled topical steroid can obviate the need for prednisone in many instances. Beclomethasone is well tolerated and often quite effective in reducing the frequency and severity of flares. Its only adverse effect has been transient candidiasis of the palate, which responds to nystatin mouthwash. Some suppression of the hypothalamic-pituitary-adrenal axis has been demonstrated in children on doses of 8 to 10 inhalations per day, but clinically significant suppression has not be demonstrated in adults whose dose is less than 20 inhalations daily. Patients already on prednisone therapy can often have their prednisone dose reduced or discontinued by making use of beclomethasone. However, patients on prednisone for over a month at daily doses in excess of 15 mg. are likely to have some degree of adrenal suppression. Thus, when beclomethasone is begun for the purpose of replacing prednisone therapy, the prednisone has to be tapered slowly over many weeks to avoid precipitating adrenal insufficiency (see Chapter 101). Oral prednisone therapy for prophylaxis is reserved for the most refractory and severe cases.

Although viral upper respiratory infections are frequent precipitants of attacks, bacterial infections are not. The presence of heavy sputum production has often been mistakenly attributed to infection, when it was actually a manifestation of the asthma itself (see Chapter 37). However, in cases where bacterial infection is documented by sputum Gram stain, prompt treatment with appropriate antibiotics is essential (see Chapter 43).

Besides the total eosinophil count, other means of *monitoring* therapy and disease activity include assessment of symptoms and signs, and determination of expiratory flow rates. Dyspnea and wheezing are obvious manifestations of active disease. Sternocleidomastoid retraction and pulsus paradoxus are important signs of very severe disease, correlating with an FEV_1 or less than 1.0 liter per second. Symptoms are not a sensitive measure of disease activity. As symptoms resolve, the FEV_1 may be only 60 to 70 per cent of normal. By the time wheezes and prolongation of the expiratory phase have disappeared, the FEV_1 has almost returned to normal; however, at this point, the maximum expiratory flow rate is still only 60 per cent of baseline values. It is felt that this residual evidence of bronchospasm is due to continued bronchoconstriction of small airways, and that failure to continue a full therapeutic program for a week or two after symptoms have resolved is responsible for the high rate of relapses that is often noted after acute flares.

PATIENT EDUCATION

Patients need to be made partners in management of their asthma, because good compliance and proper use of medication can minimize the severity and frequency of asthmatic attacks. They should be instructed in how to adjust their medication program at the onset of a flare and how to use it for prophylactic purposes. All too often, hospital admission is required because of improper use of drugs, such as excessive administration of an inhaled sympathomimetic leading to tachyphylaxis. Every patient who is capable of understanding his medications can be given instructions for initial treatment of an attack, along with strong advice to call the physician for help if relief is not obtained within hours; excessive delay in seeking assistance may lead to refractory bronchospasm. A medication booklet which lists prescribing information, side effects, and indications for use, alongside a sample of each agent, can be very helpful to patient and family.

Patients who develop bronchospasm from environmental pollution or pollens should be advised to stay indoors on particularly bad days, limit their physical activity, and make use of air conditioning. Many patients with extrinsic asthma come requesting desensitization. Although a trial of such therapy is reasonable if episodes are frequent and a single allergen is identified, it is important that the patient be made aware of the other available treatment modalities, for they are more likely to control symptoms. Patients on steroids deserve an extra measure of education and instruction (see Chapter 101) to prevent adrenal insufficiency and cushingoid side effects. Of particular importance to the success of an asthma program is careful review with the patient of his medications' side effects. Often, patients stop the wrong medication or cease therapy because they were not prepared for some of the adverse drug effects common to antiasthmatic agents.

THERAPEUTIC RECOMMENDATIONS

Prophylaxis

- Identify and advise avoidance of any known allergens and environmental irritants.
- If a single allergen is identified in a patient with severe extrinsic asthma, it is reasonable to initiate a trial of desensitization, though efficacy has not been proven conclusively.
- Maintenance therapy can be accomplished by use of an oral bronchodilator such as aminophylline (200 mg. four times daily) or terbutaline (5 mg. three times each day); dose can be adjusted downward to minimize side effects.
- If an oral bronchodilator is ineffective for prophylaxis, a 4-week trial of the inhaled corticosteroid beclomethasone should be considered. Average dose is 1 to 2 inhalations (50 to 100 mcg.) four times daily; total daily dose should not exceed 10 to 15 inhalations, because of risk of adrenal suppression at higher doses.
- Children and those with exercise-induced asthma can be given a trial of cromolyn before use of beclomethasone; an adequate trial is 4 weeks, inhaling 1 capsule four times daily.
- Only if all else fails and the patient is severely incapacitated should prednisone be resorted to for prophylaxis. An alternate day schedule of prednisone will often suffice for prophylaxis. Only the minimum dose necessary to control the disease should be prescribed; doses in the range of 10 to 15 mg. every other day are frequently adequate.
- If the patient is well controlled on oral steroids, but beclomethasone has never been tried, begin beclomethasone therapy as described above and start tapering the prednisone 1 week after initiating beclomethasone. Exert caution in tapering if the patient

has been on daily systemic steroids for over a month (see Chapter 101).

Acute Asthmatic Attacks

- If attacks are mild and infrequent, intermittent use of an inhaled sympathomimetic agent may suffice. Dose of isoproterenol in the commercially available inhaler is 1 to 2 inhalations of the 1:400 solution, repeated up to a maximum of 5 times per 24 hours. Metaproterenol in inhalation form is an alternative to isoproterenol and prescribed as 2 inhalations no more often than every 3 to 4 hours; total dosage should not exceed 12 inhalations. Only very reliable patients should be entrusted with sympathomimetic inhalers, because the risk of tachypylaxis is considerable.
- If attacks are more severe or more frequent, begin a theophylline preparation, e.g., aminophylline 200 mg. four times daily or a beta$_2$ sympathomimetic, e.g., terbutaline 5 mg. three times daily (metaproterenol 10 mg. three times daily is an acceptable alternative to terbutaline). If side effects from an agent of one class are intolerable, one can reduce dose by half and *add* to the program an agent from the other class of bronchodilators at half dose. If bronchodilation is inadequate, use full doses of both agents, rather than extreme doses of a single drug.
- For intense acute attacks, instruct the patient to come directly to the office or hospital and administer epinephrine 1:1000, 0.3 cc. subcutaneously; the dose should be repeated in 20 minutes if response has been inadequate. Two or three repeat doses may be needed to terminate an attack. An alternative to epinephrine is terbutaline 0.25 cc. subcutaneously. Hospital admission for intravenous aminophylline is indicated for patients who have not responded. If response is obtained, initiate full doses or oral bronchodilators.
- When symptoms are difficult to control in the patient on aminophylline or another theophylline preparation, obtain a serum theophylline level and increase dose to obtain a serum level in the therapeutic range of 10 to 20 mcg. per ml.
- Attacks not controlled by the above measures require hospital admission for intravenous bronchodilator therapy and systemic corticosteroids.
- Avoid use of antianxiety agents, sedatives and combination preparations that contain them. In general, avoid use of all fixed-combination preparations.
- Advise the patient to keep well hydrated.

- Once a severe attack has been brought under control, continue the full regimen for at least a week to 10 days after symptoms have resolved; then taper the program to a maintenance regimen.

INDICATIONS FOR ADMISSION

1. Patient cannot speak a full sentence over the telephone.
2. Sternocleidomastoid retraction or pulsus paradoxus is noted on physical examination.
3. FEV$_1$ is less than 1.0 liter per second.
4. Attack does not respond to subcutaneous epinephrine and oral bronchodilators.
5. Patient has a cardiac disorder with potential for serious dysrhythmias.
6. Patient is unreliable or home environment inadequate.

ANNOTATED BIBLIOGRAPHY

Bernstein, I.L., Johnson, C.L. and Tse, C.S.: Therapy with cromolyn sodium. Ann. Intern. Med., *89*:228, 1978. *(Thorough review of the use of this agent.)*

Brooks, S.M., Werk, E.E., Ackerman, S.J., *et al.*: Adverse effects of phenobarbital on corticosteroid metabolism in patients with bronchial asthma. N. Engl. J. Med., *286*:1125, 1972. *(Phenobarbital results in more rapid steroid metabolism and diminished effectiveness. Barbiturates should be prescribed with care to asthmatics on steroids.)*

Corrao, W.M., Braman, S.S., and Irwin, R.S.: Chronic cough as the sole presenting manifestation of bronchial asthma. N. Engl. J. Med., *300*:633, 1979. *(A description of a variant form of asthma in which cough was the only presenting symptom.)*

Davies G., Thomas P., Broder, I., *et al.*: Steroid-dependent asthma treated with inhaled beclomethasone dipropionate. Ann. Intern. Med., *86*:549, 1977. *(A 3-month double-blind study extended into a 9 to 11 month follow-up demonstrating efficacy of chronic use of beclomethasone and lack of endocrine suppression.)*

Horn, B.R., Robin, E.D., Theodore, J., *et al.*: Total eosinophil counts in the management of bronchial asthma. N. Engl. J. Med., *292*:1152, 1975. *(Total cosinophil count correlates with disease activity, is useful for regulating steroid therapy and helps in early detection of exacerbations.)*

Lochey, R.F., Rucknagel, D.L., and Vansclow, N.A.: Familial occurrence of asthma, nasal polyps and aspirin intolerance. Ann. Intern. Med., *78*:57, 1973. *(Describes this important triad and documents familial occurrence.)*

McFadden, E.R.: Exertional dyspnea and cough as preludes to acute attacks of bronchial asthma. N. Engl. J. Med., *292*:555, 1975. *(Presents evidence of intermittent episodes of cough and breathlessness that represent variants of asthmatic attacks.)*

————, Kiser, R., and DeGroot, W.J.: Acute bronchial asthma: Relations between clinical and physiologic manifestations. N. Engl. J. Med., *288*: 221, 1973. *(Significant airway obstruction remains even after resolution of symptoms and signs. This residual bronchospasm may serve as the basis for repeated flares if therapy is discontinued too soon.)*

Oral theophylline drugs. Medical Letter, *17*:9, 1975. *(Warns against use of fixed-dosage combination agents containing ephedrine.)*

Piafsky, K.M., and Ogilvie, R.I.: Dosage of theophylline in bronchial asthma. N. Engl. J. Med., *292*:1218, 1975. *(Excellent review of theophylline therapy.)*

Salem, H., and Jackson, R.H.: Oral theophylline preparations: A review of their clinical efficacy in treatment of bronchial asthma. Ann. Allergy, *32*:189, 1974. *(Reviews data demonstrating that chronic theophylline use prevents attacks of asthma.)*

Udfe, J.D., Tashkin, D.P., Calvarese, B., et al.: Bronchodilator effects of terbutaline and aminophylline alone and in combination in asthmatic patients. N. Engl. J. Med., *298*:363, 1978. *(Presents evidence that low doses of each agent provide bronchodilatation comparable to high-dose single-drug therapy, but with fewer side effects. Also, high doses of both drugs are effective in cases not well controlled by either drug alone.)*

Westerman, D.E., Benatar, S.R., Potgieter, P.D., and Ferguson, A.D.: Identification of the high-risk asthmatic patient. Am. J. Med., *66*:565, 1979. *(A study of 39 patients who required intubation for status asthmaticus revealed that long delay before seeking therapy, incomplete assessment of acute attacks, underuse of corticosteroids prior to admission and overuse of sedation were common in this group. Patients with labile patterns of bronchospasm or steady deterioration were at high risk of death.)*

46
Management of the Common Cold
HARVEY B. SIMON, M.D.

Upper respiratory tract infections are among the most frequent reasons for office visits, though the physician sees only a small fraction of patients with such problems, because most treat their symptoms at home with over-the-counter remedies or simply wait for the illness to pass by itself. Upper respiratory infections are the leading cause of absenteeism, accounting for an average of almost 7 days lost from work per person per year. Although a viral etiology accounts for the overwhelming proportion of cases, the physician must be alert for specifically treatable bacterial processes. In addition, familiarity with agents available for symptomatic relief is necessary because patients turn to their physicians when home remedies fail to help.

PATHOPHYSIOLOGY AND CLINICAL PRESENTATION

The upper respiratory tract is composed of two distinct types of epithelial surfaces. The oropharynx and nasopharynx are lined by a stratified squamous epithelium, and are normally teeming with a varied microbial flora. In addition, many potentially pathogenic bacteria can temporarily reside on these epithelial surfaces as "colonizers" without causing true infection. With a few exceptions, such as herpes simplex and E.B. virus, viruses are not usually long-term members of the normal flora of the respiratory tract.

Numerous host defense mechanisms protect the upper airway from infection. Mechanical defenses tend to prevent penetration of organisms from the nasopharynx and oral cavity into more vulnerable areas. These defenses include the cough, gag and sneeze reflexes, viscous mucous secretions which entrap particulate material, and ciliary action which propels such particles outward. In addition, local immunologic defenses attempt to deal with organisms which have breached the mechanical barriers. These defenses include lymphoid tissue, secretory IgA antibodies in respiratory secretions, and a rich vasculature capable of rapidly delivering phagocytic leukocytes.

Numerous viral agents including rhinoviruses, respiratory syncytial virus, adenoviruses, influenza viruses, and parainfluenza viruses can cause an identical clinical picture. Typical symptoms include coryza, pharyngitis, laryngitis, headache, malaise and fever, in various combinations. Ear and sinus discomfort is often present as well, but these symptoms are caused by mucosal edema which impairs drainage rather than by acute viral infection of these regions (see Chapters 208 and 209). Whether known as the common cold, nasopharyngitis, or the "URI," these problems generally resolve spontaneously.

Incubation periods for viral URIs range from 1 to 5 days; virus shedding lasts up to 2 weeks. Common viral upper respiratory infections rarely progress to pneumonia; most colds resolve spontaneously within 1 week, though symptoms may linger for several weeks.

PRINCIPLES OF MANAGEMENT

Once the virus has been contracted, there is no means of preventing cold symptoms. The enthusiasm that surrounded use of high-dose ascorbic acid for prophylaxis has waned as controlled studies have failed to demonstrate its efficacy. Therapeutic efforts are directed toward relieving nasal congestion, headache, and grippelike symptoms.

Millions of dollars are spent annually on over-the-counter cold remedies. Most contain a combination of ingredients, including antihistamines, sympathomimetic amines and analgesics. Some even contain more than one antihistamine or sympathomimetic. Antitussives, caffeine, vitamin C, belladonna alkaloids and expectorants are common additives as well. Antacids, laxatives, quinine, and papaverine are occasionally found.

Alpha-adrenergic agents are the most commonly used decongestants. They work by causing generalized vasoconstriction and thus reduce formation of secretions. Since they produce systemic vasoconstriction, sympathomimetics may raise blood pressure when used in doses sufficient to alleviate nasal congestion. There is no oral adrenergic agent which provides selective local vasoconstriction; nasal sprays are more effective for this purpose, but may be associated with rebound congestion after the drug effect subsides, leading to abuse of the spray. According to most authorities, nasal sprays are good for short-term therapy, while oral preparations are better when use is to continue longer than 10 days, since chronic spray applications interfere with ciliary action and irrate and dry the nasal mucosa, producing swelling.

Analgesics are quite useful for relief of the headache, fever and achiness that often accompany a cold. Aspirin and acetaminophen have similar analgesic and antipyretic effects and are key ingredients in the combination cold remedies. Salicylate derivates such as salicylamide are sometimes used, though they are much less effective than aspirin. Plain aspirin is much cheaper than any combination of agents, and is preferred.

Expectorants are included in many preparations in the belief that they stimulate the flow of mucus. There is no evidence to support this view, even though these agents are widely prescribed and requested by patients. Warm steam from a vaporizer or cold mist from a humidifier are much more effective in loosening secretions. *Cough suppressants*, including narcotics such as codeine, are effective and useful symptomatically, especially in allowing the patient to sleep uninterrupted by cough. These agents are commonly available in combination with expectorants, though they may be prescribed alone thereby saving the patient money.

Antihistamines have weak, atropine-type effects and may help to reduce secretions when used in therapeutic doses. Sleepiness is the major side effect. Combining multiple antihistamines in low amounts has no benefit over using one agent in a therapeutic dose.

Atropine, laxatives, caffeine and antacids are present in subtherapeutic doses in combination preparations; they have little impact on symptoms and only increase costs. The vitamin C included has not been shown to have any effect, even when given in gram doses.

THERAPEUTIC RECOMMENDATIONS

Relief from the symptoms of a cold is best provided by rest, fluids, aspirin and a vaporizer. A cough suppressant before bed (*e.g.*, 15 mg. codeine

sulfate) a nasal decongestant spray (*e.g.*, phenylephrine; see Chapter 212) may aid in symptomatic management and are superior to expensive combination agents which often contain irrational mixtures or subtherapeutic doses of active ingredients. Vitamin C has no proven role in prevention or alleviation of symptoms.

ANNOTATED BIBLIOGRAPHY

Coulehan, J.L., Eberhard, S., Kapner, L., *et al.*: Vitamin C and acute illness in Navajo schoolchildren N. Engl. J. Med., *295*:973, 1976. *(A double-blind trial of vitamin C and placebo in 868 schoolchildren. Vitamin C did not prove to be effective as either a prophylactic or a therapeutic agent.)*

Oral cold remedies. Medical Letter, *17*:89, 1975. *(Critiques over-the-counter oral cold remedies and warns against their high cost, irrational combination of agents, and frequent use of subtherapeutic doses of active ingredients.)*

47
Management of Tuberculosis
HARVEY B. SIMON, M.D.

Tuberculosis may be encountered by the primary care physician as either of two very different clinical problems. By far the more common presentation is the patient with a positive tuberculin skin test but no active infection; up to 7 per cent of the population in the United States today may be in this category. In contrast, only about 30,000 new cases of active tuberculosis are reported in the United States each year. One result of the declining incidence of tuberculosis is that its diagnosis and treatment have shifted from the sanatorium and the specialist to the community and the primary physician. If tuberculosis is less common today, it is still subtle due to a tremendous variety of clinical pictures. In a sense, the diagnosis of tuberculosis may actually be more difficult today because most physicians have had limited clinical experience with the disease, and are less likely to suspect its presence. In fact, it has been shown that diagnosis is delayed in many patients with tuberculosis admitted to university hospitals; some cases are recognized only at autopsy. In addition, the

management of tuberculosis has undergone such tremendous changes in the chemotherapy era that studies have demonstrated suboptimal management by many general physicians in the United States. Clearly, diagnosis and treatment of tuberculosis remain a major challenge for the primary physician.

EPIDEMIOLOGY

With the elimination of bovine tuberculosis in the United States, virtually all cases are acquired through person-to-person aerosol transmission. People with active pulmonary infection shed infected droplets, which are then airborne into the environment. Because most infectious patients discharge relatively few organisms, casual contacts have a low risk of infection, and most secondary cases occur in household members, schoolmates or other close contacts of the index case. Tuberculosis is more common in population groups where there is crowding and poverty (see Chapter 34). At present, only 10 per cent of all "new" tuberculosis diagnosed in this country results from primary infection, the vast majority representing reactivation of latent endogenous infections.

Reactivation of tuberculosis occurs in about 5 per cent of all infected individuals, the remainder having positive skin tests but no clinical illness. Reactivation is most likely to occur within the first few years of the initial infection or at times of lowered host resistance, such as adolescence or the postpartum period. However, reactivation can occur many decades after initial infection and, in fact, is now most common in the elderly. As many as one-fifth of patients with reactivated disease have histories of inadequately treated clinical tuberculosis. At times, a discrete insult to host defenses such as steroid therapy, alcoholism, malnutrition, neoplastic disease or gastrectomy can be implicated, but more often it is impossible to identify the reason for reactivation.

Atypical mycobacterial infections are probably acquired from inhalation or ingestion of organisms from sources in nature; there is no evidence for person-to-person transmission.

CLINICAL PRESENTATION AND COURSE

Primary infection. More than 90 per cent of patients are entirely asymptomatic at the time of primary infection and can be identified only through conversion of the tuberculin skin test from negative to positive. The majority of these patients have normal chest x-rays, but fibrocalcific stigmata of infection are radiographically demonstrable in others. In the past, primary infection occurred almost entirely in childhood, but as the incidence of tuberculosis has declined, primary tuberculosis is also seen in adults.

Among symptomatic patients, four broad syndromes can be identified. Most common is an *atypical pneumonia* picture, with fever and nonproductive cough. Chest x-rays may show unilateral lower lobe patchy parenchymal infiltrates and/or paratracheal or hilar adenopathy. Although such patients should receive full antituberculous chemotherapy when diagnosed, the disease usually resolves, even without treatment. Another syndrome is *tuberculous pleurisy* and effusion. These patients have fever, cough, pleuritic chest pain, and sometimes dyspnea. Chest x-rays reveal unilateral pleural effusions often without identifiable parenchymal lesions. The tuberculin test is almost always strongly positive. Diagnosis depends on examination and culture of the pleural fluid or on percutaneous needle biopsy of the pleura since sputum cultures are positive in only 30 per cent of such cases. Another syndrome is *direct progression* from primary disease to upper lobe involvement. Least common is early *systemic dissemination,* which used to be seen in children. In addition to these major manifestations, patients with primary tuberculosis may present with hypersensitivity reactions such as erythema nodosum.

Reactivation (postprimary) tuberculosis. This is the most common clinical form of tuberculosis and is seen most often in the elderly or debilitated patient. Symptoms usually begin insidiously and progress over a period of many weeks or months prior to diagnosis. Constitutional symptoms are often prominent, including anorexia, weight loss and night sweats. Most patients have low-grade fever, but higher temperatures and even chills may be seen occasionally when the disease progresses more rapidly. In addition, most patients present with pulmonary symptoms including cough and sputum production. Dyspnea is relatively uncommon in the absence of underlying chronic lung disease. A frequent complaint is hemoptysis, often in the form of bright red streaks of blood caused by bronchial irritation. Although physical examination is usually nondiagnostic, chest x-rays are highly suggestive of the diagnosis. Typical features include infiltration in the posterior apical pulmonary segments which may be unilateral or bilateral, and which progresses to frank cavitation. Apical lordotic views and chest tomography may be helpful in documenting cavitary disease. Occasionally, postprimary tuberculosis may involve the lower lung fields, and in rare instances the chest x-ray may appear normal. The tuberculin skin test is positive in about 80 per cent of patients with reactivation tuberculosis; patients with advanced disease are often malnourished and anergic.

Extrapulmonary tuberculosis. Approximately 10 per cent of all newly recognized cases of tuberculosis in the United States are extrapulmonary. While the frequency of pulmonary tuberculosis is declining, the incidence of extrapulmonary disease is remaining relatively constant. Although the clinical features of extrapulmonary tuberculosis vary widely, certain generalizations are possible. Past history is not a reliable guide to the diagnosis of extrapulmonary tuberculosis. Only 25 per cent of patients have a past history of tuberculosis; of these, virtually all have been inadequately treated. There is typically a long latent period between the first episode of infection and the extrapulmonary presentation. Approximately 50 per cent of patients with extrapulmonary tuberculosis have entirely normal chest x-rays; most of the others have stigmata of old inactive pulmonary disease, while a minority have coexisting active pulmonary infection. Although extrapulmonary disease can involve all organ systems, either singly or in various combinations, the most commonly affected areas are the genitourinary tract, the musculoskeletal system and the lymph nodes.

The most common type of extrapulmonary tuberculosis is infection of an individual organ system. Such a patient is most often afebrile and can be entirely free of constitutional complaints. Their illness typically pursues a very indolent course characterized by local organ dysfunction and eventual destruction rather than by progressive general decline. In fact, the differential diagnosis in these individuals more often suggests neoplastic disease than infection. The tuberculin skin test is almost always positive. Clinical syndromes in this category include genitourinary tuberculosis, tuberculous arthritis and osteomyelitis, tuberculous lymphadenitis and many others.

Clinical infection with *atypical mycobacteria* is not seen very often in primary care practice. Representative syndromes due to these organisms include cervical adenitis in children (scrofula), pulmonary infection, and cutaneous disease (swimming pool granuloma). Disseminated disease occasionally takes place in immunosuppressed individuals.

DIAGNOSIS

The tuberculin *skin test* is the most sensitive test for diagnosis of infection with *M. tuberculosis* (see Chapter 34); it is far more sensitive than the chest x-ray. A positive tuberculin test does not by itself prove there is active disease, but does indicate that infection has occurred. Negative tuberculin reactions have been documented in up to 20 per cent of patients with tuberculosis, particularly those individuals with overwhelming or advanced disease, malnutrition and debility. Many of these individuals are anergic, so that simultaneous skin testing with *Candida* or streptokinase-streptodornase antigens can be useful in demonstrating overall immunologic impairment.

When there is active pulmonary disease, the diagnosis of pulmonary tuberculosis can usually be confirmed by examination of the *sputum*. If patients are not able to produce sputum spontaneously, attempts should be made to induce sputum with the aid of hydration, pulmonary physiotherapy, IPPB and mucolytic agents. Bronchoscopy may be necessary for obtaining appropriate specimens. Although cultures are necessary for a positive diagnosis and are more sensitive than smears, sputum specimens should be examined microscopically either by the traditional Ziehl-Neelson (acid-fast) stain, or by the newer Truant fluorescent stain. Sputum or bronchoscopic washings should be examined both directly and after concentration by centrifugation and digestion. Carefully collected individual specimens are preferred to a 24-hour pool of sputum and saliva. Cultures of first morning fasting *gastric aspirates* are also helpful. Because gastric acid is toxic to mycobacteria, the collection bottles should contain a buffer such as sodium bicarbonate. Smears of gastric juice are misleading, because of the potential presence of saprophytic mycobacteria, and should not be performed.

Tissue biopsy is often required for diagnosis of tuberculous pleurisy or extra-pulmonary disease, since sputum and gastric samples are usually negative for organisms in these situations.

PRINCIPLES OF TREATMENT

Prophylaxis in uninfected individuals. In many parts of the world where tuberculosis is common, bacillus Calmette-Guerin (BCG) vaccine is used for the prevention of primary infection. It is intended only for prophylaxis and should not be given to patients with positive skin tests (see Chapter 34). Because the incidence of tuberculosis is relatively low in the U.S., BCG is not routinely recommended in this country. Close contacts of patients with active pulmonary tuberculosis should be considered for isoniazid (INH) therapy, particularly if they are children or adolescents (see Chapter 34).

Prophylaxis in tuberculin converters and those with latent disease. Prevention of active tuberculosis can be achieved with INH. However, the drug is not without toxicity; it can cause hepatocellular damage, particularly in older patients (see Appendix at the end of this chapter). An estimate of the risk of reactivation of tuberculosis needs to be weighed against the chances of drug-induced hepatitis in order to select patients for INH prophylaxis (see Chapter 34). In general, patients whose skin test has converted from negative to positive within the last 2 years should be considered for chemoprophylaxis. Older patients who have recovered from clinical tuberculosis but have never received chemotherapy should be evaluated to exclude active disease; if none is demonstrated, these individuals too may benefit from INH.

Although firm data are lacking, it also seems reasonable to administer INH to immunologically impaired hosts with positive tuberculin skin tests. Finally, it can be argued that all individuals below age 30 should be skin-tested at the time of routine medical evaluations, and that INH be administered to positive reactors (see Chapter 34). In contrast, patients over 35 with a positive skin test and no evidence or history of clinical tuberculosis should be followed and need not be treated, since at this age the risk of INH hepatotoxicity begins to outweigh the benefit of prophylaxis.

Patients with positive skin tests should be evaluated to exclude active infection. One needs to check for cough, fever, sputum production, pleuritic chest pain, lymphadenopathy, pleural effusion, pulmonary consolidation, and enlargement of the liver or spleen. A chest x-ray is essential, and complete blood count, differential, urinalysis and liver function tests (particularly the alkaline phosphatase) may provide clues of active disease (e.g., "sterile" pyuria or isolated alkaline phosphatase elevation). If no active infection is identified, the patient should be reassured, and the potential risks and benefits of INH therapy explained so that the patient can participate in therapeutic decision.

Treatment of patients with active tuberculosis. Antituberculous drugs are the cornerstone of therapy. Since the patient will be non-contagious shortly after starting therapy, most treatment can be administered on an outpatient basis. The chemotherapy of tuberculosis is different from other antimicrobial programs and proceeds according to a unique set of principles:

1. The use of multiple drugs is necessary to prevent the emergence of drug-resistant organisms.
2. Single daily dosages are preferred.
3. Prolonged chemotherapy is necessary. Standard multiple-drug regimens require periods of 18 to 24 months. With combinations of newer agents, shorter regimens of 6 to 9 months have been found equally effective.
4. No matter what regimen is chosen, it is important to follow patients closely to insure compliance and to monitor for drug efficacy and toxicity. The currently available antituberculous regimens are so effective that prolonged surveillance is not necessary after completion of a full course of therapy.
5. Because chemotherapy will control the organisms, surgery is reserved for the treatment of

complications such as restrictive pericardial scarring.
6. Elaborate programs of rest and diet have no place in modern treatment of tuberculosis.

Most patients with clinically active pulmonary tuberculosis should be hospitalized for the initial phases of therapy. As little as 2 weeks of multidrug therapy will greatly decrease the infectiousness of these patients, although a few mycobacteria may still be present on sputum smears or cultures. Hence, short-term admission to a general hospital is preferred, with early home care for patients who are reliable and clinically stable. Patients with extrapulmonary tuberculosis are much less infectious and can sometimes be managed entirely as outpatients.

CASE REPORTING AND PATIENT EDUCATION

All cases of tuberculosis should be reported promptly to public health authorities, so that contacts can be investigated and appropriate control measures instituted. However, it must be remembered that, particularly in elderly patients, the diagnosis of tuberculosis still carries social stigma and dire prognostic implications. Reassurance and education are therefore of great importance. It should be stressed that tuberculosis occurs in all social and economic classes, that modern chemotherapy is truly curative, that prolonged periods of hospitalization and isolation are no longer necessary.

Patients who are candidates for INH prophylaxis should understand the risks and benefits of INH therapy. If INH therapy is recommended and accepted, the patient should be instructed to discontinue the medication and report to the physician if adverse effects are noted, including skin rash, fever, fatigue, anorexia, abdominal distress, jaundice or peripheral neuropathic symptoms. The importance of full compliance with the drug regimen, be it for prophylaxis or treatment of active disease, must be stressed.

THERAPEUTIC RECOMMENDATIONS
Prophylaxis

• In the United States, BCG prophylaxis is not recommended routinely for prevention of infection, because the incidence of the disease is low. Certain high-risk groups such as children born to tuberculous mothers may merit BCG (see Chapter 34).

- Recent conversion of a tuberculin skin test to positive is an indication for INH chemoprophylaxis. Average dose is 300 mg. per day for one year. (Pyridoxine, 50 mg. per day, is given with INH to prevent peripheral neuropathy.) Positive reactors who are under age 30 should also be considered for INH prophylaxis, as should close contacts of patients with active pulmonary disease, particularly if the exposed individual is a child or adolescent. In addition, older patients who have recovered from clinical tuberculosis but have never received chemotherapy should be considered for INH therapy if they have no evidence of active disease.
- The decision to use INH for prophylaxis involves weighing the risk of drug-induced hepatotoxicity (see Appendix at the end of this chapter) with the benefit of preventing active disease. The older the patient, the greater the risk of hepatitis. Risk begins to dominate beyond age 35.

Active Disease

- Patients with active disease require combination chemotherapy. Those with mild to moderate pulmonary or extrapulmonary disease can be treated with a two-drug regimen; INH plus ethambutol for 18 to 24 months is generally preferred in these circumstances (see Appendix). Patients with far advanced cavitary disease of the lung, meningitis, pericarditis, or miliary disease require triple-drug therapy, such as INH, ethambutol and streptomycin. Because of its superior tissue penetration, rifampin may be substituted for streptomycin in the triple-drug therapy of patients with tuberculous meningitis.

1. The usual dose of INH is 5 mg. per kg. body weight, which averages 300 mg. per day for the adult. For initial therapy of life-threatening disease, doses of 10-15 mg. per kg. per day may be used. Ethambutol is available only in an oral preparation. Many authorities recommend initial therapy with 25 mg. per kg. body weight per day for the first 6 to 8 weeks of therapy, and then reduced doses of 15 mg. per kg. body weight per day for the remainder of the course. Good results have also been obtained with use of the lower dose throughout therapy. The average dose of rifampin in adults is 600 mg. per day, administered in a single dose. Streptomycin must be giv-

en parenterally. The average adult dose is 1 gm. daily for the first 2 to 8 weeks of therapy, followed by 1 gm. twice a week.

2. Standard chemotherapeutic programs requiring the use of two antituberculosis drugs should be maintained for periods of 18 to 24 months, sometimes following an initial phase of three drugs for 2 to 3 months in the very sick patient.

3. Short-course regimens, using INH, streptomycin and rifampin together for periods of 6 months are a reasonable alternative when an 18- to 24-month regimen is impractical. On this program, relapses do not exceed 2 per cent. Excellent results are also attainable from use of INH and rifampin together for 9 months, accompanied by either streptomycin or ethambutol for the first 2 months of therapy.

4. Intermittent chemotherapy is designed and should be reserved for unreliable outpatients who require supervised administration of drugs. After 3 months of standard daily treatment, these patients can be given 18 months of intermittent high-dose treatment in the format of INH 14 mg. per kg. and streptomycin 27 mg. per kg., each taken twice a week. Streptomycin toxicity, however, can be expected in up to 10 per cent of patients on this program; in such cases, high-dose ethambutol (50 mg. per kg. per dose) can be given instead.

- Hospitalization should be considered in the intial stages of active pulmonary disease to minimize risk of spread. Two weeks of chemotherapy usually suffice to render the patient noninfectious.
- With the exception of *M. kansasii* and *M. marinum,* the majority of atypical mycobacteria are drug-resistant, making therapy difficult. So-called second-line antituberculous agents are sometimes necessary (see Appendix). Consultation with a specialist in mycobacterial disease is indicated.

APPENDIX: ANTITUBERCULOUS CHEMOTHERAPEUTIC AGENTS

Chemotherapeutic agents are separated into "first-line" and "second-line" drugs. The former include INH, ethambutol, rifampin and streptomycin.

Isoniazid (INH). Introduced into clinical use in the early 1950s, INH remains the single most important antituberculous drug. Of importance is the excellent tissue penetration of this small, water-soluble molecule; the distribution of INH includes the central nervous system, tuberculous abscesses and intracellular sites. The major metabolism of INH is by hepatic acetylation. Although metabolites are excreted by the kidneys, it is not necessary to modify INH doses except in advanced renal failure. INH is available both orally and parenterally. The major toxicities of INH include:

1. Neurologic toxicity, ranging from peripheral neuropathy (which can be prevented by administration of 50 mg. of pyridoxine daily) to much less common manifestations, including encephalopathy, seizures, optic neuritis and personality changes.
2. Hypersensitivity reactions including fever, rash and rheumatic syndromes with or without positive antinuclear antibodies.
3. Hepatitis, including serious clinical hepatitis in less than 2 percent, but a transient, clinically insignificant rise in SGOT in 10 to 20 percent. Risk of clinically significant hepatitis increases with age.

The U.S. Public Health Service does not recommend routine SGOT determinations in individuals who are reliable and who are able to comply with directions for reporting symptoms of hepatitis. However, SGOT determinations can be helpful, particularly insofar as they give the physician an opportunity to briefly reinforce instructions and also because the surveillance is very reassuring to most patients. The problem with SGOT determinations is that between 10 and 20 percent of individuals receiving INH can be expected to show mild transient elevations in SGOT which will return to normal even during continued therapy and are of no clinical significance.

Although precise data are lacking, a reasonable approach is to routinely determine the SGOT at monthly intervals for the first 3 months of therapy, since most SGOT abnormalities develop during this period. In symptomatic patients with elevated SGOTs, the drug should be discontinued and liver function tests monitored. In asymptomatic individuals with mild elevations of SGOT (perhaps up to 100 units), the drug can be continued, but the patient should be monitored weekly. If the SGOT fails to return to normal in 3 to 4 weeks, it seems prudent to discontinue the INH. On the other hand, even if a patient is asymptomatic, a single, more substantial elevation of SGOT, perhaps above 200 units, may be grounds to discontinue the agent. Again, it must be

be emphasized that these are "rules of thumb" rather than precise guidelines.

Ethambutol was introduced clinically in the United States in 1967 and represented a major advance in antituberculous chemotherapy. Ethambutol penetrates tissues well, including the central nervous system when the meninges are inflamed. The drug is excreted by the kidneys. Dose modification in renal failure should be based on serum ethambutol levels (available through the manufacturer) and monitored in patients with renal failure who require the drug. The major toxicities of ethambutol include hypersensitivity reactions, such as fever and rash, and optic neuritis, which is dose-related and usually manifested first by a loss of color vision. Less common side effects include neuritis, GI intolerance, headache and hyperuricemia. The cost of ethambutol is moderate, averaging perhaps 90 cents a day.

Rifampin is the newest of the major antituberculous drugs and rivals INH in its efficacy. Rifampin is a large, fat-soluble molecule which achieves excellent tissue penetration, including the central nervous system. The drug is excreted by the liver; modification of dosage is not required in renal failure but may be necessary in hepatic insufficiency. At the present time, only an oral preparation has been approved in the United States. Unlike INH and ethambutol, rifampin is actually a broad-spectrum antimicrobial, acting against some atypical mycobacteria, *M. leprae,* many bacteria (including staphylococci, meningococci, and various gram-negative bacilli), trachoma agent, and some viruses. Patients should be cautioned to expect orange discoloration of urine, sweat, tears and saliva, which is of no clinical significance. Toxicities include hypersensitivity reactions (fever, rash or eosinophilia), hematologic toxicities (thrombocytopenia, leukopenia and hemolytic anemia), and a high incidence of hepatitis, including elevated SGOTs in up to 10 per cent. Drug interactions occur; rifampin antagonizes the effect of warfarin, oral contraceptives and methadone. Rifampin should never be used in intermittent therapy because toxic reactions (including hemolytic anemia, thrombocytopenia and hepatic failure) occur frequently. Rifampin is an expensive drug.

Although rifampin is an extremely effective antituberculous drug, we prefer to reserve the agent for patients who cannot tolerate other first-line drugs, who are treatment failures, or who have overwhelming disease. Reasons for reserving this drug include its expense and its potential for hepatotoxicity, which can be particularly confusing in a patient simultaneously receiving INH. Finally, it is often helpful to have an excellent drug such as rifampin in reserve should problems develop during the course of treatment. However, many authorities recommend rifampin in the initial treatment of tuberculosis.

Streptomycin, the first effective antituberculous drug, remains useful. Like other aminoglycosides, streptomycin has only a fair tissue distribution, being inactive at an alkaline pH in an anaerobic milieu, and penetrating the cerebrospinal fluid very poorly. Streptomycin is excreted by the kidneys, and dosage should be reduced in patients with renal failure. Major toxicities include hypersensitivity reactions and eighth nerve toxicity, especially to the vestibular division, resulting in vertigo. The cost of streptomycin is moderate. The drug is active against a variety of organisms in addition to *M. tuberculosis,* although many gram-negative bacilli have now become resistant due to widespread use over many years.

The "second-line" antituberculous drugs tend to be both less effective and more toxic than the standard agents, but occasionally are of critical importance in patients with drug-resistant tuberculosis or atypical mycobacterial infection, and in those who cannot tolerate the standard therapies. Four agents are administered orally, including para-aminosalicylic acid (PAS), pyrazinamide, ethionamide, and cycloserine. For many years, PAS was considered a first-line drug, but its relatively weak tuberculostatic action and very high incidence of gastrointestinal intolerance has now relegated it to a secondary role. Three other drugs available parenterally—kanamycin, viomycin and capreomycin—are pharmacologically similar to streptomycin.

ANNOTATED BIBLIOGRAPHY

Barlow, P.B., Black, M., Brummer, D.L., *et al.*: Preventive therapy of tuberculous infection. Morbidity and Mortality Weekly Report, *24*:71, 1975. *(The USPHS recommendations for the use of isoniazid in the "chemopropylaxis" of tuberculosis.)*

British Thoracic and Tuberculosis Association: Short-course chemotherapy in pulmonary tuberculosis: A controlled trial. Lancet, *2*:1102, 1976. *(A controlled study of 696 patients with culture-positive pulmonary tuberculosis. The authors recommend a regimen of INH and rifampin for 9 months supplemented by ethambutol for the first 2 months for treatment of pulmonary tuberculosis in Britain.)*

Daniel, T.M., Mahmoud, A.A.F., and Warren, K.S.: Algorithms in the diagnosis and management of exotic diseases. J. Infect. Dis., *134*:417, 1976. *(Despite the obvious limitations of the algorithmic approach, this paper presents an accurate, practical and concise overview of clinical tuberculosis and its management. It should be most helpful to physicians who see little tuberculosis and hence have come to regard it as an "exotic" disease.)*

East African/British Medical Research Councils: Controlled clinical trial of four short-course (6-month) regimens of chemotherapy for treatment of pulmonary tuberculosis. Lancet, *2*:237, 1974. *(An example of the British studies of short course chemotherapy which have been conducted in Africa and also in the Orient. This study demonstrated excellent results with the use of INH, streptomycin and rifampin for 6 months. Only 3 per cent of 152 patients treated with this regim relapsed. The cost effectiveness of this regimen has not been studied in the United States.)*

Hudson, L.D., and Sbarbaro, J.A.: Twice weekly tuberculosis chemotherapy. JAMA, *223*:139, 1973. *(A study of 101 manifestly unreliable outpatients with active tuberculosis which demonstrates the usefulness of intermittent chemotherapy in this setting.)*

Johnston, R,F., and Wildrick, K.H.: "State of the art" review. The impact of chemotherapy on the care of patients with tuberculosis. Am. Rev. Resp. Dis., *109*:636, 1974. *(A useful overview of the management of tuberculosis, which includes a discussion of skin testing, epidemiology and BCG as well as chemotherapy.)*

Sharbaro, J.A.: Tuberculosis: The new challenge to the practicing physician. Chest, *68* (Suppl.):436, 1975. *(A very nice overview of tuberculosis today, with an emphasis on epidemiology.)*

Stead, W.W.: Pathogenesis of the sporadic case of tuberculosis. N. Engl. J. Med., *277*:1008, 1967. *(A lucid and important overview of the "unitary concept" of the pathogenesis of tuberculosis. This excellent paper clarifies relationship between primary infection, inactive disease, and reactivation tuberculosis.)*

———., Kerby, G.R., Schlueter, D.P., and Jordahl, C.W.: The clinical spectrum of primary tuberculosis in adults. Ann. Intern. Med., *68*:731, 1968.

(A clinical study of 27 adults with primary tuberculosis, which includes an excellent summary of the wide spectrum of events that may occur following initial infection by M. tuberculosis.*)*

Wolinsky, E.: Nontuberculosis mycobacteria and associated diseases. Am. Rev. Resp. Dis., *119*:107,

1979. *(A comprehensive and authoritative review of the "atypical mycobacteria". Although this paper is very long and contains more bacteriologic detail than will interest the primary care practitioner, it is nicely subdivided so that clinically useful information is readily accessible; 592 ref.)*

48

Management of Sarcoidosis
HARVEY B. SIMON, M.D.

Sarcoidosis is a disease of unknown etiology characterized by the presence of noncaseating granulomas, often in multiple organs. The diagnosis can be based on clinical findings but often requires histologic confirmation. Sarcoidosis is ten times more prevalent in blacks than in whites. People of Scandinavian descent also have a high incidence of the disease. The incidence in females is double that in males. Although a large percentage of patients with sarcoid are asymptomatic, diverse and protean clinical syndromes may be produced, presenting diagnostic and therapeutic challenges to the primary physician. Once diagnosis is established, the major management decision involves use of corticosteroids. The primary physician needs to know the most effective, least morbid manner of establishing the diagnosis and the indications for steroids therapy.

PATHOPHYSIOLOGY, CLINICAL PRESENTATION AND DIAGNOSIS

The cause of sarcoidosis is unknown. A variety of infectious and exogenous agents have been suggested as inciting factors, but whether one or several agents are involved remains conjectural. It is possible that the granulomas and inflammatory reactions of sarcoidosis are due to an unusual immunologic response to a provocative agent in susceptible hosts.

Characteristic immunologic abnormalities occur, but it is uncertain whether they are primary or secondary. The defects in immunologic regulation involve depressed T-cell function and elevated levels of immunoglobulin, suggesting B-cell hyperactivity. Cutaneous anergy (reflecting impaired delayed hypersensitivity) and normal or elevated antibody levels are the usual immunologic findings.

Clinical manifestations of sarcoidosis reflect the sites of granulomatous inflammation. The most common presentation, especially in young adults, is bilateral hilar adenopathy, which occurs in 50 per cent and is often detected on routine chest x-ray. About 25 per cent present with bilateral hilar adenopathy and pulmonary infilrates, and 15 per cent with infiltrates alone. Right paratracheal adenopathy is seen in 50 per cent of patients with hilar disease. Disease in the hilium is not associated with invasion or compression of bronchi or nodal calcification. Erythema nodosum or uveitis (manifested by red, watery eyes) may accompany hilar adenopathy.

Some patients complain of cough, shortness of breath, wheezing, or chest discomfort as well as constitutional symptoms of fever, malaise and fatigue. Though pulmonary symptoms are the most frequent, sarcoidosis may present as peripheral adenopathy, hepatomegaly, splenomegaly or uveitis. Other presenting manifestations include fever of unknown origin, granulomatous hepatitis, salivary and lacrimal gland enlargement, arthritis, and skin lesions. Hypercalcemia due to increased sensitivity to vitamin D is reported in 10 to 30 per cent, but it is sustained in only 2 to 3 per cent. Cardiac conduction abnormalities, such as heart block, and neuropathies (including facial palsies) are each seen in about 5 per cent of cases. In addition, there are many case reports of unusual presentations.

Diagnosis of sarcoidosis is a clinical challenge. It is increasingly accepted that asymptomatic, bilateral hilar adenopathy with or without uveitis or erythema nodosum is likely to be due to sarcoidosis. In a retrospective series of 100 patients with bilateral hilar adenopathy, all 30 who were asymptomatic had sarcoid. Moreover, 50 of 52 with bilateral hilar adenopathy and negative physical examinations also had the disease. All eleven patients with neoplasm were symptomatic, and 9 had easily identifiable extrathoracic tumor upon physical examination. Among symptomatic patients, all with erythema nodosum or uveitis had sarcoid. Thus, the patient with bilateral hilar adenopathy who is asymptomatic, has a negative physical examination, or has erythema nodosum or uveitis does not necessarily require a biopsy to confirm the diagnosis of sarcoidosis. Nevertheless, some clinicians prefer to obtain a tissue diagnosis in all cases of sarcoidosis, including those with asymptomatic bilateral hilar adenopathy.

Decision to biopsy must be made viewing the potential for discovering treatable conditions and balance this probability against the risks associated with the procedure itself. For the diagnosis of hilar adenopathy, mediastinoscopy is the most direct approach and is usually well tolerated. For the documentation of pulmonary sarcoid, fiberoptic bronchoscopy with transbronchial biopsy is currently in favor. This procedure has a reported sensitivity of 60 to 80 per cent. In addition, bronchoscopy allows direct visualization of the bronchial tree so that it can be helpful in ruling out tumor and obtaining samples of secretions for laboratory study. The major complication of transbronchial lung biopsy is pneumothorax; this is infrequent in experienced hands.

In patients with extrathoracic sarcoidosis, accessible sites for biopsy include skin lesions and enlarged peripheral lymph nodes. Biopsy of conjunctivae, salivary glands and liver may reveal noncaseating granulomas, even when there is no clinical evidence of sarcoid in these tissues. Because of the low morbidity of salivary gland and conjunctival biopsies, these may be particularly useful. It must be remembered that the histologic appearance of sarcoid granulomas is not etiologically specific. Therefore, the other known causes of noncaseating granulomas must be ruled out, including tuberculosis, syphilis, berylliosis, brucellosis, Q fever, biliary cirrhosis, Wegener's granulomatosis, drug reactions and local sarcoidal reactions in nodes draining solid tumors. Hodgkin's disease is particularly difficult to exclude with mediastinoscopy in patients presenting with unilateral or asymmetric hilar adenopathy.

The Kveim test has also been used in the diagnosis of sarcoidosis. The test requires the intracutaneous injection of heat-sterilized human sarcoid tissue, usually spleen. A positive reaction consists of the development of epithelioid granulomas detected on skin biopsy of the injection site at 4 to 6 weeks. The delay period, variability of the material available for injection, and the high incidence of false-positive and false-negative results (due to impure batches of anti-gen) have limited the usefulness of the Kveim reaction.

Other abnormalities which may be present in patients with sarcoidosis include cutaneous anergy, hyperglobulinemia, abnormal liver function tests, and elevated levels of converting enzyme; none of these findings is specific, but together they are supportive of the diagnosis. Similarly, bone films of the hands may reveal changes suggestive of sarcoid.

NATURAL HISTORY

Patients with clear lungs and asymptomatic hilar adenopathy have an excellent prognosis. In one large series of untreated cases, complete remission occurred in over 75 per cent within 5 years. In 50 per cent with untreated pulmonary parenchymal involvement, complete resolution was seen within 2 years. In one third of those in whom clearing did not occur, severe fibrosis developed. Overall, at 5 years, 87 per cent were clinically well, 10 per cent had died of respiratory failure, and 3 per cent were disabled by pulmonary disease.

Hepatic granulomas are present often, but clinically symptomatic hepatitis is much less common. In occasional patients, hepatic failure or portal hypertension occurs. Cranial and peripheral neuropathies tend to occur early in the disease and are usually transient; however, in some patients, significant neurologic damage is seen. Uveitis affects about 15 per cent, comes on acutely and often resolves spontaneously. More worrisome is chronic iridocyclitis; it presents as pain and blurring of vision and may go on to produce cataracts, secondary glaucoma and blindness. As noted above, hypercalcemia persists in about 2 to 3 per cent, though it may be found transiently in up to 30 per cent. Cardiac involvement with granulomata is found in 20 per cent at autopsy, but only 5 per cent have clinically significant disorders of conduction or impulse formation. Rarely, infiltration of the myocardium produces pump failure.

PRINCIPLES OF MANAGEMENT, THERAPEUTIC RECOMMENDATIONS AND MONITORING

The goals in the treatment of sarcoid include relief of symptoms and prevention of significant impairment of organ function. The natural history of sarcoid is variable and hence the indications for therapy are often debatable. It is established that patients who present with asymptomatic bilateral hilar adenoapthy or erythema nodosum usually have a benign course, so that no treatment is indicated in the absence of symptoms.

The principal agents for the therapy of sarcoidosis are *corticosteroids*. Steroids have been shown to reduce the nonspecific inflammatory changes of the disease; but, evidence supporting steroid therapy is largely anecdotal, with few randomized, controlled, prospective studies. Steroid therapy is most effective if instituted early, because once the disease has progressed to fibrosis, the process cannot be reversed. However, there is no evidence that prophylactic therapy is worth the risk of chronic steroid use.

Treatment is usually indicated when there are pulmonary symptoms or significant and progressive deteriorations of pulmonary function tests (especially diffusion capacity) even if the patient is asymptomatic. Most authorities agree that steroids consistently produce subjective improvement in dyspneic patients with early sarcoidosis and reduce pulmonary infiltrates. Lung volumes usually improve, but not necessarily the diffusing capacity. Starting doses average 40 to 60 mg. prednisone per day and are tapered as symptoms lessen. Despite symptomatic improvement, anatomic progression is not uniformly arrested and some healing of granulomas may stimulate fibrosis. Relapses upon cessation of therapy are frequent, necessitating 12 to 24 months of treatment. Management requires close follow-up for the detection of worsening pulmonary function or progressive radiographic changes. The chest x-ray, arterial blood gases, and pulmonary function tests, including diffusion capacity tests, provide important objective measurements.

Adrenal corticosteroids are also indicated for active ocular disease. Every patient with sarcoidosis should have an opthalmologic examination, especially if ocular symptoms develop. Topical steroids may be used, but systemic therapy is usually added. Treatment is also indicated in the presence of significant or progressive involvement of any organ. Onset of hepatitis, facial nerve palsies, meningitis, myocardial conduction defects, hypercalcemia, or persistent constitutional symptoms of fever or fatigue should be treated. Therapy may be initiated with 40 to 60 mg. of prednisone. Improvement should be seen promptly, and tapering should be attempted. Treatment is usually continued for at least 6 to 8 months, but alternate-day steroids may suffice for maintenance. Objective documentation of improvement is essential. At low doses, tapering should be slow and gentle. Chloroquine, 250 to 500 mg. per day, may be useful for cutaneous or mucosal lesions. Antituberculosis therapy has no impact on sarcoidosis.

The course of patients with sarcoid may occasionally be complicated by infections such as tuberculosis, aspergillar fungus balls, candidiasis, and cryptococcosis, attributable in part to the disease and in part to the use of long-term steroid therapy.

PATIENT EDUCATION

The diagnosis of sarcoidosis is far more common than are serious consequences of the disease. The nature of the disease should be carefully explained, with emphasis on its relatively benign, self-limited nature in the asymptomatic patient. Patients who are treated with steroids should be counseled about the side effects and risks inherent in such treatment (see Chapter 101). The need for careful follow-up must be emphasized in both the asymptomatic patient (to detect the development of functional abnormalities) and the patient with symptoms (to document objective benefits of treatment). Patients should be instructed about early signs of important complications, such as red eyes, blurred vision, eye pain, and dyspnea on exertion, so that therapy is not unnecessarily delayed.

ANNOTATED BIBLIOGRAPHY

Israel, H.L., Fouts, D.U., and Begys, R.A.: A controlled trial of prednisone treatment of sarcoidosis. Am. Rev. Respir. Dis., *107*:609, 1973 *(A prospective study of 90 patients. At 3 months, those on prednisone showed improvement in all pulmonary parameters measured, but over the long term there were no significant differences between groups on prednisone and those on placebo.)*

James, D.G.: Kveim revisited, reassessed. N. Engl. J. Med. *292*:859, 1975. *(An editorial arguing that previous reports of the lack of specificity of the test were due to preparation of impure batches of sarcoid splenic suspension and that the test is actually quite specific when proper antigen is used.)*

Johns, C.J., Macgregor, M.I., Zachary, J.B., et al.: Extended experience in the long-term corticosteroid treatment of pulmonary sarcoidosis. Ann. N.Y. Acad. Sci., *278*:722, 1976. *(A series of 192 cases of severe disease treated with prednisone. Clinical improvement resulted from treatment and relapses were frequent when therapy was ter-*

minated. *In cases where relapse occurs and recurs, long-term therapy with 10 to 15 mg. of
prednisone is required, often for years.)*

Koontz, C.H., Joyner, L.R., and Nelson, R.A. Transbronchial lung biopsy via the fiber optic broncho-
sope in sarcoidosis. Ann. Intern. Med., *85:*64,
1976. *(A prospective study of 42 patients with
suspected and later proven sarcoidosis. Test sensitivity was 63 per cent. There was a higher
probability of a positive biopsy in symptomatic
patients.)*

Siltzbach, L.E., James, D.G., Neville, E., *et al.*:
Course and prognosis of sarcoidosis around the
world. Am. J. Med., *57:*847, 1974. *(A terse summary of clinical findings showing no differences
of significance among different races and ethnic
groups.)*

Smellie, H., and Hoyle, C.: Natural history of pulmonary sarcoidosis. Q. J. Med., *116:*539, 1960.
*(Data derived from a 10-year experience prior to
availability of steroids.)*

Winterbauer, R.H., Belic, N., and Moores, K.D.:
Clinical interpretation of bilateral hilar adenopathy. Ann. Intern. Med., *78:*65, 1973. *(A restro-
spective series of 100 cases. Authors argue
asymptomatic patients with bilateral adenopathy only need not undergo biopsy for definitive
diagnosis.)*

49
Techniques for the Cessation of Smoking
NANCY A. RIGOTTI, M.D.

Cigarette smoking is a major health hazard (see
Chapter 32). The evidence is detailed in the 1979
Surgeon General's report, which confirms the conclusions reached in the 1964 report and calls smoking
the "largest preventable cause of death in America
today." About one third of adult Americans (37 per
cent of men and 30 per cent of women) smoke regularly. The overall prevalence of smoking has decreased since 1964, when one half of men and one
third of women smoked. However, smoking rates are
unchanged in adolescent boys and are increasing in
teenage girls, which suggests that the rate of initiation of smoking has not decreased, since smoking
commonly begins during adolescence. The decline in
the prevalence of smoking is largely a consequence of
an increase in the number of smokers who are quitting, and is reflected in the growing prevalence of
exsmokers in the population.

According to surveys, a majority of smokers
would like to quit and have made at least one serious
attempt to do so, but only one fifth of those trying to
stop have been successful. Surprisingly, few smokers
report being specifically advised to stop smoking by
their doctor. Only 20 per cent of smokers in a British
survey recalled being told to quit. Presumably this
occurs because the physician feels that advice is futile or does not know how to help the patient to stop.
Current evidence suggest that physicians *can* be effective in getting patients to stop smoking. The primary physician has a major responsibility to take an
active role in educating and motivating the smoker
and designing a practical program for the patient
who wants to quit. Knowledge of available techniques and their efficacy is essential.

EPIDEMIOLOGY OF QUITTING

Twenty per cent of adult Americans are former
smokers. Much effort has gone into characterizing
these people and the techniques they used to quit in
hopes of finding clues to aid current smokers. Men
are more likely to stop smoking than are women, although the sex difference is less marked among
younger age groups. Lighter smokers have less difficulty quitting than do heavier smokers, while heavier
users of other drugs, notably alcohol and caffeine,
have more trouble successfully abstaining from tobacco. The smoking habits of the spouse appear to be
an important variable in predicting the success of a
smoker's attempt to quit. Those with nonsmoking
spouses are more likely to succeed than those whose
spouses smoke. The smoking behavior of other family
members, friends, and work associates has not been
shown to correlate with successful abstinence. There
is no clear-cut relationship between success at quitting and socioeconomic status or personality variables.

Reasons cited by smokers as to why they quit
have been elucidated in two recent large-scale sur-

veys, one of Americans in 1976 and another of Brit-
ons in 1972. A few common themes emerge. Health
concerns were by far the most common reason for
quitting. However, it appeared that the abstract risks
of lung cancer and heart disease were less important
than were minor smoking-related ailments such as
cough, dyspnea, or sore throat. This suggests that the
health risks of smoking must be personally relevant,
if not physically experienced, to be successful in motivating smokers to quit. It may explain why large-
scale public education programs about the adverse
effects of smoking have been more effective in
changing public opinion than in altering behavior.

The relative importance of other reasons for cessation of smoking varies among studies. Other major
reasons cited include a desire to exert self-control
over one's life, aesthetic objections to the smoking
habit, and fear of setting a bad example for others.
The cost of cigarettes appears to have little influence
among adults in the U.S.A., but is of more consequence in England. Among adolescents, reasons for
quitting are different, with lack of enjoyment being
the most common, followed by health concerns and
cost.

The methods preferred and most often used for
cessation of smoking have been the subject of large
smoking surveys. The vast majority—95 per cent—of
successful exsmokers have quit on their own, without
the aid of organized groups. There is a parallel lack
of interest in formal programs among the estimated
75 per cent of current smokers who profess the desire
to stop. Fewer than one third of them express interest
in organized programs, and only a small minority actually attend such programs when offered. This may
reflect a discrepancy between smokers who vaguely
wish to quit and those seriously intending to do so.
While the percentage of smokers interested in group
approaches is small, proponents of these programs
argue that the absolute number of potential candidates is large—15 million by a recent estimate—and
could be expected to increase if more reliable group
techniques were developed. While individual effort
may be preferred, the likelihood that even the motivated smoker will successfully quit on his own is low.
In one study, only 16 per cent of such individuals had
quit 1 year later.

Smokers who quit abruptly are more likely to be
successful than are those who try to stop gradually
by reducing the number of cigarettes smoked or by
changing to a brand lower in "tar" and nicotine. It
has been suggested that gradual reduction only prolongs the withdrawal syndrome.

OBSTACLES TO QUITTING

It is important to understand why most people
continue to smoke in spite of the weight of evidence
against smoking and the public awareness of its
health hazards. Biological and psychological hypotheses have been proposed. The biological model emphasizes the smoker's physical *addiction to nicotine*
and the unpleasant withdrawal syndrome that results
when smoking is stopped. The validity of this explanation has been clouded by years of controversy over
the existence of the withdrawal syndrome. Evidence
cited in the 1979 Surgeon General's Report strongly
supports the existence of a withdrawal syndrome,
though it remains poorly defined. The physiological
response is characterized by falls in heart rate, blood
pressure, and basal metabolic rate, and a change in
EEG rhythms and REM sleep patterns. Subjective
complaints include irritability, inability to concentrate, drowsiness, fatigue, sleep disturbances, headache, nausea, alteration in bowel habits, increased
appetite, and nicotine craving. Onset of symptoms
occurs soon after cessation of smoking, but the duration is highly variable. Severity of symptoms is dose-
dependent, being worse in heavier smokers. The
physical addiction model is also supported by the observation that regular smokers tend to smoke a cigarette every 30 to 40 minutes, which is roughly the
biological half-life of nicotine in the body, and perhaps the frequency of smoking needed to avert withdrawal.

The psychological explanation is based on social
learning theory. It regards smoking as a *learned behavior* pattern that is continued because it is emotionally rewarding for the smoker; for example, it
may reduce tension or enhance self-image. The
smoker's environment is viewed as being permeated
by cues that trigger the behavior.

Both models of smoking have provided a theoretical basis for techniques of smoking cessation. Proponents of the physical addiction model have emphasized a pharmacologic approach to lessen withdrawal
symptoms. Social learning theory has inspired a variety of behavior modification techniques which attempt to manipulate either the environmental cues
that stimulate smoking or the rewards that sustain it.

INTERVENTION STRATEGIES

The spectrum of strategies available for cessation
of smoking is broad, ranging from individualized

self-help methods to organized group programs, some employing theoretically based, experimentally tested techniques. Both commercial concerns and nonprofit organizations such as the American Cancer Society offer information and programs.

Historically, the first approaches were empirical rather than experimental, often borrowing techniques successful in combatting other bad habits. There was little emphasis on formal evaluation of programs. In the past decade, techniques based on experimentally validated hypotheses have proliferated, developed largely in clinical psychology departments interested in behavior modification. Both nonprofit and proprietary groups are now applying these techniques on a large scale.

The evaluation of smoking intervention techniques is plagued by four problems which cloud results: (1) small study populations; (2) lack of objective validation of self-reported smoking habits; (3) inadequate controls, and (4) inadequate long-term follow-up.

Inadequate follow-up is a particular problem in evaluating the true efficacy of programs, because the relapse rate is high among smokers who quit. A surprisingly common pattern of return to smoking was found among 89 studies analyzed in a 1974 review. Of those smokers who had quit by the completion of a program, regardless of technique used, only 30 per cent remained abstinent 6 months later. The relapse rate slowed after 6 months, with 25 per cent still abstinent 18 months after completing a program. A 1976 review of 200 studies found that most follow-up periods were less than 1 year. In only 5 studies had participants been followed for as long as 4 years. Given the high relapse rate, reliable conclusions can be drawn only from studies in which participants have been followed for at least 1 year after quitting smoking. The data on relapse have also inspired research interest in the development of techniques to prevent the return to smoking.

Pharmacologic methods. Attempts have been made to aid the smoker by relieving the symptoms of nicotine withdrawal. *Lobeline* (Nikoban) is a nonnicotine substitute whose systemic effects are said to mimic nicotine's. Controlled studies have found lobeline to be no better than placebo. Another approach has been to prepare nicotine in a noninhaled and presumably less harmful form. *Nicotine chewing gum* was developed to prevent withdrawal symptoms. A recent British double-blind controlled study demonstrated little advantage of gum over placebo, but did note blood levels of nicotine comparable to those achieved by smoking cigarettes. Nonspecific attempts to minimize withdrawal symptoms with *antianxiety agents* have not proven to be of benefit.

Another pharmacologic approach employs a drug in gum form which, when chewed, causes an unpleasant taste in the mouth if a cigarette is subsequently smoked. This strategy, like the analogous and older use of disulfiram (Antabuse) to prevent alcohol consumption, has the limitation of being dependent on patient compliance. In one short-term study, the gum did decrease the number of cigarettes smoked, but it did not lead to abstinence.

Behavior modification. The social learning model of smoking has inspired a host of new techniques aimed at modifying smoking behavior by manipulating environmental cues that trigger or reward smoking. *Self-control strategies* rely on the smoker's voluntary control of environmental cues. Cues are first identified by self-monitoring. The smoker typically carries a sheet with his cigarette pack and records the circumstances surrounding the smoking of each cigarette: where, when, why. From this daily cigarette log, environmental stimuli are identified. The second step is a separation of the behavior from its triggers by programmed restriction. The usual tactic is to decrease the number of situations in which smoking is allowed or to limit smoking to a predetermined time schedule. In this way, one attempts to break the association between smoking and environmental cues, while the continuation of smoking prevents the discomfort of nicotine withdrawal. At a point in the relearning process, smoking is stopped altogether.

The theory is attractive, but implementation has not produced impressive results in controlled studies. Usually a temporary reduction in smoking is achieved, but the early relapse rate is high. Smokers routinely have difficulty when they try to smoke less than 10 cigarettes per day, perhaps the level needed to prevent nicotine withdrawal symptoms.

Better results have been achieved when the technique of *contingency contracting* is added to the program. This involves the smoker's deposit of money which gets returned if prearranged conditions are met—usually the maintenance of nonsmoking or attendance at group meetings. In one small uncontrolled study, the combination of self-control and contingency-contracting techniques resulted in 84 per cent immediate abstinence and 36 per cent abstinence 18 months later. However, these results have not been duplicated. The current consensus is that contingency-contracting techniques may turn out to be most useful as a strategy for maintaining abstinence from smoking, regardless of how the abstinence is attained.

SmokEnders, a well-known commercial program, utilizes self-control techniques. Begun in 1969, the program now claims 150,000 graduates and consists of 8 weekly, 2-hour meetings run by exsmokers. Initially, self-monitoring and self-control tactics are employed to aid in a gradual decrease in smoking in preparation for total cessation after the fifth meeting. This is followed by nonspecific group support. This is the only proprietary program for which statistics on long-term follow-up have been published. In that study, 70 per cent were able to stop smoking by the end of the program; 4 years later, 39 per cent remained abstinent. However, review of the statistics by others has shown a true long-term abstinence rate of only 27 per cent, not impressively different from results achieved by other methods. The major disadvantage to the program is its considerable cost. Nonprofit organizations in a number of larger cities offer similar techniques at less expense.

Aversive conditioning techniques operate on the principle that pairing an unwanted act with an unpleasant stimulus will make the act itself unpleasant and less likely to occur. Thus, smoking is paired under controlled conditions with such aversive stimuli as electric shock and cigarette smoke. Electric shock has been paired with actual or imagined smoking or the impulse to smoke, usually in a series of treatment sessions over several days. Results have been mixed. Small uncontrolled studies have shown 50 to 80 per cent success rates at 6 months, but these findings have not been corroborated by controlled studies. It has been suggested that electric shock therapy fails because the behavior change it induces during laboratory sessions does not become generalized outside that setting.

A series of imaginative experiments has found cigarette smoke itself to be an effective aversive stimulus, which has the advantage of being repeatedly encountered by the smoker. Aversive techniques take advantage of the fact that smoke is annoying even to the heavy smoker if encountered at sufficient frequency and intensity. One technique is to blow warm stale smoke into a smoker's face as he is smoking, making an association between the unpleasant experience of breathing smoky air and smoking a cigarette. A second technique is *rapid smoking,* in which the smoker is required to inhale every 6 seconds until unable to tolerate further smoking. This

sequence is repeated at subsequent sessions until the urge to smoke is abolished. A third aversive conditioning technique is *satiation;* smokers purposely double or triple their base smoking rate or purposely chain smoke for up to a day prior to cessation. Here again the theory is to make smoking unpleasant by overdoing it.

Initial data on the aversive techniques which utilize smoke have produced some of the best results in the antismoking literature. One controlled trial reported 60 per cent abstinence at 6-month follow-up. Subsequent attempts to duplicate these results have had variable success. The rapid smoking method has become popular and is now offered by a number of commercial concerns as well as by university-based experimental groups. Controlled studies using the satiation technique have had less impressive results than those attained by other aversive methods.

Concern has been expressed in the medical literature about the physiological effects of the intense exposure to nicotine and carbon monoxide that occurs during a rapid smoking procedure. Rapid smoking acutely elevates heart rate, respiratory rate, systolic blood pressure, and blood carboxyhemoglobin concentration, and produces hypocapnia secondary to hyperventilation. The hemodynamic changes increase myocardial oxygen demand; the increased carboxyhemoglobin concentration decreases oxygen supply. It is possible that myocardial hypoxia could be induced by rapid smoking techniques in patients with coronary artery disease. Furthermore, hypocapnia-induced vasoconstriction might reduce cerebral blood flow to critical levels in smokers with cerebrovascular disease. So far, no serious complications have been reported, although symptoms of light-headedness, nausea, vomiting, and headache are commonly seen. Nevertheless, the technique of rapid smoking is not recommended in patients with cardiopulmonary or cerebrovascular disease.

Combinations of behavior modification tactics (self-control, aversive conditioning, and contingency contracting) have been particularly successful. Several of these multicomponent intervention programs have demonstrated superiority over single-component techniques, with half of smokers remaining abstinent at 6 months in well-done studies. These eclectic programs appear to offer some hope for future success in smoking intervention.

Hypnosis. This approach, usually carried out on an individual basis, employs relaxation and posthypnotic suggestion. The smoker may also be instructed in self-hypnosis exercises for use when the desire to smoke overtakes him. Great claims have been made for hypnosis, but in fact most studies are merely anecdotal, with small samples, no controls and poor follow-up. The more careful studies have shown 6-month abstinence rates of 20 to 25 per cent, no better than those of other techniques.

Individual aids. These include manuals, telephone messages, filters and nicotine-free cigarettes. They have been developed for the smoker who attempts to quit on his own, and for the most part have not been subjected to tests of efficacy. *Self-help manuals* range from pamphlets with practical tips on how to quit to books and comprehensive packages incorporating behavior modification techniques. A number of these are available free of charge from nonprofit organizations such as the American Cancer Society, American Lung Association, and American Heart Association. The National Cancer Institute offers physicians a free "Helping Smokers Quit" kit, which includes materials to distribute to patients.

Telephone messages offer education, advice, encouragement and referrals for smokers attempting to quit.

A series of progressively stronger *filters* is designed to wean the smoker from nicotine while temporarily allowing continuation of the smoking habit. Each filter is supposed to be used for 2 weeks for stepwise removal of an increasingly larger percentage of tar and nicotine from the smoker's own cigarettes. No attempt has been made to evaluate the method, but some observers skeptically note the separate availability of the strongest filter for those who do not quit smoking at the end of 8 weeks. A similar idea led to the development of *non-nicotine "cigarettes,"* which have been tried with only limited success in England; most smokers find them tasteless.

Group education techniques. A variety of group programs designed to help smokers quit use no specific techniques beyond exhortation, education, and practical advice. These have not been well evaluated. The best known is the *Five-Day Plan,* an intensive short-term program developed in 1963 in conjunction with the Seventh Day Adventist church. The program consists of 1½- to 2-hour large-group meetings held on 5 consecutive nights; participants are taught about the risks of smoking and given practical advice on reducing withdrawal effects. There is no follow-up beyond the 5 meetings. The goal of immediate, total cessation is reportedly attained by 60 to 80 per cent of participants, but half relapse within 3 months, and only 18 per cent remain abstinent for 1 year. (These figures are derived from uncontrolled studies.) The results are about the same as those achieved by individuals on their own. The Five-Day Plan is low in cost and is said to have been used by more smokers than any other organized group. The American Cancer Society has run similar group sessions with similar results reported. Behavior modification strategies have recently been added to the program, which is nonprofit and relatively inexpensive.

PHYSICIAN'S ROLE

The likelihood that a smoker will quit is increased by the occurrence of smoking-related symptoms or disease and correlates roughly with the severity of disease. Smokers often quit during an acute illness, but most relapse after recovery. The diagnosis of serious smoking-related disease in ambulatory patients can lead to long-term smoking cessation. For example, a controlled prospective natural history study of patients in New York with newly diagnosed coronary artery disease documented a dramatic and sustained decline in smoking over a 4-year follow-up period, compared to patients without symptoms. Patients hospitalized with a myocardial infarction are even more likely to quit. Numerous studies report long-term cessation in 30 per cent of such patients, even when no particular antismoking advice is given. This figure is comparable to the success achieved in ambulatory patients enrolled in specialized smoking withdrawal programs.

Patients' concern with the health risks of smoking puts the physician and other health care workers in a potentially influential but widely underutilized position to affect smoking behavior. Although three quarters of doctors in a 1975 smoking survey felt it their responsibility to convince people to stop smoking and to set an example by not smoking themselves, only 25 to 50 per cent of smokers report having been advised by their physician to quit or cut down on smoking. The failure of many physicians to advise cessation of smoking is due in part to a widely held belief that such exhortations are futile. Yet, available data indicate that a physician's advice to stop smoking can make a difference. In a well-designed study of the effect of routine antismoking advice given by London general practitioners, all smokers seen by 28 physicians during 1 month, regardless of complaint, were randomly divided into three groups: one was given no special advice and served as controls, a second was routinely advised to stop smoking, while a third was given the advice bolstered by a pamphlet and a warning to expect follow-up.

The group receiving antismoking advice showed statistically significant increases in rate of cessation at 1 month and abstinence maintained during a year of follow-up. The effect was enhanced by distribution of the leaflet and the warning about follow-up. While the percentages of patients who quit were small, they were statistically significant and confirm what previous uncontrolled studies had suggested: that simple routine advice given by physicians in ambulatory practice can be effective in motivating some smokers to quit. The effect appears easily enhanced by such simple techniques as distributing a pamphlet.

Advice by physicians to stop smoking appears even more effective when given to patients hospitalized for a smoking-related disease. In a British study, a group of survivors of myocardial infarction was given specific antismoking advice during hospitalization, with close follow-up by a special clinic and a visiting nurse. One to 3 years later, 63 per cent had stopped smoking, compared to 27 per cent of patients given no special advice.

Although the success rate of the physician's advice in the ambulatory setting does not compare with the 25 per cent long-term success rates reported by the better smoking cessation programs, the absolute number of smokers encountered by physicians is much larger. Hence, with relatively little effort, physicians could potentially change the smoking habits of a large number of patients. Advice about smoking should be a regular part of every encounter in ambulatory practice. Moreover, the physician is likely to encounter the smoker at a time of illness, when a small expenditure of effort may have maximum influence.

stresses are minimized so that quitting can be a central focus for several weeks. Periods of increased temptation, such as the holidays, are best avoided; just after New Year's Day and springtime are optimal.

- The spouse who smokes should also be advised to quit. A smoker is more likely to be successful when the spouse does not smoke or is also attempting to quit.
- The physician should be flexible in selection of a technique for cessation, realizing that different methods work for different people. No data exist on which approach is most appropriate for a particular individual. The majority of smokers will initially elect to stop on their own; such smokers will benefit from information about the withdrawal process. About one third will prefer to use an organized group. Eclectic programs utilizing a combination of behavior modification methods appear to be most effective.
- Practical advice to aid the smoker can be obtained in pamphlets and kits available from the American Cancer Society and the National Cancer Institute.
- For the smoker who prefers an organized program, the local chapters of the American Cancer Society and Lung Association are knowledgeable about available community programs and can assist in referral. If the smoker has been unsuccessful in quitting individually, a referral to a group program may be helpful.
- Follow-up is essential, because the common pattern is transient periods of abstinence followed by a high relapse rate.

RECOMMENDATIONS

- Assessment of smoking habits should be part of every medical evaluation.
- A firm statement to stop smoking should be made to all smokers.
- Motivation for quitting can be enhanced by attention to personally experienced adverse effects of smoking, whether major or minor. Quitting can also be presented in a spirit of self-improvement and responsibility for one's health, rather than as a loss of much-valued habit.
- One should set a goal of total cessation, because those who cut down but do not quit entirely are much more likely to return to baseline smoking rates.
- It is best to attempt withdrawal at a time when life

ANNOTATED BIBLIOGRAPHY

Aids for patients who want to stop smoking. Medical Letter, *20*:105, 1978. *(A brief, referenced review of the variety of commercially available individual aids and group programs.)*

Berkowitz, B., et al.: Hypnotic treatment of smoking: The single-treatment method revisited. Am. J. Psychiatry, *136*:83, 1979. *(Uncontrolled study of 40 smokers treated with hypnosis showed only 25 per cent abstinence from cigarettes at 6-month follow-up.)*

Burt, A., et al.: Stopping smoking after myocardial infarction. Lancet, *1*:305, 1974. *(Controlled prospective study of myocardial infarction survivors demonstrating the effectiveness of firm antismoking advice and education in-hospital and* good follow-up in clinic: 62 per cent of smokers stopped vs 27 per cent in a control group receiving no special antismoking message.)

Hunt, W.A., and Bespalec, D.A.: An evaluation of current methods of modifying smoking behavior. J. Clin. Psychol., *30*:431, 1974. *(This review of 89 studies finds a characteristic relapse pattern among initially successful quitters: a rapid rate of relapse over the first 3 to 6 months, with gradual progression over 18 months. It points out the importance of long-term follow-up in evaluation of ultimate efficacy of smoking intervention programs.)*

Kanzler, M., *et al.*: Long- and short-term effectiveness of large-scale proprietary smoking cessation program—A 4-year follow-up of SmokEnders participants. J. Clin. Psychol., *32*:661, 1976. *(The only published data of SmokEnders, this study finds 70 per cent immediate and 39 per cent 4-year abstinence, but the follow-up statistics have been criticized.)*

Lichtenstein, E., *et al.*: Comparison of rapid smoking, warm smoky air and attention placebo in the modification of smoking behavior. J. Consult. Clin. Psychol., *40*:92, 1973. *(A controlled study of the effectiveness of two of the average conditioning techniques, by one of the major developers of these techniques, finds that they are superior to placebo at 6-month follow-up.)*

Mausner, J., *et al.*: The influence of a physician on the smoking of his patients. Am. J. Public Health, *58*:46, 1968. *(Small study by two doctors, one of whom routinely gave antismoking advice to all patients. Six months later his patients had a slight decrease in smoking rates.)*

McAlister, A.: Helping people quit smoking: Current progress. In A.J. Enelow and J. Henderson (eds.), *Applying Behavioral Science to Cardiovascular Risk*. American Heart Association, 1975. *(A comprehensive review and evaluation of the variety of techniques applied to the problem of smoking. Emphasis is on behavior modification techniques.)*

Miller, L.C., *et al.*: Potential hazards of rapid smoking as a technic for the modification of smoking behavior. N. Engl. J. Med., *297*:590, 1977. *(Documentation of tachycardia, hypertension, hypocapnia and increased blood carboxyhemoglobin following rapid smoking session. No actual precipitation of cerebral or cardiac ischemia, but the article warns of these potential complications.)*

Russell, M.A.H.: Cigarette dependence: Doctor's role in management. Br. Med. J., *2*:393, 1971. *(Advice to the individual physician on practical ways to aid patients who want to quit smoking.)*

————, Wilson, C., Taylor, C., and Baker, C.D.: Effect of general practitioners' advice against smoking. *Brit. Med. J.* 2:231, 1979. *(A well-designed, controlled study in which routine advice to stop smoking resulted in a significant increase in cessation that was sustained over 1 year.)*

U.S. Department of Health, Education and Welfare: Smoking and Health: A Report of the Surgeon General, Washington, D.C., Government Printing Office, 1979. *(A series of comprehensive review articles on all aspects of smoking. This is the most recent update since the landmark 1964 report.)*

Wynder, E.L., and Hoffman, D.: Tobacco and health: A societal challenge. N. Engl. J. Med., *300*:894, 1979. *(A state-of-the-art review of what the authors consider the three necessary approaches to the societal problem of smoking: adult smoking cessation programs, youth programs to prevent acquisition of the habit, and development of a less harmful cigarette for those unable to quit.)*

5

Gastrointestinal Problems

50
Screening for Gastric Cancer

For unknown reasons, the incidence of gastric cancer in the United States has been decreasing at a rate of 2 to 4 per cent per year for the past several decades. During the 1930s, the death rate for gastric cancer was greater than 30 per 100,000; during the 1970s, the rate has been approximately 10 per 100,000. At present, an American has an approximately 1 per cent chance of developing gastric malignancy over his lifetime. Nevertheless, mortality remains high; approximately 85 per cent of the 20,000 Americans who develop gastric cancer each year eventually die from the disease.

The usual insidious onset of the disease and the lack of suitable screening tests have thwarted preventive measures. The primary care physician must understand the natural history of gastric cancer and the limitations of diagnostic tools in the detection of early disease.

EPIDEMIOLOGY AND RISK FACTORS

There is a marked international variation in the incidence of gastric cancer. Among countries with highest incidences are Chile, Japan, Finland, and Iceland. Incidence also varies, predictably, with age and sex. Men are twice as likely to develop gastric cancer in most countries. More than 60 per cent of cases occur in people over age 65. Fewer than 10 per cent of cases occur in people younger than age 30. The incidence among nonwhites and people in low socioeco-

nomic groups in the United States is twice that among whites and the more well-to-do.

Genetic factors do not play a major role in determining risk for gastric cancer. It has been documented that migrants from areas of high risk (e.g., Japan) in time adopt the lower rates of their new home (e.g., the United States). A genetically determined minor risk factor for gastric cancer is blood group; people with type A blood have a 10 per cent increase in risk of developing gastric cancer.

A number of environmental factors have been suggested as explanations for the geographic variability of gastric cancer incidence. Phenol, present in all smoked foods, and the high salt concentration in salted fish and meat products have been linked to the high incidence of gastric cancer in Finland, Iceland, and Japan. Talc-treated rice has been implicated in Japan and Northern China. Provinces in Chile with high gastric cancer rates are agricultural with high concentrations of nitrate present in the soil and drinking water. Nitrosamines, derived from nitrates and secondary amines, are suspected causes of gastric cancer in Chile and, to a lesser extent, in the United States where nitrates and nitrites are used as food additives in meat and fish.

A number of pathologic conditions, including gastric polyps and adenomas, have been associated with increased risk of stomach cancer. Gastric polyps are relatively infrequent; a prevalence of less than 0.5 per cent has been documented in one autopsy series. The vast majority of polyps are hyperplastic and not associated with increased cancer risk. People with adenomas, particularly villous adenomas, have the same risk of cancer when the adenomas are found in the stomach as when they are in the colon. Some authorities have argued that peptic ulcer disease predisposes patients to gastric cancer. Carcinoma is found in approximately 3 per cent of surgically resected gastric ulcers. It is likely, however, that ulceration follows carcinoma rather than *vice versa*. This association is the basis for the clinical practice of biopsying or resecting suspicious-appearing or persistent gastric ulcers.

A number of studies have demonstrated a statistical association between atrophic gastritis and gastric cancer. Achlorhydria and atrophic gastritis are common. Prevalence increases with age. An incidence of 1 per cent per year of gastric cancer among patients with atrophic gastritis has been demonstrated in one study with yearly radiographic examination. The atrophic gastritis associated with pernicious anemia is also a risk factor for gastric cancer. Evidence indicates that patients with pernicious anemia have at least a fourfold increase in risk. Some studies have found even higher rates.

NATURAL HISTORY OF GASTRIC CANCER AND EFFECTIVENESS OF THERAPY

Gastric cancer typically has an insidious presentation. The most common initial symptom is epigastric discomfort. Later symptoms include early satiety, indigestion, weight loss, and other systemic symptoms. The percentage of patients who survive 5 years has not significantly improved in recent years; it remains at 20 per cent of unselected cases. The patients who are operated on early in the course of their disease have a 60 to 90 per cent 5-year survival rate. However, despite intensive efforts at early diagnosis in Japan, fewer than 30 per cent of all cases are diagnosed early. The duration of the asymptomatic period for gastric cancer is not known, but there are many examples of very rapid, fatal courses as well as of protracted courses, which suggest a wide variability in natural history.

SCREENING AND DIAGNOSTIC TESTS

None of the tests available for the diagnosis of gastric carcinoma are suitable for wide-scale screening efforts.

Gastric Cytology. Unlike cervical cytopathology, the collection and examination of specimens for gastric cytopathologic analysis is a laborious process. Samples must be obtained either by endoscopic scraping or by gastric lavage. Examination of the resulting slides usually takes 2 to 3 hours rather than the several minutes sufficient for screening examination of cervical Pap smears. Multiple studies have demonstrated the sensitivity of gastric cytopathology studies to be approximately 90 per cent. Specificity in a laboratory with experienced personnel should be approximately 97 to 98 per cent. False-positives are often found in association with healing gastric ulcer and other gastric pathology. While cytopathology is useful for further diagnosis in documented cases of abnormality of gastric mucosa, it cannot be recommended for indiscriminate screening.

Endoscopy. Similarly, endoscopy must be considered a diagnostic rather than screening procedure. Sensitivity in making the diagnosis of gastric cancer is 90 per cent. When it is combined with scraping for cytopathology, sensitivity is increased to 98 per cent. The use of endoscopy in asymptomatic patients in Japan has had a disappointingly low yield.

Diagnostic Radiology. The sensitivity of contrast studies in the diagnosis of gastric cancer has been reported to be as high as 95 per cent. Obviously, however, it is least sensitive in cases of early disease and is too expensive and time-consuming to be considered a screening test in asymptomatic patients.

Stool analysis for occult blood (described in detail in Chap. 51) is an appropriate screening procedure for all gastrointestinal malignancies. Yearly guaiac testing has been recommended as part of the general screening for all adult patients. This is especially important for patients with identified increased risk of gastric cancer, such as those with a history of pernicious anemia or documented atrophic gastritis.

CONCLUSIONS AND RECOMMENDATIONS

- Despite a significant downward trend in incidence, gastric cancer remains a disease of high morbidity and mortality.
- The yearly analysis of stool for occult blood is indicated in all adult patients. This is especially important for those with a history of pernicious anemia, atrophic gastritis, or other gastric pathology.
- The value of gastric cytology, endoscopy, and contrast studies as routine procedures in high-risk patients is unproven. They are diagnostic procedures

and should generally be reserved for symptomatic patients or patients with occult blood demonstrated by stool analysis.

ANNOTATED BIBLIOGRAPHY

Ackerman, N.B.: An evaluation of gastric cytology: Results of a nation-wide survey. J. Chron, Dis., *20*:621, 1967. *(Survey of practices in U.S. hospitals indicating wide variation in validity of techniques. Not generally used for screening purposes but rather in response to symptoms or radiographic abnormalities.)*

Hitchcock, C.R., MacLean, L.D., and Sullivan, W.A.: Secretory and clinical aspects of achlorhydria and gastric atrophy as precursors of gastric cancer. J. Nat. Cancer Inst., *18*:795, 1957. *(Review of data indicating increase of 4.5 and 21.9 times in risk among patients with achlorhydria and pernicious anemia. Recommends frequent radiographic studies.)*

Hoerr, S.O.: Prognosis for carcinoma of the stomach. Surg. Gyn. Obstet., *137*:205, 1973. *(Five-year survivals rates ranging from 83% to 11% depending on stage; overall five-year survival rate of 18%.)*

MacDonald, W.C., *et al.*: Exfoliative cytology screening for gastric cancer. Cancer, *17*:163, 1964. *(Series of 500 patients with pernicious anemia or achlorhydria. Screening yielded 3 cases—none of which were asymptomatic, 2 of which were inoperable. The one false-positive finding resulted in an operative death.)*

Rubin, P., (ed.): Cancer of the gastrointestinal tract: C. Gastric cancer diagnosis. JAMA, *288*:883, 1974. *(Collection of 8 short articles that review the epidemiology, natural history, and diagnosis of gastric cancer.)*

51

Screening for Colorectal Cancer

Colorectal cancer is the most common malignancy found in both men and women, accounting for about 15 per cent of deaths from cancer. Americans face a lifetime probability of developing a tumor of the colon or rectum of approximately 5 per cent. This frequency, the long asymptomatic period of the disease, the availability of tests for early diagnosis, and the effectiveness of early therapy make screening for large-bowel tumors a primary care priority.

EPIDEMIOLOGY AND RISK FACTORS

Advanced age is an important risk factor. The peak age-specific incidence occurs during the seventh decade. However, about 1 per cent of colon cancers occur before age 30.

The incidence of colorectal cancer is greater in economically developed societies. Burkitt has advanced a hypothesis incriminating diets deficient in fiber and rich in refined carbohydrate. Fiber deficiency produces concentrated stool with prolonged mucosal contact. He argues that refined carbohydrate alters bacterial content and the degradation of bile salts, thereby increasing the production of carcinogens.

A positive family history is a minor risk factor. The risk in relatives with colorectal cancer is three times that of the population at large. Familial polyposis is an autosomal disease with a virtual certainty of eventual malignancy—two-thirds show evidence of malignancy at the time of diagnosis. Surveillance with cytology, sigmoidoscopy, and radiologic examination is indicated if complete colectomy is delayed.

Sporadic polyps are common lesions. The relationship of symptomatic and asymptomatic colonic polyps to cancer has been the subject of heated controversy. Some authorities have argued that at least 50 per cent of carcinomas arise from benign polyps while others have minimized their malignant potential. Much of the confusion derives from changing pathologic classifications. The clinical problem can be approached by considering a polyp, discovered endoscopically or radiologically, as a risk factor for the

Table 51–1. Polypoid Lesions of the Colon and Rectum. Relation of Size to Cancer (1116 polypoid lesions, Massachusetts General Hospital, 1954–63)

DIAMETER (CM.)	PER CENT CANCEROUS
Less than 0.5	0.5
0.5–0.9	1
1.0–1.4	1.8
1.5–1.9	6
2–2.4	10
2.5–3.4	23
3.5 or larger	29

(Behringer, G.E.: Changing concepts in the histopathologic diagnosis of polypoid lesions of the colon. Dis. Colon Rectum, *13*:116–118, 1970)

presence or development of cancer. The risk depends on the type of polyp and its size and shape. About 90 per cent of colonic lesions are small hyperplastic outcroppings rather than genuine neoplasms and are not related to carcinoma. The best estimates for prevalence of neoplastic polyps in adult populations cluster around 10 per cent. Approximately 75 per cent of these are adenomatous polyps with smaller numbers being villous adenomas and mixed villous and adenomatous lesions. Villous adenomas are generally larger and more sessile than other adenomas and often premalignant; 20 to 40 per cent have been demonstrated to contain cancers. One study found that the likelihood of malignancy in polyps 1.5 to 1.9 cm. in diameter was 6 per cent, rising to almost 30 per cent in lesions greater than 3.5 cm. (see Table 51–1).

Ulcerative colitis predisposes patients to a five to ten times greater risk of colonic cancer. The risk increases with the duration of the inflammatory disease, reaching 20 to 30 per cent in some series. Regional enteritis carries a smaller risk, though still twice that of the population at large.

Patients with previously diagnosed and resected colorectal cancers have an incidence of subsequent colon cancer approximately three times that of the general population.

NATURAL HISTORY OF COLORECTAL CANCER AND EFFECTIVENESS OF THERAPY

The most common presenting symptoms of colorectal cancer are change in bowel habits, pain, and hematochezia. These symptoms generally occur late in the course of tumor growth. Colorectal cancer grows slowly, with radiologic observations demonstrating a mean doubling time approaching two years. At the time surgery is undertaken, usually prompted by a symptomatic presentation, about 70 per cent of cancers have penetrated all layers of the bowel wall, and two-thirds of patients have regional metastatic disease.

Five-year survival rates of patients with colon cancer varies dramatically with the stage of progression at the time of diagnosis. When the tumor is limited to the submucosa (Duke's Stage A), the survival rate is about 60 per cent. Corresponding rates when lesions invade the muscularis without (Stage B) and with (Stage C) nodal metastases are approximately 40 per cent and 25 per cent respectively. As with other tumors, the importance of biologic variability (rather than delay in diagnosis) as a determinant of eventual outcome is not well understood.

SCREENING AND DIAGNOSTIC TESTS

Stool Analysis for Occult Blood. Occult intermittent bleeding has been shown to occur frequently in patients with asymptomatic lesions. The guaiac-impregnated filter paper slides (Hemoccult) in common use will regularly detect 25 ml. of blood or 10 mg. of hemoglobin per gm. of stool. More sensitive methods for blood detection provide unacceptable false-positive rates. Meat-free diets reduce false-positive rates but do not seem necessary if Hemoccult slides are used. Ascorbic acid is a common cause of false-negative results. A false-negative result may also be caused by a delay of more than 4 days in testing a sample. It is apparent that the sensitivity of occult blood determination in detecting carcinoma depends on the lesion's bleeding; a high-roughage diet is advocated to provoke bleeding from any existing lesion. Increased sensitivity can be gained by repeated guaiac testing. The specificity of guaiac testing for cancer is limited because of the high prevalence of nonmalignant bleeding lesions of the gastrointestinal tract. In the single large scale study available, 6 per cent of participants had guaiac-positive results. Of guaiac-positive patients who were fully evaluated, 10 per cent were found to have cancer.

Proctosigmoidoscopy. Traditional teaching has been that 75 per cent of carcinomas are within reach of the sigmoidoscope. Recently the number has been revised downward to 50 to 60 per cent as colonoscopy has become more prevalent. When proctosigmoidoscopic examination is performed in asymptomatic adults over age 40, the case finding rate is 0.1 to 0.3

per cent for carcinoma and 5 to 10 per cent for benign polyps. The cancer rate increases tenfold when the examinations are limited to those who present with symptoms. In one study, no cancers were found in patients younger than 50 years of age, prompting the authors to part with the recommendations of the American Cancer Society (which urges annual examinations over age 40) and to recommend the deferment of routine sigmoidoscopy until age 50. Recognizing the mean slow growth rate of colonic tumors, they also recommend biannual, rather than annual, examinations.

Radiologic Diagnosis. Contrast studies are not screening tests. The barium enema identifies lesions with a sensitivity of about 90 per cent. Lesions are most often missed in the cecum or rectosigmoid, or in the setting of ulcerative colitis or diverticulitis. Air-contrast studies are more sensitive than full-column studies for small lesions, but there is greater risk of missing larger lesions.

Colonoscopy. Colonoscopy is not a screening test. The sensitivity of colonoscopy as a diagnostic test depends on the experience of the operator. The technique also provides a method of removal with much less risk than laparotomy. This lower risk may lower the threshold for removal of small polyps.

Carcinoembryonic Antigen. Carcinoembryonic antigen is sensitive only with advanced lesions and has proven disappointingly nonspecific. Its use has been advocated in monitoring patients with previously resected tumors (see Chapter XX). It is not a suitable test for general screening.

CONCLUSIONS AND RECOMMENDATIONS

- The relatively high prevalence of colorectal cancer and characteristics of its natural history make detection in an asymptomatic stage with reduction of morbidity and mortality highly feasible. The principal risk factor for the selection of a screening population is advanced age.
- Yearly guaiac testing should be performed in adult patients. Stool testing is an inexpensive, convenient way of screening for asymptomatic disease, although sensitivity and specificity are not known. The probability of cancer (the predictive value positive) when at least one of three tests is positive, is 5 to 10 per cent in an unselected population.
- The yield of proctosigmoidoscopy in an asymptomatic population is small but significant. Resources

for examination of the asymptomatic population should be directed first at patients over 50 years of age with one or more risk factors who have not had such examinations in the previous 2 to 3 years.
- When there are no contraindications, colonic polyps greater than 1.5 cm. in diameter should be removed. If colonoscopic removal is possible, the removal of smaller lesions may be preferable to long-term followup with repeated radiologic examination.

ANNOTATED BIBLIOGRAPHY

Behringer, G.E.: Changing concepts in the histopathologic diagnosis of polypoid lesions of the colon. Dis. Colon Rectum, *13*:116, 1970. *(Data relating polyp size to presence of cancer from Massachusetts General Hospital.)*

Burkitt, D.P.: Epidemiology of cancer of the colon and rectum. Cancer, *28*:3, 1971. *(Argument for low-residue diet as a risk factor based on international variation in incidence.)*

Corman, M.L., Coller, J.A., and Veidenheimer, M.C.: Proctosigmoidoscopy—age criteria for examination in the asymptomatic patient. CA, *25(5)*:286, 1975. *(No cancers found in patients younger than 50 in a large screening study.)*

Greegor, D.H.: Occult blood testing for detection of asymptomatic colon cancer. Cancer, *28*:131, 1971. *(Five per cent of patients had a positive test; 20 per cent of those had asymptomatic tumors.)*

Hastings, J.B.: Mass screening for colorectal cancer. Am. J. Surg., *127*:228, 1974. *(Mass screening with guaiac testing produced 6 per cent positive results. Only one-third were subsequently evaluated, of these 10 per cent had cancer.)*

Jaffe, R.M., Kasten, B., Young, D.S., and MacLowry, J.D.: False-negative stool occult blood tests caused by ingestion of ascorbic acid. Ann. Intern. Med., *83*:824, 1975. *(May be a common problem unless patients are adequately instructed.)*

Morris, D.W., et al.: Reliability of chemical tests for fecal occult blood. Am. J. Dig. Dis. *21*:845, 1976. *(Provides sensitivities and specificities of available tests.)*

Ostrow, J.D., Mulvaney, C.A., Hansell, J.R., and Rhodes, R.S.: Sensitivity and reproducibility of chemical tests for fecal occult blood with an emphasis on false-positive reactions. Dig. Dis., *18*:930, 1973. *(Documents increased specificity of Hemoccult technique.)*

Powers, J.H.: Proctosigmoidoscopy in private practice. JAMA, *231*:750, 1975. *(Prevalence of colon pathology 10 times greater among patients presenting with symptoms.)*

Sherlock, P., Lipkin, M., and Winawer, S.J.: Predisposing factors in colon carcinoma. Adv. Intern. Med. *20*:121, 1975. *(More detailed treatment of epidemiologic and experimental studies of risk factors.)*

Spratt, J.S., and Watson, F.R.: The rationale of practice for polypold lesions of the colon. Cancer, *28*:153, 1971. *(Detailed consideration of natural histories of benign and malignant colonic tumors.)*

Stroehlein, J.R., *et al.*: Hemoccult stool tests. Mayo Clin. Proc., *51*:548, 1976. *(Documents substantial decrease in sensitivity when cards with stool are not tested within 4 days.)*

van Langenberg, A., and Ong,. G.B.: Carcinoma of large bowel in the young. Br. Med. J., *3*:374, 1972. *(Review of 21 cases occurring before age 25, suggesting more aggressive natural history in young adults.)*

Winawer, S.J., Sherlock, P., Schottenfeld, D., and Miller, D.G.: Screening for colon cancer. Gastroenterology, *70*:783, 1976. *(Excellent review of risk factors and screening methods. Recommends yearly guaiac testing and sigmoidoscopy in all adults over 40 years old.)*

Wolff, W.I., and Shinya, H.: Polypectomy via the fiberoptic colonoscope. N. Engl. J. Med., *288*:329, 1973. *(A series of over 1600 colonoscopies and over 300 polypectomies documenting low morbidity.)*

52

Prevention of Viral Hepatitis

Viral hepatitis is a contagious disease that afflicts over 500,000 people in the United States each year. The majority of patients experience a mild illness, but 5 to 10 per cent develop chronic hepatitis and several thousand die. Moreover, many become chronic carriers of hepatitis antigen. Outbreaks of viral hepatitis are often traced to a source of Type A virus. Many sporadic cases of hepatitis are due to type B virus, but almost 30 per cent represent non-A, non-B disease. Currently, over 90 per cent of post-transfusion hepatitis is attributable to non-A, non-B infection; the incidence of post-transfusion hepatitis due to the B virus has been greatly reduced by screening donors for B virus antigen.

Prevention of infection and prophylaxis against clinical disease are prime objectives in the management of viral hepatitis. The primary physician has major responsibility for these tasks, because patients and their contacts often present at the time of contagiousness. Prevention of viral hepatitis requires a knowledge of the common modes of viral transmission, the periods of maximal communicability, and the efficacy of gamma globulin preparations.

EPIDEMIOLOGY AND RISK FACTORS

Hepatitis A virus is shed in the feces, and transmission occurs predominantly by the fecal-oral route. Prior exposure to hepatitis A is manifested by the presence of antibody to the A virus (anti-HAV). Antibody confers lifelong immunity. More than 80 per cent of patients over age 60 are positive for anti-HAV. Since children and adolescents are least likely to have had previous exposure to the virus, they are the most susceptible to infection. Spread of infection is greatest when there are poor sanitary conditions and crowding. In a New York City study, 75 per cent of low income people had evidence of prior infection, compared to 20 to 30 per cent of residents in middle to upper income neighborhoods. There is no known carrier state.

Hepatitis B used to be considered a disease that resulted from parenteral exposure, but recent evidence suggests that nonpercutaneous transmission is a common mode of spread. Vertical transmission from mother to offspring is common in underdeveloped nations. Patients with acute hepatitis B have been found to harbor hepatitis B surface antigen (HBsAg) in saliva, semen, vaginal secretions and breast milk, as well as in the serum. Spouses of patients with acute hepatitis and people with a large number of sexual partners (e.g., male homosexuals) are maximally subjected to sources of nonpercutaneous transmission and have a markedly increased risk of contracting infection. About 0.1 per cent of healthy blood donors are positive for HBsAg, as are 5 per cent of drug addicts and over 50 per cent of patients in some dialysis units. Surgeons, laboratory technicians, oral surgeons and other medical personnel exposed to patients who are antigen-positive are at increased risk of contracting hepatitis B. Spread of infection from health personnel who are carriers of antigen is a rare event, usually explained by patient exposure to their blood from cuts or abrasions. The development and application of sensitive screening methods for detection of HBsAg has greatly reduced the incidence of post-transfusion hepatitis due to type B virus. Currently, less than 10 per cent of all post-transfusion hepatitis in the United States is due to B virus. Blood obtained from volunteer donors is less likely to contain the virus.

Non-A, non-B hepatitis often originates from transfusion of blood obtained from commercial donors. The antigenic markers for non-A, non-B hepatitis have not yet been discovered; consequently, it is impossible at present to screen donors for the disease. Over 90 per cent of post-transfusion hepatitis is currently non-A, non-B in origin. Identification of the antigen(s) associated with this form of viral hepatitis should lead to a reduction in the risk of post-transfusion hepatitis.

NATURAL HISTORY

Hepatitis A has an average incubation period of 30 days (range 15-45 days) from time of exposure to onset of symptoms. An early manifestation of disease is elevation of the serum transaminase level, which occurs about a week before onset of flulike symptoms; however, fecal shedding of hepatitis A virus (HAV) has been found to occur even before the rise in transaminases and up to 2 weeks prior to the development of symptoms. HAV disappears from stool within 2 to 3 weeks, usually coinciding with the onset of jaundice and resolution of prodromal symptoms. Fall in viral titer parallels a rise in antibody titer, which persists indefinitely. Initially, the anti-HAV is of the IgM class; during convalescence anti-HAV of the IgG class becomes predominant. No episodes of chronic hepatitis or carrier states have been found to result from hepatitis A infection. Fatalities are rare; fewer than 10 per cent of cases of fulminant hepatitis are due to type A virus infection.

Hepatitis B infection is a much more variable disease. The incubation period averages 12 weeks, with a range of 6 weeks to 6 months. About 2 to 4 weeks prior to onset of symptoms, HBsAg appears in the serum, followed by a rise in transaminase levels and symptoms. Antigen usually is cleared from the serum by 8 weeks; persistence of antigenemia beyond 13 weeks is associated with an increased risk of chronic hepatitis. Symptoms of acute hepatitis B typically last 4 to 6 weeks, but there is much variation, ranging from clinically inapparent disease to fulminant hepatocellular failure and death. Age, immunologic competence, degree of exposure, and virulence of the virus are among the determinants of disease severity. About 10 per cent of patients with syptomatic disease become chronic carriers of HBsAg; 1 to 2 per cent progress to chronic active hepatitis; 1 per cent die. Antibody to HBsAg appears at variable times after exposure, but 90 per cent eventually develop anti-HBs and it persists indefinitely.

The *e antigen* (HBeAg) has drawn attention as a predictor of infectivity. Needlestick exposure to blood from a chronic carrier that is positive for HBeAg is associated with a high risk of infection. There was speculation that finding HBeAg early in the course of illness meant an increase in the probability of developing chronic hepatitis, but this has not been borne out. HBeAg appears transiently in the early phase of all hepatitis B infections, but only in a few does it persist and signify high infectivity.

Non-A, non-B hepatitis was discovered when sera from patients with post-transfusion hepatitis were found to be negative for hepatitis A or B virus, as well as for Epstein-Barr virus and cytomegalovirus. Better identification of this variant has to await the ability of specific serologic tests. Mean incubation period is 7 weeks; like hepatitis B, the range is wide, being 3 to 15 weeks. Only a third of patients become icteric, compared to two-thirds of patients with post-transfusion hepatitis due to B virus, but over one third become chronic carriers of antigen and many progress to chronic active hepatitis.

PRINCIPLES OF PROPHYLAXIS

The principal means of prophylaxis are minimizing exposure to hepatitis virus and use of gamma globulin preparations. In many instances, gamma globulin prophylaxis does not prevent infection from occurring, but it may reduce the chances of developing clinical hepatitis. Precautions against contact with the hepatitis patient are most appropriate during the prodromal stage of illness, when the patient sheds virus most heavily. Unfortunately, there is often little clinical evidence of hepatitis at this stage, making it difficult to avoid contact with the virus. Consequently, immunotherapy emerges as the mainstay of prophylaxis.

Hepatitis A. Prophylaxis for hepatitis A can be accomplished by use of *immune serum globulin* (ISG). The gamma globulin preparation contains high titers of anti-HA and is about 80 per cent effective in preventing clinical disease. The mechanism by which ISG protects the exposed patient is believed to be passive-active immunization, in which passively administered antibody acts to minimize clinical illness, but does not prevent infection. ISG must be administered within 1 to 2 weeks of exposure in order to be most effective. Patients with a prior history of hepatitis A need not receive ISG, for they are already protected by their own anti-HA. Household contacts and small groups experiencing a common source outbreak (e.g., an athletic team) should be given ISG prophylaxis. During the early phase of clinical hepatitis when jaundice first appears, there may still be some shedding of virus; precautions such as avoiding intimate contact and careful washing of hands after contact are probably reasonable for a week or two longer. The patient should not serve food to others and may minimize transmission of virus by using disposable dishes and utensils.

Hepatitis B. The status of prophylactic therapy for hepatitis B is in a state of transition. Early study of ISG use for prophylaxis showed little effect in preventing clinical hepatitis B. Later investigations that employed ISG containing substantial titers of anti-HBs demonstrated a protective effect. *Hepatitis B immune globulin (HBIG)* was developed with the hope of attaining still better prophylaxis from a preparation that contains very high titers of anti-HBs (in

the order of 1:100,000). Controlled double-blind study comparing efficacy of HBIG against an ISG preparation that contained no anti-HBs found HBIG superior to ISG in preventing clinical hepatitis in people exposed to HBsAg from a needle stick. A similar double-blind study showed no significant difference in protective effect between HBIG and an ISG preparation that contained low to intermediate titers of anti-HBs.

The mechanisms responsible for the protection afforded by ISG and HBIG are beginning to be understood, and this understanding promises to help rationalize prophylactic therapy. Part of the protection afforded by ISG and HBIG is due to the presence of anti-HBs. The antibody seems not to prevent infection, but does limit the disease to a subclinical illness. In most instances, the greater the titer, the more protection afforded; however, retrospective analysis of data from some ISG studies does not always reveal a close correlation between ISG antibody titer and efficacy. A recent reanalysis of patient sera and ISG preparations from a major study of hepatitis B prophylaxis uncovered evidence for active immunization. As many as 36 per cent of patients given an ISG preparation that had no anti-HBs demonstrated anti-HBs in their serum. Although the ISG contained no detectable amounts of anti-HBs, it was found to have occult quantities of HBsAg complexed to antibody. The HBsAg did not cause infection in the treated patients (no core antigen was found in their sera, which argues strongly against infection), but it did result in active immunization by stimulating the patient's own production of anti-HBs. This finding might explain why ISG has often proven quite effective when given prior to exposure, but found to be variable in efficacy when administered after exposure to HBsAg.

At the present time, the indications for use of HBIG are limited because the material is very expensive and supplies are scarce. It is generally agreed that anyone with needle-stick exposure to blood that contains HBsAg should be given HBIG. Other situations in which a major exposure takes place have also been mentioned as possible indications for HBIG; e.g., sexual contact with a patient who has acute disease (provided the exposed person is not promiscuous and likely to have further contacts with other infected patients). The presence of e antigen in the HBsAg-positive source suggests increased risk of infectivity. Testing for e antigen can help determine the need for HBIG prophylaxis, provided the assay is available and the result can be obtained in less than 7 days from time of exposure, the generally assumed time limit for administration of HBIG. There are no studies available defining the maximum duration of time after exposure when HBIG can be given and still exert a protective effect, but 7 days is considered a maximum at present.

Until HBIG becomes less expensive and more widely available, ISG containing intermediate titers of anti-HBs (in the range of 1:250 or more) should suffice for moderate exposures to HBsAg. The amount of anti-HBs administered is at least partially responsible for the protective effect of ISG; the gamma globulin preparation is given in doses considerably larger than those required for hepatitis A prophylaxis. Nonintimate household contacts do not require prophylaxis, nor do casual contacts at work. Such generalizations must be qualified by the infectivity and virulence of the virus at hand as well as the consequences of infection to the exposed person. All suspected sources of hepatitis B should be tested for HBsAg, and exposed persons can be checked for presence of anti-HBs to see how susceptible to infection they are. These tests and the assay for e antigen can help define risk and the need for ISG or HBIG, but slow return of results and lack of availability of a number of these tests severely limit their usefulness at the present time. Prophylaxis should not be delayed beyond 7 days of exposure.

Reducing the spread of hepatitis B is aided by screening blood donors for HBsAg. The person discovered to be an asymptomatic carrier requires attention. If the person is a health care worker or a food handler who is genuinely free of symptoms and has normal liver function tests, he need not be removed from work unless proven to be a source of infection. Liver function should be evaluated every 4 to 6 months to rule out active disease. If such a person becomes symptomatic or shows signs of hepatitis, he should cease working temporarily until evidence of illness clears.

Risk of exposure to HBsAg ceases when antigen disappears from the bloodstream; this is usually within 6 to 8 weeks of infection. Repeat serum determinations of HBsAg can help define when precautions may be relaxed.

Non-A, Non-B Hepatitis. The principal means of reducing the incidence of this type of viral hepatitis is to use volunteer blood in preference to commercial blood. The development of means to detect antigenic markers for the non-A, non-B variants will greatly facilitate prevention of the disease. ISG and HBIG are of no use as prophylactic measures for non-A, non-B hepatitis.

RECOMMENDATIONS AND PATIENT EDUCATION

Hepatitis A Precautions (to be continued until a week after the onset of jaundice)

- Advise the patient to wash hands thoroughly after use of the toilet.
- The patient need not be confined to home, but intimate contact should be avoided.
- Prohibit the patient from handling and serving food to others.
- Advise others to avoid contact with the patient's fecal material and to wash hands thoroughly if contact is made.

Hepatitis A Prophylaxis

- Administer ISG to household contacts within 2 weeks of exposure: the dose is 0.02 ml. per kilogram; average adult dose is 2 ml. intramuscularly.
- Administer ISG for contacts in an epidemic and for travelers to areas in which hepatitis A is endemic; dose is the same as for household contacts.

Hepatitis B Precautions (to be continued until HBsAg clears from the serum)

- All blood donors should be screened for HBsAg.
- Preferentially use volunteer blood, rather than blood from commercial donors.
- Preferentially use disposable syringes and needles.
- Have patient use separate razor, toothbrush and other personal items.
- Have any materials containing HBsAg handled carefully, particularly blood samples and other bodily fluids; use of gloves is advisable.
- Recommend avoidance of intimate contact, but confinement to home is unnecessary.
- If the patient has acute disease and is sneezing or coughing productively, he should use a mask to minimize the risk of contact with saliva.
- Hands should be washed thoroughly after direct contact with the patient or with the patient's blood or feces.

Hepatitis B Prophylaxis

- Administer HBIG to persons with parenteral exposure to blood that is HBsAg-positive; if HBIG is unavailable, use 5 ml. of ISG that contains anti-HBs in titers of at least 1:250; HBIG is particularly indicated if the blood is positive for e antigen.

- Administer ISG to intimate contacts of patients with acute disease; dose is 5 ml. of a preparation that contains anti-HBs (though HBIG may soon become treatment of choice).
- Whenever ISG or HBIG is indicated, it should be given within 7 days of exposure.
- No prophylaxis is necessary for casual contacts or household contacts that are not intimate.

Non-A, Non-B Hepatitis Precautions and Prophylaxis

- Precautions are the same as those for hepatitis B, and are essentially those related to exposure to the infected patient's blood.
- There is no known means of screening for the disease.
- The best means of prevention is use of volunteer blood donors rather than commercial donors.
- ISG and HBIG are of no use in this disease.

ANNOTATED BIBLIOGRAPHY

Alter, H., Chalmer, T., Freeman, B.: Health care workers positive for hepatitis B surface antigen: are their contacts at risk? N. Engl. J. Med., *292:*454, 1975. *(A prospective controlled study that showed no evidence of spread of hepatitis to 282 patients exposed to staff positive for HBsAg. Supports view that risk is low.)*

Alter, H., et al.: Type B hepatitis: infectivity of blood positive for e antigen. N. Eng. J. Med. *295:*090, 1976. *(Presence of e antigen was found to be an important indicator of relative infectivity of HBsAg-positive serum, particularly after small volume parenteral exposure.)*

Center for Disease Control: Immune globulins for protection against viral hepatitis. Morb. Mort. Weekly Rep., *26:*425, 441, 1977. *(Recent CDC recommendations on ISG and HBIG use.)*

Deinhardt, F.: Epidemiology and mode of transmission of hepatitis A and B. Am. J. Clin. Pathol., *65:*890, 1976. *(Terse but complete review of hepatitis epidemiology with 42 references.)*

Dienstag, J.L., Feinstone, S.M., Kapikian A.Z., et al.: Fecal shedding of hepatitis-A antigen. Lancet, *1:*765, 1975 *(Most shedding occurs prior to onset of jaundice.)*

Feinstone, S.M., and Purcell, R.H.: Non-A, Non-B hepatitis. Ann. Rev. Med., *29:*356. 1978 *(Ninety per cent of post-transfusion hepatitis is due to this variant; the disease resembles type B hepatitis; good review of the subject.)*

Grady, G.F., Rodman, M., and Larsen L.H.: Hepatitis B antibody in conventional gamma globulin. J. Inf. Dis., *132:*474, 1975. *(Titers in many sera collected since 1972 have ranged from 1:100 to 1:1000.)*

Hoofnagle, J.H., Seeff, L.B., Bales, Z.B., et al.: Passive-active immunity from hepatitis B immune globulin. Ann. Intern. Med., *91:*813, 1979. *(A study of the mechanisms of immune globulin action in prophylaxis. Argues that infection is not prevented by HBIG, but clinical illness is. Suggests that ISG may cause active immunization in some instances.)*

Krugman, S., and Giles, J.: Viral hepatitis: new light on an old disease. JAMA, *212:*1019, 1970. *(Classic paper on natural history of hepatitis A and B and documentation of efficacy of gamma-globulin for prevention of hepatitis A.)*

Mosley, J.W.: Hepatitis B immune globulin (Editorial). Ann. Intern. Med., *91:*914, 1979. *(A good summary of the indications at present for ISG and HBIG as well as the areas of controversy.)*

Redeker, A.D., et al.: Hepatitis B immune globulin as a prophylactic measure for spouses exposed to acute type B hepatitis. N. Engl. J. Med. *293:*1055, 1975. *(Demonstrated high risk of hepatitis in spouses and efficacy of HBIG for prevention of clinical illness.)*

Seeff, L., et al.: Type B hepatitis after needle-stick exposure: prevention with hepatitis B immune globulin. Ann. Intern. Med., *88:*285, 1978. *(HBIG and ISG without antibody were compared in a randomized, double-blind multicenter study. HBIG was significantly more effective in preventing hepatitis. The efficacy of ISG compared to placebo was not studied.)*

Szmuness, W., Dienstag, J., Purcell, R., et al.: Distribution of antibody to hepatitis A antigen in urban populations. N. Engl. J. Med., *295:*755, 1976. *(A study of 947 randomly selected people in New York City examining the epidemiology of hepatitis A. Prevalence of antibody increases with age, decreases with rise in socioeconomic status and is unaffected by sex or race.):*

Szmuness, W., Dienstag, J., Purcell, R., et al.: Hepatitis A and hemodialysis. Ann. Intern. Med. *87:*8,

1977. *(A multicenter seroepidemiologic study of 460 patients and staff finding no evidence for parenteral spread of hepatitis A or a chronic viremic carrier state. This data support the view that parenteral spread is very rare if present at all.)*

Szmuness, W., *et al.*: On the role of sexual behavior in spread of hepatitis B infection. Ann. Intern. Med., *83*:459, 1975. *(An epidemiologic study showing a strong association between sexual pro-miscuity and serologic evidence of type B infection.)*

Villarejos, V., *et al.*: Role of saliva, urine and feces in transmission of type B hepatitis. N. Engl. J. Med., *291*:1375, 1971. *(76% of patients with acute hepatitis had antigen detectable in their saliva during the first 3 weeks after clinical onset. Urine and feces were infrequently antigen-positive.)*

53
Evaluation of Abdominal Pain

One of the most difficult problems faced by the primary physician is the outpatient assessment of abdominal pain. When the pain is acute in onset, triage decisions have to be made regarding the need for hospital admission and surgical intervention. If the pain is chronic or recurrent, the physician must design a safe, cost-effective plan for workup that will efficiently distinguish among a myriad of possible etiologies. In many instances, the exact cause of pain is not immediately evident. Nevertheless, a few basic determinations may help elucidate the underlying pathophysiology, which, in turn, can guide further assessment and decision-making. Of particular importance is the need to decide on the proper speed and extent of evaluation.

PATHOPHYSIOLOGY AND CLINICAL PRESENTATION

The major mechanisms of abdominal pain include obstruction of a hollow viscus, peritoneal irritation, vascular insufficiency, mucosal ulceration, altered bowel motility, capsular distention or inflammation, metabolic imbalance, nerve injury, abdominal wall injury, referral from an extra-abdominal site, and emotional stress.

Obstruction can cause considerable pain if the process is rapid in onset. Pain receptors in the bowel, biliary tree and ureters respond to distention. The severity of the pain is a function of the speed of onset as well as the degree of distention. Obstruction that develops slowly over weeks to months may be relatively subtle in presentation, compared to the more dramatic picture produced by acute obstruction. The pain of acute *small bowel* obstruction is typically cramping in quality, with severity greatest when the obstruction is proximal. The patient is often comfortable between bouts of pain. Severity decreases with time as bowel motility diminishes. Complete strangulation of small bowel is associated with steady pain. Vomiting is common, particularly in proximal obstruction; when the problem is distal, vomiting is less frequent, but may be feculent. Flatus and passage of small amounts of stool may occur at the outset, but soon cease if the obstruction is complete. Diarrhea is noted in some cases of partial obstruction. On examination, the patient appears restless during bouts of pain. The temperature is typically normal or only mildly elevated. The abdomen may be distended, especially when the obstruction is distal. High-pitched, hyperactive bowel sounds are characteristic, but not always present. Tenderness to palpation is not impressive, unless leakage of bowel contents has occurred, causing peritoneal soilage. The stool is usually guaiac negative.

Large bowel obstruction is, in most instances, less painful and associated with less vomiting than is obstruction of the small intestine. Constipation or change in bowel habits often precedes complete obstruction. Distention is greater than that seen in small bowel obstruction. Stools are frequently positive for occult blood, because malignancy and diverticular disease are common etiologies.

Adynamic ileus may simulate mechanical obstruction. It occurs with peritoneal irritation, acute retroperitoneal disease, hypokalemia and ischemia, as well as after operative manipulation of bowel. The patient with an ileus complains of distention, often accompanied by steady abdominal discomfort and frequent vomiting of small quantities of bile and gastric contents. On examination, there is abdominal distention; bowel sounds may be absent.

Sudden *obstruction* of the *common bile duct* or *cystic duct* by a stone produces acute pain, sometimes referred to as biliary "colic." Unlike the cramping pain of acute intestinal obstruction, the pain of biliary tract obstruction is mostly steady, lasting hours after sudden onset. In acute cholecystitis, the typical pain is maximal in the right upper quadrant radiating in the scapular region, accompanied by nausea, vomiting and fever without jaundice; at times there is only mild epigastric discomfort (see Chapter 69). In common duct obstruction, the pain is more likely to be epigastric and jaundice is noted soon after onset.

Obstruction within the *urinary tract* can present as abdominal pain. Acute ureteral blockade by a stone is extremely uncomfortable; the pain is cramping, beginning in the back and flank and radiating into the lower abdomen and groin. If acute pyelonephritis develops, upper abdominal pain, fever and chills may ensue. Acute bladder outflow obstruction presents as lower abdominal distention and pain. Symptoms of prostatism (see Chapter 131) may precede the episode.

Peritoneal irritation may cause severe pain, due to the rich innervation of the parietal peritoneum. Focal injury results in well-localized discomfort that is described as sharp, aching, or burning in quality. Spread of the irritant process leads to more generalized abdominal pain. Severity is related to the nature of the irritant and its speed of onset. There can be reflex spasm of the overlying abdominal wall musculature, producing involuntary guarding. Rebound tenderness is prominent on physical examination, bowel sounds are reduced or absent. The patient lies still, because movement exacerbates the pain. The source of peritoneal irritation need not be intra-abdominal.

Acute arterial insufficiency of the bowel may present with little more than diffuse, mild pain and hyperperistalsis that occur as a consequence of an increase in the local concentration of metabolites and mild nerve irritation. Continued ischemia leads to infarction, with signs of peritoneal soiling and shock.

Chronic arterial insufficiency may precede an acute episode of infarction, especially in cases of progressive atherosclerotic narrowing. The patient complains of episodes of cramping or dull midabdominal pain that come on 15 to 30 minutes after a meal and can last up to 2 or 3 hours. This so-called abdominal angina is greatest at times of maximal demand for blood supply to the bowel, e.g., after a large meal.

Mucosal ulceration of the upper gastrointestinal tract is accompanied by pain in over 50 per cent of cases. Although the exact mechanism of pain in ulcer disease remains incompletely understood, it is believed that acid plays a major role. This hypothesis is supported by the observation that antacid therapy often provides immediate relief. Pain pattern of duodenal ulcer disease usually parallels the acid-peptic cycle (see Chapter 64). Unless there is perforation or penetration into the pancreas, the pain is mostly confined to the epigastrium. Patients use such terms as gnawing, aching and burning to describe their discomfort.

Alteration in bowel motility may occur with *functional disturbances,* of which the irritable colon syndrome is the best example. Spasmodic, nonpropulsive segmental contractions of large bowel result in development of high intraluminal pressures and cramping lower abdominal pain. Constipation alternating with diarrhea is a characteristic presentation (see Chapter 66). Diverticular disease is also associated with altered motility and pain (see Chapter 67). *Inflammation* often results in disturbances of motility and absorption. Acute gastroenteritis and acute flares of inflammatory bowel disease (see Chapter 65) can produce cramping abdominal pain and diarrhea. In most instances, the pain is diffuse, but occasionally it is focal and can simulate appendicitis or other surgical conditions. Fever, nausea and vomiting are often prominent in the early stages of gastroenteritis; bowel sounds are usually hyperactive.

Capsular distention or inflammation results in constant, aching abdominal pain. The thin covering of connective tissue surrounding the liver and spleen is well innervated. With liver involvement, the pain localizes to the epigastrium and right upper quadrant; in the spleen, the discomfort is maximal in the left upper quadrant. If the overlying diaphragm becomes involved in the pathologic process, the patient may report pain radiating to the shoulder on the involved side. Among the most serious causes of acute splenic pain is rupture secondary to blunt trauma, as occurs in many automobile accidents. There can be a deceptive period of many hours before peritoneal signs develop if a subcapsular hematoma temporarily retards the spilling of blood into the peritoneum.

Metabolic disturbances may mimic intra-abdominal etiologies. *Porphyria* and *lead poisoning* sometimes simulate bowel obstruction, for they can cause cramping abdominal pain and hyperperistalsis. *Ketoacidosis* has been found to present with severe abdominal pain in 8 per cent of instances, and may be accompanied by emesis and an elevated white cell count. Sometimes, it can be precipitated by an acute intra-abdominal problem such as cholecystitis.

Nerve injury is a cause of pain resembling an intra-abdominal source. Irritation of a root that serves the abdomen may result from herpes infection or extrinsic compression. The pain is often lancinating and occurs in the distribution of the nerve; hyperesthesia is reported. There is no relationship between the pain and bowel function. With root irritation there may be associated rectus spasm, which is either relieved or unaffected by palpation, as opposed to the increase in spasm seen with peritoneal irritation. The pain of herpes infection often precedes the rash by several days and may persist after the skin clears, particularly in the elderly (see Chapter 184).

Abdominal wall pathology can also be mistaken for disease inside the abdominal cavity. Traumatic injury to the musculature of the wall produces pain that is constant, aching and exacerbated by movement or pressure on the abdomen. The muscles may be in spasm, simulating the involuntary guarding of peritonitis. When a generalized myositis is responsible for the muscle pain, there is discomfort in the limbs as well as in the abdomen. Occasionally, a tender mass in the wall, such as a hematoma, is found to be the source of difficulty.

Referred pain from a process originating in the chest is sometimes an etiology of abdominal complaints. Pulmonary infarction and pneumonia of the lower lobes are among the chest problems that may present as pain in the upper abdomen; at times there is even reflex muscle spasm accompanying the pain.

Upper abdominal pain, nausea and vomiting may be the principal manifestations of an acute inferior myocardial infarction. Fortunately, most intrathoracic sources of abdominal pain are accompanied by symptoms and signs of cardiac or pulmonary disease.

Psychogenic pain is among the most complex forms of abdominal pain; it is variable in presentation. Mechanisms range from simple motility disturbances found in anxious or mildly neurotic patients to intrapsychic disorders in which the pain has symbolic meaning. In general, the pain pattern differs from that typical of "organic" illness; it tends to have little relationship to physiologic stimuli; also, physical examination findings often diminish with distraction. Such features are characteristic, but by no means universal, findings. At times, it is very hard to distinguish psychogenic pain from that due to intra-abdominal pathology.

Clinical presentations of abdominal pain due to organ pathology or functional disturbances are determined, in part, by site of involvement. Although generalizations concerning the location of pain are at best crude, a few are clinically useful. Lower esophageal pain is usually subxyphoid but may be referred to the back. Gastric and duodenal disease produces epigastric discomfort, which sometimes radiates into the back. Pain from the small bowel is usually periumbilical but likely to occur in the right lower quadrant when the terminal ileum is involved. Most colonic pain is felt in the lower abdomen, particularly the left lower quadrant; with rectosigmoid problems, referral may be to the sacrum. Disease of the transverse colon may give upper abdominal discomfort. Gallbladder and common bile duct obstruction result in epigastric or right upper quadrant complaints, with characteristic radiation to the scapular region. Pancreatic pain is usually midline or to left of the epigastrium, with radiation into the back. Diffuse pain is seen with generalized peritonitis, metabolic disturbances and psychogenic illness, though all may produce focal complaints.

DIFFERENTIAL DIAGNOSIS

Since the number of possible causes of abdominal pain is large, it is helpful to consider the differential diagnosis in terms of pathophysiologic mechanisms (see Table 53–1). Etiologies causing obstruction, peritoneal irritation and vascular insufficiency are among the most dangerous. About 70 per cent of mechanical small bowel obstruction is due to adhesions

Table 53-1. Principle Mechanisms of Abdominal Pain

OBSTRUCTION	ALTERED MOTILITY
1. Gastric outlet	1. Gastroenteritis
2. Small bowel	2. Inflammatory bowel disease
3. Large bowel	
4. Biliary tract	3. Irritable colon
5. Urinary tract	4. Diverticular disease
PERITONEAL IRRITATION	**METABOLIC DISTURBANCE**
1. Infection	1. Diabetic ketoacidosis
2. Chemical irritation (blood, bile, gastric acid)	2. Porphyria
	3. Lead poisoning
3. Systemic inflammatory process	**NERVE INJURY**
	1. Herpes zoster
4. Spread from a local inflammatory process	2. Root compression
	MUSCLE WALL DISEASE
VASCULAR INSUFFICIENCY	1. Trauma
1. Embolization	2. Myositis
2. Atherosclerotic narrowing	3. Hematoma
	REFERRED PAIN
3. Hypotension	1. Pneumonia (lower lobes)
4. Aortic aneurysm dissection	
	2. Inferior myocardial infarction
MUCOSAL ULCERATION	3. Pulmonary infarction
1. Peptic ulcer disease	**PSYCHOLOGICAL STRESS**
2. Gastric cancer	1. Depression
	2. Situational stress
	3. Intrapsychic conflict

or external hernias; 90 per cent of large bowel obstruction is attributable to diverticular disease and carcinoma. Acute arterial insufficiency results most often from systemic embolization due to atrial fibrillation, severe atherosclerotic occlusive disease, and severe congestive failure with hypoperfusion. Pelvic pathology is a common extra-abdominal source of peritoneal irritation.

Other pathophysiologic mechanisms, such as nerve injury, metabolic imbalance, abdominal wall disease, disordered motility, and emotional conflict, may produce symptoms that superficially mimic a more worrisome etiology; but usually conditions associated with these mechanisms are more annoying than dangerous (an important exception is diabetic ketoacidosis). Pain referred from an extra-abdominal site is more of a problem; significant cardiac disease (e.g., inferior myocardial infarction) or pulmonary pathology (e.g., lower lobe pneumonia) may present as abdominal pain.

WORKUP

The first priority in the office evaluation of the patient with *acute abdominal pain* is to determine the likelihood of serious pathophysiology and the need for immediate hospitalization. The assessment requires examining for evidence of obstruction, peritoneal irritation, acute vascular insufficiency, and acute cardiopulmonary disease.

History. In addition to carefully obtaining a complete description of the patient's pain, checking for specific items is needed: prior abdominal surgery, previous episodes of obstruction, known gallbladder or kidney stones, presence and nature of vomitus, passage of flatus, time of last bowel movement, occurrence of diarrhea, constipation or change in bowel habits, effect of movement on pain, presence of fever and rigors, development of distention, difficulties in urination, and presence of any cardiac or pulmonary symptoms. Inquiry into symptoms of pelvic pathology, such as dyspareunia, abnormal vaginal discharge, and irregular menstrual bleeding, should be included in the assessment of every woman with abdominal pain.

On physical examination, particular attention ought to be paid to the patient's general appearance. The patient who appears reluctant to change position and keeps still is likely to have peritoneal irritation, whereas the patient with obstruction is often restless. It is important to check the vital signs for postural changes in blood pressure or heart rate, because obstruction, peritonitis, and bowel infarction can produce large losses of intravascular volume. Any hypotension, atrial fibrillation or fever should be noted; however, absence of fever does not rule out serious pathology, especially in the elderly or chronically ill patient. The skin is examined for jaundice, the sclera for icterus, the chest for splinting, a pleural friction rub, and signs of consolidation (particularly in the lower lobes), and the heart for murmurs, chamber enlargement and signs of heart failure.

One should take note of any abdominal distention, absent bowel sounds, borborygmi, focal tenderness, rebound, involuntary guarding, masses (including a distended bladder or dilated aorta) and tenderness at the costovertebral angles. If psychogenic pain is suspected, deep palpation ought to be done while the patient is distracted. Stool should be tested for occult blood, and the prostate and rectum examined for masses. Every woman with abdominal pain requires a full pelvic examination. The elderly person with an acute intra-abdominal process may at first show few signs of serious illness. Peritoneal signs may be absent or minimal. The only early clues may be unexplained mild fever, tachycardia, and vague abdominal discomfort. A high index of suspicion is needed.

Testing for nerve and muscle wall injury are often overlooked in the urgency of searching for more worrisome pathology. Two important signs of nerve involvement are pain in a dermatomal distribution and hyperesthesia. Both occur with nerve injury due to herpes zoster or nerve root impingement; however, hyperesthesia is also seen with focal peritoneal irritation. Testing is performed by gentle stroking of the skin overlying the area of pain. The rash of herpes may not appear until the time of the follow-up assessment. Abdominal wall pathology may be discovered by careful palpation of the wall for masses and muscle tenderness and by exacerbation of pain on contracting the muscles, as occurs with sitting up. Any pain on sitting up should not be confused with that due to involuntary muscle spasm from peritoneal irritation. The limbs should also be checked for muscle tenderness, which is suggestive of a generalized muscle disorder.

Laboratory tests. Relatively few are needed at the time of initial assessment. Studies are aimed at helping to determine the likelihood of obstruction, peritonitis, acute vascular insufficiency, metabolic disruption, and cardiac or pulmonary disease. The *complete blood count* (CBC) and *differential* are often helpful in confirming the presence of an acute inflammatory process. Though very nonspecific, the CBC and differential are reasonably sensitive in patients able to mount a normal acute inflammatory response. Unfortunately, the CBC may show little change in the elderly or chronically ill patient, even in an acute intra-abdominal emergency. The differential ought to be ordered even if the white cell count in "normal," because a shift to immature forms sometimes occurs without a significant elevation in the white count. At times a relatively benign condition such as viral gastroenteritis may produce an impressive elevation in the white cell count (as high as 20,000 cells per cc.) accompanied by a marked shift to immature forms, simulating the peripheral blood picture of a patient with more worrisome disease. The CBC and differential must be carefully interpreted in the context of the entire clinical picture and not used alone to decide whether or not to admit the patient.

Supine and upright *plain films of the abdomen* are essential if one suspects bowel obstruction. Multiple air-fluid levels, distention of the small bowel, and absence of gas in the large bowel are characteristic of complete small bowel obstruction; unfortunately, such findings are present in less than 50 per cent of cases of bowel strangulation, especially in the early stages of obstruction. Partial mechanical obstruction may produce some loops of bowel with air-fluid levels, but there is also gas in the colon; the same findings are found in patients with adynamic ileus. In colonic obstruction with a competent ileocecal valve, only the large bowel appears distended, but if the valve is not competent, both large and small bowel demonstrate distention and gas, mimicking the findings adynamic ileus. Distinguishing partial small bowel obstruction from ileus requires repeat films or a barium study. Suspected obstruction of the large bowel is an indication for a barium enema and a contraindication to performing an upper gastrointestinal series. Plain films of the abdomen in peritoneal irritation and acute vascular insufficiency are not very informative; a nonspecific ileus may be present. Films of the abdomen are sometimes of help in locating a stone in the urinary tract or biliary tree or in delineating a calcified aortic aneurysm. Calcification has been found on plain film of the abdomen in over 60 per cent of abdominal aneurysms.

Other simple tests can aid the initial evaluation. A *urinalysis* should be checked for pyuria, hematuria, bacteria, sugar and ketones. Mild to moderate ketonuria is common when the patient has not eaten and is unrelated to diabetes; the diagnosis of ketoacidosis requires urine ketones in large concentrations (see Chapter 98). Red cells in the urine of a patient with flank pain suggests a stone in the ureter (see Chapter 130). The *BUN, glucose* and *amylase* levels can often be obtained on a stat basis. Elevation of the serum amylase occurs not only in pancreatitis, but also in intestinal obstruction; an amylase-creatinine clearance ratio may be needed to identify the source of the elevation (see Chapter 72). Most other chemistries are not particularly helpful for immediate decision-making, because results are usually not available for 24 hours. Nonetheless transaminase, alkaline phosphatase, and bilirubin determinations can be ordered at the outset to help guide later stages of evaluation in the patient with upper abdominal pain. The initial investigation of acute upper abdominal pain should also include a *chest film* and *electrocardiogram,* looking for pleuropulmonary disease in the lower lobes and acute ischemic changes in the inferior myocardium. The patient with acute colicky pain but no signs of obstruction or inflammation may have porphyria or lead poisoning and should have urine samples checked for porphobilinogen (Watson-Schwartz test) and coproporphyrin respectively. Serum lead levels are unreliable.

Once it is determined that acute obstruction, peritonitis, bowel ischemia, and worrisome metabolic and cardiopulmonary diseases are unlikely, further evaluation can be carried out on an outpatient basis, at a more gradual pace. Among the most productive diagnostic measures is repetition of the history and physical examination. An inconsistent history raises the question of psychogenic pain; however, constancy certainly does not rule out an emotional etiology. Many serious etiologies may lead to a worsening of the clinical picture in a few days; this is particularly true for bowel ischemia, which initially may have an indolent presentation. Any patient sent home with undiagnosed acute pain requires careful follow-up and re-examination.

Selection of radiologic *contrast studies* ought to be judicious and based on the need to confirm or rule out specific diagnoses. Blind searches that involve "running the bowel" in the absence of suggestive clinical evidence are wasteful, potentially misleading, and uncomfortable for the patient. Recurrent epigastric or right upper quadrant pain in conjunction with an elevated alkaline phosphatase is an indication for a oral cholecystogram and/or ultrasound study (see Chapter 69). Epigastric pain that parallels the acid-peptic cycle or responds to food or antacids may require an upper GI series to search for an ulcer, supplemented by endoscopy, particularly if the patient is in the age range for a gastric malignancy (see Chapter 64). Episodes of lower abdominal pain in conjunction with a change in bowel habits or a guaiac-positive stool ought to be investigated by barium enema, though the young patient with a history consistent with irritable colon syndrome and guaiac-negative stools can be spared a barium study unless refractory to treatment, because the chances of malignancy are very remote (see Chapters 59, 60, and 66). At times, there is little clinical indication for a contrast study, but the patient insists on having one done. The contribution of a normal test result to the peace of mind of the patient has to be taken into account when deciding which tests to obtain.

A number of areas are worth exploring in the evaluation of the patient with *persistent* or *recurrent pain* that remains undiagnosed. Inquiry into *psychosocial issues* may prove productive. One can initiate the assessment by ascertaining the effect the pain has had on the patient's life and by exploring the patient's fears and concerns. A frontal assault on psychosocial problems can be counter-productive, especially if the patient believes the pain is not a manifestation of emotional upset. To suggest at the outset that the problem may be psychogenic before undertaking a careful medical assessment is to invite resistance and hostility. However, once a thorough

medical assessment has been concluded, it may be much easier to work with the patient in exploring areas of conflict, stress, and loss.

Occasionally a metabolic problem may simulate a psychologic etiology. The patient with acute intermittent porphyria may be mistaken for a person with neurotic or even psychotic complaints, but the diagnosis is suggested by periodic attacks of cramping pain, constipation, nausea and vomiting, and neuromuscular symptoms in conjunction with an altered psychological state. The *Watson-Schwartz test* for urinary porphobilinogen is a reliable screening test for acute intermittent porphyria in patients who are symptomatic.

Malignancy is an important diagnostic consideration in the patient with unexplained persistent pain. Upper abdominal location, radiation into the back, and impressive weight loss in a patient over age 40 suggests carcinoma of the body or tail of the pancreas. Onset of jaundice in association with chronic persistent pain is indicative of tumor in the head of the pancreas obstructing the common duct. Noninvasive diagnosis of pancreatic malignancy and other upper abdominal tumors may be greatly facilitated by *ultrasound* and *computerized tomography*. Sensitivities for each are reported to be in the range of 80 to 90 per cent. Experience with these techniques is still relatively limited, and false-positive readings are to be expected. Which test is preferable is unresolved at present, but ultrasound has the advantages of lower cost and no ionizing radiation. Because these tests are expensive, they should not be ordered without some clinical evidence for neoplasm. However, they are far less costly and morbid in comparison to exploratory surgery. Moreover a treatable condition simulating cancer, such as a pancreatic pseudocyst (see Chapter 72), may be identified. Suspected enlargement of the liver and/or spleen can be well documented by *radionuclide scanning*. Sensitivity for detection of a mass lesion in the liver by scan is 80 to 85 per cent; lesions smaller than 1.5 cm. are likely to be missed.

Therapeutic trials for diagnostic purposes are sometimes informative. Patients with suspected peptic ulcer disease can be given a course of antacid therapy or cimetidine (see Chapter 64); those with probable irritable bowel syndrome might be tried on a high fiber diet (see Chapter 66); tricyclic therapy may prove beneficial to the depressed patient with abdominal pain of unclear etiology (see chapter 215), though constipation may ensue and worsen the problem, if it is not due to depression.

The patient with chronic or recurrent abdominal

pain that defies explanation poses one of the most difficult problems in clinical medicine. In a study of 30 such patients presenting to a general internist, most had epigastric pain, distention, belching and nausea without vomiting or weight loss. Symptoms often began at the time of a personal loss or other emotional stress. Depression was commonly found. Treatment directed at depression was associated with the disappearance of pain in many instances. In a study of 64 patients with abdominal pain of unknown etiology, two thirds of patients were women. The younger the age and shorter the duration of the symptoms, the better the chances were for improvement. Older women with pain for more than 3 months were least likely to improve or to be diagnosed. Of those subjected to laparotomy, a diagnosis was obtained in only 10 per cent; the rate of improvement was the same as for those who did not undergo exploration. In 15 per cent of the total study population, a cause for the patient's abdominal pain was found, but in only 6 per cent did the condition require surgery. Thus very few patients with abdominal pain of unknown eitology are endangered by continued observation, as long as signs of serious pathophysiology are absent. Unexplained pain that is present for less than 2 weeks is likely to resolve spontaneously, but such improvement is unlikely when pain has persisted for more than 3 months.

INDICATIONS FOR ADMISSION AND REFERRAL

Any evidence suggestive of peritoneal irritation, obstruction or acute vascular compromise is an indication for immediate hospitalization and surgical consultation. Sometimes further observations made in the hospital can save the patient a surgical procedure, but no patient with the possibility of a condition that might require urgent surgery should be sent home from the office. Elderly patients are especially likely to have subtle presentations.

The patient with unexplained pain that has defied outpatient diagnostic attempts may benefit from further assessment in the hospital, especially if a need for large amounts of pain medication has developed. Admission provides an opportunity for 24-hour observation and specialty consultation. The need for further noninvasive study utilizing ultrasound, radionuclide scanning, or computerized tomography can be assessed, as can the utility of invasive investigations. Laparoscopy should be undertaken before laparotomy; it allows direct visualization of the sur-

face of the liver, gallbladder, spleen, peritoneum, diaphragm and pelvic viscera. Biopsy can be performed through the laparoscope and laparotomy may be avoided in some instances. Anything that can be done to obviate the need for an exploratory laparotomy is warranted. In an Australian study of 81 medical patients with undiagnosed abdominal pain subjected to laparotomy, 15 per cent died in the perioperative period and 40 per cent suffered morbidity from the surgery.

SYMPTOMATIC THERAPY

Patients with acute abdominal pain of unknown etiology should not be given analgesics, because important findings may be obscured. Although the patient with undiagnosed chronic pain often requests pain medication, regular use of narcotics ought to be avoided, because the risk of addiction is extremely high; many such patients have underlying psychopathology and a strong potential for narcotic abuse. The patient with terminal cancer must not be denied the relief afforded by narcotics, even if the cause of pain is not fully defined (see Chapter 89).

ANNOTATED BIBLIOGRAPHY

Cope, A.: Early diagnosis of the acute abdomen. London, ed. 14. Oxford University Press, 1972. *(A concise, systematic approach to diagnosis of acute abdominal problems. Emphasis is on history and physical findings; required reading for the primary physician.)*

DiMagno, E.P.: Pancreatic cancer: A continuing diagnostic dilemma. Ann. Intern. Med. *90*:847, 1979. (Critical editorial on available diagnostic techniques.)

Hermann, R.E., and Cooperman, A.M.: Cancer of the pancreas. N. Engl. J. Med., *301*:482, 1979. *(A short review, including discussion of methods of diagnosis; 30 refs.)*

Heukin, R.E.: Intra-abdominal imaging via nuclear medicine techniques. Radiol. Clin. North Am., *17*:39, 1979. *(Discusses the indications for use of radionuclide studies in abdominal disease; sensitivity of liver scan for detection of mass lesions felt to be 80 to 85 per cent; 39 refs.)*

Hill, O.W., and Blendis, L.: Physical and psychological evaluation of "non-organic" abdominal pain. Gut, 8:221, 1967. *(This study of 31 consecutive patients with undiagnosed abdominal pain showed a high frequency of epigastric discomfort, distention, nausea, and belching without vomiting or weight loss. Bereavement or emotional upheaval often initiated symptoms.)*

Lee, J.K., Stanley R.J., Melson, G.L., *et al.*: Pancreatic imaging by ultrasound and computed tomography. Radiol. Clin. North Am., *17*:105, 1979. *(A critical review of these 2 methods for diagnosis of pancreatic mass lesions; 50 refs.)*

Sarfeh, I.J.: Abdominal pain of unknown etiology. Am. J. Surg., *132*:22, 1976. *(Over two-thirds of cases were in women. Improvement was most likely in younger patients with symptoms of less than 2 weeks' duration. Laparotomy did not influence rate of improvement, and it established diagnosis in only 1 of 23 patients explored.)*

Scott, P.J., *et al.*: Benefits and hazards of laparotomy for medical patients. Lancet, *2*:941, 1970. *(Exploration established a diagnosis in 69 of 81 patients with extensive medical work-ups and no firm diagnosis. A remediable cause was found in 40%, but the incidence of morbidity was 45%, and perioperative mortality, 15%.)*

54
Evaluation of Nausea and Vomiting

Nausea and vomiting are extremely common. In one study of primary care practice, nausea and vomiting ranked second only to symptoms of upper-respiratory-tract infection. Not only is the problem a source of misery for the patient, it may be an early manifestation of a serious illness. Although many cases are self-limited, the discomfort produced, the possibility of important underlying pathology, and the potential for fluid and electrolyte disturbances make efficient assessment and effective control of symptoms important priorities.

PATHOPHYSIOLOGY AND CLINICAL PRESENTATION

A wide range of noxious stimuli trigger vomiting; these include gastric irritation, distention of a hollow viscus, myocardial ischemia, increased intracranial pressure, vertigo, metabolic disturbances, drugs, pharyngeal stimulation, and emotional upset. Vagal and sympathetic afferents in the pharynx, heart, peritoneum, mesentery, bile ducts, stomach, and bowel transmit impulses to the vomiting center in the medullary reticular formation. Vestibular disturbances, drugs, and metabolic derangements stimulate the chemoreceptor trigger zone in the floor of the fourth ventricle, which, in turn, activates the vomiting center. A cortical pathway to the vomiting center has been postulated. Emetic responses are mediated by the vomiting center by way of reflex arcs involving somatic and autonomic efferent fibers.

The act of vomiting is a stereotyped response that varies little regardless of cause. Even so-called projectile vomiting (which is characterized by forceful emesis without prior nausea or retching), supposedly limited to cases of increased intracranial pressure, occurs in other conditions. Moreover, nausea, retching, and nonprojectile vomiting are seen with increased intracranial pressure. Nausea and vomiting may be only one part of a symptom complex or dominate the clinical picture (as in psychogenic vomiting, early pregnancy, digitalis toxicity, and metabolic disturbances).

Early morning nausea and vomiting is quite typical of *metabolic etiologies*. Up to 75 per cent of cases of diabetic ketoacidosis are accompanied by nausea and vomiting. Emesis and nausea are found among as many as 90 per cent of patients in Addisonian crisis. Uremia may be heralded by similar symptoms; nausea often improves with correction of any associated hyponatremia, but can be refractory. Binge drinkers experience early morning nausea and dry heaves from excessive alcohol intake.

Early pregnancy is associated with mild early morning nausea and vomiting in over 50 per cent of instances. The problem is severe in less than 1 per cent, leading to electrolyte abnormalities, dehydration, and weight loss. Most cases are mild; symptoms begin after the first missed period and terminate by the fourth month. Women with severe cases often have a history of vomiting in response to psychosocial stress. The diagnosis of pregnancy is sometimes overlooked.

In contrast to the causes of early morning vomiting, symptoms can be triggered shortly after eating by psychoneurotic illness, bile reflux, peptic ulcer disease and gastritis. *Psychogenic vomiting* is characterized by years of recurrent emesis. It can often be traced back to childhood and is more frequent when there is a family history of vomiting. Patients report that symptoms appear just after eating and can be sufficiently controlled voluntarily to avoid vomiting in public. Some admit to inducing emesis; most are surprisingly untroubled by the problem. Nausea accompanies almost all episodes. A study of 20 patients with psychogenic vomiting revealed a marked predominance of women who were engaged in hostile relationships; abdominal pain and depression were uncommon.

A *pyloric channel ulcer* or *acute gastritis* may be associated with marked postprandial emesis. The vomiting in ulcer disease is believed due in part to irritation, edema and spasm of the pyloric sphincter mechanism. Concurrent bleeding can lead to vomiting of coffee-groundlike material. Patients who undergo surgery for peptic ulcer may be troubled by recurrent *bilious vomiting*, which is believed due to reflux of bile into the stomach or gastric remnant. Patients vomit bile within 15 minutes of eating; little food is present. Nausea and a bad taste in the mouth are present on awakening in the morning.

Gastric retention results in vomiting of food eaten more than 6 hours previously. A succussion splash is detectable on examination, and food is seen in the stomach on upper GI series. In chronic cases there may be gastric outflow obstruction or atony secondary to diabetic neuropathy, anticholinergic use, or gastric malignancy. Transient gastric dilatation is a frequent concomitant of pancreatitis, peritonitis, gallbladder disease, and hypokalemia.

Acute episodes of vomiting accompany a host of conditions, ranging from the self-limited to the life-threatening. The most common is *viral gastroenteritis*. After many years of attributing this illness to viral infection, investigators have finally isolated and identified the responsible viruses. Explosive bouts of nausea and vomiting in conjunction with watery diarrhea, cramping abdominal pain, myalgias, headache and fever are typical. Recovery is rapid in most instances, but symptoms may linger for 7 to 10 days.

Acute gastroenteritis that results from *food poisoning* due to salmonella or shigella infection has a similar clinical presentation and course; onset is 24 to 48 hours after exposure to the contaminated food. Domestic fowl represent the largest single reservoir of salmonella infection. Inadequate cooking is often responsible for human infection. Intake of pastries and similar items containing staphylococcal enterotoxin causes symptoms indistinguishable from viral gastroenteritis, except that onset is within 1 to 6 hours of eating the spoiled food, fever is rare, and complete clearing takes place by 24 to 48 hours. Clostridial food poisoning rarely produces prominent nausea and vomiting.

A number of intra-abdominal emergencies may precipitate acute emesis, such as peritoneal irritation and acute obstruction of a hollow viscus. Often they are accompanied by severe abdominal pain (see Chapter 53). *Intestinal obstruction*, especially of the proximal small bowel, produces marked nausea and vomiting of bilious material. Distention may be lacking, but intermittent cramping abdominal pain is characteristic. Feculent emesis is found in distal small bowel obstruction. In *acute pancreatitis*, emesis is seen in 85 per cent of patients; however, upper abdominal pain radiating into the back is the cardinal symptom, occurring in 95 per cent (see Chapter 72). Anorexia, nausea, and vomiting are early symptoms in over 90 per cent of patients with *acute appendicitis*; usually emesis clears early. As with pancreatitis, pain typically precedes other symptoms. *Acute pyelonephritis* may mimic a gastrointestinal etiology, by causing nausea, vomiting and abdominal pain. *Acute cholecystitis* sometimes triggers acute emesis, but less regularly than does *acute cholangitis* due to sudden obstruction of the common duct.

Myocardial infarction may activate vagal afferents and produce nausea, vomiting, and epigastric discomfort simulating intra-abdominal disease. A prospective series of 62 patients with acute infarction revealed nausea and vomiting at the outset in 69 per cent of those with inferior infarctions and 27 per cent of those with anterior infarctions.

Neurologic emergencies can provoke severe bouts of acute emesis. In *midline cerebellar hemorrhage*, nausea and vomiting are profuse, in association with severe gait ataxia; meningeal signs and headache are seen as well. Within a few hours the patient may become comatose and die unless promptly diagnosed and treated (see Chapter 153). One third of patients with *increased intracranial pressure* experience vomiting. When it is sudden, forceful, and not preceded by nausea it is termed "projectile," but this presentation is not specific. Concurrent bifrontal or biocciptal headache is the rule. *Migraine headaches* and *vestibular disease* are less worrisome neurologic causes of acute emesis (see Chapters 160 and 154). The former is suggested by photophobia and throbbing unilateral headache; the latter by vertigo.

Of the many *drugs* that induce vomiting, digitalis intoxication is among the most serious. Anorexia is an early sign, followed by nausea and vomiting due to stimulation of the chemoreceptor trigger zone. Visual disturbances such as colored haloes are suggestive of the diagnosis (see Chapter 27). Hypokalemia and dehydration induced by vomiting may precipitate or worsen digitalis toxicity. Unfortunately, most cancer chemotherapeutic agents produce substantial nausea and vomiting (see Chapter 88).

Drug withdrawal as well as drug excess may trigger emesis. Nausea, dry heaves, and retching beginning at about 36 hours are characteristic features of the opiate withdrawal syndrome. Sweats, chills, and restlessness precede other symptoms; the vomiting peaks by 72 hours and subsides.

Anorexia, nausea and vomiting often dominate the prodromal stage of *acute viral hepatitis* (see Chapter 70).

DIFFERENTIAL DIAGNOSIS

Table 54–1. lists some of the more common and important conditions associated with prominent nausea and vomiting. Causes of simple regurgitation are omitted from the list since they are usually manifestations of esophageal difficulties (see Chapter 57) and unaccompanied by emesis. The etiologies are listed according to clinical presentation.

WORKUP

History and physical examination supplemented by a few well-chosen laboratory studies are sufficient for diagnosis in most cases.

History should focus on such details as timing of symptoms, their relation to meals, characteristics of the vomitus, and associated complaints. Early-morning onset points to metabolic disturbances, alcoholic binge, and early pregnancy. Emesis precipitated by meals suggests psychogenic vomiting, pyloric channel ulcer, and gastritis. Onset a few hours after eating raises the possibility of gastric-outflow tract obstruction, gastric atony or bowel obstruction. Vomiting blood or coffee-ground material is indicative of gastritis and ulcer disease. Bilious vomitus means that the pyloric channel is open. When the material vomited is pure gastric juice, peptic ulcer disease and Zollinger-Ellison syndrome are suggested. Lack of acid suggests gastric cancer. Feculent material is a sign of distal small-bowel obstruction and blind-loop syndrome.

The history needs to include inquiry into abdominal pain, fever, jaundice, weight loss, abdominal surgery, external hernias, contaminated food source, family history of emesis, symptoms of diabetes, prior renal disease, ischemic heart disease, drug use (*e.g.,* digitalis, narcotics), visual disturbances, headache, ataxia, vertigo, last menstrual period, and concurrent emotional stresses and conflicts.

Physical examination requires a check for postural hypotension, malignant hypertension, irregularities of rate and rhythm, Kussmaul breathing, pallor, hyperpigmentation, jaundice, papilledema, retinopathy, nystagmus, stiff neck, abdominal distention, visible peristalsis, abnormal bowel sounds, succussion splash, peritoneal signs, focal tenderness, organomegaly, masses, flank tenderness, muscle weakness, ataxia of gait, and asterixis.

Laboratory studies. A surgical problem must be ruled out when there is acute onset of nausea and vomiting in conjunction with abdominal pain (see

Table 54–1. Some Important Causes of Nausea and Vomiting

NAUSEA/VOMITING AS PREDOMINANT OR INITIAL SYMPTOMS
ACUTE
1. Digitalis toxicity
2. Ketoacidosis*
3. Opiate use
4. Cancer chemotherapeutic agents
5. Early pregnancy
6. Inferior myocardial infarction*
7. Drug withdrawal
8. Binge drinking
9. Hepatitis
RECURRENT OR CHRONIC
1. Psychogenic vomiting
2. Metabolic disturbancies (uremia; adrenal insufficiency
3. Gastric retention
4. Bile reflux postgastric surgery
5. Pregnancy

NAUSEA/VOMITING IN ASSOCIATION WITH ABDOMINAL PAIN
1. Viral gastroenteritis
2. Acute gastritis
3. Food poisoning
4. Peptic ulcer disease
5. Acute pancreatitis
6. Small bowel obstruction
7. Acute appendicitis
8. Acute cholecystitis
9. Acute cholangitis
10. Acute pyelonephritis
11. Inferior myocardial infarction

NAUSEA/VOMITING IN ASSOCIATION WITH NEUROLOGIC SYMPTOMS
1. Increased intracranial pressure
2. Midline cerebellar hemorrhage
3. Vestibular disturbances
4. Migraine headaches

*Abdominal pain sometimes present.

Chapter 53). Acute nausea and vomiting without abdominal pain may also be a clue to serious illness. When encountered acutely in association with ataxia of gait and a stiff neck, an emergency computerized tomography scan is mandatory, since detection and prompt treatment of a midline cerebellar hemorrhage may be lifesaving (see Chapter 53).

Acute vomiting of unclear etiology without focal signs should be pursued by carefully checking medications. If a digitalis preparation is being taken, the drug should be withheld, an electrocardiogram obtained, a serum level ordered and a potassium supplement prescribed if the potassium level is below 4.0 mg. per 100 ml. (see Chapter 27).

Recurrent vomiting of unknown etiology raises the question of a psychogenic cause. The patient with psychogenic vomiting can be recognized by the characteristic history of chronic emesis, with vomiting around mealtime, partial suppressibility, and a conflict-ridden social situation. The need for additional studies in such cases is best individualized, since some patients may insist on further testing while others may be comforted by knowing that extensive studies are not necessary. Any woman of childbearing age whose vomiting is suspected to have a psychogenic cause should always have a pregnancy test before concluding that emesis is emotional in origin.

Elimination of pregnancy and psychogenic causes leaves metabolic disorders and gastric pathology among possible antecedents of recurrent emesis. Metabolic disease is suggested by vomiting that occurs in the early morning. A urinalysis and determinations of the serum BUN, creatinine, electrolytes, and glucose should be obtained. An upper GI series can confirm gastric outlet obstruction or retention. Sometimes endoscopy is necessary for assessment of the stomach (see Chapter 64). The suspicion of hepatitis can be confirmed by obtaining a transaminase level (see Chapter 70).

SYMPTOMATIC RELIEF

When treatment of the underlying condition is insufficient to control symptoms, drug therapy can provide relief, especially when it is used prophylactically. The available agents work by suppressing the vomiting center, chemoreceptor trigger zone, or peripheral receptors.

The phenothiazines are indicated for initial symptomatic treatment of vomiting caused by drugs and gastrointestinal disorders. They suppress the chemoreceptor trigger zone and probably the vomiting center and peripheral receptors as well. *Prochlorpera-*

zine (Compazine) is the phenothiazine used most often for vomiting; it can be given in doses of 5 to 10 mg. orally, every 6 hours, or 25 mg. rectally, twice daily. This class of drugs is not effective for motion sickness or vestibular disease.

The antihistamine *meclizine (Antivert)* acts on the vestibular system and the chemoreceptor trigger zone. It is best for prevention and control of motion sickness and nausea and vomiting due to vestibular disturbances. Other antihistamines with quicker onset and shorter duration of action such as *dimenhydrinate (Dramamine)* enjoy considerable popularity for motion sickness. The average dose of meclizine is 25 mg., three times daily, for vestibular disease and 25 to 50 mg., at least one hour before a trip for motion sickness. Meclizine is teratogenic in animals and not indicated for vomiting due to pregnancy. Moreover, it can cause drowsiness and should not be used prior to driving or use of machinery.

A few specific problems require elaboration:

Vomiting due to *cancer chemotherapy* is a major problem for patients being treated by drugs for malignancy. Phenothiazines sometimes suffice, but tetrahydrocannabinol has recently been demonstrated to be a potent suppressor of chemotherapy-induced nausea and vomiting (see Chapter 74).

Morning sickness is best treated with small morning feedings and support; the goal is to try to avoid use of antiemetics. If an occasional episode is particularly severe, a long-established antihistamine such as dimenhydrinate may help. The prolonged, severe form of nausea and vomiting due to pregnancy does not respond to drugs but may remit with hypnosis and/or supportive psychotherapy.

Psychogenic vomiting is best approached by attention to the conflicts troubling the patient. There are no controlled studies on effectiveness of antiemetics; fortunately, patients often do not request medication for symptomatic relief.

Phenothiazines are metabolized by the liver and in rare instances can cause jaundice; their use in controlling nausea and vomiting due to hepatitis requires close supervision.

ANNOTATED BIBLIOGRAPHY

Ahmed, S., Gupta, R., and Brancato, R.: Significance of nausea and vomiting during acute myocardial infarction. Am. Heart J., *95*:671, 1977. *(Nausea and vomiting occurred in 69% of patients with inferior infarctions, compared to 27% of those with anterior infarctions.)*

Biggs, J.: Vomiting and pregnancy. Drugs, 9:299, 1975. (A terse review of clinical presentation and therapy.)

Bordfield, P.: A controlled double-blind study of trimethobenzamide, prochlorperazine and placebo. JAMA, 196:116, 1966. (Prochlorperazine was the most effective.)

Bothe, F., and Beardwood, J.: Evaluation of abdominal symptoms in the diabetic. Ann. Surg., 105:516, 1937. (A classic study in which 75% of patients in ketoacidosis had nausea and vomiting; 8% had severe abdominal pain and elevated white counts simulating an acute abdomen. Also makes the point that intra-abdominal disease can precipitate ketoacidosis.)

Drugs for relief of nausea and vomiting. Medical Letter, 16:46, 1974. (An authoritative critique of available agents.)

Hill, O.W.: Psychogenic vomiting. Gut, 9:348, 1968. (A study comparing 20 patients with psychogenic vomiting to 22 patients with psychogenic abdominal pain. A high frequency of hostile living situations and symptoms coming on at mealtime characterized patients with vomiting.)

Kapikian, A., et al.: Human reovirus-like agent as the major pathogen associated with "winter" gastroenteritis. N. Engl. J. Med., 294:965, 1976. (An example of the isolation of such agents in acute gastroenteritis, helping to prove the link between viruses and acute gastroenteritis.)

Rimer, D.: Gastric retention without mechanical obstruction. Arch. Intern. Med., 117:287, 1966. (A good review of the problem, detailing the causes of this condition; 73 references.)

Sallen, S.E., Cronin, C., Zelen, M., et al.: Antiemetics in patients receiving chemotherapy for cancer. A randomized comparison of delta-a-tetrahydro-cannabinol and prochlorperazine. N. Engl. J. Med., 302:135, 1980. (THC proved superior to prochlorperazine in this double-blind randomized crossover trial.)

55
Evaluation of Indigestion

"Indigestion" is a vague term used by patients to denote gastrointestinal discomfort coincident with the intake and digestion of food. Symptoms include any combination of upper abdominal pain, distention, heartburn, eructation, nausea and sometimes vomiting. Almost everyone experiences such symptoms on occasion, but persistent complaints may reflect an underlying disorder of the upper gastrointestinal tract or hepatobiliary system; functional etiologies are also common.

Patients bothered by "indigestion" usually resort to a number of home remedies or over-the-counter preparations before consulting the physician. Remedies for "acid indigestion, heartburn and gas" are sold by the millions each year. The prevalence of indigestion is estimated to be as high as 250 per 1000 population, with a peak in the 25 to 44 age group and men outnumbering women by almost 2 to 1 in a British study. Because of the frequency of the problem, the discomfort it causes, and the possibility of an underlying disorder, it is important that the patient receive a thorough yet efficient evaluation. In this way a specific diagnosis can be made, etiologic therapy instituted, and proper counseling provided.

PATHOPHYSIOLOGY AND CLINICAL PRESENTATION

The term "indigestion" does not denote a specific symptom complex, but rather one or a number of gastrointestinal symptoms that may occur at any one time, depending on the underlying illness and its pathophysiology.

Heartburn is a specific manifestation of esophageal reflux. It is a retrosternal burning sensation due to incompetence of the lower esophageal sphincter. Reduced lower esophageal pressures have been recorded in response to meals high in carbohydrate and fat, coffee drinking and cigarette smoking. Antacids alleviate symptoms by neutralizing acid and raising sphincter pressure (see Chapter 56).

Eructation is a common feature of indigestion due to functional causes. Patients troubled by chronic belching have been observed to swallow air just prior to belching, thus unconsciously worsening the problem. The reason for the air swallowing (aerophagia) is unclear, although some investigators have observed that eructation seems to provide transient relief of abdominal discomfort. Anxiety and drinking of carbonated beverages can lead to aerophagia. Food gulping, gum chewing, smoking and loose dentures have also been implicated but not proven to be causes of excessive air intake.

Bloating often accompanies eructation. Controlled studies have shown that in symptomatic patients there is an exaggerated pain response to normal degrees of intestinal distention without evidence of increased gas volume or production. Retrograde movement of gas was also found, suggesting a functional disorder of intestinal motility.

Upper abdominal pain may result from the presence of gas. Acute gastric distention from swallowed air may cause sharp left-sided pain and mimic angina due to a large meal. Intake of fatty food may delay gastric emptying and contribute to the discomfort. A number of other mechanisms may be operative. Biliary, gastric, or esophageal inflammation, peptic ulceration, functional motility disturbances, and tumor have all been implicated in the upper abdominal pain of patients complaining of indigestion. These causes result in visceral pain that is typically midline, poorly localized, and described as "aching," "gnawing," "burning," or "cramping" (see Chapter 53).

Nausea and *vomiting* may be manifestations of psychogenic disease or a disorder of the stomach, duodendum, gallbladder, liver or pancreas (see Chapters 54, 64, 69 and 72).

A group of English investigators prospectively examined the presentations of 360 patients complaining of indigestion to identify the clinical findings that best distinguish the more common, yet easily confused, causes of indigestion—namely, functional disease, cholecystitis, gastric ulcer, gastric cancer, and duodenal ulcer. Some features of the clinical presentation proved helpful in identifying underlying etiology. *Pain location* limited to the right upper quadrant was almost always due to gallbladder disease, although half of patients with this condition reported only epigastric pain, as did most with functional illness, ulcer, and malignancy. *Chronicity* of complaints varied among etiologies. Pain of less than 3 months' duration showed a strong chance of being due to gastric cancer; 6 to 12 months was characteristic of gastric ulcer; 1 to 3 years, typical of gallbladder disease and functional illness; and 5 to 10 years or more, of duodenal ulcer.

Pain radiation was often nonspecific. It was referred to the back in 25 to 30 per cent of patients with ulcer and functional problems and 59 per cent of patients with gallbladder disease. Radiation to the shoulder was rather specific for cholecystitis, but occurred in only 18 per cent of patients. *Alleviating factors* were of some discriminative value. A beneficial response to food was characteristic of patients with duodenal ulcer and rare in those with other conditions. Milk provided temporary relief in 15 to 20 per cent of patients with ulcer disease and 8 per cent with functional problems, pointing out its lack of specific meaning. Antacid response was nonspecific, occurring in 37 per cent of patients with ulcers and 26 per cent of those with functional disease. Even a small fraction of those with gastric cancer (9%) and gallbladder disease (6%) obtained relief with antacids. Surprisingly, over 50 per cent of all patients in the study reported that pain was not aggravated by food intake; this feature was reported by 80 per cent of those with cholecystitis, 60 per cent with functional illness, and 50 per cent with ulcer or tumor. A relation of symptoms to fatty food intake is not unique to patients with gallbladder disease (see Chapter 69).

Pain pattern was studied. The majority of patients with continuous pain were shown to have gastric cancer. When there were pain-free periods of 1 month or more, the cause usually proved to be duodenal ulcer or functional illness. Although over 80 per cent of patients with gallbladder disease had acute attacks of pain, so did 50 per cent with functional disease, 64 per cent with gastric ulcer, and 72 per cent with gastric cancer. Pain that awoke the patient from a sound sleep was seen most often with duodenal ulcer (70%), but also reported by one-third of patients with each of the other underlying etiologies.

Age proved helpful. Gastric cancer was rare under age 50. Gastric ulcer peaked in the 50 to 59-age group; duodenal ulcer was rare after age 60, but cholecystitis peaked in the 60 to 69-age range. Most patients aged 20 to 29 had functional problems or duodenal ulcer disease.

Associated symptoms were of variable use in identifying cause. Anorexia, nausea, and vomiting were found equally among the different groups, including those who proved to have functional illnesses as well as those with an organic lesion. Jaundice and pale stools pointed to biliary tract disease, but also occurred in a few patients with gastric cancer, secondary to obstruction of the common duct. Most had normal bowel habits. Diarrhea and constipation were equally infrequent among the different groups. Weight loss greater than 7 pounds was most common in cancer patients (85%) and gastric ulcer (61%), but also seen in 25 to 45 per cent of those with functional, gallbladder, and duodenal-ulcer problems.

DIFFERENTIAL DIAGNOSIS

Common causes of indigestion include peptic ulcer (both gastric and duodenal), gallbladder disease, functional illness, and esophageal reflux. Gastric carcinoma occasionally is responsible for the symptoms; angina, gastritis and pancreatitis may be sources of acute "indigestion." In a British general practice study, fifty consecutive patients with indigestion were evaluated by upper GI series, oral cholecystogram, and endoscopy, revealing 50 per cent with ulcer, 32 per cent with functional problems, 12 per cent with gallbladder disease, and single cases of gastric carcinoma and esophageal stricture.

WORKUP

The main objective is to distinquish functional complaints from symptoms of disease within the biliary or upper gastrointestinal tract.

History. Since the term *indigestion* is vague, it must be clarified by a detailed description of symptoms. The high frequency of organic illness and the need to separate it from functional complaints make it necessary to inquire into pain pattern, timing, radiation, aggravating and alleviating factors, and associated symptoms such as heartburn, hematemesis, or jaundice.

Many traditional notions about indigestion contains numerous misconceptions. For example, fatty-food intolerance is not unique to cholecystitis, nor is pain relief by antacids specific for ulcer disease. The location, severity, and quality of pain are nondiagnostic except for the right upper quadrant localization seen in half of those with gallbladder disease. Radiation into the back is common and of little help in discriminating among causes. Although pain radiation into the shoulder points to cholecystitis, it is found only in a fraction of such cases. Weight loss, anorexia, nausea, and vomiting are also frequent nonspecific accompaniments of any etiology. In spite of these potential pitfalls, it has been shown that a carefully taken history can improve diagnostic accuracy by 20 to 30 per cent.

Physical examination is usually unrevealing, but the patient should be checked for jaundice, abdominal mass, right upper quadrant tenderness, and occult blood in the stool. Many patients experience some discomfort on deep palpation in the epigastrium, but the finding is of little diagnostic value.

Laboratory studies should be limited to those necessary to specifically test for the diagnoses suggested by the available clinical evidence, rather than subjecting every patient to a routine battery of investigations, which is wasteful, unproductive, and often misleading. When reflux is found by history, *barium swallow* is indicated, but only to rule out stricture and malignancy; the test usually does not demonstrate reflux, and there is no evidence that presence of a hiatal hernia is related to symptoms (see Chapter 56). Suspected gastric and duodenal ulcers are searched for by *upper GI series* (UGI), which will detect up to 85 per cent of ulcers. Gastric ulceration is an indication for *endoscopy* if there is suspicion of malignancy on UGI or if symptoms are refractory. The combination of UGI and endoscopy has a 95 per cent detection rate for ulceration (see Chapter 64).

Oral cholecystogram (OCG) is ordered to document suspected gallbladder disease. Failure of the gallbladder to visualize after two doses of dye indicates a diseased gallbladder in over 95 per cent of instances, after extrinsic causes of nonopacification (malabsorption, vomiting, liver disease) are excluded. *Ultrasound* can be used to detect stones in patients whose gallbladders do not visualize after the first dose of dye. The test is considerably more expensive than OCG but avoids the need to have the patient return the next day to have a second dose. In one study, ultrasound alone provided the correct diagnosis in about 93 per cent of cases. For patients allergic to dye, ultrasound could be the initial study (see Chapter 69).

Some investigators have argued that barium studies add little to clinical decision-making for patients under the age of 50 with indigestion. A study of 100 such patients who were tested by UGI and endoscopy revealed abnormal results in only 24. Signs of active or previous ulcer were noted in 16; none had evidence of cancer. Regardless of etiology, most patients were told by their physicians to take antacids, have frequent small meals, and stop smoking when they presented with indigestion. The investigators concluded that unless symptoms were refractory, cancer was suspected, or cimetidine was being considered for use, the physician could dispense with UGI and endoscopy in the patient under 50. This position requires further study, but its logic and recommendations are compelling.

X-ray negative patients need not be restudied nor undergo endoscopy unless strong clinical suspicion of cancer persists or symptoms worsen or change in pattern, suggesting a new diagnosis. X-ray negative patients with indigestion seem to have a good prognosis;

in a prospective study, 75 per cent were pain-free within 6 years, and only 3 per cent eventually developed an ulcer. Patients troubled by excessive bloating and gas may need to be tested for lactose intolerance or be given a diagnostic trial of lactose-free diet (see Chapter 66).

MANAGEMENT AND PATIENT EDUCATION

Treatment of ulcer, cholecystitis, and esophageal reflux are detailed elsewhere (see Chapters 56, 64, 69). The patient with belching and bloating should be given a detailed explanation of the mechanisms that produce symptoms. In particular, the patient needs to be reassured that the symptoms are not an indication of disordered digestion or food allergy. The patient should be instructed to avoid inducing repetitive belching, not recline after meals (which makes release of the gastric air bubble difficult), to avoid fatty foods, and to take antacids. Use of simethicone for gas has not proven to be effective. Avoidance of foods with unabsorbable carbohydrates such as beans, whole grains, and some fruits can help prevent bloating due to bacterial gas production. It may be helpful to reduce air intake as much as possible by instructing the patient not to gulp food or drink carbonated beverages.

Patients with pain and other symptoms due to functional disturbances often respond to antacids, small meals, detailed explanation, reassurance, attention to alleviating situational stresses, and occasional intemittent use of a minor tranquilizer. Indefinite use of combination agents containing a tranquilizer and an anticholinergic agent (e.g. Librax, Donnotal) should be avoided. Intake of foods which cause symptoms can be limited, but special dietary restrictions are rarely indicated.

INDICATIONS FOR REFERRAL

There are few indications for referral. In most instances diagnosis will be possible if time is taken to obtain a thorough history and become familiar with the patient. Unhurried explanation and thorough evaluation should minimize the patient's need to obtain further workup. Referral is indicated when endoscopy is needed (see Chapters 56, 57 and 64).

ANNOTATED BIBLIOGRAPHY

Bond, J.H., and Levitt, M.D.: Gaseousness and intestinal gas. Med. Clin. North Am., *62*:155, 1978. *(Reviews mechanisms of gas formation, symptoms, and management.)*

Editorial: Data base on dyspepsia. Br. Med. J., *1*:1163, 1978. *(Underscores the need for accurate history in evaluation of the patient with indigestion.)*

Gregory, D.W., *et al.*: Natural history of patients with x-ray negative dyspepsia. Br. Med. J., *4*:519, 1972. *(Patients had a benign course, with 75% pain-free in 6 years and only 3% developing ulcers.)*

Horrocks, J.C., and DeDombal, F.T.: Clinical presentation of patients with "dyspepsia." Gut, *19*:19, 1978. *(A prospective study of over 300 patients; characterizes the clinical presentations of patients with this problem. Findings are at variance with classic textbook descriptions.)*

Lasser, R.B., Bond, J.H., and Levitt, M.D.: Role of intestinal gas in functional abdominal pain. N. Eng. J. Med., *293*:524, 1975. *(Symptomatic patients had normal gas volumes, increased pain to normal degrees of distention and some retrograde gas movement.)*

Mead, G.M., *et al.*: Uses of barium meal examination in dyspeptic patients under 50. Br. Med. J., *1*:1460, 1977. *(Found UGI to be of little use in patients under 50, except in cases with refractory symptoms or when cimetidine is being considered for use.)*

56
Evaluation of Heartburn

Heartburn is experienced by almost everyone at one time or other. The term denotes a retrosternal burning sensation that moves upward and comes on or worsens with lying down, bending over, or intake of a large meal. The symptom is a specific manifestation of esophageal reflux. It can range in severity from a mild, innocuous, episodic occurrence to a disabling disease complicated by stricture or hemorrhage. The incidence of the problem among ambulatory patients ranges from 5 to 10 per cent. It was once commonly believed that heartburn resulted from a hiatus hernia, but data from recent studies have shown this not to be the case.

The primary physician needs to understand the factors that interfere with lower esophageal sphincter function so that rational assessment and therapy can be devised. One must be aware of the limitations as well as the indications for the multitude of tests currently available to study lower esophageal function.

PATHOPHYSIOLOGY AND CLINICAL PRESENTATION

The competent lower esophageal sphincter (LES) prevents reflux of stomach contents back into the esophagus. Normal pressure ranges from 12 to 30 mm Hg. In patients with reflux, pressures fall to less than 10. The presence of a hiatus hernia has no effect on LES function. LES tone is thought to be maintained by a combination of factors, including intrinsic muscle function, vagal activity, gastrin, and alpha-adrenergic stimulation. Other gastrointestinal hormones, such as prostaglandins and cholecystokinin reduce LES pressure; the latter might account for the reduction in tone noted with intake of fatty foods. Normally LES tone increases in response to increases in intra-abdominal pressure. This reflex is believed to be vagally mediated. In patients with reflux, the responses to intra-abdominal pressure and gastrin are lost.

Most cases of LES incompetence are idiopathic, but neurologic, dietary and drug factors explain some episodes. Anticholinergics, alcohol, alpha-adrenergic blockers, nitrites and diets excessive in fats or carbohydrates have been implicated. Esophageal smooth-muscle atrophy occurs with scleroderma, but even before atropy takes place, LES function is already abnormal and believed to be due to neurogenic factors. Reflux is occasionally produced by vagotomy and often results after balloon dilatation for stricture. Empirical recordings indicate that smoking, alcohol, and coffee can decrease sphincter tone. As many as 50 per cent of pregnant women experience heartburn, most during the third trimester; LES pressures are reduced, but return to normal after delivery.

Heartburn predictably occurs when reflux is present. It is distinctly rare to have significant LES incompetence and reflux without symptoms. Injury to the esophagus from repeated exposure to stomach acid can also produce dysphagia, even without demonstrable narrowing of the intraluminal diameter. Mucosal inflammation, erosion, bleeding, and scarring result from chronic, severe reflux.

The patient complains of retrosternal burning that begins within an hour of eating. Symptoms are characteristically worsened by bending over or lying down. Spicy foods, citrus juices and coffee often aggrevate or directly elicit pain. Regurgitation of food during changes in position may accompany the retrosternal discomfort. In more severe prolonged cases, even when no stricture is found, solids may become hard to swallow; the patient feels discomfort from a bolus of food temporarily caught in the esophagus. Unless there is a significant stricture or tumor, repeated efforts at swallowing will usually dislodge the food.

Some patients experience pain on swallowing liquids, reporting a dull substernal ache, less responsive to antacids than the retrosternal burning of reflux. Rarely, hematemesis results, but it may also be the presenting symptom. Subclinical blood loss from mucosal injury is a common cause of iron-deficiency anemia and guaiac-positive stools (see Chapter 60).

DIFFERENTIAL DIAGNOSIS

With a characteristic history, the chances are greater than 90 per cent that reflux is indeed present. However, vague substernal discomfort is often all the patient can report. In such instances myocardial ischemia, esophageal spasm, or, occasionally, gallbladder disease may be responsible and should be investigated. Reflux may coexist with peptic ulcer disease, functional dyspepsia, gastritis, or neoplasms of the gastroesophageal junction.

The differential diagnosis of reflux includes use of drugs that decrease LES pressure (e.g., alcohol anticholinergics, alpha-adrenergic blocking agents), diets high in fat and carbohydrate, coffee, smoking, scleroderma, surgical destruction of the LES, pregnancy, and idiopathic causes.

WORKUP

History. A characteristic history of heartburn has proven to be as reliable as any laboratory procedure for the diagnosis of reflux. The patient should be questioned carefully to identify possible aggravating factors such as fatty foods, smoking, heavy coffee consumption, and use of anticholinergics, nitrites, alpha-blocking agents or beta-adrenergic agents. History of gastroesophageal surgery or sclerodermal symptoms (e.g., Raynaud's phenomenon) ought to be sought. Relief with use of antacids may be noted.

Physical examination is usually unremarkable, but sclerodactyly, calcinosis, and telangiectasias should be noted.

Laboratory studies. When a characteristic history of reflux cannot be obtained, but reflux is still suspected, the diagnosis is best established by a combination of endoscopic esophageal biopsy or acid-infusion test, in conjunction with pH-reflux measurements. Sensitivity and specificity for the combination approach are in the range of 90 per cent; this is much better than the specificity of endoscopy or acid-infusion alone, where false-positive rates can be as high as 30 per cent. Barium swallow demonstrates reflux in only 10 to 25 per cent of symptomatic patients, but it is most helpful when dysphagia is present and stricture and tumor must be excluded. Direct measurement of the LES pressure is usually unnecessary, but indicated if surgery is contemplated in order to establish with certainty a significant reduction in LES tone.

SYMPTOMATIC THERAPY

Therapy for reflux may be divided into three stages: use of antacids to neutralize stomach acid, elevation of the head of the bed to prevent regurgitation of stomach contents, and avoidance of drugs and foods that seem to precipitate symptoms. These can be summarized as follows:

1. Small meals, especially for the evening meal
2. Elevation of the head of the bed on 6-inch blocks
3. Antacids, 30 to 60 ml., 1 hour after meals and at bedtime; calcium-containing antacid preparations (e.g., TUMS) are not to be used, since rebound hyperacidity results (see Chapter 64)
4. Avoidance of anticholinergic drugs, alcohol
5. Avoidance of smoking and foods high in carbohydrate and fat (e.g., chocolate)
6. Limiting foods that directly elicit pain; e.g., citrus juices, spices, coffee
7. Loosening of tight, binding garments (e.g., corsets) when eating and shortly afterward

This program usually suffices for most patients. When symptoms persist, a parasympathomimetic can be added. Bethanechol has been proven in double-blind studies to be effective; it significantly reduces symptoms in 60 to 70 per cent of patients. The necessary dose is 25 mg., three times a day. Patients with intractable pain, stricture, ulceration, or hemorrhage should be referred for consideration of surgery. The place of cimetidine in therapy for reflux has not been yet established, but recent studies are encouraging and suggest a role for cimetidine in patients who do not improve on antacids alone.

PATIENT EDUCATION

Successful management is dependent upon the patient's using antacids properly, eating wisely, avoiding precipitants, and elevating the bed. Thorough explanation of the mechanisms of reflux and its aggravating factors should help to provide a rational basis for the patient's action. Patients need to realize that no single measure will alleviate the discomfort of reflux, but when all are performed together, relief is extremely likely. The lack of any connection between hiatus hernia and reflux also needs to be mentioned since it is a common misunderstanding that often leads to a belief that surgery is required for treatment; this belief makes some patients reluctant to seek help.

ANNOTATED BIBLIOGRAPHY

Behar, J., Biancani, P., and Sheehan, D.G.: Evaluation of esophageal tests in the diagnosis of reflux esophagitis. Gastroenterology, *71*:9, 1976. *(A critical comparison of the major available diagnostic methods; a combination approach suggested.)*

Benz, L.J., *et al.*: Comparison of clinical measurements of gastroesophageal reflux. Gastroenterology, *62*:1, 1972. *(Report of a high correlation between reflux symptoms and induction of heartburn by acid-perfusion test.)*

Castell, D.O., and Levine, S.M.: Lower esophageal sphincter response to gastric alkalinization. Ann. Intern. Med., *74*:223, 1971. *(Antacid use results in increased sphincter tone and less reflux.)*

Cohen, S.: Diagnosis and management of gastroesophageal reflux. Adv. Intern. Med. *21*:47, 1976. *(In over 90% of patients with characteristic symptoms, there is objective evidence of reflux. This article is an excellent review of all aspects of reflux, with 99 references.)*

Cohen, S., and Harris, L.D.: Does hiatus hernia affect competence of the gastroesophageal sphincter? N. Engl. J. Med., *284*:1053, 1971. *(The presence of a sliding hiatus hernia had no effect on sphincter competence.)*

Cohen, S.: Motor disorders of the esophagus. N. Engl. J. Med., *301*:184, 1979. *(Excellent review by a major investigator; 120 refs.)*

Farrell, R., Roling, G., and Castell, D.O.: Cholinergic therapy of chronic heartburn. Ann. Intern. Med., *80*:573, 1974. *(A double-blind study with* bethanechol *vs. placebo, showing the drug reduced antacid requirements and controlled symptoms better than placebo.)*

Nebel, O.T., and Castell, D.O.: Inhibition of the lower esophageal sphincter by fat. Gut, *14*:270, 1973. *(Fatty meals decrease LES pressure and may be responsible for fatty-food intolerance.)*

Uesdrop, E., *et al.*: Oral cimetidine in reflux esophagitis. A double blind controlled trial. Gastroenterology, *74*:821, 1978. *(Efficacy documented.)*

57

Evaluation of Dysphagia

Dysphagia is the unpleasant sensation of difficulty swallowing. The patient reports that food seems to get caught before reaching the stomach. The discomfort is experienced shortly after swallowing. Because true dysphagia is an important manifestation of esophageal disease, it should be fully assessed and not misinterpreted and dismissed as psychogenic or functional in origin.

PATHOPHYSIOLOGY AND CLINICAL PRESENTATION

Dysphagia implies an abnormality in swallowing and arises from either a loss of coordinated motor activity or from mechanical obstruction, be it intrinsic narrowing or extrinsic compression. *Transfer dysphagia* (oropharyngeal dysphagia) most often occurs as a consequence of neurologic disease and presents as difficulty initiating the act of swallowing. In most instances, other neurologic symptoms (nasal speech, dysphonia, and dysarthria) dominate the clinical picture, but at times, difficulty swallowing is the major complaint. Aspiration takes places with swallowing, and fluid regurgitates into the nose. Cough following deglutition may be a manifestation of abnormal upper esophageal sphincter function. Mechanical obstruction of the pharynx or upper esophagus may also produce oropharyngeal dysphagia.

Achalasia, the most common cause of motor dysphagia, is a slowly progressive disorder with a chronic course. There is aperistalsis, partial or incomplete relaxation of the lower esophageal sphincter (LES), and increased resting LES pressure. Vigorous terti-ary esophageal contractions are seen early in the disease in young patients and may result in chest pain, but pain is not an invariable accompaniment. Lesions in the dorsal vagal nucleus, vagal trunks, and myenteric ganglia have been found; there is speculation that this perhaps represents damage caused by a neurotropic virus. As a consequence of neuron loss, the esophagus demonstrates exquisite sensitivity to gastrin and cholinergic agents. There is equal difficulty with swallowing liquids and solids, yet by eating slowly and drinking small amounts, the patient may be able to consume a full meal. Pain is reported by 70 to 80 per cent of patients, sepecially if they eat or drink rapidly. Very cold liquids or emotion may provoke symptoms. Patients find that repeated swallowing or performing a rapid Valsalva maneuver can help pass material into the stomach. Regurgitation is common and can be provoked by changes in position or by physical exercise; pulmonary aspiration sometimes results. Patients may demonstrate foul breath due to retained esophageal material. Squamous cell carcinoma of the esophagus is sometimes a complication of achalasia; it occurs in 5 to 10 per cent of patients.

Carcinoma-induced achalasia is seen with tumors at the gastroesophageal junction. Adenocarcinoma of the stomach is the most common of these neoplasms. The mechanism by which tumor induces achalasia in unclear, but manometric findings are identical to those of primary achalasia. Patients are typically over 50 and complain of marked weight loss and symptoms of dysphagia that are less than a year in duration.

Esophageal spasm is characterized by dysphagia,

sharp chest pain and high-amplitude, nonperistaltic contractions occurring with at least 30 per cent of swallows. The condition can be mistaken for angina pectoris, because the pain is substernal, can radiate into the shoulder, and responds to nitroglycerin (see Chapter 14). LES pressure and relaxation are normal in the majority of patients, and some peristaltic funtion remains. About 3 to 5 per cent of patients develop achalasia, and degenerative changes are noted in ganglia and nerves, suggesting that esophageal spasm may be an early or mild form of achalasia. Supersensitivity to gastrin and cholinergic agents can be demonstrated.

Episodic, sharp substernal chest pain and dysphagia dominate the clinical presentation; often these symptoms do not occur simultaneously. Reflux is sometimes reported and may precipitate pain. The chest pain may be severe and radiate into the shoulder; it is frequently nocturnal, awakening the patient from sleep. Chest discomfot need not occur in relation to swallowing, but sometimes can be triggered by drinking very hot or very cold liquids. Dysphagia is noted with both solids and liquids. Some asymptomatic patients manifest the radiologic and manometric criteria for esophageal spasm but rarely experience discomfort.

Scleroderma can result in a decrease in lower esophageal sphincter tone as well as a lack of propulsive motor activity. Reflux is more of a problem than is dysphagia, but as many as 20 per cent of patients may suffer some difficulty in swallowing. About 75 per cent of patients with scleroderma have esophageal involvement (see Chapter 56).

Mechanical obstruction differs clinically from motor dysfunction in that the patient has more difficulty with solids than with liquids. The duration of symptoms is shorter (less than 1 year) for patients with malignancy than it is for those with benign causes of obstruction; progression is often rapid. Most patients with tumor are over age 50 and report marked weight loss. The location of discomfort does not necessarily represent the site of obstruction, for the pain may be referred. Spontaneous pain is not a common feature of neoplasm involving the esophagus. Patients with stricture due to severe esophagitis usually have a long-standing history of reflux.

Sometimes *globus hystericus* is confused with dysphagia. The patient complains of a constant "lump in the throat." There is no actual difficulty swallowing food, even though there is a perception of something in the throat or esophagus. Symptoms are unrelated to swallowing, and esophageal function is normal.

Inflammatory lesions of the pharynx or esophagus may cause pain on swallowing; there is no disturbance of esophageal motility, but swallowing is made difficult due to pain. Even saliva may be irritating.

DIFFERENTIAL DIAGNOSIS

The causes of dysphagia can be divided into motor and obstructive categories and often subdivided according to whether they affect the upper or lower esophagus. Pharyngeal–upper-esophageal motor dysfunction is usually a consequence of a neurologic disease, such as pseudobulbar palsy, myasthenia gravis, amyotrophic lateral sclerosis, or Parkinson's disease. The important esophageal motor disorders are achalasia, diffuse esophageal spasm, and scleroderma.

Upper esophageal mechanical obstruction may be due to tumor, Zenker's diverticulum, sideropenic webs, or an enlarged thyrod. Etiologies of obstruction in the lower portion of the esophagus include carcinoma, stricture, webs and rings. Most esophageal cancers are of the squamous cell variety, though half of those in the distal half of the esophagus are adenocarcinomas, suggesting that they arise in the cardia of the stomach. Stricture occurs from chronic reflux, corrosive agents and prolonged nasogastric intubation. Causes of extrinsic esophageal compression include mediastinal tumors and aortic aneurysm.

True dysphagia must be distinguished from conditions that may produce esophageal pain without interfering with the mechanics of swallowing, as occurs with most forms of esophagitis. The patient with globus hystericus reports a constant sensation of something in the throat, but swallows normally.

There are no detailed population studies on the prevalence of dysphagia and the relative frequencies of its etiologies.

WORKUP

History. A tentative diagnosis can often be made by history. A British study found that history alone could provide an accurate diagnosis in about 80 per cent of cases. The most important historical features include the duration and progression of symptoms, relation of symptoms to solids and liquids, effect of cold on swallowing, and response to swallowing a bolus. Inquiry into these aspects of the problem help in the important task of differentiating a motor disorder from mechanical obstruction. Motor disease is suggested by gradual onset, slow progression, chronic course, equal difficulty with liquids and solids, aggravation of symptoms on swallowing cold substances, and passage of a bolus by repeated swallowing, forceful drinking, Valsalva maneuver, or throwing back head and shoulders. Mechanical obstruction is characterized by more rapid onset and progressive course, more difficulty with solids than liquids, no aggravation with cold foods, and regurgitation upon trying to swallow a bolus. The location of discomfort helps to locate the lesion only if very high or very low in the esophagus; a distal lesion may cause pain referred to the neck. Hiccups point to difficulty in the terminal portion of the esophagus.

Other historical features also have some discriminative value, including presence of pain, reflux, and neurologic defects. Pain in conjunction with dysphagia suggests spasm or achalasia, though pain may occur in these conditions without concurrent difficulty swallowing. Pain on swallowing saliva alone is characteristic of mucosal inflammation. A history of heartburn in conjunction with difficulty swallowing solids argues strongly for a stricture secondary to chronic reflux esophagitis, especially if the problem is chronic. Dysphagia that comes on only after activity, in association with motor aphasia, diplopia, or diphonia is indicative of myasthenia. Tremor or difficulty in initiating movement suggest Parkinson's disease (see Chapter 161).

The pace of illness is important to note. Rapid progression is due to tumor until proven otherwise, whereas slow progression is most consistent with a motor disorder. Weight loss may occur with any etiology and has little value in differentiating one etiology from another. The same is true for regurgitation.

On *physical examination*, the skin is noted for pallor, signs of scleroderma (sclerodactyly, telangiectasias, calcinosis), and hyperkeratotic palms and soles (a rare finding suggestive of esophageal carcinoma). The mouth should be examined carefully for inflammatory lessions, ill-fitting dentures, and pharyngeal masses. Lymph nodes are palpated in the neck and elsewhere for any enlargement suggestive of neoplasm (see Chapter 80), and the thyroid for a large goiter. The abdomen is checked for masses, tenderness, organomegaly, and occult blood in the stool (suggestive of neoplasm and esophagitis). Neurologic examination should include testing for tremor, rigidity, and fatigability as well as cranial nerve deficits.

Laboratory assessment consists of barium swallow to rule out an obstructive lesion, followed by endoscopy and/or manometry depending on the clinical and x-ray findings. Mechanically obstructing lesions will be identified by barium swallow, but some cases of gastric carcinoma may show little more than intrinsic narrowing and require endoscopy and biopsy if the history is suspicious of malignancy (rapid progression, marked weight loss). Radiologic diagnosis of motor disorders can be difficult, for early achalasia and esophageal spasm may produce few findings on barium swallow. The characteristic radiologic features of achalasia include dilatation, segmental contractions, and termination of the distal esophagus into a narrowed segment (often referred to as a "break"). If diffuse esophageal spasm occurs during barium examination, it produces multiple tertiary contractions and differs from achalasia in that there is no break. Functional assessment of dysphagia is facilitated by performing all barium studies with the patient in the supine position in order to cancel the effect of gravity, and by dipping a piece of bread into barium to better trace the movement of solid food. Ciné studies sometimes help in diagnosis of oropharyngeal dysphagia.

Failure of the barium swallow to reveal a probable etiology leaves the primary physician with the difficult decision of whether to proceed with ordering endoscopy and/or manometry. Suspicion of a motor disorder is best pursued by manometry, whereas the need to rule out tumor or another type of obstructing lesion is an indication for esophagoscopy. Consultation with a gastroenterologist skilled in evaluation of esophageal disease is useful at this point. Finding an obstructing lesion on barium examination usually requires endoscopic assessment for direct visualization, cytology, and biopsy. The high frequency of esophageal pathology in patients with genuine dysphagia is a strong argument for thorough evaluation of every patient.

SYMPTOMATIC RELIEF

Regardless of etiology and pending definitive diagnosis, all patients with dysphagia require an adequate caloric intake that can be swallowed with a minimum of discomfort. The patient suspected of having mechanical obstruction should be advised to take predominantly liquids or soft solids.

A conservative approach sometimes suffices in patients with mild motor disease. The person with achalasia is often able to manage reasonably well by eating slowly, drinking small quantities at a time, and avoiding cold foods. A trial of nitroglycerin before eating may provide some help to the patient with possible esophageal spasm and serve as a crude diagnostic test as well; anticholinergic agents are of no proven benefit, but antacids sometimes provide relief and are worth a try, especially if reflux seems to trigger symptoms. Patients with severe achalasia get little relief from dietary or drug manipulations; esophageal dilatation or myotomy is needed. Myotomy is more effective, but requires major surgery and often produces severe reflux. Consequently, esophageal dilatation is usually the first invasive procedure for treatment of severe motor disease.

Patients with mechanical obstruction often require dilatation or surgery, but there are many exceptions. The person with a lower esophageal ring is best treated by advising slow intake of small amounts; dilatation does not work very well. Restoration of adequate iron intake will reverse the pathologic changes of sideropenic dysphagia, unless a carcinoma has ensued in the pharynx. Carcinoma of the upper or middle third of the esophagus is often unresectable and best treated by radiation therapy; considerable palliation is sometimes achieved. Treatment of oropharyngeal dysphagia due to obstruction is approached surgically (e.g., removal of a Zenker's diverticulum or large goiter) whereas attention to the underlying neurologic deficit is necessary in cases due to motor dysfunction, though myotomy may help as well. The patient with globus hystericus can be given thorough reassurance, though symptoms are not likely to resolve easily.

The patient who is referred for further evaluation and therapy should continue to be closely followed by the primary physician to be certain that the patient's nutrition is not overlooked during therapy of the underlying disease and to keep the patient informed of the overall diagnostic and therapeutic plan.

ANNOTATED BIBLIOGRAPHY

Atkinson, M.: Dysphagia. Br. Med. J., *1*:91, 1977. *(An excellent discussion of the problem.)*

Castell, D.O.: Achalasia and diffuse esophageal spasm. Arch. Intern. Med., *136*:571, 1976. *(Review pathogenesis, diagnosis and treatment.)*

Cohen, S.: Motor disorders of the esophagus. N. Engl. J. Med., *301*:184, 1979. *(Authoritative review by one of the field's leading investigators; 120 refs.)*

Edwards, D.A.W.: Discriminative information in the diagnosis of dysphagia. J. Royal Coll. Physicians, *9*:257, 1975. *(Critical discussion of important historical data; diagnostic accuracy by history alone is close to 80 per cent.)*

Goyal, R.K., *et al.*: Lower esophageal ring. N. Engl. J. Med., *282*:1298, 1970. *(An uncommon but important cause of obstructions.)*

Hollis, J.B., and Castell, D.O.: Esophageal function in elderly men: a new look at presbyesophagus. Ann. Intern. Med. *80*:371, 1974. *(A careful study that finds esophageal function is rather normal in elderly people, suggesting that disordered motility is most likely caused by disease and should not be attributed to aging.)*

Hurwitz, A.L., and Duranceau, A.: Upper esophageal sphincter dysfunction: pathogenesis and treatment. Am. J. Dig. Dis. *23*:275, 1978. *(A review of the causes of oropharyngeal dysphagia and a presentation of the results of cricopharyngeal myotomy as a method of relieving symptoms; 48 references.)*

Jordan, P.H.: Dysphagia and esophageal diverticula. Postgrad. Med. *61*:155, 1977. *(An excellent review of diverticula and the etiology of the symptom dysphagia.)*

Kilman, W.J., and Goyal, R.K.: Disorders of pharyngeal and upper esophageal sphincter motor function. Arch. Intern. Med., *136*:592, 1976. *(Thorough discussion of oropharyngeal motor diseases.)*

Mukhopadhyay, A.K., and Graham, D.Y.: Esophageal motor dysfunction in systemic diseases. Arch. Intern. Med., *136*:583, 1976. *(Connective tissue disease, metabolic problems, and neuromuscular disorders are reviewed.)*

Orlando, R.C., and Bozymski, E.M.: Clinical and manometric effects of nitroglycerin in diffuse esophageal spasm. N. Engl. J. Med., *289*:23, 1973. *(Nitroglycerin can provide relief, though study is uncontrolled.)*

Parker, E.F., and Moertel, V.S.: Carcinoma of the esophagus: Is there a role for surgery. Am. J. Dig. Dis., *23*:730, 1978. *(Emphasizes the role of radiation therapy and debates the utility of surgery.)*

58
Evaluation of Diarrhea
JAMES M. RICHTER, M.D.

Diarrhea is a familiar affliction for physicians and patients alike. It is best characterized clinically as the frequent passage of unformed stools. Most episodes are brief, self-limited, and treated by patients without medical attention, but when diarrhea becomes very severe or chronic, the patient requires further assessment. The primary physician must decide when a detailed evaluation is necessary and how extensive it should be. Just as important is the need to provide symptomatic relief pending definitive measures.

PATHOPHYSIOLOGY AND CLINICAL PRESENTATION

Diarrhea is a change in a patient's bowel habits with increased stool volume, looseness, and frequency. The pathophysiologic common denominator is an increased water content of stools; this may be due to increased fluid secretion, a decreased absorption of water, or altered bowel motility. The large or small bowel may be stimulated to secrete more fluid by inflammation, hormones, or enterotoxins. Decreased reabsorption of fluid occurs with abnormalities of the bowel mucosa, loss of reabsorption surface, or presence of unabsorbable osmotically active materials in the bowel lumen, such as lactose in patients with lactase deficiency. Increased bowel motility decreases contact time with the mucosa, limiting fluid resorption, and may occur secondary to hyperthyroidism, hypergastrinemia, or previous vagotomy. Clinical presentations can be divided into acute and chronic forms.

Acute diarrheas. These are most often a consequence of *viral gastorenteritis.* These are most prevalent among children and often occur in epidemics during the fall and winter. Generally, symptoms begin abruptly after an incubation period of 48 to 72 hours, with diarrhea, nausea, vomiting, headache, low-grade fever, abdominal cramps, and malaise. Abdominal examination reveals diffuse tenderness without guarding. Bowel sounds are hyperactive. The white count is usually normal but can be elevated.

The illness usually resolves spontaneously in 24 to 48 hours.

Bacteria may cause acute diarrhea by producing a toxin in *contaminated food* or by being ingested and subsequently producing a toxin or invading the bowel mucosa. Foods contaminated by staphylococci, such as custard-filled pastries or processed meats, harbor toxin and produce nausea, vomiting, abdominal cramps, and diarrhea within a few hours of ingestion; symptoms usually last less than 12 hours. Foods that have been warmed on steam tables can become contaminated by *Clostridium perfringens;* its toxin induces diarrhea and abdominal cramps 8 to 24 hours after ingestion, lasting about 24 hours. Both conditions are distinguished by common-source outbreaks and the lack of fever. Toxigenic strains of *Escherichia coli* cause a syndrome of profuse watery diarrhea with some cramps and low-grade fever. This is the commonly experienced *traveler's diarrhea.*

Invasion of the bowel wall distinguishes the diarrheal diseases due to ingestion of salmonella, shigella, and enteropathogenic strains of *E. coli.* These are most common among children but may occur in any age group. Invasive strains of *E. coli* cause fever, severe cramps, and bloody diarrhea. Classically, *shigellosis* appears 24 to 72 hours after ingestion of organisms; there is fever, toxicity, bloody diarrhea, nausea and vomiting, and cramps. Frequently the disease is more subtle and may be difficult to distinguish clinically from other diarrheal illnesses. It usually resolves in fewer than 7 days. *Salmonellosis* presents 12 to 36 hours after ingestion, with watery diarrhea and cramps, nausea, vomiting, and fever. The illness is often nonspecific, and there is usually no blood in the stool. It typically resolves in fewer than 5 days but may persist for up to 2 weeks.

Infestation with *Giardia lamblia* is being recognized more frequently as an important cause of acute and chronic diarrhea in the United States. Giardiasis is often asymptomatic but the diarrhea may be acute, intermittent, or chronic. Stools are loose, greasy, or watery. Mucus is often present, but blood is rare. The patient may complain of upper abdominal achiness. Mild steatorrhea and malabsorption may develop when the absorptive surface of the small bowel is

Table 58-1.   A Differential Diagnosis of Diarrhea

ACUTE DIARRHEA	CHRONIC OR RECURRENT DIARRHEA
VIRUSES	*PROTOZOA*
BACTERIAL TOXINS	Giardia lamblia
Staphylococcus	Entamoeba histolytica
Clostridium	*INFLAMMATION*
BACTERIA	Ulcerative colitis
Salmonella	Crohn's disease
Shigella	Ischemic colitis
Escherichia coli	*DRUGS*
Yersinia	Laxatives
Vibrio parahaemolyticus	Antibiotics
Vibrio cholerae	Quinidine
PROTOZOA	Guanethidine
Giardia lamblia	Caffeine
Entamoeba histolytica	*FUNCTIONAL*
DRUGS	Irritable bowel syndrome
Laxatives	Diverticulosis
Antibiotics	*TUMORS*
Caffeine	Bowel carcinoma
Alcohol	Villous adenoma
FUNCTIONAL	Islet-cell tumors
Anxiety	Carcinoid syndrome
ACUTE PRESENTATIONS	Medullary carcinoma of thyroid
OF CHRONIC OR	*MALABSORPTION*
RECURRENT DIARRHEA	Sprue
	Intestinal lymphoma
	Bile-salt malabsorption
	Whipple's disease
	Pancreatic insufficiency
	Lactase deficiency
	Other disaccharidase deficiencies
	Alpha-beta lipoproteinemia
	POSTSURGICAL
	Postgastrectomy dumping syndrome
	Enteroenteric fistulae
	Blind loops
	Parasympathetic denervation
	Short bowel syndrome
	OTHER
	Cirrhosis
	Diabetes mellitus
	Heavy-metal intoxication
	Other neurogenic diarrheas
	Hyperthyroidism
	Addison's disease
	Pellagra
	Scleroderma
	Amyloidosis

extensively covered by organisms. Amebic invasion of the bowel may also be responsible for acute bloody diarrhea, particularly in endemic areas.

Chronic diarrheas. The clinical presentations of the chronic diarrheas vary widely. Fever is most consistent with an infectious or inflammatory etiology. Diarrhea at night is suggestive of an organic cause.

Blood in the stool may be a manifestation of bowel-wall involvement by neoplasm, infection, or inflammation (see Chapter 65). Mucus is a prominent finding in patients with irritable bowel syndrome (see Chapter 66). Passage of frequent, small, loose stools in association with crampy, left lower quadrant pain or tenesmus indicate disease in the left colon or rectum. The passage of large, loose bowel movements associated with periumbilical or right lower quadrant pain is suggestive of small bowel disease, as is diarrhea after meals or certain foods. Also, diarrhea after meals or certain foods is characteristic of malabsorption (see Chapter 72), an osmotic etiology, a fistula, or dumping syndrome. The presence of foul, bulky, greasy stools suggests a fat malabsorption syndrome.

Lactase deficiency is another common etiology of chronic diarrhea in adults and is particularly prevalent among blacks. Most patients observe that milk does not agree with them, and they try to avoid it. They present with nausea, bloating, cramps, and diarrhea after ingesting more lactose than usual; for example, diarrhea may develop when the patient begins drinking large amounts of milk for dyspepsia. Many drugs cause acute as well as chronic diarrheas by excessively stimulating bowel motility and reducing time for absorption of nutrients and fluids. Many antibiotics, especially ampicillin and clindamycin, are associated with diarrhea; often the diarrhea is caused by a toxin-producing clostridium which induces a pseudomembraneous colitis.

DIFFERENTIAL DIAGNOSIS

The differential diagnosis of *acute diarrhea* is dominated by infectious agents. (see Table 58-1). Viruses are the most important, frequent single cause. Staphylococcal toxin, clostridial toxin, and ingestion of salmonella, shigella, and enteropathogenic *E. coli* are common bacterial etiologies. Giardia and ameba are less frequent sources of acute diarrhea in the United States. Drugs are important and common causes of diarrhea, especially antibiotics, laxatives, magnesium-containing antacids, and other agents such as quinidine and guanethidine. Alcohol and caffeine-containing beverages should also be considered. Most causes of chronic diarrhea are capable of acute presentations.

The differential diagnosis of *chronic diarrhea* is more extensive. The infectious agents and drugs discussed under acute diarrheal disease may be responsible, but the likelihood of parasites such as ameba and giardia increases. Inflammatory bowel diseases must also be taken into account. Absorption defects due to sprue, bile-salt deficiency, lactase deficiency, intestinal lymphoma, Whipple's disease, and pancreatic insufficiency may cause chronic diarrhea. The patient who has had gastrointestinal surgery may develop diarrhea on the basis of postgastrectomy dumping syndromes, fistulae, blind loops, loss of parasympathetic innervation, or extensive bowel resection. Diarrhea may be caused directly by neoplasms, particularly villous adenoma. Diarrhea alternating with constipation raises the possibility of colonic carcinoma, irritable bowel syndrome, or diverticular disease of the bowel. A variety of extraintestinal conditions may be responsible, including cirrhosis, alcoholism, pellagra, and heavy-metal intoxications from lead, mercury, or arsenic. Occasionally, chronic diarrhea may develop with endocrinopathies such as Addison's disease, hyperthyroidism, and diabetes mellitus.

WORKUP

Acute diarrhea. The frequency and consistency of the bowel movements as well as the presence of gross blood or mucus need to be ascertained. Suddenness of onset is helpful and may point to an infectious etiology. Fever, cramps, tenesmus, and toxicity are consistent with an invasive pathogen. The ingestion of potentially contaminated food and sudden diarrhea without fever suggest staphylococcal or clostridial food poisoning. Recent travel may indicate an enterotoxigenic *E. coli* (traveler's diarrhea) or a parasitic infection. A drug history is essential.

Patients should be examined for the presence of fever and volume depletion. Temperature and postural vital signs are checked and weight is recorded for future reference. The abdomen is examined for tenderness, rebound, abnormal bowel sounds, organomegaly, or masses. Rectal examination and a stool guaiac test are mandatory. A complete physical examination may uncover signs pointing to a systemic disease.

The laboratory workup of a patient with acute diarrhea should be highly individualized. The patient who feels well except for frequent loose stools requires no laboratory testing. The patient who is ill with fever, nausea, abdominal cramps, or other systemic symptoms in addition to diarrhea should have a rectal swab or stool sample examined by methylene-blue stain or Gram stain for the presence of fecal leukocytes. If polymorphonuclear leukocytes are present in the stool, a bacterial culture should be sent and a sigmoidoscopy performed. If blood is found in the stool, a sigmoidoscopy should follow. In both instances, the appearance of the colonic mucosa must be assessed without distortion from preparatory ememas and cathartics.

If the diarrhea persists for a week or more, a secondary evaluation should be begun. Stools should once again be examined for blood and leukocytes. A second stool should be sent for bacterial culture and a fresh specimen examined for ameba or giardia. If symptoms continue to persist and the diagnosis is uncertain, the patient probably has one of the chronic or recurrent diarrheal syndromes and requires further assessment. The patient who becomes markedly dehydrated or toxic needs to be admitted to the hospital.

Chronic or recurrent diarrhea. If an acute episode of diarrhea has not resolved in 2 weeks or if a pattern of recurrent diarrhea is established, several additonal etiologies enter the differential diagnosis, and the work-up is expanded. The history is reviewed for new evidence as well as features that help distinguish small bowel disease from large bowel involvement. Rectosigmoid pathology is suggested by frequent, small, loose stools in association with crampy, left lower quadrant pain, or tenesmus. Bloody stools require investigation into neoplasm, invasive infection or inflammatory bowel disease. Small bowel disease enters into consideration when there are large, loose bowel movements associated with periumbilical or right lower quadrant pain. Any relation of the diarrhea to meals should lead to a search for malabsorption, an osmotic etiology, or a fistula; the presence of foul, bulky, greasy stools further supports the likelihood of fat malabsorption. Alternating diarrhea and constipation point to irritable colon syndrome, as does mucus in the stool. Drug use deserves careful assessment, including a check for nonprescription laxatives and caffeine-containing agents. A history of alcohol use, previous abdominal surgery, or travel needs exploration.

A complete physical examination is mandatory and may confirm suspected causes as well as establish the severity of the disease. Fever, dehydration, or cachexia should be noted. Blood pressure is checked for postural fall. The skin should be inspected for jaundice, pallor, or rash. Abdomen is noted for distention, ascites, hepatomegaly, tenderness, rebound, and masses. Rectal examination may reveal fecal impaction, perirectal fistula or a patulous anal sphincter. Stool is obtained for guaiac testing.

In most instances, the first procedure will be sigmoidoscopy performed without cleansing enemas. It should always be performed when there is blood or pus in the stool or other evidence of rectosigmoid pathology. The presence of mucosal ulcerations or bleeding should be noted and smears of the mucus carefully examined for the inflammatory cells. Mucus without inflammatory cells helps confirm the diagnosis of irritable bowel syndrome, while the finding of pus directs the diagnosis toward infection and inflammation. In cases of suspected amebiasis, fresh mucosal smears should be examined for trophozoites. Masses, ulcer margins and mucosa may be biopsied. Patients suspected of malabsorption should have stool examined qualitatively for fat by Sudan stain. Blood tests should include a complete blood count, prothrombin time, serum electrolytes, calcium, amylase, and glucose and liver function are ordered in most chronic cases; these help detect resultant electrolyte imbalance, and uncover pancreatic or hepatobiliary disease. Serum carotene may be depressed in chronic fat malabsorption and B_{12} in disease of the terminal ileum, but neither should be relied upon too greatly for diagnosis of chronic diarrhea.

Barium enema may be needed in a search for neoplasm or inflammatory bowel disease; however, it should be obtained only after three or four fresh stool specimens have been examined for parasites, since the barium will interfere with their detection. When fat malabsorption is a serious consideration, a 72-hour stool collection is analyzed quantitatively for fat. Specific tests to determine the cause of malabsorption may include a d-xylose test for small-bowel disease, a secretin-stimulation test for pancreatic insufficiency, and a lactose-tolerance test for lactase deficiency. Anatomic abnormalities such as blind loops, fistulae, or tumors may be documented by barium enema and barium study of the stomach and small bowel. If more sophisticated examinations seem indicated or if the etiology remains elusive, then a gastroenterologist should be consulted.

SYMPTOMATIC THERAPY

Acute diarrhea. The vast majority of acute diarrheal illness should be managed by maintaining *hydration* and waiting for the spontaneous resolution of the syndrome. Often, hydration can be maintained by oral fluids, even with profuse diarrhea. Solutions that containing electrolytes and sugars faciliate absorption of water; milk products ought to be avoided since acquired lactase deficiency is common. If severe dehydration or electrolyte abnormalities develop, admission to a hospital for parenteral therapy and monitoring is indicated.

Absorbent preparations are commonly used for symptomatic therapy for simple acute diarrhea. Solutions of kaolin and pectin have no proven benefit but seem to be harmless; however, they should not be relied upon in the treatment of severe diarrhea. *Opiates* such as *diphenoxylate* (dispensed as a combination with small amounts of atropine [Lomotil] in order to discourage abuse) and *loperamide* are effective in the treatment of diarrhea by directly inhibiting the motility of the intestinal smooth muscle. Diphenoxylate and loperamide are derived from meperidine but have less effect on the central nervous system. They should be used cautiously, if at all, in conditions in which toxic megacolon is possible. Their use should also be restricted in certain bacterial diarrheas, for example they may prolong the course of shigellosis. The usual dose of dephenoxylate is 2.5 to 5 mg., every 4 hours, up to 20 mg. per day. Loperamide is given as 2 or 4 mg., every 4 hours, up to 16 mg. daily. The doses can often be decreased after the initial control of the diarrhea for maintenance. Other opiates are potent antidiarrheal agents but carry a higher risk of addiction. They are particularly useful when their coincident analgesic activity is needed. Deodorized *tincture of opium* (0.5–1 ml.), *paregoric* (4 ml.), or *codeine* (30–60 mg.) are given orally every 4 hours. *Anticholinergics* are useful only for the irritable bowel syndrome (see Chapter 66).

Antibiotics should not be used routinely for acute bacterial diarrhea. They have little effect on the course of the disease and may prolong asymptomatic bacterial carrier states. However, elderly debilitated patients or those who may not tolerate bacteremia, such as those with prosthetic heart valves or sickle cell anemia, may benefit from antibiotic therapy by limiting distant complications. When antibiotics are used, ampicillin is the first choice for the treatment of shigellosis or salmonellosis. Those patients with salmonellosis who are very ill or penicillin-allergic may require chloramphenicol. Trimethoprim-sulfamethoxazole is the alternative agent for shigellosis. Traveler's diarrhea may be prevented by taking doxycycline, 100 mg., daily, prophylactically. Giardiasis is treated with quinacrine, 100 mg., three times daily, for 7 days or, alternatively, metronidazole, 250 mg., three times daily, for 7 days. The treatment of amebiasis depends on the clinical condition of the patient. Metronidazole is probably effective against trophozoites in all locations and is prescribed in doses of

750 mg., three times a day, for 10 days. Disease confined to the bowel lumen can be treated with diodohydroxyquin, 650 mg., three times daily, for 3 weeks.

Chronic diarrhea. The therapy for chronic or recurrent diarrhea is dictated by the specific etiology uncovered. Merely treating symptoms may prove ineffective or delay diagnosis of the underlying illness.

ANNOTATED BIBLIOGRAPHY

Bayless, T.M., et al.: Lactose and milk intolerance: Clinical implications. N. Engl. J. Med. 292:1156, 1975. (A study of the prevalence, characteristics, and diagnosis of lactose intolerance in adults.)

Blacklow, N.R., et al.: Acute infectious non-bacterial gastroenteritis: Etiology and pathogenesis. Ann. Intern. Med. 76:993, 1972. (This paper discusses the probable role of viral agents in producing diarrhea and histologic changes in the small bowel.)

Cummings, J.H., et al.: Laxative-induced diarrhea: a continuing clinical problem. Br. Med. J. 1:537, 1974. (A detailed review of 7 women who underwent extensive investigation to establish the diagnosis of laxative-induced diarrhea. A good review of the syndrome with emphasis on how difficult the diagnosis may be.)

DuPont, H.L., and Hornick, R.B.: Adverse effect of Lomotil therapy in shigellosis. J.A.M.A., 260:1525, 1973. (Lomotil therapy may cause fever and toxicity may be prolonged in patients with shigellosis.)

Eastham, E.J., Douglas, A.P., and Watson, A.J.: Diagnosis of Giardia lamblia infection as a cause of diarrhea. Lancet, 2:950, 1976. (Retrospective review of 31 patients found that giardia is not considered often or early enough.)

Gorbach, S.L., et al.: Traveler's diarrhea and toxigenic Escherichia coli. N. Engl. J. Med., 292:933, 1975. (Traveler's diarrhea is often due to enterotoxigenic Escherichia coli.)

Grady, G.F., and Keusch, G.T.: Pathogenesis of bacterial diarrheas (two parts). N. Engl. J. Med., 285:831, 1971. (A classic review of the pathophysiology of bacterial-induced diarrhea.)

Gurwith, M.J., et al.: Diarrhea associated with clindamycin and ampicillin therapy: Preliminary results of a cooperative study. J. Infect. Dis., 135[Suppl.]:S104, 1977. (A large prospective study of the incidence and characteristics of antibiotic-associated diarrhea.)

Harris, J.C., DuPont, H.L., and Hornick, R.B.: Fecal leukocytes in diarrheal illness. Ann. Intern. Med., 76:697, 1972. (An important article that established that fecal leukocytes indicate inflammatory causes of diarrhea, such as shigellosis, salmonellosis, typhoid fever, invasive E. coli, and inflammatory bowel disease.)

Nahmias, A.J., et al.: Newer microbial agents in diarrhea. Hospital Practice, March, 1976, p. 75. (An excellent review of infectious agents in the etiology of diarrhea, emphasizing more recently recognized microorganisms.)

Palmer, D.L., et al.: Comparison of sucrose and glucose in the oral electrolyte therapy of cholera and other severe dia(rhea. N. Engl. J. Med., 292:1107, 1977. (A discussion of the uses and limitations of oral fluid and electrolyte therapy in severe diarrhea.)

Phillips, S.F.: Diarrhea: A current view of the pathophysiology. Gastroenterology, 63:495, 1972. (An extensive review of gastrointestinal physiology and disorders causing diarrhea.)

Sack, D.A., et al.: Prophylactic doxycycline for traveler's diarrhea. N. Engl. J. Med., 298:758, 1978. (Traveler's diarrhea due to enterotoxigenic E. coli may be prevented by doxycycline, 100 mg. daily.)

Schein, et al.: Islet-cell tumors: Current concepts in management. Ann. Intern. Med., 79:239, 1973. (A complete discussion of these relatively uncommon syndromes causing diarrhea and hypokalemia.)

59
Approach to the Patient with Constipation

Constipation is a universal affliction of Western civilization, resulting in part from a diet low in crude fiber. It is among the most frequent reasons for self-medication and is particularly troublesome in the elderly. Over 200 million dollars are spent annually in the United States on laxatives; a survey of Londoners revealed 30 per cent admitting to recent laxative use.

There is no uniform definition of constipation. To some, it means movements that are too infrequent or stools that are too hard. Others complain of incomplete or difficult evacuation. Among normal people, bowel habits widely vary, and there are diverse perceptions of what constitutes normal function. Population studies show that most normal people have more than three bowel movements per week with men likely to have at least five. Stools less than 35 gm. per day are well below the lower limit of normal.

The primary physician must be able to uncover any underlying pathology as well as to provide symptomatic relief to those without a structural lesion. The prevalences of excessive laxative use and inadequate dietary fiber make it imperative that the physician be knowledgeable about the actions and adverse effects of available laxative preparations as well as dietary alternatives to their use.

PATHOPHYSIOLOGY AND CLINICAL PRESENTATION

The process of elimination of fecal waste requires two processes: filling of the rectum by colonic transport and reflex defecation of stool. Constipation may arise secondary to interference with either of these processes. The time it takes food to reach the anus is partially a function of the amount of fiber in the diet. Normal people placed on a diet containing 15 gm. of bran fiber per day have twice the number of movements per week of those on an uncontrolled diet. Patients with constipation solely on the basis of low dietary fiber usually have intermittent complaints that fully resolve with alteration of diet alone.

Exercise has an important effect on propulsion of bowel contents. Colonic transit has been observed to be significantly greater in physically active people than in those who get little exercise. Previously active persons often become constipated when put to bed on account of illness. Less dramatic, but probably no less important, is the leading of a *sedentary lifestyle*; constipation is common in inactive people.

Metabolic and endocrine disturbances can slow colonic transport. Hypokalemia, hypercalcemia, hypothyroidism, and diabetes are the most important of these in terms of frequency or potential reversibility. *Hypokalemia* can produce a generalized ileus and is most often seen in patients who take diuretics. Chronic laxative abuse may also produce hypokalemia; characteristically, there is surreptitious use of laxatives and diuretics, self-induced vomiting, pathologic desire to lose weight, and a personality disorder. Such patients present with fatigue and electrolyte disturbances. When constipation is caused by *hypothyroidism*, other manifestations of the disease are usually present, though sluggish bowel movements may be the presenting complaint. Constipation is a bothersome problem in some patients with *diabetes:* 20 per cent of those with neuropathy report severe difficulty. Significant *hypercalcemia* (serum calcium greater than 12 mg./100 ml.) can slow bowel motility.

Habitual use of *laxatives* is associated with impaired motor activity. The typical clinical picture is a long history of chronic constipation or a desire to feel "well cleaned out," followed by increasing laxative dependence, decreasing response, and ultimately a sluggish, poorly contracting bowel. Whether there is a prior underlying motor disorder or actual damage from laxative use is unsettled.

Mechanical *obstruction* from tumor, stricture, or volvulus may be responsible for the new onset of constipation. Cramping abdominal pain and distention in conjunction with a marked change in bowel habits are characteristic (see Chapter 53). Constipation occurs in over 50 per cent of patients with colonorectal cancers; it is usually a symptom of advanced disease but may be the presenting complaint.

New onset of constipation may also be precipitated by drug use. *Opiates* and agents with anticholinergic activity, such as *antidepressants* are frequently implicated. An underlying depression is often contributory, and bowel complaints may be one of many somatic symptoms (see Chapter 215). The exact mechanisms by which emotional difficulties lead to constipation remain unclear, but the fact that they play an important role is widely recognized. Experiments in patients with the irritable colon syndrome, where constipation can be an important difficulty, provide some clues regarding pathophysiology (see Chapter 66).

A lesion in the *innervation* of the bowel can result in constipation. Spinal cord pathology, transection of pelvic nerves, and ganglion abnormalities are all capable of inducing failure of normal bowel function. In most instances, other neurologic deficits are present. Disease limited to loss of neurones in the bowel wall typically presents as chronic, refractory constipation; it may date from childhood or be associated with long-standing laxative use.

A permanently damaged neuromotor apparatus is a consequence of *scleroderma*, while functional disturbances in motor activity are noted in *irritable colon syndrome* (see Chapter 66) and *diverticular disease* (see Chapter 67). Constipation results when there is an excessive degree of nonpropulsive contractions and segmentation of bowel contents. Diarrhea may quickly supervene if distal contractions cease while proximal hyperactivity continues.

Inhibition of the rectal defecation reflex has been documented in cases of local anal pathology, neurogenic disease, chronic use of laxatives and voluntary suppression. Patients with this problem are found to have stool packed into the rectal ampulla. *Voluntary suppression* of the urge to defecate is usually a concomitant of a hectic life style or deep-seated neurotic inhibitions. The resulting intermittent constipation may lead to excessive use of laxatives and enemas and damage to the reflex emptying mechanism.

Some authorities believe that substantial fluid intake is essential to normal bowel movements, though this is not well established. It is known that water is an effective means of distending the stomach and stimulating intestinal activity. The consistency of stool is a function of how much water it contains, which is due, in part, to how much is taken into it.

DIFFERENTIAL DIAGNOSIS

The causes of constipation can be grouped according to pathophysiology. *Impaired motility* can be seen with inadequate dietary fiber, inactivity, laxative abuse, irritable colon syndrome, *tumor, stricture,* inflammatory bowel disease, diverticulitis, hypothyroidism, hypokalemia, diabetes, hypercalce-

mia, pregnancy, and scleroderma. Opiates, anticholinergics (including the tricyclic antidepressants), ganglionic blockers, calcium- and aluminum-containing antacids, and antihistamines slow colonic motility. *Obstruction* may be secondary to tumor, stricture or volvulus. *Neurologic disorders* that may hinder transport include multiple sclerosis and cord lesions. *Local anorectal pathology* such as hemorrhoids and fissures, strictures, abscesses or proctitis, and voluntary suppression retard rectal emptying. Chronic laxative abuse and rectocele formation reduce the muscle strength available for defecation. Last, but not infrequent, constipation is associated with *emotional difficulties* such as depression and neurotically excessive concern with one's bowels.

WORKUP

History. Evaluation begins with definition of the size, character, and frequency of bowel movements, followed by a determination of the problem's chronicity. Acute constipation is more often associated with organic disease than is a long-standing problem. Chronic complaints that wax and wane over months and years point to a functional disturbance, often compounded by habitual laxative use. Inquiry is needed into symptoms that suggest an underlying gastrointestinal problem, such as abdominal pain, nausea, cramping, vomiting, weight loss, melena, rectal bleeding, rectal pain, and fever. Anorexia, bloating, belching, flatus, mucus, headache, depression, and anxiety should also be recorded; these symptoms may be associated with constipation of any etiology but often accompany functional disorders.

It is helpful at the first visit to take a history of working, eating, and bowel habits. Inquiry into dietary fiber intake and physical activity is essential. Laxative use and drug intake, including antacids, need to be carefully reviewed. The patient's concerns and views should be sympathetically elicited.

Physical examination should assess the patient's weight and nutritional status. Skin is noted for pallor and signs of hypothyroidism (see Chapter 100). The abdomen is examined for masses, distention, tenderness, and high-pitched or absent bowel sounds. Rectal examination includes careful inspection and palpation for masses, fissures, inflammation, and hard stool in the ampulla. The last finding rules out significant obstruction and poor colonic motility, and suggests that the problem is inadequate rectal emptying. The stool is noted for color and consistency and tested for occult blood. Anal sensitivity and reflexes are noted. Disordered innervation of the anus is indicated by finding that the anal canal opens wide when the puborectalis muscle is pulled posteriorly. Anoscopy is needed to identify internal hemorrhoids, fissures, tumors, and other local pathology. Neurologic examination should be performed to search for focal deficits and delayed relaxation phase of the ankle jerks, suggestive of hypothyroidism.

Laboratory studies. Radiologic investigation is of limited utility unless evidence from history and physical examination suggests a particular etiology. Acute onset of constipation requires ruling out obstruction and ileus, especially when accompanied by abdominal discomfort; supine and upright films of the abdomen, plus measurements of serum potassium and calcium levels are indicated. Suspicion of colonic obstruction requires a barium enema (see Chapter 53). Any hint of diabetes or hypothyrodism can be verified by urinalysis, serum glucose and thyroid-stimulating hormone determination (see Chapters 91 and 100).

An important diagnostic concern in the elderly is the possibility of constipation being due to a colonic neoplasm. Blood in the stool, weight loss, or iron-deficiency anemia mandates sigmoidoscopy followed by barium enema. Over 25 per cent of patients with colonorectal carcinomas present with constipation. However, the elderly person with no evidence of obstruction, anemia, or occult blood loss can probably be followed for a few weeks on a conservative program that includes more dietary fiber, increased exercise and monitoring of stool guaiacs, before it is decided to subject the patient to the discomfort of sigmoidoscopy and barium enema. If symptoms resolve and stools are negative for occult blood, the probability of malignancy or obstruction is low, and the patient need not undergo further testing at the present time. A return visit for repeat assessment ought to be scheduled within 4 to 8 weeks.

When the cause of constipation is obscure, it is helpful to stop all nonessential medications. The codeine in a cough suppressant, the calcium in an over-the-counter antacid, or the iron in a multiple vitamin may be responsible for an otherwise puzzling diagnostic problem.

SYMPTOMATIC MANAGEMENT AND PATIENT EDUCATION

Symptomatic management is appropriate for the patient with a functional etiology. The first intervention is careful patient education about diet and use of laxatives. Explanation is needed to reassure the patient that a daily bowel movement is not essential to good health and that comfortable patterns of elimination are dependent on good living and eating habits. The patient should stop laxatives, enemas, and non-essential drugs that may suppress colonic motility. Fiber content of the diet should be increased by adding bran, fruits, green vegetables, and whole-grain cereals and breads. Most studies show that 15 gm. of fiber per day is needed for the best effects, but the amount can be individualized. A large breakfast including bran cereal, juice, milk or coffee, and whole-grain bread is helpful. Daily exercise should be prescribed and based on the patient's physical capacity. It is important to inform the patient with chronic constipation that return of normal function may take many weeks to occur. Often immediate results are expected; when they do not appear, the patient becomes despondent, stops the program and returns to laxative and enema use.

Some patients refuse to eat bran because it makes them feel bloated and gassy. The patient can be reassured that these side effects usually resolve within a month of continued use. If dietary and exercise efforts fail or the patient insists on medication, a non-digestible fiber residue such as ground psyllium seed (Metamucil) can be beneficial. It acts to increase bulk by means of its hydrophilic properties, but it must be taken with plenty of fluids to prevent formation of an obstructing bolus; the usual dose is one teaspoon in 8 ounces of liquid, three times a day.

When fecal impaction is present, a hypertonic enema (e.g., Fleet's) will often relieve the situation. In addition, the patient can be instructed to squat over the toilet by standing on a chair in front of the bowl, providing a more favorable position for evacuating the rectum. Only rarely does one need to resort to disimpaction.

Trying to establish a convenient, uninterrupted time for defecation each day may be useful; 15 to 20 minutes following breakfast provides a good opportunity, for spontaneous colonic motility is greatest during that period. Continuing this routine each day regardless of travel or situational stress ought to be encouraged. Although there are no controlled studies proving the efficacy of this approach, it seems to help some people, though days or weeks can pass before success is noted.

Prevention of constipation during an illness that requires bed rest can be achieved by use of a high-fiber diet, bulk agents and a commode, in preference to a bed pan. Correction of any coincident hypokalemia is important (see Chapter 27). There is no evidence that prophylactic use of laxatives or stool softeners is effective. A randomized controlled study of dioctyl sodium sulfosuccinate (Colace), a popular and expensive stool softener, failed to demonstrate any effect on the quality or frequency of stools. Use of minor tranquilizers in overly anxious patients has little direct effect on constipation. When severe depression requires use of antidepressants, the least constipating agent i.e., one with minimal anticholinergic activity, should be selected. All tricyclics have some anticholinergic activity, but desipramine seems to have the least (see Chapter 215).

The importance of taking time to explain and answer questions cannot be overstated. Successful management of functional constipation is based on excellent patient cooperation. A patient who has used a particular agent for decades needs to be told why it is being removed from the program; otherwise, chances of compliance are small. Chronic laxative users should be warned that it may take 4 to 6 weeks before spontaneous movements return. Patience and sympathetic support can be rewarding, but expectations of quick results must not be raised.

(See Chapters 61, 66, 67, 68 for management of specific etiologies).

ANNOTATED BIBLIOGRAPHY

Burkitt, D., Walker, A., and Painter, N.: Effect of dietary fibre on stools and transit times and its role in causation of disease. Lancet, *2*:1408, 1972. *(Classic paper on fiber and its link to constipation and other bowel problems.)*

Connell, A., Hilton C, Irvine, *et al.*: Variation of bowel habits in two population samples. Br. Med. J., *2*:1095, 1965. *(A population study helping to define the range of normal for bowel activity and the prevalence of constipation.)*

Darlington, R.C.: Over-the-counter laxatives. J. Am. Pharm. Assoc., *6*:470, 494, 1966. *(Provides figures on spending for over-the-counter preparations; slightly dated but enlightening.)*

Goodman, J., Pang, J., and Bessman, A.: Dioctyl sodium sulfosuccinate: An ineffective prophylactic laxative. J. Chronic Dis., *29*:59, 1976. *(A randomized prospective study of patients admitted to the hospital. The drug made no difference in quality or frequency of stools.)*

Holdstock, D., *et al.*: Propulsion in the human colon and its relationship to meals and somatic activity. Gut, *11*:91, 1970. *(Physical activity was found to stimulate mass movements, and inactivity reduced them.)*

Katz, L., and Spiro, H.: Gastrointestinal manifestations of diabetes. N. Engl. J. Med., *275*:1350, 1966. *(Constipation is a frequent gastrointestinal complaint of diabetics.)*

Kirwn, W.O., and Smith, A.N.: Colonic propulsion in diverticular disease, idiopathic constipation and the irritable bowel syndrome. Scand. J. Gastroentero., *12*:331, 1974. *(Transit time is prolonged in all three, and can be significantly reduced by bran.)*

Roth, H.P., Fein, S.B., and Shurman, J.F.: The mechanisms responsible for the urge to defecate. Gastroenterology, *32*:717, 1957. *(Describes normal process of defecation and provides physiologic basis for understanding disease states.)*

Rutter, K., and Maxwell, D.: Constipation and laxative abuse. Br. Med. J. *2*:997, 1976. *(Good description of laxative abuse.)*

60

Evaluation of Gastrointestinal Bleeding

Occasionally on an office visit, a patient reports a recent episode of mild gastrointestinal bleeding. The report might be of a tarry stool, some bright red blood passed per rectum, or vomiting that produced small quantities of blood. Patients who do not feel ill may not present immediately for evaluation; often their symptoms pass. The primary physician must decide how extensively and aggressively to pursue a diagnosis in such patients. Proper decision-making requires a knowledge of the probability of a serious underlying lesion and the yields from such diagnostic tests as barium study, sigmoidoscopy, and endoscopy.

PATHOPHYSIOLOGY AND
CLINICAL PRESENTATION

Hematemesis usually represents bleeding proximal to the ligament of Treitz, though the site of blood loss may, on rare occasions, be in the jejunum. The absence of hematemesis does not rule out the possibility of active upper gastrointestinal bleeding. Melena is seen with blood loss proximal to the ileocecal valve, where hemoglobin is converted into hematin, giving the stool its tarry quality. Right colonic bleeding may also cause melena when transit is slow. Bright red blood most often originates in the colon or anorectal region, though very brisk movement of blood from more proximal sites can lead to a similar presentation.

Manifestations of blood loss are a function of quantity and rate of bleeding; patient reports are notoriously unreliable. Postural signs are important evidence of acute volume loss in excess of 1 liter; on standing the patient up from a supine position, the heart rate rises by 10 or more beats per minute and/or the blood pressure falls by at least 10 mm Hg.

DIFFERENTIAL DIAGNOSIS

The chief causes of GI bleeding can be conveniently grouped by site of blood loss. Important esophageal etiologies are esophagitis, varices, Mallory-Weiss tears, and neoplasms. Gastric lesions that bleed include ulcers, gastritis, and cancer. Duodenitis and ulceration are responsible for most bleeding from the duodendum. Sources in the small bowel and large bowel include Meckel's diverticulum, inflammatory bowel diseases, benign and malignant neoplasms, diverticulitis, hemorrhoids, and anal fissures. Vascular lesions such as hemorrhagic telagictasis, A-V malformations, and hemangiomas can occur throughout the GI tract.

Estimates of prevalence are a function of the population studied, diagnostic methods employed, and time of investigation in relation to bleeding. A recent British series of 277 cases with melena or hematemesis provided representative figures in a mixed populatin composed of both outpatients and patients seen in emergency rooms. Over 85 per cent were subjected to endoscopy; diagnosis was also made by upper GI series or at surgery: 20 per cent had duodenal ulcers; 15 per cent gastic ulcers; 12 per cent Mallory-Weiss tears; 11 per cent esophageal varices; 5 per cent gastritis, and 1 per cent gastric cancer. In 21 per cent no cause was found (half of these patients did not undergo endoscopy), and in 5 per cent multiple lesions were detected.

In a study of 311 patients who complained of anorectal bleeding and were evaluated by careful physical examination, sigmoidoscopy, and barium enema, it was found that 78.5 per cent had lesions of the anal canal, 14.5 per cent rectal and colonic disease, and 7 per cent perianal skin problems. Leading causes were hemorrhoids in 54 percent; fissure in ano, 18 per cent; neoplasm, 6.5 per cent, and inflammatory bowel diseases, 5 per cent. In 8 per cent no cause was found at time of examination. Most of the neoplasms were more than 10 cm. above the anus.

In a series of 239 patients with undiagnosed rectal bleeding subjected to colonoscopy, 40 per cent had significant lesions; 16 per cent were found to have polyps; 10 per cent inflammatory bowel disease; 9 per cent carcinomas missed by barium enema; and 3 per cent diverticular disease, hemangiomas, or other miscellaneous causes. In over 100 no cause was found.

Patients with gastronintestinal bleeding while on anticoagulant therapy are likely to have an underlying lesion. In a study examining 3800 courses of anticoagulant therapy, gastrointestinal bleeding occured in 45 patients. In 32, a source was determined: 13 had hemorrhoids; 9 peptic ulcers; and 7, neoplasms; 3 had other lesions.

Nosebleeds and respiratory-tract bleeding must be considered in the differential diagnosis of melena and guaiac positive stools. A falsely positive stool-guaiac test can be produced by use of glycerol guaiacolate, the popular expectorant. Black stools may result from bismuth (Pepto-Bismol), iron, charcoal, or spinach intake; red stools can occur from eating large quantities of beets.

WORKUP

History and physical examination often provide information regarding the location and severity of bleeding, but laboratory investigations are usually necessary to determine the exact cause. In a series of 311 cases of anorectal bleeding, history and physical examination yielded a definite diagnosis in only 28 per cent. Nevertheless, history and physical examination can play important roles that may obviate the need for more invasive testing and help in selection of an optimal procedure.

History. Before proceeding with an extensive workup, the physician ought to be certain that the history of blood loss is accurate. In particular, dark stools must not be mistaken for the black tarry ones of genuine melena. Also, the patient has to be queried specifically about nosebleeds and hemoptysis, important extraintestinal sources of gastrointestinal blood. Intake of Pepto-Bismol, iron, charcoal preparations, beets, and licorice should be investigated to be sure that the history of "bleeding" is genuine.

An approximate bleeding site can be determined by the nature of the blood loss, i.e., whether it is melena, hematemesis, or bright red blood per rectum. A crude estimate of rate and severity can be obtained by asking about postural light-headedness. The actual volume lost is not reliably obtained from the history, though extreme amounts should be taken seriously.

When the patient complains of voluminous blood loss or light-headedness, a careful check for postural change in vital signs is indicated before proceeding with a detailed office assessment. Immediate hospital admission should be arranged if blood pressure falls more than 10 to 15 mg Hg, or heart rate increases by more than 10 to 15 beats per minute when the patient stands up from a supine position. Measurement of the hematocrit in the acute phase of blood loss may show deceptively little decline if there has not been suffient time for re-equilibration of intravascular volume.

Once it is clear that the degree of blood loss does not pose an immediate hazard, office evaluation can proceed. When hematemesis is reported, sources of esophageal, gastric, and duodenal bleeding must be sought. History of heartburn, dysphagia, cirrhosis, or forceful vomiting prior to hematemesis point to esophageal etiologies. Use of aspirin, alcohol, and anti-inflammatory agents may be linked to gastric bleeding due to ulceration or gastritis. History of peptic ulcer or the presence of epigastric pain responsive to antacids or related to food raises the possibility of bleeding from a gastric or duodenal crater. However, it is noteworthy that another explanation for bleeding is often present in many patients with a history typical of ulcer disease.

When no hematemesis is noted, the source may still be from above the ligament of Treitz; however, small bowel and colonic lesions must be considered as well. Diarrhea, urgency, tenesmus, and lower abdominal cramping suggest inflammatory bowel disease (see Chapter 65). With ulcerative colitis, diverticulitis, and other forms of rectosigmoid disease, there is often some frank rectal bleeding. Weight loss or change in bowel habits raises suspicion of colonic cancer. A history of diverticular disease may be a clue to the cause of blood loss but may coexist with carcinoma, which must be ruled out. Many patients with rectal bleeding admit to past or present hemorrhoidal problems, but in almost half of cases another lesion is found to be the cause of blood loss. Anticoagulant use should be investigated.

On *physical examination* the skin is noted for pallor, ecchymoses, petechiae, telangiectasias, jaundice, and spider angiomata. The nose and pharynx are observed for sources of bleeding and the chest is auscultated and percussed for evidence of consolidation or effusion. Lymph nodes are examined for enlargement and the abdomen for organomegaly, ascites, masses, or rectal lesions. Left supraclavicular adenopathy or a rectal shelf mass points to probable bowel malignancy. The stool is checked for color and occult blood (see Chapter 51). If the patient describes recent hematemesis, a small nasogastric tube should be put down to aspirate gastric contents and test for the presence of blood.

Laboratory studies that can be of importance include *platelet count, prothrombin time,* and *partial thromboplastin time* (PTT). Tests of hematocrit, blood urea nitrogen (BUN), and creatinine are also worth ordering to help assess severity of volume depletion and chronicity of blood loss.

In the patient with rectal bleeding, the likelihood of cancer is a function of age. Less than 5 per cent of all colonrectal cancers occur in patients under age 40, and less than 1 per cent in those under age 30. Thus, if the physical examination reveals local anorectal pathology in a young patient with rectal bleeding, it is probably unnecessary to perform a sigmoidoscopy or barium enema. On the other hand, 80 per cent of colonorectal malignancies are found in patients over 50. When a person over 50 presents with rectal bleeding, he requires a through search for tumor even if a local lesion such as a hemorrhoid is discovered; 27 per cent of patients with carcinoma of the rectum and 10 per cent with carcinoma of the sigmoid have been noted to have coincidental hemorrhoids.

There are increasing amounts of data available on yields of diagnostic procedures. In a series of 311 patients with rectal bleeding subjected to history, physical examination, sigmoidoscopy, and barium enema, the history diagnosed 5 per cent, the physical examination raised the figure to 28 per cent, and the addition of sigmoidoscopy provided an answer in 90 per cent. Barium enema raised the yield in this series only another 3 per cent, probably because an unusually large number of lesions were within reach of the sigmoidoscope. Usually about 50 to 60 per cent of colonic malignancies can be viewed by sigmoidoscopy (see Chapter 51). Consequently, persons with rectal bleeding in the age group at high risk for large-bowel malignancy should undergo barium study. *Barium enema* has a sensitivity of 80 to 90 per cent for detecting carcinoma and 70 per cent for polyps greater than 5 mm. in diameter. Cancers most often missed are in the cecum or rectrosigmoid or obscured by concurrent diverticulitis or ulcerative colitis. Air-contrast techniques improve the results.

The advent of *colonoscopy* has improved the identification of bleeding sources. About 40 per cent of cases of frank rectal bleeding or occult blood loss which are associated with normal sigmoidoscopy and normal routine barium enema have been found to harbor previously undetected lesions when studied by colonoscopy. About 10 per cent have cancers; another 10 per cent, polyps, 10 per cent, inflammatory bowel disease; and 5 per cent, telangiectasis. Furthermore, carcinomas and polyps were detected in 20 per cent of patients when only diverticula were seen with barium enema. Although the role for colonoscopy is not yet settled, it seems reasonable to subject patients over age 50 to colonoscopy if they have rectal or occult blood loss in combination with normal barium enema and normal sigmoidoscopy or if they show diverticula only on barium study.

Barium studies for evaluation of upper gastrointestinal bleeding are being surpassed in utility by *endoscopy,* because the sensitivity of the UGI series is around 50 per cent, compared to almost 95 per cent for endoscopy. Esophagitis, Mallory-Weiss tears and gastritis are readily seen by endoscopy and undetectible radiologically. Moreover the swallowing of barium obscures mucosal detail and makes endoscopy impossible. Thus for suspected acute upper gastrointestinal bleeding, endoscopy is probably the procedure of first choice, with barium study as a supplementary procedure reserved for inactive bleeders or patients with normal endoscopies and unexplained blood loss. However, the improvement in detection of lesions has not yet been proven to affect outcome; neither an increase in survival not a decrease in transfusion requirements has been demonstrated. Better results require improvements in the available modalities for treatment of upper gastrointestinal bleeding.

INDICATIONS FOR ADMISSION AND REFERRAL

The patient with brisk, gross bleeding obviously requires emergency admission, as does the person with less dramatic evidence or blood loss, whose hematocrit has sharply fallen or whose vital signs show marked postural change. Workup of the patient with mild or slow blood loss can proceed safely on an ambulatory basis as long as the patient does not have serious cardiopulmonery disease and is responsible

enough to recognize and promptly report signs of worsening blood loss or volume depletion. The patient with acute hematemesis or lower gastrointestinal bleeding who has a normal barium enema and signoidoscopy ought to be seen by the gastroenterologist for consideration of endoscopy.

SYMPTOMATIC MANAGEMENT

Modest falls in hematocrit that accompany chronic low-grade gastrointestinal blood loss can be treated with oral iron (300 mg., $FeSO_4$ 3 times daily) to make up for the resulting iron deficiency (see Chapter 83). Marked but gradual decreases in hematocrit to the mid-20s are usually well tolerated unless the patient has cardiopulmonary disease. Most patients do not need transfusion unless they are symptomatic. Oral iron usually produces a prompt retriculocytosis and at least partial correction of the anemia. Patients with presumed lower-tract bleeding can be given stool softeners to decrease mechanical trauma to the lesion (see Chapter 68).

ANNOTATED BIBLIOGRAPHY

Coon, U., and Willis, P.: Hemorrhagic complications of anticoagulant therapy. Ann. Intern. Med., *133:*386, 1974. *(More than half of patients who bled on anticoagulant therapy had an identifiable underlying gastrointestinal lesion.)*

Eastwood, D.L.: Does endoscopy benefit the patient with acute upper gastrointestinal bleeding? Gastroenterology, *72:*737, 1977. *(Neither an improvement in patient survival nor a decrease in transfusion requirements could be demonstrated.)*

Foster, D.N., Miloszewski, K., and Losowsky, M.: Stigmata of recent hemorrhage in diagnosis and prognosis of upper gastrointestinal bleeding. Br. Med. J., *1:*1173, 1976. *(A series of 277 consecutive cases of hematemesis, melena and upper GI bleeding seen in emergency and outpatient settings. Duodenal ulcer, gastric ulcer, Mallory-Weiss lesions and esophageal varies led the list of causes.)*

McGinn, F., et al.: A prospective comparative trial between early endoscopy and radiology in acute upper gastrointestinal bleeding. Gut, *16:*707, 1975. *(A series of 150 patients. Endoscopy identified the source in 86% and UGI in 51%. False* positives rates were 8% for UGI and 8% for endoscopy. Use of both studies identified the source of bleeding in 91%.)

Morris, D., Levine, G., and Solomay, R.: Prospective randomized study of diagnosis and outcome of acute upper gastrointestintal bleeding: Endoscopy versus conventional radiology. Am. J. Dig. Dis. 20:1103, 1975. (Endoscope provided a definitive localization in 69% compared to 21% for UGI; the same was true for diagnosis. No differences in clinical outcome resulted, however.)

Schapiro, R.H.: The visible vessel: Curse or blessing. N. Engl. J. Med., 300:1438, 1979. (An editorial reviewing the utility of endoscopy, with emphasis on defining a high-risk group of patients with upper gastrointestinal bleeding.)

Teague, R., et al.: Colonoscopy for investigation of unexplained rectal bleeding. Lancet, 1:1350, 1978. (Provides figures on causes of bleeding in patients with normal barium enema. In over 40% a cause was found, including 10% with carcinomas.)

Tedesco, F., et al.: Colonoscopic evaluation of rectal bleeding. Ann. Intern. Med., 89:907, 1978. (Colonoscopy discovered cancers in 10% with normal sigmoidoscopies and normal barium enemas and in another 10% with diverticula alone on barium enema. As in a similar British study, almost 40% had a detectable cause of blood loss.)

Williams, J.T., and Thompson, J.P.S.: Anorectal bleeding: Study of causes and investigative results. Practitioner, 219:327, 1977. (Diagnosis was made in 90% of cases by history, physical examinations, and sigmoidoscopy. Barium enema improved yield by only 3%. In 75% the cause was local anal pathology, but most tumors were 10 cm. above the anus.)

61

Evaluation of Anorectal Problems

MICHAEL N. MARGOLIES, M.D.

Anal pain and itching are extraordinarily common complaints which cause great confusion among physicians, in part because the education of physicians and surgeons in medical centers tends to ignore the banal and emphasize the dramatic. The patient with severe anal pain has little sympathy for what he perceives as a distortion of priorities. Relief of anorectal discomfort is possible only if the primary physician is capable of discovering its causes.

Anorectal Pain

Anorectal pain may be caused by anorectal ulceration (fissure), by distention from local abscess, or by distention and edema from prolapsed or thrombosed hemorrhoids. Secondary anal sphincter spasm may prolong and intensify the pain. Malignant neoplasms of the perianal area or anorectal tract may also produce pain in late stages.

PATHOPHYSIOLOGY AND CLINICAL PRESENTATION

Fissure-in-ano is actually a more common cause of anorectal pain than hemorrhoids, but often goes unrecognized. Anal fissure begins as a traumatic lesion, usually from passage of a hard stool, and often fails to heal, partly because sphincter spasm interferes with drainage from the ulcer and makes repeated trauma more likely. Pain due to anal fissure typically worsens following a bowel movement, may be severe, and is sometimes accompanied by bleeding. On the other hand, painless or multiple fissures may be manifestations of underlying inflammatory bowel disease (see Chapter 65).

Perirectal abscess and fistula-in-ano are two stages of the same disease process, beginning as infection in the anal glands which empty into the anal crypts at the mucocutaneous junction, and subsequently spreading into the adjacent tissue. The abscess thus formed often drains through the perianal skin. Perirectal abscess is first manifested by rectal pain. Few physical signs may be apparent at the time of the first examination. In subsequent days, local swelling, erythema and tenderness become evident.

Fistula-in-ano is a communication between the anal canal and the perianal skin. It is usually nontender. The external opening may be single or multiple, with a granulation tissue bud and chronic seropurulent drainage. Occasionally, an indurated cord of tissue may be palpable, extending from the external fistulous opening toward the anal canal.

Hemorrhoids result in pain only when an external hemorrhoid is complicated by acute thrombosis or when prolapse with swelling and ischemia occurs (see Chapter 68).

Carcinoma of the perianal skin or anorectal tract may produce pain as a relatively late manifestation, especially in large ulcerated lesions, which also commonly bleed. Earlier lesions are painless nodules or plaques.

An *infected pilonidal sinus or cyst* is most common in males between ages 16 and 30. They are midline in the area of the natal cleft; multiple sinuses may be present. Recurrent secondary infections are frequent.

WORKUP

Thorough and gentle inspection of the anus and perianal region is the *sine qua non* of successful diagnosis of anal problems. Stretching the perianal skin will reveal fissures, which will come into view at the anal verge, most often in the posterior midline but occasionally in the anterior midline. In chronic fissures, there will be scarring and induration, as well as an associated hypertrophied anal papilla at the pectinate line, and a skin tag marking the external limit. Digital rectal examination in the presence of a painful fissure will almost certainly alienate the patient, and persistence in such an attempt will yield little further useful information. The same prohibition applies to anoscopy and proctoscopy in the unanesthetized patient with a fissure. On the other hand, in patients with anorectal complaints who are not acutely uncomfortable, rectal examination and sigmoidoscopy should never be deferred. Ascribing rectal symptoms to hemorrhoids without as complete an examination as permitted comfortably is a common reason for delay in diagnosis of anorectal carcinoma. When painless or multiple fissures are present, underlying inflammatory bowel disease should be con-

sidered; sigmoidoscopy and barium contrast studies are indicated. Atypical fissures or those which fail to heal should be biopsied to rule out malignancy, Crohn's disease, and chronic infection such as tuberculosis and syphilis.

If inspection reveals a painless, hard nodule or plaque in the anal region, carcinoma of the anus must be considered; biopsy will be needed for confirmation. When the lesion is ulcerated, the diagnosis is more obvious and the disease more advanced.

Crohn's disease, and less often ulcerative colitis, should be kept in mind in patients with recurrent perirectal sepsis or fistulas. Evaluation of these patients includes noting a history of abdominal pain, diarrhea, constipation, etc., and performing sigmoidoscopy and barium contrast studies (see Chapter 65). The treatment of isolated perirectal sepsis is quite different from the management of a patient with an abscess due to inflammatory bowel disease.

Infected pilonidal sinuses or cysts are distinguished from perirectal abscess by their location in or near the posterior midline in the natal cleft and by the presence of one or more skin sinuses.

SYMPTOMATIC MANAGEMENT AND INDICATIONS FOR REFERRAL

Patients with anal pain due to *fissure* should initially be treated symptomatically. Lubricants, such as mineral oil, and agents providing a soft, bulky stool, such as methylcellulose, will decrease trauma and counteract the attendant sphincter spasm. Frequent warm sitz baths provide intermittent relief of pain and spasm. Topical analgesics are of limited use and may result in skin sensitization. Systemic analgesics are sometimes necessary, but if narcotics are used, increased constipation may occur. If the pain has not improved by conservative measures in several days to weeks, the patient should be referred for surgical treatment, which has a high success rate. In general, chronic or recurrent fissures will require surgery more often than acute or superficial fissures. In patients where the pain of fissure precludes digital or instrumental examination at the first visit, these may be done at the time of surgical treatment under adequate anesthesia.

Established *perirectal abscess* will not resolve on antibiotics alone; the proper treatment is surgical drainage. Antibiotic therapy should be reserved for patients with extensive cellulitis, signs of systemic infection, immunosuppression, valvular heart disease, or intravascular prostheses. Incision and drainage of a perirectal abscess usually requires anesthesia and is not often an office procedure. Similarly, the treatment for an infected pilonidal sinus is surgical drainage, which is satisfactorily accomplished under local anesthesia.

The only successful treatment for *fistula-in-ano* is surgical. However, patients with inflammatory bowel disease should not undergo surgery for fistula as this will usually fail as long as there is any active proximal disease. Surgery is reserved for palliation of complications of fistula, i.e., drainage of recurrent perirectal abscess.

For management of hemorrhoids, see Chapter 68. Suspicion of carcinoma and need for biopsy require surgical consultation.

Pruritus Ani

Pruritus ani (chronic perianal itching) results from a variety of mechanical and inflammatory lesions and is intensified by moisture in the perianal area. Chronic itching leads to excoriation, chronic edema, thickening, fissuring, and lichenification of the perianal skin. Symptomatic relief is sought from the primary physician for this annoying problem.

PATHOPHYSIOLOGY AND CLINICAL PRESENTATION

Anatomic lesions that produce chronic discharge (such as fistulas, fissures, and hemorrhoids with intermittent mucosal eversion) can result in pruritus ani. A variety of viral, bacterial, fungal, and parasitic infections and infestations may also lead to anal itching. *Anogenital warts* (*condylomata*) are caused by a virus and are generally sexually transmitted. They may be confined to the perianal region or also involve the penis, vulva and anal canal. They are soft, filiform multiple excrescences which may enlarge, become confluent, and bleed. *Gonorrheal proctitis,* now probably the most common primary form of gonorrhea, may result in an inflammatory reaction of varying degrees with soreness, burning and purulent anal discharge. Infestation with *pinworm* (*Enterobius vermicularis*) results in perianal pruritus, especially affecting children but sometimes involving several family members. It typically occurs at night, when the female pinworm migrates downward to deposit eggs on the perianal skin. *Systemic dermatologic diseases* such as psoriasis, may be manifested in the perianal region. *Contact dermatitis* or *eczema* re-

Table 61–1.   Some Causes of Pruritus Ani

A. Anorectal Anatomic Lesions
  1. Fissure
  2. Fistula-in-ano
  3. Prolapsing hemorrhoids
B. Infections
  1. Viral warts (condylomata)
  2. Herpes simplex
  3. Syphilis
  4. Gonorrhea
  5. Erythrasma (*Corynebacterium minutissimum*)
  6. Candidiasis
  7. Trichophytosis
  8. Pinworm (*Enterobius vermicularis*)
C. Dermatologic Diseases
  1. Psoriasis
  2. Lichen planus
  3. Bowen's disease
  4. Contact eczema
D. Idiopathic

sulting from the use of a topical agent is common and can complicate the diagnosis of the original cause of pruritus; applied initially as a remedy for itching, the agent may itself cause itching due to skin sensitization.

DIFFERENTIAL DIAGNOSIS

See Table 61–1.

WORKUP

Detailed inquiry into the use of topical medications, involvement of other household members or sexual partners, and hygienic practices should be made. A few moments spent carefully inspecting the perianal area are invaluable to diagnosis. In particular, the genital region as well as the anus should be inspected for condylomata. The patient should be specifically questioned about rectal intercourse and possible gonorrheal contact when an inflamed anorectal mucosa is found; discharge should be cultured on Thayer-Martin plates. If the lesions appear as scaling plaques, one should look at the extensor surfaces of the extremities for evidence of other psoriatic lesions. Erythema or eczematous changes suggest a contact dermatitis. The patient should be asked whether topical agents have been applied to the anorectal area, including soaps, deodorants, topical anesthetics and hemorrhoidal preparations. A very anxious patient who also shows multiple excoriations over other parts of the body should lead one to consider the possibility of neurodermatitis. Low-power microscopic examination of a Scotch-tape impression of the anus will reveal the typical eggs laid by the adult female pinworm.

SYMPTOMATIC MANAGEMENT AND INDICATIONS FOR REFERRAL

Specifc therapy for pruritus ani is related to identification of a specific etiology, as for example diabetes in the patient with Candidiasis. Identification of the cause may be a challenging exercise to the primary physician. Pruritus resulting from anatomic lesions will generally remit with correction of the underlying cause. *Anogenital warts* are effectively treated with topical application of 25% podophyllin in tincture of benzoin repeated every 1 to 2 weeks. The patient is instructed to bathe between 6 and 12 hours after the application. Care should be taken to avoid applying the compound to intact skin. If anoscopy reveals intra-anal warts at the initial examination, curettage and electrocoagulation under anesthesia will be necessary.

All family members should be treated simultaneously for *pinworms*. Pyrantel pamoate (Antiminth) is the drug of choice; a one-time oral dose of 11 mg. per kg. of body weight usually suffices. Preventive measures are difficult to enforce, except for handwashing before meals and after bowel movements. The best prevention is simultaneous treatment of all members of the household.

Often, however, no specific cause is found, and pruritus appears to be a form of neurodermatitis affecting the perianal skin. However, the symptoms may often be relieved by careful attention to perianal hygiene following bowel movements, keeping the perianal skin dry with application of witch hazel, and using topical steroid ointments (0.25% hydrocortisone ointment) for several weeks to break the cycle of itching and skin changes caused by scratching. When contact dermatitis is thought to be caused by topical agents, the offending medication should be discontinued.

For treatment of gonorrheal proctitis, see Chapter 113.

PATIENT EDUCATION

When poor personal hygiene, sexual contact, irritating agents, or neurotic concerns are responsible for symptoms, the relation between the rectal discomfort and precipitants should be explained so that the patient can make corrective measures himself. Patients who obtain temporary relief of symptoms by applying topical sensitizing agents may be reluctant to halt their medication if no other therapy is advised. Daily sitz baths can be prescribed in their place.

ANNOTATED BIBLIOGRAPHY

Goligher, J.C.: Surgery of the Anus, Rectum and Colon, ed. 2. London: Bailliere, Tindell and Cassel, 1967. *(An encyclopedic description of management of anorectal problems by a surgeon.)*

William, J.A. (ed.): Clinics in Gastroenterology, vol. 4. Philadelphia: W.B. Saunders, 1975. *(Several good chapters on current evaluation of dermatologic and venereal disease problems.)*

62
Evaluation of Jaundice

The development of jaundice usually precipitates a visit to the physician. When associated symptoms are minimal, the patient is likely to present on an ambulatory basis, concerned about liver disease or cancer. The primary physician needs to assess hepatocellular function and the likelihood of an extrahepatic obstructive lesion in order to decide whether workup can proceed safely on an outpatient basis or would best be done in the hospital. Determination of the exact etiology of the jaundice is secondary to distinguishing obstruction from hepatocellular disease and other nonsurgical causes. Assessment requires familiarity with the mechanisms of jaundice and their clinical presentations, and the indications for use of noninvasive diagnostic studies available in the ambulatory setting.

PATHOPHYSIOLOGY AND CLINICAL PRESENTATION

The mechanisms responsible for jaundice include excess bilirubin production, decreased hepatic uptake, impaired conjugation, intrahepatic cholestasis, extrahepatic obstruction and hepatocellular injury. Clinically, jaundice becomes noticeable when the serum bilirubin reaches 2.0 to 2.5 mg. per 100 ml. The yellow hue may be mimicked by carotenemia, but in the latter there is no scleral icterus. Deeply jaundiced patients often demonstrate a greenish tinge due to the oxidation of bilirubin to biliverdin.

Excess bilirubin production results from accelerated red cell destruction. Occasionally, markedly ineffective erythropoiesis may be responsible. The amounts of hemoglobin and resultant bilirubin released into the bloodstream overwhelm the normal liver's capacity for uptake, and an unconjugated hyperbilirubinemia ensues. Total bilirubin rises as a result of the increased indirect fraction. All tests of hepatocellular function are normal (as are urine and stool appearances). Symptoms, signs and laboratory tests point to hemolysis or ineffective erythropoiesis (see Chapter 77).

Decreased uptake and conjugation are other mechanisms of unconjugated hyperbilirubinemia. The only evidence of hepatocellular dysfunction is an increase in unconjugated bilirubin. Frequently there is a concurrent, acquired illness such as an infection, cardiac disease or cancer. Sometimes hereditary conditions, such as Gilbert's and Crigler-Najjar syndromes are responsible. In Gilbert's syndrome, fasting and minor illness can precipitate jaundice.

Intrahepatic cholestasis may occur at a number of levels: intracellularly, (eg., hepatitis); at the canalicular level (when estrogen-induced); at the ductule (phenothiazine exposure); at the septal ducts (primary biliary cirrhosis); and at the intralobular ducts (cholangiocarcinoma). Regardless of site, there are similarities in presentation. Jaundice comes on gradually, the patient feels well, and weight loss is slow; pruritus is common. The liver is large, smooth and nontender; it may be firm but not rocky hard. Splenomegaly is unlikely except in primary biliary cirrhosis. Stools are pale and steatorrhea is present in severe cases. There is a hyperbilirubinemia, predominantly of the conjugated fraction, with marked alkaline phosphatase elevation, mild transaminase rise and normal serum albumin. Urine is dark and positive for bilirubin. Prothrombin time may be pro-longed due to malabsorption, but is reversible by vitamin K injection.

Extrahepatic obstruction occurs when stone, stricture or tumor block the flow of bile within the extrahepatic biliary tree. A history of gallstones, biliary tract surgery, or prior malignancy may be elicited. The gallbladder is sometimes palpable, especially when there is gradual development of obstruction allowing time for painless dilatation of the biliary tree. Sudden onset with pain results from passage of a stone which becomes wedged into the common duct; fever and sepsis may follow shortly thereafter, indicating cholangitis. Weight loss is a nonspecific finding, but when marked and accompanied by jaundice, it suggests carcinoma of the head of the pancreas or metastatic disease obstructing the common duct. Extrahepatic obstruction and intrahepatic cholestasis may be identical in presentation. The liver is usually enlarged; tenderness is minimal unless cholangitis or rapid distention occurs. A rock-hard mass strongly points to malignancy. As in intrehepatic cholestasis, conjugated bilirubin exhibits the greatest rise in association with a high serum alkaline phosphatase and a mild to moderate increase in the transaminase level. Any prolongation of prothrombin time is at least partially reversible with parenteral vitamin K. Urine is dark due to the conjugated bilirubinuria. Stools are pale from absence of bile.

Hepatocellular disease is typified by hepatitis, with prodromal symptoms of anorexia, nausea, abdominal pain and malaise preceding jaundice (see Chapters 52 and 70). Hepatic tenderness is notable, but there is usually less liver enlargement than with obstruction. There may be ecchymoses. Transaminases may reach dramatic levels, except in the case of alcoholic hepatitis, where the rise is no more than 5 times normal. The alkaline phosphatase rises modestly to 2 to 4 times above baseline. Urine is dark, stools

---

Table 62–1. Differential Diagnosis of Jaundice by Pathophysiological Mechanisms

A. Unconjugated Hyperbilirubinemias (urine negative for bilirubin)
   1. Increased bilirubin production
   2. Decreased hepatic uptake of bilirubin
   3. Decreased conjugation
B. Conjugated Hyperbilirubinemias (urine positive for bilirubin)
   1. Hepatocellular disease
   2. Intrahepatic cholestasis
   3. Extrahepatic obstructon

pale. There may be evidence of decreased protein synthesis. The prothrombin time is the first measure of synthetic function to become abnormal, because the half-lives of the clotting factors made in the liver are less than 7 days. If synthetic function remains depressed beyond 2 weeks, the serum albumin begins to fall. Chronic hepatocellular disease may lead to fibrosis and cirrhosis with portal hypertension, peripheral edema, ascites, gynecomastia, testicular atrophy, bleeding and encephalopathy (see Chapter 71).

DIFFERENTIAL DIAGNOSIS

The causes of jaundice are extensive but can be grouped according to major pathophysiological mechanisms and type of hyperbilirubinemia (conjugated or unconjugated) (Table 62–1). It is important to recognize that more than one mechanism can be operating in a given case. The vast majority of cases are due to obstruction, intrahepatic cholestasis, or hepatocellular injury. In young patients, hepatitis predominates. In the elderly, stones and tumor are often responsible. Drugs account for many cases of intrahepatic cholestasis, and often mimic extrahepatic etiologies.

WORKUP

History and physical examination will often suffice to provide a diagnosis or at least an indication of hepatocellular injury or obstruction. A study of 61 cases of jaundice documented by liver biopsy revealed that history and physical alone provided the correct diagnosis in 70 per cent of cases of viral hepatitis, 77 per cent of cases of obstructive jaundice and 80 per cent of cases of cirrhosis. Key historical items include presence of abdominal pain, history of alcoholism, exposure to hepatitis, and flulike onset. Of little discriminative value are histories of weight loss, pruritus, nausea and vomiting, and distaste for tobacco. Drug use, hepatitis exposure, family history of jaundice, occupation, travel, raw shellfish consumption, history of gallstones or biliary tract exploration, previous malignancy, fever, easy bruising, confusion, pale stools, and dark urine also need to be checked for. The same study examined the utility of various physical findings in diagnosis. Stigmata of cirrhosis and a palpable gallbladder were the most specific, followed by marked hepatic enlargement (6 or more cm. below the costal margin). Physical examination should include a check for any cachexia,

temperature, fetor hepaticus, pallor, depth of jaundice, purpura, spider angiomas, palmar erythema, scleral icterus, gynecomastia, lymphadenopathy, liver size and consistency, tenderness, ascites, splenomegaly, palpable gallbladder, abdominal masses, stool and urine color, edema and asterixis.

Laboratory investigation can be utilized to identify the predominant pathophysiology and to assess severity, especially when history and physical findings are nondiagnostic. Testing begins with a check of the *urine for bilirubin*. Since only conjugated bilirubin appears in the urine, its presence indicates a conjugated hyperbilirubinemia and the possibility of cholestasis, obstruction or hepatocellular injury; its absence argues for excess bilirubin production, decreased uptake and impaired conjugation. Determinations of *direct* and *indirect serum bilirubin* levels quantitatively confirm urinary findings and indicate disease severity.

An elevation predominantly of the unconjugated bilirubin fraction and a negative urinary bilirubin should initiate a search for hemolysis (see Chapter 77), ineffective erythropoiesis, hereditary causes of jaundice, and concurrent systemic illness. Standard "liver function tests" add little to the assessment of unconjugated hyperbilirubinemia; they are normal or very mildly and nonspecifically elevated.

Conjugated hyperbilirubinemia and a positive urine necessitate a check of the SGOT, alkaline phosphatase, prothrombin time and serum albumin. Mechanical obstruction and intrahepatic cholestasis are characterized by marked rises in *alkaline phosphatase* (greater than 4 to 5 times normal) and modest elevations in *transaminases* (2 to 3 times normal); the reverse is typical of hepatocellular diseases. Unfortunately, one is sometimes faced with nonspecific rises in both. The transaminases can be particularly misleading when jaundice has been present for a while, because even with pure obstruction some hepatocellular injury occurs, causing a considerable rise in the SGOT (greater than 5 times normal) and a mimicking of a nonobstructive etiology. This has been reported in about 15 per cent of cases of obstruction.

The alkaline phosphatase may also give false-positive impressions. A marked elevation in alkaline phosphatase and a cholestatic picture can occur on occasion in some forms of hepatocellular disease such as viral, alcoholic, drug-induced and chronic active hepatitides. However, a low alkaline phosphatase (under 5 Bodansky units per 100 ml.) is rarely seen in the context of extrahepatic obstruction.

Further separation of hepatocellular disease from cholestatic and obstructive conditions can be attempted by studying measures of liver synthetic function. A prolonged *prothrombin time* unresponsive to parenteral vitamin K is strongly suggestive of hepatocellular failure. Cholestasis and obstruction also may produce prolongation of the protime, but it can be reversed by vitamin K. *Serum albumin* levels fall when substantial hepatocellular injury has occurred and synthetic capacity has been suppressed for a few weeks. Interpretation of the albumin level requires consideration of dietary intake and sources of possible protein loss. In most instances, hepatocellular disease can be distinguished from cholestasis and extrahepatic obstruction on the basis of clinical data, liver function tests and response to vitamin K.* On the other hand, cholestasis and obstruction may be indistinguishable without further testing. The distinction is critical to management since mechanical blockade to flow of bile requires hospital admission and consideration of surgery. Moreover, obstruction can be a precipitant of cholangitis and sepsis.

Study of the biliary tree can be achieved by intravenous cholangiogram, ultrasound, percutaneous transhepatic cholangiogram or retrograde cannulation. *Intravenous cholangiography* is usually not helpful since the biliary cannot be visualized when the bilirubin rises above 2 to 3 mg. per 100 ml. Recently, *ultrasonography* has been studied as a noninvasive means of detecting extrahepatic obstruction. Specificity of the test is above 90 per cent; sensitivity ranges from 47 to 90 per cent and is a function of the duration and degree of bile duct obstruction. Cases of early obstruction with minimally dilated ducts may be missed unless repeat studies are performed after ducts have had a chance to increase in size. False-positives may occur from persistent ductal dilatation after relief of obstruction. Although ultrasound is a useful noninvasive method, a negative result does not rule out the possibility of extrahepatic obstruction. If obstruction is still suspected, *percutaneous skinny needle cholangiography* and/or *retrograde cannulation of the common duct* are indicated. These procedures are relatively safe and usually diagnostic, but necessitate hospital admission. A percutaneous study that is negative after three attempts virtually rules out obstruction, since dilated bile ducts are an invariable feature of obstruction. *Liver biopsy* in a case of possible obstruction is unwise,

since the risk of bile peritonitis is high and better tests are available to make an anatomic diagnosis. Once obstruction is ruled out, biopsy may provide very useful diagnostic information for assessment of hepatocellular disease.

INDICATIONS FOR ADMISSION, CONSULTATION AND REFERRAL

Admission is mandatory when jaundice is complicated by fever and peritoneal signs indicative of cholangitis. Intravenous antibiotics and surgical consultation are immediate necessities. Admission is also indicated when signs of marked hepatocellular failure such as asterixis, ascites, encephalopathy or bleeding are present (see Chapter 71). Consultation with a radiologist, surgeon and gastroenterologist experienced in hepatobiliary disease can be very useful when obstruction, cholestasis and hepatocellular injury are under consideration and cannot be readily distinguished. Choice of the best invasive means to rule out obstruction depends on the experience and techniques available locally. When liver biopsy is deemed appropriate to determine etiology, consultation with a gastroenterologist familiar with liver disease is indicated.

SYMPTOMATIC RELIEF

Mild jaundice in itself is innocuous, but more marked elevations in bilirubin may produce considerable pruritus, presumably by bile salt deposition in the skin. Cholestyramine has been used successfully to treat pruritus and is worth a try in patients who are quite uncomfortable. One 9-gm. packet of the powder containing 4 gm. of cholestyramine resin is mixed in orange juice or applesauce and taken 3 times a day. Absorption of fat-soluble vitamins may be impaired by cholestyramine, and oral or parenteral supplements of vitamins A, D, and K can be prescribed. Absorption of drugs may also be interfered with; drugs should be taken at least 1 hour before cholestyramine. Constipation or diarrhea are minor common side effects.

ANNOTATED BIBLIOGRAPHY

Datta, D., and Sherlock S.: Cholestyramine for long-term relief of the pruritus complicating intrahepatic cholestasis. Gastroenterology, *50*:323, 1966.

*Instances of anaphylaxis have been reported with intravenous use of vitamin K. Intramuscular or subcutaneous administration is preferable.

(Cholestyramine is effective; 4 to 7 days of therapy are required before relief is obtained.)

Dubin, I.: Intrahepatic bile stasis in acute nonfatal viral hepatitis: Its incidence, pathogenesis and correlation with jaundice. Gastroenterology, 36:645, 1959. *(Classic description of viral hepatitis presenting with a cholestatic picture.)*

Felsher, B., Rickard, D., and Redeker, A.: The reciprocal relation between caloric intake and the degree of hyperbilirubinemia in Gilbert's syndrome. N. Engl. J. Med., 283:170, 1970. *(An increase in unconjugated bilirubin occurred with fasting or low caloric intake—approximately 400 calories.)*

Ferrucci, J., Wittenberg, J., Sarno, R., et al.: Fine needle transhepatic cholangiography. Am. J. Roentgenol., 127:403, 1976. *(Sensitivity is 100 per cent when ducts are dilated, but falls to 75 per cent when ducts are not dilated. About 1 per cent risk of bile peritonitis, but up to 12 per cent risk of sepsis.)*

Lapis, J., Orlando, R., Mittelstaedt, C., et al.: Ultra-sonography in the diagnosis of obstructive jaundice. Ann. Intern. Med., 89:61, 1978. *(In a study of 47 cases of with cholestatic jaundice, there were no false-positives. False-negative rate was 6 per cent when bilirubin greater than 10 mg% and 53 per cent when bilirubin less than 10 mg%.)*

Levine, R., and Klatskin, G.: Unconjugated hyperbilirubinemia in the absence of overt hemolysis. Am. J. Med., 36:541, 1964. *(A series of 366 patients with a high proportion traceable to a concurrent illness rather than a hereditary condition. Cardiac disease, infection, cancer and inflammatory bowel disease accounted for over 50 per cent.)*

Schenker, S., Balint, J., and Schiff, L.: Differential diagnosis of jaundice: Report of a prospective study of 61 proved cases. Am. J. Dig. Dis., 7:449, 1962. *(A study of the merits of clinical features and laboratory tests in the differential diagnosis of jaundice.)*

63

Approach to the Patient with an External Hernia

MICHAEL N. MARGOLIES, M.D.

PATHOPHYSIOLOGY AND CLINICAL PRESENTATION

Abdominal hernias are exceedingly common, often causing occupational disabilities and posing the risk of incarceration and strangulation of bowel. Fortunately, adequate evaluation can usually be performed in the office by means of history and physical examination. The primary physician must distinguish between patients who require surgical referral and those who may be managed expectantly.

A hernia is a defect in the normal musculofascial continuity of the abdominal wall that permits the egress of structures not normally passing through the parietes. In general, the significant feature of hernia is not the size of the protrusion or the sac, but the size and rigidity of the defect in the abdominal wall. Fixation and rigidity of the hernial ring are the features which permit incarceration and strangulation. The distinction between congenital and acquired hernia is not often clear, as many hernias that appear following trauma or straining represent a congenital predisposition, such as indirect inguinal hernia in the adult. This distinction has little bearing on management, although it may make considerable difference to the patient who may be compensated if the hernia can be attributed to trauma at work. Some of these hernias are incidental to, and antedate the perceived injury.

Disorders resulting in increased intra-abdominal pressure may contribute to the appearance of a hernia and affect the postoperative management as well. For example, chronic cough due to cigarette smoking or bronchitis can precipitate or worsen herniation; the same is true of symptomatic prostatism.

The symptoms of an uncomplicated or reducible external hernia are related not to its size but to the degree of pressure on its contents. Patients with large scrotal hernias containing much intestine may have few symptoms other than a dragging sensation. A mass appears upon standing which reduces when the patient is supine. Pain may be intermittent, disappearing when the hernia is reduced. Patients with small hernias containing an entrapped knuckle of bowel may have rather severe pain and nausea. Many patients with femoral, umbilical, or epigastric hernias may be entirely unaware of their existence.

An *irreducible* or *incarcerated hernia* is one in which the contents cannot be replaced into the abdomen. Here the mass remains palpable with the patient relaxed and in the supine position. A *strangulated hernia* is an irreducible one in which the blood supply to the entrapped bowel loop has been compromised, resulting in small bowel obstruction and infarction. These patients will complain of colicky abdominal pain, nausea and vomiting and will have signs of small bowel obstruction with distention, tympany and hyperperistalsis. In addition, careful examination will demonstrate a tender, irreducible groin or ventral hernia.

Indirect inguinal hernias, which account for one-half of hernias in adults, pass through the internal abdominal inguinal ring along the spermatic cord through the inguinal canal, and exit through the external inguinal ring. In the male, these can descend into the scrotum. *Direct inguinal hernias* pass through the posterior inguinal wall medial to the inferior epigastric vessels, through Hesselbach's triangle. *Femoral hernias* pass through the femoral canal inferior to the inguinal ligament and become subcutaneous in the fossa ovalis. It is often difficult to distinguish between these three forms, especially when there is incarceration and the sac is large.

Indirect inguinal hernias are 8 to 10 times more common in men than in women, while femoral hernias are 3 to 5 times more common in women than in men. Nevertheless, the most common hernia in women is the indirect inguinal type. The diagnosis is less often made in women because physical examination of the external inguinal ring is more difficult. Direct hernias increase in incidence with advancing age and are the least likely of the external hernias to incarcerate or strangulate. Strangulation is frequent in femoral hernias.

The majority of patients with strangulated inguinal hernias are aware of the hernia prior to strangulation. In contrast, nearly half of those with strangulated femoral hernias are unaware of the hernia prior to strangulation. In addition, groin pain and tenderness are absent in a significant percentage of cases of strangulated femoral hernia.

The commonly encountered ventral hernias include umbilical, epigastric, and incisional varieties. Ventral hernias are often more obvious with the patient standing. *Umbilical hernias* pass through the umbilical ring and represent failure of the ring to obliterate after birth. In the infant, these often close spontaneously within the first 2 years of life. In the adult, they are more common in women and are associated with obesity, multiparity and cirrhosis with ascites. Umbilical hernias are often missed because they are obscured by subcutaneous fat. There is a high risk of incarceration and strangulation and a greater mortality than with inguinal hernia because large bowel is frequently entrapped.

Incisional hernias are those which develop in the scar of a previous laparotomy or in a drain site. They are associated with a previous postoperative wound infection, dehiscence, malnutrition, obesity and smoking. They are more common in vertical than in transverse scars. Incisional hernias often have multiple defects and several rings. They are frequently irreducible or only partially reducible because of adhesions within the sac. Patients with very large incisional hernias may be remarkably free from symptoms of intestinal obstruction, although incarceration is common; strangulation is relatively uncommon because of the usually large size of the defects.

Epigastric hernias occur through the linea alba between the xiphoid process and the umbilicus. They may be quite difficult to detect in the obese and must be looked for in patients with epigastric pain. Incarcerated epigastric hernia may produce symptoms which mimic peptic ulcer disease or biliary colic.

DIFFERENTIAL DIAGNOSIS

Recognizing a hernia usually presents little difficulty, although distinguishing one type of inguinal hernia from another can sometimes be complicated. Differential diagnosis of an entrapped femoral hernia includes not only inguinal hernia but femoral lymphadenopathy, saphenous varix, psoas abscess and hydrocele. On occasion it is impossible to differentiate an incarcerated femoral hernia from a single enlarged femoral lymph node (the lymph node of Cloquet).

EVALUATION

Diagnosis and evaluation of external hernias require no more than a brief history and careful physical examination; laboratory and radiologic studies are unnecessary unless major complications have resulted.

History. The patient is questioned about groin pain, swelling, ability to reduce the hernia, circumstances of onset, and aggravating and alleviating factors, such as exacerbation on standing, straining or coughing. Acute onset of colicky abdominal pain, nausea and vomiting suggests entrapment and strangulation in a patient with a known hernia.

Physical examination is directed toward distinguishing among (1) hernias that are uncomplicated and require no therapy, (2) those which can be repaired electively, and (3) those in which emergency surgery is the safest course. The physical examination is also important in distinguishing the anatomic type of hernia, because prognosis and likelihood of incarceration and strangulation differs among the various types. The patient with a reducible hernia should be examined in both the supine and standing positions. Inspection is often as important as palpation for detection. Examination should include a Valsalva maneuver to increase intra-abdominal pressure. In the male, small inguinal hernias are looked for by invaginating the scrotal skin while the patient is standing. To detect ventral hernias, the patient should be supine and then asked to lift the head from the examining table and to bear down in order to tense the abdominal wall.

If a hernia is irreducible, the physician should look for local tenderness, discoloration, edema, fever, and signs of small bowel obstruction. It is often difficult to distinguish a simple incarceration from early strangulation; for this reason these two lesions are managed identically by immediate referral to a surgeon. Surgical exploration is the only way to be certain that there is no compromised bowel trapped in the hernia sac. Conversely, when signs of small bowel obstruction are present, it is essential to examine thoroughly for a strangulated femoral hernia because groin pain and tenderness may be absent.

A few conditions are believed to have more than a chance association with hernias, and some argue that they should be screened for. Whether or not the adult patient with a recent hernia is more likely to have an occult carcinoma of the colon remains a source of controversy. It had been suggested that patients undergo routine sigmoidoscopic examination and barium enema. However, if the patient reports no change in bowel habits and the stools are repeatedly guaiac-negative, it is probably unnecessary to submit him to more extensive investigation for occult malignancy. Symptoms and signs of prostatism are frequently present in the elderly male with hernia and may require relief prior to herniorrhaphy. The entire abdomen ought to be examined for masses, hepatomegaly, and ascites, which are sometimes associated with hernia formation.

PRINCIPLES OF MANAGEMENT AND INDICATIONS FOR REFERRAL

Patients with *symptomatic reducible inguinal hernias* should undergo elective repair for relief of symptoms and prevention of strangulation. Reduction by means of a truss is unsatisfactory even in patients with relative medical contraindications to surgery. Moreover, surgical repair can be done under local anesthesia in the high-risk patient.

In patients with a nontender incarcerated inguinal hernia of recent onset, but without signs of inflammation or bowel obstruction, it may be safe to attempt gentle reduction ("taxis"). This is best accomplished with the patient supine and the hips and knees flexed. If gentle pressure over the hernial sac fails to reduce the mass further, efforts should be abandoned and the patient referred for surgery forthwith. Often the patient has more experience in reducing his own hernia than the physician. Patients with evidence of strangulated groin hernias should be subjected to immediate operation regardless of medical contraindications; if untreated, death will result from bowel necrosis.

Patients with *reducible femoral hernias* should undergo prompt elective repair because of the high incidence of strangulation. Whenever there is a question of an incarcerated femoral hernia, it is safest to proceed immediately with surgical exploration.

In umbilical hernias, surgery is unnecessary if on physical examination there is a small asymptomatic fascial defect without protrusion. When herniation is detected, however, umbilical defects should be repaired, as there is a high risk of incarceration and strangulation. The danger of strangulation is compounded by the greater likelihood of colonic entrapment with a resultant higher mortality rate than in hernias in which small intestine is strangulated. Therefore, all incarcerated umbilical hernias should be managed as if they were strangulated. Elective umbilical herniorrhaphy should be avoided in patients with ascites; instead, efforts should be directed toward reducing the ascites (see Chapter 71). The problem in patients with cirrhosis and ascites is made more difficult when the skin overlying the sac thins out and poses the risk of rupture.

Patients with small neck incisional hernias or tender incarceration should undergo repair on an urgent basis. Patients who have trophic changes or ulceration in the skin overlying incisional hernias are also candidates for urgent surgery. In some instances, cellulitis of the skin overlying the hernia sac occurs and is difficult to distinguish from strangulation of the contents of the sac. Management of large incarcerated incisional hernias that occur in the abdomen in very obese patients is a particular problem. Major efforts should be directed toward weight reduction prior to repair if it is possible to procrastinate. If there is doubt, however, as to the presence of intestinal obstruction or viability of the contents of the sac, the advice of a surgeon should be sought promptly.

Factors contributing to hernia formation should be corrected if possible. Prostatectomy is occasionally required following repair of hernia, and the patient with symptoms of prostatic obstruction should be advised of this possibility. Patients with chronic bronchitis and emphysema, or with chronic cough due to cigarette smoking, should be urged to stop smoking promptly to diminish symptoms due to the hernia and to decrease the possibility of postoperative complications.

PATIENT EDUCATION

Patients who are to be managed conservatively must be taught to watch for signs of complications. It is the responsibility of the physician to instruct the patient in the symptoms of incarceration and strangulation and in the urgency of seeking help should they occur. If the patient is deemed incompetent to make such observations and to obtain help promptly, a strong case can be made for proceeding with surgery. Patients scheduled for elective surgery also require instruction, because incarceration occasionally occurs prior to the planned operation.

Many patients with asymptomatic or mildly symtomatic reducible hernias will be reluctant to undergo surgery because their symptoms are minimal. If they fall into the high-risk group, e.g., femoral or small neck incisional hernias, they should be informed of the strong likelihood of strangulation and the minuscule morbidity and mortality associated with surgery.

ANNOTATED BIBLIOGRAPHY

Anson, B., and McVay, C.B.: *Surgical Anatomy*, ed. 5. Philadelphia: W.B. Saunders, 1971, vol. I, pp. 461. *(Extensive description of the anatomy of the inguinal and femoral regions.)*

Brendel, T.H. and Kirsh, I.: Lack of association between inguinal hernia and carcinoma of the colon. N. Engl. J. Med., 284:369, 1971. *(One view of the relationship of hernia to colon carcinoma. See also Terezis, et al., below.)*

Clain, A.: *Hamilton Bailey's Physical Signs in Clinical Surgery*, ed. 15. Chicago: Year Book Medical Publishers, 1973. *(Details the differential diagnosis of hernia based on physical signs.)*

Dunphy, J.E., and Botsford, T.W.: *Physical Examination of the Surgical Patient: An Introduction to Clinical Surgery*, ed. 4. Philadelphia: W.B. Saunders, 1975, p. 117. *(A concise, well-illustrated approach to physical examination of patients with hernia.)*

Terezis, N.L., Davis, W.C., and Jackson, F.C.: Carcinoma of the colon associated with inguinal hernia. N. Engl. J. Med., 268:774, 1963. *(A view opposite to that of Brendel and Kirsh, above.)*

64

Management of Peptic Ulcer Disease

Peptic ulcer disease is a common affliction. Epidemiologic studies provide prevalence estimates of 5 to 10 per cent and a 1 to 3 per cent incidence rate. Males outnumber females by 2 to 1. Peak prevalence of duodenal ulcer occurs in men aged 45 to 54; in gastric ulcer, men aged 55 to 64. Duodenal ulcers account for four fifths of cases. For unexplained reasons, the frequency of peptic ulcer disease is declining, yet it still remains a source of considerable morbidity, although mortality is minimal. Recent developments in pharmacologic therapy have produced new methods of medical management. The primary physician should be able to manage most patients presenting with peptic ulcer disease. The goals are to alleviate pain, promote healing, and minimize chances of recurrence and complications. The clinician needs to know the details of antacid use, the effects of dietary and pharmacologic agents, and the indications for the new histamine H_2-receptor antagonists. As the physician of first contact, the primary care doctor must also be able to identify all patients who require endoscopy and surgical referral.

PATHOPHYSIOLOGY AND CLINICAL PRESENTATION

The pathophysiology of gastric and duodenal ulcers is incompletely understood, but the common denominator is acid-induced injury to the mucosa. Duodenal ulcers occur in patients with *increased gastric acidity*. It is postulated that these patients have increased parietal cell mass, increased acid production at rest and in response to stimulation, inability to turn off acid production, and increased rates of gastric emptying with acid more rapidly delivered to the duodenum. It is also speculated that duodenal defenses are reduced. Although available data point to acid as the prime pathophysiological abnormality inducing ulceration, the precise pathophysiological alterations are still incompletely defined.

The pathophysiology of gastric ulcer has been conceptualized into a logical explanation that still lacks confirmation. The current theory is that *pyloric sphincter incompetence* permits reflux of bile salts and lysolecithin, which break down the gastric mucosal barrier allowing back diffusion of hydrogen ions, cellular injury and ulceration. Exogenous agents such as aspirin also damage the mucosal barrier and permit back diffusion. It is noteworthy that gastric ulcers usually occur in the lesser curvature, at the junction of the antrum and the acid-secreting part of the stomach. The significance of this observation is not yet known. Patients with gastric ulcers are not hypersecretors of acid.

The clinical presentations of gastric and duodenal peptic ulcers are somewhat similar but rather nonspecific. Patients may present with pain, bleeding, or obstruction, or they may be symptom-free. Epigastric pain, relieved by antacids and occurring in clusters of daily symptoms for a few weeks separated by pain-free periods of months, is characteristic of peptic disease. Duodenal ulcer pain is classically relieved by food, absent before breakfast, and responsible for awakening the patient at night; it starts 2 to 3 hours after a meal. However, careful studies of patients with documented duodenal ulcers have shown that in some individuals pain is often worsened by meals, present before breakfast, and continuous rather than periodic. Gastric ulcer pain is more likely to be precipitated by food and often radiates from the epigastrium to the back or substernal region. It, too, can awaken the patient and be relieved by food. In both conditions, the pain may be dull, aching, gnawing or burning in quality, consistent with its visceral quality.

CLINICAL COURSE

Studies of the natural history of ulcer disease are marred by the fact that a substantial number of patients undergo surgery. Nevertheless, available data show that most ulcers heal completely by 4 weeks, though large ones may take up to 12 weeks. The majority of patients become pain-free within the first 4 weeks. There is a poor correlation between presence of pain and existence of an ulcer crater. Pain cannot be used alone as an indicator of disease activity.

Recurrences are frequent; for gastric ulcer, the 5-year recurrence rate is 30 to 50 per cent. The patient with more than two or three repeat gastric ulcers is rare, whereas multiple recurrences are not unusual with duodenal ulcer disease. There is no correlation between recurrence rate and ulcer size, duration of symptoms or location. Recurrent ulcers heal just as rapidly and completely as original lesions. The incidence of recurrence after gastrectomy is reported to be in the range of 5 to 10 per cent.

For duodenal ulcer, the rate of developing a major complication such as hemorrhage, perforation, or obstruction is less than 1 per cent per year. There is no evidence that elective surgery reduces the mortality rate. The risk of elective surgery seems to equal the risk of the disease itself. Bleeding is frequent; almost 15 per cent of patients experience at least one hemorrhagic episode. Bleeding is slightly more common from duodenal ulcers than from gastric ones. Bleeding is 2 to 3 times more frequent than perforation.

PRINCIPLES OF THERAPY

Acid secretion and mucosal susceptibility to injury are the common pathophysiological determinants of gastric and duodenal peptic ulcer disease. Although each of these factors may differ in its relative importance in each site, both seem to be central to ulcer formation. The approach to countering gas-

Table 64–1. Neutralizing Capacities and Sodium Content of Popular Liquid Antacids

ANTACID	CONTENTS	MEQ/30 ML.	ML/140-MEQ DOSE	SODIUM CONTENT MG./30 ML.
Mylanta II	Mg-Al hydroxides	124	34	8
Maalox	Mg-Al hydroxide gel	78	54	15
DiGel	Mg-Al hydroxides	76	58	Not available
Riopan	Mg-Al hydroxides	66	64	4
Amphojel	Al hydroxide gel	58	74	23
Gelusil	Mg-trisilicate Al hydroxide gel	40	108	5

tric acid production involves neutralizing acid with antacids, inhibiting acid production by use of H_2-receptor antagonists and anticholinergics, and avoiding excessive postprandial acid secretion by dietary manipulation. Agents which may break down the mucosal barrier are eliminated from daily intake.

Antacids are the mainstay of therapy, because they are effective, relatively inexpensive, and safe. When used in a dose sufficient to buffer gastric acid (e.g., 140 mEq, 1 hour after a meal), they have been shown endoscopically to be more effective than placebo in promoting healing of duodenal ulcers. Lower doses have been demonstrated by endoscopy to promote healing of gastric ulcers. These agents are no more effective than placebo for reliving pain due to duodenal ulcer, although they are better than placebo in gastric ulcers.

The buffering capacities of liquid antacid preparations vary considerably, ranging from 6 to 128 mEq per 15 ml. Liquids are superior to tablets in buffering capacity. Calcium carbonate preparations are among the most potent in neutralizing capacity, but their usefulness is limited by the fact that they stimulate rebound acid secretion. The most effective liquid antacids contain magnesium and aluminum hydroxides. When the aluminum hydroxide mixes with acid, nonabsorbable aluminum salts are formed which by themselves are constipating. The magnesium salts formed are poorly absorbed but frequently cause diarrhea, an effect which may not be completely canceled by the constipating action of the aluminum. Many of the liquid antacids contain considerable amounts of sodium. A low-sodium preparation is sometimes needed to avoid sodium excess in patients who must restrict salt intake. Table 64–1 lists relative strengths of common antacids and their sodium content.

Studies correlating healing with acid neutralizing capacities indicate that substantial doses of antacids are needed. Previous failures to demonstrate the effectiveness of antacids may have been due to inadequate doses. About 140 mEq at a time seems to be

necessary to bring the gastric pH into the 3.5 to 5.0 range. Typical 30-ml. doses of many popular antacids provide only 60 mEq. Even though contents listed on labels of weak and strong antacid preparations are similar, the relative amounts and solubilities of ingredients do vary, accounting for differences in potency.

The timing of the antacid dose affects degree of acid neutralization. If given with a meal, the antacid is wasted, since food is a perfectly adequate buffer. When antacid is given 1 hour after eating, gastric acidity is kept at zero for another 1½ to 2 hours, countering the food-induced stimulation of acid secretion. A second dose 3 hours after a meal provides another hour of acid neutralization and tides the patient over to the next meal.

Problems associated with antacid use are relatively few, but important to recognize. Diarrhea is common due to the cathartic effect of insoluble magnesium salts. Treatment is to alternate therapy with an antacid containing only aluminum hydroxide. Antacids enhance the absorption of dicumarol and L-dopa and decrease absorption of phenothiazines, sulfonamides, INH and penicillin. Phosphate depletion is a rare occurrence in patients using an aluminum-containing antacid; insoluble aluminum phosphate forms. Excess sodium absorption has already been mentioned. Magnesium-containing antacids should be avoided in renal failure; the small amounts of magnesium absorbed cannot be eliminated. Calcium can be absorbed and precipitate hypercalcemia if renal function is depressed. Calcium also triggers rebound acid secretion, making such antacids irrational choices.

Diet. Contrary to common beliefs, there is no evidence that any particular dietary manipulation promotes healing or reduces acidity. The one exception is that avoidance of eating before bedtime probably reduces nocturnal acid levels by removing the postprandial stimulus to acid secretion. Otherwise, bland diets, frequent feedings, small feedings, and avoidance of spices, fruit juices, and acidic foods have never been shown to result in significant reduction in acid secretion or to change the course of disease. Milk also provides no advantages; in fact, it stimulates acid secretion by virtue of its protein content. Some patients claim certain foods "disagree" with them, and these can be avoided, but not for the sake of altering acid secretion. Although coffee—decaffeinated as well as caffeine-containing—stimulates acid secretion, as do other caffeine-containing beverages, there is no epidemiologic evidence proving that intake is associated with increased incidence of peptic ulcer.

Anticholinergics achieve only a 30 per cent reduction in food-stimulated acid secretion, but provide a 50 to 60 per cent reduction in nocturnal secretion. It was believed these agents had to be used in near toxic doses to lower acid levels, but a recent study has shown that low-dose propantheline (15 mg.) is just as effective as the so-called optimal dose (48 mg.). Anticholinergics have a limited role in ulcer therapy. Since they suppress nocturnal acid secretion, these agents may be tried in an adjunctive role for better control of nocturnal pain. When combined with cimetidine, there is a synergistic effect. Further study of their use with H_2-receptor antagonists is needed and should be watched for. Since anticholinergics reduce lower sphincter tone, they may cause or worsen reflux. Moreover, they should not be used in suspected gastric outlet obstruction.

Cimetidine, a histamine H_2-receptor antagonist, represents a new development in peptic ulcer therapy. The drug blocks histamine stimulation of parietal cell acid production. European studies have shown marked improvement in healing of duodenal ulcers compared to placebo; however, in a U.S. multicenter double-blind study, the incidence of healing was similar to placebo, perhaps because patients were also allowed to use antacids as needed. Antacid use in the cimetidine group was half that of the placebo users. When compared to a high-dose antacid regimen (30 ml. Mylanta II given 1 and 3 hours after meals), cimetidine proved equally effective in healing duodenal ulcers. Its effectiveness in gastric ulcer disease is less extensively studied but seems to be similar.

Although it appears that cimetidine is an important advance, it is too early to determine its exact role in treating peptic ulcer disease. Antacids have finally been proven effective in healing duodenal ulcers, are less expensive, are relatively free of adverse effects, and should be the mainstay of any ulcer regimen. Cimetidine is best reserved for the refractory or complicated case, and perhaps for prevention of recurrence. Preliminary evidence from Scandinavian studies suggests efficacy in reducing the rate of recurrence.

The standard dose of cimetidine is 300 mg. with each meal and before bed; this schedule inhibits food-induced and nocturnal acid secretion. Reduction in acid production of approximately 80 per cent is achieved and lasts 4 to 6 hours. So far, few adverse effects have been noted; reported are gynecomastia in 0.3 per cent and reversible minor elevations of serum creatinine in 10 per cent and of transaminases in 5 per cent. Neither of these laboratory abnormalities requires stopping the drug. Cimetidine has been reported to potentiate the hypoprothrombinemic effect of warfarin by about 20 per cent in some patients; close monitoring is warranted. In the elderly, mental confusion may occur with cimetidine use. The literature should be watched closely for further developments in this exciting area, particularly the efficacy of cimetidine in preventing recurrence and complications and in speeding the healing process.

Avoidance of agents which damage the mucosal barrier (allowing back diffusion of hydrogen ions and ulceration) is an important component of ulcer therapy. Of the many agents implicated, only *unbuffered aspirin* has been unequivocally proven to have this effect. *Ethanol* also damages the mucosal barrier and can cause gastritis, but has never been associated with an increased incidence of ulcer formation. Its correlation to ulcer disease has been its relation to smoking, but never as an independent determinant of risk. *Indomethacin, phenylbutazone, ibuprofen* and *naproxen* can cause mucosal erosions, but do not result in back diffusion or in increased formation of ulcers. *Corticosteroids* have long been felt to be ulcerogenic. The association derives in part from the observation that there was an increased incidence of ulcer disease in those taking prednisone for rheumatoid arthritis. Prospective controlled studies have failed to document any relation between prednisone and ulcer, though many clinicians believe there is a cause-and-effect relationship, especially at high doses.

There is definitely an epidemiologic relation between *smoking* and peptic ulcer, but the mechanism is unknown. Smoking does not weaken the mucosal barrier, nor does it stimulate acid secretion, but it does delay healing.

The role of *emotional stress* in ulcer disease is supported by (1) a higher incidence of chronic stress in ulcer patients compared to controls; (2) increased acid production triggered by acute stress; and (3) more prolonged course and poorer prognosis in those with chronic severe anxiety. These findings do not imply that peptic ulcer disease is universally associated with emotional distress, but that it may be an important factor in some patients. Treatment of such individuals needs to include attention to the issues producing anxiety and perhaps use of minor tranquilizers (see Chapter 214). Hospitalization of the extremely anxious ulcer patient speeds healing by removing him from a stressful environment, but only stays of 4 weeks or more have been shown to be effective, making this form of therapy rather impractical in most cases.

Prevention of recurrence by medical therapy is an important goal of therapy, but an elusive one. Chronic use of antacids or cimetidine has not yet been conclusively proven effective, although there is some suggestive evidence for cimetidine in doses of 2 tablets at bedtime. Avoidance of aspirin is obvious. It is believed prudent to cut back on caffeine, smoking and stress, though the utility of such maneuvers is unproven.

PATIENT EDUCATION

A major part of the therapeutic effort is to overcome much of the mythology surrounding ulcer disease so that a rational plan can be carried out. Many patients will put themselves on bland diets, increase milk and cream intake, and purchase calcium carbonate antacid tablets in efforts at self-treatment. Some even take aspirin for the pain. Careful explanation of what does and does not stimulate acid secretion and cause mucosal damage is essential.

Many physicians insist that coffee-drinking be stopped, though this may cause more difficulty than is warranted by its role in pathogenesis. The same is probably true for alcohol use and smoking, though there are numerous other excellent health reasons to halt these habits; the presence of an ulcer may be a good opportunity to motivate the patient to quit.

It is essential to inform the patient that there is little relation between pain and presence of the ulcer. Many stop their antacids when pain resolves, only to delay healing and risk complications and recurrence of pain. Stressing proper antacid use is worth considerable effort. Many individuals prefer tablets and purchase popular calcium carbonate preparations such as Tums, rather than use a prescribed liquid antacid. When liquids are impractical to carry about

during the day, tablet forms of the liquid preparations are available. Although less efficacious, they are a reasonable alternative to calcium carbonate or no antacid at all. Diarrhea also deters some from their program; it is worthwhile to provide a supply of aluminum hydroxide antacid to have on hand if diarrhea sets in.

Those with stressful home or work situations may benefit from detailed discussion of ongoing conflicts. The opportunity to ventilate one's feelings may itself lessen tension and help point the way to a solution. However, solutions need not be extreme; there is no evidence that major changes in job or family situation contribute to healing. Discussion can be supplemented by teaching the patient simple relaxation techniques, especially when there are otherwise refractory situational stresses.

The patient needs to be taught to watch for complications of ulcer disease. In particular, the manifestations of gastrointestinal bleeding should be well understood so that there is no delay in seeking help. If the question of elective surgery arises, the patient should be made a full partner in the decision, since there are few definite guidelines for operation. A value judgment is necessary, and the costs and benefits of surgery versus continued medical therapy need to be discussed.

MONITORING THERAPY AND INDICATIONS FOR REFERRAL AND ADMISSION

If gastric ulcer is detected by x-ray, a repeat study should be done at 4 weeks to document decrease in size and continued signs of benignity. If ulcer was documented only by endoscopy, repeat examination by the gastroenterologist at 4 weeks is warranted for similar reasons. If complete healing has not occurred, follow-up study at 6 weeks is needed, since most ulcers should have healed or should be more than 90 per cent healed by that time. If healing of a small ulcer is still not complete at 6 weeks, endoscopy for biopsy and cytology is indicated. If the ulcer was very large to begin with, endoscopy can be postponed and a final check made in 12 weeks; large ulcers may take up to 3 months to heal completely. Delay or failure to heal requires consultation with the gastroenterologist to review the medical program and the chances of cancer.

Since duodenal ulcer is far less likely to represent malignancy, monitoring by x-ray and endoscopy is reserved for documenting a suspected complication such as bleeding. Periodic repetition of studies is unnecessary and expensive, even when there is recurrence of typical symptoms, unless a different course of therapy such as surgery is contemplated. Following stool guaiacs and blood counts can help detect bleeding, as can careful questioning of the patient.

Refractoriness to therapy is an indication for referral to the gastroenterologist. Admission is mandatory when symptoms of hemorrhage, penetration, perforation or gastric outlet obstruction are present; both surgeon and gastroenterologist need to be consulted.

A most difficult issue is when and whom to select for *elective surgery*. Much has to do with the patient's preferences; gross generalizations are meaningless. Clearly those with recurrent major bleeds, gastric outlet obstruction, or evidence of malignancy need to be seen by the surgeon. Seventy-five per cent of patients with intractable pain obtain relief when treated surgically, but subgroups with alcohol abuse, character disorders or severe neuroses do poorly when operated on. The decision to resort to elective surgery for recurrent disase should be made in conjunction with the patient, weighing the small risk of operative mortality and the morbidity of postgastrectomy syndrome against the mobidity and cost of recurrent pain, time lost from work, and need for chronic drug therapy.

Refinement in surgical therepy has occurred. Development of the highly selective vagotomy with transsection of fibers to the parietal cell mass produces results comparable to vagotomy and drainage procedure while avoiding most of the side effects. Vagotomy with antrectomy is associated with fewer recurrences, but the patient is subjected to greater operative risk and such long-term difficulties as the dumping syndrome.

THERAPEUTIC RECOMMENDATIONS

- Advise patient to omit all salicylates.
- Advise patient to omit bedtime snacks but to consume three meals daily.
- Encourage cessation of smoking and alcohol use.
- Advise patient to decrease use of coffee and other caffeine-containing beverages; complete cessation is unnecessary.
- Tell the patient to avoid only those foods which cause discomfort. Do not restrict any other foods or utilize bland diet. Frequent small feedings are unnecessary.
- Begin liquid antacid program with a noncalcium-

containing antacid, giving doses at 1 and 3 hours after meals and before bed, in amounts sufficient to provide 70 MEQ. of buffering capacity per dose for gastric ulcer and 140 MEQ. per dose for duodenal ulcer.
- Continue therapy for at least 4 to 6 weeks.
- Use an aluminum hydroxide preparation intermittently if there is diarrhea.
- Give cimetidine 300 mg. h.s. or propantheline 15 mg. h.s. for nocturnal pain.
- Add cimetidine 300 mg. with each meal and before bed to the antacid program in severe or refractory cases.
- Nonsalicylate anti-inflammatory agents such as prednisone and indomethacin need not be discontinued if there is no bleeding and they are absolutely necessary.
- Attend to anxiety-related issues, but advice to make major job or geographic changes is unwarranted.
- Repeat x-ray or endoscopic examination for gastric ulcer at 4 weeks and again at 6 and 12 weeks until healing is demonstrated. No repeated examinations are needed for uncomplicated duodenal ulcer beyond initial documentation at onset of illness.
- Treat recurrences in similar fashion. No definitive medical measures for preventing recurrences are known at present, but avoidance of salicylates and reduction in smoking are reasonable measures. Follow the literature for the role of cimetidine in prevention of recurrent ulcers.

ANNOTATED BIBLIOGRAPHY

Binder, J.H., Cocco, A., Crossley, R., *et al.*: Cimetidine in treatment of duodenal ulcer: A multicenter double-blind study. Gastroenterology, *74*:380, 1978. *(There was no significant difference between efficacy of cimetidine and placebo, but concomitant antacid use was allowed as needed, which may account for lack of statistically significant difference.)*

Buchman, E., Kaung, D.T., Dolank, et al.: Unrestricted diet in treatment of duodenal ulcer. Gastroenterology, *56*:1016, 1969. *(Dietary restrictions made little or no difference in treatment of duodenal ulcer.)*

Conn, H.O., and Blitzer, B.L.: Nonassociation of adrenocorticosteroid therapy and peptic ulcer. N. Engl. J. Med., *294*:473, 1976. *(Refutes the argu-*

ment that steroids are a cause of ulcers and finds no evidence to support the notion that high doses are more ulcerogenic than lower ones.)

Feldman, M., Richardson, C.T., Peterson, U.L., *et al.*: Effect of low-dose propantheline on food-stimulated gastric acid secretion. N. Engl. J. Med., *(Low-dose [15 mg.] anticholinergic therapy was just as effective in reducing acid secretion as the traditional "high-dose" therapy [48 mg.]. Moreover, when combined with cimetidine, suppression was greater than obtainable with either agent alone.)*

Fortran, J.S.: Placebos, antacids, and cimetidine for duodenal ulcer. Editorial. N. Engl. J. Med., *298*:1081, 1978. *(A critical appraisal of current therapies for duodenal ulcer, arguing that the place for cimetidine is uncertain at present and that it is not yet definitively superior to other forms of therapy already available.)*

Fortran, J.S., Morawski, S.G., and Richardson, C.T.: In vivo and in vitro evaluation of liquid antacids. N. Engl. J. Med., *288*:923, 1973. *(Reviews the neutralizing capacities of various antacids.)*

Friedman, G.D., Siegelaub, A.B., and Seltzer, C.: Cigarettes, alcohol, coffee and peptic ulcer. N. Engl. J. Med., *290*:469, 1974. *(An epidemiologic study from the Kaiser-Permanente organization showing an increased prevalence of ulcer disease in smokers. Coffee consumption and alcohol were correlated with cigarette smoking, but were not independent determinants of prevalence of ulcer disease.)*

Fry, J.: Peptic ulcer: A profile. Br. Med. J., *2*:809, 1964. *(A study of over 200 patients with peptic ulcer followed in the outpatient setting for 5 to 15 years. Source of statistics on natural history, rate of complications, and efficacy of surgery.)*

Gugler, R., *et al.*: Cimetidine for anastomotic ulcers after partial gastrectomy. N. Engl. J. Med., *301*:1077, 1979. *(A randomized controlled trial showing cimetidine superior to placebo in preventing recurrences.)*

Levant, J.A., Walsh, J.H., and Isenberg, J.: Stimulation of gastric secretion and gastrin release by single oral doses of calcium carbonate. N. Engl. J. Med., *289*:555, 1973. *(Calcium carbonate causes rebound acid hypersecretion, even though it is a good neutralizing agent.)*

Levy, M.: Aspirin use in patients with major upper gastrointestinal bleeding and peptic ulcer. N. Engl. J. Med., *290*:1158, 1974. *(A report from the Boston Drug Surveillance Project showing a statistically significant association between heavy long-term aspirin use and peptic ulcer disease in patients presenting to the hospital.)*

Mahl, G.F.: Anxiety, HC1 secretion and peptic ulcer etiology. Psychosom. Med., *12*:158, 1950. *(Acute anxiety raises acid secretion.)*

Peterson, W.L., Sturdevant, R.A., Frankl, H.D., *et al.*: Healing of duodenal ulcer with an antacid regimen. N. Engl. J. Med., *297*:341, 1977. *(Documents the efficacy of high-dose [1000 MEQ: per day] antacid therapy in healing duodenal ulcers compared to placebo. Also shows a surprisingly high rate of pain relief by placebo and delay in healing in cigarette smokers.)*

Rutter, M.: Psychological factors in short-term prognosis of physical disease. 1. Peptic ulcer. J. Psychosom. Res., *7*:45, 1963. *(Severe anxiety prolongs recovery and makes relapse more likely.)*

Spiro, H.M.: Moynihan's Disease? The diagnosis of duodenal ulcer. N. Engl. J. Med., *291*:567, 1974. *(Argues for attending more to the patient than to the ulcer itself with repeat endoscopies and barium studies.)*

65

Management of Inflammatory
Bowel Disease
JAMES M. RICHTER, M.D.

Ulcerative colitis and Crohn's disease are the most common chronic inflammatory diseases of the bowel, usually characterized by bloody diarrhea and abdominal pain. Their manifestations may be subtle or dramatic, and initially they may be difficult to distinguish from acute diarrheal diseases and from each other (see Chapter 58). The management of patients with inflammatory bowel disease rests on establishing a secure diagnosis, being aware of the waxing and waning nature of the illness, understanding the potential complications, and providing symptomatic relief and support skillfully.

PATHOPHYSIOLOGY, CLINICAL PRESENTATION AND COURSE

Ulcerative colitis is an idiopathic, diffuse inflammatory disease of the bowel mucosa. The disease typically begins in adolescence or young adulthood, but may occur at almost any age. Caucasians are affected more often than blacks. Prevalence is highest among Jews. The cardinal symptoms are bloody diarrhea and abdominal pain; in severe cases, fever, anorexia, and weight loss are present as well. The variability of presentations is remarkable, ranging from malaise and no symptoms referable to the colon, to fever, prostration, abdominal distention and passage of large volumes of liquid stool.

The disease need not be confined to the bowel; extracolonic manifestations include arthritis, uveitis, jaundice and skin lesions. The course is characteristically chronic, recurrent and unpredictable. An insidious presentation in no way indicates a benign course, and a fulminant onset may be followed by long, relatively asymptomatic periods.

Ulcerative colitis almost always involves the distal colon and rectum, making diagnosis possible by sigmoidoscopy. The mucosa becomes edematous, obscuring the fine network of submucosal vessels. The moist, glistening mucosal surface is lost, and a granular appearance develops. The bowel wall is friable, bleeding spontaneously or when touched with a swab. In advanced cases, pseudopolyps and discrete ulcers may be seen. Smears of mucus show polymorphonuclear leukocytes. Barium enema documents extent of disease. Findings range from mucosal denudation to frank ulceration, with loss of haustral markings and a tubular appearance. There are no skip areas.

Liver involvement occurs in the form of pericholangitis and fatty infiltration; these are common histologic findings in ulcerative colitis, but are seldom symptomatic. Much less frequently, chronic active hepatitis, cirrhosis or sclerosing cholangitis is seen. A migratory, monoarticular arthritis affecting the large joints develops in 10 per cent of patients. This arthritis often coincides with an exacerbation of colitis and resolves with control of the underlying disease. Ankylosing spondylitis also occurs, but runs a course independent of the colitis. Uveitis or episcleritis may be seen at any time during the course of the disease. Erythema nodosum, pyoderma gangrenosum and oral aphthous ulcerations are found in about 5 per cent of patients, usually during active colitis.

Patients with ulcerative colitis develop carcinoma of the colon about 10 times more often than the general population. The risk of developing carcinoma increases with the extent and duration of colitis. Patients with ulcerative proctitis probably are not at increased risk, while individuals with pancolitis have a twentyfold increase in the chance of developing cancer. Although cancer may develop at any point in the course of the disease, the risk becomes substantial after seven years. At 7 years, the annual incidence of carcinoma is 1 per cent and increases to 2 per cent after 25 years of disease.

Ulcerative proctitis. The patient with ulcerative proctitis is often a young adult who presents with rectal bleeding and tenesmus. Typically the bleeding is mistakenly attributed to hemorrhoids, and is not severe. Diarrhea or constipation may be present, but often there are small, frequent bowel movements with a small amount of mucus. On sigmoidoscopy, an edematous, friable rectal mucosa is observed. Barium enema is normal above the rectosigmoid. Bacterial cultures for gonorrhea and shigella and smears for amebae are negative.

Ulcerative proctitis is a variant of ulcerative colitis, distinguished principally by its good prognosis and paucity of serious complications. Relapses are common, but less than 15 per cent progress to generalized ulcerative colitis. The distant complications of colitis are unusual, and carcinoma of the rectum develops no more commonly than in an unaffected individual.

Crohn's disease. This condition is a chronic, relapsing inflammatory disorder of the alimentary tract, usually beginning in early adulthood. The inflammation is granulomatous and may extend through all layers of the bowel wall. It is characteristically discontinuous, with diseased segments separated by normal bowel. The condition often affects the distal ileum and right colon; less frequently it involves only the small bowel or colon. It may be seen in any portion of the alimentary tract, from the buccal mucosa to the anus.

Symptoms vary, depending on the location and extent of disease. Diarrhea and abdominal pain are cardinal symptoms, occurring in almost 80 per cent of patients. Weight loss, vomiting, fever, perianal disease and bleeding are common. Fistulas, constipation or abdominal mass may be early manifestations. Symptoms can develop quite subtly or present as a fulminant disease with systemic toxicity.

Physical examination may reveal a discrete abdominal mass, but usually a normal abdomen or doughy loops of bowel are found. Fistulous tracts involving the abdomen or perianal area are seen in up to 10 per cent of cases. Arthritis, ankylosing spondylitis, uveitis, erythema nodosum, aphthous oral ulcers and pyoderma gangrenosum occur in Crohn's disease as in ulcerative colitis. In addition, cholelithiasis and nephrolithiasis have a higher incidence than in the general population.

Sigmoidoscopy is abnormal in less than 20 per cent of cases; fistulas or discrete ulcers are found. Granulomas may be demonstrated by biopsy. Barium enema and upper gastrointestinal series often show segmental involvement of large and small bowel as well as strictures, fistulas or ulcers. Because the primary abnormality in Crohn's disease is submucosal,

the x-rays sometimes appear normal. In those cases, colonoscopy helps by demonstrating segmental disease and ulcerations which may be missed on barium studies.

PRINCIPLES OF MANAGEMENT AND THERAPEUTIC RECOMMENDATIONS

Successful management of inflammatory bowel disease is dependent on accurate diagnosis. Responses to therapy differ according to etiology. Assessment of the patient with suspected inflammatory bowel disease is an ongoing process requiring confirmation of the diagnosis and determination of the extent of disease.

Ulcerative colitis. The condition is diagnosed when the clinical symptoms are supported by characteristic findings at sigmoidoscopy and, if necessary, rectal biopsy. The disease almost invariably affects the distal bowel and rectum and may extend proximally throughout the colon, thus making the examination of the rectum an essential part of the workup. Sigmoidoscopy should be performed without any preparation, so as not to distort the mucosal appearance. Sigmoidoscopy can be performed without delay; barium enema should be postponed until disease activity has subsided, since there is a risk of perforation. Barium enema is used to provide support for the diagnosis and document the proximal extent of disease. Some patients have entirely normal barium enemas, but in most there is mucosal denudation and loss of haustral markings; in some, the colon has a rigid, tubular appearance. Rectal biopsy below the peritoneal reflection can be used to confirm the diagnosis when it is in doubt.

Other conditions need to be ruled out. Crohn's disease of the colon is differentiated from ulcerative colitis by the absence of discontinuous colonic involvement, significant small bowel involvement, fistula formation and granulomas on biopsy. Amebiasis is excluded by examination for trophozoites of swabs taken from the edge of ulcers. When a high-quality parasitology laboratory is not available, a serological test for amebiasis should be sent. An acute bacillary dysentery, such as shigellosis, should always be excluded by stool cultures. Radiation proctitis, pseudomembranous colitis and Behçet's syndrome need to be considered in evaluating these patients.

Symptomatic relief of diarrhea can be provided

with hydrophilic colloids and opiates. One or 2 tablespoons of *psyllium hydrophilic colloid* in water daily often helps to bind the stool. *Diphenoxylate hydrochloride*, 2.5 to 5.0 mg (Lomotil, 1 or 2 tablets), or *codeine*, 15 to 30 mg., four times a day, may help patients with severe daytime or nocturnal diarrhea. These drugs should be used cautiously in acutely ill patients, since they may contribute to toxic colonic dilatation.

No specific *diet* improves or exacerbates ulcerative colitis. Patients should be instructed in the principles of good nutrition and encouraged to maintain hydration during exacerbations. Some patients with ulcerative colitis seems to have increased incidence of lactose deficiency. A trial of a milk-free diet or a lactose tolerance test may help identify such patients. Those who are anemic from blood loss need oral or parenteral iron supplementation (see Chapter 75).

The role of *psychotherapy* in the treatment of ulcerative colitis has been extensively debated and remains unresolved. Probably all patients benefit from a close therapeutic alliance with a primary physician who can meet their medical needs and provide supportive psychotherapy. Certainly some patients benefit from formal psychiatric therapy.

Pharmacologic control of the underlying disease is accomplished by use of sulfasalazine and corticosteroids. Ambulatory patients with mild to moderate disease may respond to *sulfasalazine* 2 to 4 gm. daily in four divided doses. The drug is used to decrease steroid requirements in those with moderate disease, produce remissions in those with mild disease, and prolong remissions in asymptomatic patients. Most patients should be continued on sulfasalazine indefinitely.

Steroids, both systemic and topical, counter the inflammatory process. Rectal steroids in the form of enemas or suppositories may produce prompt remissions in those whose disease is limited to the left colon. Steroid suppositories containing 15 or 25 mg. of hydrocortisone can be used one to three times daily. Alternatively, a retention enema containing 100 to 200 mg. of hydrocortisone may be given at night. Local steroids are probably partially absorbed but cause fewer long-term problems than oral steroids.

Oral steroids should be begun in high doses when there is moderate to severe active disease with systemic symptoms. Starting dose is at the level of 60 mg. per day of prednisone, which is tapered to the lowest dose necessary to maintain control of symptoms. Few patients will respond to alternate-day steroids. Hospital admission for observation and moni-

toring is often indicated when the patient is ill enough to require oral steroid therapy. Individuals whose disease is limited to the distal colon and is unassociated with systemic symptoms may be treated with steroids on an ambulatory basis.

When uveits and colitis flare together, oral steroids are often effective for both. In the absence of active colitis, the uveitis may be treated locally with steroids and mydriatics. Treatment of erythema nodosum, pyoderma gangrenosum, or oral aphthous ulcerations is directed toward control of the colitis.

All patients, especially those with pancolitis, who have disease of greater than 7 years duration should be examined for the development of cancer. Yearly proctosigmoidoscopy with musocal biopsy to look for dysplasia is indicated, as is an air contrast barium enema. If available, colonoscopy should replace barium enema every other year. When mucosal dysplasia is found or a suspicious lesion is seen on barium enema, colonoscopy is mandatory.

Probably the most difficult issue in the ambulatory care of patients with ulcerative colitis is the need for and timing of *surgery*. Total colectomy offers patients a complete cure of the disease and most systemic complications. In each patient the morbidity of active disease and the threat of cancer must be weighed against the risks of major surgery and the inconvenience of a permanent ileostomy. Many individuals welcome an ileostomy after years of painful bloody diarrhea. Any patient with pancolitis for more than 10 years should be considered for surgery, since risk of cancer is substantial (see above).

The primary physician should prepare each patient for surgery and subsequent ileostomy with a frank but sensitive discussion. Many patients have fears and anxieties which they will not discuss unless their physician mentions the subject. It is very helpful to have a person of the same age and sex who has had an ileostomy discuss the procedure with the patient.

Ulcerative proctitis. In light of its good prognosis, treatment should be principally symptomatic. In mild cases patients will obtain relief with *psyllium hydrophilic colloid* (Metamucil) alone. *Sulfasalazine* 2 to 4 gm. daily will provide a satisfactory response when there is more active disease. In troublesome cases, *rectal steroids* can provide help. Steroid suppositories containing 15 or 25 mg. of hydrocortisone can be used one to three times daily. Alternatively, a retention enema containing 100 to 200 mg. of hydrocortisone, may be given at night. Systemic steroids are not indicated in ulcerative proctitis. The therapeutic response can be measured symptomatically and confirmed by proctosigmoidoscopy.

Crohn's disease. Most patients can be helped on an outpatient basis by judicious use of medications and careful follow-up. A working alliance between the patient and his primary physician is essential, since the disease is chronic and often difficult to manage. Symptomatic relief of diarrhea can also be provided by diphenoxylate or codeine, but these may worsen obstructive symptoms in some patients. *Psyllium hydrophilic colloid* adds some substance to the stool and may help control diarrhea, though it too may worsen obstruction.

Sulfasalazine has been used for years for diarrhea and abdominal pain in doses of 2 to 4 gm. daily. The National Cooperative Crohn's Disease Study has conclusively demonstrated its efficacy in acute disease of the colon. No improvement was observed in patients whose disease was confined to the small bowel. Sulfasalazine was not efficacious in maintaining remissions when given chronically.

When a patient is acutely ill or if moderate measures are not effective in a week or two, *steroids* may be needed. High doses, such as 60 mg. of prednisone, should be used initially with a response expected in a few days. The dose may then be decreased to the minimum level necessary to control symptoms.

Eventually, 70 per cent of all patients will require *surgery.* The decision to operate must be carefully considered when full application of all available medical therapy fails to control the disease. Surgery is to be considered when there is severe debilitating disease, persistent fistulas, obstruction, abscess or severe bleeding. The principle of surgical therapy is to remove the grossly involved bowel and spare as much normal-appearing bowel as possible. Most patients will have many productive years after surgery; however, the recurrence rate is 30 to 50 per cent.

Nutrition is central to the therapy of patients with Crohn's disease. Adequate protein and calories must be provided. There is nothing special about elemental diets, but they may add the extra nutrition needed during exacerbations. Some patients who have had ileal surgery may need vitamin B_{12} supplementation. Other patients who have diarrhea after ileal resection may improve on cholestyramine or fat restriction. Obstructive symptoms may be improved by lowering roughage intake. Some patients with diarrhea may have lactose deficiency and respond to a milk-free diet.

Acutely ill patients often need hospitalization for good supportive care, close observation and the management of complications. Repeat radiographic and endoscopic studies are not necessary, except for planning surgical therapy. Clinical criteria are sufficient to judge the course of disease and document improvement.

ANNOTATED BIBLIOGRAPHY

Dissanayake, A.S., and Truelove, S.C.: A controlled therapeutic trial of long-term maintenance treatment of ulcerative colitis with sulfasalazine. Gut, *14*:923, 1973. *(A series of patients with ulcerative colitis treated with maintenance sulfasalazine had one-fourth the relapse rate of patients receiving placebo.)*

Dobbins, W.D.: Current status of the precancer lesion in ulcerative colitis. Gastroenterology, *73*:1431, 1977. *(A study of 453 total colectomies revealing a precancerous lesion in 66 per cent of rectal specimens from patients with cancer and a 33 per cent chance of cancer if there was a rectal precancer.)*

Farmer, R.G., Hawk, W.A., and Turnbull, R.B.: Clinical patterns in Crohn's disease: A statistical study of 615 cases. Gastroenterology, *68*:627, 1975. *(An extensive review outlines the various clinical presentations of Crohn's disease and its course.)*

Farmer, R.G., Hawk, W.A., and Turnbull, R.B.: Indications for surgery in Crohn's disease. Gastroenterology, *71*:245, 1976. *(The extensive experience of a referral center with surgical therapy of Crohn's disease.)*

Folley, J.H.: Ulcerative proctitis. N. Engl. J. Med., *282*:1362, 1970. *(A succinct clinical description of ulcerative proctitis, its course and therapy.)*

Glotzer, D.J., et al.: Comparative features and course of ulcerative and granulomatous colitis. N. Engl. J. Med., *282*:582, 1970. *(A clinically useful review of the distinction between ulcerative colitis and Crohn's colitis and their common features.)*

Goldman, P., and Peppercorn, M.A.: Sulfasalazine. N. Engl. J. Med., *283*:20, 1975. *(A review of the pharmacology and clinical application of sulfasalazine.)*

Greenstein, A.J., Janowitz, H.D., and Sacher, D.B.:

The extraintestinal complications of Crohn's disease and ulcerative colitis: A study of 700 patients. Medicine, *55*:401, 1976. *(An extensive review of the extraintestinal complications of inflammatory bowel disease.)*

Lennard-Jones, J.E., *et al.*: Cancer in colitis: Assessment of the individual risk by clinical and histological criteria. Gastroenterology, *73*:1280, 1977. *(The cancer risk among patients with ulcerative colitis is correlated with duration of the disease and mucosal dysplasia. A protocol for detecting patients at high risk for developing carcinoma is proposed.)*

National Cooperative Crohn's Disease Study: Gastroenterology, *77*:825, 1979. *(Demonstrated the efficacy of sulfasalazine in acute disease of the colon. No improvement was observed in patients whose disease was confined to the small bowel.)*

Whittington, P.F., Barnes, H.V., and Bayless, T.M.: Medical management of Crohn's disease in adolescence. Gastroenterology, *72*:1338, 1977. *(The special problems of Crohn's disease in adolescence are reviewed and a therapeutic plan applicable to all patients is proposed.)*

66
Management of the Irritable Bowel Syndrome

The irritable bowel syndrome is a prevalent disease in modern society, reportedly accounting for half of gastrointestinal complaints seen by physicians and ranking as a major cause of industrial absenteeism. The condition has been referred to by many names, including "irritable colon syndrome," "mucous colitis" and "spastic colon." It can be defined as a functional disturbance of intestinal motility, strongly influenced by emotional factors. Patients seek help because of gastrointestinal symptoms, fear of serious illness, and psychological problems. Irritable bowel can mimic organic disease, often goes unrecognized, and results in extensive workups and frustrating attempts at therapy. The primary physician must become expert in the diagnosis and management of this very common condition in order to avoid unnecessary investigations and to initiate effective symptomatic therapy.

PATHOPHYSIOLOGY AND CLINICAL PRESENTATION

Irritable bowel syndrome is a disturbance of bowel motor activity. Nonpropulsive colonic contractions and slow-wave myoelectric patterns at 2 to 3 cycles per minute constitute about 40 per cent of electrical and contractile activity at rest in patients with irritable bowel syndrome, compared to 10 per cent in normals. These contractions are felt to impede propul-

sion of stool, and when excessive, they account for the constipation and discomfort so prevalent in this condition. The diarrhea often seen in the syndrome is believed to occur as a result of increased contraction in the small bowel and proximal colon and diminished activity in the distal large bowel, creating a pressure gradient and causing accelerated movement of intestinal contents. Meals cause an increase in colonic contractions, but controlled study has shown that patients with irritable colon syndrome have a significantly exaggerated increase in response to food compared to normals.

Emotional stress has long been considered an important contributing factor. Hypermotility in response to stress has been documented, and a high prevalence of psychiatric illness has been uncovered. A psychological study of 29 patients with irritable bowel syndrome and 33 controls found that 72 per cent of the former had a psychiatric illness, compared to only 15 per cent of the controls. Psychiatric symptoms usually preceded bowel compaints. Hysteria and depression were the most frequent emotional disorders. A hospital-based epidemiologic study of 102 patients with irritable colon syndrome revealed a significantly higher frequency of life stresses in this group than among 735 individuals in the control group.

Laboratory experiments correlating response to a stress interview with sigmoid motility and symptoms have shown that when patients expressed coping behavior, they had heightened sigmoid contractions and were most often troubled by constipation and abdominal pain; when exhibiting depressive behavior, they had diminished sigmoid activity and diarrhea.

The commonly encountered syndrome of diarrhea alternating with constipation may reflect the different responses to stress that an individual may manifest. Moreover, laboratory study of normal individuals subjected to experimentally induced stress showed similar bowel responses, suggesting that irritable colon physiology is a nomal reaction to severe stress. What seems to characterize the patient persistently bothered by irritable colon symptoms is the greater prevalence of serious situational stresses, psychopathology and perhaps learned visceral responses to threatening situations. This psychophysiological response to stress may be altered by agents affecting gut motility, such as anticholinergics.

Clinical presentation is illustrated by a series of 50 patients treated in an outpatient unit. Most patients (62 per cent) experienced onset of symptoms before age 40; 50 per cent were under 30 at time of onset; and one-quarter were under 20. Chronicity was the rule, with little change in symptoms over time, except for waxing and waning. Duration was in years. Only 14 per cent actively carried a diagnosis of irritable bowel syndrome. Abdominal pain was present in 90 per cent, mucous stools in 36 per cent, pelletlike stools in 38 per cent, diarrhea alone in 10 per cent, excessive flatus in 36 per cent. Fifty per cent considered their symptoms related to stress; 34 per cent denied this; 66 per cent manifested symptoms of anxiety or depression. The abdominal pain was most often in the left lower quadrant or lower abdomen (62 per cent), but in 28 per cent there were multiple sites of pain. Upper abdominal involvement occurred in 38 per cent. The pain was typically achy rather than crampy, often relieved by a bowel movement or passage of flatus. It was unusual for the pain to awaken the patient. Radiation was variable, and even extended into the left chest and arm when gas was trapped in the splenic flexure.

Small, hard, infrequent stools and an empty rectal ampulla characterize the constipation. Prolonged retention of stool allows for full absorption of intestinal water content. The diarrhea is typically small in volume, associated with visible amounts of mucus, and may follow a hard movement by a few hours. There may be urgency. Dyspepsia and excessive gaseousness are also reported (see Chapter 55). Weight loss is rare; symptoms usually parallel situational stresses.

CLINICAL COURSE

Irritable bowel syndrome is a chronic, relapsing condition with no evidence of significant morbidity or mortality. A prospective British study providing follow-up at 2-month intervals over 3 years found that severity waxed and waned, but the constellation of symptoms remained remarkably constant. At 1 year, 50 per cent were unchanged, 36 per cent improved, 12 per cent symptom-free and 20 per cent worse. The symptom-free period was usually less than a few months. One third of employed patients lost time from work. There was no correlation between time lost and number of visits to the doctor; 40 per cent made five or less visits, and 46 per cent made none at all. At 2 years, a similar pattern was found. Only one patient remained symptom-free from the first year.

Studies on clinical course identified groups of patients with different prognoses. The group with symptoms triggered by a major life stress enjoyed long symptom-free periods after the acute problem abated, whereas those with continuous intestinal complaints in response to daily living rarely became asymptomatic.

PRINCIPLES OF MANAGEMENT

Successful therapy requires recognition of the psychophysiological nature of the problem. Physiological manipulations may provide temporary symptomatic relief, but attention to the patient's emotional needs and life situation are essential to successful long-term management.

The therapeutic value of close follow-up and *supportive therapy* is illustrated by the prospective British study cited above. Most patients reported feeling better, less concerned about their bowels, and more able to cope with their symptoms and the stresses of daily life. Even though there were frequent relapses, these seemed to be of less importance when they occurred in the context of close medical support.

In the context of a thorough medical evaluation, the clinician needs to collect full details of the patient's life situation, aspirations, accomplishments, frustrations and losses. Descriptions of fears, concerns and expectations should be encouraged so these can be addressed. It is also very important that one be compassionate, interested and able to accept the complaints as real. It is not useful for the physician to undermine the patient's symptoms by trying to convince him that it is a totally emotional problem. Rather, one needs to identify important life stresses and relate these to triggering of changes in bowel physiology.

When specific underlying emotional illness is identified, treatment should be directed toward it. In a study of 67 patients with irritable bowel syndrome, 56 were felt to be depressed and received a *tricyclic antidepressant.* Over 50 per cent became symptom-free, 33 per cent improved, and 20 per cent showed no benefit. Conversely, when bowel symptoms are not due to a well-defined psychiatric illness, use of psychotropic agents is less effective. A double-blind controlled study of 52 patients manifesting nonspecific anxiety showed that *diazepam* had no effect on bowel complaints compared to placebo. However, patients bothered predominantly by diarrhea have been found to be more neurotic than those with constipation and perhaps might respond to psychotherapy.

Dietary manipulations have been incompletely successful and remain controversial. There is no evidence that a low-residue diet is of any use, but there are conflicting data regarding bran. In a double-blind trial óf 50 patients eating a standardized bran biscuit or placebo biscuit, there was no difference in effect. Both groups reported subjective improvement in over 50 per cent of individuals. A more recent controlled, but unblinded British study of 26 patients showed significant improvement in symptoms and colonic motor activity in the bran-fed group compared to controls.

Many patients complain of "food allergies," but no changes in colonic motor activity have been found to occur on intake of the offending food. However, lactose intolerance may go unrecognized, even by routine lactose tolerance testing. As a result, a trial of restricting dairy products is worthwhile in those bothered by excessive flatus and diarrhea. In general, diet should be attractive, balanced and unrestricted.

Symptomatic relief is often necessary before some patients will turn their attention to the stresses precipitating symptoms. *Anticholinergics* have been tried in such circumstances. Although these agents have been shown to inhibit the postprandial increase in nonpropulsive colonic contractions, their clinical effectiveness is unproven. The consensus is that they are worth a try in cases where abdominal pain and constipation are the major compaints and routine measures have failed. Such patients should first receive a hydrophilic colloid or bulk preparation (see Chapter 59) and a diet with *increased fiber* to com-

bat the constipation before an anticholinergic such as propantheline is added. Disabling diarrhea may require small doses of diphenoxylate for brief periods.

An essential part of management is establishment of a supportive *doctor-patient relationship* providing reassurance, explanation and advice (see Chapter 1). The irritable bowel syndrome is one of many diseases without a simple resolution, and success in its management will depend significantly on the physician's relationship to and interaction with the individual patient. A great deal of effort needs to be directed at helping the patient to understand and to cope with his life situation. The modalities of education, diet and drugs are available to the physician. No single approach has been proven successful in randomized, placebo-controlled, double-blind studies. The major principle of therapy is to implement each measure sequentially, minimizing risk to the patient while providing close support. Attempts aimed at complete relief of symptoms are bound to be met with frustration and excessive, even dangerous use of pharmacologic agents. Emphasis should be on a sympathetic approach that moves the patient toward a more healthy adaptation to his environment.

THERAPEUTIC RECOMMENDATIONS

- Stop all nonessential medicines which may affect bowel function, especially laxatives.
- Provide thorough reassurance after eliciting concerns and fears; address issue of cancer.
- Sympathetically obtain details of life stress, living situation, losses and frustrations.
- Identify and treat specifically any underlying depression or other psychiatric illness.
- For the patient bothered predominantly by constipation, increase dietary fiber and exercise; add Metamucil, 1 rounded teaspoon in 8 oz. of water 3 times daily, if constipation is still troublesome. Stronger laxatives are not indicated.
- Resort to anticholinergic agents only if all else has failed and constipation and pain are intolerable. Propantheline 15 mg. can be administered before each meal and titrated to achieve mild anticholinergic side effects such as dry mouth.
- For the patient with diarrhea, increased dietary fiber is worth a try first; if symptoms are disabling, a brief course of diphenoxylate 5 mg. t.i.d. can be given.
- No dietary restrictions are indicated unless diar-

rhea is disabling; and then a trial of a lactose-free diet should be initiated for 1 week. Dairy products are avoided.

- Sedatives and tranquilizers are of little use for relief of bowel symptoms.
- Initiate supportive psychotherapy, aimed at sympathetically helping the patient to adapt and manage his life situation.
- Avoid attempts aimed at complete suppression of symptoms.
- See the patient at regular intervals, and be available for help at times of increased stress.

INDICATIONS FOR REFERRAL AND ADMISSION

This is one condition where a continuous relationship is essential, and any perceived need for referral should be acted upon only after thorough discussion with the patient. In general, referral is helpful when there are refractory disabling symptoms, such as uncontrollable diarrhea, or when serious psychopathology is encountered. A hospital admission may, in rare circumstances, be appropriate and very beneficial in helping the patient to learn new means of coping with stress and providing a respite from an intolerable living situation.

PATIENT EDUCATION

The major lesson to be mastered in this condition is the relationship between stress and symptoms. Techniques which may help in this effort include having the patient keep a diary of daily events and symptoms, as well as thoroughly discussing major losses, frustrations and conflicts, and their connection to the bowel problem. Patients also need to know that their symptoms are not manifestations of a serious underlying condition such as cancer or inflammatory bowel disease, a frequent misconception. Emphasis must be placed on learning to adapt to one's living situation, changing it where possible, and coping better when the problem is more intransigent. Patients must understand that symptoms will wax and wane, as will their emotional stresses. Total relief is not possible, but improvement in function is achievable.

ANNOTATED BIBLIOGRAPHY

Almy, T.: Experimental studies on the irritable colon. Am. J. Med., *10*:60, 1951. *(Classic experiments on relation of stress to bowel activity.)*

Deutsch, E.: Relief of anxiety and related emotions in patients with gastrointestinal disorders. Am. J. Dig. Dis., *16*:1091, 1971. *(Diazepam relieved anxiety but did not improve bowel symptoms any better than did placebo.)*

Drossman, D.A., Powell, D.W., and Sessions, J.T., Jr.: The irritable bowel syndrome. Gastroenterology, *73*:811, 1977. *(A superb review emphasizing motility factors, diagnosis, treatment and prognosis of this difficult syndrome. Eighty-six references.)*

Esler, M., and Goulston, K.: Levels of anxiety in colonic disorders. N. Engl. J. Med., *288*:16, 1973, *(Patients with predominant diarrhea were significantly more anxious and more neurotic by psychometric testing than normals or those with constipation and pain.)*

Hislop, I.: Psychological significance of the irritable colon syndrome. Gut, *12*:452, 1971. *(Fifty-six of 67 patients with irritable colon syndrome were treated with tricyclic antidepressants. Over 80 per cent reported significant improvement.)*

Ivey, K.J.: Are anticholinergics of use in the irritable colon syndrome? Gastroenterology, *68*:1300, 1975. *(A careful review of the use of anticholinergic drugs that concludes that although the evidence is dubious, they appear to be of some benefit in patients with pain or constipation as their major syndrome. Use is advised when patients fail to respond to routine measures. Fifty-three references.)*

Manning, A., Heaton, K., Harvey, R., et al.: Wheat fibre and irritable bowel syndrome. Lancet, *2*:417, 1977. *(A controlled but unblinded study of 26 patients showing significant improvement in symptoms and colonic motor activity in the bran-treated group only.)*

Soltoft, J., Krag, B., Hoyer, E., et al.: A double-blind trial of the effect of wheat bran on symptoms of irritable bowel syndrome. Lancet, *1*:270, 1976. *(No difference in effect over 6 weeks between bran and placebo; over 50 per cent improved in each group. Dose of bran was 30 gm. per day.)*

Sullivan, M., Cohen, S., and Snape, W.: Colonic

myoelectric activity in irritable bowel syndrome. N. Engl. J. Med., *298*:878, 1978. *(Patients with irritable bowel syndrome and abnormally prolonged increase in postprandial motor activity, which was reduced by an anticholinergic agent.)*

Waller, S., and Misiewicz, J.: Prognosis in the irritable bowel syndrome. Lancet, *2*:754, 1969. *(Symptoms wax and wane with little permanent resolution, but supportive therapy helps patients to cope.)*

Wangel, A., and Deller, D.: Intestinal motility in man. III. Mechanisms of constipation and diarrhea with particular reference to the irritable colon syndrome. Gastroenterology, *48*:69, 1965. *(A motility study of the large bowel, demonstrating increased proximal and distal activity aggravated by food and emotion in patients with constipation and pain, and diminished distal activity in those with diarrhea.)*

Young, S., Alper, D., Norland, C., *et al.*: Psychiatric illness and the irritable bowel syndrome. Gastroenterology, *70*:162, 1970. *(Seventy-two per cent of patients with irritable bowel syndrome in a general group practice have an underlying psychiatric illness; only 28 per cent were properly recognized and diagnosed.)*

67

Management of Diverticular Disease

Diverticula, abnormal herniations of colonic mucosa through the muscularis, are extremely common and increase with age. Autopsy studies estimate their presence in 20 per cent of people over 40 and in 70 per cent of those over 70. About 15 per cent of people with the condition develop attacks of diverticulitis. It is possible that the recent emphasis on increasing the fiber content of the diet will reduce the incidence of diverticulosis in Western countries. The primary physician encounters many elderly patients with gastrointestinal complaints referable to diverticular disease. The physician must effectively and economically recognize and treat mild manifestations of disease, reduce the chances of complications, and decide when admission and surgical intervention are necessary.

PATHOPHYSIOLOGY, CLINICAL PRESENTATION AND COMPLICATIONS

Increased intracolonic pressure causes herniation of colonic mucosa. Consequently, diverticula occur most frequently in the sigmoid where the colon is narrowest and pressure highest. Diverticula show a predilection for points of relative weakness in the muscularis where branches of the marginal artery penetrate the colonic wall. Current research indicates that the low fiber content of modern diets has a causal role, producing less bulky stool and increased intracolonic pressure. Conditions associated with abnormal colonic activity and segmentation, such as irritable colon syndrome, may contribute to the pathogenesis of diverticula; this remains speculative. The possibility of muscular degeneration has been suggested but remains unproven.

The diverticular sac can become inflamed when undigested food residues and bacteria get trapped in the thin-walled sac; blood supply is mechanically compromised and bacterial invasion ensues. Microperforations can occur producing peridiverticular and pericolonic inflammation.

Most diverticula are asymptomatic and discovered incidentally on barium enema. However, sometimes colonic motor activity is disturbed, and intermittent left lower quadrant pain results. Constipation is common, and occasionally there is tenderness or a palpable, thickened colon. Diverticulitis is characterized by left lower quadrant pain, tenderness, fever and leukocytosis in a patient with known diverticulosis.

The major complications of diverticular disease are perforation, obstruction and bleeding. Perforations may lead to abscess formation. The abscesses may spontaneously drain into bowel or erode into an adjacent organ, forming fistulas. Perforations that fail to become walled off may cause peritonitis. Chronic inflammation can thicken the bowel wall and lead to obstruction. Erosion into a blood vessel may result in brisk rectal hemorrhage. The incidence of hemorrhage, obstruction or perforation was 15 per cent in a 15-year study by the Lahey Clinic.

PRINCIPLES OF MANAGEMENT

The goals of therapy are prevention of symptoms, relief of pain and avoidance of complications. Since diverticular disease is felt to be, in part, a manifestation of a low-fiber diet, *bran* has been tried in therapy. Prospective British studies of bran use have shown reversal of abnormal bowel physiology and reduction in symptoms in over 90 per cent of cases. The average amount of bran needed to achieve an effect is 15 gm. per day. Some individuals are bothered by flatulence and bloating during the first 2 to 3 weeks of bran use, but this usually resolves.

Patients unable to tolerate bran may be treated with bulk agents such as *psyllium* (Metamucil). Irritant laxatives should be avoided. The efficacy of *anticholinergics* is controversial; painful spasm may be lessened, but the risk of constipation is increased, raising the likelihood of inspissation of fecal material. Undigestible materials (e.g., seeds) which may block the mouth of a diverticulum should be omitted from the diet.

Diverticulitis can be treated at home when symptoms are mild. The aim of therapy is to markedly reduce bowel activity in order to lessen the chance of perforation. *Rest* and clear *liquids* usually suffice. Strong analgesics and antipyretics should not be prescribed because they may mask signs of worsening inflammation. Broad-spectrum oral *antibiotics* such as ampicillin are customarily used, especially when fever exceeds 101°F.

An important decision in the therapy of diverticulitis is whether to treat the patient medically or opt for elective *surgical resection* of the involved bowel after initial resolution of symptoms. Proponents of surgical therapy argue that the frequency of complications warrants prophylactic operation once a patient experiences an attack of diverticulitis. The courses of 132 patients at Yale-New Haven Hospital with documented uncomplicated diverticulitis were analyzed. Of the 99 treated medically and 33 treated surgically, the rates of recurrence were almost identical. Moreover, three-quarters never had more than one attack. The increased length of hospitalization and postoperative morbidity were not balanced by a marked reduction in rate of recurrence or complications. However, the presence of abscess, perforation or obstruction is an indication for surgery. Although controlled data are lacking, most authorities recommend treatment with a high-fiber diet after acute symptoms have ceased.

THERAPEUTIC RECOMMENDATIONS AND PATIENT EDUCATION

For the patient with known diverticula and occasional pain or constipation:

- Increase fiber content of the diet. The best sources are bran, root vegetables (particularly raw carrots and fruits with skin). Bulk laxatives like psyllium hydrophilic mucilloid (Metamucil) can be used in patients who cannot tolerate bran, but are relatively expensive.
- Inform patients that any bloating or flatulence due to bran intake usually resolves with continued use.
- Advise patients to avoid foods with seeds or undigestible material that may block the neck of a diverticulum, such as nuts, corn, popcorn, cucumbers, tomatoes, figs, strawberries and caraway seeds.
- Have patients avoid laxatives, enemas, and opiates since they are potent constipating agents.
- Use of anticholinergics should be reserved for refractory cases.
- Instruct patients to report fever, tenderness or bleeding without delay.

For patients with mild diverticulitis (temperature less than 101°F, white cell count below 13,000 to 15,000):

- Prescribe bed rest and clear liquid diet.
- Use mild nonopiate analgesics for pain.
- Begin a broad-spectrum antibiotic such as oral ampicillin 500 mg. four times daily or tetracycline 500 mg. four times daily.
- Monitor temperature, pain, abdominal exam for signs of peritonitis, and white count for elevation.

INDICATIONS FOR ADMISSION AND REFERRAL

The development of a temperature greater than 101°F, persistence of pain for more than 3 days and increasing pain indicate need for admission. A markedly elevated white count may be the only clue of a deteriorating situation, for many patients with diverticulitis are elderly and may not demonstrate much in the way of fever, abdominal pain or signs of peritonitis. The management of a patient with bleeding, abscess or perforation requires surgical consultation; operative intervention may be urgent.

ANNOTATED BIBLIOGRAPHY

Almy, T., and Howell, D.A.: Diverticular disease of the colon. N. Engl. J. Med., *302*:324, 1980. *(An authoritative review; 119 refs.)*

Boles, R., and Jordan, S.: Clinical significance of diverticulosis. Gastroenterology, *35*:579, 1958. *(An analysis of 294 patients with diverticulosis; mean duration of follow-up was 15 years. Frequency of hemorrhage, obstruction or perforation was 15 per cent.)*

Horner, J.L.: Natural history of diverticulosis of the colon. Am. J. Dig. Dis., *3*:343, 1958. *(A study of 503 patients followed in the ambulatory setting for 1 to 18 years [mean 8 years]. Incidence of diverticulitis was about 15 per cent.)*

Larson, D., Masters, S., and Spiro, H.: Medical and surgical therapy in diverticular disease. Gastroenterology, *71*:734, 1976. *(A report of 132 patients followed for a mean of 9.8 years [range 6 to 12 years] after medical or surgical therapy for acute diverticulitis. There was no significant difference in outcome; in about 75 per cent of instances no further problems occurred among those in either group.)*

Painter, N., Almeida, A., and Colebourne, K.: Unprocessed bran in treatment of diverticular disease of the colon. Br. Med. J., *2*:137, 1972. *(Seventy patients treated with bran in a prospective but uncontrolled study. Over 90 per cent showed marked improvement in symptoms.)*

Taylor, I., and Duthie, H.: Bran tablets and diverticular disease. Br. Med. J., *2*:988, 1976. *(A crossover trial of bran tablets, high roughage diet and a bulk agent with an antispasmodic; 20 patients. All agents improved measurements of bowel function, but bran was most effective in relieving symptoms and normalizing colonic motor activity.)*

68
Management of Hemorrhoids

Hemorrhoids are a source of much misery though they are of no consequence unless they cause discomfort or bleeding. Therapy is directed toward relief of symptoms, and should be accomplished with a minimum of discomfort, cost and time lost from work. Simple approaches to pain relief and sensible modification in bowel habits to prevent progression constitute the essentials of medical therapy. The primary physician must be certain that symptoms are attributable to hemorrhoids, alleviate any anxiety about neoplasm, provide conservative medical therapy and decide on the need and timing of surgery.

PATHOPHYSIOLOGY AND CLINICAL PRESENTATION

Theories explaining the etiology of hemorrhoids invoke a number of mechanisms, including increased venous pressure secondary to upright posture and straining at stool, arteriovenous communications in rectal tissue, and prolapsed cushions of tissue secondary to loss of support. Clinically, hemorrhoids are associated with pregnancy, portal hypertension and constipation. The relative absence of hemorrhoids in African populations that have high-residue diets has led to the suggestion that an increase in dietary fiber might prevent the development of hemorrhoids.

Hemorrhoids may be classified by presentation as first degree when they merely bleed, second degree if they prolapse upon high pressure but return spontaneously, and third degree when the anal suspensory ligament is stretched to the point of permanent prolapse. Hemorrhoids are considered to be *internal* when derived from the superior hemorrhoidal plexus above the dentate line, and *external* when located below the dentate line and covered by squamous epithelium.

Pain, incomplete defecation, constipation, excessive moisture, rectal itching, bleeding or detection of a prolapsed mass are the common presentations. Hemorrhoids are regularly encountered as incidental findings on physical examination. Skin tags are evidence of previous hemorrhoids that have thrombosed, leaving connective tissue. The complications of hemorrhoids include bleeding, prolapse and thrombosis.

PRINCIPLES OF MANAGEMENT

It is not necessary to remove hemorrhoids in order to treat them effectively. Symptomatic relief and prevention of progression can usually be provided by use of simple local measures and change in bowel habits. Cold packs at onset, followed by hot sitz baths, often suffice to alleviate pain. Topical anesthetics can supplement the effort when pain is severe. Softening of the stool to diminish straining is essential and acheived in part by increasing dietary fiber and by temporary use of stool softeners such as dioctyl sodium sulfosuccinate. Irritant laxatives should be avoided (see Chapter 59). Stubborn itching and inflammation respond to topical steroids; hydrocortisone suppositories are quite adequate and the least expensive. Many clinicians advise aggressive treatment for thrombosed hemorrhoids, but conservative methods often suffice.

If symptoms become intractable, referral for surgical treatment is indicated. This requires knowledge of the risks and benefits of the therapeutic alternatives and the resources available in the community. Hemorrhoids may be treated definitively by surgical removal, but effective alternatives with less morbidity have been developed in recent years. The common objective of the alternative surgical approaches is removal of the hemorrhoid without prolonged hospitalization or disability. Impressive published results exist for several alternate methods. The alternatives include forced anal dilatation, rubber band ligation, and cryosurgery. Conventional hemorrhoidectomy requires hospitalization and general anesthesia; it is quite painful. Injection of sclerosing agents has fallen out of favor since it may cause scarring of the anal canal. Forced dilatation requires anesthesia, but produces results similar to hemorrhoidectomy with less pain and less time lost from work. The major complication is incontinence and, therefore, it should not be used in patients who are elderly or whose main complaints are soiling or incontinence. Rubber band ligation is simply a ligation suture of redundant tissue which can be done on outpatient basis, though 3 or 4 visits may be required. Cryosurgery does not require anesthesia and is relatively painless; the main disadvantage is development of a foul-smelling discharge for a week following the procedure; occasionally, stricture is a late occurrence.

THERAPEUTIC RECOMMENDATIONS

- Advise frequent hot sitz baths for relief of pain. At the initial recognition of pain, the patient can apply a cold pack for the first few hours, then take hot baths 3 or 4 times a day.
- Topical anesthetics may be useful for the acute relief of severe pain. Lidocaine (Xylocaine) ointment is preferred because it is less allergenic than benzocaine.
- If inflammation and itching are present, prescribe a suppository preparation containing a steroid, e.g., hydrocortisone.
- Treat constipation by having patient increase dietary fiber and use a stool softener, e.g., dioctyl sodium sulfosuccinate, 100 mg. t.i.d. Following resolution of acute symptoms, the high-fiber diet should be continued.
- For thrombosed hemorrhoids:
  1. Instruct the patient to lie prone with ice applied to the thrombosed hemorrhoid.
  2. Prescribe oral analgesics; codeine may be required.
  3. Prescribe stool softeners.
  4. Conservative therapy should be successful in 3 to 5 days; otherwise refer the patient for surgical removal of the clot, which will relieve pain promptly.
- Intractable symptoms require surgical therapy. The specific method chosen is dependent on the surgical expertise available in the community.

PATIENT EDUCATION AND PREVENTION

Instruction in proper diet and bowel habits is extremely helpful.

- Advise the patient to increase the intake of dietary fiber; suggest bran, carrots, green vegetables and fruits with skin. Some people find foods such as chili, onions and alcohol irritating. If this applies to your patient, suggest avoidance.
- Emphasize the importance of providing a regular time to have bowel movements. After bowel movements, the patient should avoid vigorous wiping; patting ought to suffice, and it minimizes irritation.

- Instruct the patient not to linger on the toilet or strain at stool. Long periods of standing should be avoided.
- Caution the patient against use of irritant laxatives.
- At the first sign of recurrent symptoms, institute frequent hot sitz baths.

ANNOTATED BIBLIOGRAPHY

Anscombe, A.R., et al.: A clinical trial of the treatment of hemorrhoids by operation and Lord procedure. Lancet, 2:250, 1974. (A prospective study of 2 groups of 100 patients comparing hemorrhoidectomy and dilatation. Success rates were 98 per cent and 84 per cent, respectively, with dilatation producing fewer days of disability.)

McCaffrey, J.: Lord treatment of hemorrhoids. Lancet, 1:133, 1975. (A 4-year follow-up revealed 75 per cent of 50 patients treated by the Lord techniques of manual dilatation were symptom-free.)

Outpatient treatment of hemorrhoids. (Editorial.) Br. Med. J., 2:651, 1975. (An editorial emphasizing that it is unnecessary to completely remove hemorrhoids to relieve symptoms. The excellent results and cost-saving of "ambulatory proctology" are noted.)

Prasad, G.C., et al: Studies on etiopathogenesis of hemorrhoids. Am. J. Proctol. 27(3):33, 1976. (An excellent review of the pathogenesis of hemorrhoids.)

Taggart, R.E.B.: Hemorrhoids and palpable anorectal problems. Practitioner, 212:221, 1974. (A succinct, complete review of the current alternatives in treating hemorrhoids. Other anal lesions, infection, fissure, fistula, pruritus and prolapse are discussed.)

To tie; to stab; to stretch, perchance to freeze. (Editorial.) Lancet, 2:645, 1975. (Concludes that hemorrhoidectomy should be reserved for failure of other methods.)

Treatment of hemorrhoids. Medical Letter, 17:7, 1975. (A one-page summary of new methods, calling attention to the possibility of nonsurgical therapy.)

What are hemorrhoids? (Editorial.) Br. Med. J., 4:365, 1975. (A review of the theories concerning pathogenesis of hemorrhoids.)

69
Management of Asymptomatic Gallstones and Chronic Cholecystitis

Gallbladder disease affects over 15 million Americans, and more than 350,000 cholecystectomies are performed each year. Many patients with stones are asymptomatic, while others suffer from chronic cholecystitis, with recurrent bouts of abdominal discomfort. The occurrence of asymptomatic gallstones or chronic cholecystitis requires that the primary physician determine who is a candidate for cholecystectomy and who can be managed conservatively.

CLINICAL PRESENTATION AND COURSE

Gallbladder disease may be asymptomatic or manifested by recurrent pain. Characteristically, the pain of biliary colic is rather sudden in onset, builds to a maximum within 1 hour, is steady, localized to the right upper quadrant or epigastrium, lasts 2 to 4 hours, and occasionally radiates to the left or right scapula. There is often nausea and vomiting. Dyspeptic symptoms, fatty food intolerance, belching and bloating have also been attributed to chronic gallbladder disease, but the association has not been proven. Prospective studies have shown that such symptoms are just as frequent in middle-aged women without gallstones as in those with them. When patients with these symptoms are operated on, the dyspepsia often persists after cholecystectomy. Reflux of bile into the stomach has been noted in such individuals.

The rare patient with biliary colic, who has a normal gallbladder study on routine oral cholecystogram and ultrasound, may have acalculous gallbladder disease, an uncommon condition, or multiple small stones undectable by conventional methods. These subtle forms of gallbladder disease may be discovered by observing delayed gallbladder emptying in response to a fatty meal or cholecystokinin.

The clinical course of untreated gallbladder disease is not known with precision. Two prospective studies, totalling 1300 patients who had at least one bout of pain, showed that over a follow-up period of 5 to 20 years, 30 per cent had recurrence of pain, and 20 per cent experienced complications such as jaundice, cholangitis or pancreatitis; half remained asymptomatic. Those with nonvisualizing gallbladders on oral cholecystogram had twice the rate of complications. Since all patients in these studies had pain requiring a hospital admission, and almost 70 per cent had nonvisualizing oral cholecystograms, this patient population probably represented a group with a greater likelihood of complications than one with a predominance of visualizing gallbladders and asymptomatic stones. The skewed nature of the study population is suggested by a screening study of asymptomatic men which revealed that only 15 per cent of those with gallstones had gallbladders which failed to opacify. Thus prognosis seems in part related to the functional status of the gallbladder, as measured by its ability to concentrate dye.

Although there is no certainty that the onset of complications will be preceded by episodes of biliary pain, a study of 600 patients found that over 90 per cent of patients who suffered a complication of gallbladder disease had prior warning symptoms of biliary colic, thoough these were often mild and ignored. Most patients with pain on presentation had similar patterns of pain on follow-up. When 112 patients with asymptomatic stones were followed without surgery for 10 to 20 years, 27 per cent eventually complained of dyspepsia, 19 per cent had biliary colic, and 4.5 per cent experienced transient jaundice. There were no deaths due to delay of surgery.

In sum, the patient with gallstones and visualizing gallbladder seems to have a relatively favorable prognosis. Individuals with nonvisualizing gallbladders and recurrent pain have twice the rate of complications. Increased risk is also associated with stones larger than 2.5 cm., age over 60, and diabetes. Some authorities believe there is a cause-and-effect relationship between gallstones and carcinoma of the gallbladder. The cancer occurs mostly in older women. The association with stone formation is based on circumstantial autopsy data and is not unversally accepted.

PRINCIPLES OF THERAPY

Patients with recurrent biliary colic and nonvisualizing oral cholecystograms should undergo *elective cholecystectomy*, since the risk of complications is far greater than the risk of surgery. This is especially true for diabetics. However, there is no evidence that the vast numbers of patients with asymptomatic stones would benefit from surgery. Even though surgical mortality is only 0.5 per cent, the risk of conservative management is not much different and involves far less expense and morbidity. Surgical mortality rises to 4.2 per cent for patients over age 60, as does risk of complications from gallbladder disease. The decision to operate on elderly patients and those with serious illness has to be individualized. Operating on all women over 65 with stones in order to prevent carcinoma would result in more death from surgery than lives saved.

Medical therapy with *chenodeoxycholic acid* is still in the investigational stages. A national multicenter study is underway, though smaller, controlled studies have been done. The agent reduces the cholesterol content of bile to achieve an unsaturated composition. It has been shown to dissolve cholesterol-containing gallstones over 6 to 24 months of therapy. Calcified stones are not affected. Patients with nonfunctioning gallbladders do not respond well. The therapeutic effect is dose-related and lasts up to 9 weeks after therapy is stopped. Adverse effects include diarrhea and minor elevations in serum transaminase levels. The elevations usually disappear, even with continued therapy. Biliary colic and jaundice have occurred, presumably due to passage of partially dissolved stones, though the rate is less than that for untreated patients. Recurrence of stones has been documented after discontinuation of the drug, making chronic therapy necessary. The feasibility of intermittent therapy is under study, as is the safety of chronic use of this agent. No changes have been noted in serum cholesterol concentrations; surprisingly, triglycerides decrease by about 20 per cent.

The role of chenodeoxycholic acid in treatment of gallstones is unsettled at the moment. Among the best candidates for therapy are patients with asymptomatic large cholesterol stones and those who are too sick to undergo surgery. The cost of therapy at present is over $350 per year, making the drug too expensive for mass use on a chronic basis. Therapy is contraindicated in inflammatory bowel disease and peptic ulcer disease, because the drug increases bile acids which may be harmful to colonic or gastric mucosa.

A few preventive measures are worth noting. Increased incidence of gallstone formation has been noted with use of oral contraceptives and clofibrate. Patients taking these agents should be monitored for gallstones and taken off the drugs if any evidence of stone formation or cholecystitis develops. There is no evidence that dietary measures such as a low-fat diet or avoidance of particular foods has any effect on biliary colic. Dyspepsia responds to antacids in about 25 to 50 per cent of cases (see Chapter 55), and even surgery sometimes relieves such symptoms, though not with any consistency.

THERAPEUTIC RECOMMENDATIONS

- Patients who are completely asymptomatic and have a visualizing gallbladder should be followed and need not undergo cholecystectomy unless they are in the high-risk group, e.g., are diabetic, have a stone larger than 2.5 cm. The decision regarding elective surgery in the elderly has to be individualized.
- Patients with recurrent biliary colic and a nonvisualizing gallbladder should undergo elective cholecystectomy, provided they are otherwise surgical candidates.
- Patients who should undergo cholecystectomy but cannot, due to advanced age or concurrent illness, might be given a trial of chenodeoxycholic acid, beginning with 1,000 mg. per day; dose is adjusted downward if diarrhea or SGOT elevations develop. (Follow literature for results of a soon-to-be-completed national multicenter study.)
- Clofibrate and oral contraceptives should be stopped, or dosages decreased, in patients with stone formation.
- There is no need to alter diet or restrict fats in the treatment of biliary colic; anticholinergics are of no benefit.
- Dyspeptic symptoms should be treated with antacids. Avoidance of foods which precipitate symptoms may be worth a try. Severe refractory dyspepsia occasionally responds to surgery when gallstones or a nonopacifying gallbladder is present.

PATIENT EDUCATION

The asymptomatic patient needs to be reassured of the benign nature of his illness and should not be pushed into surgery or unnecessary dietary restriction. Dyspepsia may respond to antacids, and, thus, careful instruction in their use is indicated. The reluctant person at high-risk for complications of gallbladder disease requires thorough explanation of the chances of complications and of the relatively low risk of elective surgery. However, the choice of elective surgery is the patient's, and initial refusal should be respected. In such instances, a trial of medical therapy and/or approaching the patient at a later date about surgery may produce better results than simply discharging the patient because he refuses elective operation. On the other hand, the very anxious patient with asymptomatic gallstones who steadfastly insists on surgery out of concern for future complications might be allowed to undergo elective cholecystectomy in order to provide peace of mind, provided there are no medical contraindications to undergoing surgery.

ANNOTATED BIBLIOGRAPHY

Bennion, L.J., and Grundy, S.M.: Risk factors for development of cholelithiasis in man. N. Engl. J. Med., *299*:1161, 1978. *(Authoritative review, of current knowledge.)*

Carveth, S.W., Priestley, J.T., and Gage, R.: Size and number of gallstones in acute and chronic cholecystitis. Mayo Clin. Proc., *34*:371, 1959. *(Stones larger than 2.5 cm. are more likely to precipitate attacks of cholecystitis than are smaller stones.)*

Cole, W.H.: The false normal oral cholecystogram. Surgery, *81*:121, 1977. *(Stones and gallbladder disease are missed in 2 to 4 per cent of studies due to the small size of stones or presence of acalculous disease. Thus, false-negative rate is 2 to 4 per cent for oral cholecystograms.)*

Comfort, M.W., Gray, H.K., and Wilson, J.M.: The silent gallstone: A ten- to twenty-year follow-up study of 112 cases. Ann. Surg., *128*:931, 1948. *(There were no deaths in this group attributable to delay of surgery, and only 19 per cent had episodes of colic during the period of follow-up.)*

Dunn, F.H., et al.: Cholecystokinin cholecystography. J.A.M.A., *228*:997, 1974. *(Controlled evaluation in the diagnosis of patients with acalculous disease.)*

Iser, J.H., Dowling, R.H., Moh, H., et al.: Chenodeoxycholic acid treatment of gallstones. N. Engl. J. Med., *293*:378, 1975. *(A prospective study of 70 patients, examining the factors influencing outcome. Those with cholesterol stones and visualizing gallbladders did best. One hundred per cent of those whose bile became unsaturated responded. Dissoluation of stones took from 6 to 24 months.)*

Mujahad, Z., Evans, J.A., and Whalen, J.P.: The nonopacified gallbladder on oral cholecystogram. Radiology, *112*:1, 1974. *(Persistent nonvisualization of the gallbladder after second dose has a sensitivity of more than 95 per cent for detecting diseased gallbladders.)*

Newman, H.F., Northrup, J.D., and Rosenblum, M., et al.: Complications of cholelithiasis. Am. J. Gastroenterol., *50*:476, 1968. *(Over 90 per cent of those who experienced complications had one or more prior episodes of colic.)*

Price, W.H.: Gallbladder dyspepsia. Br. Med. J., *3*:138, 1963. *(Frequency and severity of dyspeptic complaints are unrelated to presence or absence of gallstones.)*

Rhine, J.A., and Watson, L.: Gallstone dyspepsia. Br. Med. J., *1*:32, 1968. *(Of 32 patients undergoing cholecystectomy for dyspepsia, 13 still had similar symptoms after surgery.)*

Schein, C.J.: Acute cholecystitis in the diabetic. Am. J. Gastroenterol., *51*:511, 1969. *(Cholecystitis can be a lethal disease in the diabetic; documents increased risk in this subpopulation.)*

Thistle, J.L., et al.: Chenotherapy for gallstone dissolution: I. efficacy and safety. J.A.M.A., *239*:1041, 1978. *(A summary of current clinical experience with chenodeoxycholic acid.)*

Wenckert, A., and Robertson, B.: The natural course of gallstone disease. Gastroenterology, *50*:376, 1966. *(About 30 per cent of patients managed medically and followed 5 to 20 years had attacks of colic, and another 20 per cent had complications. These high figures are due in part to the fact that all were hospitalized initially, and well over half had nonvisualizing gallbladders, a sign of more advanced disease.)*

70
Management of Viral Hepatitis

Over half a million cases of viral hepatitis occur in the United States each year. Type B virus accounts for about 50 per cent. The newly appreciated non-A, non-B variety of viral hepatitis is probably responsible for over 90 per cent of posttransfusion cases. Mortality from all types is well under 1 per cent, but a definite percentage of patients progress to carrier states or chronic hepatitis. The latter is associated with increased risks of cirrhosis and death.

The primary physician needs to be skilled in the management of viral hepatitis, because the problem is frequently encountered in the outpatient setting. The goals of therapy are to provide symptomatic relief, prevent spread, and minimize the consequences of chronic hepatitis should it occur. Effective outpatient management requires knowledge of the natural history of hepatitis, the methods for monitoring disease course, the indications for prophylaxis (see Chapter 52), the means of distinguishing between chronic active and chronic persistent forms of the illness, and the indications for steroid therapy.

CLINICAL PRESENTATION AND
NATURAL HISTORY
(see Chapter 52)

Acute viral hepatitis. In most instances this is usually a self-limited disease, with 85 per cent of hospitalized individuals and over 95 per cent of outpatients making full recoveries within 3 months. The majority of patients never become jaundiced; their illness is mistakenly labeled "viral syndrome" unless a transaminase is ordered. Some are even asymptomatic. When the patient is elderly or is immunologically compromised, the prognosis is more guarded and the illness often more severe and prolonged.

The patient notes onset of prodromal symptoms after an incubation period of 2 to 6 weeks for Type A viral infection, 6 to 24 weeks for Type B disease, and 3 to 18 weeks for non-A, non-B hepatitis. Characteristically, there are 7 to 14 days of malaise, anorexia, nausea, vomiting, low-grade fever, right upper quadrant discomfort and fatigue. Transaminase elevations precede onset of symptoms. If jaundice develops, it

usually does so as prodromal complaints begin to subside. Persistence of prodromal symptoms is seen in more severe cases. By 6 to 8 weeks, most patients are well on their way to full recovery, although persistence of isolated, mild transaminase elevations after clinical recovery is sometimes noted; this "transaminitis" has no prognostic significance if it resolves by 3 to 6 months.

There are a number of variations on the classical clinical presentation. In some cases of Type B infection, the prodromal phase may by accompanied by a serum-sicknesslike illness with urticaria, arthralgias, and polyarticular arthritis. In other patients, a cholestatic picture supervenes with marked jaundice and pruritus lasting 2 to 6 months. About 5 to 15 per cent of patients with viral hepatitis suffer mild relapses during convalescence, usually without developing chronic hepatitis.

Progression to chronic hepatitis varies according to type of infection. There are no documented cases of chronic hepatitis due to Type A virus. On the other hand, 1 to 2 per cent of patients with hepatitis B infection develop chronic hepatitis, and 5 to 10 per cent become chronic carriers of hepatitis B surface antigen (HBsAg). Some chronic carriers progress to chronic hepatitis. About 20 to 30 per cent of patients with non-A, non-B hepatitis run a prolonged course, developing evidence of chronic hepatitis on biopsy. Progression to chronic hepatitis is often manifested by little more than persistence of mild symptoms and biochemical abnormalities for 6 months. Many patients are anicteric. In the case of Type B disease, continued antigenemia and failure to develop antibody to B virus are associated with increased risk of chronicity. There are no early predictors of chronicity; reports regarding e antigen as an early sign of risk for chronic hepatitis have not been borne out.

Chronic hepatitis. There are two forms of chronic hepatitis: chronic persistent and chronic active. The distinction is histologic and requires liver biopsy, because clinical manifestations may be identical. *Chronic active hepatitis* is identified by the presence of significant periportal necrosis ("piecemeal necrosis"); marked round cell infiltration and fibrous septae extending into the lobules are also characteristic.

In contrast, *chronic persistent hepatitis* shows almost no periportal involvement, being limited to a round cell infiltrate in the portal tract. Differentiation between the two types of chronic hepatitis is important for both prognosis and treatment, for chronic persistent disease is a benign illness, while chronic active hepatitis is associated with an increased risk of cirrhosis and/or death.

Although progression to cirrhosis and death is a distinct possibility in some forms of chronic active hepatitis that are not treated, it is not inevitable in all cases and seems to be at least partly a function of disease severity. Studies have demonstrated that patients with marked symptoms, sustained transaminase elevations of greater than 10 times normal, gamma globulin levels twice normal, or bridging or multilobular necrosis on biopsy (regardless of how minor clinical manifestations may be) are at increased risk. Patients fulfilling the biochemical criteria of severe disease were found in a prospective study to have a 40 per cent 6-month fatality rate. In those with bridging or multilobular necrosis, cirrhosis developed in 40 per cent and death occurred in 20 per cent after 5 years. The incidence of cirrhosis in patients with minimal symptoms and necrosis limited to the periportal region was less than 3 per cent and no deaths occurred.

Whether etiology is a prognostic factor remains unresolved and the subject of ongoing investigation. At present, there are only small-scale observations available regarding differences in natural history for antigen-positive and antigen-negative disease.

PRINCIPALS OF MANAGEMENT

Acute viral hepatitis. The disease is generally a benign and self-limited illness; it can be managed on an outpatient basis in most instances. Hospitalization should be reserved for high-risk patients (the elderly and the immuno-compromised) and those in whom marked prothrombin time prolongation ($>$ 15 seconds), encephalopathy, edema or severe discomfort develops. At present, no treatment has proved to alter the course or prevent the sequelae of acute viral hepatitis. Goals of care are to maintain adequate nutrition, avoid further hepatocellular insults from drugs and alcohol, prevent spread, and minimize the discomfort of prodromal and jaundice phases. These objectives are achieved by a commonsense approach to management of the uncomplicated case. Specific dietary manipulations, steroid therapy, and strict bed rest have no effect on course or prognosis of acute,

uncomplicated viral hepatitis. Oral contraceptives need not be stopped, but alcohol intake should be omitted and use of other drugs known to cause hepatic injury discontinued or monitored carefully. Exercise does not hinder recovery; patients should be allowed to engage in as much activity as they feel comfortable with, so long as they avoid excessive tiring. Prophylactic measures require consideration (see Chapter 52).

Symptoms may be quite incapacitating. Nausea and vomiting can be controlled by cautious use of prochlorperazine (phenothiazines cause a cholestatic hepatitis in 1 per cent of patients, so careful monitoring is necessary). Small frequent feedings, especially in the morning when nausea wanes, can assure adequate caloric intake. No foods need be restricted. Mild pruritus can be treated with antihistamines, but severe cases often require cholestyramine (see Chapter 62).

Chronic hepatitis. Treatment of chronic hepatitis depends on the type and severity of disease. The goals are to relieve symptoms, prevent cirrhosis and reduce the chances of mortality. Since *chronic persistent hepatitis* has an excellent prognosis, no treatment is indicated beyond simple symtomatic and preventive measures. Chronic active hepatitis is a more ominous condition. *Severe chronic active hepatitis* manifested by bridging, multilobular necrosis or the combination of high transaminase levels ($>$ 10 times normal), globulin levels twice normal and marked symptoms has a poor prognosis, as described above. Controlled prospective trials, such as a major study performed at the Mayo Clinic, have demonstrated clinical, biochemical and histologic resolution of severe chronic active disease in 80 per cent of cases treated with prednisone or prednisone plus azathioprine. Remission of histologic changes to those of chronic persistent disease or to normal were seen within 6 to 36 months. Intervention in cases with severe symptoms and advanced pathologic changes on biopsy was associated with a significant decrease in mortality. It is important to note that most patients in the Mayo study and similar studies were negative for hepatitis B surface antigen. There is some uncontrolled evidence that antigen-positive patients who are severely ill are less responsive to corticosteroids than patients who are antigen-negative.

Patients with *mild chronic active hepatitis* pose a therapeutic dilemma at the present time, because the probability of morbidity and mortality in such cases is less well established and must be balanced by the significant complications of long-term steroid therapy (see Chapter 101). Two-thirds of patients on steriods in the Mayo study experienced at least one serious complication attributable to prednisone. Patients with less severe disease had very low death rates, regardless of whether they received prednisone or placebo. Moreover, since most were antigen-negative, it is unclear what the prognosis is for antigen-positive patients with mild disease; available evidence suggests that this form of disease runs a benign course and is not an indication for steroids. Controlled study of this question is being pursued.

At the present time, the markedly symptomatic patient with biochemical and histologic evidence of severe disease should be treated with corticosteroids, or steroids plus azathioprine if the patient cannot tolerate high-dose prednisone due to age or underlying illness. Those with symptoms but less advanced histologic findings might also benefit from therapy, perhaps a shorter course which minimizes risk of steroid side effects. Patients with minimal symptoms and early histologic changes are probably not in need of immediate therapy, but do require close monitoring. There are no data on treatment of the asymptomatic patient with biopsy-proven chronic active hepatitis, though some argue by analogy that individuals with multilobular necrosis should be treated.

There are two equally effective therapeutic regimens: *high-dose prednisone* or *reduced-dose prednisone in combination with azathioprine.* The latter is preferred by some, since it produces fewer side effects, though long-term adverse effects of azathioprine are unknown at present. Alternate-day prednisone reduces biochemical abnormalities, symptoms and mortality, but does not achieve symptomatic relief or histological remission as predictably or as completely as daily prednisone therapy.

Severe complications from steroid therapy usually become manifest by 18 months. When azathioprine is used in combination with prednisone, the rate of steroid-induced complications falls from 40 per cent to 10 per cent. Problems are more likely to occur in those with hypoalbuminemia or hyperbilirubinemia.

Therapy is initiated with 30 mg. prednisone plus 50 mg. azathioprine, or with 60 mg. prednisone, reducing the prednisone by 5 to 10 mg. at a time as symptoms and signs abate. A maintenance dose of 7.5 to 15 mg. of prednisone is common. This program is continued until there is objective evidence of true remission, i.e., transaminase falls to less than twice normal and piecemeal necrosis disappears from liver biopsy. Other indications for cessation of

therapy are signs of unacceptable drug toxicity (worsening liver injury, hepatotoxicity, intolerable gastrointestinal upset, leukopenia, thrombocytopenia, compression fractures) or failure to respond. Symptoms usually improve within 6 months, transaminase levels within 12, and histology within 24. Rarely, more than 36 months are necessary to achieve remission.

Upon remission, a trial of phasing out therapy may be undertaken, while monitoring closely for signs of relapse. Gradual reduction in medication is performed over 6 weeks until treatment is terminated. Relapses occur in 50 per cent; they are especially common in patients with cirrhosis, often necessitating prolonged therapy for many years or multiple courses of treatment. About 20 per cent of patients fail on conventional doses but may respond to higher doses. Relapses usually occur early; patients with remissions which last for more than 6 months have only an 8 per cent relapse rate. Most cases of relapse are accompanied by symptoms and marked transaminase elevations, but in 10 per cent there is no evidence other than change in biopsy. Rates of repeat remission and relapse are 80 per cent and 50 per cent, respectively. Failure to respond is most often due to incorrect diagnosis or inadequate doses of medication.

MONITORING COURSE AND RESPONSE TO THERAPY AND INDICATIONS FOR REFERRAL AND ADMISSION

Acute viral hepatitis. The patient can be followed by observing symptoms and monitoring hepatocellular function. A transaminase level once monthly is useful to judge presence of ongoing disease, though the absolute level is not a particularly sensitive determinant of disease severity in the acute phase of illness. Prothrombin time is a good measure of hepatocellular synthetic function and is worth checking when the patient first presents and when there is suspicion of worsening. Serum bilirubin also correlates with severity. A fall in serum albumin indicates hepatocellular failure, but may take a while to occur since its half-life is 28 days. Alkaline phosphatase and LDH add little to monitoring.

An office visit 2 weeks after first presentation is often helpful to be sure there is no worsening and that the patient is managing satisfactorily. Thereafter, follow-up depends on how well the patient feels. At 3 months, a repeat transaminase, bilirubin, albumin, prothrombin time and hepatitis B surface antigen should be performed to ascertain disease activity, severity and clearing of antigen.

If symptoms and laboratory evidence of activity persist after 3 months, repeat evaluations at monthly intervals are indicated. Referral for liver biopsy is indicated if the illness has not resolved by 6 months. It is particularly important to obtain help from a gastroenterologist or pathologist experienced in interpreting biopsy material obtained from patients with chronic hepatitis; diagnosis depends on histologic appearance and can be difficult.

Chronic hepatitis. Patients with mild *chronic persistent hepatitis* may be followed casually, but those who are symptomatic deserve careful monitoring and periodic reassessment to be sure there are no signs of progression. When *chronic active hepatitis* has been identified, very close follow-up is vital. If prednisone and azathioprine are used, weekly and later biweekly platelet and white cell counts are required. Transaminase, bilirubin, and gamma globulin levels ought to be obtained at 2 weeks, 3 months, and then every 6 months to monitor response and identify treatment failure. A complete evaluation should be performed every 6 months, including a liver biopsy if clinical and biochemical remission has occurred. Admission to the hospital is indicated for worsening mental status, bleeding, refractory ascites, or poor home environment. Patients with mild chronic active disease who do not receive therapy should be monitored in similar fashion and rebiopsied if symptoms or biochemical parameters worsen.

PATIENT EDUCATION

Hepatitis often affects previously vigorous people accustomed to full activity. The prolonged course and magnitude of malaise commonly precipitate a reactive depression. Thorough explanation of the disease's course, design of a sensible treatment program which actively involves the patient and family, and close follow-up can maximize compliance and minimize depression.

Instruction concerning diet and activity is central to a comprehensive treatment program. In particular, it is important to prevent unnecessary restriction of activity and to assure adequate nutrition. Patients can be told to do as much as they feel like doing, so long as they avoid overtiring themselves. Small, frequent meals, especially in the morning, are best tol-

erated. No foods need be restricted, but carbohydrates seem to be the best tolerated food when nausea is pronounced.

THERAPEUTIC RECOMMENDATIONS*

Acute Viral Hepatitis

- Maintain adequate caloric intake and a balanced diet. Small feedings are best tolerated, especially in the morning. No foods need be restricted.
- Assure adequate rest, but activity need not be unduly restricted if the patient feels capable of it.
- Omit potentially hepatotoxic agents, especially alcohol.
- Treat severe pruritus with cholestyramine, though antihistamines may suffice for less troublesome cases (see Chapter 62).
- Treat severe nausea and vomiting with a cautious trial of prochlorperazine (e.g., 10 mg. t.i.d. p.r.n.). The drug is capable of producing cholestasis and should be discontinued at the first sign of worsening jaundice.
- Admit if signs of marked worsening of hepatocellular function occur, e.g., encephalopathy, bleeding, prolongation of prothrombin time beyond 15 seconds. Also consider admission for maintaining adequate caloric and fluid intake when symptoms are severe.
- Check transaminase, prothrombin time, bilirubin, albumin/globulin and HBsAg at onset and at 2 and 12 weeks. Any patient with evidence of persistent symptoms or laboratory abnormalities should be retested every 4 weeks and referred for liver biopsy if clearing has not taken place by 6 months.

Chronic Hepatitis

- Follow patients with chronic persistent hepatitis at regular intervals and rebiopsy if there are signs of marked worsening. Otherwise treat symptomatically. Steroids are not indicated.
- Begin high-dose prednisone (60 mg. daily) or combination prednisone (30 mg.) plus azathioprine (50 mg.), also given daily, in patients with severe chronic active hepatitis manifested by multilobular or bridging necrosis, disabling symptoms, and marked transaminase and globulin elevations. Combination therapy is preferred for the elderly, diabetics and others who cannot tolerate long-term high-dose steroids.

* See Chapter 52 for prophylactic measures.

- Taper prednisone by 5 to 10 mg. at a time until a minimum daily maintenance dose is established that is effective in controlling symptoms and signs.
- Monitor transaminases, bilirubin and globulins at 2 weeks, 3 months, and 6 months; then every 6 months. If the patient is taking azathioprine, obtain platelet and white cell counts weekly for 3 months; biweekly to triweekly thereafter.
- Continue maintenance therapy for at least 24 to 36 months; then consider attempting discontinuation of therapy with a 6-week period of phasing out medication.
- Failure to achieve clinical improvement within 2 to 8 months of initiating therapy is an indication for consultation and consideration of high-dose treatment.
- Treat relapses in the same manner as new cases.
- Perform full evaluation every 6 months, including liver biopsy when there is evidence of clinical improvement or worsening.
- Patients who are HBsAg-positive but asymptomatic probably need not be treated. The same applies to those with minimal clinical disease, antigen negativity and necrosis limited to the periportal region. These individuals should be seen regularly and rebiopsied if symptoms and chemistries worsen.
- Patients with multilobular necrosis but minimal or absent symptoms may be treated with prednisone-azathioprine, but indications in this setting are not well established.
- Admit to the hospital when there is evidence of marked worsening of hepatocellular function.

ANNOTATED BIBLIOGRAPHY

Berk, P.D., *et al.*: Corticosteroid therapy for chronic active hepatitis. Ann. Intern. Med., *85*:523, 1975. *(An editorial which argues that not all forms of chronic active hepatitis have the same prognosis, and that selectivity should be exercised in treating, because therapy has a high morbidity associated with it.)*

Boyer, J.L.: Chronic hepatitis—A perspective on classification and determinants of prognosis. Gastroenterology, *70*:1161, 1976. *(Correlates histology with prognosis; a critical review with 66 refs.)*

Czaja, A.J., and Summerskill, W.H.J.: Chronic hepatitis: To treat or not to treat? Med. Clin. North. Am., *62*:71, 1978. *(A discussion of the factors influencing the decision to treat. Severity of disease is the most important factor.)*

Dienstag, J.L., *et al.*: Etiology of sporadic hepatitis B surface antigen-negative hepatitis. Ann. Intern. Med., *87*:1, 1977. *(As many as 25 per cent of antigen-negative sporadic cases in the community unrelated to transfusion may be due to non-A, non-B disease. Not all non-A, non-B infection is derived from transfusion.)*

Feinstone, S.M., and Purcell, R.H.: Non-A, non-B hepatitis. Ann. Rev. Med., *29*:359, 1978. *(Ninety per cent of post-transfusion hepatitis is due to non-A, non-B infection. The condition is associated with a high frequency of progression to chronic hepatitis.)*

Koretz, R., Suffin, S., and Gitnick, G.: Posttransfusion chronic liver disease. Gastroenterology, *71*:797, 1976. *(A prospective study of 47 patients with posttransfusion hepatitis. Chronic hepatitis, manifested by transaminase elevations for 20 weeks, developed in over 50 per cent. About half of these individuals had the chronic active variety. Age, sex, number of units transfused, presence or absence of symptoms and underlying illness were unrelated to risk of chronic hepatitis. Many had non-A non-B disease.)*

Krugman, S., *et al.*: Viral hepatitis type B: Studies on natural history and prevention re-examined. N. Engl. J. Med., *300*:101, 1979. *(An updated and detailed evaluation of natural history, utilizing advances in immunologic techniques to re-examine sera collected in classic natural history studies.)*

Nefzger, M., and Chalmers, T.: The treatment of acute infectious hepatitis: Ten year follow-up study of the effects of diet and rest. Am. J. Med., *35*:299, 1963. *(A classic prospective study on the impact of diet and rest in 460 servicemen; no particular diet or activity program made any difference in long-term outcome.)*

Nielsen, J., Dietrickson, O., Elling, P., *et al.*: Incidence and meaning of persistence of Australia antigen in patients with acute viral hepatitis. Development of chronic hepatitis. N. Engl. J. Med., *285*:1157, 1971. *(A prospective study of 112 patients with hepatitis B, which was among the first to demonstrate the significance of persistent antigenemia, showed persistence of antigen beyond 13 weeks in 4.3 per cent; all developed chronic hepatitis; 8 of 11 had the chronic active variety.)*

Soloway, R., Summerskill, D., Baggenstoss, A.H., *et al.*: Clinical, biochemical and histologic remission of severe chronic active liver disease. Gastroenterology, *63*:820, 1972. *(The Mayo Clinic prospective double-blind randomized trial showing that prednisone or prednisone plus azathioprine was superior to placebo and azathioprine alone in treatment of severe disease. Relapse was frequent but easily treated.)*

Werner, B., and Blumberg, B.: E antigen in hepatitis-B-virus-infected dialysis patients: Assessment of its prognostic value. Ann. Intern. Med., 89:310, 1978. *(HBeAg is a useful indicator of infectivity but is of no clear prognostic value in predicting chronicity of infection.)*

Wright, E.C., et al.: Treatment of chronic active hepatitis: An analysis of 3 controlled trials. Gastroenterology, *73*:1422, 1977. *(A critique of the major studies. Concludes that they do demonstrate a reduction in cirrhosis and mortality for patients with severe antigen-negative disease who are treated with steroids.)*

71
Management of Cirrhosis

Although cirrhosis represents an irreversible stage of chronic liver disease, the cooperative patient can be kept rather comfortable and active in the ambulatory setting. Not infrequently, prognosis can be reasonably favorable if the insult which resulted in cirrhosis abates and preventable complications and further hepatocellular injury can be avoided. The primary physician is often faced with responsibility for long-term management of the cirrhotic patient and needs to know how to control ascites and edema, prevent encephalopathy, treat infection, manage diet, and determine need for a shunt procedure.

NATURAL HISTORY

The course of cirrhosis depends on the nature, extent and activity of the underlying hepatocellular disease. Patients with Laennec's cirrhosis who abstain from alcohol have a 5-year survival rate of 60 per cent, but if they continue to drink, survival falls to 40 per cent. Onset of jaundice or ascites reduces 5-year survival to 30 per cent. For patients with postnecrotic cirrhosis, the 5-year survival rate is around 25 per cent, with death due to variceal bleeding, encephalopathy or hepatoma. In primary biliary cirrhosis, death ensues within 5 to 10 years of onset of symptoms. Variceal bleeding and infection are common precipitants of end-stage hepatocellular insufficiency.

Portal hypertension, fluid retention and encephalopathy are the major sequelae of cirrhosis; they lead to varices, splenomegaly, ascites, edema and coma. Variceal bleeding has been found to occur in over 50 per cent of cirrhotics, and 50 per cent die of advanced encephalopathy.

PRINCIPLES OF THERAPY

The first objective is to halt further *hepatocellular injury*. Cessation of drinking is essential to management of Laennec's cirrhosis (see Chapter 216). Corticosteroid therapy in alcoholic hepatitis has been inconclusive, but steroids can limit progression to cirrhosis in some patients with severe chronic active hepatitis (see Chapter 70). Prednisone does not alter the course of primary biliary cirrhosis. The development of secondary biliary cirrhosis can be halted if the obstruction to bile flow can be removed or bypassed.

Ascites and edema result from increased portal pressure, salt and water retention and hypoalbuminemia. In itself, ascites is not a hazard, though it is uncomfortable and can compromise respiratory mechanics when massive. The best initial approach is, if possible, to strictly *limit salt intake* to 250 mg. per day and water intake to 1,500 ml. daily, and to ensure a daily protein intake of 50 gm. If encephalopathy is present as well, protein intake must be limited to 20 to 30 gm. per day. Such a program will often result in a diuresis of 300 to 500 ml. per day of ascitic fluid without precipitating hyponatremia or dehydration. Moreover, serum albumin can be maintained as long as some hepatocellular synthetic function remains. This program requires a cooperative patient and a very conscientious family.

If attempts at salt and free water restriction do not suffice, a *diuretic program* can be instituted, but there is a limit to the amount of ascitic fluid that can be mobilized from the peritoneal cavity each day. Studies have demonstrated that compartmentalization of ascitic fluid occurs such that a maximum of only 900 ml. per can be lost by diuresis, regardless of how much total body fluid loss is induced. Additional fluid losses are drawn from peripheral stores of edema fluid; once these are depleted, losses come from intravascular volume and may result in severe volume depletion.

If a diuretic program is deemed necessary, careful control and monitoring are essential, especially after peripheral edema has resolved. Spironolactone is often a first choice, because it induces a mild diuresis and counters the hyperaldosteronism and hypokalemic alkalosis commonly seen in patients with ascites. Use of very potent diuretics (e.g., furosemide) may precipitate serious hypovolemia and hepatorenal syndrome. Failure to maintain diuresis is not an automatic indication for prescribing a stronger diuretic; rather, it is a warning of possible hypovolemia, as is the presence of postural changes in blood pressure and pulse. Rapid intake of a few hundred milliliters of free water can help confirm the presence of hypovolemia, since urine output will rise temporarily. *Paracentesis* is rarely indicated for treatment of ascites; reaccumulation of fluid quickly follows, often at the expense of intravascular volume. Only patients with truly disabling and refractory ascites should be referred for consideration of a *peritoneo-venous (LeVeen) shunt*. Infection and coagulopathy have limited its utility.

Encephalopathy is a manifestation of the liver's inability to detoxify nitrogenous metabolites. Excess dietary protein and gastrointestinal bleeding are important precipitating factors; sedatives and hypokalemic alkalosis also contribute. Prevention and management of encephalopathy require restriction of dietary protein, avoidance of excessive diuretic use, discontinuation of tranquilizers and sedatives, induction of bowel cleansing, and inhibition of urea-splitting microorganisms. *Dietary protein* is limited to 30 to 40 gm. per day. *Neomycin* has been used to reduce the population of urease-containing microorganisms. Unfortunately, chronic use of doses in excess of 4 gm. per day may result in considerable gastrointestinal absorption and achievement of significant serum levels of this nephrotoxic and ototoxic antibiotic, especially in patients with renal disease.

Lactulose is a useful addition to the treatment of encephalopathy. When given orally, this indigestible sugar reaches the colon intact and becomes acted upon by bacterial lactulases, resulting in an acidified stool, increased bowel motility, and shifts in bacterial flora to a predominance of lactobacilli. The net result is lessened ammonia production and absorption. Although lactulose *per se* does not inhibit urea-splitting organisms, it does reduce their population by fostering proliferation of lactobacilli. Lactulose can be given orally or as an enema; the latter route gives clinical improvement within 12 hours, whereas after oral administration, 24 to 48 hours may elapse before the patient improves. Side effects are diarrhea, bloating and cramping. Dosage is adjusted to avoid marked diarrhea, which can worsen encephalopathy. A double-blind, controlled study comparing lactulose and neomycin found them to be equally effective. Data on combined use are scantly, though one would expect the neomycin to kill lactobacilli and limit the utility of the lactulose.

The question of a *shunt procedure* often arises as a means of controlling the consequences of portal hypertension. Over the past decade, prospective studies have more clearly defined the indications for portasystemic shunts. At the present time, a few generalizations are possible: (1) the likelihood of variceal bleeding is significantly reduced by portacaval shunting and probably by splenorenal shunts as well; (2) patients who have had documented variceal bleeding may benefit from an elective shunt procedure since risk of death from bleeding is reduced; (3) patients with varices that have never bled should not undergo prophylactic portacaval shunt; since the probability of encephalopathy and fatal coma rises substantially, life may not be prolonged; (4) the main determinant of survival after shunt is underlying hepatocellular function; the more compromised the hepatocytes, the greater the risk of coma and death; (5) side-to-side portacaval anastomoses or splenorenal shunts are best for relief of truly intractable ascites, but have the usual attendant risk of precipating encephalopathy.

THERAPEUTIC RECOMMENDATIONS AND MONITORING

- The patient should maintain a caloric intake of at least 2000-3000 Kcal. per day.
- Use of alcohol or any other hepatoxic agents must be totally prohibited.
- Avoid use of tranquilizers and sedatives.
- For ascites, the patient should be instructed to restrict sodium intake to 250 mg. per day and fluids to 1500 ml. per day and to ensure 50 gm. of protein daily. Patient and family will require consultation with the dietician for specific menus and food lists.
- If salt and fluid restrictions do not suffice to control ascites, begin spironolactone, 25 mg. four times daily. If after 1 week there is no significant improvement, increase the daily dose by 100 mg. each week until a maximum of 400 mg. per day is achieved.
- Diuresis of peripheral edema and ascites should be limited to 1 to 2 pounds per day when peripheral edema is present and to no more than 1 pound per day once peripheral edema has resolved.
- A further increase in diuresis can be attempted with a thiazide (e.g., 50 mg. hydrochlorothiazide per day); monitoring for hypokalemic alkalosis is necessary. Use of potent diuretics (e.g., furosemide) should be undertaken with extreme caution and only after milder diuretics have proven ineffective, because irreversible hepatorenal syndrome may be precipitated.
- Watch for early signs of volume and potassium depletion. Monitor serum potassium, BUN and creatinine frequently and check for postural changes in blood pressure and pulse on each examination. Halt diuretic program at first sign of intravascular volume depletion.
- Regularly replace potassium losses due to hyperaldosteronism and diuretic use, starting with daily 20- 40-meq doses of KCl elixir and adjusting according to serum potassium level. If a potassium-sparing diuretic is being employed, potassium supplements should be stopped unless hypokalemia persists.
- Restrict protein intake to 20 to 30 gm. per day at the first sign of mild encephalopathy; check for asterixis on each office visit. Measuring venous NH_3 level gives only a very crude estimate of encephalopathic state, but is worth doing occasionally. False-positive elevation can occur when a tourniquet is left on too long.
- When protein restriction is insufficient to control mild encephalopathy, begin oral lactulose, 30 to 50 ml. three times daily with meals, adjusting dose to minimize diarrhea; or oral neomycin 1,000 mg. four times daily, reducing the dose to 2 gm. per day if possible if long-term therapy expected.
- Monitor prothrombin time, albumin and bilirubin to assess severity and course of hepatocellular function.
- Check stools at each visit for evidence of occult bleeding.

INDICATIONS FOR REFERRAL AND ADMISSION

The patient with worsening encephalopathy, gastrointestinal bleeding, or significant volume depletion requires prompt hospitalization. Stubborn cases of marked ascites may respond to elective admission and strict limitation of sodium. Consultations with both a gastroenterologist and an experienced surgeon are in order when elective portosystemic shunt is considered.

PATIENT EDUCATION AND SUPPORT

It should be emphasized to the patient and family that prognosis can be improved and symptoms lessened by careful adherence to the prescribed medical program. In particular, dietary discipline and omission of alcohol are central to a successful outcome and need to be stressed. Many of these patients are chronic alcoholics with low self-esteem. A nonjudgmental, sympathetic physician can be instrumental in providing support and improving chances of compliance. Depression is a frequent accompaniment of the later stages of chronic liver disease and is manifested by failure to comply and outright expressions of wanting to die. Treatment is very difficult. Antidepressant drugs may cause oversedation and thus are risky. There are no simple measures, but interest and support from the physician can help enormously.

ANNOTATED BIBLIOGRAPHY

Conn, H.O.: Rational management of ascites. Prog. Liver Dis., 4:269, 1972. *(Argues for use of high-dose spironolactone in treating ascites, since the drug counters the associated hyperaldosteronism.)*

Conn, H.O., et al.: Comparison of lactulose and neomycin in the treatment of chronic portal-systemic encephalopathy. Gastroenterology, 72:573, 1977. *(A double-blind controlled study showing both drugs to be of equal efficacy and very low in toxicity.)*

Hoyumpa, A.M., et al.: Hepatic encephalopathy. Gastroenterology, 76:184, 1979. *(A thorough and practical review; 40 refs.)*

Malt, R.A.: Portasystemic venous shunts. N. Engl. J. Med., 295:24, 1976. *(Excellent, terse, critical review of types of shunts and the indications for their use.)*

Management of hepatic ascites. (editorial). Lancet, 1:311, 1978. *(A critical assessment of therapeutic measures, including peritoneovenous (LeVeen) shunting. Argues that a shunt operation should rarely be necessary.)*

Sehar, L., Ching, S., and Gabuzda, G.: Compartmentalization of ascites and edema in patients with hepatic cirrhosis. N. Engl. J. Med., 282:1391, 1970. *(Documents the differing maximal rates of reabsorption for peripheral edema and ascites. Warns of the need to limit diuresis to ½ to 1 lb. per day in patients with ascites and no edema, so as to avoid depletion of intravascular volume.)*

72

Management of Pancreatitis
JAMES M. RICHTER, M.D.

The primary physician may encounter pancreatitis in three forms which lend themselves to ambulatory management: (1) recovery phase of acute pancreatitis, (2) chronic, mild relapsing pancreatitis presenting as recurrent abdominal pain, and (3) pancreatic insufficiency, with diarrhea and weight loss.

In the United States, most cases of pancreatitis are a result of excess ethanol ingestion or biliary tract disease, chiefly among middle-aged alcoholic men and elderly women with gallstones, respectively. A penetrating duodenal ulcer, trauma, hypercalcemia, hypertriglyceridemia, vascular disease, tumor, heredity, ampullary stenosis, and drugs such as thiazide diuretics, glucocorticosteroids, azathioprine and sulfasalazine are also associated with pancreatitis. Frequently, no etiology is found. The course, response to therapy, and prognosis are in part functions of the etiology.

The primary physician must be able to distinguish acute pancreatitis from other causes of acute upper abdominal pain, and chronic pancreatitis from pancreatic carcinoma. Objectives of management include relief of pain, removal of precipitants, and assurance of adequate nutrition.

CLINICAL PRESENTATION AND COURSE

Acute pancreatitis. The manifestations of acute pancreatitis disease are produced by inflammatory breakdown of pancreatic architecture, with release of digestive enzymes into the intersititium of the gland, leading to autolysis. Classically, acute pancreatitis produces constant epigastric, periumbilical or left upper quadrant pain radiating to the back, often increased by food and decreased by upright posture. Vomiting can be quite persistent. Examination reveals abdominal tenderness and may include decreased bowel sounds, distention and fever. The diagnosis of acute pancreatitis is supported by elevated serum amylase, serum lipase, and an amylase-creatinine clearance ratio greater than 5 per cent. The *se-*

rum amylase is elevated principally in pancreatic disease but may also be high in renal insufficiency, salivary gland disease, and biliary tract disease as well as other intra-abdominal diseases without detectable pancreatitis. The *serum lipase* is more specific but less sensitive than the serum amylase. The *amylase creatinine clearance ratio* is also more specific than the serum amylase and is almost as sensitive. In addition to pancreatic disease, the clearance ratio may be elevated in renal insufficiency, diabetic ketoacidoses, and cutaneous burns. When the diagnosis is uncertain, ultrasonography may show edema in the gland, and radiographic constrast studies of the gallbladder, stomach, and duodenum help to rule out biliary and peptic ulcer disease.

The course of acute pancreatitis depends on severity of the disease and the underlying etiology. In a patient recovering from acute pancreatitis, symptoms are reliable indicators of disease activity. Elevated enzymes in an otherwise asymptomatic patient are usually of no significance. The serum amylase routinely falls to normal within several days, but some asymptomatic patients may have elvevated enzymes for weeks after an uncomplicated illness. In rare instances, persistently elevated enzymes in an asymptomatic individual may be a clue to the presence of a silent pseudocyst. If a mass is palpable or pain arises, a pseudocyst should be ruled out; ultrasonography of the upper abdomen is the procedure of choice.

Chronic pancreatitis characteristically presents and proceeds as bouts of mild to severe recurrent epigastric pain, ofter occurring in chronic alcoholics after years of excessive drinking. Sometimes chronic pancreatitis is heralded by a severe attack of acute pancreatitis. At other times there may be constant mild pain or simply the painless insidious onset of exocrine insufficiency and diabetes. The pain of chronic pancreatitis is not precisely constant and often varies in intensity over days to weeks. There may be exacerbations of pain, nausea, and vomiting after eating or drinking alcohol. Elevated serum amylase and amylase-creatinine clearance ratios are helpful, but the incidence of normal values is greater than in acute pancreatitis.

Individuals who present with chronic recurrent abdominal pain and a history of relapsing pancreatitis are not often difficult diagnostic problems, but the patient without such a history requires more extensive assessment. A plain film of the abdomen may reveal pancreatic calcification, a late finding in alcoholic pancreatitis. Ultrasonography may demonstrate a diffusely enlarged gland, local mass or pseudocyst.

If ultrasound evaluation is normal and pancreatic disease is strongly suspected on clinical grounds, pancreatic function testing or computerized axial tomography should be done. Two normal studies correctly predict a normal pancreas in 90 per cent of cases. An abnormal finding in any one study warrants further evaluation to distinguish between chronic pancreatitis and pancreatic carcinoma. At institutions where the technology exists, endoscopic retrograde pancreatography has proven to be an effective diagnostic techinque. Abdominal angiography may be helpful when retrograde pancreatography is unavailable or fails.

The course of chronic pancreatitis is variable and depends on removal of causative factors. Presently it is not known how cholelithiases causes pancreatitis, but successful and early surgical therapy almost always prevents recurrent or chronic pancreatitis. With recurrent disease, pancreatic insufficiency may gradually develop over years, manifested by weight loss and steatorrhea. Onset of clinical diabetes is a very late complication and a sign of far advanced disease, though mild glucose intolerance is seen early on.

Pancreatic insufficiency. Patients with pancreatic exocrine insufficiency complain of weight loss and frequent, greasy bowel movements. Weight loss is often striking but nonspecific in this population, which tends to substitute alcohol for other forms of nourishment. Objective evidence of maldigestion may be obtained by a qualitative examination for stool fat with Sudan stain. Rarely, more complicated studies are indicated to document deficient pancreatic secretion; when the question does arise, a secretin stimulation test can be employed to demonstrate exocrine insufficiency. A small group of patients do not give a prior history of recurrent abdominal pain; they deserve evaluation for hemochromatosis and cystic fibrosis in addition to investigation for the usual causes of pancreatitis.

PRINCIPLES OF MANAGEMENT

Acute pancreatitis. Patients recovering from acute pancreatitis generally tolerate a full diet prior to discharge from the hospital, although a diet moderately restricted in fat is often recommended to lessen the degree of pancreatic stimulation. Cimetidine, antacids and anticholinergics are frequently given with the hope of reducing the stimulus to pancreatic secretion, but are of unproven efficacy. If a patient returns with severe pain and vomiting, acute in-hospital therapy should be reinstituted. Patients with mild pain and no vomiting may be treated on an ambulatory basis with restriction of fat and protein and careful follow-up.

Knowledge of the specific cause of the pancreatitis is essential to successful therapy; an etiologic diagnosis should be fully pursued. The alcoholic often understates his alcohol consumption. With increased comfort and confidence in his physician, the patient may revise his previous estimate upward if questioned again. It is often helpful to ask the patient's family about his drinking. Of the conditions associated with pancreatitis, alcoholism is the most difficult to deal with and is often associated with treatment failure. Even the pain of pancreatitis often does not persuade the dedicated drinker to turn away from the bottle. Nevertheless, the treatment of alcoholism should be undertaken with considerable effort (see Chapter 216), since there is much to gain by the cessation of drinking.

All patients who have had pancreatitis should undergo evaluation of the biliary tract. However, the oral cholecystogram may not visualize until 4 to 6 weeks after a bout of acute pancreatitis. After an acute episode, a serum calcium should be repeated, since it is often depressed during the acute disease, masking hypercalcemia. Repeatedly elevated fasting triglyceride determinations may lead to the diagnosis of a treatable etiology.

Chronic pancreatitis. Treatment of chronic pancreatitis consists of removing the causative factor and instituting analgesia. Again, many of these patients are confirmed alcohol abusers. The young patient without demonstrable gallbladder disease or alcoholism who has chronic pancreatitis or at least two episodes of acute pancreatitis may be helped by biliary exploration or an ampullary sphincteroplasty. Low-fat diets, anticholinergics, and antacids theoretically decrease pancreatic secretion but do not reliably lessen the pain. Aspirin should be tried; unfortunately, narcotic analgesia is often required. Methadone is well suited for long-term outpatient use.

Numerous surgical procedures have been designed to relieve the pain of the patient suffering from chronic pancreatitis. When biliary tract disease and a pseudocyst are excluded, surgery should be reserved for the severely symptomatic patient, who may respond to a 95 per cent pancreatectomy. Aggressive surgical procedures other than sphinctero-plasty aimed at relieving ductal obstruction do not reliably relieve pain.

Pancreatic insufficiency. Management of pancreatic insufficiency begins with a therapeutic trial of oral pancreatic enzymes to judge efficacy of therapy. The patient who benefits from use of exogenous enzymes will tolerate their unpleasant taste and the mild discomfort they cause and will take them faithfully, while the patient who does not benefit will discontinue them. Pancreatic enzymes are available as extracts of hog pancreas. Pancreatin contains trypsin, amylase and some lipase, while pancrealipase contains trypsin, amylase and extra amounts of lipase. The response to therapy is not uniform. The usual dose is 0.5 to 2.5 grams with each meal. Because enzyme preparations are partially inactivated by gastric acid or need increased alkalinity in the duodenum, they may work better when given with antacids, bicarbonate or cimetidine. Medium-chain triglycerides are often helpful, for they can be absorbed in the absence of lipase. Therapy can be assessed by monitoring symptoms, weight and qualitative stool fat determinations. Clinically significant fat-soluble vitamin deficiencies are uncommon, perhaps because intact bile secretion prevents complete fat malabsorption.

Most patients with chronic pancreatitis have abnormal glucose tolerance tests, but few develop frank diabetes mellitus. Mild glucose intolerance can be watched, but insulin dependence may occur. Hypoglycemia may be a problem, but ketoacidosis is rare. The vascular complications of diabetes seldom appear, perhaps because most patients do not survive long enough.

THERAPEUTIC RECOMMENDATIONS

Recovery Phase of Acute Pancreatitis

- Begin feedings with food rich in carbohydrates, low in protein and fat. Gradually increase amount of protein in diet as tolerated, followed by slow resumption of fat intake.
- Oral cholecystogram should be obtained after 4 to 6 weeks.
- Repeat serum calcium and triglycerides.

Chronic Pancreatitis

- Treat inciting cause, e.g., alcoholism, biliary tract disease, hypercalcemia, hyperlipidemia.

- Readmit for recurrent acute pancreatitis.
- Temporarily limit fat intake.
- Begin with mild analgesics for pain control, such as aspirin or acetaminophen 600 mg. q. 4h.
- Pain unrelieved by mild analgesia is an indication for a course of narcotic analgesics, such as methadone 5 or 10 mg. q. 6 or 8 h.
- Further evaluation is needed to rule out carcinoma, pseudocyst, and biliary tract disease.

Pancreatic Insufficiency

- Give oral pancreatic extract with each feeding in doses of 0.5 to 2.5 gm. (2 to 8 tablets) with full meals and 0.5 gm. with snacks. Lack of effect may require addition of an antacid (e.g., 60 cc. of Mylanta with each meal) or cimetidine to neutralize gastric acid and prevent enzymes from becoming inactivated.
- Provide high calorie diet rich in carbohydrate and protein.
- Supplement diet with a medium-chain triglyceride preparation. Restrict fat in symptomatic steatorrhea.
- Monitor glucose tolerance and treat clinical diabetes, if present, with insulin.

PATIENT EDUCATION

Most patients know little about the pancreas and its role in digestion. Moreover, few are aware of the connection between alcohol abuse and pancreatitis. Patient cooperation regarding diet, alcohol intake and use of enzyme extracts may be facilitated by a better understanding of the function of the pancreas and the nature of pancreatitis. Also, patients with acute pancreatitis who are making good recoveries can be comforted by the fact that recurrence is not common when the underlying cause is treated.

The patient with intractable pain and narcotic dependence poses one of the most difficult problems encountered in clinical medicine. A major pitfall is the development of an adversary relationship between patient and physician concerning the need for narcotics. Although there are no simple solutions, it is essential to elicit, understand, and respond to patient concerns, fears, and needs at the very outset. A well-informed patient who has confidence in his physician and in himself requires less pain medication than one who is scared, feels abandoned, and is in conflict with his doctor.

ANNOTATED BIBLIOGRAPHY

Bank, S., Marks, I.N., and Vinik, A.I.: Clinical and hormonal aspects of pancreatic diabetes. Am. J. Gastroenterol., *64*:13, 1975. *(A clinical description of pancreatic diabetes, its therapy and its distinctive properties.)*

Banks, P.A.: Acute pancreatitis. Gastroenterology, *61*:382, 1971. *(This article is a general review of pancreatitis, its pathophysiology, clinical features, differential diagnosis, and therapy.)*

Brooks, F.P.: Testing pancreatic function. N. Engl. J. Med., *286*:300, 1972. *(A practical review of the methods and utility of pancreatic stimulation tests and stool examination.)*

Di Magno, E.P., *et al.*: A prospective comparison of current diagnostic tests for pancreatic cancer. N. Engl. J. Med., *97*:737, 1977. *(A prospective clinical study demonstrating the utility of ultrasonography, pancreatic function testing, and endoscopic retrograde pancreatography in the evaluation of the patient with chronic abdominal pain suggestive of pancreatic carcinoma or chronic pancreatitis.)*

Ferrucci, J.T., and Eaton, S.B.: Radiology of the pancreas. N. Engl. J. Med., *288*:506, 1973. *(A brief review of the radiologic approach to pancreatic disease emphasizing pancreatic scanning, hypotonic duodenography, ultrasonography, angiography, and endoscopic pancreatocholangiography.)*

Frye, W.J., and Child, C.G.: Ninety-five percent distal pancreatectomy for chronic pancreatitis. Ann. Surg., *162*:543, 1965. *(First description of a surgical procedure that regularly provided pain relief for patients with chronic pancreatitis, short of the radical Whipple procedure.)*

Kosta, J.M., Nardi, G.L., and Sevantos, F.: Distal pancreatic duct inflammation. Ann. Surg., *172*:256, 1970. *(Demonstrates the success of ampullary sphincteroplasty in selected patients with chronic pancreatitis.)*

Salt, W.B., and Schenker, S.: Amylase, its clinical significance: A review of the literature. Medicine, *55*:269, 1976. *(A thorough review of the pathophysiology of the serum amylase and the urinary amylase clearance.)*

Saunders, J.H.B., and Wormsley, K.G.: Pancreatic extracts and the treatment of pancreatic exocrine insufficiency, Gut, *16*:157, 1975. *(Provides a de-*

tailed review of pancreatic extracts, pancreatic replacement therapy, and the assessment of the efficacy of pancreatic replacement.)

Warshaw, A.L., and Fuller, A.F.: Specificity of increased renal clearance of amylase in diagnosis of

acute pancreatitis. N. Engl. J. Med., *292*:325, 1975. *(A useful discussion of the use of the amylase creatinine urinary clearance ratio in the differential diagnosis of the elevated serum amylase.)*

73

Management of Gastrointestinal Cancers

JACOB J. LOKICH, M.D.

Recent developments in combining chemotherapy and radiation therapy with surgery for treatment of gastrointestinal cancer have added substantially to palliation and potential for cure, although mortality is still high (50 to 80 per cent). Moreover, improvements in management of the gastrointestinal complications of cancer, such as obstruction, ascites, and cachexia, have improved the quality of life for these patients (see Chapter 74).

Gastrointestinal malignancies are among the most common tumors found in adults. The treatment of local disease is the province of the surgeon, but management of advanced disease is a responsibility coordinated by the primary physician. It is important to know the indications and limitations of available treatment modalities in order to make best use of therapies offered by the surgeon, radiation therapist, and oncologist.

Gastric Cancer
EPIDEMIOLOGY, CLINICAL PRESENTATION AND COURSE (See Chapter 50)

There are about 23,000 new cases of gastric cancer eacy year, with the incidence decreasing slightly in the last decade; nevertheless, mortality remains relatively unchanged (80 per cent at 5 years). Gastric carcinomas may be silent for long periods of time. Abdominal pain, gastric ulceration, bleeding, weight loss, and obstruction are among the possible clinical manifestations of the disease.

PRINCIPLES OF MANAGEMENT

Symptom palliation is achieved most often by surgery. In spite of the presence of metastatic disease or extensive size of the regional tumor, a palliative "debulking" resection is generally worthwhile. This type of surgery appears to prolong survival significantly, especially when it is used in conjunction with combination chemotherapy (5-fluorouracil [5-FU] and a nitrosourea). Prospective therapeutic studies are in progress, using combination chemotherapy in addition to regional radiation therapy. (The reader should follow the literature closely for the results of these trials.)

Pancreatic Cancer
EPIDEMIOLOGY

Less than 5 per cent of patients will survive pancreatic cancer. There are over 22,000 new cases annually. Most patients are over age 40.

CLINICAL PRESENTATION AND COURSE

The tumor is usually occult until regional extension occurs. When the head of the pancreas is involved, obstructive jaundice commonly results. The tumor characteristically extends to liver and retroperitoneum. When it involves the paraspinal nerve plexus, back pain results, which clinically may herald the disease.

PRINCIPLES OF MANAGEMENT

Total pancreatectomy or Whipple procedure may be curative if the disease if very localized, which is, however, rare. Surgical management is predominantly confined to palliative bypass of the biliary tree or a gastroenterostomy. Additional palliative therapy involves a combined approach of radiation therapy with 4000 or 6000 rads in combination with the drug 5-FU. Prospective therapeutic trials have demonstrated that 5-FU improves both survival rate and functional status. In spite of this apparent therapeutic effect, however, the median period of survival for patients with regional pancreatic cancer is less than 1 year.

Colon Cancer (Excluding Rectal Cancer)
EPIDEMIOLOGY (see Chapter 51)

Colon cancer is among the leading malignancies of adults. There are 70,000 new cases annually. Survival has remained unchanged in the past 20 years, and almost 50 per cent die each year.

CLINICAL PRESENTATION AND COURSE
(see Chapter 51)

Manifestations are related to the site of the tumor. Tumors of the ascending colon may be relatively silent until they are far advanced, producing little more than mild iron-deficiency anemia or intermittently guaiac-positive stools. Tumors of the descending colon and sigmoid often appear earlier owing to rectal bleeding or melena. At the time of surgery, 50 to 75 per cent of patients demonstrate tumor which has penetrated the bowel wall and 60 per cent show regional metastases. Survival is a function of extent of penetration and spread. Once tumor has invaded serosa and nodes, 5 year survival is no more than 20 to 40 per cent.

PRINCIPLES OF MANAGEMENT

The chemotherapy of colon cancer either as an adjuvant to surgery or for metastatic disease has not advanced substantially since the introduction of 5-FU in 1956. Although the use of 5-FU in advanced disease is associated with a modicum of tumor regression in approximately one fifth of patients, it has not improved survival in the overall group.

Adjuvant chemotherapy has been advocated, including the use of short-term 5-FU or combined immunotherapy with bacillus Calmette Guerin (BCG) and 5-FU. To date, all prospective randomized and controlled studies of adjuvant therapy for colon cancer have failed to demonstrate any advantage for such treatment. Patients do not routinely receive adjuvant chemotherapy unless they are participating in a prospective trial.

The early trials of multiple-drug therapy that used 5-FU in combination with a nitrosourea and vincristine demonstrated a high response rate in patients with metastatic disease. Subsequent studies, however, have failed to confirm these data, and new combination chemotherapy regimens are being explored. Patients should be considered for chemotherapy only if they have symptomatic metastases and require palliative therapy.

Sequential monitoring of plasma carcinoembryonic antigen (CEA) levels is an essential component of patient management; lack of change or a rise in the CEA level is indicative of resistant progressive disease, justifying the discontinuation of therapy. On the other hand, treatment can be continued if there is a decrease in the CEA level, particularly if it is associated with symptomatic or objectively apparent tumor regression, indicative of an antitumor effect.

Rectal Cancer
EPIDEMIOLOGY

There are 30,000 new cases of rectal cancer annually. Mortality is similar to that of colon cancer; only 50 per cent are cured.

CLINICAL PRESENTATION AND COURSE

Rectal cancer commonly presents with occult or obvious rectal bleeding, with or without an alteration in bowel habits. The presence of tenesmus is often a late sign, reflecting extension of the tumor beyond the bowel wall. Rectal or perianal pain is a consequence of invasion of the pararectal structures and the sacral plexus. An important component of the routine rectal examination should be to check circumferentially into the rectal pouch following palpation of the prostate; a major proportion of carcinomas of the rectum may be localized to the posterior rectal wall and may be at the periphery or tip of the examining finger.

Rectal cancer differs from colon cancer in that it tends to invade locally and to recur in the pelvis alone or in association with distant metastases in the liver or peritoneal surfaces. The tendency to recur locally has resulted in the development of adjunctive therapies, particularly radiation in conjunction with surgery, which may augment the local control of such lesions.

PRINCIPLES OF MANAGEMENT

Preoperative radiation therapy in patients with large lesions may be used in order to reduce the size of the local tumor and to allow for resection. In multiple series involving radiation of these patients, the pathologic stage has been significantly reduced to a more superficial level (i.e., from the Duke's C category to Duke's A and B categories). In addition, frequency of local recurrence has been decreased, and survival rates extended beyond historical controls. Postoperative radiation therapy is given to patients with locally advanced tumor that has been totally resected as well as to patients with advanced local disease that involves lymph nodes or serosal penetration. The local recurrence rate has been markedly diminished.

The use of chemotherapy for rectal cancer is similar, if not identical, to that for colon cancer, with a disappointing rate of tumor response.

ANNOTATED BIBLIOGRAPHY

Carter, S.K., and Comis, R.L.: The integration of chemotherapy into a combined modality approach for cancer treatment (pancreas adenocarcinoma). Cancer Treat. Rev., 2:193, 1975. (A comprehensive review of the surgical radiation therapy and chemotherapy approach to pancreas carcinoma and a rational approach to multiple modality treatment for this tumor.)

Dewys, W.D.: Anorexia in cancer patients. Cancer Res. 37:2354, 1975. (A review of the mechanisms of cachexia in cancer patients and the potential application of hyperalimentation. This is one of a series of articles in the journal which contains papers presented at a Nutritional Symposium related to cancer.)

Gunderson, L.L., and Sosin, H.: Areas of failure found at reoperation (second or symptomatic look) following "curative surgery" for adenocarcinoma of the rectum: Clinicopathologic correlation and implications for adjuvant therapy. Cancer, 34:1278, 1974. (This important retrospective study established that the biologic behavior of rectal cancer was characteristic in that local recurrence was a prominent feature and therefore serve as a strong rationale for the use of adjuvant local radiation therapy.)

Higgins, G.A., Humphrey, E., Juler, G.L., LeVeen, H.H., McCaughan, J., and Keehn, R.J.: Adjuvant chemotherapy in the surgical treatment of large bowel cancer. Cancer, 38:1461, 1976. (This definitive summary of more than 1,000 patients entering these studies employing 5-FU and FUDR for short or long term courses fails to establish a role for 5-FU, but does indicate that therapeutic trends continue to stimulate future and prospective randomized trials.)

Kligerman, M.M.: Preoperative radiation therapy in rectal cancer. Cancer, 36:691, 1975. (This summary of the use of radiation therapy as a preoperative modality contains a review of the literature as well as supporting rationale for such an approach.)

Li, M.C., and Ross, S.T.: Chemoprophylaxis for patients with colorectal cancer: Prospective study with five-year follow-up. JAMA, 235:2825, 1976. (An inadequate study from the standpoint of experimental design which nonetheless suggests an advantage for adjuvant chemotherapy in regional colon cancer. This study is the singular study which has demonstrated such an effect and all prospective randomized trials have failed to determine a role for 5-FU as in adjuvant.)

Lokich, J.J.: Tumor markers: Hormones, antigens, and enzymes in malignant disease. Oncology, 35:54, 1978. (The general considerations of tumor markers as specific monitors of malignancy are reviewed and specific recommendations regarding the realistic application of tumor markers are presented.)

Lokich, J.J., Skarin, A.T., Mayer, R.J., Henderson, I.C., Blum, R., and Frei, E., III: Lack of effectiveness of combined 5-fluorouracil and methyl CCNU in advanced colorectal cancer. Cancer, 40:2792, 1977. (An example of the development of the combination chemotherapy regimen for colon cancer, which although initially enthusias-

tically proposed, was subsequently found with increasing experience to be relatively ineffective. The article emphasizes the lack of success with any of the therapeutic modalities presently employed in colon cancer and the need to explore new forms of treatment.)

Moertel, C.G.: Carcinoma of the stomach: Prognostic factors and criteria of response to therapy. M.J. Staquet (ed.): Cancer Therapy, Prognostic Factors and Criteria of Response. New York: Raven Press, 1975. *(A summary of the experience at the Mayo Clinic in over 300 patients with* *gastric cancer; discusses the natural history and lack of impact of chemotherapy on survival.)*

Moertel, C.T., Childs, D.S., Reitemier, R.J., *et al.:* Combined 5-fluorouracil and supervoltage radiation therapy of locally unresectable gastrointestinal cancer. Lancet, 2:875, 1969. *(The original prospective randomized trial which established improved survival as a consequence of the addition of chemotherapy to routine radiation therapy for regionally extensive upper gastrointestinal cancer.)*

74

Gastrointestinal Complications of Cancer
JACOB J. LOKICH, M.D.

Palliative management of gastrointestinal complications is often a vital part of cancer care, contributing markedly to patient comfort and nutrition. Gastrointestinal problems result from primary disease, metastases, the toxic effects of therapy, and metabolic disturbances. Important complications include biliary obstruction, pain, portal hypertension, malignant ascites, cachexia, nausea, vomiting and bowel obstruction. Some of these problems mandate surgical intervention, but ascites, cachexia, pain, nausea, and vomiting are problems requiring the attention of the primary physician.

Table 74–1. Management of Hepatic Metastases

MODALITY	INDICATION OR RESULTS
Surgery	
Resection	For localized tumor with long free interval
Dearterialization	For palliation of tumor confined to but diffuse in the liver
Chemotherapy	
Systemic infusion	Response rate, 20%
Arterial infusion	Response rate, 40–60%
Embolization	Similar to dearterialization
Radiation	For pain or obstructive jaundice only

HEPATIC METASTASES

The liver is the predominant site of metastases from gastrointestinal cancers. Also, lung and breast cancers frequently metastasize to the liver. Metastases may produce jaundice if biliary tract obstruction occurs, pain if there is distension of Glisson's capsule, or portal hypertension if the portal vein is blocked. Obstruction of the portal circulation results in increased portal vein pressure which, in turn, can cause bleeding varices, hepatic encephalopathy, and ascites. The first two complications of portal hypertension are extraordinarily rare complications of malignancy. Only 50 or so patients have been reported in whom hepatic metastases caused esophageal varices; only 20 patients have been reported with hepatic coma as a consequence of hepatic metastases. Ascites is a much more common occurrence with gastrointestinal tumors and is mechanically induced either by portal hypertension or by diffuse peritoneal implants with secondary exudation of fluid.

Modalities for management of hepatic metastases include surgery, chemotherapy, and radiation (see Table 74–1). Surgical approaches that involve *hepatic resection* are reserved for patients with a long free interval and solitary metastases, primarily from colon lesions. *Dearterialization* is a surgical procedure that involves hepatic artery ligation as well as selective identification and ligation of ancillary arterial vessels supplying the liver surface. The rationale for dearterialization is that the tumor's blood supply is derived predominantly from the hepatic artery while the blood supply to liver parenchyma is also provided by the portal venous system. Therefore, dearterialization does not permanently compromise the normal hepatic tissue, although transient ischemic hepatitis occurs in most patients. Tumor regression has been observed in a substantial proportion of patients treated by dearterialization, although improvement in survival rates has not been established. The use of dearterialization along with controlled, induced hepatic artery embolization may be a major palliative approach to hepatic metastases.

Radiation therapy has been employed as a palliative measure only for patients with *hepatic pain* due to massive hepatic distension. It is successful in a surprising proportion of patients, even though the radiation dose is reduced to 2500 rads to preclude radiation hepatitis. This dose is substantially smaller than that customarily used to combat tumor. *Narcotics* are often needed as well (see Chapter 89).

Radiation therapy has also been used in patients with *obstructive jaundice* due to tumor in the porta hepatis. When the tumor is particularly radiosensitive (e.g., breast cancer or lymphoma), the response to radiation may be prolonged. Because of this response, it is important in the evaluation of cancer patients with jaundice to search for an obstructive cause.

The *chemotherapy* for hepatic metastases from any site may be administered by systemic infusion, by the oral route, or by direct arterial infusion using a surgically or radiographically placed catheter. The use of 5-fluorouracil (5-FU) as the primary drug results in response rates of about 20 per cent when it is administered intravenously and 40 to 60 per cent when selective arterial infusion is used.

Not uncommonly, hepatic metastases are discovered at the same time or even prior to discovery of the primary tumor, as is often the case with cancer of the colon. *Synchronous metastases* may represent up to 15 per cent of new cases of colon cancer. The management of synchronous metastases is being developed. In the presence of symptoms that are specifically derived from the primary tumor, such as bleeding or obstruction, a primary surgical resection is often undertaken if the patient has a life expectancy (on the basis of the hepatic metastases) that exceeds 2 months. In the presence of an asymptomatic primary tumor in the bowel, however, therapeutic efforts are directed first at the metastatic disease; if successful, a surgical approach to the primary tumor may be undertaken. This approach assumes that the median survival for patients with hepatic metastases does not exceed 6 months; therefore, in patients not responding to chemotherapy, the likelihood of dying of distant disease far exceeds the likelihood of significant complications from the primary tumor site.

MALIGNANT ASCITES

Ascites may occur as a complication of diffuse peritoneal implantation or secondary to portal venous hypertension. Occasionally, ascites may be the most debilitating symptom as a consequence of abdominal distention and pain; but often a significant clinical effect is the marasmus that occurs as a consequence of sequestration of the protein-rich fluid in the abdomen.

A surgical *shunt procedure* that employs a one-way valve catheter which is placed in the peritoneal cavity and run subcutaneously into the jugular venous system (the so-called LeVeen or peritoneal-jugular venous shunt) has been employed in patients with nonmalignant ascites and more recently in patients with neoplastic effusions. Excellent control of the ascites due to malignancy has been achieved, as increased abdominal pressure and a negative intrathoracic pressure cause ascitic fluid to move across the one-way valve into the venous sytem. This system allows for the restitution of body stores of amino acids and proteins and improves nutritional status, as well as decreases abdominal distention. One complication from use of these shunts has been the development of disseminated intravascular coagulation in some patients due to the presence of thromboplastin-like material in the ascitic fluid. Patients with prolonged prothrombin times are at particular risk for this complication; consequently, candidates should have a prothrombin time obtained.

The use of surgical drainage for ascites is not as effective as it is for effusions of the pleural space. Similarly, intra-abdominal instillation of chemotherapeutic agents and radioisotopes has been relatively ineffective. Sclerosing drugs and irritants to seal the peritoneal space are not recommended, since an irritant effect on the bowel may result in necrosis, perforation, or secondary fibrosis and adhesions leading to obstruction.

CANCER CACHEXIA

Weight loss, inanition, and protein depletion with marasmus are common systemic effects of primary as well as metastatic cancer. These are a consequence of anorexia, taste distortion, vomiting, maldi-

Table 74–2. Factors that Determine Weight Loss in Cancer Patients

FACTOR	MECHANISM	TREATMENT
Anorexia	Associated with hepatic metastases and possibly mediated by a para-neoplastic polypeptide suppressing appetite center	Appetite stimulant
Taste Distortion	Dysgeusia or irritant effect of drugs	None
Vomiting	Emesis secondary to therapy (drugs, radiation)	Intermittent chemo-therapy schedule Prochlorperazine te-trahydrocannabinol
Oral Stomatitis	Secondary to chemotherapy	Topical anesthesia
Maldigestion	Secondary to enzymatic insufficiency	Pancreatic enzyme
Malabsorption	Secondary to obstruction or alteration of mucosal surface	Antitumor measures
Malutilization	Metabolic derangement related to tumor secretion or a consequence of mechanisms that compensate for limited nutrient availability	Antitumor measures

gestion, malabsorption, and malutilization (see Table 74–2). Such factors combine to induce the self-perpetuating and debilitating cycle of food rejection secondary to tumor growth, which simultaneously weakens host immune mechanisms and promotes tumor growth. Moreover, host tolerance to radiation and chemotherapy is compromised, thus restricting the ability to tolerate therapeutic doses of either form of treatment.

The mechanism(s) responsible for anorexia are not well defined. Anorexia may be due to a tumor-induced polypeptide which affects the satiety center or chemotherapy agents causing taste distortion or an irritant effect. Maintaining nutrition in the face of anorexia often requires the use of protein-rich, *high-calorie supplements* (e.g., eggnog, milkshakes, Sustacal), frequent small feedings, and blenderized meals in patients unable to eat solids. The use of corticosteroids to promote euphoria may also increase appetite, but this effect is transient and not worth the major side effects which develop as a consequence of the dosage necessary to promote appetite. The marijuana derivative, tetrahydrocannabinol, seems to have a potent appetite stimulant effect, but is not yet available for general use.

Chemotherapy-induced gastrointestinal effects include vomiting, painful stomatitis, and ulcerative enteritis. Chemotherapy programs often employ intermittent schedules in order to minimize the chronic nausea and vomiting associated with treatment. More often than not, the treatments are associated with self-limited vomiting of a few hours' duration. Treatment programs are designed so that there are no more than 2 to 3 episodes per month. Palliation of nausea can be achieved in part with simultaneous use of a phenothiazine, such as *prochlorperazine* (see Chapter 88); at times, the drug does not suffice. Recent double-blind controlled studies of tetrahydrocannabinol given experimentally to patients with

nausea secondary to chemotherapy have shown the drug to be at least as good as and often better than prochlorperazine in ameliorating chemotherapy-induced emesis. The use of the drug is still experimental. The management of chemotherapy-induced stomatitis is generally conservative, employing *topical paste anesthetics.* Viscous lidocaine preparations are of little use; paste preparations are more helpful in that the duration of analgesia is protracted. Unfortunately, taste distortion occurs as a consequence of the topical anesthetic effect.

Disorders of digestion, absorption and caloric utilization are generally a consequence of metabolic effects of the tumor or the unavailability of appropriate enzyme resources such as pancreatic enzymes or adequate gastric acid. Chemotherapy *per se* has no specific effects on metabolism or other processes involved in digestion, absorption or caloric utilization. The use of exogenous *enzyme preparations* in patients with previous pancreatectomy and the use of liquid saliva to promote deglutition in patients with salivary glands compromised by radiation are examples of supportive measures which may be necessary in patients with cancer cachexia.

Hypokalemia and hypercalcemia may also lead to anorexia, nausea, vomiting, or constipation. Correction of these electrolyte imbalances may lessen symptoms. Radiation and chemotherapy may produce enteritis with mucosal ulceration, resulting in diarrhea and vomiting. The effect is transient and generally the entire mucosal surface reconstitutes within 7 days.

ANNOTATED BIBLIOGRAPHY

Harmon, D.C., *et al.*: Disseminated intravacular coagulation with peritoneovenous shunts. Ann. Intern. Med., *90*:774, 1979. *(Documents this im-*

portant complication, which is particularly frequent in patients with prolonged prothrombin times.)

Sallen, S.E., *et al.*: Antimetics in patients receiving chemotherapy for cancer: A randomized comparison of tetrahydrocannabinol and prochlorperazine. N. Eng. J. Med., *302*:135, 1980. *(Tetrahydrocannabinol proved to be effective and safe.)*

Proceedings of the National Cancer Institute National Conference on Nutrition in Cancer. Cancer, *43*: Supplement, 1979. *(An excellent collec-tion of papers on all aspects of cancer cachexia and its management.)*

Straus, A.K., *et al.*: Peritoneovenous shunting in management of malignant ascites. Arch. Surg., *114*:489, 1979. *(Of 37 patients shunted, 27 achieved palliation that lasted until death.)*

Turck-Maischeider, M., and Kazem, I.: Palliative irradiation for liver metastases. JAMA, *232*:625, 1975. *(An example of the use of radiation therapy in reduced doses of 1600 to 2500 rads for symptomatic relief of pain.)*

6

Hematologic and Oncologic Problems

Section A: Hematology

75
Screening for Anemia

Anemia is a sign of underlying abnormality rather than a diagnosis in itself. The incidental finding of a low hematocrit or hemoglobin level is often an important clue to the diagnosis of an underlying condition that may be either trivial or life-threatening. Patients with fatigue or other subjective symptoms often ask about their "blood count." In such cases, the absence of anemia is reassuring. But is the otherwise well patient likely to benefit from either the identification or treatment of asymptomatic anemia? The answer to this question depends on the prevalence of conditions most likely to cause asymptomatic anemia and the relationship between hemoglobin level and those symptoms that are often attributed to anemia.

EPIDEMIOLOGY AND RISK FACTORS

By far the most common cause for asymptomatic anemia is iron deficiency due to inadequate dietary replacement of iron lost from the body. Daily iron requirements for males and postmenopausal females are between 0.5 and 1 mg. Because additional iron is needed by menstruating and pregnant women, their daily requirements are 2 mg. and 2.5 mg. respectively. Since only 5 to 10 per cent of the 10 to 20 mg. of the iron contained in the average adult diet is ab-

sorbed, it is not surprising that iron deficiency is common in women of childbearing age. Population studies have found 10 to 20 per cent of menstruating women to have abnormally low concentrations of hemoglobin (usually less than 12 gm. per 100 ml.). Between 20 and 60 per cent of pregnant women have hemoglobin levels below 11 gm. per 100 ml. Anemia is less likely to occur in women taking birth control pills and more likely to occur in women with intrauterine devices. Iron deficiency is rare in adult males; if present, it is a clear indication for diligent investigation of the gastrointestinal tract. Absorption of iron may be decreased after gastrectomy or in the presence of achlorhydria.

Sideroblastic and megaloblastic anemias are much less common. Pernicious anemia, the most common form of B_{12} deficiency, has a prevalence of 0.1 per cent in individuals of Northern European extraction. It is much less common among other ethnic and racial groups. Folate deficiency is common during pregnancy and in patients with alcoholic liver disease, when it is often accompanied by sideroblastic anemia. Anticonvulsant drugs including phenytoin, primidone, and phenobarbital may interfere with folate absorption with resulting megaloblastic anemia. Thalassemia minor is a common cause of mild anemia in patients of Mediterranean or Far Eastern extraction. Sickle cell disease and trait, by far the most

315

common hemoglobinopathy, is discussed in the following chapter.

That old age is not in itself a risk factor for anemia related to deficiency states has been documented in a British study. Two per cent of males and 4 per cent of females had hematocrits below 36 per cent. There were no cases of macrocytic anemia despite moderate prevalence of folate or B_{12} levels below commonly accepted reference levels.

NATURAL HISTORY OF ANEMIA AND EFFECTIVENESS OF THERAPY

Obviously, the natural history of anemia depends on the underlying cause. What symptoms can mild or moderate anemia itself be expected to cause? The hyperkinetic symptoms that follow compensatory increases in cardiac stroke volume and heart rate are rarely present before hemoglobin levels have fallen to 7.5 gm. per 100 ml. Other highly subjective symptoms including irritability, fatigue and headache have been attributed to milder degrees of anemia. A British survey, however, found no relationship between the frequency of such symptoms and the level of hemoglobin (ranging from 8 to 12 gm. per 100 ml.) among women found to have iron deficiency anemia during a screening program. There was indirect evidence that levels under 8 gm. per 100 ml. were associated with symptoms severe enough to prompt presentation to a physician. Among the asymptomatic women identified by screening, no benefits from treatment were detected. Another report from Britain demonstrated a prevalence of anemia of 10 per cent among screened women. There was a noteworthy absence of treatable underlying conditions other than iron deficiency and, again, no demonstrable benefits from treatment. It has been noted by some investigators that symptoms occur earlier, with higher hemoglobin concentrations, in megaloblastic anemia, but supporting evidence is fragmentary.

SCREENING AND DIAGNOSTIC TESTS

The laboratory measurements of hematocrit and hemoglobin concentrations are straightforward. Automated methods are reliable and reproducible when specimens are properly handled. It must be remembered, as with all continuous laboratory varia-

bles, that the choice of a reference value for defining normality is arbitrary. This is particularly true in light of the unclear relationship between significant symptomatology and mild "anemia."

CONCLUSIONS AND RECOMMENDATIONS

- Anemia is a common condition. It may be secondary to serious underlying disease or simple dietary deficiency. Determination of hemoglobin concentration or hematocrit is recommended as part of the evaluation of many varied presenting complaints.
- Iron deficiency anemia is common among women of childbearing age, particularly those who are pregnant.
- There is no clear relationship between degrees of mild to moderate anemia and significant symptoms. No clearly measurable benefits following the treatment of mild anemia have been identified in screening studies.
- While determination of a complete blood count may provide clues to the presence of early treatable disease such as GI malignancy, more specific alternatives such as stool testing for occult blood are available. Routine screening for anemia in nonpregnant, asymptomatic patients is not recommended.

ANNOTATED BIBLIOGRAPHY

Committee on Iron Deficiency: Iron deficiency in the United States. JAMA, 203:407, 1968. *(Reviews prevalence studies of iron deficiency anemia.)*

Elwood, P.C., Shinton, N.K., Wilson, I.L., Sweetnam, P., and Frazer, A.C.: Haemoglobin, Vitamin B_{12} and folate levels in the elderly. Br. J. Haematol., 21:557, 1971. *(Ten per cent of males with hemoglobin less than 13 gm./100 ml, 10 per cent of females less than 12.5 gm./100 ml. No megaloblastic anemia found.)*

Elwood, P.C., Waters, W.E., Greene, W.J.W., Sweetnam, P.M., and Wood, M.M.: Symptoms and circulating haemoglobin level. J. Chron. Dis., 21:615, 1969. *(Symptoms not correlated with hemoglobin level in those found anemic on screening.)*

Elwood, P.C., Waters, W.E., Greene, W.J., and Wood, M.M.: Evaluation of a screening survey for anemia in adult nonpregnant women. Br. Med. J., 4:714, 1967. *(Not very extensive follow-*

up but no serious underlying disease detected among anemic women.)

Zadeh, J.A., Karabus, C.D., and Fiedling, J.: Hemoglobin concentration and other values in women

using an intrauterine device or taking corticosteroid contraceptive pills. Br. Med. J., *4*:708, 1967. *(Hemoglobin levels fall with IUD use. Increase with birth control pill use.)*

76
Screening for Sickle Cell Disease and Sickle Cell Trait

Sickle cell disease is the most common of the clinically significant hemoglobinopathies. In the United States, the disease and trait occur almost exclusively among blacks. During the late 1960s and early 1970s, sickle cell disease received a great deal of attention in the medical and lay press. The importance of screening for individuals with disease and trait was stressed. Some states legislated mandatory screening programs.

Sickle cell disease (the SS hemoglobin homozygous state) is usually identified during childhood. Patients whose anemia is not identified by screening are often diagnosed after presentation with impaired growth, increased susceptibility to infection or painful crisis. Screening of adults is aimed at the identification of asymptomatic carriers of sickle trait (the AS hemoglobin heterozygous state). The principal objective is to reduce the prevalence of the homozygous condition by means of genetic counseling. Whether or not screening benefits the people screened has been debated. Screening performed without subsequent education and counseling can be harmful. An understanding of the natural history of sickle cell trait and disease, sensitivity to the concerns of affected patients, and selective use of available screening tests are all necessary if such harmful effects are to be avoided.

EPIDEMIOLOGY AND RISK FACTORS

Sickle cell disease has a prevalence of about 0.15 per cent among black children in the United States. Double heterozygotes including those with hemoglobin SC or S-beta-thal are even less common. Prevalence of sickling disease is lower among adults, since the life span of SS homozygotes and double heterozygotes is decreased.

Screening surveys have documented a prevalence

of sickle trait of 7.4 percent among black veterans and 8.7 percent in the black community of San Francisco. Some studies have shown regional differences in prevalence. Prevalence does not decrease with age. Sickle cell trait is present in low frequency in Southern Italy and higher frequency in parts of Greece. It remains a very rare finding in Americans of Mediterranean extraction.

NATURAL HISTORY OF SICKLE CELL DISEASE AND EFFECTIVENESS OF THERAPY

The natural history of sickle cell disease is variable. Most children exhibit failure to thrive and suffer frequent infections. Anemia is usually moderate but can become severe, often as a result of infection or folate deficiency. The course is punctuated by painful crises precipitated by infection, dehydration, or hypoxia. Organ infarction, congestive heart failure, cholelithiasis and skin ulcers are some of the complications of chronic disease. Because supportive care has been improved, life expectancy for patients with sickle cell disease has increased. However, it remains significantly shortened.

In contrast, life expectancy is not affected by sickle cell trait. AS red blood cells sickle at much lower oxygen tension than SS cells. The only clinical abnormality that occurs with any frequency among patients with sickle cell trait is painless hematuria, presumably the result of small infarcts of the renal medulla where red cells are particularly susceptible to sickling.

The vastly different health implications of sickle cell trait and sickle cell disease have been lost on some screened individuals and, unfortunately, some physicians. Concern about risk of sudden death has been raised by four case reports of army recruits previously unknown to have sickle trait who died during basic training at a moderately high altitude. Increased risk of sudden death among people with sickle cell trait has not been confirmed. On the contrary, extensive examinations of people with sickle cell trait have disclosed no differences in x-rays, ECG findings, spirometry, blood chemistries, and psychological factors when compared to controls matched for age, sex and race. Sickle cell trait is not significantly less frequent among black athletes, including professional football players, than it is among blacks in general.

If the principal reason for screening adults is to provide genetic counseling, it is important to consider the effectiveness of such counseling. Evidence suggests that identification and counseling of heterozygotes do not alter marriage and parenthood decisions. The individual who does not wish to make such decisions on the basis of carrier status is not likely to benefit from screening. Some families have been traumatized by questions of paternity raised by indiscriminate screening. Because of the confusion among patients and physicians about differences between sickle cell disease and trait, unnecessary anxiety may be the most common result. Surveys have demonstrated that many internists and general practitioners do not sufficiently understand the implications of screening test results to properly counsel patients.

SCREENING AND DIAGNOSTIC TESTS

Screening tests for sickle cell trait are inexpensive and reproducible. Tests for sickling, including the use of 2 per cent metabisulfite solution and the more expensive commercial methods, are positive in the presence of hemoglobin S but do not distinguish between homozygotes, heterozygotes, and double heterozygotes (hemoglobin S combined with thalassemia or hemoglobin C). Hemoglobin electrophoresis can also be performed inexpensively.

CONCLUSIONS AND RECOMMENDATIONS

- Sickle cell disease is a serious health hazard that usually presents during early childhood.
- Sickle cell trait is associated with minimal risk of morbidity. The principal reason for screening adults for the presence of sickle trait is to facilitate genetic counseling.
- Indiscriminate screening followed by inadequate counseling may be harmful and is not likely to provide benefits to individuals who will not revise mar-

riage and parenthood decisions on the basis of test results.
- Screening for sickle trait should be offered to black adults in reproductive age groups. Implications of test results should be fully explained before testing is performed.

ANNOTATED BIBLIOGRAPHY

Barnes, M.G., Komarmy, L., and Novack, A.H.: A comprehensive screening program for hemoglobinopathies. JAMA, *219*:701, 1972. *(Describes screening program based on simple, inexpensive electrophoresis.)*

Jones, S.R., Binder, R.A., and Donowho, E.M.: Sudden death in sickle-cell trait. N. Engl. J. Med., *282*:323, 1970. *(Four cases of sudden death among 4000 black army recruits undergoing basic training at high altitude.)*

Kellon, D.B., and Beutler, E.: Physician attitudes about sickle cell disease and sickle cell trait. JAMA, *227*:71, 1974. *(An editorial based on responses to a questionnaire that suggest misunderstanding of screening implications by a significant proportion of internists and family practitioners.)*

Motulsky, A.G.: Frequency of sickling disorders in U.S. blacks. N. Engl. J. Med., *288*:31–33, 1973. *(Estimates prevalence of double heterozygotes as well as SS disease at birth [1 in 625 with SS; 1 in 833 with SC; and 1 in 1667 with S-beta-thal] and in the population.)*

Murphy, J.R.: Sickle cell hemoglobin in black football players. JAMA, *225*:981, 1973. *(The rate of Hb AS among black football players in the NFL was 6.7 percent.)*

Petrakis, N.L., Wiesenfeld, S.L., Sams, B.J., Collen, M.F., Cutler, J.L., and Siegelaub, A.B.: Prevalence of sickle-cell trait and glucose-6-PD-deficiency. N. Engl. J. Med., *282*:767, 1970. *(An 8.7 prevalence of sickle trait among over 4,000 San Francisco blacks.)*

Sears, D.A.: The morbidity of sickle cell trait. Am. J. Med., *64*:1021, 1978. *(Extensive review with 296 references concluding that while certain abnormalities do occur with increased frequency in sickle cell trait, survival is not impaired.)*

Whitten, C.F.: Sickle-cell programming—An imperiled promise. N. Engl., J. Med., *288*:319, 1973. *(Lists the arguments against indiscriminate screening.)*

77
Evaluation of Anemia

Anemia is a frequent problem in primary care practice. A study of a London general practice of 5000 patients revealed an annual incidence of 17.5 new cases per 1000 patients. Other surveys have shown that the average primary physician comes across 40 to 50 new cases each year. The condition is not a diagnosis but rather a sign of underlying disease, particularly in men and in the elderly, in whom readily detectable pathology is found in over 50 per cent of instances.

The definition of anemia is quantitative, based on a reduction in hematocrit or hemoglobin concentration to levels at least two standard deviations below the mean for healthy individuals of similar age, sex and altitude of residence. Mean hematocrit for adult men at sea level is 46 per cent, with a range of 41 to 51 per cent; for women the mean is 42 per cent, and the range 37 to 47 per cent. Slight differences may be noted when automated techniques are used to measure the hematocrit. Normal mean hemoglobin concentration is approximately 16 gm. per 100 ml., for men, with a range of 14 to 18 gm. per 100 ml.; for women the mean is 14 gm. per 100 ml., and the range is 12 to 16 gm. per 100 ml. In men over 65, the mean falls to 13.5 gm. per 100 ml.; in women over 65, 13.1 gm. per 100 ml. Anemia is defined in terms of concentration, because it is easier to measure than the total red cell mass. If plasma volume is expanded, a spurious anemia may be diagnosed; if plasma volume falls below normal, a true anemia may be masked. Thus, the diagnosis of anemia must be considered in the context of the patient's volume status.

A systematic approach is necessary for the evaluation of anemia, because the number of possible etiologies and diagnostic tests are great.

PATHOPHYSIOLOGY AND CLINICAL PRESENTATION

The pathogenesis of anemia is conceptually straightforward. There is either marked blood loss, excessive destruction or inadequate production; often two or more factors are operating simultaneously. Excessive destruction can result from membrane disorders, abnormal hemoglobins, enzyme deficiencies and a host of extrinsic problems such as mechanical or antibody-mediated disruption. Decreased production occurs when there are defects in stem cell proliferation and differentiation, DNA synthesis, hemoglobin synthesis or a combination of these.

Clinical presentation of the patient with anemia depends on abruptness of onset, severity, age and ability of the cardiopulmonary system to compensate for the decrease in blood volume and oxygen-carrying capacity. When onset is gradual, symptoms may be minimal due to adequate time for compensatory adjustments to decreased hemoglobin. Important responses to anemia include an increase in 2,3-DPG (facilitating oxygen delivery to tissues) and expansion of the plasma volume.

There are few symptoms when the hematocrit is above 30, the anemia gradual in onset, and the patient otherwise healthy. However, if the hematocrit falls still further, dyspnea and mild fatigue may begin to appear upon strenuous exertion. Greater reductions in hematocrit result in cardiopulmonary symptoms that come with lesser activity. Age and cardiopulmonary reserve are also important determinants of symptoms. A potpourri of nonspecific complaints frequently accompanies anemia, including headache, tinnitus, poor concentration, palpitation, vague abdominal discomfort, anorexia, nausea and diarrhea or constipation. Tachycardia and diminished peripheral resistance occur as the hemoglobin falls below 7.5 gm. per 100 ml.; a systolic flow murmur due to high output is common. Pallor is an obvious finding best seen in the conjunctivae, but it is of little quantitative significance. More specific clinical features are a function of etiology. Anemias can be classified according to red cell morphology.

Microcytic anemias. Iron deficiency is often characterized by slow development and vague complaints. In mild cases the relation between the anemia and symptoms is tenuous. Fatigue, headache and irritability are frequently noted by women with iron deficiency, but a community study of 295 anemic patients showed no correlation between symptoms and hemoglobin concentration. The headache, paresthesias and burning tongue sometimes occurring in this condition have been thought to be caused by low tissue levels of cellular iron. Double-blind studies examining the effect of iron vs. placebo in relieving symptoms are conflicting. Menorrhagia is another complaint attributed by some investigators to instances of iron deficiency, but this is disputed by others. Pica and dysphagia (due to an esophageal (web) are classic, though rare, features today.

The physical findings which occur in iron deficiency are a bit more specific than are symptoms. Atrophic glossitis is commonly found, as is cheilitis. Koilonychia, with spooning, ridging and thinning, are rare. Other physical findings and symptoms are manifestations of the underlying cause. The earliest laboratory changes are depletion of marrow iron stores and a corresponding fall in serum ferritin. These are followed by a decrease in serum iron and an increase in transferrin, producing in many cases a reduction in the per cent saturation to below 16 per cent. The first change in the peripheral blood is a drop in the hematocrit and hemoglobin. Only with increasing severity (hemoglobin below 9 gm. per 100 ml.) do red cells become microcytic and eventually hypochromic.

Chronic blood loss is the most frequent cause of iron deficiency in adults. Malabsorption of iron and inadequate dietary intake are seldom major factors, though heavy antacid use and gastrectomy can inhibit iron uptake. Most menstruating women show depletion of iron stores, since the equivalent of 20 mg. of iron is lost each month, and 500 mg. iron is lost with each pregnancy, while daily normal iron intake provides only 1 mg.

In the *anemia of chronic disease*, symptoms are those of the causal illness. Chronic inflammatory diseases, chronic infections and neoplasms are the most common etiologies. The anemia is usually moderate with hemoglobins in the 7 to 11 gm. per 100 ml. range. Both serum iron and iron binding capacity are reduced; marrow iron stores and ferritin are normal or increased. The smear is most often normocytic, but can be hypochromic and even microcytic, mimicking iron deficiency. The serum iron falls before anemia sets in; per cent saturation may be less than 16 per cent, again simulating iron deficiency.

Thalassemia minor is typically asymptomatic and discovered during evaluation of a microcytic hypochromic anemia which does not respond to iron. Many persons with this hereditary condition are of Mediterranean ancestry. There are no characteristic physical findings. The red cell count is elevated, and the smear may reveal targeting and basophilic stippling in addition to some polychromatophilia, poikilocytosis and anisocytosis. The hemoglobin A_2 level is elevated, which helps to identify the thalassemia trait.

Sideroblastic anemias are a heterogeneous set of disorders, including a primary type which may be a preleukemic state, a pyridoxine-responsive variant, and other variants associated with rheumatoid arthritis, polyarteritis, malabsorption, chronic alcoholism, cancer, porphyria, lead poisoning and true pyridoxine deficiency. In the primary type, patients are typically over age 60; liver and/or spleen are palpable in over 50 per cent. The smear is dimorphic; since some cells are normochromic and others hypochromic; confusion with iron deficiency can result. Anisocytosis and poikilocytosis are pronounced. Serum iron is elevated, and iron binding is capacity reduced. Marrow iron stains show many abnormal ringed sideroblasts.

Macrocytic Anemia. *Vitamin B_{12} deficiency* results most frequently from reduced gastric production of intrinsic factor, as occurs in pernicious anemia. The more than chance association with Hashimoto's thyroiditis and vitiligo has suggested an autoimmune mechanism. Blind loop syndrome, total gastrectomy and terminal ileal disease are other causes. Dietary lack is very rare, since B_{12} is available in everyday foods and body stores contain a 3-year reserve. Onset is gradual; in pernicious anemia, symptoms usually become evident in the sixth decade. Sore tongue and numbness and tingling in the extremities are classic symptoms of B_{12} deficiency, but anorexia, diarrhea and other gastrointestinal complaints may predominate. The neurologic manifestations also include disturbances of position and vibratory sense, due to lesions in the posterior columns of the spinal cord, and incoordination, spasticity and up-going toes indicative of damage to the corticospinal tract. The neurologic syndrome is uncommon, but may present in the absence of anemia. Mild memory loss, depression and irritability sometimes appear as well.

By the time the anemia is discovered, it may be quite severe. Hypersegmented polymorphonuclear leukocytes are an early finding specific for the megaloblastic anemias. Oval macrocytes are also characteristic, though poikilocytosis is considerable. The MCV rises above 100, and serum B_{12} falls below 100 pg/ml. In pernicious anemia, achlorhydria is found on histamine stimulation.

Folate deficiency is more likely to follow inadequate dietary intake than is B_{12} deficiency, because bodily stores are limited to a 3-month reserve. Chronic alcohol abuse is the classic setting. Increased demand for folate, as in pregnancy, hemolysis, malignancy and severe psoriasis, is another precipitant. Malabsorption syndromes, such as sprue, and drugs which inhibit folate uptake, such as phenytoin and other anticonvulsants, also can precipitate the anemia. The same is true for folate antagonists such as methotrexate, trimethoprim and triamterene. Hematologic features resemble those of B_{12} deficiency; there are no neurologic deficits.

Normochromic, Normocytic Anemias. Hemolytic anemias are a diverse group. Inherited forms are due to intrinsic red cell defects; acquired types depend primarily on extra-erythrocytic mechanisms such as immunologic or mechanical injury. Clinical presentations vary according to rate of destruction, compensatory adaptations, and underlying etiology. Jaundice sets in when the liver's capacity to conjugate the excess bilirubin from hemoglobin breakdown is exceeded; the serum level of unconjugated bilirubin climbs. Splenomegaly evolves as trapping of damaged red cells progresses. Sudden fever, chills, headache, back and abdominal pain, and hemoglobinuria characterize severe acute hemolysis.

The peripheral smear is normochromic normocytic, but may be macrocytic due to release of immature forms during rapid red cell destruction and regeneration. Polychromatophilia is typical, and nucleated red cells, stippling, spherocytes, schistocytes and Howell-Jolly bodies are often noted. The reticulocyte count is elevated unless there is an accompanying marrow defect.

Sickle cell disease is the most prevalent hemolytic condition in the black population. *Sickle cell trait* is asymptomatic and anemia is absent, though mild hematuria due to sickling in the hypertonic renal medulla sometimes occurs. The peripheral smear is normal except for an occasional target cell. Hemoglobin electrophoresis reveals less than 50 per cent of total hemoglobin to be of the S variety. *Sickle cell anemia* is a less benign problem. Painful aplastic crises, leg ulcers, hepatomegaly, hematuria, renal concentrating defects, and mild jaundice can occur; a cardiac flow murmur is common. Painful crises are precipitated by stress and characterized by pain in the lower extremities, back or abdomen. Fever and leukocytosis may be present as well. Attacks last up to a week and then resolve spontaneously. Aplastic crises are due to a concurrent illness that suppresses erythropoiesis, leading to marked worsening of anemia. The smear is normochromic; sickled cells may be noted as well as target forms. Hemoglobin electrophoresis reveals a predominance of hemoglobin S (see Chapter 76).

Drug-induced hemolysis is being recognized more frequently. Three mechanisms have been identified: (1) adsorption to the red cell of drug-antibody complexes, as occurs with quinidine; (2) drug adsorption to the red cell, followed by binding of antidrug antibody, as found with penicillin; (3) induction of a red cell "autoantibody," noted with long-term methyldopa use, but rarely causing significant hemolysis. The hallmark of most drug-related hemolytic episodes is a positive direct Coombs test.

Aplastic anemias are usually idiopathic, but they may be linked to a chemical agent or an idiosyncratic drug reaction. Onset is gradual, with fatigue and bleeding noted first; infection is a later problem. There is no organomegaly. The smear appears normochromic normocytic, but the number of platelets is diminished. There are no signs of increased red cell production. The reticulocyte count is zero, and a pancytopenia is present.

The *anemia of chronic renal failure* is due to reduction in both production and survival or red cells. Lack of erythropoietin and metabolic injury to erythrocytes are postulated mechanisms. The severity of the anemia parallels the degree of azotemia. The smear is normochromic normocytic; burr cells are sometimes prominent.

Hypothyroidism is associated with a number of anemic states. Iron deficiency may occur secondary to heavy menstrual bleeding. Also, a macrocytic picture that clears upon administration of exogenous thyroid hormone is not uncommon. A true megaloblastic anemia due to B_{12} deficiency occurs in about 10 per cent of hypothyroid patients with a macrocytic smear; the relation between hypothyroidism and pernicious anemia is unresolved, but an autoimmune mechanism is postulated. More typical of hypothyroidism is a mild normochromic normocytic anemia.

Liver disease is responsible for a host of anemias, especially when accompanied by alcoholism and poor diet. Folate deficiency, marrow suppression, hypersplenism, bleeding and bile salt alteration of the red cell membrane all contribute. The smear shows considerable poikilocytosis with spiculated red cells and some macrocytes; if folate deficiency occurs, a megaloblastic picture is superimposed.

DIFFERENTIAL DIAGNOSIS

A practical method for organizing the many causes of anemia is to group them according to (1) the appearance of the Wright-stained smear of the peripheral blood and (2) the electronically determined red cell indices. This method allows for classi-

Table 77-1.   Differential Diagnosis of Anemia by Morphology

Normochromic-Normocytic (MCV 82-92, MCHC 32-36)
1. Hemorrhage
2. Hemolysis
3. Aplastic anemia, pure red cell aplasia
4. Marrow infiltration
5. Hypothyroidism
6. Chronic disease
7. Chronic renal failure
8. Cirrhosis
9. Early iron deficiency

Macrocytic (MCV > 100, MCHC 32-36)
1. B_{12} deficiencies
2. Folic acid deficiencies
3. Antimetabolites
4. Accelerated erythropoiesis (acute hemolysis, hemorrhage)
5. Increased membrane surface area (liver disease)
6. Myxedema
7. Aplastic anemia

Microcytic (MCV 50-82, MCHC 24-32)
1. Iron deficiency
   a. Chronic blood loss
   b. Inadequate intake
   c. Inadequate absorption
   d. Excess demand
2. Abnormal hemoglobins
3. Thalassemia
4. Sideroblastic anemia
5. Chronic disease

fication of etiologies into normochromic-normocytic, hypochromic-microcytic, and macrocytic categories (see Table 77-1) and facilitates workup.

The majority of patients who present with anemia have iron deficiency. The London general practice study mentioned earlier revealed that 95 per cent of women and 50 per cent of men with anemia had an iron deficiency picture. In males and the elderly, this is very likely to be due to occult bleeding from an underlying lesion. In the London study, 95 per cent of men with iron deficiency had blood loss from a gastrointestinal source. In a British study of anemia in the elderly, 110 patients over age 65 who presented with anemia were evaluated; 70 per cent had iron deficiency and about half had evidence of gastrointestinal blood loss. In 40 per cent of these cases, the etiology was listed as "undetermined," but many patients did not undergo full workup because of advanced age. Prevalence of iron deficiency anemia among premenopausal women is conservatively estimated to be 15 per cent, rising to over 30 per cent during pregnancy.

In the London survey, anemia was attributed to chronic disease in 4 per cent (probably an underestimate) and to B_{12} deficieny in 8 per cent. The British

study of elderly patients reported 14 per cent had folate deficiency and 9 per cent had a low B_{12} level.

WORKUP

The diagnosis of anemia is based on measurement of the *hematocrit* and/or *hemoglobin concentration* of venous blood. Any abnormal test result should be repeated for confirmation before further evaluation is undertaken. Proper interpretation requires consideration of the patient's volume status. An overly expanded plasma volume will dilute the red cell mass and lead to a false positive diagnosis of anemia. Conversely, dehydration may mask an underlying anemia by causing an artificially elevated reading.

A *Wright-stained smear* of the peripheral blood and the red cell indices should be obtained and studied in order to categorize the anemia (see Table 77-1) and facilitate diagnosis.

It is of utmost importance that the physician personally review the peripheral smear; reliance on indices alone or laboratory reports of the smear can be misleading. The smear and indices should be examined in conjunction with one another, for there can be discrepancies. For example, a mixed anemia produces a dimorphic population of macrocytes and microcytes on smear, but the average of the two populations results in normal red cell indices by electronic counter. Cells which easily flatten out (as in liver disease) may appear larger on smear than they actually are; correlating indices with morphology helps to avoid misinterpretation. The nucleus of the mature small lymphocyte is a good reference for normal red blood cell size on smear. One can also make a control smear of known blood to help judge abnormalities. Once a morphologic categorization is made, further evaluation can commence, often with careful review of the appearances of all blood elements on smear.

Microcytic Hypochromic Anemias

The basis for classification is hypochromia and microcytosis as manifested by small red cells with an increase in the area of central pallor on smear, a mean corpuscular hemoglobin concentration below 32, and a mean corpuscular volume below 82. In early stages, not all features may be present. History should focus on any abnormal blood loss, change in bowel habits, melena, heavy aspirin use, family history of anemia (especially in those of Mediterranean descent), concurrent malignancy, symptoms of chronic infection or chronic inflammatory process, number of pregnancies, pica, dysphagia, history of lead exposure, dietary iron intake, quantity of menstrual blood loss, gastric resection, changes in nails and soreness of the tongue. Physical examination includes checking for glossitis, cheilitis, koilonychia, splenomegaly, rectal mass, guaiac positivity, pelvic mass and signs of chronic infectious, inflammatory or neoplastic disorders.

The most useful tests in evaluation of microcytic hypochromic anemias are the *serum iron, total iron-binding capacity* (TIBC) and calculation of the *per-cent saturation* [(Fe/TIBC) × 100]. Percent saturation is a sensitive measure of iron deficiency. In a study of 132 patients with documented iron deficiency, including 17 with normochromic normocytic smears, all had percent saturations of 16 per cent or less. However, the specificity of the test is limited by the finding that some patients with the anemia of chronic disease also have per cent saturations which fall below 16 per cent. The more typical pattern in anemia of chronic disease is a low iron and low TIBC in contrast to the low iron and increased TIBC characteristic of iron deficiency.

When it is unclear whether the cause of the anemia is iron deficiency or chronic disease, a determination of marrow iron stores by *needle aspiration* or *serum ferritin* level will settle the issue, since these are the most sensitive and specific tests of iron deficiency. Iron stores are very low or absent in iron deficiency and normal or increased in anemia of chronic disease; serum ferritin follows a similar pattern. Previously, it was necessary to do a bone marrow aspiration on such patients. However, the development of a sensitive immunoradioassay for serum ferritin and the demonstration that levels below 12 ng/per ml. correlate with absence of marrow iron stores suggest that marrow study can be avoided. A simple alternative to ferritin or marrow study is to prescribe a clinical trial of oral iron, monitoring the reticulocyte count over a week to 10 days. A significant rise in the reticulocyte count is strong evidence for the diagnosis of iron deficiency. Microcytic anemias with low serum irons which fail to respond can then be studied by ferritin or marrow evaluation.

In thalassemia, serum iron is normal or increased, and the iron-binding capacity and the per cent saturation are normal. In hemoglobinopathies, the serum iron and iron-binding capacity are normal as well. In sideroblastic anemias, the serum iron is increased and the total iron-binding capacity decreased.

If serum iron and iron-binding capacity are *normal* and the patient is of Mediterranean extraction, a *hemoglobin A_2 determination* can help make the di-

agnosis of thalassemia trait. Similarly, *hemoglobin electrophoresis* can help detect an abnormal hemoglobin. If the serum iron is *increased,* a check of the hemoglobin A_2 level is needed to rule out thalassemia; a *marrow aspirate,* in which increased numbers of abnormal sideroblasts are sought, is also needed.

To summarize:
1. The important initial tests in the evaluation of microcytic hypochromic anemia are a determination of the serum iron, total iron-binding capacity, and percent saturation.
2. When percent saturation is below 16 per cent, a diagnositc trial of iron therapy can be tried.
3. Alternatively, a serum ferritin determination and/or bone marrow aspiration can be ordered.
4. Hemoglobin electrophoresis and A_2 determination and, occasionally, bone marrow study supplement the workup when serum iron is normal or increased.

Macrocytic Anemias

The criteria for inclusion in this group are a mean corpuscular volume greater than 100, a normal mean corpuscular hemoglobin concentration, and macrocytes on smear. (Often the latter are hard to detect in mild cases.) Marked macrocytosis identified electronically is clinically significant. For example, in a study of 100 patients with mean corpuscular volumes (MCV) greater than 115, over half had folate and/or B_{12} deficiency; another 25 per cent had liver disease or alcoholism accompanied by liver disease.

The first objective is to distinguish megaloblastic from nonmegaloblastic causes. The *peripheral smear* is the single most helpful test. Hypersegmented polymorphonuclear leukocytes are the earliest and most specific sign of a megaloblastic anemia, seen in over 65 per cent of cases. Oval macrocytes are also characteristic. An increase in hypersegmented polys can be screened for by counting the number of neutrophils with five or more lobes in a routine 100-cell differential. Finding three neutrophils with five lobes or even one with six is strong presumptive evidence for megaloblastic anemia. *Bone marrow aspiration* may be needed in confusing situations, but in most instances a peripheral smear should do. It must be remembered that megaloblastic marrow changes can revert to normal within 12 to 24 hours of therapy, and thus treatment should be delayed if marrow examination is anticipated. However, neutrophil hypersegmentation may persist for up to 2 weeks after onset of vitamin replacement.

If the anemia has been identified as megaloblastic, the next step is to determine whether it is due to folate or B_{12} deficiency. History and physical examination can give important clues. A history of gastric surgery or raw fish intake, or symptoms of terminal ileal disease, vitiligo, hypothyroidism, steatorrhea, glossitis or subacute combined system disease suggest B_{12} deficiency. Alcoholism, poor nutrition, pregnancy, blood dyscrasias, sprue, severe psoriasis, and anticonvulsant intake suggest folate lack. Antimetabolite therapy with folate antagonists such as methotrexate can cause a megaloblastic picture with normal serum folate levels.

Obviously, *serum folate* and *B_{12} determinations* are helpful, but there are a number of pitfalls in interpreting the results. Many assays for B_{12} levels are bioassays; recent antibiotic intake can interfere with them. Recent green vegetable intake can cause a false rise in the folate level. Also, B_{12} levels may be low in patients with folate deficiency alone; thus, both folate and B_{12} levels must always be measured together.

A *therapeutic trial* of folate or B_{12} (they should never be given simultaneously) can be used when serum assays are unavailable or the results confusing. The hematocrit and reticulocyte counts are measured twice prior to administration, then followed every few days up to 10 days after a small but effective dose of B_{12} (*e.g.,* 100 mg. I.M.) or folate (1 mg. I.M.) is given. The trial is positive if a significant rise in reticulocyte count occurs within 10 days. Large doses are not used because they can cause a nonspecific reticulocytosis in patients with megaloblastic anemias.

To distinguish B_{12} deficiency due to malabsorption from that due to lack of intrinsic factor, an *oral Schilling test* with and without intrinsic factor is used. An unlabeled intramuscular dose of 1,000 μg of B_{12} is given to saturate binding sites prior to the oral radioactive dose. Both urine and plasma levels of labeled B_{12} are measured to maximize accuracy. The difficulty with the test is that B_{12} deficiency can itself cause malabsorption, confusing test interpretation. Thus, the test should be postponed until the deficiency is corrected. In malabsorptive states there will be no improvement with intrinsic factor, whereas there will be in pernicious anemia. Currently, there is no reliable test widely available for determining folate malabsorption.

Nonmegaloblastic macrocytic cases can be divided into subgroups in which marrow activity is increased, normal or decreased. To make this determination, a *reticulocyte count* is needed. The normal range is 0.8 to 2.5 per cent in males and 0.8 to 4.1 per cent in females. To correct for the degree of anemia, the reticulocyte count is multiplied by the hematocrit and divided by 0.45. Increased reticulocytes are due to hemorrhage or hemolysis. Normal or decreased levels occur in myxedema, liver disease, myelophthisic states, chronic disease and hypoplastic anemia. The patient should be questioned and examined carefully for symptoms of any of these conditions, and the smear studied again. In myelophthisic processes, there may be a particularly large number of teardrops on peripheral smear; a *bone marrow biopsy* will confirm the diagnosis.

To summarize:
1. Peripheral smear is examined for hypersegmented polys and oval macrocytes.
2. If they are present, serum B_{12} and folate levels are ordered.
3. Alternatively, a diagnostic trial of a small dose of B_{12} or folate can be performed, monitoring reticulocyte count.
4. When B_{12} deficiency is detected, a Schilling test is helpful to differentiate between lack of intrinsic factor and malabsorption.
5. The reticulocyte count and peripheral smear examination are important to evaluation of nonmegaloblastic cases; bone marrow biopsy is indicated if a myelophthisic process is suspected.

Normochromic Normocytic Anemias

This category encompasses a diverse group of conditions which can be classified according to marrow response. A *reticulocyte count* is obtained. If increased, it suggests hemolysis or recent hemorrhage. If there is no history of recent hemorrhage. A careful drug history, an examination for splenomegaly, and determinations of bilirubin, haptoglobin, and lactic dehydrogenase (LDH), and a Coombs test should be undertaken to assess the possibility of hemolysis. Common drugs implicated in the different types of drug-induced immune hemolytic anemias include quinidine, penicillin, methyldopa and the cephalosporins. Bone marrow examination in cases of hemolysis is unnecessary.

If the reticulocyte count is not appropriately elevated, a search for metabolic causes of marrow suppression, such as renal failure, myxedema, Addison's disease and alcoholic liver disease is in order. In addition, early iron deficiency may present as a normochromic, normocytic anemia, as can the anemia of chronic disease. A serum iron and total iron-binding capacity should be checked and a calculation of the per cent saturation made. If the *peripheral smear* shows considerable numbers of teardrop forms and fragmented cells, suggesting a myelophthisic process, a *bone marrow biopsy* is indicated (an aspiration of the marrow may only yield a dry tap).

A very low or absent reticulocyte count is suggestive of an aplastic anemia, especially if accompanied by evidence of pancytopenia on peripheral smear and cell counts. History of drug use (e. g., chloramphenicol, phenylbutazone, antimetabolites, gold), toxin exposure (benzene, insecticides) or recent viral illness may provide a clue to etiology. In the majority of instances, the history is unrevealing. Bone marrow biopsy is diagnostic.

To summarize:
1. The reticulocyte count is checked.
2. If the count is elevated, evidence for recent hemorrhage or hemolysis is sought.
3. If the reticulocyte count is not elevated, a search for underlying renal, endocrine or liver disease should be undertaken, as well as an evaluation for early iron deficiency anemia and anemia or chronic disease.
4. If the peripheral smear shows many teardrop forms and fragmented cells, a marrow biopsy is indicated.
5. If the reticulocyte count is practically zero and the peripheral blood count and smear show a pancytopenia, a marrow biopsy is necessary.

SYMPTOMATIC THERAPY

Few patients who present with an anemia of gradual onset require immediate correction of the anemia. The one exception is the patient with angina who may be compromised by the decrease in oxygen-carrying capacity. In almost all other instances, evaluation should proceed in an orderly manner and therapy withheld until a specific diagnosis can be made and a specific therapy implemented (see Chapter 83). The all too common practice of simultaneously prescribing multiple hematinics can obscure important findings. The elderly and others with symptoms and limited cardiopulmonary reserve should be admitted for inpatient evaluation and consideration of transfusion therapy.

PATIENT EDUCATION

Patients commonly think an anemia is due to vitamin or iron deficiencies. Many try self-treatment prior to seeing a physician; others request vitamin therapy. A common error among both patients and physicians is to attribute symptoms of depression, such as fatigue and listlessness, to an underlying anemia. Unless the hematocrit is well below 30, or the patient has very little cardiopulmonary reserve, this attribution is unjustified (see Chapter 5).

The patient needs to be told to what extent his anemia accounts for his symptoms, what the possible causes are, and what the appropriate workup will involve. Attention to these details is likely to enlist patient cooperation, lessen anxiety, and foster a better working relationship between doctor and patient.

ANNOTATED BIBLIOGRAPHY

Bainton, D., and Finch, C.: The diagnosis of iron-deficiency anemia. Am. J. Med., *37*:62, 1964. *(A classic study examining the specificity and sensitivity of the serum iron, TIBC and percent saturation.)*

Cartwright, G.: The anemia of chronic disorders. Semin. Hematol., *3*:351, 1966. *(Excellent review with 73 references.)*

Committee on Iron Deficiency: Iron deficiency in the United States. JAMA, *203*:407, 1968. *(Documents the absence of hypochromia in microcytosis early in the course of iron deficiency. The earliest findings are loss of stainable iron in the marrow and fall in the serum iron with rise in the total iron-binding capacity. Good review of epidemiology and workup.)*

Conrad, M., and Crosby, W.: The natural history of iron deficiency induced by phlebotomy. Blood, *20*:173, 1962. *(Anemia is the earliest change in peripheral blood; microcytosis and hypochromia follow.)*

Edwin, E.: The segmentation of polymorphonuclear neutrophils in hypovitaminosis B_{12}. Acta Med. Scan., *182*:401, 1967. *(Sixty-four per cent of patients with B_{12} deficiency exhibited hypersegmentation on smear. Good discussion of errors in counting lobes.)*

Entisham, M., and Cape, R.: Diagnosing and treating anemia. Geriatrics, *32*:99, 1977. *(Good summary of studies of anemia in the elderly.)*

Fairbanks, V.: Diagnostic tests for iron deficiency. Ann. Intern. Med., *75*: 640, 1971. *(A study of the utility of the serum iron, TIBC, per cent saturation and marrow.)*

Frank, M.M. et al: Pathophysiology of immune hemolytic anemia. Ann. Intern. Med., *87*:210, 1977. *(A lucid review of types and their mechanisms.)*

Fry, J.: Clinical patterns and course of anemias in general practice. Br. Med. J., *2*:1732, 1961. *(Clinical epidemiology of anemia as seen in a London general practice.)*

Lindenbaum, J.: Small intestinal function in B_{12} deficiency. Ann. Intern. Med., *80*:326, 1974. *(Provides evidence for malabsorption due to, rather than as a cause of, B_{12} deficiency.)*

Lipschitz, D., Cook, J., and Finch, C.: A clinical evaluation of serum ferritin as an index of iron stores. N. Engl. J. Med., *290*:1213, 1974. *(A study correlating serum ferritin levels with iron stores; a level of less than 12 ng./ml. was specific for iron deficiency.)*

McPhedran, P., et al: Interpretation of electronically determined macrocytosis. Ann. Intern. Med., *78*: 677, 1973. *(The finding of an MCV greater than 115 was associated with folate or B_{12} deficiency in over 50 per cent and with liver disease in another 25 per cent.)*

Nath, B.J., Lindenbaum, J.: Persistence of neutrophil hypersegmentation during recovery from megaloblastic granulopoiesis. Ann. Intern. Med., *90*: 757, 1979. *(Hypersegmentation may persist up to two weeks after onset of therapy.)*

Taymor, M., Sturgis, S., and Yahia, C.: The etiological role of chronic iron deficiency in production of menorrhagia. JAMA, *187*:323, 1974. *(A double-blind study documenting iron superior to placebo in improving menorrhagia.)*

Tudhope, G., and Wilson, G.: Anemia in hypothyroidism. Q. J. Med., *29*:513, 1960. *(A detailed hematologic study of 116 cases of hypothyroidism revealing anemia in over 30 per cent; pernicious anemia occurred in 7 per cent.)*

Van der Weyden, M., Rother, M., and Firkin, B.: Metabolic significance of reduced B_{12} in folate deficiency. Blood, *40*:23, 1972. *(Low B_{12} levels can occur in folate deficiency; the reduction is usually moderate and improves with folic acid replacement.)*

Victor, M., and Lear, A.: Subacute combined degeneration of the spinal cord. Value of serum B_{12} determinations. Am. J. Med., *20*:896, 1956. *(The neurologic deficits may occur in the absence of anemia.)*

Wood, M., and Elwood, P.: Symptoms of iron deficiency anemia: A community survey. Br. J. Prev. Soc. Med., *20*:117, 1966. *(In 295 patients studied, there was little correlation between symptoms and serum hemoglobin concentration.)*

78
Evaluation of Polycythemia
BEVERLY WOO, M.D.

An elevated red cell count, hemoglobin concentration, or hematocrit often occurs as an unexpected finding, noted coincidentally on obtaining an automated complete blood count. The upper limit of normal for a hematocrit is 52 per cent for males, 47 per cent for females. In the context of marked dehydration or severe lung disease, the elevation comes as no surprise; but in the absence of such concurrent disease, a search for an underlying cause is warranted. Possible etiologies include polycythemia vera, occult malignancy, right-to-left shunts, and hemoglobinopathies. The finding may even be spurious. In most instances, the primary physician should be able to distinguish among the variety of etiologies on clinical grounds, aided by a few simple laboratory studies.

PATHOPHYSIOLOGY AND CLINICAL PRESENTATION

True polycythemia, as opposed to relative or spurious polycythemia, is defined as an absolute increase in red cell mass. It may represent a stem cell defect, as in polycythemia vera, or be triggered by excess erythropoietin production, as in the secondary polycythemias.

Polycythemia vera is a myeloproliferative disorder. The etiology is not completely understood, but the disease appears to occur secondary to an intrinsic cellular defect and is not dependent on erythropoietin. It is characterized by abnormal proliferation of all blood elements in the bone marrow and extramedullary sites, producing absolute erythrocytosis, leukocytosis, thrombocytosis, splenomegaly, a hypercellular bone marrow and, often, myeloid metaplasia and myelofibrosis. Polycythemia vera is an uncommon disease, with an incidence in the United States of 4 to 5 cases per million per year, or about 1000 new cases in the U.S. per year. However, the prevalence of the disease is relatively higher because of the long life span in the majority of patients. The peak age of onset is 50 to 60.

A small percentage of patients with polycythemia vera have a relatively benign course, with red cell volume controlled by occasional phlebotomy, and pruritus and hyperuricemia controlled by medication. Polycythemia vera can evolve into a malignant, disordered condition with the development of myeloid metaplasia, myelofibrosis and acute leukemia.

It is not surprising that the presence of true polycythemia is often unsuspected, since symptoms develop gradually and are frequently vague and rather nonspecific. Most are attributable to hyperviscosity, hypervolemia and consequent sluggish blood flow which take place when the hematocrit rises above 55. Headache, dizziness, vertigo, tinnitus, fullness of the head, and blurred vision are among the common neurologic symptoms. Patients may complain of angina pectoris or claudication when there is coexisting atherosclerotic disease. Generalized weakness, fatigue, sweating and lassitude are frequently reported. Gastrointestinal complaints may predominate—for example, fullness, belching, epigastric discomfort. In polycythemia vera, a classic symptom is pruritus after bathing, believed due to abnormal histamine release. Also, gouty joint complaints occur in the context of marked secondary hyperuricemia caused by increased cell turnover. Left upper quadrant discomfort is a manifestation of the significant splenomegaly usually seen in polycythemia vera.

Hemostasis is disturbed in polycythemia vera due to hyperviscosity and defects in platelet function. Patients may present with bleeding in uncommon sites, such as hepatic, mesenteric or retinal veins, or with bleeding in the form of epistaxis, menorrhagia, easy bruisability or oozing from the gums.

On examination, the patient has a deep red appearance; peripheral cyanosis and ecchymosis may be noted. Blood pressure is usually normal. Hepatomegaly is present in 40 per cent and splenomegaly in 70 per cent.

Secondary polycythemia (erythrocytosis) represents the majority of cases of increased red cell mass. The increase is usually an appropriate physiological response to tissue hypoxia, and occurs when the PaO_2 falls chronically below 55 mm. Hg or, more precisely, when the arterial oxygen saturation (SaO_2) drops below 92 per cent. Obvious mechanisms of hypoxia include residence at high altitudes and severe pulmonary disease, but cyanotic heart disease, increased carboxyhemoglobin from heavy cigarette smoking, and hemoglobinopathies with high affinities for oxygen can have a similar deleterious effect on tissue oxygenation.

Decreased tissue oxygenation is thought to be detected in the kidneys, causing release of erythrogenin, which acts enzymatically on a plasma protein substrate to form erythropoietin. There also seems to be a less sensitive nonrenal system for detecting tissue hypoxia and producing erythropoietin. Erythropoietin is a glycoprotein hormone which stimulates RNA synthesis, causing hematopoietic precursor cells to proliferate and differentiate into early erythroblasts. These cells mature at a faster than normal rate; early release of reticulocytes from the marrow and increased heme synthesis results. The increase in red cell mass improves tissue oxygenation, to the extent that hyperviscosity does not compromise it.

Pathologic secondary polycythemia results from inappropriate erythropoietin production, occurring autonomously in the absence of generalized tissue hypoxia. Renal diseases and a host of malignancies have been implicated. Inappropriate erythropoietin levels due to renal disorders and malignancies are very unusual occurrences, but it is important to be aware of them since polycythemia may be a clue to their existence. About 1 to 3 per cent of renal cell carcinomas have erythrocytosis as a manifestation. Hydronephrosis and renal cystic diseases are occasionally associated with elevations in erythropoietin; the mechanism is felt to be a reduction in blood flow to normal tissue due to compression. Huge uterine myomas, cerebellar hemangiomas and hepatomas are also causes, although the mechanisms are unclear; up to 10 per cent of hepatoma patients in one series had erythrocytosis.

Relative polycythemia refers to an increase in hemoglobin concentration or hematocrit which occurs without a rise in red cell mass. It results from severe volume depletion, as encountered in burns, protracted diarrhea or vomiting, etc. *Spurious polycythemia*, also known as stress erythrocytosis or Gaisbock's syndrome, is a variant of relative polycythemia, associated with a low-normal plasma volume and high-normal red cell mass. Most patients with spurious polycythemia are middle-aged men with obesity, hypertension and stress. The basis for the abnormality is unknown.

DIFFERENTIAL DIAGNOSIS

Patients with polycythemia can be separated into three diagnostic categories: (1) polycythemia vera, (2) secondary polycythemia, and (3) relative or spurious polycythemia. Secondary polycythemia may present as a physiological response to tissue hypoxia, as in high altitude living, cyanotic congenital heart disease, severe pulmonary disease, hemoglobinopathies and cigarette smoking. Secondary polycythemias which occur without a hypoxic stimulus are seen in some cases of renal cell carcinoma, hydronephrosis, renal cystic disease, uterine myoma, cerebellar hemangioma and hepatoma. Relative polycythemia can be caused by any condition producing severe volume depletion, for example, protracted vomiting, persistent diarrhea or excessive diuretic use. Spurious polycythemia is an idiopathic condition.

WORKUP

History. The first objective is to differentiate patients with polycythemia vera from those with secondary polycythemias. Important historical points suggesting a secondary polycythemia include high altitude residence, known congenital heart disease, history of heart murmur and cyanosis, smoking more than two packs per day, symptoms of chronic lung disease, familial occurrence, and history of renal cystic disease. Patients with polycythemia vera are free of such history and should be checked for symptoms of hyperviscosity or bleeding, such as lassitude, headache, pruritus, sweating, easy bruising, abdominal pain, menorrhagia and epistaxis. History of diuretic use, vomiting, diarrhea, hypertension and stress suggest relative or spurious polycythemias.

Physical examination includes checking for hypertension, cyanosis, clubbing, ecchymoses, signs of chronic lung disease, heart murmurs, hepatic en-

largement, splenomegaly, and abdominal and pelvic masses.

Laboratory evaluation should begin with a *complete blood count, platelet count* and *peripheral blood smear examination*. Two-thirds of patients with polycythemia vera have an elevated WBC count, usually to 12,000–25,000/mm^3, and occasionally as high as 50,000–100,000/mm^3, with increased immature forms and basophils. Half of polycythemia vera patients have thrombocytosis, with platelet counts in the 450,000 to 1,000,000 per mm^3 range. Large, bizarre platelets and megakaryocytic fragments may be seen on the blood smear. In secondary and spurious polycythemia, the WBC, platelet count and blood smear are normal. In polycythemia vera, red cell morphology becomes abnormal with progression of disease. With the development of myeloid metaplasia, anisocytosis and poikilocytosis with teardrop forms, ovalocytes, elliptocytes and nucleated red blood cells are seen.

An *arterial blood gas* with *oxygen saturation* (SaO$_2$) determination is important in the assessment of less obvious cases. A PaO$_2$ less than 55 mm. Hg and a SaO$_2$ less than 92 per cent indicate significant hypoxemia. In two-pack-per-day cigarette smokers, the SaO$_2$ determination that is calculated from the measured PaO$_2$ and a standard blood oxygen dissociation curve may be misleading. This method will given an erroneously high SaO$_2$ if carboxyhemoglobin levels are elevated; polycythemia due to increased carboxyhemoglobin will be missed. This problem can be avoided by ordering an SaO$_2$ determination that is measured directly rather than calculated from PaO$_2$.

The diagnostic criteria for polycythemia vera are an elevated total red cell volume, normal SaO$_2$ and splenomegaly. In the absence of splenomegaly, at least two of the following should be present: an elevation in platelet count (over 400,000/mm^3), white cell count (over 12,000/mm^3), leukocyte alkaline phosphatase, serum B$_{12}$ level, or unbound B$_{12}$-binding capacity.

If polycythemia vera and hypoxia-induced secondary polycythemia are ruled out, one should look for signs and symptoms of renal lesions and tumors, especially renal cell carcinoma. An *IVP* with *nephrotomograms* may be diagnostic. When there is a strong family history of polycythemia, one should obtain a hemoglobin electrophoresis in search of a mutant hemoglobin with an abnormally high oxygen affinity.

The patient suspected to have a spurious polycythemia can usually be identified clinically (middle-aged male with hypertension, obesity and stressful life-style). The measurement of total red cell volume should be reserved for the unresolved case in which polycythemia vera cannot be distinguished from spurious erythrocytosis.

SYMPTOMATIC THERAPY

The therapy of polycythemia is aimed at elimination of the primary cause when possible, for example, correction of a right-to-left shunt. The cessation of cigarette smoking (see Chapter 49) will normalize carboxyhemoglobin levels. For selected patients with severe chronic obstructive pulmonary disease, chronic oxygen therapy may normalize arterial oxygen saturation (see Chapter 44). When tumors or renal lesions are removed, secondary polycythemia often disappears.

When the cause of polycythemia cannot be removed, blood volume should be controlled by phlebotomy. Up to 500 cc. of blood can be removed as often as every 2 to 3 days to lower the hematocrit below 55 and alleviate the symptoms due to hyperviscosity and hypervolemia. In patients who are elderly or have a compromised cardiovascular system, smaller volumes of blood should be removed once or twice per week. Replacement with plasma volume expanders is usually unnecessary. Patients should not undergo surgery unless blood volume has been controlled adequately. Phlebotomy can provide gratifying relief of hyperviscosity symptoms and prevent the thromboembolic and hemorrhagic complications of polycythemia in patients with secondary polycythemia and indolent polycythemia vera.

Control of polycythemia vera with phlebotomy alone is possible when platelet and WBC counts are relatively normal. Pruritus can usually be minimized with cholestyramine (4 gm. t.i.d.) or cyproheptadine (4 to 16 mg. per day), and gout can be prevented with allopurinol (see Chapter 149). Most cases of polycythemia vera require treatment with radioactive phosphorus (^{32}P) or alkylating agents, because phlebotomy fails to control thrombocytosis, reduce painful splenomegaly, or keep up with very active disease. Control has been achieved in more than 80 per cent of cases with the use of chlorambucil or ^{32}P. The International Polycythemia Vera Study Group indicates that for patients over 40 years of age, carefully administered myelosuppressive therapy supplemented by phlebotomy will give the most favorable prognosis. The influence of phlebotomy, ^{32}P therapy and chemotherapy on survival and development of acute leukemia is under investigation.

PATIENT EDUCATION AND INDICATIONS FOR REFERRAL

Patient education is essential to encourage smokers to give up cigarettes (see Chapter 49) and chronic obstructive pulmonary disease patients to follow a maximal program for improving oxygenation (see Chapter 44). The patient's understanding of the basis of his disease and its prognosis should help in achieving compliance (see Chapter 1). When polycythemia vera is diagnosed, patients should be referred to a hematologist for design of a treatment program. Referral is also appropriate when diagnosis is difficult and measurement of red cell mass or bone marrow biopsy are being considered.

ANNOTATED BIBLIOGRAPHY

Adamson, J.W.: Familial polycythemia. Semin. Hematol., *12*:383, 1975. (*Molecular and physiological mechanisms of familial polycythemias.*)

Balcerzak, S.P., and Bromberg, P.A.: Secondary polycythemia. Semin. Hematol., *12*:353, 1975. (*Excellent review of pulmonary physiology related to tissue hypoxia-induced polycythemia and other classes of secondary polycythemia.*)

Berlin, N.I.: Diagnosis and classification of the polycythemias. Semin. Hematol., *12*:339, 1975. (*Reviews differential diagnosis and workup of polycythemia.*)

Brown, S.M.: Spurious (relative) polycythemia: A nonexistent disease. Am. J. Med., *50*:200, 1971. (*Patients with this condition were men with high normal red cell masses and low normal plasma volumes.*)

Modan, B.: An epidemiological study of polycythemia vera. Blood, *26*:657, 1965. (*Incidence was 4 per million; median age was 60. Sex ratio was close to 1:1.*)

Smith, J.R., and Landaw, S.A.: Smokers' polycythemia. N. Engl. J. Med., *298*:6, 1978. (*Occurs in heavy smokers and resolves when smoking is stopped.*)

Thomas, D.J., et al.: Cerebral blood-flow in polycythemia. Lancet, *2*:161, 1977. (*Documents marked reduction in blood flow that returns to normal after repeated phlebotomies.*)

Wasserman, L.R.: The treatment of polycythemia vera. Semin. Hematol., *13*:57, 1975. *(The natural history of P. vera and preliminary findings of the P. vera study group.)*

Weinreb, N.G., and Shih, C.F.: Spurious polycythemia. Semin. Hematol., *12*:397, 1975. *(Review of the topic and results of study of 69 patients.)*

79

Evaluation of Thrombocytopenia

Thrombocytopenia is not a common problem in office practice, but may be encountered in the context of evaluating a patient who presents with petechiae, purpura, or a bleeding problem. A normal platelet count ranges from 150,000 to 300,000 per mm³. Counts below 100,000 are considered abnormal, but spontaneous bleeding rarely occurs until the count falls below 20,000. The first determination to be made is whether there is a significant risk of severe hemorrhage mandating urgent hospital admission. If severe hemorrhage is not imminent, outpatient evaluation can commence.

PATHOPHYSIOLOGY AND CLINICAL PRESENTATION

Thrombocytopenia may result from increased platelet destruction, decreased production, or abnormal pooling. *Increased destruction* of platelets is the most common cause of thrombocytopenia. The primary mechanism is immunologic, induced either by drugs, viruses, lymphoproliferative disorders or systemic lupus erythematosus. For example, certain drugs are believed to act as haptens; they bind to serum proteins to form the antigen and stimulate antibody production. The platelet is destroyed when it adsorbs the antigen-antibody complex. Thrombocytopenia following viral infection generally occurs 1 to 2 weeks after viral illness, suggesting the formation of antibodies that either damage the platelet or cause formation of platelet antibodies.

Among the important causes of increased platelet destruction is *idiopathatic thrombocytopenic purpura* (ITP). The condition is more common in young adults, children and women and is different in adults than in children in that the course is a chronic waxing and waning one with few spontaneous remissions. The spleen is usually not palpable, though it might be slightly enlarged. There is no lymphadenopathy, hepatomegaly, or sternal tenderness. Mild fever is sometimes seen.

Drug-induced thrombocytopenia is an idiosyncratic reaction, with quinidine among the most frequently involved agents. Rapid fall in platelet count to levels below 10,000 are not uncommon, and acute hemorrhage may ensue. Prompt return of the count to safe levels is typical as soon as the responsible drug is withheld.

The thrombocytopenias associated with *chronic lymphocytic leukemia* (CLL) and *systemic lupus erythematosus* (SLE) follow clinical patterns similar to ITP. In addition, lymphadenopathy and splenomegaly are found in the majority of patients with CLL, and 25 per cent have hepatomegaly as well. In SLE, arthritis and arthralgias are reported in 90 per cent, skin rash in 70 per cent, lymphadenopathy in 60 per cent and renal disease in 50 per cent (see Chapter 139). Platelet counts below 100,000 are not frequent, being reported in about 15 per cent of cases.

Decreased production implies bone marrow failure. The bone marrow may be suppressed by drugs, depressed after a viral infection, or replaced by tumor (see Chapter 77). Thrombocytopenias due to conditions causing *marrow failure* or a *myelophthisic process* usually occur in the context of a generalized pancytopenia. On occasion, individual drugs cause selective *inhibition of platelet production*. Chlorothiazide, tolbutamide, and ethanol are among the best documented. Megakaryocyte production suffers in *megaloblastic anemia* and quickly improves with replacement therapy. Transient thrombocytopenia may follow influenza, hepatitis, rubella, and other diseases.

Increased pooling can be seen in disorders associated with an abnormally enlarged spleen. Splenomegaly results in excessive trapping and a fall in number of circulating platelets.

Regardless of etiology, there are a few characteristic features of the blood loss due to thrombocytopenia. Typical are the appearance of petechiae and slow oozing after trauma, rather than brisk bleeding. Mucosal bleeding is common and menorrhagia or epistaxis may be presenting complaints.

Table 79–1. Important Causes
of Thrombocytopenia

Decreased Production
  1. Drugs (e.g., thiazides, alcohol)
  2. Viral infection (e.g., influenza, hepatitis)
  3. Megaloblastic anemia
  4. Generalized marrow failure
  5. Myelophthisic process
Accelerated Destruction
  1. Drug-induced immunologic injury (e.g., quinidine, methyldopa, sulfonamides, phenytoin, digitoxin, barbiturates)
  2. Systemic lupus erythematosus
  3. Chronic lymphocytic leukemia
  4. Infection
  5. Idiopathic thrombocytopenic purpura
Increased Sequestration
  1. Hypersplenism

DIFFERENTIAL DIAGNOSIS

The causes of thrombocytopenia can be grouped according to pathophysical mechanisms, i.e., increased destruction, decreased production or sequestration (Table 79–1). Drug reactions and ITP are the most frequent etiologies encountered in adults.

WORKUP

History. It is essential to obtain a complete drug history. All nonessential drugs should be stopped and essential medications changed if possible while the patient is evaluated. Failure of platelets to return to normal 7 days after cessation of medication rules out a drug etiology. A history of viral infection and symptoms suggestive of lupus (see Chapter 139) should be sought.

Physical examination can be used to define the extent of bleeding by checking for postural signs and examining the mouth, nose, urine, and stool for evidence of blood loss. Petechiae and purpuric lesions ought to be noted and if prominent, outlined with a marking pen so that progress, regression, or appearance of new lesions can be monitored. The lymph nodes, liver and spleen need to be palpated for enlargement. Joints are examined for signs of arthritis, suggestive of lupus; hemarthrosis is not characteristic of thrombocytopenia.

Laboratory studies begin with a complete blood count, platelet count and peripheral smear examination. The finding of megathrombocytes on peripheral smear suggests accelerated platelet production in response to increased peripheral destruction. When a drug-induced thrombocytopenia seems obvious, a bone marrow biopsy need not be done; otherwise, biopsy is essential to distinguish increased peripheral destruction from decreased marrow production. If marrow examination reveals abundant megakaryocytes, a diagnosis of increased peripheral destruction is established, while the absence of megakaryocytes suggests failure of platelet production. Examination of the bone marrow may also reveal a specific cause of impaired production, such as megaloblastic anemia, aplastic anemia, or tumor replacement. If there is active bleeding, bone marrow biopsy should be deferred until hemostasis can be assured; sternal aspiration may be substituted.

In patients with a presumed immunologic etiology, a Coombs test to check for an associated hemolytic anemia and an antinuclear antibody determination to exclude the diagnosis of lupus are indicated. Detection of antiplatelet antibody titers is available as a research tool and may in time provide clinically important information. Currently it is not an essential diagnostic test.

INDICATIONS FOR ADMISSION

The decision to hospitalize should be based on evidence of clinical bleeding, not solely on the platelet count. In most healthy patients with decreased platelets, the entire workup can be safely accomplished on an outpatient basis. The presence of bleeding, so-called wet purpura, or a platelet count below 20,000 is an indication for hospital admission.

PATIENT EDUCATION

The outpatient with a marginal platelet count should be advised to (1) avoid dangerous activity, particularly contact sports, (2) stop all nonessential medications, (3) report any bleeding, (4) come to the doctor when any sign of infection occurs (because platelet count and platelet function may be reduced by infection) and (5) use stool softeners to avoid straining and a soft toothbrush to prevent bleeding.

ANNOTATED BIBLIOGRAPHY

Clancy, R., et al.: Qualitative platelet abnormalities in ITP. N. Engl. J. Med., *286*:622, 1972. *(Study demonstrated impaired platelet aggregation in 9 of 11 patients with chronic ITP.)*

Cowan and Hines. Thrombocytopenia of severe alcoholism. Ann. Intern. Med., *74*:37, 1971. *(Alcohol depresses production and decreases platelet survival.)*

Evans, R.S.: Primary thrombocytopenic purpura and acquired hemolytic anemia. Arch. Intern. Med., *87*:48, 1951. *(The original description of Evan's syndrome.)*

Garg, S.K., et al.: Use of megathrombocyte as an index of magakaryocyte number. N. Engl. J. Med., *284*:11, 1971. *(This article showed that megathrombocytes in the peripheral smear are an index of bone marrow megakaryocyte activity.)*

Karpatkin, S.: Autoimmune thrombocytopenia pur-

pura. Am. J. Med. Sci., *261*:127, 1971. *(Excellent review.)*

Karpatkin, S.: Drug-induced thrombocytopenia. Am. J. Med. Sci., *262*:69, 1971. *(A case of aldactone-induced thrombocytopenia plus a review finding quinine, quinidine, chlorothiazide, and acetazolamide the most common offenders.)*

Karpatkin, S., et al.: Cumulative experience in the detection of antiplatelet antibody in 234 patients with idiopathic thrombocytopenic purpura, systemic lupus erythematosus and other clinical disorders. Am. J. Med., *52*:776, 1972. *(Antibody was detected in 65 per cent of ITP patients.)*

Miescher, P.A.: Drug-induced thrombocytopenia. Semin. Hematol., *10*:31, 1975. *(A good review.)*

80
Evaluation of Lymphadenopathy
HARVEY B. SIMON, M.D.

Of the nearly 600 lymph nodes throughout the body, only a few are normally palpable, including small nodes in the submandibular, axillary and inguinal regions. Nevertheless, lymphadenopathy is a very common presenting symptom. Most often, adenopathy indicates benign, self-limited disease; this is particularly true in children and young adults, who are more prone to reactive lymphatic hyperplasia. Despite this, patient concern is often substantial, due to worry about acute infectious processes on one hand and neoplastic diseases on the other. A systematic evaluation of lymphadenopathy will provide reassurance as well as a correct diagnosis.

PATHOPHYSIOLOGY AND CLINICAL PRESENTATION

Small lymph nodes in the neck, axilla and groin may be palpable in normal individuals. Palpable nodes in other regions or any node exceeding 1 cm. in size should be regarded as potentially abnormal. Inflammation and infiltration are responsible for pathologic enlargement. Although size alone is not itself diagnostic, nodes in excess of 3 cm. suggest neoplastic disease. Localized lymphadenopathy may represent spread of disease from an area of drainage. Of particular importance are palpable supraclavicular

nodes. The left one, which is sometimes referred to as the "sentinel" node, is in contact with the thoracic duct, which drains much of the abdominal cavity. The right supraclavicular node drains the mediastinum, lungs, and esophagus.

In addition to lymphadenopathy, abnormalities of the lymphatic system may present in other ways. Lymphangitis, appearing as red, warm streaks along the course of superficial lymphatic networks, suggests an acute inflammatory response to pyogenic infection in the drainage area; staphylococci and streptococci are frequently responsible. Lymphadenitis, presenting as a tender, warm, soft, rapidly enlarging node, has similar significance and often reflects acute pyogenic infection of the node itself. Lymphedema results from interruption of lymphatic drainage; surgical node dissection, radiotherapy or fibrosis due to chronic infections such as filariasis or lymphogranuloma venereum are causes of lymphedema.

DIFFERENTIAL DIAGNOSIS

The causes of lymphadenopathy can be conveniently considered in terms of location of the enlarged nodes (see Table 80–1). In children and young adults, most adenopathy is due to reactive hyperplasia and less likely to represent serious pathology than is its occurrence in adults.

Table 80-1. Important Causes of Lymphadenopathy

GENERALIZED LYMPHADENOPATHY	LOCALIZED LYMPHADENOPATHY
Infections	*Anterior Auricular*
Mononucleosis	Viral conjunctivitis
Other viral illnesses	Trachoma
Toxoplasmosis	Cat-scratch disease
Secondary syphilis	*Posterior Auricular*
Hypersensitivity Reactions	Rubella
Serum sickness	Scalp infection
Phenytoin and other drugs	*Submandibular or Cervical (Unilateral)*
Vasculitis (systemic lupus, rheumatoid arthritis)	Buccal cavity infection
Metabolic Disease	Pharyngitis (can be bilateral)
Hyperthyroidism	Nasopharyngeal tumor
Lipidoses	Thyroid malignancy
Neoplasia	Lymphoma, Hodgkin's disease
Leukemia	Metastatic tumor
Hodgkin's disease (advanced stages)	*Cervical Bilateral*
Non-Hodgkin's lymphoma (advanced stages)	Mononucleosis
	Sarcoidosis
	Toxoplasmosis
	Lymphoma
	Leukemia
	Pharyngitis
	Tuberculosis (can be unilateral)
	Coccidiomycosis
	Supraclavicular, Right
	Plumonary malignancy
	Mediastinal malignancy
	Esophageal malignancy
	Supraclavicular, Left
	Intradominal malignancy
	Renal malignancy
	Testicular or ovarian malignancy
	Axillary
	Breast infection or malignancy
	Upper extremity infection
	Epitrochlear
	Syphilis (bilateral)
	Hand infection (unilateral)
	Inguinal
	Syphilis
	Genital herpes
	Lymphogranuloma venereum
	Chancroid
	Lower extremity or local infection

WORKUP

A number of fundamental questions should be raised in every case of lymph gland enlargement.

History and physical examination often provide critical information and the answers to many of these queries.

1. Is the palpable mass indeed a lymph node? A variety of other structures, including enlarged parotid glands, cervical hygromas, thyroglossal and branchial cysts, hemangiomas, abscesses, lipomas and other tumors may on occasion be confused with lymphadenopathy.

2. Is the lymphadenopathy acute or chronic? Clearly, lymph node enlargement due to acute viral or pyogenic infections becomes less likely as the days and weeks pass, and granulomatous inflammation (sarcoid, tuberculosis, fungal infection) and neoplastic disease become greater worries. Even so, chronicity alone is not always a harbinger of serious disease, for on occasion reactive hyperplasia can persist for many months.

3. What is the character of the enlarged node itself? Tender, mobile nodes most often reflect lymphadenitis or lymphatic hyperplasia in response to acute inflammation. Firm, rubbery, nontender nodes may be found in lymphoma. Painless, stone-hard, fixed, matted nodes suggest metastatic carcinoma.

4. Is the adenopathy localized or generalized? Numerous systemic processes, including *infections* (infectious mononucleosis and other viral infections, toxoplasmosis, secondary syphilis, etc.); *hypersensitivity reactions* (serum sickness, reactions to phenytoin [Dilantin] and other drugs, and vasculitis, including systemic lupus erythematosus and rheumatoid arthritis); *metabolic diseases* (hyperthyroidism and various lipidoses), and *neoplasia* (especially leukemia) can produce generalized lymphadenopathy. However, Hodgkin's disease is usually unicentric in origin and spreads to contiguous regional nodes, so that generalized adenopathy is rare except in very advanced disease. While certain non-Hodgkin's lymphomas may be multicentric, generalized adenopathy is also a late finding and is usually asymmetric, unlike the earlier and more symmetric adenopathy of some leukemias, such as chronic lymphocytic leukemia.

Localized adenopathy should raise additional possibilities, depending on the area involved. For example, *submandibular* lymphadenopathy, which is perhaps the most common type of adenopathy, fequently results from pharyngitis (viral, streptococcal, gonococcal) or head and neck or intraoral infection. While these benign processes vastly predominate, it should be remembered that patients with Hodgkin's disease most often present with cervical lymphadenopathy. *Preauricular* adenopathy may be a component of "occuloglandular fevers" due to adenoviral conjunctivitis, sarcoidosis, tularemia, cat scratch disease and other processes. *Posterior auricular* or *posterior cervical* adenopathy frequently reflects infections of the scalp, but may also be prominent in systemic processes, such as rubella or toxoplasmosis. While *anterior cervical* lymphadenopathy often results from head and neck infections, isolated supraclavicular node enlargement is more indicative of metastatic malignancy; the *right supraclavicular* nodes drain the mediastinum, esophagus and thorax, while *left supraclavicular* adenopathy (Virchow's node) is suggestive of primary intra-abdominal neoplasia. *Axillary* nodes become enlarged in response to upper extremity infection, but breast cancer must be considered as well. Although enlarged *epitrochlear* nodes are traditionally associated with secondary syphilis, this finding reflects generalized lymphadenopathy in lues; epitrochlear lymphadenopathy can be seen in many other systemic processes, as well as in response to hand infections. *Inguinal* lymphadenopathy is much more common. Inguinal nodes are palpable in most normal individuals, but they can enlarge substantially in infections of the genitalia or perineum, as well as in lower extremity infections.

5. Are there associated systemic or localizing symptoms or signs? Fever, rash, weight loss, sore throat, dental pain, genital inflammation and infections of the extremities are clues which may be particularly helpful. A careful examination of the skin for a primary inoculation site may provide the clue to a diagnosis of processes such as cat scratch disease or tularemia. Careful examination for scalp infections, dermatophytes and scabies may be rewarding. Similarly, the finding of hepatomegaly, splenomegaly, or both may be of great significance (e.g., mononucleosis, sarcoidosis). Sternal tenderness can be present in leukemia.

6. Are there unusual epidemiologic clues? To cite a few examples, patients exposed to cats may develop cat scratch disease or toxoplasmosis, which may also result from eating poorly cooked meat. Travel to the southwest United States may suggest the possibility of plague. An appropriate travel history or exposure to bird droppings may suggest fungal infection, as may lacerations sustained while gardening, in the case of sporotrichosis. Contact with wild rodents may result in tularemia, as may tick bites. A history of exposure to tuberculosis may be an important clue to scrofula. More commonly, community outbreaks may provide clues to the diagnosis of streptococcal pharyngitis or rubella, while a history of sexual exposure may raise the question of gonorrhea, syphilis, genital herpes or lymphogranuloma.

Laboratory studies need not be very elaborate. A *complete blood count* with *differential* is almost always indicated and may be a valuable clue to detection of infectious mononucleosis, other viral processes or toxoplasmosis (lymphocytosis, atypical lymphocytosis), pyogenic infection (granulocytosis), hypersensitivity states (eosinophilia), or malignancies (anemia, abnormal granulocytes).

If pharyngitis or cervical or submandibular adenopathy is present, a *throat culture* is mandatory; it should be remembered that while these are routinely processed for streptococci, special Thayer-Martin medium must be used as well if gonococci are suspected. *Urethral* or *cervical cultures* and smears should also be obtained if gonorrhea is a potential cause of inguinal lymphadenopathy. Blood cultures are indicated in the rare cases of suspected plague, tularemia or brucellosis or if the clinical picture suggests staphylococcal or streptococcal lymphadenitis.

Serological tests may be of great value; the *heterophil* and *serological tests for syphilis* are obvious examples. In addition, a serum sample can be frozen during the acute phase of the illness to be submitted with a later convalescent phase serum specimen for *antibody titers* of various viruses, fungi and Toxoplasma. Brucellosis may also be diagnosed serologically. Serological tests, including *antinuclear antibodies* and *rheumatoid factor,* may suggest a noninfectious process such as collagen-vascular disease. A different form of immunologic test, the delayed *hypersensitivity skin test,* can be useful in the evaluation of possible tuberculous lymphadenitis. Reliable skin tests are available for coccidioidomycosis and tularemia. On the other hand, cutaneous anergy may suggest sarcoidosis or lymphoma, but is nonspecific. If available, a Kveim skin test may be helpful in the evaluation of sarcoidosis (see Chap. 48). Skin testing may be very helpful in the diagnosis of cat scratch disease, but like the Kveim test, the necessary antigen is available only on a research basis in selected centers.

A variety of blood chemistries may help in selected cases. Elevations of *uric acid* may reflect lymphoma or other hematologic malignancies. Liver function tests are of particular value; while abnormalities may be present in a great variety of illnesses which produce lymphadenopathy (ranging from mononucleosis to sarcoidosis to malignancy), they do provide an additional parameter to follow, and may suggest liver involvement, which can be further evaluated by biopsy.

Among radiologic studies, the *chest x-ray* is particularly valuable, since hilar adenopathy may be present in patients with enlargement of peripheral nodes. Hilar adenopathy may also be detected on chest x-rays in the absence of peripheral lymphadenopathy. Sarcoidosis, lymphoma, fungal infection, tuberculosis or metastatic carcinoma (particularly from a lung primary) should be among the diagnostic considerations. Mediastinoscopy may be required for diagnosis. On occasion, lymphomatous retroperitoneal or intra-abdominal nodes may enlarge enough to present as an abdominal mass. When lymphoma is a serious possibility, or when staging is necessary in known lymphoma or Hodgkin's disease, studies such as intravenous pyelography, lymphangiography, abdominal ultrasound, or gallium scanning can be used to detect enlargement of the retroperitoneal nodes; bone marrow biopsy can also be helpful (see Chapters 81, 82).

In addition to the studies outlined above, careful *observation* over a period of time may be very useful diagnostically, since in many cases benign lymphadenopathy will regress spontaneously even if no etiologic diagnosis has been made. But if adenopathy persists over a period of weeks, if the nodes are enlarging, or if neoplastic disease seems likely, biopsy should be performed.

Lymph node biopsy should be considered as the most direct approach to the diagnosis of lymphadenopathy. Although the majority of such procedures are technically easy and can be accomplished under local anesthesia, this is an invasive test and should be employed only when simpler approaches have failed to provide a diagnosis. In the case of fluctuant nodes, *needle aspiration* can be used to diagnose infectious processes in some cases.

The node to be biopsied should be selected with care; if generalized adenopathy is present, it is best to avoid inguinal or axillary nodes when possible, because reactive hyperplasia in these areas may make interpretation difficult. In general, enlarged supraclavicular nodes have the highest diagnostic yield. When possible, excisional biopsy is preferred. At the time of biopsy, tissue should be submitted for appropriate bacteriologic smears and cultures, as well as for histologic study. Touch preps may be useful. Special stains for bacteria, mycobacteria and fungi may be helpful, as may specific stains for unusual processes such as PAS stains for Whipple's disease or lipidosis, and Congo red stains for amyloid. Interpretation of lymph node pathology can be quite difficult and requires careful study by experienced observers. With such study, benign processes such as toxoplasmosis or cat scratch disease can be suspected histologically, and detailed analysis of serial sections may reveal lymphomas which are not diagnosed with less intensive pathologic study. Finally, if pathologic study reveals reactive hyperplasia or is nondiagnostic, patients should be followed carefully, since up to 25 per cent may eventually exhibit an illness responsible for the lymphadenopathy, most often lymphoma.

ANNOTATED BIBLIOGRAPHY

Greenfield, S., and Jordan, M.C.: The clinical investigation of lymphadenopathy in primary care practice. JAMA, *240*:1388, 1978. (*A systematic algorithmic approach to the workup of peripheral lymphadenopathy in the ambulatory setting.*)

Lalle, A.M., and Oski, F.A.: Peripheral lymphadenopathy in childhood. Am. J. Dis. Child., *132*:357, 1978. (*A retrospective study of 75 lymph node biopsies in patients younger than 18. Fifty-five per cent were nondiagnostic, 28 per cent showed granulomatous inflammation, and 17 per cent showed lymphoproliferative disorders. Clinical findings correlated poorly with pathologic diagnosis.*)

Saltzstern, S.L.: The fate of patients with nondiagnostic lymph node biopsies. Surgery, *58*:659, 1965. (*A retrospective study of lymph node biopsies in 177 adult males. In 68 patients, the indication for biopsy was lymphadenopathy; 52 per cent of these were nondiagnostic, but 17 per cent of patients with nondiagnostic biopsies subsequently developed lymphoma. Supraclavicular node biopsies had the highest diagnostic yield.*)

Sinclair, S., Beckman, E., and Ellman, L.: Biopsy of enlarged superficial lymph nodes. JAMA, *228*:602, 1974. (*A retrospective pathologic study of 135 lymph node biopsies performed because of undiagnosed lymphodenopathy. Sixty-three per cent of the biopsies were diagnostic; 50 patients had lymphoma, 14 carcinoma, 6 tuberculosis, 1 histoplasmosis, 7 acute lymphadenitis, and 1 Dilantin sensitivity. Of the 50 patients with nondiagnostic biopsies, 25 per cent developed a disease related to the indications for biopsy, which was most often lymphoma, and which usually occurred within 8 months of the initial biopsy.*)

81

Approach to the Patient
with Hodgkin's Disease
JACOB J. LOKICH, M.D.

Hodgkin's disease must be considered an uncommon malignancy in that the annual incidence is approximately three cases per 100,000 population, or a total of approximately 7,000 cases annually. However, the disease affects young people and is often curable. Peak incidence is between the ages of 20 and 40 (with a second peak over 60). The primary physician has an important role in staging the disease, coordinating plans for management and delivering follow-up care on an outpatient basis.

PATHOLOGY, CLINICAL PRESENTATION AND COURSE

The histology of Hodgkin's disease incorporates four categories: lymphocyte predominance, nodular sclerosis, mixed cellularity and lymphocyte depletion. *Lymphocyte predominance* occurs in 10 to 15 per cent of patients, *nodular sclerosis* in 20 to 50 per cent, mixed cellularity in 20 to 40 per cent, and *lymphocyte depletion* in 5 to 15 per cent. In about 15 per cent of cases, classification is difficult and requires expert interpretation of the histology. In all instances the *sine qua non* of diagnosis is the pathognomonic Reed-Sternberg cell.

The clinical presentation of the disease most commonly involves cervical or mediastinal adenopathy which is asymmetrical and asymptomatic; however, any area containing lymph nodes may be the site of presentation, including the axilla and the inguinal region. The nodes are firm and nontender; they often are matted, but may be discrete and freely movable. Fever, weight loss, night sweats, or alcohol-induced pain may develop and almost always represents advanced stage disease.

Conceptually, Hodgkin's disease is unicentric in origin and progresses by contiguous extension along lymphatic pathways. This pattern of evolution is in contrast to non-Hodgkin's lymphomas, which are multicentric and associated with more advanced stages of disease at initial presentation.

The differential diagnosis of Hodgkin's disease includes infectious mononucleosis and other nonbacterial adenopathies in the young (see Chapter 80). In the elderly, other malignancies are a common diagnostic consideration; they are particularly suspect in the presence of a fever of unknown origin.

Staging at time of presentation is important to a determination of prognosis and choice of therapy (see Table 81-1). *Stage I* is defined as disease confined to a single node-bearing area; *stage II* involves two contiguous node-bearing areas on the same side of the diaphragm; *stage III* is nodal involvement on both sides of the diaphragm; and *stage IV* represents visceral (liver, lung parenchyma, bone) lesions. The special category designated *E* (for extranodal) was created because of data which indicate that involvement of an organ contiguous to a lymph node-bearing area has a distinctly better prognosis than does visceral involvement that is hematogenous. Nonetheless, the prognosis is not as good as it would be if there were no organ involvement.

Early (stages I and II) and advanced (stages III and IV) Hodgkin's disease are relatively equally distributed in terms of frequency. More sophisticated staging by pathologic as well as clinical procedures generally tends to advance the stage of disease. Approximately 20 per cent of patients will have fever, night sweats, or a significant loss of weight. These systemic symptoms are incorporated into the staging system because they are important determinants of prognosis. When absent, the designation is A; when any of the three is present, the designation is B. Patients with pruritus only are no longer included in the B group.

The prognosis of Hodgkin's disease has improved dramatically with the advent of careful staging and improved radiation technology and chemotherapy programs. Five-year survival and 5-year relapse-free figures indicate 80 per cent 5-year overall survival and 60 per cent relapse-free survival, when all stages of disease are combined (see Table 81-1).

Table 81–1. Hodgkin's Disease: Stages, Relative Incidences, and Prognosis

STAGE	DEFINITION	RELATIVE INCIDENCE (%)	THERAPY	5-YEAR SURVIVAL (%)*	5-YEAR RELAPSE-FREE (%)*
Stage I	Confined to single node-bearing area	30	Radiation	86.0	72.5
Stage II	Confined to two contiguous node-bearing areas; on one side of diaphragm	25	Radiation	93.6	69.0
Stage III	In nodal areas on both sides of the diaphragm	25	Radiation and chemotherapy	81.3	61.1
Stage IV	Visceral lesions (liver, lung) *not in* continuity with nodes	20	Chemotherapy	39.0	26.9
Special Categories					
E	Visceral extranodal disease in continuity with nodes. For example, lung mass extending out from hilum		Radiation +/− chemotherapy		
B	Symptoms of fever, weight loss, or sweats		Chemotherapy +/− radiation		

Survival and disease-free figures for each stage combine patients with A and B disease. (From Kaplan, H.S., and Rosenberg, S.; Management of Hodgkin's disease. Cancer, *36*:796, 1975.)

PRINCIPLES OF MANAGEMENT

Staging

Staging is critical to design of a therapeutic program and estimation of prognosis. History should ascertain presence of fever, night sweats, or weight loss. Careful palpation of all lymph nodes and assessment of liver and spleen size are important, though enlargement by physical examination does not necessarily indicate involvement by the disease. One-half of patients with a palpable spleen do not have histologic splenic involvement, and one-quarter with normal-sized spleens do.

The specific staging procedures indicated in Hodgkin's disease are outlined in Table 81–2. Since some of the most common forms of Hodgkin's disease involve the mediastinum, a *chest radiograph* is essential. Routine use of *tomography* to evaluate the lung fields is not indicated in the absence of hilar or mediastinal adenopathy, since identification of pulmonary nodules in the absence of hilar or mediastinal disease is not common. However, use of tomography to identify tracheal compression in patients with mediastinal lesions is critically important in those who are to undergo laparotomy; compromised airway may result in a mortality when intubation for general anesthesia is attempted. Therefore, all patients with mediastinal mass lesions who are to have a staging laparotomy should have midline tracheal tomograms, both AP and lateral, to evaluate the air flow column.

Lymphangiography was developed to detect occult disease below the diaphragm by visualizing the retroperitoneal nodes. Unfortunately, the test has a low sensitivity, with a false-negative rate of 20 per cent; this limits its utility for staging. When strict radiologic criteria for nodal involvement are used, specificity reaches 95 per cent, with less than 5 per cent false-positives noted. Thus, a positive study is helpful, but a negative lymphangiogram does not rule out disease below the diaphragm and requires use of a more definitive staging procedure. Moreover,

Table 81–2. Staging Procedures for Hodgkin's Disease

STUDY	INDICATION
Radiographic Studies	
Chest Radiograph	All patients; tomograms if mediastinal or hilar disease
Lymphangiogram	*Only if* (a) no clinical evidence of infradiaphragmatic disease, (b) no mass or lung disease, or (c) no advanced stage signs or symptoms (B)
Surgical Studies	
Laparoscopy	Preferable to laparotomy in presence of B symptoms. To identify liver pathology
Laparotomy	Stage I or II disease and no symptoms
Hematologic Studies	
Bone Marrow Biopsy	Only if clinical Stage IIB or more
Liver Function Tests Complete Blood Count ESR, Serum Copper, Leukocyte Alkaline Phosphatase	Usefulness unclear

even if the test is positive, it does not detect involvement of the liver or spleen, which is an important determinant of therapy. Lymphangiography carries a small risk of pulmonary insufficiency related to extravasation of dye in the lung parenchyma, and it should not be performed in those with severe lung disease. Lymphangiography should be performed in all patients with clinical stage I or II disease without B symptoms, particularly those patients in whom laparotomy is scheduled, in order to identify the lymph nodes to be removed. About 25 per cent of patients classified clinically are reclassified on the basis of lymphangiogram results.

The use of *computerized tomographic scanning* to evaluate the abdominal extent of disease will undoubtedly have some of the same limitations as lymphangiography. Microscopic disease within retroperitoneal nodes will be undetectable, contributing to the false-negative rate, but specificity should be high.

The *staging laparotomy* includes wedge biopsy of the liver, splenectomy and examination of the lymph nodes in contiguous chains, exclusive of mesenteric nodes. The operation has a low mortality rate (0.5 per cent) and negligible early morbidity. However, patients who receive radiation and chemotherapy after splenectomy are at some risk (21 per cent in one series) for fulminant sepsis, with its attendant 50 per cent mortality; those who undergo splenectomy but do not receive combination therapy appear to be much less vulnerable to serious infection.

The staging laparotomy has the advantage of allowing more precise definition of the extent of disease, thereby guiding more rational therapeutic approaches. Laparotomy frequently results in reclassification of patients into different disease stages and consequent alterations in therapeutic programs. In a series of 114 patients who underwent staging laparotomy, 18 received less irradiation, 10 received more, 2 were given radiation instead of chemotherapy, and 4 received chemotherapy instead of radiation. Two other advantages of laparotomy with splenectomy are that radiation to the left upper quadrant can be avoided and the ovaries can be moved out of the way of a radiation therapy portal. At the present time, laparotomy is indicated in all patients with stage I or II disease without symptoms. In clinical stage III disease, the issue of laparotomy is controversial. Chemotherapy is being employed more commonly in stage III, so that pathologic confirmation by laparotomy may not be necessary for determining choice of therapy.

Laparoscopy has been advocated as a less invasive means of identifying liver involvement in patients with a high probability of disease below the diaphragm, for example, those with B symptoms. Liver biopsy specimens are taken from suspicious areas under direct visualization. Laparoscopy is superior to percutaneous liver biopsy (20 per cent yield vs. 5 per cent), but its yield does not quite match that of open biopsy performed during staging laparotomy. Few patients with Hodgkin's disease that involves the liver are free of systemic complaints; on the other hand, neither hepatomegaly upon physical examination or scan nor elevated alkaline phosphatase levels identify patients likely to have positive biopsies.

Bone marrow biopsy in patients with systemic symptoms or disease beyond stage II is positive in up to 20 per cent of patients. Since disease in the marrow is often focal, multiple biopsies are necessary to avoid sampling error. Marrow aspiration is never useful. A positive marrow classifies the disease as stage IV, and makes laparotomy unnecessary. Patients with stage I or IIA disease clinically have never been reported to have positive marrow biopsies, but stage IIB is associated with marrow involvement in 9 per cent of patients.

Many other tests for staging of Hodgkin's disease lack sensitivity and/or specificity. Such is the case for liver and spleen scans, bone scans and gallium scans, which are not indicated in routine staging. Complete blood count, alkaline phosphatase, and sedimentation rate are similarly nonspecific. The use of the erythrocyte sedimentation rate, serum copper, and leukocyte alkaline phosphatase as indices of disease activity and extent is promoted by various investigators, but all of these tests represent nonspecific approaches to evaluating the patient with Hodgkin's disease.

In sum, the history is reviewed for characteristic systemic symptoms; the physical examination focuses on lymph-node-bearing areas. If the patient is clinically in stage I or II and would be treated by radiation, a staging laparotomy should be performed to identify disease below the diaphragm. Until it becomes possible to predict more accurately who is likely to have occult disease in the abdomen, one must reply on the laparotomy. In instances where systemic symptoms are present, a laparoscopy and bone marrow biopsy can be performed as preliminary studies; if either is positive, the need for laparotomy is obviated. Lymphangiography produces too many false negatives to be relied upon without intra-abdominal evaluation and, even if positive, fails to provide information about the liver and spleen which is necessary for selecting radiation therapy, chemotherapy, or both.

Treatment

Therapy for Hodgkin's disease has resulted in a cure rate which is substantial in all stages. For patients with stage IA and IIA disease, *local radiotherapy* to contiguous node-bearing areas has resulted in an 85 to 90 per cent cure rate. *Total nodal radiation therapy* has been used in Stages IB and IIB, delivered at a dose of 3500 to 4500 rads over a 3- to 4-week period through a portal referred to as the "mantle" for chest radiation and the "inverted Y" for intra-abdominal lymph nodes. This total nodal form of radiation therapy is most effective when cobalt or linear accelerator machines are used to maximize the therapeutic effect in the lymph nodes and to spare normal tissues, including the skin. Radiotherapy as a single modality has been employed for patients with stage III disease, particularly in asymptomatic stage IIIA disease, and the cure rate is in the range of 50 to 60 per cent. More recently, Hodgkin's disease distributed on either side of the diaphragm (stage III) has been treated with a combined approach of radiation therapy and chemotherapy or with chemotherapy alone.

The *chemotherapy* of Hodgkin's disease is a milestone in the development of cancer therapy. The Mustargen, Oncovin, prednisone, procarbazine *(MOPP)* therapeutic program developed in 1965 at the National Cancer Institute has served as a prototype for the development of combination chemotherapy as it is known today for many malignant diseases. The program is based on the identification of four agents with individually distinctive mechanisms of antitumor acitivity. Their side effects are nonadditive, thus minimizing drug-related morbidity. Response rates for stage IIIB and IV disease are in the 80 per cent range, and complete remission of disease is the rule.

By manipulation of dosages and schedules of drugs, sophisticated chemotherapy can be delivered conventiently to outpatients. Potentially curative therapy in patients with advanced disease in the stage IV category has become possible for approximately 50 per cent of the patients who enter complete remission. MOPP therapy is administered according to the dosage schedule outlined in Table 81–3 for a finite period of 6 months, at which time restaging is carried out; in the absence of residual disease, therapy is discontinued.

Over 50 per cent of patients *relapse* after complete remission with MOPP therapy. Retreatment with MOPP may induce a second remission if the disease-free interval was over 12 months. An alternative chemotherapeutic approach was developed for the substantial numbers of patients who *relapse* after radiation and subsequent MOPP therapy. The combination referred to as ABVD incorporates Adriamycin, bleomycin, vinblastine and DTIC, or diaminotriazenoimidazole (Carboxamide). This noncrossresistant regimen is employed in patients who are MOPP-resistant, and, more recently, in combination with MOPP either as an alternative sequence or as a compact therapy following a course of MOPP therapy. The response rate is comparable to that achieved with MOPP therapy; the durability and potential for cure are not yet established.

Prophylaxis agaihst pneumococcal septicemia is an important consideration in splenectomized patients. The efficacy of the *pneumococcal vaccine,* (see Chapter 4) in patients who undergo splenectomy

Table 81–3.   Chemotherapy of Hodgkin's Disease

DRUGS	DOSAGES		RECYCLE
	Day 1	*Day 8*	
MOPP			28 days
Mustargen (nitrogen mustard)	6 mg./M²	6 mg./M²	
Oncovin (vincristine)	1.4 mg./M²	1.4 mg./M²	
Prednisone	40 mg./M²/d × 14 days		
Procarbazine	100 mg./M²/d × 14 days		
	Day 1	*Day 14*	
ABVD			28 days
Adriamycin	25 mg./M²	25 mg./M²	
Bleomycin	5 mg./M²	5 mg./M²	
Vinblastine	6 mg./M²	6 mg./M²	
DTIC	250 mg./M²	250 mg./M²	

for staging of Hodgkin's disease is unresolved. There is some evidence that treatment for Hodgkin's disease impairs the antibody response to the vaccine. The literature should be followed for more data.

MONITORING THERAPY

Periodic examination of involved nodes is the simplest means of judging response to therapy. Many laboratory parameters have been developed but offer little advantage over physical examination and chest x-ray. The need for periodic restaging is a judgment to be made in consultation with the oncologist. Patients receiving MOPP require close surveillance (see Chapter 88). Patients being treated with radiation should be watched for bone marrow suppression, and, when lung fields are involved, radiation pneumonitis.

INDICATIONS FOR CONSULTATION AND REFERRAL

Hodgkin's disease is an excellent example of a condition requiring the advice and coordination of many specialists. The primary physician needs to consult the oncologist, surgeon and radiation therapist to plan staging and selection of a therapeutic program; yet, with their help, he can provide the major portion of ongoing care.

PATIENT EDUCATION

Many patients will greet the diagnosis of Hodgkin's disease with dread, equating it with carcinoma and a fatal outcome. Without raising false hopes, the physician can point to the excellent 5-year survival rates and the high percentage of individuals who are disease-free after 10 years. Patients who have undergone splenectomy should be advised to have polyvalent pneumococcal vaccine before undergoing chemotherapy or radiation, which inhibits immune response. Since chemotherapy can cause permanent sterility, it is important to review this prospect with the patient and family before embarking on treatment. Pretherapy sperm storage has been advocated, but specimens are suboptimal.

ANNOTATED BIBLIOGRAPHY

Aisenberg, A.: The staging and treatment of Hodgkin's disease. N. Engl. J. Med., *299*:1288, 1978. *(In a series of 75 patients with clinical Stage I or II disease, one third were reclassified to clinical Stage III on the basis of a positive lymphangiogram, and another one third on the basis of a staging laparotomy.)*

Bagley, C., Roth, J., Thomas, L., and DeVita, V.: Liver biopsy in Hodgkin's disease. Ann. Intern. Med., *76*:219, 1975. *(Yield of percutaneous biopsy was half that obtained via laparoscopy or laparotomy.)*

DeVita, V., Canellos, G., and Moley, J.: A decade of combination chemotherapy of advanced Hodgkin's disease. Cancer, *30*:1495, 1972. *(The earliest experience with MOPP therapy developed by the National Cancer Institute is reviewed in the perspective of a long follow-up period and new programs.)*

Ellman, L.: Bone marrow biopsy in the evaluation of lymphoma, carcinoma and granulomatous disorders. Am. J. Med., *60*:1, 1976. *(Terse review of utility of bone marrow exam for staging.)*

Fisher, R.I., DeVita, V.T., Hubbard, S.P., *et al.*: Prolonged disease-free survival in Hodgkin's disease with MOPP reinduction after first relapse. Ann. Intern. Med., *90*:761, 1979. *(Patients who relapse after at least 12 months of remission induced by MOPP may respond with another remission to retreatment with MOPP.)*

Greenberg, L.H., Wong, Y.S., Richardson, A.P., Jr., and Dollinger, M.R.: Combination chemotherapy of Hodgkin's disease in private practice. JAMA, *221*(3):261, 1972. *(This unusual report of the application of sophisticated combination chemotherapy in the private practice of medicine attests to the safety and comparability of therapeutic results to the more complex large institution trials.)*

Kadin, M.E., Glatstein, E., and Dorfman, R.F.: Clinicopathologic studies of 117 untreated patients subjected to laparotomy for the staging of Hodgkin's disease. Cancer, *27*:1277, 1971. *(A follow-up of the initial report of the use of laparotomy in staging patients with Hodgkin's disease, which has become a standard procedure. The use of laparotomy as a determinant of therapy is not specifically emphasized, but the low complication rate is indicated.)*

Kaplan, H.S.: Role of intensive radiotherapy in the management of Hodgkin's disease. Cancer, *19*:356, 1966. *(The early experiences subsequently borne out by progressively more sophisticated randomized trials are reviewed in detail.)*

Kaplan, H.S., and Rosenberg, S.: Management of Hodgkin's disease. Cancer, *36*:796, 1975. *(A comprehensive review of Hodgkin's disease by the world's authority on the clinical and therapeutic aspects.)*

Schimpff, S.C., O'Connell, M.J., Green, W.H., and Wernik, P.H.: Infections in 92 splenectomized patients with Hodgkin's disease. Am. J. Med., *59*:695, 1975. *(This article indicates a relatively low incidence of sepsis in splenectomized patients; however, there is a 50 per cent mortality with pneumococcal sepsis.)*

Siber, G.R., Weitzman, S.A., Aisenberg, A.C., *et al.*:

Impaired antibody response to pneumococcal vaccine after treatment for Hodgkin's disease. N. Engl. J. Med., *299*:442, 1978. *(Patients who underwent splenectomy and were given the vaccine after the initiation of therapy showed a markedly impaired antibody response.)*

Silverman, S., DeNardo, G., Glatstein, E., and Lipton, M.: Evaluation of the liver and spleen in Hodgkin's disease. I. Value of hepatic scintigraphy. II. Value of splenic scintigraphy. Am. J. Med., *356*:362, 1972. *(Liver scan was sensitive but not specific; spleen scan lacked sensitivity and specificity.)*

82

Approach to the Patient with Non-Hodgkin's Lymphoma

JACOB J. LOKICH, M.D.

Non-Hodgkin's lymphoma is approximately twice as common as Hodgkin's disease, with 15,000 new cases annually and an incidence of six per 100,000 population. In contrast to Hodgkin's disease, non-Hodgkin's lymphoma represents a composite of at least three or more pathologic categories, each based on specific immunologic and pathologic features and having distinctive clinical course and therapeutic response. Non-Hodgkin's lymphoma strikes much later than Hodgkin's disease; peak incidence is in the fifth decade. Prognosis is much less favorable in terms of long-term cure, although survival and responsiveness to therapy are substantial.

The role of the primary physician is to carry out staging, coordinate design of a therapeutic program, and deliver long-term outpatient care (including chemotherapy) in conjunction with the oncologist.

the time of pathologic analysis. Two patterns are separable: nodular and diffuse. The *nodular* pattern within the lymph node histologically indicates a favorable prognosis (see Table 82–1) and a substantial likelihood of response to a variety of modalities, including total body irradiation, and also single-drug chemotherapy. In contrast, *diffuse* histology is associated with shorter survival, even though the response rate to complex chemotherapy regimens is significant and much higher than that achieved by single-agent therapy. The diffuse histologic pattern is, however, characteristic of at least one disease of long-duration, chronic lymphatic leukemia.

The *cell type* or differentiation also influences prognosis and, therefore, the therapeutic approach. Of the three cell type categories (lymphoblastic, histiocytic and mixed lymphohistiocytic), only the *histiocytic* type has been established as being potentially

PATHOLOGY, CLINICAL PRESENTATION AND PROGNOSIS

In contrast to Hodgkin's disease, the pathologic classification of non-Hodgkin's lymphoma is a crucial determinant of therapy. The categories outlined in Table 82–1 represent a composite of categorizations based on those of Rappaport, Lukes and Butler, Dorfman and others. These categories are still somewhat controversial, and establishment of specific survival expectations is difficult.

A major determinant of response to therapy is the *architecture* of the tumor within the lymph node at

Table 82–1. Pathologic Categories in Non-Hodgkin's Lymphoma

CATEGORY	RESPONSE TO CHEMOTHERAPY	SURVIVAL
Architectural Distribution		
Nodular	40–50%	Long
Diffuse	60–80%	Short
Cell Type (Differentiation)		
Lymphoblastic	60–80%	Unestablished
Histiocytic	50–60%	20% Long-term
Mixed	60–80%	Unestablished
Variants		
Immunoblastic	Variable	Unknown
Hairy cell	Variable	Long

curable with complex chemotherapy. The complete response rate in this group of patients is high (40 to 60 per cent) and the survival curve appears to parallel the normal population at approximately two years for 20 to 30 per cent of patients. The clinical course of the better differentiated *lymphocytic* type resembles that of chronic lymphatic leukemia, and, in fact, pathologic and clinical distinctions between chronic lymphatic leukemia and lymphosarcoma are often difficult. *Immunoblastic lymphomas* are in a special category referred to as *immunoangioblastic lymphomas* by Rappaport. These clinical lesions are variably responsive to chemotherapy, and their prognosis is unpredictable. The *hairy cell* lymphomas are generally associated with splenomegaly, a leukemic phase, and an excellent prognosis.

Immunologic characterization of the lymphoma is possible; specific anti-immunoglobulin markers are used to identify B-cells and special *in vitro* assays (for E rosettes) to identify T-cells. The distinction between B- and T-cell lymphomas is of importance pathophysiologically, but its clinical significance has not yet been established.

Non-Hodgkin's lymphomas occur in nodal or extranodal sites or both. The disease is usually disseminated at the time of clinical presentation. Localized or regional lymphoma is relatively uncommon, stage I and II lymphomas accounting for less than 10 per cent of all cases. Also unlike Hodgkin's disease, extranodal disease is often solitary and likely to be confined to the organ of origin. Waldeyer's ring, bone and upper gastrointestinal tract are the most frequently involved extranodal sites, accounting for up to 16 per cent of cases. Extranodal lymphoma can have a favorable prognosis, particularly in the absence of nodal disease. Five-year survival rates are as high as 30 to 50 per cent, independent of pathologic type.

PRINCIPLES OF MANAGEMENT

Staging

Staging helps to determine prognosis and affects the selection and intensity of treatment modalities. Staging for non-Hodgkin's lymphoma is distinctly different from that for Hodgkin's disease, because advanced disease is more common in the former. Hodgkin's disease is conceptually unicentric in origin and progresses via contiguous lymph node extension. Non-Hodgkin's lymphoma, in contrast, is multicentric in origin and appears in discontinuous lymph node chains. Physical examination should include evaluation of all node-bearing areas, including unusual sites such as the epitrochlear area, Waldeyer's ring and preauricular nodes. Liver and spleen are commonly enlarged. Routine staging procedures, including chest radiographs and bone marrow biopsies are indicated in all patients. In contrast to Hodgkin's disease, the staging system for the non-Hodgkin's lymphomas does not include a category for symptoms or a designation for contiguous visceral involvement or splenic disease. Patients with clinical stage I or II disease (confined to one regional area) should also have a *lymphangiogram* if the disease is above the diaphragm. For lymphangiography, the false-negative rate is 8 to 33 per cent and the false-positive rate 11 to 17 per cent.

Bilateral or multiple *bone marrow biopsies* can identify occult stage IV disease. In a series of 131 patients with non-Hodgkin's lymphoma, 37 per cent had positive biopsies when more than one site was sampled. Aspiration is inadequate since the false-negative rate is 30 per cent; biopsy producing a solid bone marrow specimen is essential.

Whole body gallium scanning is particularly useful for staging histiocytic lymphoma, because these tumors appear to accumulate the isotope selectively. False-positive rate is low and ranges from 5 to 18 per cent, but the false-negative rate is about 50 per cent, meaning that a negative scan does not rule out disease. The utility of the scan is in obtaining a positive result.

Staging laparotomy is not indicated in non-Hodgkin's lymphoma because the yield from lymphangiogram and bone marrow biopsy is high and because changes in stage based on laparotomy findings are not of therapeutic significance, in that the majority of patients are treated with chemotherapy.

Therapy

The therapeutic approach to the non-Hodgkin's lymphomas, in contrast to that in Hodgkin's disease, is based predominantly on chemotherapy. *Radiation therapy* is confined almost exclusively to regional disease localized to a single nodal area (stage I or II). Total body irradiation for patients with nodular histopathology in stage III is investigational. *Chemotherapy* may be administered in the form of a single agent or as complex, multi-drug regimens. The simpler and more innocuous single-drug regimens have been advocated for nodular histopathology and the lymphoma variants which are consistent with chronic lymphatic leukemia, since survival is not influenced by more aggressive therapy. In contrast, for lymphomas in the histiocytic category, the multidrug regimens are essential to prolonged survival and potential cure (Table 82–2).

The original three-drug regimen, COP (cyclo-

Table 82–2.   Chemotherapy of Non-Hodgkin's Lymphoma

DRUGS	DOSAGES	RECYCLE	INDICATION
CVP		21 days	Nodular lymphoma
Cyclophosphamide	100 mg./M²/d/ po × 10 days		
Vincristine (Oncovin)	1 mg./M²/d days 1 and 8		
Prednisone	50 mg./M²/d × 10 days		
BVAP		21 days	Second line
Bleomycin	5 mg./M² weekly to maximum dose 200 mg./M²		
Vinblastine	5 mg./M²		
Adriamycin	45 mg./M²		
Prednisone	50 mg./M²/d × 5 days		
BACOP		28 days	Histiocytic lymphoma
Bleomycin	5 mg./M² weekly		
Adriamycin	45 mg./M² day 1		
Cyclophosphamide	500 mg./M² day 1		
Oncovin	1.0 mg./M²		
Prednisone	50 mg./M² × 5 days		
C-MOPP		28 days	Histiocytic lymphoma
Cyclophosphamide	100 mg./M²/d/ po × 10 days		
Oncovin	1.4 mg./M² days 1 and 8		
Procarbazine	100 mg./M²/d × 10 days		
Prednisone	50 mg./M²/d × 10 days		

phosphamide, Oncovin and prednisone), is administered at 3- to 4-week intervals, and employs either oral or intravenous cyclophosphamide. In patients who fail to respond to COP or who relapse after initial response, secondary therapy may employ non-cross-resistant drugs such as bleomycin and doxorubicin (adriamycin). One such second-echelon regimen is BVAP (bleomycin, vinblastine, Adriamycin, prednisone). Secondary responses are invariably shorter in duration. A more intensive first-echelon combination chemotherapy regimen employs all the active drugs in a five-drug regimen referred to as BACOP. The drug scheduling in such a regimen is designed to allow for continuous therapy, maximize the number of complete remissions, and enhance the duration of remission. In histiocytic lymphoma, this regimen appears to be particularly effective in inducing response; it also achieves cure in a finite group of patients in spite of advanced disease. The so-called C-MOPP combination is a recently developed regimen which employs cyclophosphamide in place of nitrogen mustard and may achieve similar responses without the addition of bleomycin and Adriamycin.

MONITORING THERAPY

Judging response to the therapy is similar to that for Hodgkin's disease (see Chapter 81). Close surveillance is needed for the patient on chemotherapy (see Chapter 88).

PATIENT EDUCATION

The strong likelihood that chemotherapy-induced sterility will occur, at least temporarily, needs to be discussed with the patient. Fortunately, this disease occurs more frequently in older age groups (in contrast to Hodgkin's disease) where reproductive capacity is less likely to be an issue. Return of spermatogenesis is seen in some patients, beginning about 2 years after completion of chemotherapy. Potency and libido are unaffected.

The encouraging results of chemotherapy, even in patients with advanced disease, provide new hope. As with Hodgkin's disease, the patient can be given a fairly accurate assessment of his prognosis after careful histologic study and staging have been carried out. Often the prognosis is far better than the patient's fearful expectations and can be shared profitably.

INDICATIONS FOR REFERRAL

Management of the patient with lymphoma needs to be a cooperative venture from the start, with the primary physician working closely with the oncologist experienced in lymphoma. Selection of treatment modality requires the judgment of one who is familiar with available protocols, which are still undergoing revision. Although consultation and referral are essential, the primary physician can assume responsibility for long-term management as soon as a treatment plan is devised. Working closely with the oncologist, the patient's personal physician can administer and monitor the chemotherapy program on an outpatient basis, maintain continuity, and provide psychological support.

ANNOTATED BIBLIOGRAPHY

Aisenberg, A.: Malignant lymphoma. N. Engl. J. Med., *288*:883, 1973. *(The first part of this excellent review provides a terse summary of clinical presentation, histology and staging. 84 refs.)*

Brunning, R., Bloomfield, C., McKenna, R., and Peterson, L.: Bilateral trephine bone marrow biopsies in lymphoma and other neoplastic diseases. Ann. Intern. Med., *82*:365, 1975. *(Reports a 37 per cent yield on bilateral samples; 11 of 50 samples were positive only on one side, emphasizing need for bilateral procedure.)*

Castillino, R., Billingham, M., and Dorfman, R.: Lymphographic accuracy in Hodgkin's disease and malignant lymphoma with a note on the "reactive" lymph node as a cause of most false-positive lymphograms. Invest. Radiol., *9*:155, 1974. *(A prospective study with 114 non-Hodgkin's lymphoma patients. The false-negative rate was 8 per cent and false-positive rate 11 per cent. Most false-positives resulted from misreading a reactive lymph node.)*

Chabner, B.A., *et al.*: Sequential nonsurgical and surgical staging of non-Hodgkin's lymphoma. Ann. Intern. Med., *85*:149, 1976. *(Helps define approach to staging, based on studies at the National Cancer Institute.)*

DeVita, V.T., Chabner, B., Hubbard, S.P., Canellos, G.P., Schein, P., and Young, R.C.: Advanced diffuse histiocytic lymphoma, a potentially curable disease. Lancet, *1*:248, 1975. *(This was the first report of cure in non-Hodgkin's lymphoma and appeared to be paradoxical in that the most aggressive lymphoma was singled out as having a finite curability potential.)*

Ezdinli, E., *et al.*: Comparison of intensive versus moderate chemotherapy of lymphocytic lymphomas: A progress report. Cancer, *38*:1060, 1976. *(Emphasizes the importance of nodular vs. diffuse histologic pattern and in a relatively large group of patients [273], demonstrates the potential need for conservative single agent therapy in some patients.)*

McCaffery, J., Rudders, R., Kohn, P., *et al.*: Clinical usefulness of [67]gallium scanning in the malignant lymphomas. Am. J. Med., *60*:523, 1976. *(The false-positive rate was low [5 per cent] but the false-negative rate was high [45 per cent].)*

Proceedings of the National Conference on Lymphomas and Leukemias: Cancer (Suppl.), *421* (2), August, 1978. *(A comprehensive review of the state of the art of diagnosis and therapy in the hematologic neoplasms including Hodgkin's and non-Hodgkin's lymphomas as viewed from the perspective of individuals who have been most influential in developing concepts in management.)*

Sherins, R., and DeVita, V.: Effect of drug treatment for lymphoma on male reproductive capacity. Ann. Intern. Med., *79*:216, 1973. *(Azoospermia is not uncommon [10 of 16 in this series] after chemotherapy. Potency and libido are maintained; spermatogenesis may return, but only after more than 2 years after drug therapy.)*

83
Management of Iron Deficiency Anemia

Iron deficiency anemia is extremely common, occurring in about 10 to 15 per cent of premenopausal woman. The condition is a sign of underlying disease, particularly when found in men and the elderly (see Chapter 77). The first priority is to detect and treat the cause of the anemia. Empirical use of iron without attention to the cause of the iron deficiency reflects failure to comprehend the significance of the anemia. However, there are instances where iron replacement can be helpful. It is important to know the indications for iron therapy as well as the most economical and effective forms of replacement.

CLINICAL PRESENTATION AND COURSE

In menstruating women, the balance between dietary iron intake (1 mg. per day) and loss (15 mg. per month) is precarious. Low-grade anemia, especially when losses from pregnancy (approximately 500 mg.) are not made up, is common. However, the many vague complaints in otherwise healthy menstruating women that are attributed to "low iron" have not been found to correlate with the severity of the anemia or to respond to its correction in controlled studies.

Iron deficiency anemia is usually slow in onset, allowing for compensatory changes such as increases in 2,3-DPG and cardiac output to minimize symptoms. When blood loss has been rapid or the anemia severe (hemoglobin below 7 gm./100 ml.), patients are likely to become symptomatic, especially if cardiopulmonary reserve is limited. Replacement therapy is required in such cases, regardless of etiology. Also, the occasional patient with severe iron deficiency who presents with glossitis, angular stomatitis, koilonychia or esphageal web improves upon correction of the deficiency. Whether or not the menorrhagia sometimes seen with iron deficiency is corrected by iron is a subject of debate. Patients who have undergone subtotal gastrectomy and gastrojejunostomy have up to a 60 per cent chance of incurring iron deficit due to loss of acid-secreting capacity, rapid gastric emptying, and bypass of the duodenum. Pregnancy is almost certain to produce iron deficiency, since a net loss of over 500 mg. of iron occurs.

Unless the cause of the iron deficiency is removed, recurrence rates are high, even when treatment is prescribed. In a series of 100 cases, 29 relapses were noted; in 24 instances, inadequate iron was being taken; in 12, blood loss continued in excess of iron therapy, and in 4, malabsorption was documented.

PRINCIPLES OF MANAGEMENT

The importance of identification and treatment of the underlying etiology cannot be overremphasized, especially when the anemia is found in a man or an elderly patient (see Chapter 77). The severity of the anemia does not indicate the seriousness of the cause. Indications for iron replacement are tempered by the fact that symptoms are often minimal and the morbidity from a mild anemia is low. Moreover, as noted above, correction of the iron deficit is not certain to alleviate the host of vague complaints often attributed to it. Nevertheless, replacement therapy makes sense when (1) the patient is symptomatic and has a limited cardiopulmonary reserve, (2) the anemia has become moderately severe (hemoglobin 8–9 gm. per 100 ml.), (3) the patient is pregnant, (4) the patient had a subtotal gastrectomy and gastrojejunostomy, (5) continued heavy blood loss is anticipated, or (6) the patient is recovering from megaloblastic anemia.

Oral iron is preferred; the ferrous form is better absorbed than the ferric one. Absorption occurs best under conditions of low pH in the proximal small bowel. Phytates and phosphates found in food bind iron and reduce absorption. When iron tablets are taken with meals, a 40 per cent drop in absorption can be demonstrated. Absorption also varies according to the severity of the deficit. About 20 per cent of an oral dose is taken up initially, but absorption falls to 5 per cent after 1 month of therapy, even though the anemia remains incompletely corrected.

Most ferrous salts have equivalent rates of absorption and produce similar rates of hemoglobin replenishment. Choice is a matter of cost and side effects; the degree of gastrointestinal upset is a function more of the iron content of the tablet than of the form of ferrous salt used. Slow-release preparations have been touted as producing fewer side effects and requiring only once-daily administration. However, they dissolve slowly and can bypass the proximal small bowel before significant absorption has occurred. There is no evidence they are worth the extra cost, which is about ten times that of ferrous sulfate. Some preparations contain ascorbic acid with the claim that the acid facilitates absorption, especially in patients with achlorhydria; such patients respond quite adequately to ferrous sulfate alone, probably because of the excess amount of iron available.

The recommended dose for iron deficiency is 300 mg. of ferrous sulfate, three times daily. Although taking iron with a meal reduces absorption, it also lessens disagreeable gastrointestinal symptoms such as nausea and epigastric discomfort. Constipation and diarrhea are frequently reported as well, but are less a function of the amount of iron available for absorption. About 25 per cent of patients report side effects.

The response to iron is apparent within 10 days of initiating therapy; a reticulocytosis is first noted, followed by a rise in the hemoglobin concentration of 0.1 to 0.2 gm. per 100 ml. per day. Several weeks of therapy are required to bring the hemoglobin level back up to normal, and replenishing iron stores may take months. However, speed is not an issue unless blood loss is rapid, in which case blood transfusion rather than iron therapy is the treatment of choice. The response to parenteral iron therapy is no more rapid than that seen with oral preparations.

Parenteral iron has a very limited role. It should be used only in patients who have had an adequate trial of oral iron and shown a genuine intolerance to all available preparations. Patients with inflammatory bowel disease may require parenteral iron due to the irritant effect of oral iron and the need to take large doses in order to keep up with blood loss. Parenteral iron has also been suggested for patients with malabsorption, but most are able to absorb a sufficient amount of oral iron. Intramuscular administration has been associated with development of sarcomas at injection sites and should be avoided. Fatal anaphylatic reactions and asthma have been produced by all parenteral forms of iron administration. If parenteral iron must be used, it should be administered by the intravenous route, beginning with a very small test dose and continuing with a slow drip; a syringe with epinephrine should be drawn up at the same time and kept on hand.

PATIENT EDUCATION AND PREVENTION OF IRON DEFICIENCY

Patients need to be instructed on the best means of minimizing gastrointestinal side effects in order to maximize compliance. Starting with a small dose, e.g., 300 mg. per day, of ferrous sulfate and building to 900 mg. per day avoids initial intolerance. Taking iron just after eating may also help. It needs to be made clear that therapy has to be continued on a regular basis for weeks and often months.

Prevention of iron deficiency is most important in those with increased needs, i.e., pregnant women and young children. The average American diet contains 12 mg. of iron per 2000 calories. Twenty per cent is absorbed by markedly iron-deficient patients and 5 to 10 per cent by others; thus, about 0.6 to 1.2 mg. is taken up under normal circumstances each day. Daily requirement for men and postmenopausal women is 0.5 to 1.0 mg. per day, indicating that dietary intake should suffice. However 1.5 mg. per day is needed by menstruating women and 2.5 mg. per day by pregnant women. Iron-rich foods can be used to avoid the need for iron supplements. Fish, meat (particularly liver) and iron-enriched cereals and bread are excellent sources. Eggs and green vegetables are also high in iron, but the iron is unavailable for absorption because it is bound to the phosphates and phytates present in these foods.

When diet alone seems inadequate and needs are very high, as in pregnancy, a once-daily dose of 150 to 300 mg. of ferrous sulfate is recommended to avoid significant iron deficiency. It must be emphasized that most people who eat a balanced diet do not require iron supplements. Taking widely promoted tonics which contain iron, vitamins and minerals is expensive and unnecessary in most instances.

ANNOTATED BIBLIOGRAPHY

Adverse effects of parenteral iron. Medical Letter, *19*:35, 1977. *(Recommends extreme caution in use of these agents due to risks of sarcomas with intramuscular injection and anaphylaxis reported with all parenteral forms of therapy.)*

Brise, H., and Hallberg, L.: Influence of meals on iron absorption in oral iron therapy. Acta Med. Scand. (Suppl.), *171*:376, 1962. *(Absorption fell 40 per cent when oral iron was taken with meals.)*

Crosby, W.: Who needs iron? N. Engl. J. Med., *297*:543, 1977. *(Terse review of iron requirements and need for supplements.)*

Elwood, P., and Williams, G.: A comparative trial of slow-release and conventional iron preparations. Practitioner, *204*:812, 1970. *(No therapeutic advantage found for the slow-release preparations.)*

Fry, J.: Clinical patterns and course of anemias in general practice. Br. Med. J., *2*:1732, 1961. *(Recurrence rate of iron deficiency was 30 per cent after treatment.)*

Kerr, D., and Davidson, S.: Gastrointestinal intolerance to oral iron preparations. Lancet, *2*:489, 1958. *(An early description of GI side effects of oral preparations.)*

Oral iron. Medical Letter, *20*:45, 1978. *(Menstruating and pregnant women may need iron supplements; ferrous sulfate is least expensive and no less effective or less well tolerated than other preparations.)*

Wood, M., and Elwood, P.: Symptoms of iron deficiency anemia: A community survey. Br. J. Prev. Soc. Med., *20*:117, 1966. *(The correlation between hemoglobin concentration and symptoms was poor. Iron therapy produced no statistically significant improvement in complaints.)*

84
Outpatient Oral Anticoagulant Therapy

Oral anticoagulant therapy with coumarin derivatives has become a major therapeutic tool in the prevention of fibrin thrombus formation. Approximately 300,000 patients are stricken annually by thromboembolism; over 50,000 die. A great deal of morbidity and mortality could be avoided by timely anticoagulation. It is important to know (1) indications for therapy, (2) how to initiate and maintain patients on oral anticoagulants in the outpatient setting, (3) common complications, and (4) drugs and conditions which interfere with or potentiate the anticoagulant's effect.

MECHANISM OF ACTION

Warfarin and other coumarin derivatives inhibit vitamin K-dependent synthesis of clotting factors II, VII, IX and X. Since both intrinsic and extrinsic clotting cascades are affected, the prothrombin time (PT) and the partial thromboplastin time (PTT) are prolonged. The half-lives of factors II, VII, IX and X range from 5 hours for factor VII to 100 hours for Factor II. Full anticoagulant effect is not achieved until the patient has been on warfarin for about 5 days, even though prolongation of PT and PTT may be noted after a few days of therapy.

INDICATIONS

Therapy is indicated in conditions having a high risk of thrombus formation and subsequent embolization. Well-controlled studies documenting conditions associated with a high incidence of thromboembolism that can be significantly reduced by oral anticoagulant therapy are few in number. The consensus is that mitral stenosis complicated by atrial fibrillation (see Chapter 23), deep vein throbophlebitis (see Chapter 30), pulmonary embolization, systemic embolization and implant of an artificial prosthetic heart valve are indications for oral anticoagulant therapy. Other conditions felt by many to be indications for oral anticoagulant therapy, but less well established, include transient ischemic attacks (see Chapter 159), chronic and paroxysmal atrial fibrillation in the elderly (see Chapter 23), congestive cardiomyopathy (see Chapter 27), and ventricular aneurysm. There is no evidence that atherosclerotic heart disease is prevented by use of coumarin anticoagulants.

CONTRAINDICATIONS

Contraindications to the use of oral anticoagulants need to be considered in the context of urgency of anticoagulation, risk and seriousness of potential complications, and duration of therapy. Patients with previous central nervous system bleeding, recent neurosurgery or frank bleeding should not receive warfarin. Important relative contraindications include active peptic ulcer disease, chronic alcoholism, blindness (unless in supervised situations), bleeding diathesis, and severe hypertension. When taken early in pregnancy, coumarins may cause birth defects; when they are used at delivery, fetal hemorrhage can occur. Heparin should be used in place of warfarin during early pregnancy and childbirth. Embarking on oral anticoagulant therapy is unwise when follow-up cannot be readily maintained, when laboratory facilities for accurately measuring the prothrombin time are inadequate, or when the patient is unreliable.

METHODS OF INITIATING AND MONITORING THERAPY

Patients with acute pulmonary embolization, deep vein thrombophlebitis, or acute systemic embolization should be admitted for immediate parenteral administration of heparin to be followed by oral warfarin therapy. Other patients are in less urgent need of immediate full anticoagulation and can be safely started on a warfarin program as outpatients. One method of initiating outpatient therapy is to prescribe 10 mg. of warfarin daily for the first 3 days;

the prothrombin time is measured on the third day. At 10 mg. per day, it takes a mean of 5 days to reach therapeutic range. The dose is subsequently adjusted or maintained to achieve a prothrombin level of 1.5 to 2 times control. When there is a small theoretical risk of central nervous system bleeding, as in moderate hypertension, therapy can be adjusted to maintain a range of 1.4 to 1.6 times control.

Once the desired level of anticoagulation is achieved, the PT is measured once every 3 weeks. In about 85 per cent of patients, dosage adjustments over time are unnecessary; in 15 per cent, they are. Since it is impossible to predict who will and who will not need adjustments, the PT is checked every 3 weeks, the schedule being rigorously enforced.

There are many possible methods of dosage adjustment. One which is designed to maximize safety and avoid wide swings in prothrombin time utilizes 10 per cent changes in weekly dose, unless PT is grossly out of range. For example, if the patient is taking 7.5 mg. per day, the weekly dose is 52.5 mg. If the prothrombin time is too low, the dose is increased so that on 2 of the 7 days, the patient takes 10 mg., and 7.5 the other 5 days. The prothrombin time is then measured weekly for the next 2 weeks.

Outpatient anticoagulation requires facilities for accurate prothrombin time measurement, reliable collection of samples, and the ability to contact patients promptly. Careful monitoring and follow-up are essential to the safety and success of any outpatient anticoagulation program. At the beginning of therapy, patients can benefit considerably from a session with a nurse who can instruct them in the use of warfarin, answer questions, test understanding, and provide informative booklets for them to take home. The importance of close monitoring and patient education cannot be overemphasized. If the patient fails to keep his appointment for a prothrombin time test, he should be contacted immediately. A computer system can provide reminders so that no patient is lost to follow-up. To further simplify therapy and avoid confusion, scored 5-mg. tablets of sodium warfarin can be used exclusively. Commercial laboratory services are sometimes employed to draw samples at home for patients who have difficulty coming to the office for frequent PT determinations.

COMPLICATIONS

Bleeding is the obvious complication of therapy. In one large series involving over 3500 courses of therapy, acute or gross bleeding occurred in 6.8 per cent, with 4 deaths. Frequency of bleeding correlated with degree of prolongation of the prothrombin time, advanced age and use of a large loading dose. Major bleeding in the central nervous system and gastrointestinal tract was responsible for morbidity and mortality.

Patients with prothrombin times in therapeutic range (i.e., 1.5 to 2 times control), who bleed from the urinary tract, rectum or vagina while on anticoagulant therapy should be considered to have an underlying pathologic process until proven otherwise. In the series noted above, a lesion was found to be responsible for the bleeding in over 50 per cent; occult malignancy in the bladder and colon was not uncommon.

In rare instances, hemorrhagic necrosis of skin has been reported in women, and cyanotic toes in men; all with prothrombin times in therapeutic range.

CONDITIONS AND MEDICATIONS WHICH INCREASE AND DECREASE ANTICOAGULANT EFFECT OF WARFARIN (TABLE 84–1)

Drugs which *potentiate* the effect of warfarin may do so by preventing synthesis or absorption of vitamin K, displacing warfarin from binding sites, inhibiting microsomal degradative enzyme activity, increasing catabolism of clotting factors, or impairing platelet function. Hepatocellular failure results in impaired synthesis of clotting factors and albumin; cholestasis makes for less efficient absorption of vitamin K. Both conditions are capable of prolonging the prothrombin time and potentiating the effects of warfarin.

Anticoagulant effects are *decreased* by agents which induce microsomal enzymes, decrease absorption of warfarin, or increase synthesis of clotting factors or binding proteins. Moreover, coumarins will cause a decrease in the metabolism of tolbutamide and phenytoin by competing for the same degradative enzymes. The prothrombin time should be measured when any change in drug program is made, and it should be followed closely thereafter.

INDICATIONS FOR CONTINUATION AND TERMINATION OF THERAPY

Therapy should be continued indefinitely in patients with valvular disease with atrial fibrillation,

Table 84–1. Common Drugs Which Interact with Oral Anticoagulants

DRUG	MECHANISM
Agents *potentiating* the anticoagulant effect of warfarin	
Alcohol	Decreased metabolism during acute intoxication
Allopurinol	Inhibition of microsomal enzymes
Anabolic steroids	Unknown
Chloral hydrate	Displacement of binding sites
Chloramphenicol	Inhibition of microsomal enzymes
Clofibrate	Displacement from binding sites
Indomethacin	Impairment of platelet function
Phenylbutazone	Displacement from binding sites
Salicylates	Impairment of platelet function
Sulfonamides	Unknown
Thyroxine	Increased catabolism of clotting factors
Agents *decreasing* the anticoagulant effect of warfarin	
Barbiturates	Induction of microsomal enzymes
Cholestyramine	Decreased absorption
Oral contraceptives	Increased synthesis or activity of some clotting factors
Gluthethimide	Induction of microsomal enzymes
Rifampin	Induction of microsomal enzymes

systemic embolization, and artificial heart valves. In other instances, there are few data on proper duration of therapy. In deep venous thrombosis, most experts recommend continuation of therapy for approximately 3 to 6 months; the same is true in pulmonary embolization. Deep vein thrombophlebitis or pulmonary emboli that recur after 6 months of treatment are usually followed by retreatment for a period of 12 months. If a serious bleeding problem develops in a patient on anticoagulant therapy, the prothrombin time can be corrected promptly by administration of fresh frozen plasma. This is the preferred mode of therapy. Parenteral administration of vitamin K is also effective, though it may take longer to have an effect (up to 5 hours) and can cause refractoriness to warfarin if prompt reinstitution of anticoagulant therapy is attempted. The decision to discontinue anticoagulant therapy in the context of bleeding needs to be individualized. The risk of hemorrhage has to be balanced against the risk of serious embolization.

PATIENT EDUCATION

Avoidance of unnecessary morbidity depends on thorough patient education. Prior to initiation of outpatient therapy, the patient and responsible family members need to learn the name of the medication, the dose, time of day to be taken, need for routine check of PT, necessity of avoiding alcohol and aspirin-containing compounds, and recognize signs of bleeding such as melena and spontaneous ecchymoses. Teaching undertaken by the nurse, as well as distribution of helpful booklets detailing proper use of the drug, are essential components of the patient education effort. Any patient who is incapable of understanding the instructions or deemed unreliable should not be placed on therapy, since the risks of hemorrhage probably outweigh any possible benefits. The one exception is the patient who can be closely supervised by family members or health care professionals.

ANNOTATED BIBLIOGRAPHY

Coon, W.W., and William, P.W.: Hemorrhagic complications of anticoagulant therapy. Arch. Intern. Med., *133*:386, 1974. *(A review of 3800 courses of anticoagulant treatment, detecting bleeding in 6.8 per cent. Frequency of bleeding increased with intensity of treatment as reflected in prothrombin time. More than half of the patients with bleeding had an identifiable lesion responsible for the bleeding.)*

Deykin, D: Warfarin therapy. N. Engl. J. Med., *283*:691, 1970. *(Excellent discussion of warfarin's actions, metabolism and interactions with other drugs.)*

Duration of anticoagulant therapy for thromboembolism. Medical Letter, *13*:69, 1971. *(Three to 6 months for deep vein thrombosis and first episode of pulmonary embolization. Recurrences are treated for 12 months; guidelines are all based on opinions of consultants; controlled studies are nonexistent.)*

Feder, W., and Auerback, R.: Purple toes: An uncommon sequela of oral coumarin drug therapy. Ann. Intern. Med., *55*:911, 1961. *(A complication seen in 1 per cent of patients, all men with PT in range.)*

Koch-Weser, J., and Sellers, E.M.: Drug interaction with coumarin anticoagulants. N. Engl. J. Med.,

285:487, 1971. *(Good summary of the many possible potentiating and inhibiting interactions.)*

Mackie, M., and Douglas, A.: Oral anticoagulants in arterial disease. Br. Med. Bull., 23:177, 1978. *(Critical review of the evidence for coumarin use in coronary, cerebral, rheumatic and peripheral vascular disease; 95 refs.)*

O'Reilly, R.A., and Aggeler, P.M.: Studies on coumarin anticoagulation: Initiation of therapy without a loading dose. Circulation, 38:169, 1968. *(At 10 mg. per day, it took a mean of 5.2 days to achieve therapeutic range; using 15 mg. per day, it took 2.7 days. No bleeding problems were encountered compared to frequent problems when larger [25 mg.] initial doses are used.)*

Ramsay, D.M.: Thromboembolism in pregnancy.

Obstet. Gynecol., 45:129, 1975. *(Warfarin therapy is associated with birth defects early in pregnancy and fetal hemorrhage at the time of delivery. Heparin is preferred when anticoagulation is necessary, though warfarin can be used in mid-pregnancy.)*

Verhagen H: Local hemorrhage and necrosis of skin and underlying tissues during anticoagulant therapy with dicumarol. Acta. Med. Scan., 148:453, 1954. *(A very rare but important complication, occurring in women whose PTs were in range.)*

Wessler, S.: Anticoagulant therapy. JAMA, 228:757, 1974. *(Argues that the only established indications for anticoagulant use are atrial fibrillation with mitral stenosis, prosthetic heart valve, deep vein thrombophlebitis, pulmonary emoblization and systemic emoblization.)*

Section B: Oncology

85

Evaluation of the Unknown Primary Tumor

JACOB J. LOKICH, M.D.

An unknown primary cancer is found in up to 15 per cent of all patients presenting with malignancy. It often prompts an extensive search for the site of origin, undertaken in the hope that a treatable form of cancer will be found. The term "unknown primary" has particularly specific meaning; it is meant to denotes a lesion that is a metastasis and not a primary tumor of the organ within which it is found. It is most often an incurable lesion, but treatment options are nonetheless available. A tumor is designated as an unknown primary tumor or tumor of unknown origin (TUO), after meeting the following two criteria: the tissue is histologically confirmed, determined to be an epithelial, mesenchymal, or lymphomatous malignancy, and a primary tumor of the organ is ruled out. In addition, routine screening must fail to identify the primary source, and the possibility of a metachronous metastasis must be eliminated. The latter is particularly important since metastases may develop after a long dormant phase in patients with a variety of tumors, including breast cancer, melanoma, and renal-cell tumors; solitary metastases of these tumors are not uncommon.

The most common sites for unknown primary tumors are the lung, bone, liver, and lymph nodes. The primary care physician is often the first to discover these lesions and must have an effective diagnostic approach.

The TUO can represent an expensive and uncomfortable diagnostic workup for the patient. Assessment should be guided by the basic principle of attempting to identify a treatable tumor. Confirmation by histopathologic diagnosis and application of sophisticated pathologic techniques to clarify the site of origin are essential before undertaking a search for a primary tumor. Extensive staging is usually unwarranted, since the tumor is already metastatic.

CLINICAL PRESENTATION

A TUO may present in the lung as a solitary nodule or recurrent pleural effusion (see Chapters 39 and 40). Mediastinal TUOs, often present with catastrophic secondary complications, such as dysphagia, stridor or respiratory difficulty, or superior vena cava syndrome. In bone, TUO may appear as a lytic or blastic lesion of axial skeleton, long bones, or skull.

An isolated hard lymph node is another common presentation (see Chapter 80), as is a hepatic nodule or focal defect on liver scan.

DIFFERENTIAL DIAGNOSIS*

In patients without a prior malignancy, the new pulmonary nodule indicative of tumor may represent a primary tumor of the lung or a synchronous metastasis from another site (see Chapter 40). The same is true for a nodule in patients with a prior malignancy (see Chapter 42). If breast cancer is the previous malignancy, there is a 70 to 80 per cent chance that the pulmonary shadow on radiographic examination represents a synchronous metastasis; if colon cancer is the previous malignancy, 50 per cent of such patients will have a new primary tumor in the lung; and, finally, if Hodgkin's disease is the previous primary tumor, the pulmonary lesion will be Hodgkin's disease in almost all instances.

Recurrent pleural effusions are a common complication of mesothelioma and various metastatic pleural lesions (see Chapter 39). Mediastinal tumors are usually from lung or breast or spread of lymphoma. In bone, osteoblastic lesions are observed primarily with breast, prostate, and lung cancers and, less commonly, with thyroid cancer and lymphoma. These must be distinguished from osteogenic sarcoma, chondrosarcoma, and Ewing's sarcoma, which are the treatable primary bone tumors. Focal defect on liver scan may be due to granulomatous disease, benign hepatomas, and primary hepatic malignancies, as well as a metastatic lesion. High cervical nodes may be associated with submucosal nasopharyngeal tumor or may represent a site of metastasis from a tumor within the oral cavity. Axillary adenopathy suggests a metastasis from the ipsilateral breast, and inguinal nodes develop metastases from the genitalia or perineal structures (see Chapter 80).

WORKUP

The most important general principle in evaluation of a patient with TUO is to search carefully for treatable tumor. In men, the most treatable tumor is prostatic cancer; in women the most amenable to therapy are breast and ovarian cancers. Patients with undifferentiated carcinoma must be evaluated for lymphoma, which also responds to treatment.

A number of other tumors are routinely sought,

* See individual chapters noted for full differential diagnoses of each of these entities.

even though they are untreatable or respond less than optimally to chemotherapy or radiation. These include pancreatic cancer, gastric and colonic cancer, and renal-cell carcinoma. Recognition and treatment of the asymptomatic primary tumor does not improve longevity. The expense and discomfort incurred by the many diagnostic studies ordered in search of them can be avoided if the physician remembers to look primarily for the treatable malignancy (see Table 85–1).

The second major principle in evaluation of a TUO, is that, after a metastatic lesion has been identified, it is unnecessary to stage the patient for other sites of metastases since the incurable nature of the tumor has already been revealed. Thus, the patient who presents with a pulmonary nodule and is found to have breast cancer as a primary source does not require a liver scan to document the presence of liver disease. Treatment in patients with cancer is determined first and foremost by stage of disease, but once metastases have been identified, the tumor is sufficiently staged. The prime consideration for therapy becomes the presence of symptoms.

Before investigation for a treatable primary tumor is initiated, a *histologic diagnosis* of tumor must be made on tissue obtained from the metastatic site. Most commonly, a specific tissue type is identified, although the histopathologic origin of the tumor may be undifferentiated carcinoma, or simply malignant tumor. It must be noted that biopsied tissue fixed in formalin and sectioned reveals architectural relationships as well as its histologic detail. On the other hand, the cytologic examination of an aspirated fluid or of an aspirated solid mass lesion, yields malignant-appearing cells without any architectural relationships. Cytologic preparation also may misrepresent nuclear and cytoplasmic abnormalities, which can be induced by inflammation or drugs. Therefore, in patients with serositis and pleural or peritoneal effusions, the cytologic diagnosis should be confirmed by tissue diagnosis.

The histologic designation of *adenocarcinoma* does not definitively establish the primary source of the tumor. Any organ may develop a glandular malignancy. The distinction on histologic grounds between an adenocarcinoma of the ovary, the stomach, the lung, or the breast is possible, but other methods may be needed. The estrogen receptor protein (ERP) assays are useful because ERP has been identified only in breast cancer and in a small number of non-mammary tumors. At present, though, no other receptor proteins are available for routine use.

The histologic designation *undifferentiated carcinoma* presumes a level of anaplasia, which cannot be used to reliably identify the origin of the malignancy.

Additional tissue should be obtained in order to define the tumor more precisely by electron microscopy, surface marker typing, and special histochemical staining for intracytoplasmic and intranuclear inclusions.

The patient with a *solitary pulmonary nodule* is often evaluated for the presence of tumor outside the lung before it is determined that the nodule represents a tumor. The first task is to confirm the diagnosis of malignancy; this involves consideration of transpulmonary needle aspiration vs. bronchoscopic fiberoptic brushing vs. thoracotomy (see Chapters 40 and 42). Whether the tumor is associated with a prior malignancy or not, thoracotomy is generally indicated when it is necessary to maximize the histopathologic information, as well as to remove all known tumor, or to stage and establish the extent of disease by direct observation. A needle aspiration may yield cytologic information but does not identify the tumor site of origin. Furthermore, the tissue obtained cannot be evaluated by electron microscopy, surface marker typing, or special staining.

Pleural effusions due to malignancy can be diagnosed cytologically, though there are pitfalls. Mesothelioma, a primary tumor of the pleura, may be mistaken for adenocarcinoma when cytologic specimens are used. Often a pleural biopsy in conjunction with aspiration is more informative, especially when granulomatous disease is also under consideration (see Chapters 39 and 47). A diagnosis of adenocarcinoma in cytologic fluids does not identify the primary source; for these patients, diagnosis should be approached by searching for treatable tumors.

Mediastinal malignancies that produce symptoms of dysphagia, respiratory difficulty, or superior vena cava syndrome are almost invariably due to primary lung cancer, metastatic breast cancer, or lymphoma. All can be rather well managed by local radiation therapy and do not warrant extensive evaluation and search for the primary tumor.

The identification of a *bony lesion* that is radiographically characteristic of neoplasia should be followed up with a biopsy of the area. If the lesion is inaccessible or is amenable to biopsy only with difficulty, an alternate first step is to obtain a routine bone marrow biopsy from the iliac crest. The vast majority of patients with bony metastases have multiple lesions that often invade the bone marrow. The second crucial step is to obtain a bone scan in order to identify other sites of tumor that may be more easily accessible to a fluoroscopically-guided biopsy. Having established a histologic diagnosis of malignancy in the bone, the search for the primary should, as always, be confined to focusing on treatable tumor.

Bony metastases are generally not treated systemically; for the most part they are palliated locally by radiation therapy when symptoms arise. Therefore, in the absence of symptoms, the bone lesions may simply be monitored unless a definitively responsive tumor, such as prostate or breast cancer, can be identified.

Hepatic TUOs are usually diagnosed by liver biopsy. Most are adenocarcinomas. Once an adenocarcinoma in the liver has been identified, it is unnecessary for therapy to order an upper GI series, small bowel follow-through, barium enema, colonoscopy, pancreatic endoscopy, or gallbladder series. None of the tumors that arise in any of these sites, once metastatic to the liver, are sufficiently treatable with systemic therapy to warrant establishing the diagnosis. Furthermore, patients with hepatic metastases have a life expectancy of less than six months. Prophylactic surgery of the primary tumor is not indicated unless significant antitumor effect can be demonstrated in the metastatic disease. Assessment for antitumor effect should be scheduled to occur at 4 to 6 weeks, if cytotoxic chemotherapy is utilized. Only if marked response is documented is search for the primary tumor warranted.

Lymph nodes in the cervical, axillary, and inguinal sites occasionally harbor an unknown primary tumor. For the most part, lymph node lesions are drainage areas for a TUO in a contiguous organ (see Chapter 80).

Cervical lymph nodes are first biopsied to determine the histopathologic category of tumor. If an epidermoid carcinoma is found, then extensive otolaryngological evaluation of the nasopharynx, retropharynx, and oral cavity must be performed, including blind biopsies of the base of the tongue and the nasopharynx. If no definite primary is identified, the carcinoma must be managed by either radiation or lymph node dissection on the ipsilateral site. The carcinoma is cured in 20 to 35 per cent of patients. Other tumors that may be metastatic to cervical nodes include those of the sinuses and salivary glands; if the histopathology is adenocarcinoma, the sinuses or the salivary glands may be the primary source. If the histologic studies indicate lymphoma, then the diagnosis and staging approach are altogether different (see Chapters 81, 82).

Axillary nodes that histologically manifest adenocarcinoma are most commonly associated with mammary cancer. Even in the presence of a normal mammogram, mastectomy may be necessary because

Table 85-1.   Categories of Tumor Treatability and Drug Management

TUMOR	RESPONSE RATE (%)	TREATMENT
Responsive		
Choriocarcinoma	90-100	Methotrexate, actinomycin
Testicular cancer	80	Vinblastine sulfate, bleomycin and platinum
Lymphoma (including Hodgkin's disease)	50-70	COP, MOPP, BACOP
Breast cancer	40-60	Hormones, cyclophosphamide (Cytoxan), and doxorubicin (Adriamycin)
Prostate cancer	40-60	Hormones
Ovarian cancer	40-60	Cyclophosphamide (Cytoxan), and doxorubicin (Adriamycin)
Sarcoma	30-50	Doxorubicin (Adriamycin) combinations
Neurosecretory (endocrine tumors)	20-30	Streptozotocin
Marginally Responsive		
Colon and other GI tumors	10-15	5-Fluorouracil
Melanoma	10-15	DTIC
Unresponsive		
Lung, kidney, liver, pancreas, brain		

identification of the primary tumor can be difficult. The diagnosis may be assisted by performing ERP assays on any tissue obtained from the axilla that appears to be a carcinoma (see Chapter 118).

Inguinal adenopathy is approached diagnostically and therapeutically in much the same manner as cervical adenopathy. The presence of an epidermoid carcinoma or adenocarcinoma may be treated by local radiation therapy bilaterally if there is no evidence of an anal or prostatic lesion on blind biopsy. If inguinal node biopsy identifies a lymphoma, there is no need for lymphangiography, particularly in the presence of adenopathy at sites above the diaphragm. Lymphangiography alone is never a diagnostic procedure and only occasionally a staging procedure, since it generally cannot determine therapy. It invariably requires histologic confirmation, particularly in the presence of lymphangiographically positive lymph nodes (see Chapters 81, 82).

TREATMENT

The most treatable metastatic tumors are outlined in Table 85-1. Based on pathologic and clinical criteria, the therapeutic approach to the patient may be based on a prudent estimate of the most likely treatable tumor. If the pathologic type is indeterminate (undifferentiated), treatment is directed toward the most responsive tumor in this class, namely, lymphoma. Metastatic adenocarcinoma in men should be treated as metastatic prostate cancer, and in women as metastatic ovarian or breast cancer, since these are the most treatable tumors. Metastatic prostate cancer has a 40- to 60-per cent response rate to hormonal therapy (see Chapter 137). Carcinoma of the breast has a similar response rate to therapy; modalities include hormonal treatment for some patients and chemotherapy for others (see Chapters 87 and 118)

ANNOTATED BIBLIOGRAPHY

Copeland, E. M., and McBride, C. M.: Axillary metastases from unknown primary sites. Ann Surg., *178*:25, 1972. *(The breast is the most common primary source in woman with an undifferentiated axillary lesion, but alternatives include primary melanoma or adnexal tumors of the extremity.)*

Fitzpatrick, P. J., and Kotalik, J. F.: Cervical metastases from an unknown primary tumor. Ther. Radiol., *110*:659, 1974. *(Radiation therapy for cervical lymph nodes in an unknown primary tumor may result in a cure rate of more than 40 per cent, in spite of inability to identify the primary tumor source. Emphasis on the site of cervical node involvement and the technique of radiation therapy produces optimal therapeutic effect.)*

Lokich, J. Tumor of unknown origin. In Lokich, J. (ed.): Clinical Cancer Medicine. Boston: G. K. Hall, 1979. *(A pragmatic and comprehensive approach to the unknown primary tumor emphasizing pathologic and diagnostic techniques in relationship to establishing treatable tumors.)*

Moertel, C. G., Reitemeier, R. J., Schutt, A. J., and Hahn, R. G.: Treatment of the patient with adenocarcinoma of unknown origin. Cancer, 30:1469, 1972. (This is a singular series from the Mayo Clinic of more than 150 patients with adenocarcinomas treated with 5-fluorouracil. The response rate in the collective series was approximately 15 per cent and the primary tumor site in those patients coming to autopsy was predominantly pancreas.)

Nystrom, J.S., Weiner, J. M., et al.: Metastatic and histologic presentations in unknown primary cancer. Semin. Oncol., 4:53, 1977. (The PCS or primary cancer site is identified on the basis of the development of a discriminate function in a homogeneous series from a single university of over 250 patients. The most common primary tumor site above the diaphragm was the lung and below the diaphragm was the pancreas.)

Smith, P. E., Krementz, E. T., and Chapman, W.: Metastatic cancer without a detectable primary site. Am. J. Surg., 113:633, 1967. (In more than 70 per cent of the cases, a primary tumor site was not established, in spite of extensive diagnostic evaluation. The survival was longest in those patients with undifferentiated tumor.)

Zaren, H. A., and Copeland, E. M., III: Inguinal node metastases. Cancer, 41:919, 1978. (One per cent of more than 2,200 patients with inguinal node metastases had an unknown primary tumor; in them, survival and possible cure was obtained in 50 per cent by surgical excision alone. In only one of the 22 patients with an unknown primary tumor was the primary tumor found.)

86

Approach to Staging and Monitoring

JACOB J. LOKICH, M.D.

Staging and monitoring are essential components of cancer management. Staging is performed to assess the extent of disease, and it is used to help determine prognosis and therapy. Monitoring serves to detect the reappearance or progression of cancer and contributes importantly to updating prognosis and revising treatment plans. Staging and monitoring procedures are determined by tumor type, its natural history, response to therapy, and characteristic pattern of spread. The frequency and duration of monitoring depend on the rate of disease recurrence.

If the primary physician is to be responsible for the management of the cancer patient, he must be able to stage and monitor disease. This task requires knowledge of the indications for and limitations of the many available laboratory tests and radiological procedures, so that important decisions about test and procedure selection can be made effectively, and unnecessary expense and discomfort avoided.

STAGING TERMINOLOGY

The general classification of staging is based on the anatomic distribution of disease. It is broadly categorized as *local* (confined to a visceral site); *re-gional* (extension within the local site, with or without involvement of contiguous lymph nodes); or *distant* (generally hematogenous metastases beyond the regional scope which precludes treatment that uses local surgical removal). This staging system is translated into T for tumors, N for nodes and M for metastases. Subcategories may be developed depending upon the size of the tumor (T-1 to 3); the number or fixation of the lymph nodes (N-1 to 2); and the presence of lack of metastases (M-0 or 1).

PRINCIPLES AND PROCEDURES OF STAGING

Staging procedures are selected predominantly on the basis of the malignancy's characteristic pattern of local and metastatic spread. The type of tumor and the natural history of its rate of growth are other determinants of the staging strategy. For example, sarcomas metastasize hematogenously, usually to lung, and rarely proceed to lymph nodes. Thus, lung tomography is an important staging tool for sarcomas, while lymphangiography is not.

Two other important factors in the selection of a staging procedure are the sensitivity and specificity

Table 86–1. Radiographic Procedures in Staging Cancer

PROCEDURE	TUMOR TYPES	FALSE-POSITIVE (%)	FALSE-NEGATIVE (%)	COMMENT
Tomography	Sarcoma, testicle, Hodgkin's	5–10	10	False negative directly related to size of lesion False positive due to identification of benign lesions
Lymphangiography	Hodgkin's lymphoma, prostate, ovary	20	10	Nondiagnostic changes
Radionuclide scans				
Liver	GI, breast, lung	20	10	Rarely abnormal without clinical signs or biochemical changes
Bone	Breast, lung, GU	10	<5	Incidence of positive scans related to stage of 1° tumor
Gallium	Melanoma	10	30	Infection (abscess) causes positive scan
Brain	Melanoma, renal, breast, lung	<5	<10	Supplemental CAT scan
Lymphoscintography	Ovary, breast	In development		
Metastatic series	Breast, lung, GU	10	20–50	
Angiography		Not standard		
Intravenous pyelogram		Not useful		
Ultrasonography	Retroperitoneum	10–20*	10–20*	Resolution to 4 cm.; distinguish cystic from solid mass

*Estimated

of the test (see Chapter 2) for the particular tumor in question.

Radiographic Procedures. X-ray studies are most frequently used for determining the extent of disease and include tomography, lymphangiography, radionuclide scans, metastatic series, angiography, intravenous pyelography, and ultrasound (Table 86–1).

Tomography, more specifically, full-lung tomography is rarely helpful in the detection of occult metastases, but rather, is most applicable in delineating an abnormality found on standard chest film. However, full-lung tomography is routinely employed in the preoperative evaluation of sarcomas and testicular cancers, because these tumors commonly metastasize to the lungs, and the presence of a metastasis obviates the need for amputation or retroperitoneal node dissection (see Chapter 137). Depending on the size of the lesion and the distance between individual tomography pictures, the tomographic assay may have a significant false-negative rate. In at least 10 per cent of patients with established pulmonary nodules, the total number of nodules is underestimated.

Lymphangiography (LAG) was developed primarily for the evaluation of retroperitoneal lymph nodes in the staging for Hodgkins's disease, but it has similarly been employed for lymphoma. The usefulness of this test for staging has declined in recent years, because treatment no longer depends heavily on LAG findings, (see Chapters 81 and 82). An additional factor that limits the usefulness of the study is the necessity for histologic confirmation because of a high false-positive rate. Recently, staging of prostatic and ovarian cancers has been performed using LAG, but this still remains controversial. In fact, ovarian tumors generally metastasize to peritoneal surfaces, and prostatic lesions transfer to pelvic lymph nodes, neither of which would be evaluated adequately by LAG, which delineates mostly the iliac and para-aortic nodes.

Radionuclide scanning has achieved increasing levels of sophistication. Scanning is best used for detection rather than for monitoring; even then tissue confirmation is needed. Liver and bone scans are among the most frequently ordered staging procedures, but they are often performed unnecessarily.

Hepatic scanning is employed in staging of gastrointestinal cancers. However, the liver scan rarely detects disease that is not predicted on the basis of abnormal liver function tests or clinical hepatomegaly. Furthermore, a large percentage of hepatic scans demonstrate abnormalities that are not necessarily consistent with cancer and may be related to secondary drug effects or incidental inflammatory disease. Because true-positive scans are found in less than 1 per cent of patients with otherwise operable primary

Table 86-2. Surgical Procedures in Staging Evaluation of Cancer

PROCEDURE	TUMOR	COMMENTS
Scalene node biopsy	Lung, testicle, cervix	Diagnostic; 10% positive in stage II disease
Lymphadenectomy	Breast, melanoma, head and neck	May be therapeutic but more specifically prognostic
Laparoscopy	Hodgkin's disease, esophagus, ovary	Allows limited access to abdominal contents; has high false-negative rate
Laparotomy	Hodgkin's disease, melanoma, ovary	Definitively evaluates the abdomen and allows for debulking and splenectomy

breast or colon cancer, routine liver scanning for metastases is not warranted in these conditions.

Bone scanning is an exquisitely sensitive means of detecting abnormalities of bone physiology, but in all instances diagnostic confirmation by standard radiographs and, occasionally, by biopsy is necessary. The advantage of bone scanning is earlier detection of disease than is possible by standard x-ray metastatic series, but early detection is not necessarily translated into prolonged survival. Therefore, bone scanning should be used primarily in response to symptoms or in the evaluation of the therapeutic approach to primary tumors. Studies have demonstrated that in patients with Stage I breast cancer (tumor of less than 5 cm. confined to the breast) the bone scan is positive in less than 5 per cent of patients, which does not justify the routine application of bone scanning to screen for metastases.

Gallium scanning was developed to provide a specific agent that would localize within tumors. There is, however, a high false-negative rate (30 per cent). In addition, a high proportion of patients may have false-positive scans because ^{67}Ga localizes within inflammatory masses. It has been applied more specifically to two tumor classes: melanoma and lymphoma. It is also being evaluated as a test for the detection of premorbid bleomycin pulmonary toxicity. The discomfort of the test, which involves frequent enemas, and the high false-negative rate generally relegate gallium scanning to infrequent use.

Standard radiographs, such as *metastatic series,* have a high false-negative rate and are relatively insensitive, but the false-positive rate is low. *Contrast studies,* such as intravenous pyelography, venography, and angiography, are infrequently applied in the staging evaluation, although they may aid in planning surgery.

Ultrasonography is not useful as a quantitative monitor of intra-abdominal tumor, but it is quite effective as a means of detecting lesions greater than 4 cm. in the pancreas or the retroperitoneum and al-

lows for distinguishing cystic from solid masses. *Computerized axial tomography (CAT),* both of the brain and now of the entire body, is available not only as a means of identifying retroperitoneal, intrathoracic, or intracerebral pathology, but also as a means of quantitative evaluation. The resolution power of these scanning procedures makes early detection possible, but histologic confirmation is still necessary. These scans may well revolutionize detection capabilities, but specific guidelines for the cost-effective application of CAT scanning are yet to be established.

Surgical Procedures. Surgical staging of cancer has evolved from *lymph node dissection* procedures. Lymphadenectomy was initially undertaken in patients with breast cancer and malignant melanoma to eliminate contiguous sites of disease. For both tumors, however, it has been demonstrated that lymphadenectomy at the time of surgery for the primary lesion does not extend survival, but does serve as a prognostic determinant (Table 86–2).

Lymph node evaluation of distant disease has become a recognized staging procedure. For example, scalene node biopsy is sometimes performed in patients with primary tumors of the cervix or testicle. In a small proportion of patients, metastases to distant lymph node sites are demonstrated; the identification of distant metastases is important to the management of the primary tumor (see Chapter 137).

Laparotomy and *laparoscopy* have been used in the evaluation of Hodgkin's disease and, more recently, in the evaluation of ovarian cancer to detect abdominal disease. Laparotomy and splenectomy are recommended for the staging of Hodgkin's disease in patients with potential disease below the diaphragm, helping to delineate the radiation portals as well as to move the ovaries out of the port of radiation therapy. For patients who already have evidence of disease below the diaphragm (positive lymphangiography, palpable inguinal nodes, or splenomegaly), the evalua-

Table 86–3.   Periodicity of Follow-up Examination Following Local Surgery for Colon (Dukes B$_2$ and C) and Breast (Stage II) Cancers

TUMOR	INCIDENCE OF SUBSEQUENT METASTASES (%)	INCIDENCE OF NEW (SECOND) 1° (%)	EXAMINATION	FREQUENCY OF EXAMINATIONS
Colon	70	5	Barium enema	Every 2 years
			Sigmoidoscopy or colonoscopy	Every 3 years
			CEA	Every 6 months
			Liver scan	Not indicated
Breast	70	10	Mammogram	Every 1–2 years
			Bone scan	Not indicated
			Metastatic series	Not indicated

tion of the abdomen should be confined to laparoscopy and biopsy of the liver. Patients with clinical disease below the diaphragm and, particularly, patients with B symptoms have a high incidence of secondary complications following laparotomy and splenectomy (see Chapter 81).

Biochemical and immunological markers have begun to be utilized in staging and monitoring, although in general they remain crude indicators. *Acid phosphatase* elevations occur when prostatic carcinoma spreads to bone; recent improvements in fractionation have improved the test's sensitivity and specificity (see Chapter 137). *Alpha-fetoprotein* is helpful in confirming diagnoses of hepatoma and embryonal testicular tumor and monitoring their responses to therapy. Sequential *carcinoembryonic antigen (CEA)* levels correlate with the extent of tumor burden and the likelihood of relapse after surgery for tumors of the breast and gastrointestinal tract (see Chapters 51 and 118). However, CEA lacks specificity. An isomeric species of CEA, designated CEA-S, has been found to produce fewer false-positives and to be more specific for colonic cancer. *Estrogen receptors* are found in breast cancers that are most likely to respond to hormonal manipulation. Their detection can be extremely useful in planning therapy, since the lack of estrogen receptors practically rules out the probability of response to hormonal treatment. The presence of progesterone receptors improves the chance of therapeutic response (see Chapter 118).

PRINCIPLES AND PROCEDURES OF MONITORING DISEASE

Once the extent of disease is determined and treatment initiated, monitoring begins. As noted earlier, the frequency and duration of monitoring are dependent upon the rate of disease recurrence. The procedures selected are based in part on tumor type, response to therapy, stage of disease, and pattern of metastasis. Test sensitivity and specificity are also important.

Local or Regional Disease. Patients with local or regional disease may be monitored by routine physical examinations supplemented by careful examination of the disease site at 3-month intervals for the first year following operation, and at 4-month intervals for the second year. Thereafter, follow-up may be accomplished at 6-month intervals for a minimum of 5 years. By and large, most tumors will recur at a maximum rate during the first 2 years following the initial operation—if in fact they are destined to recur. Three malignancies are notorious for late recurrence: breast carcinoma, melanoma, and renal cell carcinoma. In some patients with these tumors, the lag period before the development of detectable metastases may extend beyond 10 years from initial diagnosis.

Periodic evaluation of patients with regional disease who have undergone curative primary therapy should be directed less at detecting the presence of asymptomatic metastases, and more at finding new primary tumors in the involved organ (Table 86–3). Identification of asymptomatic metastases by radionuclide scanning is of little use, because the early detection and treatment of asymptomatic metastatic disease does not necessarily improve survival.

Metastatic Disease. Follow-up examinations for patients with metastatic disease who receive systemic therapy should be performed at intervals determined by the time expected for an objective clinical response. For hormonal therapy of breast cancer, clinical evidence of response may take as long as 3 months to appear. The effects of cytotoxic chemotherapy may be seen rapidly, for example, within two courses of treatment or 4 to 6 weeks. This is particularly true for exquisitely responsive tumors such as breast, testicular, ovarian, and oat-cell carcinomas.

Patients with metastatic disease receiving palliative systemic therapy should be examined for evidence of new disease. Unnecessary chemotherapy-induced morbidity can be avoided if ineffective palliative systemic therapy is discontinued at the first signs of new disease. Response to therapy may be objectively demonstrated after a predictable interval, but new growth or spread may be noted on earlier examination.

An important corollary to the monitoring of patients with metastatic disease on systemic therapeutic regimens is to define the most objective site of disease to be followed and to avoid additional staging procedures if they do not alter the therapeutic plan. For example, a patient with hepatic metastases from primary breast cancer need not endure a bone scan unless there is bone pain or fracture. The tumor is already established as being incurable, and therapy is determined by the presence of liver metastases. Alternatively, the patient with bony metastases that are difficult to monitor may undergo selective staging in order to identify a more measurable marker of metastatic disease, such as plasma carcinoembryonic antigen.

ANNOTATED BIBLIOGRAPHY

Galasko, C.S.B.: The value of scintography in malignant disease. Cancer Treat. Rev., 2:225, 1975. *(A comprehensive assessment of the technical features of scintography and its application to monitoring malignant disease. The identification of tumor specific, tumor searching agents is reviewed in relationship to other uses of radionuclide scanning in malignant disease.)*

Lokich, J.J.: Carcinoembryonic antigen (CEA): A monitor of therapy for breast and colon cancers. Am. Fam. Physician, 17:173, 1978. *(The author promotes the application of CEA as a tumor associating antigen in specific clinical settings with specific tumor categories.)*

Lokich, J.J.: Tumor markers: Hormones, antigens, and enzymes in malignant disease. Oncology, 35:54, 1978. *(The general considerations of tumor markers as specific monitors of malignancy are reviewed and specific recommendations regarding the realistic application of tumor markers are presented.)*

O'Connell, M.J., Wahner, H.W., Ahmann, D.L., Edis, A.J., and Silvers, A.: Value of preoperative radionuclide bone scan in suspected primary breast carcinoma. Mayo Clin. Proc., 53:221, 1978. *(It is emphasized that localized disease uncommonly reveals a positive bone scan which would be a determinant of future therapy. Specific guidelines for the timing of bone scans in breast cancer are outlined.)*

Sears, H.F., Gerber, F.H., Sturtz, D.L., and Fouty, W.J.: Liver scan and carcinoma of the breast. Surg. Gynecol. Obstet., 140:409, 1975. *(The specific lack of usefulness of liver scans in 100 patients with carcinoma of the breast in this series may be extended to other tumors. It is, therefore, rarely useful to employ liver scans in patients who have other sites of documented extension of their disease or who lack hepatomegaly, liver pain or abnormal liver function tests.)*

Veronesi, et al.: Inefficacy of immediate node dissection in melanoma of the limbs. N. Engl. J. Med., 297:627, 1977. *(This specific reference to the use of lymphadenectomy in malignant melanoma as a prognostic, rather than as a therapeutic procedure is an example which may be extended to other tumors in which lymph node dissection is employed routinely as a staging device.)*

Wittes, R.E., and Yeh, S.D.J.: Indications for liver and brain scans: Screening tests for patients with oat cell carcinoma of the lung. JAMA, 238:506, 1977. *(The lack of usefulness of liver and brain scans in the staging of patients with oat cell carcinoma is reviewed in a singular experience.)*

87

Approach to the
Treatment of Cancer

JACOB J. LOKICH, M.D.

The treatment of cancer has become multifaceted, involving the interdigitation of physician support with surgery, radiation, cytotoxic agents and, most recently, immune stimulation. The role of the primary physician is pivotal; most cancer patients can remain at home with their families and receive optimal therapy on an outpatient basis when there is a primary physician working closely with a cancer center or local specialist in cancer management. Only when radiation therapy, blood product transfusions, or experimental protocols are used is it essential for the patient to go to a cancer treatment center.

Curative treatment that focuses on the primary tumor site has traditionally been the province of surgery, with radiation and chemotherapy relegated to palliative roles. More recently, radiation and chemotherapy have been employed as adjuvants for local disease, enhancing the capability of surgery to cure. Moreover, radiation therapy has proved to be curative in early Hodgkin's disease (see Chapter 81) and cervical cancer (see Chapter 137). The role of immune therapy is currently undergoing clinical trial.

In order to provide effective care to the cancer patient, the primary physician should have a thorough understanding of the natural history of the tumor in question and its potential responsiveness to surgery, radiation and drug therapy. Skillful management requires proper staging and monitoring (see Chapter 86), knowledge of the indications, limitations and adverse effects of each treatment modality (see Chapters 88 and 89), formation of a supportive alliance with patient and family (see Chapter 90), and access to expert advice.

COMMUNICATION AND SUPPORT

The task of educating the patient while simultaneously providing hope and support for the patient and family begins at the crucial point of informing the patient of the diagnosis (see Chapter 90). Many families may insist that the diagnosis be withheld from the patient; only rarely is this warranted. For the vast majority of patients, their knowledge of the diagnosis is crucial to management. The patient and his family may need to resolve preexisting differences that the critical illness may magnify. Importantly, too, the patient's willingness to accept a treatment that may be associated with some morbidity often depends on his understanding the diagnosis and prognosis. Finally, the physician and the medical staff are vastly better able to deal with the patient if there is candor which facilitates the development of trust (see Chapter 1).

Common misconceptions about cancer include the certainty of death, intractable pain, and erosive, disfiguring disease. In order to avoid needless worry, it is essential at the outset to address these common concerns directly, even if the patient does not express them. When confronted with the diagnosis and the prognosis, some patients may reject or deny the information. It may even be necessary periodically to reinforce or repeat the facts of the situation, particularly if the patient has expectations and plans that are unrealistic, such as planning for college or becoming pregnant. However, constantly reminding the patient of the prognosis, particularly when life expectancy is measured in weeks, is unnecessary; support is more important (see Chapter 90).

The family certainly needs full and frequent apprisal of the patient's status and prognosis. Patients often pass through a sequence of emotions that have been characterized by Kubler-Ross. These include periods of denial, hostility, anger, hope, depression, and finally acceptance. The physician often has much impact in determining the length of any one phase before the patient accepts living with cancer. The physician's role in this aspect of treatment is as important to maintaining the patient's quality of life as is any other therapeutic modality (see Chapter 90).

LOCAL TUMOR THERAPY: SURGERY AND RADIATION

Surgery has traditionally assumed the dominant role in the management of cancer. Diagnosis is established and confirmed by surgical biopsy, and cure may be effected by operation. Nonetheless, there has recently been a shift in emphasis toward minimizing surgical procedures, particularly when the prognosis is determined by factors such as distant metastases, and when salvage by secondary local modalities can be accomplished. Four standard surgical operations have been scaled down in many cases to less radical procedures to lessen chances of morbidity:

1. Lymph node dissection for malignant melanoma
2. Limb amputation for osteogenic sarcoma
3. Ostomy and AP resection for rectal cancer (see Chapter 75)
4. Radical mastectomy for breast cancer (see Chapter 118)

Although controversial, the surgical approach to these lesions may be modified by the addition of local therapy (e.g., radiation) or systemic therapy (e.g., cytotoxic agents).

Radiation therapy has become more effective due to development of high-energy linear accelerators and technical improvements in delivery, which have lowered rates of morbidity and increased rates of survival and local control. There are at least two tumors for which radiation therapy is now the local therapy of choice: early stages of Hodgkin's disease (see Chapter 81) and carcinoma of the cervix (see Chapter 137). Radiation in conjunction with surgery may be curative in some tumors when administered pre- or postoperatively. In other malignancies the combined application of radiation and either surgery or chemotherapy may promote palliation and chances for long-term survival, although rarely achieving cure (see Table 87–1).

Radiation therapy does not have an established role in the therapy of some tumors. In at least three kinds of malignancies, the role of radiation therapy either alone or in conjunction with surgery must still be considered controversial (see Table 87–1).

ADJUVANT OR COMBINED THERAPY OF LOCAL OR REGIONAL CANCER

Adjuvant therapy involves the addition of chemotherapy or radiation to surgical procedures. The rationale for adding radiation therapy is primarily to

Table 87–1. Tumors for Which Radiation Therapy is the Primary Essential Modality

Radiation therapy alone is curative
  Hodgkin's disease
  Cancer of the cervix
  Seminoma or dysgerminoma
Radiation therapy plus other therapy is curative
  Rectal cancer (pre- or post-operative)
  Head and neck cancer (pre- or post-operative)
  Uterine (endometrial) cancer (pre- or post-operative)
  Soft tissue sarcoma
Radiation therapy plus other therapy is palliative
  Cancer of the pancreas
  Brain tumors
  Lung cancer
  Cancer of the prostate
Controversial or unestablished palliative or curative
  Breast cancer
  Ovarian cancer
  Testicular cancer

promote local control of presumed residual microscopic tumor. In theory, chemotherapy functions as an adjuvant modality because of the possibility that tumor cells are released into the circulation at the time of surgery. In addition, adjuvant chemotherapy may be effective because it affects existing micrometastases at a time when they are rapidly proliferating and likely to be quite drug sensitive.

Adjuvant therapy has been proposed or is part of ongoing trials for treatment of a number of cancers (see Table 87–2); at present it is a proven and established therapy for carcinomas of the breast and rectum. In breast cancer, premenopausal women with positive lymph nodes and pathologic stage II disease have benefited from the addition of chemotherapy. It has reduced the incidence of recurrence and prolonged disease-free survival to 4 years (see Chapter 118). Patients with rectal cancer that extends beyond the bowel wall (so-called Duke's B_2 or C lesions) have shown reduced local recurrence rates and possibly increased survival time with the use of radiation therapy (see Chapter 75). The role of preoperative radiation therapy in comparison to postoperative radiation therapy has not been definitely established (see Table 87–2).

For the vast majority of tumors, local or regional disease is incurable in spite of adjuvant modalities. Only 15 per cent of patients with stage II malignant melanoma survive 5 years; less than 5 per cent of patients with lung, renal cell, and pancreatic cancers that are regionally advanced show long-term survival. Thus chemotherapy, immune therapy and radiation are not generally employed as adjuvant modalities for these tumors, unless used investigationally.

Table 87-2. State and Category of Tumors that Require Adjuvant Chemotherapy or Radiotherapy

TUMOR	STAGE	ADJUVANT MODALITY	STATUS
Breast cancer	II	Chemotherapy (CMF)	Established for pre-menopausal women
Lung cancer	I	Immune therapy	Unestablished
Colon cancer	B_2/C	Chemotherapy (5-fluorouracil + nitro-sourea) Immune therapy	Unestablished; clinical trials ongoing
Rectal cancer	B_2/C	Radiation	Established for post-operative radiotherapy; preoperative radiotherapy speculative
Ovarian cancer	I, II	Chemotherapy and radiation	Unestablished; ongoing trials
Testicular cancer	II	Chemotherapy (vinblastine, bleomycin, 1-CPDD)	Unestablished; ongoing trials

For rare tumors such as testicular cancer (see Chapter 137), osteogenic sarcoma, or Hodgkin's disease (see Chapter 81), the role of ancillary modalities is important in extending survival time and limiting morbidity of regional disease.

With the advent of more effective cytotoxic drugs and the use of radiation to sterilize local sites of tumor with minimal morbidity, the combined approach to local, regional, and even advanced cancers should become an increasing part of standard management. Currently, the application of forms of therapy ancillary to surgery must await the outcomes of ongoing clinical trials.

MANAGEMENT OF ADVANCED METASTATIC CANCER

The management of advanced disease is largely palliative, and involves systemic therapy provided by *cytotoxic drugs.* Chemotherapeutic regimens have become increasingly sophisticated and complex, but also more effective due to development of new agents and multiple-drug regimens (see Chapter 88). Decisions concerning use and timing of cytotoxic therapy in advanced disease are difficult, because of the potential morbidity associated with such therapy and the frequent lack of established benefit in promoting cure or even in prolonging survival. The decision to use chemotherapy in advanced disease is often a philosophical one, based on the feelings of patient, family and physician.

Any decision to employ chemotherapy should involve an analysis of host tolerance as well as potential tumor responsiveness. Most important, the use of chemotherapy must be preceded by informed consent of the patient, who should be aware of the side effects as well as the potential for response. A common

misconception is that the drugs invariably create morbidity and prolong life only at the cost of agonizing discomfort. In fact, when effective, chemotherapy can improve the quality of life as well as prolong it and, when it is ineffective, it will not necessarily induce more than transient morbidity.

In addition to these considerations, the primary indications for the use of chemotherapy in advanced disease include:

1. A probability of tumor responsiveness to chemotherapy greater than 30 per cent for a partial response and greater than 5 per cent for a complete response
2. Progressive tumor growth during a period of observation (e.g., pulmonary nodules doubling in less than 30 days)
3. Symptomatic metastatic disease (e.g., pleural effusion)

Within these guidelines, cytotoxic therapy can be administered with a reasonable risk-benefit balance.

The use of *experimental drug therapy* should be reserved for:

1. Patients who have failed with known effective drugs (i.e., those drugs with a response rate > 30 per cent and established ability to prolong survival)
2. Patients who wish to have or insist on a new form of treatment
3. Patients who have a measurable parameter to monitor for judging effectiveness of therapy

Immune therapy, utilizing agents such as BCG, is a new form of systemic treatment, designed to promote a generalized response that can affect tumors at any site. It is often included in the classification of chemotherapy, which is also systemic. Immune therapy remains a highly experimental form of treatment, to be administered predominantly, if not exclusively, as a part of clinical trials at regional cancer centers. The use of intralesional immune therapy may be effective in small, superficial cutaneous lesions.

ANNOTATED BIBLIOGRAPHY

Frei, E., III. Combination cancer therapy. Cancer Res., *32*:2593, 1972. *(Experimental and conceptual development of the concept of multiple-drug therapy.)*

Gilbert, H.A., *et al.*: Evaluation of radiation therapy for bone metastases: Pain relief and quality of life. Am. J. Roentgenol, *129*:1095, 1977. *(A study of 158 patients, revealing considerable success in achieving palliation. Mean survival was 1 year after therapy, indicating that relief of pain was worthwhile, since patients lived for a considerable period of time.)*

Kaplan, H.S.: Radiotherapeutic advances in the treatment of neoplastic disease. Isr. J. Med. Sci., *13*:808, 1977. *(A comprehensive discussion and review of the applications of radiation therapy in treatment of cancer.)*

Schabel, F.M., Jr.: Rationale for adjuvant chemotherapy. Cancer, *39*: (Suppl.) 2875, 1977. *(Discusses the biologic reasons for use of adjuvant therapy.)*

Staquet, M.: Cancer Therapy: Prognostic Factors and Criteria of Response. New York: Raven Press, 1975. *(A comprehensive interpretation of the natural history of solid tumors and hematologic malignancies and the impact of therapy on survival as well as objective tumor regression.)*

Weichselbaum, R., Goebbels, R., and Lokich, J.: Complications of therapy. In Lokich, J. (ed.): Clinical Cancer Management. Boston: G.K. Hall, 1979. *(A comprehensive review of the acute as well as chronic effects of chemotherapy and radiation therapy and a discussion of the reversibility of such effects as well as the mechanism of induction.)*

88
Principles of Cancer Chemotherapy
JACOB J. LOKICH, M.D.

The availability of chemotherapy for the cancer patient represents an important contribution to patient management. However, because the drugs are not selective, it is necessary to consider the adverse effects of therapy as well as their antitumor effects. The judicious use of chemotherapy involves a delicate balance of the two.

Chemotherapy has become a concern of the primary care physician as more cancer patients are managed on drug regimens outside of the hospital. Design of the chemotherapy program requires the expertise of the oncologist, for drug regimens are constantly being revised and new agents developed. However, it is often the primary physician who must follow the patient on a day-to-day basis and manage the entire range of medical and emotional problems encountered (see Chapter 74, 89, 90) even though close cooperation with the oncologist is important. The role of the primary physician requires that he know the general indications for chemotherapy and the major toxic and adverse side effects of the commonly employed agents. He must evaluate response to therapy and alleviate side effects. In some instances, he may be called upon to administer chemotherapeutic agents, necessitating familiarity with proper dosage, route and technique.

PRINCIPLES OF THERAPY

There are three principle applications for chemotherapy: as a preoperative therapy, as adjuvant or postoperative therapy, and as palliative therapy for advanced disease. *Preoperative chemotherapy* is used to treat tumors that are moderately sensitive and responsive to drugs. The goal is to decrease the tumor bulk and make possible a more conservative surgical approach than would otherwise be possible. Determining the responsiveness of the individual tumor to drug therapy may also provide a more rational basis for long-term adjuvant treatment. *Postoperative adjuvant therapy* has not yet been established as a

Table 88-1. Combination Chemotherapy Regimes in Management of Cancer

PROGRAM	TUMOR	DOSE SCHEDULE	RESPONSE RATE (%)
CMF	Breast	See Chapter 118	
Cytoxan-Adriamycin	Ovary, breast	See Chapter 118	60-80, 40-60
MOPP	Hodgkin's disease	*Every 28 days* M, 6 mg./m², Day 1 and 8 O, 1 mg./m², Day 1 and 8 P, 100 mg./m² for 10 days Pr, 50 mg. for 10 days	80
COP; CVP	Non-Hodgkins lymphoma	*Every 30 days* C, 100 mg./m² for 10 days O, 1 mg/m², Day 1 and 8 P, 50 mg. for 10 days	60
ABVD	Hodgkin's disease	*Every 28 days* A, 25 mg./m² B, 10 mg./m², day 1 and 14 V, 6 mg./m² D, 200 mg./m²	80
VBP	Testicular	*Every 28 days* V, .02 mg./kg., Day 1 and 2 B, 15 mg./m², Day 1 and 8 Pt, 20 mg./m², Day 1 to 5	80-100

M = Mustargen; O = Oncovin, P = Prednisone, Pr = Procarbazine, C = Cyclophosphamide
A = Adriamycin, B = Bleomycin, V = Vinblastine, D = DTIC, Pt = Cis-platinum.

standard form of treatment for most tumors; it is undergoing assessment (see Chapter 87).

Cancer chemotherapy has evolved from a palliative role to a curative one, as a part of combination therapy involving radiation and surgery. This change has resulted from the discovery of increasingly effective chemotherapeutic agents and the development of *multi-drug regimens* that have increased not only the response rate, but also the duration of the response and the percentage of patients who enter a complete clinical remission. Single agent regimens are still being employed, but mostly as adjuvant therapy or when a cancer is uniquely sensitive to a single drug, such as dactinomycin (Actinomycin D) for choriocarcinoma (see Chapter 137).

The most active drugs in the management of cancer are the alkylating drugs and doxorubicin (Adriamycin). The combined use of these drugs, may be effective in a broad section of tumors, including lung, breast, and ovarian cancer, as well as in the hematologic malignancies. Consequently, for desperately ill patients with an ill-defined tumor, the combination may be employed as a first-line chemotherapy with a salutary effect.

The component drugs of combination regimens share important characteristics: they are each active against the specific tumor, have different modes or mechanisms of action on the tumor, have variant tox-icities, and act at different sites in the cell cycle. This has permitted increased effectiveness without increased toxicity.

The treatment of advanced disease with chemotherapy has been variably successful; there are a number of effective tumor-specific regimens (see Table 88-1). In the absence of an established therapy (or research protocol), the asymptomatic patient should not be a candidate for chemotherapy, especially if the disease or the lesion cannot be measured by standard criteria. For the most part, the role of chemotherapy in advanced disease remains palliative. Patients who have an objective response, with at least partial tumor regression, usually live longer than those who achieve no response. Patients whose disease stabilizes according to objective criteria fare no better than patients who achieve no response. Therefore, when it can be objectively determined that a tumor has not regressed by 50 per cent or more, therapy should be stopped or changed to an alternative drug regimen; the patient is unlikely to benefit from continued therapy.

Meaningful response to chemotherapy is usually observed within two courses of treatment. Only rarely does continued treatment in the absence of initial response result in an increased appreciation of response; usually, more therapy is unwarranted. To determine whether or not chemotherapy may be effective, one should schedule initial follow-up to take place within 2 months of the initiation of treatment.

Sequential therapy has been found to be associated with a lower response rate than is maximal therapy that employs all active agents simultaneously at the outset of therapy. When chemotherapy is introduced sequentially or when second-line drugs are employed after failure of an initial program or a relapse, response is less likely.

The principal factor prohibiting the generalized application of chemotherapy is that the majority of cytotoxic drugs have a relative lack of selectivity for the tumor cell, resulting in a narrow therapeutic index. This factor, combined with the fact that there is a steep dose-response relationship for most cytotoxic effects generally results in some form of host toxicity.

Cytotoxic drugs can adversely affect normal cell populations with rapid turnover, such as those of the bone marrow, hair follicles, and gastrointestinal mucosa. Bone marrow suppression, alopecia, and gastroenteritis are frequentially encountered shortly after initiation of chemotherapy. For example, onset of acute marrow suppression is common 7 to 10 days after therapy and may last about one week.

The most common chronic effect of cytotoxic therapy is cumulative *suppression of the bone marrow.* Among patients who are now living as a consequence of more effective therapy, marrow suppression represents a universal phenomenon that affects the stem-cell population and may lead to chronic thrombocytopenia, anemia, and leukopenia.

Alopecia is a concomitant effect of only four drugs: nitrogen mustard, cyclophosphamide, vincristine, and doxorubicin. It is usually partial, but with doxorubicin the hair loss is generally total. Alopecia begins approximately 2 weeks after initiation of treatment and is complete by 4 to 6 weeks. Alopecia is always transient, and hair often grows during the course of treatment; however, total restitution does not take place until chemotherapy is stopped.

The *gastrointestinal toxicity* of chemotherapy can be debilitating; nausea and vomiting are common. Hoever, with the judicious use of antiemetics, sedatives, behavioral conditioning, and compassionate support, the adverse gastrointestinal effects can be minimized. The chemotactic trigger zone of the brain stem is exquisitely sensitive to a variety of chemotherapeutic agents and activates the emesis center, resulting in the nausea and vomiting. The best approach to the vomiting, therfore, is to suppress the trigger zone and emesis center. Phenothiazines and other antimetics are used for this purpose (see Chapter 74).

The most serious risks of chemotherapy are *leukopenia* leading to overwhelming sepsis and *thrombocytopenia* resulting in hemorrhage. Uniformly, leukopenia and thrombocytopenia are dose-related and may be prevented or lessened by dose adjustment in patients who have marginal marrow reserve due to marrow invasion, age, or prior therapy. Nonetheless, the goal of most chemotherapeutic regimens is to induce some degree of leukopenia, for it serves as a measure of cytotoxic effect and as a guideline to dosage.

Of concern is the increasing evidence that *secondary malignancies,* such as acute leukemia, may develop in patients treated with alkylating agents. Although the accumulating evidence grows increasingly compelling, the risk of treatment remains outweighed by its benefits.

Cytotoxic Chemotherapeutic Agents. Cytotoxic drugs have been grouped into five categories based on their mechanism of action or the chemical derivation of the drug (Table 88–2).

The alkylating agents are a large group that include cyclophosphamide, nitrogen mustard, chlorambucil (Leukeran), phenylalanine mustard (L-PAM, Alkeran), and mitomycin C. All of the alkylating drugs are commercially available. The most commonly used drug in this class is *cyclophosphamide,*

Table 88–2.   Cytotoxic Chemotherapeutic Drugs

CLASS	PROTOTYPE	ADMINISTRATION	ADVERSE EFFECTS
Alkylating drug	Cyclophosphamide	Intravenous, oral	Hemorrhagic cystitis
Antimetabolite	5-Fluorouracil	Intravenous	Gastrointestinal
Antibiotics	Doxorubicin (Adriamycin)	Intravenous	Cardiomyopathy
	Bleomycin	Intramuscular, intravenous	Interstitial pneumonitis
Plant alkaloid	Vincristine	Intravenous only	Neurotoxicity
Miscellaneous	Nitrosoureas	Intravenous, oral	Marrow failure
	Cis-platinum	Intravenous	Renal failure

which may be administered intermittently either by injection at 3-week intervals or as a 7- to 10-day course of oral medication. The alkylating agents in general have a broad spectrum of antitumor activity, and cyclophosphamide has been effective against many tumors. The alkylating agents with the fewest side effects (except for myelosuppression) are L-PAM and chlorambucil. There is no known advantage of one schedule or route of drug administration over another.

The *antimetabolites* include 5-fluorouracil, methotrexate, and the antileukemic drugs cytosine arabinoside, hydroxyurea, and 6-mercaptopurine. These drugs interfere with synthesis of DNA and, therefore, have greatest effect on rapidly growing cells. The antimetabolites are uniformly and rapidly metabolized or excreted in the urine and, therefore, must be administered frequently. They are most effective when administered as a 24-hour or continuous infusion. 5-fluorouracil is the prototype and has been extensively applied in gastrointestinal cancer. The drug is best administered intravenously for 5 to 7 days, and repeated at 5- to 6-week intervals.

The *antibiotics* include dactinomycin and more recently developed drugs such as doxorubicin and bleomycin. Doxorubicin (*Adriamycin*) is an anthracycline antibiotic with a spectrum of activity comparable to the alkylating drugs. In combination with the alkylating drugs, doxorubicin appears to be synergistic in antitumor effect. The drug has a cumulative toxic effect on the heart that results in a cardiomyopathy, limiting the maximum cumulative dose to 500 mg. per m.^{2} *Bleomycin,* a polypeptide antibiotic mixture, causes pulmonary fibrosis, an effect that may be dose-related or, occasionally, idiosyncratic. As a result, the maximum cumulative dose for bleomycin is 200 mg. per m.^{2}

The *plant alkaloids* are mitotic inhibitors. They are primarily the vinblastine and vincristine derivatives of the periwinkle plant. These drugs are always administered intravenously and most commonly on a weekly basis. Their chief adverse effects are cumulative neurotoxicity (seen with vincristine), which recedes slowly with drug withdrawal, and marrow suppression (vinblastine).

Miscellaneous or mixed mechanism agents include two important drugs: nitrosoureas and cis-platinum. The *nitrosoureas* are alkylating drugs that cross the blood-brain barrier. They have a unique, delayed marrow-suppressive effect that necessitates a specific drug schedule with a long hiatus between administered courses (6 weeks). *Cis-platinum* has primary activity in testicular and ovarian cancer and

Table 88–3. Drugs that Require Slow Intravenous Administration and the Careful Avoidance of Extravasation

Actinomycin D
Doxorubicin
Mitomycin C
Cis-platinum
Nitrogen mustard
Vincristine

probably squamous tumors. It is administered at 3- to 4-week intervals primarily in combination with other drugs. It can cause renal failure in patients inadequately hydrated.

MANAGEMENT RECOMMENDATIONS

Administration of cancer chemotherapeutic drugs by the primary care physician requires a specific understanding of routes of administration and particularly the potential hazard of extravasation associated with certain intravenously administered agents (see Table 88–3). In each instance, extravasation results in tissue irritation and secondary inflammation leading to ulceration and necrosis, which not uncommonly require surgical grafting and débridement. In the event of extravasation, the local area may be injected with cortisone preparation, and ice applied. The actual inflammation and necrosis may not occur for 3 to 10 days following injection, although pain is generally present early on. Repeated intravenous use of such drugs, often results in sclerosis and endothelial deterioration, particularly when small-caliber veins are used for infusion. The agents used should go into large-bore veins in the antecubital fossa or higher.

Multiple drug regimens are designed first and foremost for convenient outpatient administration. The dose and schedule of the component drugs are adjusted to minimize side effects (see Table 88–1).

Suppression of chemotherapy-induced vomiting requires identifying the pattern of emesis. Some agents cause vomiting that begins approximately 30 to 45 minutes following injection. In other regimens, particularly Cytoxan and Adriamycin, the vomiting begins 4 to 5 hours after injection. The approach, to antiemetic use should be based on time of emesis. An important cause of vomiting, which in time becomes more severe than that induced by drug therapy, is the conditioned vomiting response. This pattern of vomiting develops following the second or third course of emesis-inducing cancer treatment; it is

Table 88–4. Schematic for Management of Chemotherapy-Induced Emesis

Day prior to therapy
  Mild tranquilizer with or without tricyclic compound
Day of therapy
  Phenothiazine spansule or suppository
  Normal food intake (to minimize retching on an empty stomach, which produces muscle cramps and pain)
  1 hour prior to anticipated emesis, 200 to 400 mg. barbiturate plus phenothiazine to sedate
  Phenothiazine at 3- to 4-hour intervals if vomiting exceeds four discharges per hour

characterized by anxiety and anorexia the day before therapy and a conditioned response that may be precipitated by little more than driving down the street on which the therapy center is located. This form of emesis is best treated by tranquilizers for 1 to 2 days prior to treatment. Other forms of antiemetic support being developed include hypnosis and the use of tetrahydrocannabinol (see Chapter 74). In many instances, sedation and phenothiazines suffice for chemotherapy-induced emesis (see Table 88–4). Within 24 hours, vomiting usually has completely ceased, but anorexia and a feeling of extreme fatigue may persist as a consequence of the vigorous exertion involved in emesis.

Management of *bone marrow suppression* requires adjustments in dose and timing of chemotherapy. Generalized marrow suppression is common. The pattern of suppression is a function of the type of drug, its dose and schedule (see Table 88–5). Nitrosoureas, for example, induce thrombocytopenia more often than leukopenia and do so in delayed fashion at 21 days, with recovery sometimes not achieved until Day 35.

In monitoring patients on chemotherapeutic regimens, the anticipated nadir days for blood counts are the most crucial times to obtain follow-up complete blood counts. In patients who develop leukopenia, the observation period ought to be intensified, depending upon the level of the count and the presence of associated fever or sepsis (see Table 88–6). Dose adjustment for the subsequent course of therapy is therefore based on the nadir level. The goal of treatment should be to maintain intermittent white blood counts at between 2000 and 3000 cells/mm.[3] Dose escalation or reduction is not necessary if a blood count is maintained at this level at nadir time. A small number of drugs have absolutely no effect on the bone marrow (see Table 88–5), but the majority have some impact with variation in the time of the nadir count and the duration of marrow suppression.

EVALUATION OF RESPONSE TO THERAPY

Monitoring patients on chemotherapeutic regimens for adverse effects is performed in concert with evaluation of the effectiveness of treatment. Objective tumor measurements are often difficult to define, but generally the oncologist depends on them to gauge response to therapy (see Table 88–7).

The criteria of response are often difficult to evaluate because partial responses may be influenced by nontumor factors. In addition, some forms of metastatic disease simply cannot be measured, such as osseous metastases and, particularly, osteoblastic lesions. There are established criteria for some metastatic patterns, such as hepatomegaly where the criterion for response is a 30 per cent decrease in the sum of measurements made below the costal margin at the midclavicular and midxiphoid lines. Peritoneal masses, pleural effusions, and skin ulcerations are not considered amenable to evaluation. The availability of ultrasound and computerized body tomography may promote the ability to quantify lesions in the retroperitoneum, but at present this method of evaluation is limited.

Tumor markers as measurements of response have been established only for human chorionic gonadotropin in patients with choriocarcinoma. Recent-

Table 88–5. Chronologic Patterns of Marrow Suppression Secondary to Chemotherapy

AGENT	NADIR DAY	DURATION
Non-Suppressive Drugs		
Bleomycin		
Vincristine		
Streptozotocin		
Corticosteroids		
DTIC		
Marrow-Suppressive Drugs		
1. Alkylating drugs		
Cyclophosphamide		
Nitrogen mustard	5–8	Variable
Mitomycin C	Delayed	Cumulative
2. Antibiotics		
Doxorubicin	12–14	5 days
Dactinomycin		
3. Antimetabolites		
5-Flourouracil	5–10	<5 days
Cytosine arabinoside		
Methotrexate		
4. Natural products		
Vinblastine	8–12	3 days
5. Others		
Nitrosoureas	14–28	Cumulative
Hydroxyurea	Variable	
Procarbazine	Variable	

Table 88-6.   Management of Leukopenia and Chemotherapy

WHITE BLOOD COUNT (WBC) AT NADIR	MONITORING SCHEDULE	CHEMOTHERAPY DOSE
1000-2000	Repeat in 1 week	Allow recovery to >3000, treat with 100% dose
500-1000	Observe on outpatient basis daily until WBC is same on consecutive days	Allow recovery to >3000, treat with 50% dose
100-500	Hospitalize for observation	Allow recovery to >4000, treat with 25% dose

ly, the use of carcinoembryonic antigen monitored sequentially has been applied to colon cancer and to breast cancer with varied success. Also, better fractionation of acid phosphatase has improved its specificity in prostatic cancer. Other biochemical parameters, such as alkaline phosphatase and the various hepatic enzymes, have been uniformly inadequate to evaluate the effectiveness of treatment (see Chapter 86).

ANNOTATED BIBLIOGRAPHY

Chabner, B.A., *et al.*: The clinical pharmacology of antineoplastic agents. N. Engl. J. Med., *292*:1107, 1159, 1975. *(Excellent review of pharmacokinetics, toxicities and drug interactions.)*

Frei, E. III: Combination cancer therapy. Cancer Res., *32*:2593, 1972. *(Experimental and concep-*

Table 88-7.   Criteria of Response to Therapy

Survival

Measured from time of diagnosis, metastasis, or initiation of treatment in days, weeks, or months, to be compared by median (as opposed to mean) to a randomized control or historical control not receiving treatment or receiving alternative treatment. Survival as a measurement of time may also be supplemented by a time measurement of diagnosis to point of recurrence and is translated as disease-free survival

OBJECTIVE REDUCTION IN TUMOR

Partial response

Equals a 50% reduction in the product of the maximum perpendicular diameters of the most easily measurable lesion without increase in other lesions and wth a minimum duration of 4 weeks.

Complete response

Equals a 100% reduction in all evidence of tumor for minimum of 4 weeks without appearance of new lesions.

Stable disease

Equals a less than 25% decrease in measurable disease without development of other lesions.

No response (progressive disease)

Equals a more than 25% increase in the size of the lesion or the development of new lesions.

Improvement

Equals a 25-50% reduction in the product of maximum perpendicular diameters lasting at least 4 weeks.

tual development of the concept of multiple drug therapy.)

Golden, S., Horwich, A., and Lokich, J.: Chemotherapy and You. Department of Health and Welfare Publication No. (NIH) 76-1136. *(This pamphlet originally produced at the Sidney Farber Cancer Institute is available for patient use from the National Cancer Institute and serves as a layman's introduction to the concept of chemotherapy and its potential effects.)*

Sallen, S.E., *et al.*: Antiemetics in patients receiving chemotherapy for cancer: A randomized comparison of tetrahydrocannabinol and prochlorperazine. N. Engl. J. Med., *302*:135, 1980. *(Tetrahydrocannabinol proved to be effective and was often preferred to prochlorperazine for relief of drug-induced emesis.)*

Schein, P.: Long-term effects of cytotoxic and immune suppression therapy. Ann. Intern. Med., *82*:84, 1978. *(A detailed review of the mechanisms and durations of adverse effects of cytotoxic agents on various organ systems.)*

Wasserman, T.H., *et al.*: Tabular analysis of clinical chemotherapy of solid tumors. Cancer Chem. Rep., *3*:6:399, 1975. *(Cross-referencing of the single-agent chemotherapy effect on solid tumors by each tumor category is reviewed incorporating data in the literature as well as unpublished reports available only at the National Cancer Institute. This uncritical compilation represents an important resource for detailing which drugs have been employed; this is not reliable as a resource for the level of activity of individual drugs in the tumor because of the heterogenity of the data base.)*

Weichselbaum, R., Goebbels, R., and Lokich, J.: Complications of therapy. *In* Lokich, J. (ed.): Clinical Cancer Management. Boston: G.K. Hall, 1979. *(A comprehensive review of the acute as well as chronic effects of chemotherapy and radiation therapy and a discussion of the reversibility of such effects as well as the mechanisms of induction.)*

89
Management of Cancer-induced Pain
JACOB J. LOKICH, M.D.

Relief of pain is certainly an essential objective in the treatment of the cancer patient, although Osler, in a review of more than 500 patients with terminal cancer, found that less than 10 per cent of preterminal patients required analgesia. Yet, it is indeed a tragic situation when relentless pain is superimposed upon a fatal outcome. In most instances, effective amelioration of pain can be achieved with proper use of analgesics. Unfortunately undertreatment of pain is common.

The primary physician is the person to whom the patient most often turns for pain relief. One must know not only the appropriate treatments and their limitations, but also how to support the cancer patient and minimize the emotional suffering that is invariably interwined with the perception of pain (see Chapter 90).

PATHOPHYSIOLOGY AND CLINICAL PRESENTATIONS

The pain syndromes associated with cancer can be separated into acute and chronic clinical states, and the acute pain syndromes further subdivided (see Table 89-1). The major pain syndromes are more often than not a prelude to the incureable stage of illness, but may precede the terminal phase by a substantial interval.

Peripheral Nerve Compression Syndromes. The relatively uncommon nerve compression syndromes result in pain in the shoulder or arm (brachial plexus), buttocks and perineum (sacral plexus), lumbar area (paraspinal nerves), and mouth or face (trigeminal nerve). All are secondary to nerve entrapment and, occasionally, nerve invasion by tumor growth.

Nerve Root Compression Syndromes. Pain originating in the back and radiating down an extremity is characteristic of root compression. When there is an associated neurologic deficit, it suggests the possibility of evolving cord compression. The tumor most commonly extends either from the retroperitoneal

space or from a contiguously involved bony structure. Bone scans or radiographs often demonstrate lytic or blastic lesions. Compression syndromes may also occur as a consequence of vertebral body collapse secondary to tumor without direct tumor compression of the nerve.

Osseous Pain Syndromes. Metastases to the bony skeleton may cause pathologic fractures; the development of pain in a bony site is invariably secondary to interruption of the cortex, which may or may not be observed radiographically. Common sites are vertebra, long bones, pelvis and skull.

Another form of osseous metastasis involves the bone marrow or medullary cavity. Intramedullary tumor is characteristic of leukemia, but also may be observed in some solid tumors, particularly malignant melanoma. These produce a pain syndrome characterized by diffuse bone sensitivity in the presence of normal bone x-rays.

Abdominal Pain Syndromes. Abdominal pain may develop as a consequence of intestinal obstruction, cramping pain is characteristic (see Chapter 53). Ascites can be uncomfortable as a consequence of abdominal distention. Hepatic metastases may cause pain by distending the liver capsule or irritating the peritoneal surface secondary to tumor necrosis. The latter is often associated with a friction rub.

Thoracic Pain Syndromes. Pain associated with thoracic disease is generally a consequence of local invasion of the intercostal nerves. Pleuritic pain may develop if the malignancy spreads to involve the pleura. Direct invasion of a contiguous bony structure may result in local or referred pain.

Special Pain Syndromes. The *phantom limb syndrome* characteristically develops following amputation in patients with osteogenic sarcoma, especially in those who have endured the tumor over a long period. Persistence of phantom limb pain may lead to narcotic dependence. It is only after a protracted period of time that the reverberating neural circuit is eventually exhausted.

Table 89-1. Classification and Types of Cancer-related Pain

SYNDROME	CAUSES OR ANATOMIC SITE	COMMON CANCERS
Peripheral nerve compression or entrapment	Brachial plexus Sacral plexus Paraspinal nerves Trigeminal nerve	Breast Rectum Pancreas Mouth
Nerve root compression	Paraspinal tumor or vertebral collapse	Breast Lung Myeloma
Osseous lesions	Pathologic fractures or intramedullary expansion	Breast Prostate Lung
Abdominal lesions	Obstruction Hepatic metastases Ascites	GI tumors
Thoracic lesions	Pleuritis or intercostal neuritis	Lung
Special pain forms		
Phantom limb	Reverberating neurocircuit	Sarcoma
Herpes zoster	Neuralgia	Hodgkin's disease
Hypertrophic pulmonary osteoarthropathy	Periarticular distal extremities	Lung Sarcoma

Herpes zoster (shingles) occurs in patients with hematologic malignancies, particularly Hodgkin's disease, the non-Hodgkin's lymphomas and chronic lymphatic leukemia. Postherpetic pain may persist in the absence of typical skin lesions; herpes zoster should be suspected in patients complaining of pain in a dermatomal distribution (see Chapter 185).

Hypertrophic pulmonary osteoarthropathy (HPO) produces a periarticular pain syndrome which develops in patients with primary or metastatic tumors of the lung and mesotheliomas. The mechanism of the periarticular pain is unclear (see Chapter 41).

fective pain relief as are tumor control and proper analgesic use (see Chapter 90).

Control of Tumor. For pain directly related to the tumor, the most important therapeutic maneuver is the introduction of *tumor-specific therapy*. Surgery and radiation therapy are the principal modalities for the treatment of localized malignancy. Adjuvant therapy, employing chemotherapy or radiation, is also being utilized. Advanced metastatic cancer is treated with cytotoxic drugs for palliation of symptoms (see Chapter 87).

Even if disease is widespread, *local surgical excision* may be necessary for tumors which cause pain

PRINCIPLES OF MANAGEMENT

Optimal selection of pain relief measures requires identification of the pathophysiologic process responsible for the discomfort. Rational therapy can then be instituted. Often a multifaceted approach is necessary. Psychological support, control of tumor, analgesics, neurosurgical procedures, and behavioral methods are among the important modalities for treatment of cancer-induced pain (see Table 89–2).

Support. The importance of psychological support from both physician and family cannot be overemphasized. The personal role of the primary physician is vital to successful control of pain. The understanding and concern given are as central to ef-

Table 89-2. Approaches to Therapy of Cancer-related Pain

1. Psychological support
2. Tumor control
3. Drug therapy
   a. Nonaddictive analgesics (anti-inflammatory drugs)
   b. Narcotic analgesics
   c. Psychotropic drugs
4. Neurosurgical ablative procedures
   a. Dorsal rhizotomy
   b. Sympathectomy
   c. Percutaneous cordotomy
   d. Chemical hypophysectomy
5. Unproven methods of pain management
   a. Hypnosis
   b. Acupuncture
   c. Behavior modification

Table 89–3.   Analgesic Drugs*

LEVEL	DRUG	DOSAGE	SCHEDULE	COMMENT
I	Aspirin Phenacetin Acetaminophen	2 tabs.	Every 4–6 hours	Inhibits platelet activity Nephrotoxic when used chronically Overdose can cause GI toxicity
II	Oxycodone-aspirin-phenacetin-caffeine (Percodan)	1 or 2 tabs.	Every 4–6 hours	Addicting
	Codeine sulfate	30–60 mg.	Every 4–6 hours	
III	Meperidine	100 mg.	Every 4–6 hours	Ineffective orally at <100 mg.
	Hydromorphone (Dilaudid)	4 mg.	Every 4–6 hours	
	Morphine	10 mg. SQ	Every 2–4 hours	
	Heroin	Variable	Variable	Unavailable
IV	Brompton solution	1 tsp.	Constant schedule	Euphoria without somnolence, controversial superiority to standard drug therapy

*Listed in order of increasing potency and side effects.

because of size, fixation of underlying muscle, distention of the subcutaneous tissue, or localized secondary infection. For example, patients with fungating tumors of the breast may benefit from removal of the breast ("toilet mastectomy"); this achieves a modicum of pain control and minimizes secondary infection.

Lesions of the extremities producing similar local complications (i.e., pain, disfigurement, secondary infection or poor function) may be considered for local surgical control; amputation is rarely justified or necessary. Local cryosurgery or electrocautery and more recently laser treatment will remove the lesion with a minimum of morbidity and permit maintenance of the limb.

Drug Therapy. Control of cancer pain often requires use of narcotics and psychotropic drugs. To withhold narcotics or use them in subtherapeutic doses makes little sense in patients with limited life expectancies. If narcotics are deemed necessary, they should be used in full pharmacologic doses as often as needed to provide relief. Analgesics are often inadequate when emotional distress is prominent; concurrent measures are needed to alleviate anxiety and depression. Since pain is often maximal at night, an increase in the bedtime dose can be helpful.

Analgesics can be classified on the basis of effectiveness (see Table 89–3). *Aspirin* and *acetaminophen* are employed initially for mild pain. Aspirin is especially helpful when there is an inflammatory component. Intermediate preparations contain *codeine* or one of its derivatives, often in combination with nonnarcotic analgesics. *Stronger narcotic agents* are used in relatively equivalent doses (see Table 89–4). The synthetic preparations offer the advantage of

being less nauseating and constipating, but they lack the euphoric effect of the naturally-occurring preparations. Partial antagonists (e.g., pentazocine) may actually inhibit pain relief when used with other narcotics.

The development of an agent that has the analgesic effects of narcotics and the ability to induce euphoria without causing somnolence has been a major goal of physicians caring for cancer patients. When single narcotics are used for management of extreme pain, the doses necessary often leave the patient semiconscious, at best. *Brompton solution* (Table 89–5) is a mixture of cocaine, alcohol and morphine (or heroin). It has been suggested that the mixture may add substantially to patient's comfort without producing excessive sedation. Such solutions are not commercially available, but can be easily prepared by a pharmacist.

No patient should have to endure pain if effective analgesia is available. Patients may require 10 mg. or more of morphine as often as every hour to control intractable pain. The dose should be administered on a schedule (not p.r.n.) and increased as tolerance de-

Table 89–4.   Relative Potency of Narcotic Algesics

DRUG	TRADE NAME	EQUIVALENT DOSAGES (MG.)
Morphine sulfate	———	10
Heroin	———	3
Hydromorphone	Dilaudid	1–5
Oxycodone	In Percodan	15
Meperidine*	Demerol	100 (orally)
Methadone*	Dolophine	10
Codeine	———	60
Pentazocine*	Talwin	50

*Synthetic narcotic.

Table 89–5.　Brompton Solution No. 1

Morphine sulfate	0.5 gm.
Cocaine HC1	0.5 gm.
Citric acid	2.0 gm.
Propylene glycol	100.0 ml.
Alcohol U.S.P. 95%	300.0 ml.
Sorbitol solution 70%	250.0 ml.
Saccharin sodium	0.5 gm.
Berry-citrus blend	4.0 ml.
Water q.s. ad. 1000 ml.	

Dissolve morphine sulfate, cocaine HC1 and citric acid in 100 ml. of water.

Add sorbitol solution, propylene glycol and alcohol, in that order.

Dissolve saccharin in 50 ml. of water. Add with constant stirring to above solution.

Adjust to 900 ml. Assay morphine and cocaine. Add flavor.

q.s. ad. with water to make 1000 ml. Filter.

velops. Patients endure their condition much better when they know that maximum pain relief is available to them. All members of the health care team and family need to be informed of the patient's analgesic needs in order to avoid reluctance on the part of pharmacist, nurse or family to dispense the necessary type and amount of medication.

In addition to employing analgesic drugs, *psychotropic agents* are often helpful to counter the intense anxiety/depression that frequently accompanies chronic pain and reinforce the sensory perception (see Table 89–6).

Neurosurgical Procedures. A proportion of patients with metastatic cancer will have a slowly growing tumor which may be associated with chronic refractory pain in conjunction with prolonged survival. In these patients, determining the source of pain and controlling it with analgesics are often difficult. In such cases, neurosurgical procedures are resorted to. Before such extreme measures are utilized, it is important to characterize the pain as precisely as possible to avoid mistaking a psychogenic component for an organic one. Treating the latter while ignoring the former is bound to end in failure and unnecessary suffering. When there is confusion as to the nature of the pain, a *nerve blockade* can serve an important diagnostic function. There are three types of blocks: sensory, sympathetic and motor. By employing control solutions of normal saline in addition to titered solutions of anesthetic, the physician can determine the source of pain and, if organic, classify it into sensory, sympathetic or motor nerve involvement.

Neurosurgical procedures are indicated only

when (1) pain is uncontrolled by narcotic analgesics, (2) tumor control allows prediction of substantial longevity, and (3) functional status is significantly compromised by pain.

Rhizotomy is successful in 50 per cent of patients with malignancy; efficacy is not necessarily predicted by the success of a peripheral nerve block. *Chordotomy* is presently done percutaneously, avoiding general anesthesia and allowing for precise delineation of the pain tracts. Electrical chordotomy or radiofrequency chordotomy achieves long-term pain control in 40 to 70 per cent of patients. However, chordotomy, particularly the open surgical approach, is associated with potential functional loss, necessitating a discussion with the patient of the risks involved. Lateralization or regionalization of the pain syndrome makes chordotomy an important therapeutic option.

Finally, *hypophysectomy* induced by a chemical injection procedure (so-called alcohol-induced adenolysis) has been employed in limited numbers of patients in this country. Pain control may be related to the opioid peptides or endorphins in the hypothalamic area and is not necessarily related to the responsiveness of the tumor to hormonal ablation.

Behavioral therapies for pain control are a new approach to treatment. The influence of operant conditioning on the threshold for perception and tolerance to pain is well-established. *Behavior modification* or deconditioning may, therefore, have a role in pain control. Other investigational methods are *hypnosis* and *acupuncture,* which have been demonstrated to have some effect, particularly in the relief of chronic pain syndromes.

Many considerations are important when behavioral methods are introduced. First, one needs to be certain that specific organic causes and the anatomic

Table 89–6.　Ancillary Psychotropics and Sedatives

DRUG	USE
Phenothiazines	May be synergistic when used concomitantly with narcotics to augment pain control
Antihistamines	Same
Tranquilizers	For patients in whom anxiety decreases the pain threshold
Sedatives or soporifics	For pain-induced insomnia
Mood elevators	For patients in whom depression reinforces the pain syndrome

lesion are attended to. Behavioral therapy should never be the singular treatment, but it may help when applied in conjunction with more standard forms of treatment. Second, the effects of these therapies are usually transient and require reinforcement. The pain syndrome becomes refractory unless a concomitant deconditioning or unlearning process is occurring. Finally, the identification of appropriate patients is crucial. Those unlikely to respond tend to be older, more control-oriented, committed to religious or rigid ideals, cynical or hostile. Younger patients and those involved in meditation or astrology are likely to be sympathetic to and benefit from a behavioral approach.

MANAGEMENT RECOMMENDATIONS FOR SPECIFIC PAIN SYNDROMES

Peripheral Nerve Compression. The specific therapeutic approach to all such syndromes is the application of local antitumor therapy (for the most part, radiation treatment) to induce regression of the tumor. The nerve compression syndromes are, however, generally associated with a resistant tumor which has invaded along the nerve sheaths, and palliation is often only temporary.

Nerve Root Compression. The distinction between direct tumor compression and osseous inpingement on the nerve is often difficult, but local radiation is the treatment of choice. The absence of improvement following radiation therapy suggests that bony compression is the major component. Structural support by orthopedic measures, including brace or corset splinting, may be salutary.

Bone Pain and Pathologic Fractures. Fractures of weight-bearing bones should be prophylactically immobilized by surgery in conjunction with radiation therapy that is instituted for therapy of bone pain. Pathologic fractures of nonweight-bearing sites with or without symptoms should be managed with radiation therapy. In either instance, rapid healing follows treatment of responsive tumors such as those of breast or prostate.

Abdominal Pain. In most instances of intra-abdominal pain, the effectiveness of the antitumor treatment is limited, making analgesic drug therapy essential. Obstruction is an indication for surgery.

Thoracic Pain. When there is invasion into a local bony structure, radiation therapy is indicated.

Neurosurgical procedures may be needed later. Hypertrophic pulmonary osteoarthropathy can cause considerable discomfort, but rapid resolution of the pain is achieved with removal of the intrathoracic process either by surgery or radiation therapy. The narcotic requirement in patients with HPO is inordinate and generally necessitates thoracic surgical intervention, regardless of the presence of metastases.

ANNOTATED BIBLIOGRAPHY

Bonica, J. (ed.): International Symposium on Pain. In Advances in Neurology, Vol. 4. New York: Raven Press, 1974. *(An extensive review of the basic biology and pathophysiology of pain mechanisms, including the diagnosis and therapeutic approaches to pain. A review of the psychologic approaches, including hypnosis, operant conditioning, and behavioral modification adds to the comprehensive nature of the symposium.)*

Brechner, V. L., Ferrer-Brechner, T., and Allen, G. D.: Anesthetic measures in management of pain associated with malignancy. Semin. Oncol., 4:99, 1977. *(A general and practical review of the neurosurgical approaches to pain as well as the local anesthetic approach. Specific emphasis on the pain due to perineal, Pancoast, and pancreatic tumors, presented in sequential management steps.)*

Catalano, R. B.: The medical approach to management of pain caused by cancer. Semin. Oncol., 2:379, 1975. *(Thorough review of pathophysiology and detailed discussion of available narcotics.)*

LaRossa, J. T., Strong, M. S., and Melby, J. C.: Endocrinologically incomplete transethmoidal trans-sphenoidal hypophysectomy with relief of bone pain in breast cancer. N. Engl. J. Med., 298:1332, 1978. *(A possible clinical translation of the data developing with regard to encephlan localization in the hypophysis. The lack of a hormonal mechanism for analgesia suggests an intrinsic mechanism in the hypophysis as the vehicle for analgesia, thus implicating a role for encephlans.)*

Marks, R. M., and Sachar, E. J.: Undertreatment of medical inpatients with narcotic analgesics. Ann. Intern. Med., 78:173, 1973. *(Provides evidence suggesting that "refractory" pain is often due to the prescribing of subtherapeutic doses of narcotics.)*

Snyder, S. H.: The opiate receptor and morphine-like peptides in the brain. Am. J. Psychiatry, *135*:6:645, 1978. *(A comprehensive review of the basic and experimental data on the identification of endomorphans and encephlans in brain substance.)*

90
Management of the Psychological Aspects of Cancer

JACOB J. LOKICH, M.D.

For most patients, the diagnosis of cancer evokes images of pain, suffering, mutilation, and certain death. These basic fears are so intertwined with the word "cancer" that confirmation of the diagnosis places extreme emotional stress on the patient and his family. It is in managing this anguish that the physician plays a most important role. The physician often represents the one person to whom the patient and family can turn and must be not only the source of scientific and medical expertise but also the provider of emotional support and understanding. It is important to recognize that cancer affects not only the patient but also his family, who must grieve and resolve their own fears and anxieties. The physician is frequently obliged to deal with many members of the family, often at differing levels of need for information and support. By virtue of his long-standing relationship with the patient and family, the primary physician is in an ideal position to provide effective support.

The three most important times of stress for the patient are the time of diagnosis, the time for initiation of treatment, and the preterminal phase when it is apparent to both patient and family that all hope is lost. This is not to say that inordinate psychological reactions to cancer are not observed and not without significance in patients with curable cancer; however, these patients are inclined to resolve their concerns with time, and the stress is less forceful when there are no symptoms.

COMMUNICATING THE DIAGNOSIS

It is not uncommon for physicians to avoid telling the patient the diagnosis in accurate terms and to resort to the use of euphemisms such as "tumor" or "lesion" or "lump." The family often insists that the spouse, parent or child not be told the diagnosis, with the well-meaning intention of avoiding depression. It is rare that ignorance of the diagnosis or minimizing the prognosis is helpful for the patient or the family. The patient who is told, for example, that his tumor is totally removed and need not worry, becomes confused when he is informed that he may need chemotherapy or radiation therapy. Such a patient is likely to become noncompliant and may refuse therapy or develop significant adverse affects simply as a consequence of his inability to comprehend the need for therapy when the tumor has been completely removed (see Chapter 1).

More important, the patient who is unaware of the diagnosis and prognosis may not resolve important issues in his life. He may continue to have persistently uncomfortable relationships with other members of his family, which might otherwise be resolved if all were to understand the prognosis. Similarly, the uninformed family is unable to express its grief gradually over time, and death may appear to be sudden. The resulting unresolved grief may profoundly affect the surviving family members (see Chapter 215).

The goal in communicating the diagnosis and prognosis is to be accurate without destroying all hope. First and foremost, the words "cancer" and "malignant tumor" should be used at the outset of the interview and not avoided, although constant repetition of the terms is usually unnecessary. The term "fatal" ought to be omitted in discussions of prognosis, for it implies little hope of control. When informed of an incurable malignancy, the patient and family want to know "how much time is left?" A rough estimate may be necessary if the patient must arrange his affairs, but, if possible, the physician should avoid indicating a specific period of time, because it is apt to be inaccurate. Preferably, the physician should focus the patient toward realistic therapeutic approaches and reinforce his role in living instead of dying.

PATIENT AND FAMILY REACTIONS

Patient reactions at the time of presentation of the diagnosis depend on preconceived ideas about cancer and what the specter of cancer suggests to them. Denial, hostility, rejection of loved ones, regression to immaturity, and withdrawal represent the most common reactions.

Hostility is occasionally an early reaction to the diagnosis. Anger may be directed against the medical team for the delayed diagnosis or for inadequate attention, as well as toward family members, who may be viewed as not particularly upset and happy to finally "get their way." This phase is generally transient, receding as the patient comes to recognize the reality of the situation and the need for family and physician. Hostility is difficult for both patient and doctor and may be intense enough to lead the physician and family to reject the patient emotionally. If recognized, this reaction should be allowed to run a natural course without withdrawing support.

Infantile regression is an accentuated response commonly occurring in the patient with a dependent personality. It also develops as a reaction-formation in patients who were overly independent before their illness. If it is more than transient, infantile regression must be mitigated by providing a parental figure who will be, on the one hand, supportive and, on the other hand, stern and demanding. Infantile regression places an inordinate burden on the family who are called upon to provide extraordinary amounts of support.

Withdrawal is an extreme form of regression, often tinged with elements of hostility. Direct confrontation is essential for the patient who withdraws; constant encouragement and the setting up of goals for achievement (such as ambulation, planning trips, or visiting friends) are critical.

Denial of the diagnosis is generally a transient reaction. When denial is mild, the physician may need only to reinforce his remarks with re-presentation of the facts or provision of objective and tangible evidence. However, in some patients, denial is extreme and functions as a crude psychological defense mechanism, necessary for sustaining the psyche. A constant onslaught of evidence and reinforcement of the diagnosis or prognosis may be counterproductive and is not justified.

The reactions of the family are critical to the patient's well-being and to aiding the health care team in providing maximum support. Thus, the physician must be concerned with the family's responses to the patient and to the diagnosis. Not uncommonly, complete families—wives, husbands, and children—may be alienated by the patient, who disallows them the opportunity to resolve their confusion. Such alienation, which may approach pathologic proportions, can be understood with the help of the physician. A frequent family reaction is to provide smothering protection in compensation for guilt over previous misunderstandings with the patient and the need to resolve such differences. Again, the physician can help alleviate such pathologic reactions.

PSYCHOLOGICAL REACTIONS TO CANCER TREATMENT

The patient who enters treatment for cancer is subjected to a reinforcement of the diagnosis and a rekindling of the fears regarding threats to self-esteem and self-image. The latter may be particularly demoralizing if the cancer treatment involves bodily disfigurement or a physical limitation that is either cosmetically mutilating or functionally disabling. Thus, the patient who requires a mastectomy, jaw resection, amputation, or colostomy faces a significant and frightening change in self-image. The distortions that are incorporated into the patient's unconscious perhaps as a result of real or imagined experiences with friends, are potentially devastating. Often these distortions are unrealistic and unsubstantiated, but, more importantly, they may be unexpressed. The physician must inquire into the patient's concerns and offer a realistic appraisal in order to minimize unnecessary anguish (see Chapter 1). Patient education is a most important component of the approach to dealing with the stress of therapy. It additionally serves to cushion the stress by allowing the patient to intellectualize about the disease and its treatment. In this "demythologizing process" patient fears are identified and dealt with openly. Often the result is a more acceptable view of one's illness and treatment. Educational materials may facilitate the task. For example, booklets are available from the National Cancer Institute (NCI) that address questions that the patient may have about various types of therapy (e.g., *Chemotherapy and You,* NCI-HEW Publication No. 76-1136). Detailed explanation of the therapy in terms of its effect on the tumor as well as its potential side effects allows the patient to approach treatment realistically.

MANAGEMENT OF THE PRETERMINAL PHASE

"Terminal cancer" is an expression commonly employed by both patients and physicians but with distinctly different definitions. Strictly defined, "terminal cancer" means that death will ensue within a 4-week period. The physician should avoid using the term "terminal" in talking with the patient or family. Not infrequently, patients may absorb the label and yet live for months or even years. The term imposes upon the family and the patient a tremendous stress, often resulting in withdrawal.

The physician's role in the terminal phase is a crucial one. It is essential to remain sensitive to all the patient's needs and specifically, to the patient's need to know that his physician is always available. If the patient is at home, frequent home visits may be enormously appreciated. It may be helpful to allow the patient to come to the office once or twice a week, even though there are no specific medications to be administered.

It is not incumbent upon the physician to reinforce the inevitability of death to patients who have entered a preterminal or terminal state and are sustaining hope for a reversal of the tumor. More important, however, during this period, the family must be apprised precisely in order to allow them to pass through the grieving process successfully.

The approach to preterminal care has begun to include more emphasis on comfort measures and care at home or in a hospice, where hospital routines and studies are omitted in favor of psychologic and symptomatic support.

PSYCHOTROPIC DRUG THERAPY

The use of psychotropic drugs for cancer patients has not been scientifically evaluated, but in many instances such drugs have a beneficial effect. For example, tricyclic antidepressants may be helpful in alleviating somatic symptoms of depression. If there is no contraindication, they should not be withheld on the basis of the common clinical misconception that "the patient is appropriately depressed, considering the diagnosis and prognosis" (see Chapter 215).

In recent years, hallucinogens and other consciousness-altering drugs have been used in terminal patients to promote euphoria and an acceptance of death. Such drugs are currently under investigation for use in terminal illness. The literature should be followed for developments in this very interesting area.

ANNOTATED BIBLIOGRAPHY

Cullen, J.W., Fox, B.H., and Isom, R.N. (eds.): Cancer: The Behavorial Dimensions. New York: Raven Press, 1976. *(Three papers focusing on coping with cancer and the difficulties of the physician and the patient in the presentation and the confrontation with the diagnosis of cancer represent an extensive personal experience by the three authors [J.C.B. Holland, M.J. Krant, and J.N. Vettese]. This is a useful introduction to the experience of patient issues in dealing with cancer.)*

Gates, C.: Psychodynamics of the Cancer Patient. In Lokich, J. (ed.): Primer of Cancer Care. Boston: G.K. Hall, 1978. *(Based on the central concept that self-esteem is the singular aspect of the ego which must be supported and maintained. The impact of cancer on the ability of the patient to relate to his surroundings, to his closest friends and family members, and to his own goals and aspirations is assessed. The author specifically identifies a means of recognizing the anxiety states associated with cancer diagnosis and awareness.)*

Gates, C. and Hans, P.: Psychologic complications of cancer and its treatment. In Lokich, J. (ed.): Clinical Cancer Medicine. Boston: G.K. Hall, 1979. *(Case histories detail patient reaction to the process of dying and living with cancer and the inherent difficulties in enduring treatment. The practical use of psychotropic drug therapy is described.)*

Golden, S., Horwich, C., and Lokich, J.: Chemotherapy and You. Department of Health and Welfare Publication No. (NIH) 76-1136. *(This pamphlet originally produced at the Sidney*

Farber Cancer Institute is available for patient use from the National Cancer Institute and serves as a layman's introduction to the concept of chemotherapy and its potential effects.)

Krant, M.J.: The hospice movement. N. Engl. J. Med., 299:547, 1978. *(A thoughtful presentation of the methods and issues involved with this approach to terminal care.)*

Lokich, J.: Telling the diagnosis. In Lokich, J. (ed.): Primer of Cancer Care. Boston: G.K. Hall, 1978. *(Through the use of multiple examples, the author describes a selected group of patient reactions to the diagnosis of cancer and clarifies the pro's and con's of the informed patient emphasizing the need to increase awareness in order to allow the patient and the family to resolve differences and to settle at some point of equilibrium.)*

7

Endocrinologic Problems

91
Screening for Diabetes Mellitus

Diabetes is, after obesity and thyroid disease, the most common metabolic disorder encountered by the primary physician. Concern on the part of the patient about requirements for parenteral therapy and vascular complications make diabetes one of the most feared diagnoses. Diabetes screening is commonly requested by the patient, as detection campaigns and advertising have heightened public awareness of the disease. However, while there is no question that treatment effectively reduces symptoms associated with the metabolic derangements induced by diabetes, benefits of treatment initiated in the asymptomatic phase have not been demonstrated. Uncertainty about the natural history of diabetes does not allow definitive recommendations regarding screening or treatment of early disease. The nonspecificity of screening tests, particularly as predictors of subsequent vascular complications, must be kept in mind.

EPIDEMIOLOGY AND RISK FACTORS

Diabetes mellitus is heterogeneous. It is likely that a number of pathophysiological mechanisms are responsible for the decrease in beta cell production of, or decreased peripheral response to, insulin. Reports of diabetes prevalence depend heavily on definitions of glucose intolerance and case-finding methods. Overall prevalence in the United States is approximately 2 per cent. Since the noninsulin-dependent, or maturity-onset, form of diabetes is five to times more common than the insulin-dependent, or juvenile-onset, form, overall prevalence increases dramatically with age. While the incidence of insulin-dependent disease peaks during the second decade and is low after age 30, noninsulin-dependent diabetes is rare before the fifth decade and peaks after age 65. Overall prevalence is about 2 per cent in the third and fourth decades, 4 per cent during the fifth and sixth, and 8 per cent during and after the seventh decade.

While a genetic predisposition to diabetes mellitus has been clearly established, the mode of inheritance is not well defined. Concordance in identical twins has been shown to be greater than 90 per cent when onset is after age 40 in the index twin. A concordance rate of approximately 50 per cent is the rule when disease occurs before age 40. Only 20 per cent of patients with insulin-dependent diabetes (most with onset before age 40) have a first degree relative with a diabetic history. While these family studies establish the importance of inheritance, they also suggest an etiologic role for infection and other acquired conditions in the genetically predisposed individual.

Epidemiologic studies have demonstrated at least a temporal relationship between viral infections and increased risk of development of insulin-dependent diabetes. Coxsackie group B, mumps and rubella are among the viruses most clearly implicated. That autoimmune mechanisms may be involved has been suggested by the association of pernicious anemia and thyroiditis with insulin-dependent diabetes.

377

The importance of obesity as a risk factor for noninsulin-dependent diabetes cannot be overstated. Overnutrition and resulting obesity diminish sensitivity of peripheral tissues to insulin. Carbohydrate intolerance and diabetes follow. Eighty per cent of adult diabetics are obese or have a history of obesity. Among adults who are at least 25 per cent over their ideal body weight, one out of every five has elevated fasting blood sugar levels, and three out of every five have abnormal glucose tolerance tests.

Pregnancy also increases the risk of either transient or, presumably in predisposed individuals, permanent diabetes. Diabetes may also be induced or unmasked by other stressful situations or by the administration of corticosteroids. A number of other drugs, including benzothiadiazine diuretics, growth hormone, epinephrine, and thyroxine, can also impair glucose tolerance.

NATURAL HISTORY OF DIABETES AND EFFECTIVENESS OF THERAPY

Since diabetes mellitus is heterogeneous and is defined on the basis of varying degrees of glucose intolerance, descriptions of its natural history are difficult. A number of terms describing the stages in the natural history of diabetes have gained common usage. *Prediabetes* or potential diabetes is a term that can be applied with certainty only in retrospect. *Latent* or *stress diabetes* refers to the condition of individuals who have normal glucose tolerance but in whom glucose intolerance has been known to occur in relation to pregnancy, infection, obesity, or other periods of stress. *Chemical diabetes* describes the asymptomatic but detectable stage of the disease. *Clinical diabetes* is usually heralded by polyuria, polydipsia, polyphagia, and weight loss. When diabetes is noninsulin-dependent and occurs late in life, onset in usually insidious. In insulin-dependent cases, onset is more often precipitous and associated with ketoacidosis.

Data concerning progression from one stage of diabetes to another are fragmentary. When the customary liberal criteria are used to define chemical diabetes (oral glucose tolerance test results of 160 mg. per 100 ml. at one hour or 120 mg. per 100 ml. at two hours), a minority of patients with glucose intolerance progress to clinical diabetes. Approximately 30 per cent of women with chemical diabetes diagnosed before age 50 progressed over a 10-year period to the clinical stage. A prospective study of young subjects with chemical diabetes demonstrated an incidence of clinical disease of only 10 per cent during 16 years of follow-up.

Vascular and neurologic complications occur in an unpredictable pattern, reflecting again the heterogeneity of diabetes. The incidence of complications clearly tends to increase with the duration of clinical diabetes. This is reflected in mortality rates for diabetics. When compared with age-matched nondiabetics, rates for diabetics increase with duration of known disease. In one study of patients followed for up to 25 years, the increase in risk with duration was greater after age 40 and among women. Long-term studies of patients followed for as long as 40 years, however, have indicated that clinical evidence of microvascular disease, atherosclerosis, or neuropathy may occur in only 20 to 40 per cent of insulin-dependent patients. Complications, in general, occur with similar frequency in patients with noninsulin-dependent disease if duration of known disease is considered.

Coronary artery disease is the most common cause of death among diabetics. Autopsy studies indicate that coronary disease is two to three times more common among diabetics that nondiabetics. Not surprisingly, coronary disease is more prevalent in patients who have had the disease longer. Peripheral vascular disease is also very common among diabetics; clinical studies have indicated a prevalence of about 60 per cent. Diabetics in Framingham were shown to be four to five times more likely to have intermittent claudication and two to three times more likely to suffer the morbid consequences of stroke than nondiabetics. Complications seem to be more clearly related to duration than to severity of diabetes.

Data regarding the incidence of retinopathy among diabetics are conflicting, presumably reflecting both differences in populations studied and definitions of retinal abnormalities. In general, the incidence of retinopathy increases with duration regardless of age at onset. Prevalence ranges of 40 to 80 per cent have been reported among patients with known diabetes lasting 20 to 30 years. Neovascularization or malignant retinopathy is more common among long-term, younger insulin-dependent diabetics.

Renal disease has been reported in 15 to 80 per cent of autopsies among diabetics. Renal failure is the cause of death in 6 to 12 per cent of diabetic patients. While prevalence estimates vary widely from study to study, it is clear that the risk of glomerulosclerosis with clinically evident functional impairment increases dramatically with the duration of the disease.

While duration of glucose intolerance and associated metabolic abnormalities can be related to many of the complications of diabetes, the variability of the natural history must be kept in mind. It has been argued that all complications, including specific microangiopathic changes, have been identified in patients without evident glucose intolerance. Whether or not the morbidity and mortality associated with the complications can be influenced by therapy is a matter of long-standing debate. Some have argued that close control of glucose levels results in fewer and later complications. Others point out the heterogeneity of diabetes and the variable incidence of complications independent of glucose control. It has been argued that close control may involve selection of cases in which complications are less likely to develop because of the milder nature of the diabetes itself (see Chapter 98, Management of Diabetes). Regarding screening, there is no evidence that therapy of asymptomatic patients with chemical diabetes offers any benefit.

SCREENING AND DIAGNOSTIC TESTS

The simplest screening test is analysis of urine obtained 1 to 2 hours after a heavy carbohydrate meal. The *sensitivity* and *specificity* of this procedure depend on both the renal threshold for glucose and the validity of the chemical reaction used to detect glycosuria. Glucose usually begins to appear in the urine when the arterial blood level reaches the 150 to 180 mg. per 100 ml. range. This renal threshold is often lower during late pregnancy and with some chronic diseases. A higher threshold may be present in old age. Renal glycosuria, Fanconi's syndrome and rare nonglucose forms of melituria (assuming a copper reduction test) may produce positive urine reactions in the absence of elevated blood glucose levels. Copper reduction tests (e.g., Clinitest) detect all forms of melituria except sucrose. Glucose oxidase enzyme strips (Clinistix, Tes-tape) are specific for glucose.

More sensitive and specific is the direct measurement of serum or whole blood glucose. The precise values of sensitivity and specificity depend on criteria used for a positive test result. One-hour postprandial blood levels greater than 170 mg. per 100 ml. are generally considered indicative of diabetes. There is,

however, wide disagreement among experts; many physicians consider values greater than 160 mg. per 100 ml. positive while others require levels as high as 200 mg. per 100 ml. Regardless of which reference value is used, it must be kept in mind that plasma glucose levels are approximately 15 per cent higher than corresponding blood glucose levels, and a downward adjustment should be made when these measurements are used. Fasting blood glucose levels can be quite specific, but again definitions of abnormal vary. Some physicians would diagnose diabetes on the basis of fasting blood glucose levels greater than 100 mg. per 100 ml. Others require higher levels. The predictable increase in fasting and postprandial glucose levels with age should be considered when evaluating test results.

CONCLUSIONS AND RECOMMENDATIONS

- Diabetes mellitus is a common but heterogeneous condition. Family history and, in the adult, obesity are principal risk factors.
- Because diabetes mellitus is heterogeneous and defined on the basis of varying degrees of glucose intolerance, its natural history has not been well defined. The incidences of diabetic complications tend to increase with the duration of disease but are unpredictable in individual patients.
- Whether or not close control of glucose levels with conventional insulin therapy influences the incidence or severity of vascular and neurologic complications is a matter of debate. Because there is no evidence that therapy of asymptomatic patients with chemical diabetes offers benefit, the routine measurement of blood glucose levels to screen asymptomatic individuals for chemical diabetes is not recommended.

ANNOTATED BIBLIOGRAPHY

Burditt, A.F., Caird, F.I., and Draper, G.J.: The natural history of diabetic retinopathy. Q. J. Med., *37*:303, 1968. *(Statistical treatment of observations in 2000 diabetics suggesting glucose level may be related to development of retinopathy but not to its progression.)*

Craighead, J.E.: Current views on the etiology of insulin-dependent diabetes mellitus. N. Engl. J. Med., *299*:1439, 1978. *(Reviews possible inter-*

play among genetic, infectious and immunologic mechanisms.)

Ellenberg, M.: Diabetic complications without manifest diabetes. JAMA, *183*:926, 1963. *(Early review. Virtually any of the common "complications" can precede detectable abnormalities in carbohydrate metabolism.)*

Garcia, M.J., McNamara, P.M., Gordan, T., and Kannell, W.B.: Morbidity and mortality in diabetics in the Framingham population. Diabetes, *23*:105, 1974. *(Insulin-dependent diabetic women have the greatest relative mortality. Increased mortality among diabetics is not entirely explained by associated obesity, hypertension and hyperlipidemia.)*

Hirohata, T., MacMahon, B., and Root, H.F.: The natural history of diabetes. I. Mortality. Diabetes, *16*:875, 1967. *(Excess mortality of diabetes increases with age of onset and is higher in females than males.)*

Knowles, H.C., Guest, G.H., Lampe, J., Kessler, M., and Stillman, T.G.: The course of juvenile diabetes treated with unmeasured diet. Diabetes, *14*:239, 1965. *(Uncontrolled prospective study following treated diabetics without rigidly controlled diets establishing risk of complications.)*

O'Sullivan, J.B.: Age gradient in blood glucose levels: Magnitude and clinical implications. Diabetes, *23*:713, 1974. *(Mean fasting levels increase 2 mg. per 100 ml. per decade, postprandial at 4 mg. per 100 ml. per decade.)*

O'Sullivan, J.B., and Mahan, C.M.: Prospective study of 352 young patients with chemical diabetes. N. Engl. J. Med., *278*:1038, 1968. *(Only 32 per cent of those with chemical diabetes by Fajans and Conn criteria progressed to overt diabetes within 10 years.)*

Paz-Guevara, A.T., Hsu, T-H, and White, P.: Juvenile diabetes mellitus after 40 years. Diabetes, *24*:559, 1975. *(Insulin-induced hypoglycemia was the most common complication. The prevalence of complications were: significant visual impairment in 50 per cent; nephropathy in 59 per cent; neuropathy in 50 per cent; peripheral vascular disease in 40 per cent; and major cardiac complications in 20 per cent.)*

Siperstein, M.D.: The glucose tolerance test: a pitfall in the diagnosis of diabetes mellitus. Adv. Intern. Med., *20*:297, 1975. *(Excellent review of the nonspecificity of the glucose tolerance test. Recommends relying on fasting values.)*

Takazakura, E., Nakamato, Y., Hayakawa, H., *et al.*: Onset and progression of diabetic glomerulosclerosis: A prospective study based on serial renal biopsies. Diabetes, *24*:1–9, 1975. *(Serial biopsy data with equivocal results. Progression of renal disease seemed more determined by the type of diabetes rather than the degree of control of blood glucose.)*

Valleron, A., Eschwege, E., Papoz, L., and Rosselin, G.E.: Agreement and discrepancy in the evaluation of normal and diabetic oral glucose tolerance test. Diabetes, *24*:585, 1975. *(Compares criteria for positive GTT. Only 48 per cent of subjects were classified the same way by all criteria. The 2-hour value was best discriminator between universally recognized diabetics and nondiabetics.)*

Winegrad, A.I., and Greene, D.A.: The complications of diabetes mellitus. N. Engl. J. Med., *298*:1250, 1978. *(A brief review of variability of complications and implications for etiologic hypotheses.)*

92
Screening for Thyroid Cancer

Cancer of the thyroid is a relatively rare disease with a low mortality rate. Approximately 8000 cases are diagnosed each year in the United States; the number of deaths caused by the tumor is about 1000 annually—only 0.25 per cent of cancer deaths. Nevertheless, this disease has major significance for the primary physician because of its iatrogenic relationship to childhood irradiation of the head and neck. A high prevalence of thyroid cancer, diagnosed after a long latent and/or asymptomatic period, has repeatedly been documented among patients exposed to such irradiation. The appropriate approach to the evaluation and management of exposed patients having various degrees of thyroid abnormalities remains a subject of debate. Public awareness of the problem has increased in recent years.

CHILDHOOD IRRADIATION AND THYROID CANCER

Generally, the incidence of thyroid cancer increases with age. This is particularly true of tumors with anaplastic or follicular histopathologies and of the medullary carcinomas derived from the parafollicular cells. The most common tumors, with papillary histopathology, have a bimodal age-specific incidence with peaks in the 30s and late in life. Thyroid tumors occur approximately twice as frequently in females. Whites seem to be at greater risk than blacks. Approximately 20 per cent of the rare medullary carcinomas are familial.

The major identifiable risk factor for the development of thyroid cancer is a history of external irradiation of the head and neck. External irradiation was used as early as 1907 to shrink an enlarged thymus in infancy. During the 1920s and subsequently until the 1950s, it was used extensively for treatment of enlarged tonsils and adenoids, cervical adenitis, mastoiditis, sinusitis, hemangiomas, tinea capitis, and acne. Concern about ill effects began to mount in 1950 when a history of neck irradiation was noted in 9 of 28 cases of childhood thyroid cancer with a latency period of 5 or more years. Further documentation followed, and radiation to the neck was discontinued. In 1973, attention focused on the issue again when 40 per cent of a series of adults with thyroid cancer were found to have a history of irradiation. Clearly, the latent period between exposure and diagnosis of cancer could be measured in decades. It was also clear that the exposed population at risk was substantial—estimates ranged from one million to two million individuals—and largely unidentifiable.

Successive reports focused on the risk among exposed individuals. Large studies indicated that more than 25 per cent had detectable thyroid abnormalities; the prevalence of cancer was estimated at 7 to 9 per cent. These figures must, however, be considered in light of information available regarding the prevalence of thyroid carcinoma in the general population.

NATURAL HISTORY OF THYROID CANCER AND EFFECTIVENESS OF THERAPY

The prevalence of occult carcinoma of the thyroid is not well defined. Autopsy studies have indicated that prevalence ranges from 5 to 13 per cent. An often quoted study showing an overall prevalence of 5.7 per cent found highest age-specific rates in the fifth and sixth decades.

A high prevalence of asymptomatic thyroid cancer is not surprising in light of the benign clinical course of most thyroid tumors after diagnosis. Follow-up studies have determined that probability of survival depends on tissue type and age of the patient. For localized papillary carcinoma, survival approximates that of age-matched controls; in one large study, there were no deaths among patients under 40 during 10 to 15 years of follow-up. The course of follicular cancer is only slightly more aggressive. Anaplastic tumors, on the other hand, run a rapid clinical course to death.

The relatively high prevalence of occult thyroid cancer presumed to be present, in general, raises a number of questions about the significance of tumors found during the evaluation of patients with radiation exposure. It is worth noting that in the largest study, conducted at Michael Reese Hospital in Chicago, 47 per cent of the tumors identified after surgery was recommended because of palpable or scan abnormalities were incidental findings. That is, 29 of 60 cancers were not found in or near the benign nodule that prompted surgery. There is no evidence indicating that these tumors are more likely to result in morbidity or mortality than occult tumors found in the general population.

SCREENING AND DIAGNOSTIC TESTS

The sensitivity of history-taking in identifying individuals at risk is not known. Many who were irradiated during early childhood may be unaware of their exposure. Physical examination of the thyroid gland is often difficult, and the palpable nodule is a nonspecific finding. Thyroid scan is more sensitive in detecting thyroid abnormalities, but, since it fails to distinguish between benign and malignant disease, is even less specific. The hazard of additional radiation exposure, particularly when ^{131}I scanning is performed, must be considered, as well as the expense incurred. It should be noted, however, that a number of studies indicate that physical examination itself becomes more sensitive after scanning is performed and the physician is aware of scan results.

Large studies utilizing both multiple examination and ^{99m}Tc scanning indicate that 60 per cent of thyroid abnormalities (identified by either or both modalities) will be identified by palpation alone. Scanning alone will be more than 95 per cent sensitive. However, palpable abnormalities appear to be more specific for cancer. In one study of patients with palpable nodules who ultimately had thyroidectomy, the prevalence of cancer was 34 per cent, compared with 19 per cent among patients who went to surgery on the basis of scan abnormalities alone. Physical examination was nearly 80 per cent sensitive in identifying thyroids containing cancers. Cancers found in glands with scan abnormalities alone were often incidental, unrelated to the scan abnormality.

Attempts to use measurements of serum thyroglobulin as a screening test for thyroid cancer have not been successful. Despite poor specificity, thyroglobulin abnormalities are disappointingly insensitive.

When abnormalities are detected on examination or scan, additional diagnostic steps are indicated. The palpable nodule accompanied by a hypofunctioning area on scan is considered by some an indication for surgery. In some centers, needle biopsy of the nodule has become the preferred approach to patients with, as well as those without, a history of irradiation. While some physicians would operate on the basis of scan abnormalities alone, careful follow-up examination with reservation of surgery for palpable abnormalities has been recommended as a prudent alternative. An alternative explanation for scan abnormalities should be considered and thyroid function and the status of antithyroid antibodies determined. Needle biopsy is generally recommended in cases of diffuse thyroid enlargement when it is important to rule out thyroiditis or when the patient is a poor surgical risk (see Chapter 93).

When physical examination or scan findings are questionable, some physicians have used suppression of the thyroid for 3 to 6 months in an effort to shrink normal thyroid tissue, thereby increasing the sensitivity of the examination for autonomous nodules. On the basis of animal experiments, long-term thyroid suppression as prophylaxis for thyroid cancer has also been advocated for all patients with an exposure history or, more selectively, those with questionable scans.

CONCLUSIONS AND RECOMMENDATIONS

- Childhood irradiation is an important risk factor for thyroid carcinoma that may be diagnosed as long as 35 years after exposure.
- The prevalence of thyroid abnormalities among the estimated one to two million patients with an exposure history is about 25 per cent. The prevalence of thyroid cancer has been estimated to be 7 to 9 per cent.
- The significance of occult thyroid cancer in exposed patients is not known. There appears to be a high prevalence of occult tumors in the general population.
- Identification of patients at risk is an important part of history-taking.
- Patients at risk should be carefully examined yearly or at least every two years. Scanning is not necessary in the absence of palpable abnormalities. If scanning is performed, low radiation dose methods should be used (^{99m}Tc or ^{123}I).
- In general, surgery should be reserved for patients with palpable abnormalities of the gland. Needle biopsy may be preferred in cases where a single nodule has been identified. Multiple examinations by experienced examiners may be necessary. Thyroid suppression may increase the sensitivity of thyroid palpation. Repeat examination of patients with normal examination but abnormal scan should be performed yearly.

ANNOTATED BIBLIOGRAPHY

Arnold, J., Pinsky, S., Ryo, U.Y., et al.: ^{99m}Tc-pertechnetate thyroid scintigraphy in patients predisposed to thyroid neoplasms by prior radiotherapy to the head and neck. Radiology, 115:653, 1975. (Documents higher sensitivity but very low specificity of technetium scanning.)

Crile, G., Jr., Esselstyn, C.B., Jr., and Hawk, W.A.: Needle biopsy in the diagnosis of thyroid nodules appearing after irradiation. N. Engl. J. Med., 301:997, 1979. (An important editorial citing data that support a conservative approach for those with nodules.)

DeGroot, L., and Paloyan, E.: Thyroid carcinoma and radiation: A Chicago endemic. JAMA, 225:487–491, 1973. (Reported that 40 per cent of patients with thyroid carcinoma had a history of childhood irradiation to the neck.)

Favus, M.J., Schneider, A.B., Stachura, M.E., *et al.*: Thyroid cancer occurring as a late consequence of head-and-neck irradiation. Evaluation of 1056 patients. N. Engl. J. Med., *294*:1019, 1976. *(An important paper. Of 1056 patients, 16.5 per cent had nodular disease on palpation, another 10.7 per cent on technetium scanning. Estimated prevalence of carcinoma of 9 per cent.)*

Duffy, B.J. Jr., and Fitzgerald, P.J.: Cancer of the thyroid in children: A report of 28 cases. J Clin Endocrinol., *10*:1296, 1950. *(The initial cluster report.)*

McKenzie, A.D.: The natural history of thyroid cancer. A report of 102 cases analyzed 10 to 15 years after diagnosis. Arch. Surg., *102*:274, 1971. *(Mortality associated with histologic type and age—higher in older age groups.)*

National Cancer Institute: Information for physicians on irradiation-related thyroid cancer. Ca, *26*:150, 1976. *(Good summary with recommendations.)*

Nelson, R.L., Wahner, H.W., and Gorman, C.A.: Rectilinear thyroid scanning as a predictor of malignancy. Ann. Intern. Med., *88*:41, 1978. *(Documents a low sensitivity [54 per cent] and notes the low specificity of hypofunctioning with either ^{99m}Tc or ^{131}I scanning.)*

Refetoff, S., Harrison, J., Karanfilski, B.T., *et al.*: Continuing occurrence of thyroid carcinoma after irradiation to the neck in infancy and childhood. N. Engl. J. Med., *292*:171, 1975. *(Reports findings in 100 patients with irradiation histories; 26 had palpable abnormalities, 7 carcinoma.)*

Sampson, R.J., Woolner, L.B., Bahn, R.C., *et al.*: Occult thyroid carcinoma in Olmstead County, Minnesota: Prevalence of autopsy compared with that in Hiroshima and Nagasaki, Japan. Cancer, *34*:2072, 1974. *(Prevalence of 5.6 per cent among 157 autopsies of clinically occult thyroid Ca. Highest age specific prevalence between 40 and 60.)*

Schneider, A.B., Favus, M.J., and Stachura, M.E.: Plasma thyroglobulin in detecting thyroid carcinoma after childhood head and neck irradiation. Ann. Intern. Med., *86*:29, 1977. *(Thyroglobulin levels not found to be very useful.)*

Schneider, A.B., Favus, M.J., Stachura, M.E., *et al.*: Incidence, prevalence and characteristics of radiation-induced thyroid tumors. Am. J. Med., *64*:243, 1978. *(Further follow-up from Michael Reese Hospital and Medical Center demonstrating a high [36 per cent] incidence of new thyroid tumors after surgery. Thyroid suppressive therapy appeared to prevent recurrences.)*

Walfish, P.G., and Volpe, R.: Irradiation-related thyroid cancer. Ann. Intern. Med., *88*: 261, 1978. *(Editorial focusing on diagnostic and management issues.)*

Woolner, L.B., Beahrs, O.H., Black, B.M. *et al.*: Classification and prognosis of thyroid carcinoma: A study of 885 cases observed in a 30-year period. Am. J. Surg., *102*:354, 1961. *(Noninvasive disease without significant morbidity or mortality.)*

93

Evaluation of Thyroid Nodules

Thyroid nodules are an extremely common phenomenon, both clinically, and histologically. A palpable thyroid nodule can be detected in up to 4 per cent of the adult population; the prevalence of nodules in autopsy series approaches 50 per cent. The incidence increases with age and is 6 to 9 times greater in women than in men. Frequently at issue is whether biopsy or surgical excision is required to rule out carcinoma. The primary physician must be skilled in the detection of thyroid lesions by physical examination and must be able to plan a cost-effective evaluation of a palpable thyroid nodule.

PATHOPHYSIOLOGY AND CLINICAL PRESENTATION

The pathophysiology of thyroid nodules is varied and incompletely understood. It has been demonstrated that nodules, even autonomously functioning ones, have histochemical similarities to tissue stimulated by TSH, and will respond to TSH. Autonomously functioning thyroid nodules have the capacity for growth and function independent of trophic hormones. Radiation of the thyroid or adjacent areas has been shown to induce both benign neoplasms and well-differentiated papillary and follicular carcinomas. A 10- to 35-year latent period has been found for onset of thyroid neoplasms after low-dose head and neck irradiation. Observations of victims exposed to atomic bomb fallout have supplied further evidence that thyroid neoplasms can be induced by radiation.

Simple goiters may undergo degenerative changes such as infarction, hemorrhage, or fibrosis leading to nodularity, which may be solitary or multiple. Nodules may develop from simple goiters when colloid accumulates in hyperplastic cells producing so-called colloid cysts.

Benign and malignant thyroid nodules are usually asymptomatic and discovered by the patient or examining physician. Large nodules may cause a cosmetic problem or compress an adjacent structure. The nodules are usually painless unless rapid growth, inflammation, or hemorrhage occurs and produces significant discomfort.

Most *benign adenomas* are follicular. They are usually unifocal and present as solitary nodules both by examination and on scan. Growth is typically slow over many years; ^{131}I uptake in the early stages is moderate. Later, if the nodule's function becomes autonomous, it suppresses TSH, and concentrates ^{131}I; the remainder of the gland atrophies, and a "hot" nodule appears on scan, with no radioactive iodine uptake in the remaining thyroid tissue. Most cold nodules represent adenomas that have undergone hemmorhagic necrosis. Most thyroid cysts are benign nodules that have necrosed and degenerated. Rarely a malignant lesion degenerates in a similar fashion.

Thyroid *carcinomas* are uncommon; the current incidence is 2.5 per 100,000 population per year. They are more frequent in women than in men. *Papillary carcinomas* are the most common and account for 60 to 70 per cent of all thyroid malignancies. The lesions are slow-growing, spread to local lymph nodes, and metastasize late; as a result, prognosis is good. *Follicular carcinomas* make up another 15 to 20 per cent of thyroid cancers. Lymph node metastases may occur without invasion of the thyroid capsule; this occurrence does not alter prognosis. Hematogenous spread is early and initial presentation is often from a metastasis to lung or bone.

Anaplastic carcinomas comprise another 10 to 12 per cent of cases; these are very invasive, usually inoperable and fatal within 1 year.

Medullary carcinomas, derived from the parafollicular cells of the thyroid, may occur as an autosominal dominant disease, as in familial medullary cancer and multiple endocrine neoplasia types II and III in conjunction with pheochromocytoma. The malignancy often presents as a thyroid nodule located in the upper half of the thyroid gland. It can be multicentric, especially in the familial forms. At least 50 per cent of medullary carcinomas of the thyroid occur sporadically. Calcitonin, produced by the parafollicular or "C" cells, is a tumor marker for medullary carcinoma.

Subacute thyroiditis and *chronic thyroiditis* can present as nodular glands that may be tender (subacute) or rubbery (chronic) in quality, though there is a great deal of variation (see Chapter 99).

DIFFERENTIAL DIAGNOSIS

The differential diagnosis of the thyroid nodule includes benign adenoma, cyst, primary thyroid carcinoma, metastatic carcinoma (e.g., lymphoma), subacute thyroiditis and chronic thyroiditis. The vast majority of nodules are benign. In rare instances, sarcoidosis or tuberculosis is to blame.

WORKUP

History can help determine the risk of malignancy. Although definitive assessment cannot be made by history and physical examination alone, these elements of the evaluation can provide important information regarding risk and need for biopsy or excision. Age and sex are most helpful. The incidence of malignancy among patients with thyroid nodules is considerably higher in males than in females, although women make up a greater proportion of those with thyroid cancer. Moreover, the incidence of thyroid cancers in patients with nodules is greatest in those under age 40, especially if they have previously been subjected to head or neck irradiation. Hoarseness or dysphagia of recent onset or family history of pheochromocytoma or medullary carcinoma also raises the probability of malignancy. Conversely, a history of living in an iodine-deficient area, goiter, or ingestion of goitrogens such as lithium, turnips or beets, as well as female sex, family history of goiter, and age greater than 40, favor a benign lesion.

Symptoms of hypo- or hyperthyroidism argue against malignancy, as does sudden growth or sudden onset of neck pain, which points to subacute thyroiditis or hemorrhage into a benign adenoma.

Physical findings suggestive of cancer include a firm, irregular large nodule (greater than 2 cm.) that is fixed—reflected by failure to move with swallowing. Multiple nodules suggest a benign condition, such as multinodular goiter. The consistency of the tissue may not be diagnostic because malignancy may be present in soft nodules, e.g., papillary carcinomas which have undergone cystic degeneration. A general physical assessment should be made of skin, hair, eyes, heart rate, blood pressure, temperature, and reflexes for evidence of hyper- or hypothyroidism.

Laboratory studies. Scan and ultrasound are currently the most commonly employed means of assessment. A nodule which takes up ^{131}I is rarely malignant. The finding of little or no uptake, i.e., a "cold" or "cool" nodule, is suggestive of thyroid carcinoma, but not diagnostic, for only 20 per cent of such nodules prove to be malignant. If the nodule is cold, *ultrasound* is helpful in distinguishing cystic from solid lesions; the former are for the most part benign except for the rare papillary carcinoma that has degenerated. The limits to ultrasound include an inability to detect a lesion smaller than 1 cm. or greater than 4 cm. or to differentiate a benign from a malignant solid nodule.

An alternative approach that has been advocated is *aspiration needle biopsy,* foregoing scan and ultrasound. Its yield and accuracy parallel excisional biopsy results. A fine needle is used. The older method of excisional biopsy is not utilized unless the patient has a high risk of malignancy, i.e., a young male with a cold solid nodule. The safety of fine-needle biopsy has been established, and the procedure is a reasonable alternative to scan and ultrasound if a physician skilled in the technique is available. Moreover, the procedure can be used to treat cysts and obtain material for cytologic examination.

Other laboratory studies have only ancillary utility. *Thyroid indices* may reveal hypo- or hyperfunctioning gland, which is evidence against carcinoma. In rare instances, a plain film of the neck may demonstrate punctate calcifications indicative of the psammona bodies seen in papillary carcinoma or shell-like calcification characteristic of a benign lesion. A very high *erythrocyte sedimentation rate* accompanying a tender gland is very suggestive of subacute thyroiditis.

In sum, one should either obtain a fine-needle biopsy or attempt to determine if the nodule is cold and solid before proceeding to excisional biopsy. Although cystic cold nodules are usually, but not always, benign, they should be assessed for presence of cancer by aspiration and subsequently by biopsy if the cyst cannot be fully decompressed and a residual nodule remains. Response to TSH suppression is not a reliable diagnostic test, because carcinomas as well as adenomas may shrink when TSH secretion is inhibited.

When suspicion of medullary carcinoma arises (e.g., there is a strong family history), a *calcitonin level* should be obtained; elevation is virtually diagnostic. Occasionally, provocative testing with infusion of calcium or pentagastrin is necessary to demonstrate an elevated calcitonin level.

SYMPTOMATIC THERAPY

Patients with benign lesions who are otherwise healthy can be given a trial of exogenous thyroid hormone therapy in an attempt to decrease the size of the nodule. Approximately 10 to 30 per cent of patients with nontoxic nodular goiters will show a decrease in nodule size when treated with doses of L-thyroxine sufficient to suppress TSH. The rationale is that suppression of TSH should diminish nodule size in those lesions that are TSH responsive, e.g., follicular adenomas. The required dose of L-thyroxine is often slightly supraphysiologic, i.e., 0.2 to 0.3 mg. daily. Thyroid hormone therapy is not indicated in the elderly or in those with underlying coronary disease. It is unknown whether therapy prevents increase in nodule size in patients who have not achieved a decrease.

Multinodular goiters often do not shrink much because they are composed of a great deal of fibrous tissue. Bothersome large cysts require surgical removal, but smaller ones can be aspirated as necessary.

PATIENT EDUCATION

The primary care physician should counsel and closely follow patients with previous head or neck radiation (see Chapter 92). Regular follow-up is important in any patient with a nodule, and the patient should be instructed to call if there should be a change in size, development of lymphadenopathy, pain, dysphagia or hoarseness.

ANNOTATED BIBLIOGRAPHY

Burman, K.D., Earll, J.M., Johnson, M.C., *et al.*: Clinical observations on the solitary autonomous thyroid nodule. Arch. Intern. Med., *134*:915 1974. *(Of 54 patients with solitary autonomous thyroid nodules, only one or perhaps two manifested any evidence of hyperthyroidism.)*

Gershengorn, M.C., McClung, M.R., Chu, E.W., *et al.*: Fine-needle aspiration cytology in the preoperative diagnosis of thyroid nodules. Ann. Intern. Med., *87*:265 1977. *(Thirty-three patients who had aspiration biopsy and excisional biopsy were assessed. Satisfactory aspiration specimens were obtained in 97 per cent. The diagnosis of malignancy was made in nine, seven were correct, and there was one false-positive and one occult carcinoma unrelated to the clinical nodule. Eighteen aspirations were interpreted as benign. There was one false-negative.)*

Hamburger, J.I.: Solitary autonomously functioning thyroid lesions: Diagnosis, clinical features, and pathogenetic mechanisms. Am. J. Med., *58*:740, 1975. *(A review of 164 patients with autonomously functioning thyroid lesions; 140 were nontoxic and 24 were toxic. Observation is advised for patients with nontoxic nodules unless toxicity appears imminent.)*

Mortensen, J.D., Woolner, L.B., and Bennett, W.A.: Gross microscopic findings in clinically normal thyroid glands. J. Clin. Endocrinol., *15*:1270, 1955. *(A Mayo Clinic autopsy study of 821 patients without clinical thyroid disease, demonstrating 406 patients with single or multiple nodules; a 4.2 per cent incidence of carcinoma in the nodular glands.)*

Wang, C.A., Vickery A.L., Jr., and Maloof, F.: Needle biopsy of the thyroid. Surg. Gynecol. Obstet., *143*:365, 1976. *(Ninety patients were biopsied with a large-bore [Vim-Silverman] needle. The needle biopsy was correct in 90 per cent. Of the remaining nine patients, four thought to have embryonal adenomas, and five thought to have lymphocytic thyroditis, had carcinomas, a false-negative rate of 10 per cent. Complications included four hematomas, two cases of tracheal puncture, two of transient laryngeal nerve palsy, and one of needle tract implantation.)*

Warner, S.C.: Modalities of medical therapy for nodular goiter. In Warner, S., and Ingbar, S. (eds.): The Thyroid. New York: Harper and Row, 1978, p. 525. *(A critical discussion of thyroxine therapy.)*

94

Evaluation of Asymptomatic Hypercalcemia

The proliferation of automated multichannel analyzers has resulted in the discovery of many patients with asymptomatic elevations of serum calcium. The serum calcium concentration is the sum of calcium bound to protein, diffusible calcium complexes, and ionized calcium. The level is tightly regulated, with 95 per cent of people having values between 9.5 and 10.5 mg. per 100 ml. and 99 per cent having values between 8.3 and 10.9 mg. per 100 ml.

Although the actual definition of true hypercalcemia requires an increase in the ionized fraction of calcium, this determination is not widely used due to technical difficulties in measurement. For practical purposes, hypercalcemia is arbitrarily defined as a level of total serum calcium 2 standard deviations or more above the mean. To account for variability in protein available for binding and to avoid falsely low readings, the serum calcium is corrected for a low serum albumin (0.8 mg. per 100 ml. is added to the measured serum calcium for every 1 gm. per 100 ml. fall in serum albumin below 4.0 gm. per 100 mg.).

As is true for any quantitative test, the definition of an abnormal level is a statistical one and thus somewhat arbitrary. The probability that underlying pathology exists is far greater than if the level were normal, but one elevated random determination in an asymptomatic individual is not tantamount to diagnosis of a disease state (see Chapters 2 and 3). There is much variability in the assay for serum calcium; over 50 per cent of first-time elevations in serum calcium are not confirmed on repeat determination. On the other hand, early hyperparathyroidism and other conditions may present solely as a silent, minor elevation in calcium.

The primary physician must be able to interpret an abnormal calcium determination, decide how extensively to evaluate the symptom-free patient, and in particular decide how aggressively to pursue diagnoses of early hyperparathyroidism and occult malignancy.

PATHOPHYSIOLOGY AND CLINICAL PRESENTATION

In primary care practice, hypercalcemia is usually noted as an incidental laboratory finding subsequent to multiphasic screening. *Hyperparathyroidism* is overwhelmingly the most likely etiology for hypercalcemia in the asymptomatic patient. In a recent population survey in Sweden, 15,903 people were screened for elevated calcium levels; 95 had hypercalcemia on repeat testing. Hyperparathyroidism was suspected in 88 patients, 59 of whom underwent neck explorations; parathyroid adenomas were identified in 57. The presentation of primary hyperparathyroidism is notoriously nonspecific. The textbook picture: "stones, bones, abdominal groans and psychic moans" has given way to a far more subtle and less specific presentation. The patient is either symptom-free or complains of fatigue, irritability and mild gastrointestinal symptoms such as nausea or constipation. Among 31 patients with hypercalcemia detected in a medical clinic population study, only 8 presented with specific symptoms or signs; most of the remaining 23 admitted to some fatigue and irritability which disappeared after removal of a parathyroid adenoma.

Hyperparathyroidism increases with age, peaking in the fourth to sixth decade, and is twice as common in females as in males. There is little evidence that extrinsic factors predispose to hyperparathyroidism, though the possibility that head and neck irradiation contributes has been suggested. The hypercalcemia of hyperparathyroidism results from excess parathormone causing bone reabsorption and a decrease in renal excretion of calcium. The vague symptoms of fatigue, irritability and constipation have been attributed to the elevation in calcium. Hyperparathyroidism is due to adenoma in 80 per cent of cases, to generalized hyperplasia in 15 per cent and to carcinoma in less than 5 per cent.

Reports of "normocalcemic hyperparathyroidism" have appeared. Adenomas have been found in patients with "normal" calcium levels, but these patients often have episodes of definite hypercalcemia and baseline calcium levels that are at the upper limits of normal. These probably represent early cases of hyperparathyroidism. Instances of hyperparathyroidism without any evidence of hypercalcemia have yet to be documented.

Hyperparathyroidism may exist concurrently with other endocrinopathies in the multiple endocrine adenomatosis (MEA) syndromes. The combination of hyperparathyroidism, pituitary adenoma, and pancreatic tumor is designated MEA-I; when hyperparathyroidism coexists with pheochromocytoma and medullary carcinoma of the thyroid, the designation is MEA-II.

Neoplasia is the second most frequent cause of hypercalcemia and the most common in inpatient settings. Breast cancer accounts for most cases; it is estimated that 10 to 12 per cent of women with breast cancer will have hypercalcemia at some point in their illness, due to the high frequency of *skeletal metastases*. The mechanism of the hypercalcemia is postulated to involve the local release of substances which produce bone resorption. Myeloma is associated with induction of an osteoclast-activating factor. In some instances the hypercalcemia of malignancy is due to production of *ectopic parathormonelike substances* by the neoplasm. Epidermoid or large cell anaplastic tumors of the lung and renal cell carcinomas are the most frequently implicated and account for about 20 per cent of all tumor-related cases of hypercalcemia. Other factors implicated in neoplastic hypercalcemia include prostaglandins, osteoclastic activating factors, and certain therapeutic agents, particularly the hormonal therapy used in breast cancer (see Chapter 118). Dehydration, anorexia and immobilization can exacerbate the hypercalcemia of malignancy. Higher levels of hypercalcemia (greater than 13.8 mg. per 100 ml.) are more often associated with neoplasia than with hyperparathyroidism. Symptoms are a function of the rate of development of hypercalcemia as well as the degree of elevation. Among 25,847 patients screened in a general medical clinic in the early 1950s, 67 persons with abnormal serum calcium levels were detected, 31 of whom had hyperparathyroidism and 17 malignancy. In only 4 of the patients with malignancy was hypercalcemia the presenting finding. In a series of 100 patients in Canada, gastrointestinal symptoms occurred in 75 per cent, though it was difficult to separate the influence of the underlying tumor from that of hypercalcemia.

Increased absorption of calcium is responsible for the hypercalcemia due to vitamin D intoxication, sarcoidosis, and milk-alkali syndrome. *Vitamin D intoxication* results from many months of ingesting massive amounts of vitamin D (100,000 units or more per day). In severe cases of *sarcoidosis* with evidence of systemic involvement, there can be increased intestinal sensitivity to vitamin D, stimulating calcium absorption. Patients with *milk-alkali syndrome* characteristically consume extraordinary amounts of milk and absorbable calcium-containing antacids. They put themselves at risk for hypercalcemia and renal failure.

Transient elevations in serum calcium are often noted at the onset of administration of *thiazide diuretics;* the effect usually lasts only 10 days, but in some patients it may persist and continue even after cessation of therapy. The mechanism has not been elucidated, but persistent elevation is sometimes a manifestation of occult hyperparathyroidism. Significant hypercalcemia has been noted in rare cases of *thyrotoxicosis,* but mild elevations have been reported in 14 to 27 per cent of individuals with hyperthyroidism, presumably due to accelerated turnover of bone. A similar mechanism exacerbated by immobilization may in rare instances, lead to hypercalcemia in patients with severe Paget's disease.

DIFFERENTIAL DIAGNOSIS

Primary hyperparathyroidism probably accounts for more than half of cases, certainly the majority of asymptomatic patients discovered on routine screening. Neoplasia is the next most common etiology, dominated by breast cancer, but also seen in up to 40 per cent of patients with myeloma and in cases where tumors produce parathyroid hormone (PTH) or PTH like substances, such as epidermoid carcinoma of the lung and renal cell carcinoma. Hypercalcemia caused by immobilization and thyrotoxicosis involves accelerated bone turnover. Among the exogenous causes of hypercalcemia are megadoses of calcium carbonate antacids in conjunction with excessive milk consumption, vitamin D intoxication, and rare instances of lithium carbonate use. Severe cases of sarcoidosis with evidence of systemic involvement are sometimes complicated by hypercalcemia. Thiazide diuretics sometimes produce transient elevations in serum calcium, as can Addison's disease.

WORKUP

Before an extensive evaluation commences, a *repetition of the serum calcium* determination is essential. The frequency of false-positive readings is as high as 50 per cent, resulting from variability in the serum calcium assay and spurious elevations due to venous stasis induced by prolonged application of the tourniquet at the time the blood sample is drawn. The repeat sample should be obtained after an overnight fast, and measurements of serum albumin and phosphate should be carried out concurrently. Phosphate levels fall after a meal and may be mistaken for the hypophosphatemia of hyperparathyroidism. The calcium concentration is corrected for any decrease in albumin. Before the calcium determination is repeated in the patient with a single elevation in serum calcium, he should be instructed to cease using any calcium-carbonate-containing antacids, exogenous vitamin D, thiazide diuretics, lithium carbonate, or unusual calcium preparations such as bone meal (used by some health food advocates). In the case of thiazides, 2 weeks should be allowed to pass before reassessment.

History. Once true hypercalcemia has been confirmed, further evaluation can commence. Even if the patient is "asymptomatic," inquiry is needed into some of the more subtle manifestations of hypercalcemia, such as mild fatigue, weakness, irritability, anorexia and constipation. The patient should also be asked about items pertinent to etiology such as a history of bone pain, breast masses, breast cancer, other malignancies, peptic ulcer disease, abdominal pain, heat intolerance, weight loss and other manifestations of hyperthyroidism, lymph node enlargement, hemoptysis, cough, dyspnea, kidney stones, flank pain and hematuria.

Physical examination in the asymptomatic patient is unlikely to be very revealing, but a few findings are worth checking for. The blood pressure should be noted, because it is sometimes elevated in hypercalcemia. The eyes are examined for gross evidence of band keratopathy (very rare), nodes for enlargement, breasts for masses, abdomen for tenderness and organomegaly, and bones for focal tenderness.

Laboratory studies. A few simple tests ordered at the outset may be informative, particularly a *fasting calcium, albumin, phosphate, chloride* and *alkaline phosphatase.* An elevated serum calcium in conjunction with a low phosphate and a chloride-to-phosphate ratio of greater than 33 are very suggestive of hyperparathyroidism; however a normal serum phosphate does not rule out the diagnosis. The phosphate level is usually normal in hypercalcemia due to malignancy. A markedly elevated alkaline phosphatase is typical of bony metastases as well as active Paget's disease. In hyperparathyroidism, the alkaline phosphatase is normal or mildly elevated.

Other simple studies can contribute to assessment. A *complete blood count* and *sedimentation rate (ESR)* are often informative. Anemia and a very high sedimentation rate in the context of hypercalcemia raise the possibility of malignancy, especially myeloma, which should be checked for with a *serum immunoelectrophoresis (IEP)*. If the serum IEP is negative, a urine IEP should be obtained, because occasionally the serum IEP is negative in cases of myeloma. A chest x-ray may reveal lung tumor or bilateral hilar adenopathy and pulmonary infiltrates suggestive of sarcoidosis (see Chapter 48).

Simultaneous determinations of the serum calcium and *parathyroid hormone (PTH)* are needed for the diagnosis of hyperparathyroidism in the asymptomatic patient. PTH measurement by radioimmuno assay is available from many commercial laboratories. In hyperparathyroidism, there is an inappropriately high PTH level for the amount of calcium in the serum. It is important to recognize that this PTH level may be "within normal limits" for PTH levels of patients who are normocalcemic, but this same amount is inappropriately high for the degree of calcium elevation that is present. If PTH is undetectable, hyperparathyroidism is excluded. Some commercial assays also detect ectopically-made PTH as well as PTH that originates in the parathyroid gland; unfortunately, these assays cannot distinguish between the two. Any inappropriate elevation in PTH detected by such an assay requires ruling out a tumor capable of ectopic PTH production before a diagnosis of hyperparathyroidism can be made; a chest x-ray and intravenous pyelogram should be obtained to search for a renal or pulmonary source of PTH.

A history of breast cancer, bone pain, or a markedly elevated alkaline phosphatase is an indication for a *bone scan* to detect skeletal metastases. Evaluation of thyroid or adrenal function should be restricted to cases where clinical signs and symptoms of endocrinopathy are present.

When hyperparathyroidism has been diagnosed, the issue of anatomic localization arises because definitive therapy requires surgical removal. In some centers, arteriographic and venous catheterization techniques have been perfected to help define the responsible lesion preoperatively; however, these methods are not widely available, and neck exploration by an experienced surgeon usually suffices. Angiography should be reserved for patients in whom initial surgery was unsuccessful.

SYMPTOMATIC MANAGEMENT

The genuinely asymptomatic patient requires little more than a good fluid intake (2 to 3 liters per day) and liberal salt use, which often suffice to lower mild elevations in serum calcium. Furosemide can be used to supplement hydration and salt when the hypercalcemia does not adequately respond. More aggressive treatment and hospitalization are needed for severe symptomatic hypercalcemia.

There is some evidence that prostaglandin inhibitors, such as aspirin and indomethacin, might be beneficial for treatment of hypercalcemia due to cancer in patients who have evidence of increased prostaglandin excretion. However, definitive therapy requires treating the malignancy. Sarcoidosis complicated by hypercalcemia often responds to corticosteroids, which are also indicated for other systemic manifestations of the disease (see Chapter 48).

INDICATIONS FOR REFERRAL

The circumstances under which to recommend surgery for mild, asymptomatic hyperparathyroidism are not clearly defined. The decision is one that is dependent on the patient's preferences, his access to skillful surgical therapy, and the physician's assessment of the patient's ability to undergo major surgery. The primary physician should explain to the patient that a conservative approach without surgery requires regular follow-up, and there is roughly a one-in-five chance that an operation will become necessary over the next 5 years. The natural history of asymptomatic hyperparathyroidism has not been well defined, though a prospective study from the Mayo Clinic has revealed that approximately 20 per cent of asymptomatic patients required surgery within a 5-year period because of progression of the disease. Unfortunately, no criteria were found useful for early identification of individuals who would need surgical intervention.

Surgery is usually recommended in patients with decreased renal function, a history of calcium stones, or x-ray evidence of marked bone reabsorption. Bone densitometry, which can detect loss of bone much earlier than standard bone films, has been suggested as a way to refine the decision about whether to employ surgery, but is not widely available. Among the data that must be considered in deciding whether or not to recommend surgery are the facts that many patients with untreated hyperparathyroidism do well for many years and that the surgical procedure is a technically difficult one for which an experienced surgeon must be available.

Additional prospective studies defining the natural history of asymptomatic hyperparathyroidism are needed to determine whether the individual patient with mild disease (serum calcium 10.5 to 11.5 mg.

per 100 ml.) will benefit from being operated on in the asymptomatic phase. In the elderly patient with mild elevations, a conservative approach is probably indicated. In younger patients with mild disease and limited access to an experienced parathyroid surgeon, expectant follow-up may be preferable. When excellent parathyroid surgical therapy is available, the cure rate for first neck exploration by experienced surgeons is over 90 per cent. On the other hand, one must consider the difficulties inherent in a second exploration when an inexperienced surgeon fails to obtain a cure at first operation.

PATIENT EDUCATION

Though not definitive, a number of simple recommendations can help lessen difficulties associated with mild hypercalcemia of any etiology. All agents that can raise the serum calcium should be discontinued, including vitamin D, thiazides and calcium-containing antacids. Vigorous hydration for prevention of stone formation and renal tubular damage is sessential; a minimum fluid intake of 2 to 3 liters per day should be encouraged. Liberal salt use in conjunction with high fluid intake facilitates calcium excretion. Patients should be encouraged to remain as active as possible and avoid immobilization, particularly if they have Paget's disease.

ANNOTATED BIBLIOGRAPHY

Besarab, A., and Caro, J.F.: Mechanisms of hypercalcemia in malignancy. Cancer, *41*:2276, 1978. *(A review of the more important mechanisms.)*

Bone, H.G., Snyder, W.H., and Pak, C.Y.: Diagnosis of hyperparathyroidism. Ann. Rev. Med., *28*: 111, 1977. *(Emphasizes the changing clinical presentation of the disorder resulting from detection of the disease in the asymptomatic or early phases.)*

Boonstra, C.E., and Jackson, C.E.: Hyperparathyroidism detected by routine serum calcium analysis—Prevalence in a clinic population. Ann. Intern. Med., *63*:468, 1965. *(In a population of over 25,000, 67 patients with hypercalcemia were identified. Thirty-one had hyperparathyroidism, though only 8 were symptomatic. In only 4 was hypercalcemia the presentation of an underlying malignancy.)*

Christensson, T., Hellstrom, K., Wengle, B., et al.: Prevalence of hypercalcemia in a health screening in Stockholm. Acta Med. Scand., *200*:131, 1976. *(In a population of over 15,000, 95 patients were confirmed to have hypercalcemia, with probable hyperparathyroidism in 88.)*

Myers, W.P.: Differential diagnosis of hypercalcemia and cancer. CA, *27*:258, 1977. *(A well-written review for the clinician.)*

Palmer, F.J., Nelson, J.C., and Bacchus, H.: Chloride phosphate ratio in hypercalcemia. Ann. Intern. Med., *80*:200, 1974. *(The chloride-to-phosphate ratio was greater than 33 in 96 per cent of patients with primary hyperparathyroidism.)*

Purnell, D.C., Scholz, D.A., Smith, L.H., et al.: Treatment of primary hyperparathyroidism. Am. J. Med., *56*:800, 1974. *(A 5-year follow-up on a prospective Mayo Clinic study revealing that surgery was necessary in 20 per cent of previously asymptomatic primary hyperparathyroid patients.)*

Seyberth, H.W., et al.: Prostaglandins as mediators of hypercalcemia associated with certain types of tumors. N. Engl. J. Med., *293*:1278, 1975. *(Aspirin or indomethacin lowered serum calcium in 6 patients with evidence of increased urine prostaglandin excretion.)*

Stowt, R.M., Smith, L.H., Wilson, D.M., et al.: Hydrochlorothiazide effects on serum calcium and immunoreactive parathyroid hormone concentrations. Ann. Intern. Med., *77*:587, 1972. *(A study of normal subjects; total serum calcium increased significantly after 1 day of thiazide, and ionized calcium increased after 17 days. Both remained elevated 2 weeks after cessation of therapy.)*

95
Evaluation of Hypoglycemia

Stimulated by articles in the lay press, patients with a host of functional complaints such as fatigue, weakness, light-headedness, inability to concentrate, palpitations and anxiety come to physicians wondering if they have "hypoglycemia." Many seek a medical explanation to account for their difficulties, although a substantial portion have underlying emotional problems and attendant psychophysiological symptoms unrelated to serum glucose levels.

Hypoglycemia is defined statistically as a plasma glucose concentration less than 45 mg. per 100 ml., but glucose levels may reach 35 mg. per 100 ml. in normal asymptomatic women. A low serum sugar becomes a clinical problem only if symptoms of neuroglycopenia occur; unfortunately, some of these symptoms are very nonspecific and resemble complaints expressed by anxious patients, e.g., light-headedness, nervousness, irritability, palpitations, tremulousness.

The primary physician should be able to recognize the occasional patient likely to have symptoms on the basis of hypoglycemia from the vast numbers of people with functional complaints unrelated to a low blood sugar. Clinical identification is necessary to avoid unnecessary glucose tolerance testing and distraction away from other etiologies.

PATHOPHYSIOLOGY AND CLINICAL PRESENTATION

Hypoglycemia can result from increased insulin secretion, enhanced glucose utilization, or inadequate functioning of one or more compensatory glucoregulatory mechanisms. When hypoglycemia occurs, the liver responds with increased glycogenolysis and gluconeogenesis, stimulated by glucagon and epinephrine, which activate hepatic phosphorylase. In addition, the pituitary secretes growth hormone (which inhibits utilization of glucose by muscle and enhances lipolysis) and ACTH (which promotes adrenal glucocorticoid production). The increased cortisol acts to stimulate gluconeogenesis and diminish muscle uptake of glucose.

The clinical presentation of chemical hypoglycemia depends on the rapidity of the fall in blood sugar, age, and adequacy of compensatory mechanisms. Symptoms are usually classified as neuroglycopenic or catecholamine-mediated. Neuroglycopenic symptoms result in part from depressed central nervous system activity, due to the inadequate supply of glucose to the brain; the physiologic state is similar to cerebral anoxia. Other symptoms are manifestations of autonomic responses to hypoglycemia. The earliest signs of hypoglycemia are hunger, sweating, restlessness and palpitations. Very severe falls in serum glucose (as with insulin reactions) are accompanied by an altered mental status, with slow mentation, stupor or seizures. Chronic fatigue, constant anxiety, and lethargy are not parts of this picture.

Establishment of an absolute correlation between clinical presentation and serum glucose levels is difficult because there are substantial variations among individuals and because the rate of decline in serum sugar is an important factor in the genesis of symptoms. Parasympathetic responses such as hunger may occur as glucose drops below 70 mg. per 100 ml. followed by sympathetic reactions causing tachycardia, diaphoresis and tremor at approximately 35 mg. per 100 ml. It must be recognized that many people with blood sugars between 35 and 45 mg. per 100 ml. are completely asymptomatic. In fact, 23 per cent of the normal population demonstrate serum sugars below 50 mg. per 100 ml. during glucose tolerance testing.

The hypoglycemias can be classified pathophysiologically as postprandial or fasting. In the *postprandial* variety, the fall in glucose results from an abnormal response to the intake of food. *Functional reactive hypoglycemia* is a commonly encountered postprandial form, which is frequently detected in individuals with emotional problems, probably because they come complaining of "hypoglycemia" and often undergo glucose-tolerance testing. Oral glucose tolerance testing (OGTT) reveals normal patterns during the first 2 hours, with symptomatic hypoglycemia occurring 2 to 5 hours after eating. In some, secretion of insulin is exaggerated, but often this is not the case, and the cause of the excessive fall in glucose remains unknown. This functional syndrome has little relationship to the future development of diabetes, but heavy consumption of sweets is sometimes associated with the condition.

Adult-onset diabetes may also result in postprandial hypoglycemia. A diabetic glucose tolerance curve is noted on OGTT during the first 2 to 3 hours, followed by transitory hypoglycemia between hours 3 and 5. Insulin release is found to be sluggish, with levels inappropriately high for the level of serum glucose at hand. Fortunately, the majority of adult-onset diabetics do not experience reactive hypoglycemia on glucose tolerance testing.

About 10 per cent of *postgastrectomy* patients are bothered by postprandial hypoglycemia. Rapid entry of glucose into the small bowel excessively stimulates still unidentified gut factors which trigger release of too much insulin. Hypoglycemia and neuroglycopenic symptoms appear 2 to 3 hours postprandially—earlier than in reactive hypoglycemia.

Fasting hypoglycemias that result from autonomous insulin secretion, overuse of exogenous insulin, or defects in glycogenolysis and gluconeogenesis, and generally worsen with fasting or exercise. *Insulinomas* represent a rare but important cause of uncontrolled insulin production. Over 85 per cent of insulinomas are benign islet cell tumors. The clinical presentation can be confusing, and levels of serum glucose are not always low after an overnight fast. In a series of 39 patients with proven islet-cell tumors, just about half had glucose levels above 60 mg. per 100 ml. after 10 hours of fasting; in 20 per cent, this level persisted for a full week with the patient on a regular diet. Thus it should be no surprise that clinical presentations may be highly variable in timing and severity. For example, in a Mayo Clinic series of 60 patients with insulinomas, the timing of symptoms was equally divided between early morning, late afternoon, and several hours following a meal. The only valid generalization is that fasting and exercise may precipitate symptoms; profound degrees of hypoglycemia may result. In the Mayo Clinic series, a combination of diplopia, blurred vision, sweating, palpitations and weakness occurred in 85 per cent. Confusion or abnormal behavior occurred in 80 per cent, amnesia occurred in half, and 10 per cent experienced seizures.

Other causes of fasting hypoglycemia include excess doses of *exogenous insulin, sulfonylurea* administration, and defects in glycogenolysis or gluconeogenesis (as in severe pituitary or adrenal insufficiency, end-stage liver disease, and severe alcoholism complicated by poor nutrition).

Two groups of nonhypoglycemics must be differentiated from patients manifesting genuine falls in glucose in conjunction with symptoms. One group is composed of anxious and depressed individuals who have multiple bodily complaints of a functional or psychophysiological nature (see Chapter 218). The most common symptoms include fatigue, headache, spasms, palpitations, numbness, sweating, and mental dullness. They attribute their symptoms to "hypoglycemia" in order to explain their difficulties and avoid the psychosocial issues at hand. Requests for glucose tolerance testing are frequent. A second group is bothered by postprandial symptoms very similar to those experienced by patients with reactive hypoglycemia, yet in the context of normal serum sugar levels. The pathophysiology of this alimentary variant is unknown.

DIFFERENTIAL DIAGNOSIS

The differential diagnosis of true hypoglycemia can be organized around whether it is fasting or postprandial. The hypoglycemias most commonly encountered in the outpatient setting are postprandial and include functional reactive hypoglycemia, postgastrectomy syndrome, and adult-onset diabetes. The most common forms of fasting hypoglycemia are due to excessive doses of insulin or sulfonylureas. End-stage liver disease, alcoholism complicated by poor nutrition, Addison's disease, and hypopituitarism are causes of impaired glycogenolysis or gluconeogenesis that may result in hypoglycemia. Rare etiologies include insulinomas and pelvic or retroperitoneal neoplasms. In rare cases of severe hypothyroidism or chronic renal failure, there may be hypoglycemia.

WORKUP

History. The physician is often urged by many anxious or depressed patients to investigate their suspicions of hypoglycemia. It is important to be able to select on clinical grounds those individuals most likely to have hypoglycemia in order to avoid wasteful or misleading laboratory studies. Inquiries into symptoms of depression (see Chapter 215) and chronic anxiety (see Chapter 214) and questioning about any concurrent family, job or financial stresses are critical to assessment when the patient reports multiple functional complaints. Patients admitting to chronic fatigue, lethargy, loss of vitality, constant nervousness, sleep disorders and related symptoms should be informed that hypoglycemia does not present in such fashion and that investigation would best proceed in other directions to ferret out the etiology of the fatigue and other somatic symptoms (see Chapters 5 and 218). Further investigation into hypoglycemia should be reserved for patients without evident emotional problems who are troubled by paroxysmal or postprandial sweating, palpitations, hunger, visual disturbances, or restlessness. One needs to establish the timing of symptoms, especially in relation to eating, fasting and exercise in order to separate fasting from postprandial etiologies.

If symptoms are unrelated to meals, one should check for use of insulin or sulfonylurea agents. Cases in which the fasting hypoglycemia is due to end-stage liver disease, adrenal insufficiency, marked hypopituitarism, or severe hypothyroidism are usually self-evident, with other symptoms dominating the clinical picture. If symptoms occur postprandially, it is important to inquire into a history of diabetes, gastric surgery, or heavy use of sweets (some authorities believe that consumption of candy and other foods rich in mono- and disaccharides is associated with functional reactive hypoglycemia).

Physical examination usually contributes little, but ought to be checked for postural hypotension, hyperpigmentation, visual field defects, and signs of hepatocellular disease (see Chapter 62). In obscure cases, a search for a pelvic mass might be helpful.

Laboratory studies. The initial objective is to document the correlation between symptoms and a low serum glucose concentration. Without such documentation, one cannot make the diagnosis of hypoglycemia. If the patient's story is suggestive of postprandial hypoglycemia, an *oral 5-hour GTT* can be performed. It is essential that samples be taken not only at regular hourly intervals, but also and particularly when symptoms are reported. If the oral GTT is abnormal and if hypoglycemia is believed due to rapid gastric emptying, an *intravenous GTT* can be performed, becaue the intravenous test will be normal and differentiate the condition from the other forms of postprandial hypoglycemia.

Fasting hypoglycemias can be identified by withholding food and exercising the patient. An *overnight fast* of 10 hours will often cause a fall in the glucose levels to less than 60 mg. per 100 ml. in the majority of patients with fasting hypoglycemias, but not in those with the reactive types. Extending the fast 4 more hours causes a drop below 50 mg. per 100 ml. in a greater percentage of patients, and by 24 hours, glucose level is about 35 mg. per 100 ml. in most. Occasionally, *72 hours of fasting* are required for demonstration of hypoglycemia. Since exercise promotes a fall in serum glucose, it may be used in conjunction with fasting to bring out hypoglycemia and precipitate symptoms. Two-thirds of the patients with insulinomas will develop hypoglycemia within 24 hours; and fewer than 5 per cent will have to fast for 72 hours.

Concurrent determination of *plasma insulin lev-*els when the patient is symptomatic will help document that excess insulin is the etiologic factor. When there is a question of factitious hypoglycemia due to self-administration of excess insulin, a *"C"-peptide* assay can be helpful if available. In the synthesis of endogenous insulin, the C-peptide is formed as proinsulin is split. Low C-peptide levels in the presence of high serum insulin concentrations indicate exogenous insulin use.

Need for additional studies in the patient with fasting hypoglycemia depends on suspicion of other etiologies. Cortisol and ACTH determinations are indicated if hypopituitarism or adrenal insufficiency is suggested by clinical findings. Extensive liver function tests may be superfluous if the patient is floridly jaundiced, but the prothrombin time and serum albumin are good measures of hepatocellular function and are worth obtaining (see Chapter 62).

SYMPTOMATIC MANAGEMENT

Treatment of most fasting hypoglycemias requires attending directly to the underlying etiology. Patients on sulfonylurea agents will require adjustment of dose and recognition that the drug's effects may be potentiated by phenylbutazone, probenecid, aspirin, warfarin, or alcohol. Cases induced by heavy alcohol abuse will resolve with cessation of drinking and return of adequate food intake, as long as heptatic function remains adequate; there is little one can do in end-stage liver disease.

The treatment of reactive functional hypoglycemia is dietary. Patients should be instructed to have five or six small feedings a day. Some have advocated that the diet should be high in protein, with fewer than 30 per cent of the calories derived from simple sugars and starches. Weight loss is useful in obese latent diabetics (see Chapter 98). Patients with alimentary hypoglycemia due to rapid gastric emptying have been treated with anticholinergics without impressive results. Some advocate adding guar gum and pectin to the diet because they slow glucose absorption. Further study is needed of the value of such treatments.

PATIENT EDUCATION

It is essential that the physician avoid mislabeling a patient as hypoglycemic, especially when an individual already misattributes his symptoms to "low sugar." The incidental discovery of a blood sugar level below 60 mg. per 100 ml. on a random determination certainly does not warrant the diagnosis. In all likelihood, the patient is normal. The diagnosis requires concurrent demonstration of symptoms and very low serum glucose levels. Patients without clinical evidence of hypoglycemia or its causes should be told that glucose tolerance testing is not indicated. A few will insist that they undergo the GTT and probably should have the test to avoid their roaming from one doctor to another.

A number of patients will initially refuse to accept the fact that hypoglycemia is not responsible for their symptoms; the attribution had served to explain a variety of functional symptoms for the patient. One needs to explore with these people their concerns and discuss other causes that might be responsible, including anxiety and depression (see Chapters 214 and 215).

ANNOTATED BIBLIOGRAPHY

Chaiyapon, C., Freinkel, N., Nagel, T.C., et al.: Plasma C-peptide and diagnosis of factitious hyperinsulinism. Ann. Intern. Med., 82:201, 1975. (The finding of low C-peptides is helpful in diagnosing factitious hyperinsulinism.)

Fajans, S.S., and Floyd, J.C.: Fasting hypoglycemia in adults. N. Engl. J. Med., 294:766, 1976. (A physiologically oriented review of fasting hypoglycemia with a table of causes organized around pathophysiological mechanisms.)

Freichs, H., and Creutzfeldt, W.: Hypoglycemia 1. Insulin-secreting tumors. Clin. Endocrinol. Metabol., 5:747, 1976. (Well done, current review.)

Jung, Y., Khurana, R.C., Corredot, D.G., et al.: Reactive hypoglycemia in women: Results of a health survey. Diabetes, 20:435, 1971. (A discussion of the criteria that should be used to make the diagnosis of reactive hypoglycemia.)

Marks V: Hypoglycemia 2. Other causes. Clin. Endocrinol. Metabol., 5:769, 1976. (Well done, current review of some of the less common etiologies.)

Megyesi, K., Kahn, C.R., Roth, J., et al.: Hypoglycemia in association with extrapancreatic tumors: Demonstration of elevated plasma NSILA-s by a new radioreceptor assay. J. Clin. Endocrinol. Metabol., 38:931, 1974. (The description of an NSILA, an inhibitor of insulin degradation, as a possible cause of nonpancreatic-tumor-associated hypoglycemia.)

Merimee, T.J., and Tyson, J.E.: Stabilization of plasma glucose during fasting—Normal variations in two separate studies. N. Engl. J. Med., 291:1275, 1974. (Established that women have lower blood sugars and may normally have blood sugars in the 40s. Glucose levels must fall below 35 mg. per 100 ml. to be significant.)

Permutt, M.A., Kelly, J., and Bernstein, R., et al.: Alimentary hypoglycemia in the absence of gastrointestinal surgery. N. Engl. J. Med., 288:1206, 1973. (Hypoglycemia due to increased insulin secretion is possibly an abnormality of endocrine regulation.)

Rutsky, E.A., McDaniel, H.G., Tharpe, D.L., et al.: Spontaneous hypoglycemia and chronic renal failure. Arch. Intern. Med., 138:1364, 1978. (Description of four patients on dialysis in whom hypoglycemia developed.)

Yeager, J., and Young, R.T.: Nonhypoglycemia as an epidemic condition. N. Engl. J. Med., 291:907, 1974. (A succinct discussion of how to manage patients with self-diagnosed "hypoglycemia.")

96
Evaluation of Hirsutism
SAMUEL R. NUSSBAUM, M.D.

Hirsutism in women is characterized by excessive hormone-dependent growth of pubic, axillary, abdominal, chest and facial hair. A patient may present for evaluation of hirsutism when her hair growth is regarded as excessive or as coarser or longer than that of individuals in her societal, geographic or racial environment. For example, Mediterranean women are among the more hirsute of Caucasians, yet, in their country of origin, the excess hair is rarely considered unattractive and few seek medical advice. However, women of the same Mediterranean background living in the United States occasionally present to physicians complaining of their appearance; for them hirsutism may connote loss of femininity or sexuality in a society preoccupied with stereotyped perceptions of beauty. Virilization is characterized by temporal hair recession, deepening voice, increased muscle mass and clitoromegaly; in contrast to hirsutism, it represents more significant endocrine pathology. When dealing with excessive hair growth, the primary physician needs to decide whom to evaluate for underlying endocrine disease, and whom to simply reassure and, if need be, treat symptomatically.

PATHOPHYSIOLOGY AND CLINICAL PRESENTATION

Hair follicles are found over the entire body except for the palms and soles. Hair growth is of two types: lanugo or vellus, which is soft, unpigmented and rarely more than 2 cm. long, and terminal, which is coarse, pigmented, and grows in excess of 2 cm. A survey of college women revealed that one-quarter had easily noticeable facial hair, one-third reported hair extending along the linea alba from the pubic area (male escutcheon) and 17 per cent had chest hair. Three quarters of women over 60 have a measurable growth of facial hair. Hirsutism has familial and racial patterns. Mediterranean women are more hirsute than Scandinavians, white women are more hirsute than black women, and black women are more hirsute than Asian women.

The stimulus for hair growth is a testosterone metabolite, 5-alpha dihydrotestosterone. Hirsute women have elevated production rates of either relatively weak androgens such as androstenedione, or of the more potent androgen, testosterone; at times, the serum concentration of androstenedione or testosterone is frankly elevated. The source of enhanced androgen production may be the ovary, the adrenal or both. In hirsute women, a greater proportion of testosterone, which is usually synthesized from adrenal androstenedione and dehydroepiandrosterone, is secreted directly by the ovary. The majority of women with idiopathic hirsutism demonstrate ovarian overproduction of androgens, when selective ovarian and adrenal vein catheterizations are performed.

DIFFERENTIAL DIAGNOSIS

The vast majority of patients with isolated hirsutism have an inherited condition reflecting an idiopathic increase in adrenal or ovarian androgen production. In the virilized patient, whose levels of testosterone often exceed 200 ng. ml., the likelihood of a testosterone-producing tumor is enhanced. Such lesions include an arrhenoblastoma, hilar cell tumor,

stromal hyperthecosis and Leydig cell hyperplasia. Virilization may be a component of Cushing's syndrome, especially if the underlying etiology is adrenocortical carcinoma or ectopic ACTH production. Other etiologies of Cushing's syndrome are more likely to cause excess hair growth and typical cushingoid features without true virilization.

In the absence of virilization, hirsutism in association with obesity and oligomenorrhea or amenorrhea is suggestive of the polycystic ovary syndrome (see Chapter 107). These patients have elevated and dysynchronous luteinizing hormone (LH) secretion and elevated testosterone levels, occasionally only appreciated when the unbound serum testosterone is measured.

Drugs are sometimes responsible for hirsutism, particularly oral contraceptives containing androgenic progestins (see Chapter 115). Phenytoin is occasionally implicated, and androgenic steroids will result in excess hair growth. Manipulation of and trauma to the hair follicle, e.g., from tweezing hairs, may be responsible for local coarse growth.

WORKUP

The initial objective is to identify the hirsute patient who is likely to have an underlying endocrine disorder and to be in need of detailed investigation. The paramount concern in evaluating the hirsute woman is to exclude significant endocrine pathology. History-taking should include inquiry into symptoms of virilization (voice change, hair recession, acne, clitoral enlargement), changes in menstruation, progression of hirsutism, and development of obesity, hypertension, or infertility. A detailed drug history, covering use of oral contraceptives, androgens or phenytoin, should be obtained. A family history of hirsutism in mother, grandmother, aunts and sisters is reassuring.

Physical examination is studied for evidence of virilization, i.e., temporal hair recession, deep voice, acne, increase in muscle mass and clitoromegaly. In assessing the patient, Cushing's syndrome should be suspected when centripetal obesity, violaceous striae, and muscle wasting are encountered. Patients with oligomenorrhea or amenorrhea, obesity and hirsutism require careful pelvic examination for the presence of bilaterally enlarged nodular ovaries indicative of polycystic ovary disease. However, as many as 50 per cent of patients with polycystic ovaries will not have clinically palpable ovarian abnormalities.

A young woman of Mediterranean ancestry who complains of excess facial hair yet has regular menses and a strong family history of similar degrees of hirsutism need not undergo extensive endocrine studies. Patients with virilization, amenorrhea, cushingoid appearance, hypertension, or progressively worsening hirsutism deserve more extensive assessment.

When amenorrhea, obesity and hirsutism occur, especially in the context of infertility, one needs to rule out polycystic ovary disease. Since pelvic examination may not reveal palpably enlarged ovaries, laboratory testing is indicated to help select patients for diagnostic laparoscopy. Testosterone and LH secretions are typically increased. Because gonadotropin secretion may be episodic, three serum samples taken 15 to 20 minutes apart should be pooled for assay. Measurements of serum LH and FSH (follicle-stimulating hormone) usually show an increased LH:FSH ratio. Such patients are the best candidates for laparoscopy.

Patients having a cushingoid appearance should be screened for Cushing's syndrome by an overnight dexamethasone suppression test. The patient is given 1 mg of dexamethasone at midnight; a plasma cortisol level is obtained at 8:00 a.m. the following day; it should be suppressed to less than 5 micrograms per 100 ml. If the cortisol level is not suppressed to less than 5 micrograms per 100 ml., formal dexamethasone suppression testing should be carried out. The 24-hour urinary free cortisol, if available, is greater than 100 micrograms per 24 hours in Cushing's syndrome.

When virilization is suspected, serum testosterone and urinary 17-ketosteroids should be measured. Serum testosterone will often be in the male range (greater than 300 ng. per 100 ml.) in women with masculinizing ovarian or adrenal neoplasms. Measurement of 24-hour urinary 17-ketosteroids will detect elevated adrenal androgens such as androstenedione and dehydroepiandrosterone; 17-ketosteroids will be elevated in adrenal adenomas, adrenocortical carcinomas, and in inherited biochemical defects in cortisol biosynthesis. Testosterone is not measured as a 17-ketosteroid, so 17-ketosteroids will be normal in the majority of masculinized patients.

SYMPTOMATIC MANAGEMENT AND PATIENT EDUCATION

Alternative approaches to the symptomatic management of hirsutism include (1) supportive reassurance without specific therapy, (2) cosmetic manipulation such as bleaching, waxing, electrolysis and depilatories, (3) medical therapy directed at suppressing androgen production, and (4) definitive therapy of underlying diseases such as Cushing's syndrome or masculinizing ovarian neoplasms.

Many women can be effectively cared for by reassurance that their hirsutism has no serious underlying cause and will not impair fertility or sexuality. If a woman remains concerned about her appearance, cosmetic manipulation or medical suppressive therapy is appropriate. Hair may be bleached with 6 per cent hydrogen peroxide solution, alkalinizing the solution with 20 drops of ammonia for each ounce of peroxide.

Shaving removes unwanted hair, but because hair is clipped at the skin surface and grows at an average rate of 1 mm. a day, "stubble" appears within a day or two. Epilation with tweezers or hot wax may retard hair growth for several months; however, these methods are associated with a risk of low-grade folliculitis. Use of chemical depilatories also requires application of a nonfluorinated topical steroid to prevent irritation. Electrolysis, the only permanent method of hair removal, involves electrocoagulating and destroying the hair root; however, it is a costly and time-consuming process and should be performed by a licensed, trained electrologist.

Suppression of ovarian and adrenal androgen production may be achieved with oral contraceptives, such as progestogen-dominant combination pills containing 2 mg. norethindrone and 0.1 mg. mestranol (Norinyl 2 mg. or Ortho-Novum 2 mg.) or estrogenic-type contraceptives containing 2.5 mg. norethynodrel or 1 mg. ethynodiol diacetate and 0.1 mg. mestranol (Enovid or Ovulen). Side effects of these drugs, including increased risks of thromboembolism, stroke and myocardial infarction, must be reviewed with the patient (see Chapter 115). A decrease in hirsutism is usually not evident for at least 6 to 12 months; a decrease in the rate of hair growth is noted first, followed by transformation to lighter, fine, downy hair.

Adrenal suppression with supraphysiologic doses of glucocorticoids, such as dexamethasone given at bedtime, may cause a decrease in hirsutism, but iatrogenic hypothalamic-pituitary-adrenal suppression will result (see Chapter 101) and subject the patient to the risk of adrenal crisis. This therapy should be reserved solely for hirsute women with elevated ketosteroids and normal testosterone determinations, if it is used at all.

New approaches to the medical management of hirsutism utilizing cyproterone acetate (an androgen antagonist) and medroxyprogesterone and spironolactone have been reported. Because androstenedione is converted to testosterone in fatty tissue, weight reduction is an adjunct to all therapies for hirsutism.

INDICATIONS FOR REFERRAL

Patients with virilization and elevated testosterone or 17-ketosteroid levels require evaluation by the endocrinologist and gynecologist, since a virilizing tumor may be present. If polycystic ovaries are palpated or the LH:FSH ratio and testosterone are increased, referral for laparoscopy is appropriate. At times, after a thorough evaluation by the primary physician, a patient found to have hereditary hirsutism will want a second opinion regarding a possible underlying etiology; in such instances a referral to the endocrinologist may facilitate care.

ANNOTATED BIBLIOGRAPHY

Bardin, C.W., and Lipsett, M.B.: Testosterone and androstenedione blood production rates in normal women and women with idiopathic hirsutism or polycystic ovaries. J. Clin. Invest., 46:891, 1967. (A higher secretion of ovarian testosterone occurs in PCO and hirsute women when contrasted to nonhirsute women who have testosterone produced from conversion of androstenedione.)

Barnes, G.W., et al.: Cyproterone actetate: A study involving two volunteers with idiopathic hirsutism. Clin. Endocrinol., 4:65, 1975. (Antiandrogen therapy is demonstrated to be effective in combination with ethinyl estradiol in 2 women with severe hirsutism.)

Correa de Oliveira, R.F., Novaes, L.P., Lima, M.B., et al.: A new treatment for hirsutism. Ann. Intern. Med., 83:817, 1975. (Medroxyprogesterone is reported as an effective treatment for hirsutism.)

Ettinger, B., Goldfield, E.D., Burrill, K.C., et al.: Plasma testosterone stimulation-suppression dynamics in hirsute women; correlation with long-term therapy. Am. J. Med., 54:195, 1973. (An article showing the effectiveness of estrogen-progestagen combinations in the treatment of hirsutism.)

Forbes, A.P.: Endocrine function in hirsute women. N. Engl. J. Med., 294:665, 1976. (Editorial which accompanies the paper by Kirschner, Zuker, and Jespersen [see below].)

Givens, J.R.: Hirsutism and hyperandrogenism. Adv. Intern. Med., 21:221, 1976. (A comprehensive review of androgen excess in the production of hirsutism.)

Kirschner, M.A., and Bardin, C.W.: Androgen production and metabolism in normal and virilized women. Metabolism, 21: 667, 1972. (An excellent review of androgens, their metabolism and the differential diagnosis and evaluation of the virilized woman.)

Kirschner, M.A., Zuker, I.R., and Jespersen, D.: Idiopathic hirsutism—An ovarian abnormality. N. Engl. J. Med., 294:637, 1976. (Although 20 of 44 women had suppression of plasma testosterone and androstenedione with dexamethasone, the ovaries were the predominant source of androgen production.)

McKnight, E.: The prevalence of "hirsutism" in young women. Lancet, 1:410, 1964. (An epidemiologic study showing prevalence of hirsutism among college students.)

Ober, K.B., and Hennessy, J.F.: Spironolactone therapy for hirsutism in a hyperandrogenic woman. Ann. Intern. Med., 89:643, 1978. (A case report showing the antiandrogenic effect of sprionolactone benefiting hirsutism.)

97

Evaluation of Gynecomastia

Gynecomastia is defined as enlargement of the male breast due to increse in glandular tissue. It is unilateral in a third of cases and may cause pain. It must be distinguished from simple obesity. Some patients are concerned about loss of masculinity or the possibility of breast cancer. Others may not have recognized the change and come to the physician at the suggestion of friends or family. Gynecomastia is a transient physiological event in 70 per cent of pubertal boys; its prevalence in adults is less than 1 per cent. The physician must thoroughly investigate the cause, allay fears and help the patient decide about treatment.

PATHOPHYSIOLOGY AND CLINICAL PRESENTATION

Gynecomastia can result from increased testicular or adrenal secretion of estrogens, increased conversion of testosterone and androstenedione to estradiol and estrone, estrogen-producing tumors, gonadotropin-producing tumors, and estrogen ingestion. Klinefelter's syndrome is an example of increased estrogen secretion. In heart failure, there is increased shunting of testosterone and androstenedione to the periphery where they are converted to estrogens. In cirrhosis and hyperthyroidism, there is also increased peripheral conversion. Much of the conversion takes place in fatty tissue. HCG-producing tumors stimulate testicular production of estradiol. Teratomas of the testes and carcinomas of the lung, pancreas, and colon are known sources of ectopic HCG. Spironolactone is one of the more commonly used drugs with estrogenic effects. The gynecomastia of puberty is believed to be linked to a high estradiol:progesterone ratio, though this is controversial. Numerous other drugs are associated with gynecomastia, operating directly through hormonal stimulation or indirectly by inhibiting androgen production or effect.

The clinical presentation is usually a noticeable increase in breast tissue. Tenderness may be noted in a third of patients, but actual pain is less frequent. Enlargement is usually central and symmetrical, though it is occasionally eccentric. Idiopathic and drug-induced gynecomastias are usually unilateral, while pubertal and hormonal etiologies often cause bilaterial change. It may be that asymmetry is a more accurate description than unilateral enlargement, judging from the prevalence of bilaterally histologic but not clinically evident gynecomastia in autopsy series.

There are a few distinctive clinical presentations. In Klinefelter's syndrome, gynecomastia develops around puberty in a patient with long limbs, small, firm testes, infertility, and normal or deficient secondary sex features. In cirrhosis, patients present with loss of libido, loss of body hair and testicular atrophy (see Chapter 71). Carcinoma of the male breast is distinct from gynecomastia; it is characterized by a unilateral, eccentrically located firm mass which may be fixed. Male breast cancer is rare; it is

generally not more frequent in patients with gynecomastia, though there is a higher incidence in Klinefelter's syndrome.

DIFFERENTIAL DIAGNOSIS

Seventy per cent of healthy pubertal males have transient gynecomastia which regresses in 1 to 2 years. Testicular or adrenal tumors are rare in this age group. The gynecomastia of Klinefelter's syndrome also presents around puberty. In one series, 15 per cent of all young patients with gynecomastia had primary hypogonadism.

The two most common causes of gynecomastia in adults are drugs and alcohol-related liver disease. Estrogens, androgens, spironolactone, digoxin, phenothiazines, amphetamines, reserpine, methyldopa, isoniazid, imipramine, phenytoin, heroin, cimetidine, and marijuana have all been associated with gynecomastia, although the association is tenuous in some. In one series, 22 per cent of patients had a history of taking a drug associated with gynecomastia, and 26 per cent had alcoholic liver disease.

Recovery from malnutrition due to severe illness, as seen with hemodialysis or congestive heart failure, may be associated with breast changes. A number of hyperthyroid patients have gynecomastia. Tumor-related gynecomastia is feared, but rare; tumors capable of HCG production include those of lung, liver, pancreas, colon and stomach. Feminizing adrenal, testicular and pituitary tumors are very rare causes of gynecomastia. In just under 10 per cent of cases, a probable cause is not identified. Gynecomastia must be distinguished from carcinoma of the male breast.

WORKUP

History. Onset, location, duration and course deserve note. The most important aspect is a detailed inquiry into drug use, including alcohol consumption and marijuana use. Any symptoms of hyperthyroidism (see Chapter 99) or changes in libido, skin, voice, testicles or hair should be elicited. Weight loss, change in bowel habits, history of heart failure or dialysis, headaches and visual field disturbances should be ascertained.

Physical examination often provides helpful clues. Arm span greater than height suggests Klinefelter's syndrome. One needs to look at the skin for jaundice, spider angiomas, pallor, changes in texture, and decreases in pubic and axillary hair. The eyes are checked for exophthalmus, and the neck is palpated for goiter. The breast examination requires distinguishing the glandular texture of true gynecomastia from the fatty consistency of breast enlargement related to obesity; asymmetry or nodules deserve note. The question of malignancy in the breast tissue must always be considered in gynecomastia. If the enlargement is unilateral and eccentric, or if the breast feels particularly firm or nodular, biopsy should be performed. Any signs of heart failure (see Chapter 27) and hepatocellular disease (see Chapter 62) should be noted. The abdomen must be palpated for masses, and the stool tested for occult blood. The testicles are examined for atrophy and nodules.

Laboratory studies. Gynecomastia not due to puberty or drugs may require further testing. A free T_4 should be obtained in the patient with signs or symptoms suggestive or hyperthyroidism, and SGOT, albumin and prothrombin time are indicated in the patient with a history of alcohol consumption or physical findings suggestive of hepatocellular failure. When Klinefelter's syndrome is strongly suspected on the basis of clinical appearance, a buccal smear can help confirm the diagnosis by revealing Barr bodies. If there is no evident etiology, a serum human chorionic gonadotropin (HCG) determination should be obtained; it may indicate the possibility of an HCG-producing tumor. If the HCG level is elevated, a chest x-ray and stool test for occult blood are needed to search for a tumor. Again, biopsy is mandatory for a firm, nodular breast mass.

SYMPTOMATIC MANAGEMENT AND PATIENT EDUCATION

Removal of the offending drug usually produces regression of breast enlargement within a month or two. Gynecomastia that accompanies puberty or refeeding after starvation is a transient phenomenon which can be managed by providing reassurance. Treatment of hyperthyroidism will usually improve gynecomastia. Gynecomastia attributable to alcoholic liver diease or Klinefelter's syndrome is not likely to respond to any treatment. When HCG-secreting tumors are discovered, resection of the tumor is indicated if possible.

The persistence of gynecomastia may produce cosmetic problems. Patients who are considerably bothered by breast enlargement may elect to undergo mastectomy, but this should be accomplished only after the etiology has been elucidated. There is no evidence that antiestrogen drugs such as clomiphene are useful in adults, though they may have a role in puberty.

When a benign etiology such as drug-induced gynecomastia is discovered, it is comforting to reassure the patient that the condition is not a reflection of loss of maleness or a carcinomatous process. It must be remembered that some conditions that produce gynecomastia may reduce potency; this situation must be confronted and discussed with the patient. There is no evidence of carcinomatous degeneration in gynecomastia except in Klinefelter's syndrome. Pain, irritation or social problems that may arise should be dealt with symptomatically and sympathetically.

ANNOTATED BIBLIOGRAPHY

Bannagan, G.A. and Hajdu, S.I.: Gynecomastia: Clinicopathologic study of 351 cases. Am. J. Clin. Pathol., *57*:431, 1972. *(The histologic appearance of fibrous gynecomastia relates to duration, irrespective of etiology. Idiopathic and drug-induced gynecomastias are usually discrete and unilateral, while endocrine and pubertal gynecomastias are bilateral.)*

Braunstein, G.D., Vaitukaitis, J.L., Carbone, P.P. *et al.*: Ectopic production of human chorionic gonadotropin by neoplasms. Ann. Intern. Med., *78*:39, 1973. *(HCG was found in 60 of 828 patients with established neoplasms.)*

Gordon, G.G., *et al.*: Effect of alcohol (ethanol) administration on sex-hormone metabolism in normal men. A Engl. J. or ed., *295*:797, 1976. *(Alcohol caused a decrease in testosterone production as well as limiting the LH response.)*

Knott, D., and Bidlingmaier, R.: Gynecomastia in male adolescents. J. Clin. Endocrinol, Metab. *4*:187, 1975. *(Discussion of mechanisms.)*

Rose, L.I., Underwood, R.H., Newmark, S.R., *et al.*: Pathophysiology of spironolactone-induced gynecomastia. Ann. Intern. Med., *87*:398. 1977. *(A review of mechanisms of spironolactone-induced gynecomastia.)*

Williams, M.W: Gynecomastia, its incidence, recognition and host characterizations in 447 autopsy cases. Am. J. Med., *34*:103, 1963. *(An interesting pathologic study, revealing a 40 per cent incidence of histologic gynecomastia, though only four cases involved clinically obvious enlargement.)*

98
Approach to the Patient with Diabetes Mellitus

Diabetes mellitus is the most common endocrinologic problem encountered by primary care physicians. In one community study, the incidence was found to be 133 new cases per 100,000 population per year. Prevalence figures range from 12 to 18 cases per 1000, with slightly higher rates in women and the elderly. Tasks and decisions central to management include (1) designing a therapeutic program that is practical safe, and acceptable to the patient, (2) determining when drug therapy is needed to supplement weight reduction, (3) choosing between insulin and oral agents and (4) deciding how closely to control blood sugar.

PATHOPHYSIOLOGY, CLINICAL PRESENTATION, AND COURSE

Idiopathic diabetes mellitus is a heterogeneous condition. In the juvenile variety, there is often total loss of insulin-secreting ability and possibility of ketoacidosis. Adult-onset diabetes is characterized by preservation of some insulin production (albeit abnormal in amount and timing of release) and consequently little risk of ketone body formation.

The pathogenesis of diabetes is incompletely understood. Although there is a genetic determinant in both juvenile diabetes and adult-onset disease, studies of monozygotic twins suggest that exogenous factors may play a more important role in juvenile-onset diabetes than in maturity-onset disease. In those predisposed to glucose intolerance, clinical diabetes may be precipitated or worsened by obesity, infection, stress, thiazides, glucocorticosteroids or pregnancy. Conditions associated with excess secretion of growth hormone, cortisol, epinephrine or glucagon may also result in glucose intolerance. Hemochromatosis, chronic pancreatitis, and cystic fibrosis are capable of destroying a substantial part of the pancreas and leading to absolute deficiency of insulin.

Most adult-onset diabetics present without symptoms of hyperglycemia; often their diabetes is discovered on routine screening or during evaluation for an unrelated problem. The textbook description of polyuria, polydipsia, and polyphagia occurs in only a minority of adult patients. At times, the initial manifestation of diabetes is one of its complications, such as neuropathy, retinopathy, or nephropathy.

The pathophysiology of diabetic *neuropathy* is incompletely understood, but appears related to insulin deficiency. Myoinositol, a phospholipid component of the nerve cell membrane, becomes depleted, resulting in prolonged conduction times. In addition, hyperglycemia leads to accumulation of sorbitol in tissues with a polyol pathway for metabolism of glucose. Schwann cells have such a pathway; the excess sorbitol may induce swelling by its osmotic effect and compromise nerve function. Microangiopathic changes may contribute to the neuropathy by decreasing blood supply to the nerve and causing Wallerian degeneration of myelin sheaths. Peripheral neuropathy commonly reduces sensation in the lower extremities and may produce pain. Autonomic neuropathy may present as impotence, gastrointestinal motility disturbances, orthostatic hypotension, or urinary retention; it is usually permanent.

Diabetic *nephropathy* is primarily due to microvascular disease, which is thought to be related to abnormal platelet function and induction of increased basement membrane formation. The thickened basement membrane seen with diabetes is believed related to the degree and duration of hyperglycemia. Proteinuria is the first clinical manifestation. Mean duration of disease at the onset of proteinuria has been found to be about 17 years; progressive deterioration of renal function usually follows over the next 2 to 4 years. Interestingly, a recent study found that very tight control of blood glucose could reduce the spilling of protein in patients with long-standing, insulin-dependent diabetes who did not have renal failure or significant proteinuria; this suggests that improved control may reduce the chances of nephropathy. However, the precise relationships between microangiopathy, renal disease, and severity and duration of diabetes remain controversial.

Increased *susceptibility to infection* results from impaired polymorphonuclear leukocyte function. Cellulitis and candidiasis occur with increased frequency. Urinary tract infections are common in patients with urinary retention. *Eye complications* include reversible changes in lens configuration associated with rapid fluctuations in glucose concentrations, cataracts, and retinopathy (see Chapter 200).

PRINCIPLES OF MANAGEMENT

The goals of therapy in diabetes are normalization of carbohydrate metabolism and prevention of multisystem complications. The optimal degree of *control of blood sugar* remains a subject of heated debate among diabetologists. The controversy centers on whether attempts to restore glucose to near normal will reduce the serious consequences of diabetes. The proponents of loose control support their positions by citing results of the University Group Diabetes Project (UGDP) study; insulin treatment was found to be no better than diet in preventing death from cardiovascular complications. The studies that show a relationship between microangiopathic complications and degree of control are discounted by those favoring loose control; their criticism is that these studies reflect different degrees of disease rather than treatment.

There are no unbiased, randomized, prospective studies demonstrating that the rate of complications is decreased in "tightly" controlled diabetics, but carefully performed laboratory studies have shown reversal of renal lesions following pancreatic transplantation in diabetic rats. Moreover, there are preliminary reports of diminished proteinuria and decreased retinopathy in diabetics whose blood sugars are closely controlled. Although normalization of blood sugars to nondiabetic fasting and postprandial levels is the ideal objective, it is difficult to achieve with available means. Most agree that some degree of control is necessary, but the cost of tight control is an increase in the risk of hypoglycemic reactions. Whether the risk is outweighed by the benefits of stringent control remains unresolved at the present time. The literature should be followed for new data on this important issue.

Diet. The cornerstone of therapy for all diabetics is reduction of excess weight through dietary restriction of caloric intake. Weight loss has been shown to enhance the sensitivity of peripheral insulin receptors to endogenous insulin and to reduce requirements for exogenous insulin. It is impossible to predict the exact effect that will result from each pound lost, but a reduction of even 7 to 10 pounds often provides measureable improvement in glucose tolerance.

Most stable *adult-onset diabetics* can be adequately controlled by diet alone. The main goal of dietary therapy in diabetics who do not require insulin is achievement of ideal body weight. Ideal body weight can be estimated for women by figuring 100 pounds for the first 5 feet of height and adding 5 pounds for each additional inch. For men the calculation, is 106 pounds for the first 5 feet and 6 pounds for each addtional inch. Patients with small frames require a 10 per cent subtraction; those with large frames, a 10 per cent addition.

To achieve ideal weight, one must restrict caloric intake. The amount of reduction necessary can be determined by estimating the patient's daily caloric needs. Basal caloric needs equal the ideal weight times 10. If the patient is sedentary, one adds 3 times the desired body weight to the basal caloric need to obtain the total number of calories consumed each day. If the patient is moderately active, one adds 5 times the ideal body weight; if engaged in strenuous activity, one adds 10 times the ideal weight to the basal requirement. A reasonable goal is the loss of 1 or 2 pounds per week. This necessitates a deficit of 3,500 to 7,500 calories per week or 500 to 1,000 calories daily.

For the diabetic who does not require insulin, the goal is reduction in calories. The diet ought to be well adapted to the patient's life-style (see Chapters 221, 222). Of lesser importance is ingestion of particular percentages of carbohydrate, fat, and protein. The view that restriction of carbohydrate is essential has been challenged by recent evidence showing that a diet high in carbohydrate and fiber actually improved glucose tolerance. There is no need to severely limit the intake of simple or refined sugars, because there is no evidence that such forms of carbohydrate are in themselves diabetogenic. Data purporting to show such a relation often demonstrate little more than a link with obesity. High-fiber diets may reduce postprandial hyperglycemia and avoid wide fluctuations in serum glucose.

Patients who are not taking insulin do not require elaborate exchange systems, careful timing of meals, or other special dietary accomodations. However, such measures are appropriate for patients who require insulin. Exercise may help lessen glucose intolerance by increasing cellular uptake of glucose and improving tissue response to insulin by contributing to weight loss.

For *insulin-dependent diabetics,* the essential aspect of dietary therapy is the timing of meals. Three meals, supplemented by snacks before bed and some-times in midmorning and midafternoon, are often needed. The timing of meals must be designed to match the periods of peak insulin effect and the pa-tient's activity schedule; increased exercise requires a snack to prevent hypoglycemia. Simple sugars are re-stricted because they may worsen postprandial hy-perglycemia but the patient should carry a source of simple sugar for use in case of an insulin reaction.

Drug Therapy. When reduction to ideal weight fails to achieve reasonable control or when the pa-tient is unable to lose weight, drug therapy is indicat-ed. Many adult-onset diabetics used to be given *oral hypoglycemia agents,* often before much effort was made to lose weight. The safety of the sulfonylurea oral agents has been called into question by the find-ings of the University Group Diabetes Program (UGDP) study, which revealed an increased rate of cardiovascular sudden death in patients on long-term tolbutamide therapy. This unexpected result gave rise to considerable controversy and a series of refu-tations which attacked the design of the UGDP study. Independent biometric review of the study's design and data analysis concluded that the burden of proof is on the critics of the UGDP study to show that sulfonylureas are safe. The biguanide class of oral hypoglycemics also have been found to cause se-rious side effects; phenformin has been linked to the production of fatal lactic acidosis. Another important drawback of oral agents is their frequent lack of long-term efficacy.

At the present time, the available oral hypoglyce-mic agents have only a limited role in the treatment of diabetes. Sulfonylureas can be of some help in pa-tients with symptomatic hyperglycemia who cannot take insulin because of infirmity, blindness, or abso-lute unwillingness. These agents can provide short-term control of symptoms in obese patients who are entering a weight reduction program; their use should be regarded as a temporizing measure only, which will have to be abandoned in favor of insulin, if weight loss fails.

Insulin is the drug of choice for diabetics who are prone to ketosis and for those symptomatic adult-on-set patients who cannot be adequately controlled by diet alone. Since 1971, "single peak" insulin, a purer preparation of insulin than had been used previously, became widely available; it is termed "single peak" because of the pattern it creates on chromatography. It contains 99 per cent insulin or insulinlike materi-als. Most commercial insulin that is routinely used

today is of this type, and is a mixture of beef and pork insulins purified by passage through a molecu-lar sieve. A more highly purified insulin preparation is termed "single component;" it contains 99 per cent pure insulin. This latter form has few advantages over single peak insulin, unless the patient has insulin allergy or lipoatrophy. To facilitate insulin adminis-tration, insulin preparations are now standardized to the U100 concentration.

Insulin preparations are available in short-, inter-mediate-, and long-acting forms. The intermediate forms (NPH and lente) are the preparations most commonly used. Peak activity is 6 to 12 hours. The short-acting forms (CZI and semilente) peek at 2 to 4 hours. The majority of diabetics can be controlled with a single dose of intermediate-acting insulin in the morning before breakfast.

About 10 per cent of insulin-dependent diabetics are early or type "A" responders; they become hy-poglycemic in the early afternoon, because they ex-perience their peak insulin effect after 5 or 6 hours; they often become hyperglycemic later in the day. Their insulin treatment needs to be adjusted, with the intermediate insulin dose split into two-thirds given in the morning and one-third before supper. Occasionally, supplementation with a small dose of short-acting insulin is necessary in the morning and evening.

Another 10 per cent of diabetics on insulin are late or type "C" responders. They experience the peak effect of insulin in the late evening or early morning. Such patients require a reduction in in-termediate-acting insulin and the addition of a short-acting preparation to the morning dose. An ad-ditional small evening dose of short-acting insulin be-fore the evening meal may be necessary if postpran-dial hyperglycemia is a major problem in the early evening.

It has been suggested that patients who respond adequately to intermediate-acting insulin, so-called type "B" reactors, may also achieve greater control by dividing their total daily dose into injections be-fore breakfast and before supper. This schedule is sometimes supplemented by small amounts of short-acting insulin, to further improve control and mini-mize wide swings in serum glucose. An important disadvantage of multiple doses is the inconvenience to the patient (although one can mix short- and in-termediate-acting preparations in the same syringe). The risk of hypoglycemia may actually be lessened by minimizing wide swings in the blood sugar through use of a divided daily dose of intermediate insulin, but attempts to tighten control still further may increase the possibility of an insulin reaction from severe hypoglycemia.

Initiation of insulin therapy can be carried out on an ambulatory basis as long as the patient is reliable, nonketotic, and not severly hyperglycemic. Treatment can be initiated with 10 to 15 units of an intermediate-acting insulin and increased by 3 to 5 units per day, based on urine and blood sugar determinations. Prior to initiation of insulin therapy, simultaneous serum and double-voided urine glucose determinations should be obtained to facilitate interpretation of urine tests. The concentration of insulin preparations has been standardized; U-100 is now used exclusively to simplify administration of proper dose. Injection sites are rotated to minimize the small risk of sterile abscesses, and the dose is injected subcutaneously. The abdomen is the preferred site of insulin administration, because insulin injected into the arm or leg is utilized more rapidly than normal when the limb is exercised. Insulin is best stored in the refrigerator, but can be left at room temperature for 12 hours without any loss of potency.

Although most diabetologists agree that one should attempt to achieve as much control as is possible, the question remains whether close control can be accomplished safely with the means of insulin administration currently available and the limitations to patient compliance inherent in a program which requires constant vigilance and repeated injections. Intelligent, well-motivated, reliable individuals can be taught to regulate their daily insulin doses within predetermined limits according to the results of urine testing, level of activity, caloric intake, and timing of meals. Less adept patients risk insulin reactions when tight control is attempted, and one must settle for less stringent regulation in the interest of avoiding serious hypoglycemic episodes. Reasonable control might be considered attainment of a fasting serum glucose of less than 150 mg. per 100 ml., a 2 hour postprandial level of less than 200 mg. per 100 ml. and avoidance of hypoglycemia at 4 p.m.

Worsening hyperglycemia in a patient taking a previously adequate insulin dose deserves prompt attention. Dietary indiscretion and failure to take insulin or use it properly are common etiologies, but occult infection, especially of the urinary tract or skin, may be responsible and must be ruled out. Emotional stress, pregnancy, and corticosteroid use are other precipitants of worsening hyperglycemia.

In rare instances, *insulin resistance* is encountered. Insulin resistance is arbitrarily defined as an insulin requirement of greater than 200 units per day for a period of more than 2 days. The mechanism involves antibody formation to insulin or, in rare instances, to peripheral insulin receptors. Prevalence is about 0.1 per cent of patients on insulin, and about two-thirds of cases occur within a year of initiating therapy. Most patients are over age 40, and there is no sex predilection. Onset is over several weeks, and the course is self-limited, ending by 6 to 12 months in over 75 per cent of cases. The severity of the problem does not correlate with prior dose. Therapy involves escalating dose as needed, switching to pure pork insulin, and, in refractory cases, employing prednisone on an every-other-day basis.

Rebound hyperglycemia (the *Somogyi effect*) may be mistaken for inadequate control. The problem is due to administration of excess insulin, precipitating very low serum sugars during sleep. Compensatory mechanisms result in rebound hyperglycemia, so in the morning, the patient finds increasing glycosuria. The condition is most prevalent in patients who take an excess of 40 units of insulin per day. Diagnosis of the condition is often difficult because the hypoglycemia usually occurs in the early morning and is hard to document. Reports of nightmares and finding trace to 1+ amounts of glucose and large ketones in the first morning voided urine are suggestive. The best means of identifying the problem is to be aware of the potential for it; one reduces dose by a few units each day rather than increasing the dose, if large doses are already being utilized and yet control seems to be deteriorating.

Insulin reactions occur when food intake is delayed, unusual physical activity is undertaken, or insulin dose is excessive. Symptoms vary with the type of insulin used. With short-acting preparations, onset is rapid, with hunger, sweating, abdominal discomfort, palpitations, tremor, weakness, and restlessness. Symptoms resolve within 10 to 20 minutes of taking carbohydrate. If autonomic neuropathy is present or the patient is taking propranolol (a beta-adrenegic blocking agent), mental confusion may be the only symptom. Intermediate- and long-acting insulin preparations cause a less precipitous decline in glucose and a less pronounced catecholamine response to hypoglycemia. Headache, blurred vision, tremor, yawning, and confusion are the predominant early neuroglycopenic symptoms. Severe reactions may lead to loss of consciousness.

The use of insulin requires attention to diet and the timing of caloric intake. The presence throughout the day of circulating exogenous insulin necessitates regular provision of glucose substrate. The most commonly utilized ADA diets recommend eating two ninths of the total calories at breakfast and lunch, four-ninths at dinner, and one-ninth as an evening snack. The total number of calories is not nearly as essential to the insulin-dependent diabetic as is consistency in the timing of meals and their individual caloric content. During exercise, more glucose is utilized; an increase in caloric intake is preferable to a reduction in insulin dose.

Management of Complications. Since it is uncertain whether controlling hyperglycemia will halt the progression of all complications, it is important that associated risk factors be attended to. For example, cigarette smoking should be stopped (see Chapter 49); hypertension (see Chapter 21) and hypercholesterolemia (see Chapter 22) need to be brought under control in attempts to lessen the chances of atherosclerotic disease.

Although the progression to *renal failure* may be inexorable once heavy proteinuria (greater than 3 gm. per day of albumin) occurs, the risk of preventable kidney impairment due to pyelonephritis and papillary necrosis can be minimized by prompt identification and aggressive treatment of urinary tract infections (see Chapter 129). Patients with urinary retention due to autonomic insufficiency are at increased risk of infection and in need of therapy to improve elimination of urine (see Chapter 126). Treating hypertension should also help preserve renal function. Intravenous pyelography (IVP) may precipitate acute renal failure in diabetics; dehydration, preexisting renal impairment, and old age increase the likelihood of this complication. Any diabetic being considered for IVP needs to be well hydrated prior to and following the procedure.

Foot care is essential to prevention of *cellulitis, osteomyelitis* and *amputation.* Feet must be kept clean, interdigital spaces dry, callus pared down, and toenails carefully trimmed. Frequent inspection for skin breakdown and signs of cellulitis need to be stressed, as does the importance of wearing properly fitting shoes and not walking barefooted. The older patient who is incapable of self foot care should be scheduled to see the podiatrist regularly.

Optimizing glucose regulation is the principal means of limiting *neuropathy.* Neuropathic pain has been treated with phenytoin, carbamazepine, and combinations of tricyclic antidepressants and phenothiazines, but no singularly effective program has emerged in controlled trials. The postural hypotension, impotence, and urinary retention associated with autonomic neuropathy are usually permanent. If sexual performance is limited by impotence, careful evaluations should be carried out to assess neuropathic and psychogenic contributions (see Chapters 126, 217). Often anxiety and depression are superimposed on neurologic dysfunction. Patients who are severely incapacitated sexually can be considered for implantation of a prosthetic device.

Gastrointestinal motility problems can be difficult to treat. There is no curative therapy. Small frequent feedings and cholinergic agents such as metoclopramide or bethanechol may help lessen symptoms due to gastroparesis. Patients with diarrhea due to bacterial overgrowth in the bowel can be treated with a trial of a broad-spectrum antibiotic. Nocturnal diarrhea is not related to bacterial overgrowth and is refractory to most forms of therapy. Fortunately, it often resolves spontaneously.

Diabetics should be encouraged to have regular dental examinations, because they have a higher incidence of *pyorrhea* and *abscesses;* also, minor dental infections may be responsible for worsening hyperglycemia.

Retinopathy and other eye problems require ophthalmologic assessment (see Chapter 200).

MONITORING THERAPY

On office visits, one should concentrate on treatable aspects of diabetes and prevention of complications. One ought to measure the blood pressure and weight, examine the eyes for retinopathic changes, inspect the feet for any signs of pressure damage or infection, and reemphasize the need to control coexisting risk factors for vascular disease (hypertension, smoking). Laboratory monitoring should include a blood sugar, urinalysis, BUN, and creatinine. The role of the hemoglobin A_1C determination in monitoring is not yet fully established, but it may have the advantage of giving an indication of integrated glucose control over the previous 3 to 4 weeks. Hemoglobin becomes glycosylated when synthesized in the context of hyperglycemia. At present, a review of the reliable patient's urine testing reports probably suffices for estimating control between examinations.

Patients on intermediate-acting insulin should be advised to test their urine before breakfast and before supper; those on short-acting preparations need to check urine before lunch or at bedtime, depending when they take their dose. All patients require instruction in how to test their urine; the double-voiding technique for collection of the sample ought to be reviewed to maximize the accuracy of urine testing. Tape or tablets can be used; the choice is an individual one for the patient, though some feel that tablets are more accurate. Instruction in proper performance of the urine testing method chosen is probably more important than which particular method is used.

PATIENT EDUCATION

The success of any program for metabolic control depends on patient compliance. Because diet is the cornerstone of therapy in diabetes, thorough instruction on the rationale and workings of the dietary program must be provided to patient and family. Sample diets or charts can often be obtained from local nutritionists or the American Diabetes Association. Fad diets or self-imposed restrictions should be discouraged. For the adult-onset diabetic who is obese and does not require insulin, emphasis ought to be placed on reduction of total calories and not on the amount of carbohydrate that is consumed. Obsessive concern over the use of sugar is unwarranted. Inclusion of the family in all dietary instruction will make the patient's adaptation easier.

The patient receiving insulin requires intensive and continuous education. Careful instruction is needed in injection technique. The physician or nurse must be sure the patient can see well enough to fill the syringe properly. Prefilled syringes should be supplied or someone else made responsible for preparing the insulin if there is any question of the patient's ability. The patient and family must be cognizant of hypoglycemic reactions, including symptoms and appropriate therapy. A syringe with glucagon is given by some physicians to the patient's family for intramuscular injection in the event the patient becomes unconscious. Often a hypoglycemic patient is unable to take oral sugar, and forcing liquid orally may result in aspiration.

Intelligent, reliable patients who are motivated to attain the tightest glucose control possible can be provided with guidelines for adjusting their own insulin doses based upon urine testing. Such patients can use a combination of short- and intermediate-acting insulins to advantage.

The importance of skin and foot care must be emphasized. Regular appointments with a podiatrist are indicated for the elderly diabetic who cannot see

well; others should be taught to pare down callus and keep feet dry and free of trauma.

INDICATIONS FOR ADMISSION AND REFERRAL

Any insulin-dependent diabetic who cannot take in food or fluids because of protracted vomiting requires admission. If cellulitis develops in the foot, admission for intravenous antibiotic therapy is needed. Referral to an endocrinologist is suggested for insulin resistance and other difficulties in attaining safe control. The guidelines for ophthalmologic referral are presented in Chapter 200. Recurring urinary tract infections or incomplete bladder emptying are indications for urologic evaluation; proteinuria greater than 3 gm. per day and worsening renal insufficiency should be evaluated in conjunction with the nephrologist.

ANNOTATED BIBLIOGRAPHY

Arky, R.: Current principles of dietary therapy of diabetes mellitus. Med. Clin. North Am., *62*:655, 1978. *(Excellent summary of dietary methods for control of diabetes.)*

Boden, G., et al.: Monitoring metabolic control in diabetic outpatients with glycosylated hemoglobin. Ann. Intern. Med. *92*:357, 1980. *(This study found that H6A$_1$ was useful during periods of stability or rapid deterioration.)*

Colwell, J.A., Halushka, P.V., Sarji, K.E., et al.: Vascular disease in diabetes: Pathophysiological mechanisms and therapy. Arch. Intern. Med., *139*:225, 1979. *(A good, succinct review; 66 refs.)*

Committee for the Assessment of Biometric Aspects of Controlled Trials of Hypoglycemica Agents: Report. JAMA, *231*:584, 1975. *(A review of the UGDP study; supports UGDP findings.)*

Davidson, J.K.: Plasma glucose lowering effect of caloric restriction in obesity-induced insulin treated diabetes mellitus. Diabetes, *26* (Suppl.): 355, 1977. *(Caloric restriction can reduce insulin requirements.)*

Davidson, M.B.: The case for control in diabetes mellitus. West. J. Med., *129*:193, 1978. *(A well-reasoned argument advocating 2 daily doses of intermediate-acting insulin and small supple-*

ments of short-acting insulin to achieve tight control.)

Ellenberg, M.: Sexual function in diabetic patients. Ann. Intern. Med., 92:331, 1980. (A brief review of the problem. Points out there is no evidence of sexual dysfunction in diabetic women.)

Fraser, D.M., and Campbell, I.W.: Peripheral and autonomic nonfunction in newly diagnosed diabetes mellitus. Diabetes, 26:546, 1977. (Significant impairment of conduction velocity was found in newly diagnosed diabetics; it improved with treatment.)

Gabbay, K.H.: Hyperglycemia, metabolism and complications of diabetes mellitus. Adv. Intern. Med., 20:521, 1975. (The sorbitol pathway's role in mediating diabetic complications is described.)

Ganda, O.P., and Soeldner, J.S.: Genetic, acquired and related factors in the etiology of diabetes mellitus. Arch. Intern. Med., 137:461, 1977. (Review of pathogenic mechanisms.)

Jenkins, D.J.A., and Leeds, A.R.: Decrease in postprandial insulin and glucose concentrations by guar and pectin. Ann. Intern. Med., 86:20, 1977. (An interesting approach undergoing study.)

Kamdar, A., Weidmann, P., Makoff, D.L., et al.: Acute renal failure following intravenous use of radiographic contrast dyes in patients with diabetes mellitus. Diabetes, 26:643, 1977. (Seven diabetic patients with IVP-dye-induced renal failure; all recovered within 4 weeks. An analysis of these patients and those in the interim identified old age, existing renal impairment, vascular complications and dehydration as predisposing factors in acute renal failure.)

Katz, L.A., and Spiro, H.M.: Gastrointestinal manifestations of diabetes. N. Engl. J. Med., 275:1350, 1966. (Classic review, detailing diarrheal disorders due to diabetes as well as other gastrointestinal difficulties; 88 refs.)

Koivoske, V.A., Felig, P.: Effects of leg exercise on insulin absorption in diabetic patients. N. Engl. N. Med., 298:79, 1978. (Injections in the abdomen avoid accelerated absorption of insulin with leg exercise and prevent exercise-induced hypoglycemia.)

Kussman, M.J., Goldstein, H.H., and Gleason, R.E.: The clinical course of diabetic nephropathy.

JAMA, 236:1861, 1976. (Mean duration of disease at onset of proteinuria was 17 years; all had progressive deterioration thereafter.)

Lebovitz, H.E., and Feinglos, M.N.: Sulfonylurea drugs: Mechanism of antidiabetic action and therapeutic usefulness. Diabetes Care, 1:189, 1978. (Extensive review of sulfonylureas.)

Mirande, P.M., and Horwitz, D.L.: High fiber diets in treatment of diabetes mellitus. Ann. Intern. Med., 88:482, 1978. (Diabetics on constant calorie regimen were treated with high and low fiber diets. Lower glucoses were achieved with 20-gm. fiber diet; the approach may have some promise.)

Molnar, G.D.: Clinical evaluation of metabolic control in diabetes. Diabetes, 27 (Suppl.); 216, 1978. (A critical review of methods for assessing control, including urine and serum glucose levels, hemoglobin A_1C and other techniques.)

Schiavi, R.C.: Psychological treatment of erectile disorders in diabetic patients. Ann. Intern. Med., 92:337, 1980. (Points out that impotence in diabetics is often a combination of psychological and physiological difficulties, rather than an either/or situation. Treatment must attend to both components.)

The University Group Diabetes Program: A study of the effects of hypoglycemic agents on vascular complications in patients with adult-onset diabetes. Diabetes, 19 (Suppl. 2); 747, 1970. (The famous UGDP study which found an increased mortality in patients using tolbutamide.)

Viberti, G.C., Pickup, J.C., Jarrett, R.J., et al.: Diabetic control and renal function. N. Engl. J. Med., 300:638, 1979. (Continuous subcutaneous insulin infusion significantly reduced urinary albumin excretion in 7 patients with long-term insulin-dependent diabetes.)

Winegrad, A.I., and Greene, D.A.: Diabetic polyneuropathy: The importance of insulin deficiency, hyperglycemia, and alteration in myoinositol metabolism in its pathogenesis. N. Engl. J. Med., 195:1416, 1976. (Decreased intracellular myoinositol may mediate neuropathy.)

Zonana, J., and Remoin, D.L.: Inheritance of diabetes. N. Engl. J. Med., 293:603, 1976. (Genetic reviews conclude heredity is a factor, but precise transmission unknown.)

99
Management of Hyperthyroidism

Hyperthyroidism is the clinical expression of a heterogeneous group of disorders that produce elevations of free thyroxine (FT_4) and/or triiodothyronine (T_3). Well-recognized forms of hyperthyroidism are diffuse toxic goiter (Graves' disease), toxic multinodular goiter, and toxic uninodular goiter. The prevalence of hyperthyroidism is not precisely known, but the condition occurs in women 8 times more often than in men. Approximately 15 per cent of recognized cases occur in persons over the age of 60; the clinical presentation of hyperthroidism in the elderly is often atypical. The primary physician should be able to recognize hyperthyroidism and design a therapeutic program appropriate to the patient's age, clinical condition, and personal preferences. The indications and limitations of surgery, radioiodine therapy and antithyroid agents must be understood.

PATHOPHYSIOLOGY, CLINICAL PRESENTATION, AND COURSE

The primary physiological alteration in hyperthyroidism is excess secretion of thyroid hormone, which stimulates calorigenesis, catabolism, and enhanced sensitivity to catecholamines. This produces the classic picture of heat intolerance, nervousness, tremor, increased appetite, weight loss, excessive sweating, lid lag, stare and muscle weakness.

In *Graves' disease*, an autoimmune mechanism is postulated, involving chronic stimulation of the gland's TSH receptors by a thyroid-stimulating immunoglobulin (TSI). The disease accounts for close to 90 per cent of hyperthyroidism in those under the age of 40. Infiltrative exophthalmos and pretibial myxedema are among the most specific physical manifestations; interestingly, the eye findings may predate other evidence of hyperthyroidism and sometimes worsen after treatment. The gland is diffusely enlarged and a bruit can be heard in severe cases. Tachycardia, nervousness, tremor and brisk reflexes are common; the skin is velvety and hair silky. Onycholysis, vitiligo, and gynecomastia sometimes accompany Graves' disease and are suggestive of the diagnosis. Cardiac complications are uncommon because of the relative youth of the patient population. The clinical course is a wax-ing and waning one, with exacerbations and remissions of unpredictable duration. After many years, mild hypothyroidism may ensue.

Toxic multinodular goiter (Plummer's disease) accounts for most cases of hyperthyroidism in middle-aged and elderly persons. The condition is often associated with a long-standing simple goiter. The gland is clinically and pathologically indistinguishable from that of nontoxic multinodular goiters. Cardiovascular symptoms may dominate the clinical presentation; new onset of heart failure, atrial fibrillation or angina is not uncommon and reflects the high prevalence of coexisting organic heart disease in this older population. In a series of 85 hyperthyroid patients between ages 60 and 82, two-thirds experienced heart failure and 20 per cent reported angina. Only a minority evidenced the more typical symptoms of hyperthyroidism; for example, less than 11 percent had polyphagia. On the other hand, 33 per cent suffered from anorexia, and constipation was as prevalent as diarrhea. Lid lag may be noted on occasion, but exophthalmos does not occur. Sometimes apathy and weight loss are the most prominent clinical features and can be so profound as to suggest occult malignancy or severe depression.

The autonomously funtioning *single toxic nodule* presents clinically much like the toxic multinodular goiter. The major differentiating factor is the finding of a "hot" nodule surrounded by suppressed gland on radioiodine thyroid scan.

T_3 *thyrotoxicosis* is an important entity to consider when patients with clinically apparent hyperthyroidism have normal T_4 levels. The condition has been reported in association with both diffuse and nodular goiters. Its clinical presentation is no different from hyperthyroidism due to elevations in T_4.

Transient hyperthyroidism may occur in association with subacute or chronic thyroiditis, due to uncontrolled release of hormone. The clinical manifestions of hyperthyroidism are usually mild. The course is self-limited, and hypothyroidism often ensues. *Subacute thyroiditis* typically follows a viral illness, producing a tender multinodular gland. The occasional case associated with hyperthyroidism is abrupt in onset in conjunction with thyrotoxic symptoms. The erythrocyte sedimentation rate is high and thyroid scan characteristically shows little or no uptake of radioiodine. *Chronic thyroiditis (Hashimoto's)* is a common cause of goiter, but hyperthyroidism is neither frequent nor permanent. Etiology is thought to involve an immunologic mechanism; there are high titers of antibodies to microsomes and thyroglobulin. Prevalence is highest in middle-aged women. The gland feels rubbery and is enlarged, sometimes asymmetrically. Hypothyroidism eventually develops in a substantial number of cases.

The occurrence of clinical hyperthyroidism in the context of a small gland raises the possibility of certain unusual causes of hyperthyroidism, such as pituitary neoplasms, HCG-producing trophoblastic tumors, struma ovarii and excess intake of exogenous thyroxine or iodide.

PRINCIPLES OF THERAPY

The goal of therapy is to correct the hypermetabolic state with a minimum of side effects and with the smallest incidence of hypothyroidism. For definitive therapy, one must choose among antithyroid drugs, radioiodine and thyroidectomy.

Recognition of hyperthyroidism has been facilitated by reliable assays for free T_4 and total T_3. The ability to measure T_3 has made detection of T_3 toxicosis possible, whereas in the past there may have been only a borderline or even normal T_4 level in the context of clinical hyperthyroidism. TRH stimulation testing has also aided the interpretation of equivocal thyroxine levels. In patients with genuine hyperthyroidism, the TSH response to TRH stimulation is minimal or absent. This reflects suppression of the pituitary by elevated levels of thyroid hormone. The TRH stimulation test is unnecessary in most instances, but has a diagnostic role in difficult cases, e.g., apathetic hyperthyroidism.

Hyperthyroidism should not go untreated, particularly in the elderly who are at risk for cardiovascular complications. Moreover, not only are symptoms uncomfortable, but thyrotoxic crisis may occur if the untreated patient is unexpectedly exposed to a severe acute stress, such as emergency surgery or sepsis.

Acute, symptomatic relief from hyperthyroidism can be achieved by use of *propranolol*, taking advantage of its beta-blocking action in order to minimize catechol-mediated manifestations. The drug is also believed to exert its effect by preventing peripheral conversion of T_4 to T_3. It is also given for atrial fibrillation (see Chapter 23) or angina (see Chapter 25)

due to hyperthyroidism. In the presence of concurrent congestive heart failure, it should be used with extreme caution, if at all, due to its negative inotropic effect (see Chapter 27). Propranolol needs to be prescribed in conjunction with other treatment modalities for more definitive therapy of hyperthyroidism, because it does not interfere with thyroid hormone secretion. Propranolol is used in doses that range from 40 to 320 mg. per day.

The *antithyroid drugs* methimazole and propylthiouracil (PTU) can be used in most patients, with the exception of pregnant or lactating women (these agents cross the placenta and also appear in the milk). PTU acts by interfering with synthesis of thyroxine and blocking peripheral conversion of thyroxine to T_3, though at conventional doses this latter effect is probably not clinically important. Methimazole does not have an effect on peripheral monoiodination, but is more potent; the doses used are one-tenth those of PTU. Biochemical response to the antithyroid drugs is generally apparent within 1 to 2 weeks, although a clinical response takes longer. Initial PTU therapy averages 300 mg. per day, given in divided doses every 8 hours. When clinical and biochemical control are attained, the dose is tapered to the lowest amount needed to maintain a euthyroid state. The thyroid-blocking agents are associated with a low risk of inducing hypothyroidism, but a high rate of recurrence once therapy is stopped. Usually, treatment is continued for 12 to 24 months, then halted to see if relapse occurs. PTU induces remission in approximately 50 per cent of patients with Graves' disease treated for 1 to 2 years, but a third to a half of those who respond will relapse. A recent study found that the remission rate after only 3 to 5 months of therapy was 40 per cent, suggesting that tapering could begin as soon as control is well established.

Side effects of the antithyroid agents include dermatitis, arthralgias, elevated transaminases, fever, and lymphadenopathy. Leukopenia occurs in up to 10 per cent of patients. If polymorphonuclear leukocyte count falls to 1500 per mm³, the drug should be withheld. Agranulocytosis is rare, affecting fewer than 2 per 1000.

These antithyroid agents are useful for treatment of Graves' disease, preoperative control of thyrotoxic patients, therapy prior to and following radioiodine ablation, and long-term treatment of children, adolescents and young adults. Patients who relapse or fail to achieve remission need to be considered for ^{131}I or surgical ablation.

Iodides interfere with the release of thyroxine.

They have been used to prepare patients for thyroidectomy, but their clinical role has generally been superseded by the combined use of PTU and propranolol.

Radioiodine treatment is one form of ablative therapy. [131]I was introduced in 1942 and is widely used today. It is indicated in Graves' disease when antithyroid drugs do not suffice, when there is toxicity or intolerance to antithyroid agents, when the patient is elderly or noncompliant, and when medical problems or patient preference contraindicates surgery. Pregnant women should not be given ^{131}I because the drug crosses the placenta and is concentrated by the fetal thyroid. The major disadvantages of ^{131}I therapy are a delay in controlling symptoms and a high incidence of hypothroidism.

The period prior to onset of clinical improvement is variable, but usually is about 2 to 3 months. Patients often require propranolol and/or antithyroid drugs in the meantime to achieve early clinical control.

Induction of hypothyroidism is the most frequent problem with ^{131}I therapy. With high-dose treatment, hypothyroidism occurs in 70 per cent by 1 year; lower doses of radioiodine cause only 10 to 15 per cent of patients to become hypothyroid in the first year; an additional 3 to 6 per cent become hypothyroid annually. The risk of eventual hypothyroidism requires that patients be regularly reevaluated, generally at 6-month intervals. Controversy exists over the use of high-dose radioiodine, which provides predictable relief but a high incidence of hypothyroidism, versus low-dose regimens, which involve lower early risk of hypothyroidism but lesser control of the disease. The concern that ^{131}I would lead to long-term radiation injury has not been borne out. There is no evidence of increased rates of birth defects or thyroid carcinoma.

Surgery represents the most direct ablative approach to hyperthyroidism, but involves several complications. The objective is to reduce thyroid mass sufficiently to cure the hypermetabolic state without inducing a hypothyroid condition. Unfortunately, there is a substantial incidence of permanent hypothyroidism, and smaller but perceptible risks of hypoparathyroidism and laryngeal paralysis. Moreover, hyperthyroidism may recur despite subtotal thyroidectomy in Graves' disease. Prior preparation of the patient with antithyroid drugs is required to avoid precipitating thyroid storm. Surgery is particularly useful for relieving esophageal obstruction; cosmesis and pregnancy are other indications. It is also a choice when antithyroid drugs fail or produce complications, or when patients are noncompliant. However, ^{131}I is increasingly replacing surgery, because it is a less expensive and less morbid therapy.

Hyperthyroidism due to thyroiditis can be managed symptomatically with propranolol, because spontaneous resolution is the rule. Aspirin, and occasionally corticosteroids, are indicated in subacute thyroiditis to control inflammatory symptoms. The treatment of Graves' disease complicated by infiltrative exophthalmos requires caution; if hypothyroidism is precipitated, it may worsen the ophthalmopathy. Severe exophthalmos may require using very high doses of prednisone of (120 to 150 mg. per day) or surgical decompression of the orbit. Solitary toxic nodules respond well to ^{131}I or ablative surgery, but since the rest of the gland may be inactive, it is important to assess its response to TSH prior to therapy.

INDICATIONS FOR REFERRAL AND ADMISSION

Patients who are candidates for ^{131}I therapy should have a thyroid scan and be seen by the endocrinologist or radiation therapist for calculation of the dose of ^{131}I to be administered. Consultation with an endocrinologist is also indicated in the management of the pregnant or lactating hyperthyroid patient and the individual with severe exophthalmos. Referral for consideration of surgical therapy is indicated when the patient is pregnant, has obstruction to swallowing, desires cosmetic improvement, or fails antithyroid drug therapy. Hospital admission is needed if heart failure, rapid atrial fibrillation, or angina develops.

THERAPEUTIC RECOMMENDATIONS

- Begin propranolol for immediate control of symptoms. Typical starting dose is in the range of 80 mg. per day, given in divided amounts; greater doses are needed if symptoms are very severe or not initially controlled by 80 mg. per day.
- Initiate definitive therapy by adding an antithyroid drug (e.g., propylthiouracil 100 mg. t.i.d. or methimazole 10 mg. t.i.d.). Adjust dose after 2 weeks according to the serum free T_4 level and symptoms, using the lowest possible dose to maintain biochemical and clinical control. Antithyroid drug therapy can be used as the initial definitive treatment modality for most patients, with the exception of pregnant or lactating women.
- Continue antithyroid therapy until control is accomplished (usually 3 to 5 months). Tapering at this time can be attempted to see if remission has

been achieved. If a relapse of symptoms occurs, consideration of another form of definitive therapy should be undertaken; however, many authorities would recommend continuing antithyroid therapy for 12 to 24 months before tapering.

- Monitor patients on antithyroid drug therapy with periodic white blood counts, and stop therapy if the neutrophil count falls below 1500 per mm³.

- Utilize ¹³¹I therapy for patients who are poor operative risks (e.g., the elderly) and those who cannot be maintained on antithyroid agents. If ¹³¹I therapy is used, continue antithyroid therapy and/or propranolol for 2 or 3 months after administration. After ¹³¹I therapy, evaluate the patient every 6 months for development of hypothyroidism.

- Refer patients with obstructive symptoms, pregnancy, cosmetic concerns, and failure or refusal of antithyroid or radioiodine therapy for surgical evaluation. If surgery is contemplated, continue antithyroid and/or propranolol therapy into the preoperative period.

- Treat patients with transient hyperthyroidism due to thyroiditis symptomatically with propranolol.

ANNOTATED BIBLIOGRAPHY

Brown, J., et al.: Autoimmune thyroid disease—Graves' and Hashimoto's. Ann. Intern. Med., 88:279, 1978. (A review of recent developments in pathogenesis, diagnosis and threrapy.)

Greer, M.A., Kammer, H., and Bouma, D.J.: Short-term antithyroid drug therapy for the thyrotoxi-cosis of Graves' disease. N. Eng. J. Med., 297:173, 1977. (Patients were treated until they became clinically euthyroid; this required 3 to 5 months of therapy. The remission rate was 40 per cent, which is close to the rate achieved with 1 to 2 years of treatment.)

Irvine, W.J., et al.: Spectrum of thyroid function in patients remaining in remission after antithyroid drug therapy for thyrotoxicosis. Lancet, 2:179, 1977. (In some patients, spontaneous euthyroidism or hypothyroidism followed discontinuation of therapy, suggesting that the natural history of the disease may include spontaneous remission or even development of hypothyroidism.)

Kaplan K.M., and Utiger, R.D.: Diagnosis of hyperthyroidism. Clin. Endocrinol. Metab., 7:97, 1978. (Critical review of diagnostic tests. Diagnosis is usually possible by utilizing a few simple tests.)

Utiger, R.D.: Treatment of Graves' disease. N. Engl. J. Med., 298:643, 1978. (Argues for antithyroid drug therapy as the initial treatment modality for most patients; critically reviews other forms of therapy.)

Zonszein, J., et al.: Propranolol therapy in thyrotoxicosis: A review of 84 patients undergoing surgery. Am. J. Med., 66:411, 1979. (Administration of propranolol alone provided rapid, safe and effective preparation of thyrotoxic patients undergoing emergency or elective thyroid or nonthyroid surgery.)

100
Management of Hypothyroidism

The development of accurate and relatively inexpensive techniques for diagnosis of hypothyroidism and the availability of levothyroxine have greatly facilitated management of hypothyroidism. The majority of hypothyroid patients have primary disease of the thyroid gland, with chronic (Hashimoto's) thyroiditis, idiopathic thyroid atrophy, previous ¹³¹I therapy, and subtotal thyroidectomy being the leading causes. Less frequent etiologies include neck irradiation, iodide administration and use of lithium or para-aminosalicylic acid. Pituitary insufficiency can result in secondary hypothyroidism. Rarely, hypothalamic disease is the source of difficulty. The prevalence of hypothyroidism increases with age. Women are more frequently affected than are men. Not infrequently, a patient comes for evaluation, having been prescribed a thyroid preparation for unclear reasons; a decision is necessary regarding continuation of the drug. The primary physician should be capable of determining when replacement therapy is indicated and of providing it with safety and precision.

PATHOPHYSIOLOGY, CLINICAL PRESENTATION, AND COURSE

The clinical manifestations of hypothyroidism reflect the decreases in metabolic rate and sensitivity to catecholamines that result from insufficient circulating thyroid hormone. Early symptoms are gradual in onset and nonspecific. The patient typically complains of fatigue, heavy menstrual periods, slight weight gain, or cold intolerance. These symptoms are followed over the next few months by reports of dry skin, coarse hair, hoarseness, continued weight gain (though appetite is minimal) and slightly impaired mental activity. Later, depression may be evident.

In late stages, hydrophilic mucopolysaccharide accumulates subcutaneously, producing the myxedematous changes which characterize this severe form of the disease; the skin becomes doughy, the face puffy, tongue large, expression dull, and mentation slow, even lethargic. Muscle weakness, joint complaints, diminution in hearing, and carpal tunnel syndrome are also found.

On examination, the thyroid gland is not palpable unless there is a goiter, which may be due to thyroiditis, hereditary defects in thyroxine synthesis, or use of iodides, PAS or lithium. The heart may show signs of dilatation or an effusion. Bowel sounds are diminished, and the relaxation phase of the deep tendon reflexes is slowed or "hung up." A mild anemia may be present (see Chapter 77) and hypercholesterolemia is often noted. In severe cases of myxedema, dilutional hyponatremia occurs as a result of inadequate renal blood flow. A warning of impending myxedema coma is a rise in arterial pCO_2, which takes place as respiratory drive weakens.

In secondary hypothyroidism there may be signs of concurrent ovarian and adrenal insufficiency, such as loss of axillary and pubic hair, amenorrhea, and postural hypotension. Myxedematous changes tend to be less marked than with primary hypothyroidism.

The onset of hypothyroidism is usually gradual and its course progressive. At times, hyperthyroidism precedes hypothyroidism (see Chapter 99), but eventually the disease or its treatment decreases thyroid reserve. Drugs which have an antithyroid effect produce rapid but reversible forms of hypothyroidism.

PRINCIPLES OF THERAPY

The first step is to stop all thyroid and antithyroid medications in order to confirm the diagnosis when it is in question. Patients who are taking a thyroid preparation, yet lack documentation of hypothyroidism, can be taken off their medication without serious risk. Abrupt cessation of exogenous thyroid hormone therapy is not dangerous as long as there is no prior history of severe hypothyroidism, because there are adequate and prompt (though submaximal) pituitary and thyroid gland responses to halting of hormone intake. It takes about 5 weeks for full function to return, at which time testing for hypothyroidism can be carried out.

The diagnosis of primary hypothyroidism is readily achieved by demonstrating a low free T_4 and an increased TSH; the TSH is the more sensitive indicator of primary hypothyroidism. The range of normal for the free T_4 is wide; the test may not detect the patient who has a moderate decline in thyroid function, because the free T_4 level may still be within the range of "normal." Nevertheless, the free T_4 is a better measure of thyroid function than is the T_4, because the former is not affected by changes in protein binding. The radioactive iodine uptake and the serum cholesterol contribute little to diagnosis. Secondary hypothyroidism is identified by a TSH level that is not appropriately elevated in the setting of inadequate thyroid function. To test pituitary reserve, TRH can be given and TSH response noted. In primary hypothyroidism and in hypothalamic disease, a surge of TSH is produced, but not in secondary hypothyroidism.

Treatment of mild to moderate hypothyroidism is best done in gradual fashion, because hypothyroid patients are very sensitive to the effects of thyroxine. An excessive rate of replacement may cause palpitations, tremor, nervousness, or even angina. Full replacement doses of L-thyroxine average between 150 and 200 mcg. per day. Schedules for treatment depend on age, presence of cardiac disease, and severity of symptoms. Young, otherwise healthy patients can be started on 50 mcg. per day of thyroxine. This dose can be increased in 25-to 50-mcg. increments every 2 weeks until a euthyroid state is achieved.

In patients over age 50 who are at risk for coronary disease, more cautious replacement is indicated. Thyroid medication may produce angina, sinus tachycardia or arrhythmias (particularly atrial fibrillation) in patients with underlying coronary artery disease. It may be necessary to initiate therapy in these patients with 25 mcg. per day. If angina or cardiac symptoms occur, the dose of thyroid hormone should be reduced; when increments are resumed, the dose should be increased more slowly. The concurrent administration of propranolol has been advocated by some to protect the heart from overstimulation by thyroid replacement. This may be of particular use in patients with angina.

L-thyroxine is now the agent of choice, on the basis of uniform bioavailability, cost, safety and ease of monitoring therapy (the serum T_4 level directly reflects the dose utilized). The onset of effect is gradual; the agent's half-life is about 24 hours, making once-a-day therapy possible. Some of the drug is converted peripherally to T_3, making it unnecessary to use the more expensive preparations which contain mixtures of T_4 and T_3. The use of exogenous T_3 is considered inadvisable for replacement purposes, especially in older patients, because it causes rapid increases in metabolic rate and oxygen demand, and can precipitate angina. Moreover, its short half-life produces wide swings in T_3 levels and requires frequent administration. For these reasons, many physicians find it best to switch patients from older thyroid hormone preparations and T_3 to L-thyroxine.

Adequate replacement should result in resolution of fatigue, loss of excess weight, and reversal of autonomic symptoms. The first signs of response are modest loss of weight, increase in pulse rate, and resolution of constipation. Myxedematous skin changes, pleural and pericardial effusions, and elevated creatine phosphokinase levels also normalize, but require more time. Most patients feel better within 2 weeks, and clinical resolution is usually complete by 3 months.

Laboratory monitoring of replacement therapy involves measurement of TSH and free T_4. TSH is best for determining if sufficient thyroxine is being given to avoid hypothyroidism but cannot distinguish excessive from physiologic thyroxine doses; a free T_4 level will detect excesses. Once a stable dose is achieved, twice-yearly assessments are probably sufficient. Any upward adjustments in dose should be made in small increments.

The treatment and monitoring of *secondary hypothyroidism* must take into account the lack of TSH response and probable coexistence of adrenal and ovarian hypofunction. Because thyroid replacement and the resultant rise in metabolic rate can precipitate addisonian crisis, adrenal function should be assessed with an ACTH stimulation test prior to prescribing replacement therapy in any patient suspected of having secondary hypothyroidism. Treatment with cortisone acetate should precede L-T_4 replacement.

Therapy for primary hypothyroidism is continued indefinitely.

THERAPEUTIC RECOMMENDATIONS

- Stop any exogenous thyroid or antithyroid medication if reason for use is unclear.
- Confirm the diagnosis of hypothyroidism with TSH and free T_4 determinations.
- If the TSH is not appropriately elevated, test for pituitary insufficiency.

Primary Hypothyroidism

- If possible, stop all potential antithyroid agents (e.g., iodides, PAS, lithium) and the antithyroid drugs methimazole and propylthiouracil if they are being used (see Chapter 99).
- Begin replacement with L-thyroxine, initiating therapy with 50 mcg. per day in most patients, but using 25 mcg. in those with clinical coronary disease.
- Increase dose by 25 to 50 mcg. every few weeks, according to clinical response, tolerance of side effects (e.g., tremor, angina or arrhythmias) and TSH and free T_4 levels. Elderly patients and those with coronary disease may require smaller, more gradual increments in dose.
- Average replacement doses are in the range of 150 to 250 mcg. per day of L-thyroxine. L-thyroxine is the drug of choice. Combination preparations containing T_3 are unnecessary, since T_4 is converted peripherally to T_3.
- Therapy can be monitored by measurement of TSH and free T_4. The TSH is needed to detect undertreatment, and the free T_4, overtreatment.

Secondary Hypothyroidism

- Perform ACTH stimulation test to assess adrenal reserve. If low, give cortisone acetate *before* providing thyroid replacement.
- Replace thyroid hormone as for primary hypothyroidism.
- Monitor therapy by following clinical signs and free T_4.

PATIENT EDUCATION

Euthyroid patients who are placed on exogenous thyroid inappropriately for treatment of fatigue or obesity are often reluctant to give up the medication. Documenting that their thyroid status is perfectly normal is an essential first step to successfully taking them off the medication. Often a request from the physician to temporarily halt thyroid hormone for 5 weeks in order to measure TSH and free T_4 is agreed to. Usually there is little change in how the patient feels, and this helps to convince the patient that exogenous hormone is unnecessary.

Hypothyroid patients need to be warned of the danger of increasing their medication too rapidly or of taking more than is prescribed. Unfortunately, some patients adjust their doses on the basis of other symptoms which they mistakenly attribute to hypothyroidism, e.g., those of depression. All patients should be instructed to regularly measure and record their weight and report to the physician any unexplained change of 5 or more pounds.

It is imperative that the patient and family be instructed in the signs of worsening hypothyroidism. Hypothyroid patients have been known to stop taking their thyroid medication. The importance of continuing therapy indefinitely must be emphasized to the patient and persons close to him.

ANNOTATED BIBLIOGRAPHY

Brown, J. (moderator): Thyroid physiology in health and disease. Ann. Intern. Med., *81*:68, 1974. *(A good review of pathophysiology.)*

Inada, M., *et al.*: Estimation of thyroxine and triiodothyronine distribution and the conversion rate of thyroxine to triiodothyronine in man. J. Clin. Invest., *55*:1337, 1975. *(Most T_3 derives from peripheral conversion of T_4, both in normals and in hypothyroid patients. These data suggest that replacement therapy using T_3-T_4 mixtures is unnecessary and that L-thyroxine should suffice.)*

Krugman, L., Hershman, J., Chopra. I., *et al.*: Patterns of recovery of the hypothalamic-pituitary-thyroid axis in patients taken off chronic thyroid therapy. J. Clin. Endocrinol Metab., *41*:70, 1975. *(Full recovery of pituitary and thyroid responsiveness to TRH occurred in euthyroid patients 5 weeks after withdrawal of chronic thyroid hormone therapy.)*

Rootwelt, K., and Solberg, H.E.: Optimum laboratory test combinations for thyroid function studies, selected by discriminant analysis. Scan. J. Clin. Lab. Invest., *38*:477, 1978. *(The free T_4 and TSH are the best studies for detection of hypothyroidism; serum cholesterol, RAI uptake and other tests commonly ordered were of little use.)*

Stock, J., Sarks, M., and Oppenheimer, J.: Replacement dosage of L-thyroxine in hypothyroidism. N. Engl. J. Med., *290*:529, 1974. *(Mean replacement dose needed was 169 ug, as determined by return of TSH levels to normal. T_3 levels were close to normal after use of T_4, demonstrating peripheral conversion of T_4 to T_3 and lack of need to supply T_3.)*

101
Glucocorticosteroid Therapy

The therapeutic potency of glucocorticosteroids has led to their widespread and, sometimes, indiscriminant use. A number of questions must be addressed prior to the initiation of steroid therapy. (1) Is the underlying disorder of such severity that the benefits of therapy outweigh the substantial risk of serious side effects? (2) Will prolonged treatment be required, or will a brief limited course suffice? (3) Have alternative, less morbid therapies been maximally utilized? (4) Does the patient have any underlying condition which will worsen on steroid therapy or predispose him to drug-induced complications? (5) Can alternate-day therapy be utilized?

The primary physician must decide when and how to institute steroid therapy, whether to use daily or alternate-day treatment, and how to withdraw chronic glucocorticoid treatment safely.

ADVERSE EFFECTS

The adverse effects of glucocorticosteroid therapy are a function of dose and duration of use. A few are irreversible; fortunately most resolve within several months of terminating therapy.

Suppression of the hypothalamic-pituitary-adrenal (HPA) axis is among the most important consequences of chronic glucocorticoid use. An incompletely resolved issue is how long and at what dose must therapy be given in order to suppress the HPA axis to a clinically significant degree. Adrenocortical atrophy has been noted as early as 5 days after initiation of steroid treatment, as has reduced responsiveness to exogenous ACTH stimulation and metyrapone. Most data suggest that 20 to 30 mg. of prednisone or its equivalent given on a daily basis for 10 days or more can induce clinically significant HPA suppression.

Daily physiologic doses of glucocorticosteroids (eg., 5 to 7.5 mg. prednisone) given in the morning do not cause suppression of any consequence, but if the same doses are given at night, normal diurnal cortisol secretion is inhibited. Doses just above the physiologic range are suppressive after about a month of use. Alternate-day therapy and ACTH treatment do not induce clinically significant HPA suppression. A single daily pharmacologic dose of glucocorticoid produces less HPA suppression than does the same dose given in divided fashion over the course of the day.

After chronic use of pharmacologic doses, it takes about 12 months for full recovery of the HPA axis to occur (as measured by response to exogenous ACTH, metyrapone, or insulin tolerance testing). Hypothalamic-pituitary function returns first, beginning 2 to 5 months after cessation of suppressive therapy, and is manifested by appropriate plasma ACTH levels that demonstrate a normal diurnal pattern. Signs of adrenal recovery become evident at 6 to 9 months, with return of the baseline serum cortisol to normal; maximal adrenal response to ACTH does not reappear until 9 to 12 months.

Laboratory data on suppression and recovery of HPA activity are relatively abundant, compared to the scant amount of clinical information available on how long a patient is at risk for serious adrenal insufficiency after cessation of steroid use. Guidelines for replacement therapy in times of stress are based on the results of laboratory investigation. There is no proven method for accelerating the restoration of normal HPA function once inhibition has occurred. The administration of ACTH does not appear to speed adrenal recovery.

There are a number of other important metabolic and endocrinologic problems that result from chronic corticosteroid use. *Negative nitrogen balance* (due to inhibition of protein synthesis and enhancement of protein catabolism) is believed to be partially responsible for reduced muscle mass, weakness, thinning of the skin, and striae formation. *Glucose intolerance* is common. Mechanisms include increases in peripheral insulin resistance, gluconeogenesis, glucagon secretion, and substrate availability. Usually the glucose intolerance is mild, does not lead to ketosis, and resolves upon cessation of therapy. In patients who develop carbohydrate intolerance, the effect appears to be dose-related. *Fat redistribution* accounts for the characteristic truncal obesity and cushingoid appearance. This change is minimized with alternate-day therapy or when daily physiologic doses are taken each morning, but not when ACTH or daily pharmacologic glucocorticoid doses are used.

There is *enhanced susceptibility to infection* resulting from the anti-inflammatory and immunosuppressive actions of corticosteroids. Bacterial infections are common. Candidiasis and aspergillosis sometimes result. Herpes zoster, varicella, vaccinia, and cytomegalovirus are the principle viral infections encountered in patients on steroids. Reactivation of tuberculosis is a well-recognized risk (see Chapter 47).

Osteoporosis develops when large steroid doses are used over prolonged periods. The incidence is unknown because it is difficult to measure skeletal mass accurately and inexpensively. The precise relation between dose, duration of use and risk of osteoporosis remains unclear. Patients with a predisposition to osteoporosis, such as menopausal women and immobilized individuals, appear to be among the most susceptible. The axial skeleton is affected more than the limbs, and vertebral compression fractures may result. *Aseptic necrosis* of the femoral head and other bones is a well-recognized but rare skeletal complication; sometimes it may be due to the underlying illness for which corticosteroids are being given, as is the case in rheumatoid arthritis.

The issue of *peptic ulceration* and steroid therapy remains unresolved. Early clinical reports that corticosteroid therapy increased the risk of ulcer disease were uncontrolled and did not take into account the severity and nature of the underlying illness. Recent reviews of available data have not uncovered a statistically significant relationship between ulcer disease and steroid use. Most controlled studies omit patients with previous ulcer disease because they are a high-risk group, but in doing so avoid addressing the issue of whether this important subgroup is adversely affected. Nevertheless, it is felt by many clinicians that prolonged use of large doses increases the risk of ulceration.

Myopathy may be seen in patients on chronic therapy when large doses are utilized. Proximal muscle wasting and weakness of the lower extremities are characteristic; patients complain of difficulty climbing stairs. Average time of onset is 5 months into treatment. Muscle enzymes are normal; the condition is reversible.

Psychological and *behavioral changes* are of considerable importance, and are particularly frequent in the elderly. The reported incidence is as high as 25 to 40 per cent of patients receiving steroid therapy. Increased appetite, mild euphoria, and changes in sleep patterns are rather common at the onset of treatment. Psychoses, which are not predictably related to dose or duration of therapy, can occur; they slowly respond to reduction or cessation of steroid use. Some clinicians argue that the patient's premorbid personality plays a role, while others deny this. Steroid therapy can exacerbate previous psychiatric disease.

Posterior subcapsular cataracts are reported in 10 to 35 per cent. They are usually dose- and duration-dependent. A few require removal; most do not. *Hypertension* and *fluid retention* with peripheral edema are more frequent when agents with mineralocorticoid effects are used (see Table 101–1), and are not dependent on preexistence of elevated blood pressure. Again dose and duration of therapy are important factors. *Electrolyte derangements* are common, especially hypokalemia. *Acute pancreatitis* is noted with increased frequency in patients taking corticosteroids. *Acne* is seen more often with ACTH use than with glucocorticoids, due to stimulation of ad-

Table 101–1.   Commonly Used Glucocorticoids

DURATION OF ACTION	GLUCOCORTICOID POTENCY*	EQUIVALENT GLUCOCORTICOID DOSE (MG.)	MINERALOCORTICOID ACTIVITY
Short-acting			
Cortisol (hydrocortisone)	1	20	Yes†
Cortisone	0.8	25	Yes†
Prednisone	4	5	No
Prednisolone	4	5	No
Methylprednisolone	5	4	No
Intermediate-acting			
Triamcinolone	5	4	No
Long-acting			
Betamethasone	25	0.60	No
Dexamethasone	30	0.75	No

* The values given for glucocorticoid potency are relative. Cortisol is arbitrarily assigned a value of one.
† Mineralocorticoid effects are dose-related. At doses close to or within the basal physiologic range for glucocorticoid activity, no such effect may be detectable.
(Adapted from Axelrod, L.: Glucocorticoid therapy. *Medicine, 55*:39, 1976.)

renal androgen production, but the problem does bother patients on corticosteroids. *Panniculitis* is unique to iatrogenic Cushing's syndrome.

PRINCIPLES OF THERAPY

The cardinal principle of steroid therapy is to obtain the maximal therapeutic benefit while minimizing the complications and potential problems inherent to interfering with normal hypothalamic-pituitary-adrenal function. Steroids usually do not cure disease or alter its natural history; rather they suppress the inflammatory response or modify the immunologic abnormality. Steroid treatment is in some sense symptomatic, and therefore one must carefully weigh the perceived therapeutic benefit against the potential risks.

Once it has been determined that the potential benefits outweigh the probable risks of therapy, the physician faces the task of deciding which agent to use, for how long, at what dose, and in what schedule. Minimizing HPA suppression is a major consideration and best accomplished by utilizing a short-acting agent (see Table 101–1), on an alternate-day schedule, at the smallest possible dose for the shortest period of time. It is also preferable to use a preparation that has the least mineralocorticoid activity (see Table 101–1), and it is certainly important to continue using maximal nonsteroidal therapy so that the steroid dose prescribed is the lowest one possible.

Although ACTH does not cause clinically significant HPA suppression or adrenal atrophy, it must be given parenterally, and there is no way to know how much glucocorticoid effect is obtained from a given dose. These disadvantages, as well as induction of mineralocorticoid and androgenic effects, limit its usefulness. ACTH has not been shown to be superior to prednisone.

Most conditions which require corticosteroid treatment can be adequately managed with *alternate-day therapy*, although it is often necessary to begin with a program of daily steroids when symptoms are severe and the disease very active. Important advantages of alternate-day treatment are avoidance of significant HPA suppression and minimization of cushingoid side effects, without a substantial loss of anti-inflammatory activity. It appears that the anti-inflammatory effects of glucocorticosteroids persist longer than the undesirable metabolic effects. Other adverse effects that are reduced or eliminated by an alternate-day schedule include inhibition of delayed hypersensitivity, susceptibility to in-

fection, negative nitrogen balance, fluid retention, hypertension, and psychological and behavioral disturbances.

Alternate-day therapy by itself will not prevent HPA suppression if a long-acting steroid preparation is used (e.g., dexamethasone). Moreover, therapy must be truly alternate-day, with the total dose given first thing in the morning every other day; intermittent therapy or doses given throughout the day every other day do not preserve HPA responsiveness.

Although daily steroid therapy is often required to bring florid disease under control, alternate-day treatment is as effective or nearly as effective in maintaining control. Only temporal arteritis and case reports of fulminant ulcerative colitis and pemphigus vulgaris have been found to require daily steroid doses to maintain control of symptoms and disease activity. In fulminant ulcerative colitis, high-dose, alternate-day therapy has not been tried in a systematic fashion. Among the conditions found to respond well to alternate-day corticosteroids are certain forms of the nephrotic syndrome (see Chapter 123), sarcoidosis, myasthenia gravis, and asthma.

Once daily steroid treatment has achieved control of disease activity, it is advisable to attempt switching the patient to alternate-day therapy. The objective is to maintain the same total steroid dose while gradually increasing the dose on the first day and decreasing it on the second day, so that a point is reached where a double dose is given every other day, with no drug given in between. The rapidity with which the changeover can be made is variable and depends on the activity of the underlying disease, duration of therapy, degree of HPA suppression, and the patient's cooperativeness. A rough guideline for switching to alternate-day therapy is to make changes in increments of 10 mg. of prednisone (or its equivalent) when the daily prednisone dose is greater than 40 mg., and in 5 mg. increments when the daily dose is between 20 and 40 mg. Below 20 mg. per day, the change ought to be in amounts of 2.5 mg. The interval between changes ranges from 1 day to several weeks and is determined empirically, based on clinical response. It is important to keep in mind that most patients who have been on a daily steroid program for more than 2 weeks probably have some degree of HPA suppression.

When *daily therapy* is necessary, HPA suppression can be minimized by having the patient take the entire dose first thing in the morning and by using a short-acting glucocorticoid at the lowest possible dose. Daily single-dose regimens may be as effective or nearly as effective as divided dose regimens in controlling underlying illness; however, in contrast to alternate-day therapy, manifestations of Cushing's syndrome are not prevented.

Withdrawing patients from daily steroid therapy can precipitate adrenal insufficiency, flare of the underlying illness, or a withdrawal syndrome. There is no way to speed HPA recovery, nor are there specific schedules for reducing dose. One must monitor disease activity and decrease dose empirically in small amounts, watching for flare of disease or signs of adrenal insufficiency such as hypotension and gastrointestinal distress.

One approach to reducing the dose toward physiologic levels is to make changes in decrements of 10 mg. of prednisone or its equivalent every 1 to 3 weeks, as long as the dose is above 40 mg. Below 40 mg., the decrement is 5 mg. Once a physiologic dose of prednisone is reached (5 to 7.5 mg. per day), the patient can be switched to 1-mg. prednisone tablets or the equivalent dose of hydrocortisone so that further reductions in dose can be made in smaller steps than is possible using 5-mg. prednisone tablets. Weekly or biweekly reductions can then be carried out in steps of 1 mg. of prednisone at a time, as permitted by disease activity.

Some patients develop a *steroid withdrawal syndrome* during the tapering process, characterized by depression, myalgias, arthralgias, anorexia, headaches, nausea and lethargy. Studies have failed to show a relationship between these symptoms and low cortisol or 17-hydroxycorticosteroid levels. In most instances, complaints are reported when levels are normal or even elevated, but falling rapidly. HPA responsiveness has also been found to be normal in many of these patients. The mechanisms responsible for this syndrome are unknown, but seem linked to the rapidity with which dose is tapered.

At times of anticipated stress, such as preoperatively, when it is necessary to know what the status of the HPA axis is and whether supplementary steroid therapy is needed, an ACTH stimulation test can provide an indication of adrenal reserve. Since adrenal response is the last component of the HPA system to return, testing of suppression can be done with ACTH stimulation. A test injection of synthetic ACTH is given intravenously; if in 1 hour the serum cortisol is greater than 18 mcg. per 100 ml., there is no need to supplement for stress. The response of the serum cortisol to intravenous ACTH stimulation corresponds to the cortisol level that can be expected from such stresses as general anesthesia and surgery.

If the patient cannot mount an adequate cortisol response or testing is impractical because of urgency or unavailability of agents or assays, corticosteroid supplementation should be given for acute stress. Even minor illnesses such as gastroenteritis, influenza, or pharyngitis are indications for an additional 100 mg. of hydrocortisone per day in divided doses. This will also suffice for minor surgical procedures such as dental extraction. During major stress, such as trauma or surgery, the patient should be given 100 mg. of hydrocortisone every 6 to 8 hours. The need to continue supplementation can be evaluated by repeat ACTH stimulation testing.

PATIENT EDUCATION

Steroids should be used with caution in patients whose reliability or intelligence is in question, because of the risk of HPA suppression and adrenocortical insufficiency. Patients on suppressive doses of steroid should be informed of the need for steroid supplementation when there is stress or illness and should wear an identification bracelet which states that they take a corticosteroid. Patients must understand the need to contact the physician and to increase steroid dosage when subjected to physiological stress. The family can be given a prepackaged syringe containing dexamethasone phosphate, 4 mg., to be injected intramuscularly if the patient should become unconscious or so ill as not to be able to take steroids by mouth.

Many patients are fearful or reluctant to be taken off chronic steroid therapy out of concern for recrudescence of the underlying illness or because malaise is experienced as the drug is tapered. A detailed review of the side effects of prolonged therapy is necessary so that the rationale for reducing dose and the desirability of eventually discontinuing corticosteroids are understood and appreciated. Any change in dose and schedule should be written out. When chronic, daily, high-dose therapy is required, the psychological impact of adverse effects (e.g., cushingoid features) can be lessened by forewarning the patient of their likelihood and at least partial reversibility.

THERAPEUTIC RECOMMENDATIONS

- Utilize glucocorticoids only when other forms of therapy have been used in maximal doses and proven inadequate, and when the risks of steroid use are outweighed by the therapeutic benefit expected.
- Add the least possible dose of cortocosteroid to the

ongoing treatment program, but *do not replace previous therapy* with steroid treatment when there is partial benefit from nonsteroidal agents.

- Use a short-acting preparation with the fewest possible mineralocorticoid effects (e.g., prednisone). ACTH offers few advantages and a number of disadvantages; it must be given parenterally and it stimulates mineralocorticoid and androgen production.

- Try initiating therapy on an alternate-day basis if symptoms are not severe; HPA suppression and cushingoid effects are thus avoided. Most conditions respond as well or nearly as well to alternate-day doses as to daily ones.

- If alternate-day therapy is not successful or symptoms are severe, daily therapy ought to be used. Try to give the entire dose in the morning to minimize HPA suppression.

- Since HPA suppression may occur after as little as 20 to 30 mg. prednisone given daily for 7 to 10 days and may not completely return to normal for 9 to 12 months, patients on daily pharmacologic doses should be advised of the need to supplement their steroid intake when under stress or experiencing an acute illness; 100 mg. per day of hydrocortisone or its equivalent should be prescribed in divided doses. It usually suffices for minor illnesses; 100 mg. hydrocortisone every 8 hours is needed for trauma or surgery. Give the patient's family a prepackaged syringe containing 4 mg. dexamethasone for intramuscular emergency use. ACTH stimulation testing can be performed to assess the adequacy of adrenal reserve.

- Initiate withdrawal of steroids by moving from a divided-dose schedule to a once-daily morning dose and from daily dose schedules into alternate-day therapy. Condensing divided doses into a single daily dose can usually be done rather quickly, but moving from daily to alternate-day therapy must be gradual and requires monitoring for flare of underlying disease and adrenal insufficiency.

- To switch from a daily to an alternate-day corticosteroid program, one increases the dose on the first day and decreases the dose on the second day by the equivalent of 10 mg. of prednisone if the daily dose is above 40 mg., and by 5 mg. if the daily dose is below 40 mg. Below 20 mg., the increment is 2.5 mg. The interval between changes in dose is determined empirically, based on clinical status of the patient. The end point of switching occurs when the previous entire 2-day dose is given once every other day.

- Tapering of alternate-day therapy can proceed in

10-mg. decrements when dose is above 40 mg., and 5-mg. steps when it is below 40 mg. Rapidity of tapering is limited by recrudescence of disease activity and development of symptoms of withdrawal or adrenal insufficiency; it is determined empirically. Once the dose is down to 5 mg. of prednisone, switch to 20 mg. hydrocortisone or 1-mg. prednisone tablets and reduce dose in decrements of 2.5 mg. hydrocortisone or 1 mg. prednisone.

- At a dosage level of 10 mg. hydrocortisone, check 8:00 a.m. cortisol level. If it is greater than 18 mcg. per 100 ml., stop exogenous steroids; otherwise, continue therapy and do ACTH stimulation testing to determine if it is safe to taper.

- If withdrawal symptoms are a problem on alternate-day therapy, a small morning dose of hydrocortisone, 10 to 20 mg., given on the off day may help alleviate symptoms without prolonging HPA suppression.

ANNOTATED BIBLIOGRAPHY

Axelrod, L.: Glucocorticoid therapy. Medicine, 55:39, 1976. *(A superb review concentrating on the duration of suppression of the pituitary-adrenal axis, the relative merits of single-dose therapy, alternate-day therapy, and the fact that ACTH has not been demonstrated superior to orally administered glucocorticoids; 188 references.)*

Byyny, R.L.: Withdrawal from glucocorticoid therapy. N. Engl. J. Med., 295:30, 1976. *(A protocol for withdrawal is suggested which is eminently reasonable and feasible.)*

Dale, D.C., Fauci, A.S., and Wolff, S.M.: Alternate day prednisone, leukocyte kinetics and susceptibility to infections. N. Engl. J. Med., 291:1154, 1974. *(An important study establishing that alternate-day steroid therapy leaves leukocyte counts, inflammatory responses and neutrophil half-life normal, as compared to daily steroid therapy which causes significant reductions).*

Graeber, A.L., Ney, R.L., Nicholson, W.E., et al.: Natural history of pituitary adrenal recovery following long-term suppression with corticosteroids. J. Clin. Endocrinol. Meta., 25:11, 1965. *(A classic paper which showed that patients on glucocorticoids for 1 to 10 years had full restoration of function generally within 1 year, that hypthalamic-pituitary function was restored during the initial 2 to 5 months, that 17-hydroxy-*

corticosteroids returned to normal during months 6 to 9 [probably a response to supranormal levels of ACTH], and that from 9 months on all responses to testing were essentially normal. The study provides no information about recovery following shorter courses of glucocorticoids.)

Meikle, A.W., and Tyler, F.H.: Potency and duration of action of glucocorticoids. Effects of hydrocortisone, prednisone and dexamethasone on human pituitary-adrenal function. Am. J. Med., 63:200, 1977. *(A paper that demonstrates the prolonged suppressive effect of desamethasone on the pituitary-adrenal axis. The intrinsic potency and relative rate of disappearance from plasma are the two most important factors determining the relative potency of orally administered glucocorticoids.)*

Streetend, H.P.: Corticosteroid therapy complications and therapeutic implications. JAMA, 232:1046, 1975. *(A short review of the likely complications associated with the therapeutic use of glucocorticoids.)*

8

Gynecologic Problems

102
Screening for Breast Cancer

Carcinoma of the breast is the most common malignancy in women. Internationally, its incidence varies widely, in that rates in North America and Northern Europe are 5 to 6 times higher than those in Asia and Africa. The incidence among American women over 35 years of age is about two new cancers per 1,000 women per year. The lifetime probability that an American woman will develop breast cancer is between 7 and 8 per cent. Most women overestimate this probability, probably because nearly 80 per cent have known someone with the disease. Only about 25 per cent of treated women are cured; nearly 30,000 women die of the disease each year in the United States. Despite diagnostic and therapeutic advances, these figures have changed little in the past 30 years. The high incidence and the degree of illness and deaths associated with the disease, coupled with the importance of the breasts to women's self-image, make carcinoma of the breast one of the most feared tumors. The primary care provider deals with breast tumor diagnosis or associated fears on a daily basis.

EPIDEMIOLOGY AND RISK FACTORS

Assessment of risk for the individual patient depends on the following epidemiologic characteristics:

Age. Risk increases throughout life for American women. Seventy-five per cent of breast cancers occur after the age of 40. In Boston, the annual incidence per 100,000 women approaches 300 at age 80, four times the rate at age 40.

Reproductive History. Generally, there is an inverse relationship between breast cancer risk and parity, but it seems that age at first full-term pregnancy is the key variable. First pregnancy must occur before age 30 to provide a protective effect. The risk in women who deliver before age 20 is about half that of nulliparous women and one third that of women whose first child is born after age 35. An aborted pregnancy does not seem to reduce risk. The effect of lactation on risk, if any, is minor.

Menstrual History. Both late menarche and early natural menopause reduce breast cancer risk. Women whose menarche occurred after age 16 have half the risk of those whose menarche occurred earlier. Women in whom menopause occurred before age 45 have half the risk of those in whom menopause occurred after age 55. Women in whom early menopause is surgically induced seem to be similarly protected.

Family History. A family history of breast cancer, whether among maternal or paternal relatives, increases risk to 2 to 3 times that of the general population. Relatives of women with bilateral disease have an even higher risk.

History of Benign Breast Disease. The risk of breast cancer is increased approximately fourfold in women with chronic cystic mastitis. Acute breast diseases associated with lactation do not appear to affect risk.

History of Previous Malignancy. Contralateral lesions, most of which are second primaries, subsequently develop in approximately 10 per cent of women with breast cancer. Women with endometrial carcinoma have slightly increased risk.

Drugs. The role of drugs is controversial. Retrospective studies that have since been challenged have suggested a two- to fourfold increased risk of breast cancer in older women with a history of resperpine use. An increased risk of breast cancer with either oral contraceptive or postmenopausal estrogen use has not been conclusively demonstrated.

Mammographic Findings. Recently, the prominance of ductal patterns on mammography has been identified as a risk factor for subsequent breast carcinoma. To date, however, there is still disagreement about the reproducibility of mammographis classification schemes and their prognostic significance.

NATURAL HISTORY OF BREAST CANCER AND EFFECTIVENESS OF EARLY THERAPY

Little can be said with certainty about the natural history of breast cancer. The few observational studies of untreated breast cancer have shown widely variable tumor doubling times ranging from less than a week to more than 6 months. The mean duration of the preclinical phase of the disease has been estimated to be 20 months. Estimates of lead time, from the Health Insurance Plan (HIP) of Greater New York screening trial, have been 7 months at the initial screening examination and approximately 1 year for subsequent screenings at yearly intervals.

It is particularly difficult to judge the benefit of early treatment of breast cancer because of the widely variable course of the disease after diagnosis at any stage. Biologic determinism as the major influence on outcome has been widely debated. Many studies have shown that there is not a clear relationship between survival rates and the length of time the patient delayed seeking medical attention after becoming aware of the tumor, despite the drop in 5-year survival rates from 85 per cent to about 50 per cent when there is nodal involvement.

Data from the HIP randomized breast cancer screening trial, however, suggest substantial benefits of screening. After 7 years of follow-up, breast cancer mortality was 30 per cent lower in the study group. This reduction was evident in women over 50 but not in those between 40 and 49.

SCREENING METHODS

Breast self-examination has been the mainstay of prevention programs; through the years, 90 per cent of tumors have consistently been detected by patients. Nevertheless, the effectiveness of self-examination in the early detection of disease is a matter of ongoing debate. This effectiveness depends on size and other characteristics of the breast. Small or poorly supported pendulous breasts are most suitable. Examination of large, well supported breasts is difficult for both patients and physicians. All women should be taught self-examination techniques; they should be emphasized in those who are at risk and have breasts that are anatomically suitable.

Physical examination is extremely important and should never be neglected. A recent study indicates that the proportion of lesions confined to stage I at the time of diagnosis is higher for tumors discovered during routine physical examination than for those found during breast self-examination. Early data from the HIP study indicate that physical examination is more sensitive than mammography in all age groups, particularly in women under 50. Newer mammographic techniques may be relatively more sensitive. Nevertheless, the presence of any solitary dominant nodule is an indication for biopsy regardless of mammography results.

Mammography is a valuable aid in the diagnosis of breast masses and as a screening test in high-risk populations. Its use as a general screening test is more controversial. There is no question that benefits can be substantial—one third of HIP breast cancers found were detected by mammography alone. Costs are also substantial—65,000 mammograms on 20,000 women detected only 44 HIP cancers—including the risks of repeated radiation exposure. However, newer methods require significantly less radiation exposure.

Compared to physical examination, mammography is least sensitive in patients under age 50. Mammography has a particular advantage in women with large, difficult-to-examine breasts.

Currently, *thermography* is neither sensitive nor specific, its role needs to be further delineated.

CONCLUSIONS AND RECOMMENDATIONS

- A number of easily assessed factors allow an estimate of the risk of breast cancer in the individual patient.
- The benefit of early diagnosis appears to be significant.
- Self-examination should be taught to all women by the primary care provider. The technique should be emphasized when the woman is at high risk and has breasts that are suitable for effective self-examination.
- Physical examination may be the most sensitive detector of breast cancer, particularly in younger women. It should be performed in all women at yearly intervals, more frequently in high-risk populations.
- Mammography contributes independently to cancer detection. It is, however, expensive, and repeated examinations involve some risk of radiation-related carcinogenesis. Mammography should be performed in all women with palpable breast mass or masses, discharge, or other abnormalities. Indications for mammographic screening of asymptomatic women remain controversial. It should be performed at age 50 in all women with a significant risk factor and in those whose breasts are difficult to examine. Repeated yearly mammographic examination should be reserved for those with prior cancer or with two or more risk factors. Examination every 2 to 3 years would be appropriate for women with a single risk factor, including difficult-to-examine breasts. Some argue that more widespread mammographic screening, including women in younger age groups, is indicated, but the risk-benefit ratios for such patients remain uncertain.

ANNOTATED BIBLIOGRAPHY

Bailar, J.C.: Mammography: A contrary view. Ann. Intern. Med., *84*:77, 1976. *(Looks at HIP data, analyzes radiation risk, concludes that routine mammography "may eventually take almost as many lives as it saves.")*

Boston Collaborative Drug Surveillance Program: Surgically confirmed gallbladder disease, venous thromboembolism and breast tumors in relation to postmenopausal estrogen therapy. N. Engl. J. Med., *290*:15, 1974. *(No strong associations between estrogens and breast cancer.)*

Henderson, I.C., and Canellos, G.P.: Cancer of the breast: The past decade. N. Engl. J. Med., *320*: 17, 1980. *(Extensive review that notes the importance of natural history in measuring effectiveness of screening and therapy.)*

Hoover, R., Gray, L.A., Cole, P., and MacMahon, B.: Menopausal estrogen and breast cancer. N. Engl. J. Med., *295*:401, 1976. *(Retrospective population study showing 30 per cent increased risk with borderline statistical significance.)*

MacMahon, B., Cole, P., and Brown, J.: Etiology of human breast cancer: A review. J. Natl. C. Inst., *50*:21, 1973. *(Extensive review of risk factors [excluding drug history] as well as etiologic hypotheses with 178 references.)*

Mahoney, L.J., Bird, B.L., and Cooke, G.M.: Annual clinical examination: The best available screening test for breast cancer. N. Engl. J. Med., *301*: 315, 1979 *(Eighty-six percent of 30 new breast cancers among high-risk patients were detected on clinical examination.)*

Moore, F.D.: Editorial. Breast Self-examination. N. Engl. J. Med., *299*:304, 1978. *(Comments on two papers in same issue that try to quantify the effectiveness of breast self-examination. Dr. Moore remains skeptical.)*

Moskowitz, M., Milbrath, J., Gartside, P., et al.: Lack of efficacy of thermography as a screening tool for minimal and Stage I breast cancer. N. Engl. J. Med., *295*:249, 1976. *(True-positive rate less than false-positive rate.)*

Sadowsky. N.L., Kalisher, L., White, G., and Ferrucci, J.T.: Radiologic detection of breast cancer. N. Engl. J. Med., *294*:379, 1976. *(Recommendations for screening and diagnostic uses of xeromammography and thermography.)*

Sayler, C., Egan, J.F., Raines, J.R., and Goodman, M.J.: Mammographic screening: Value in diagnosis of early breast cancer. JAMA, *238*:872, 1977. *(Results from Cancer Demonstration Project suggesting improved sensitivity of mammography.)*

Shapiro, S., Goldberg, J.D., and Hutchinson, G.B.: Lead time in breast cancer detection and implications for periodicity of screening. Am J. Epidemiol., *100*:357, 1974. *(Average duration of preclinical disease previously estimated to be 20 months. Lead time estimated to be 1 year—7 months at initial exam and 11–13 months at subsequent screenings.)*

Strax, P., Venet, L., Shapiro, S., Gross, S., and Venet, W.: Breast cancer found in repetitive examination in mass screening. Arch. Environ. Health, *20*:758, 1970. *(HIP initial examination results—55 cancers detected on initial exam., 44 per cent were found in clinical exam alone, 38 per cent on mammography alone and remainder on both.)*

Thier, S.O.: Breast cancer screening: A view from outside the controversy. N. Engl. J. Med., *297*:1063, 1977. *(Editorial by a member of the NIH/NCI consensus development panel.)*

Thiessen, E.V.: Breast self-examination in proper perspective. Cancer, *28*:1537, 1971. *(Suitability depends on breast size and characteristics.)*

Venet, L., Strax, P., Venet, W., and Shapiro, S.: Adequacies and inadequacies of breast examination by physicians in mass screening. Cancer, *28*:1546, 1971. *(Contribution of physical examination greatest in younger age groups. Mammography most useful after 50.)*

103

Screening for Cervical Cancer

Cancer of the cervix is the second most common malignancy among women. In the United States, the incidence of invasive cervical cancer is 20,000, and annual mortality is 8,000. There is a very long asymptomatic period during which cytologic detection is possible. Early therapy is often curative. Appropriately, the Pap smear is one of the most widely used cancer screening tests.

socioeconomic factors are controlled. It has been estimated that a history of first intercourse prior to age 18, parity of 5 or more, multiple sex partners (4 or more), poverty, or prior venereal disease increases the risk of cervical cancer three- to fourfold.

The most compelling risk information comes from the Pap smear itself, in that the risk of carcinoma is 100 times greater in women with dysplasia than in those with a normal cervix.

EPIDEMIOLOGY AND RISK FACTORS

Age and sexual activity are the principal risk factors for cervical cancer.

The age-specific prevalence rates for carcinoma *in situ* follow a bimodal distribution with the dominant, first peak of about 6 per 1,000 women occurring in the 30 to 45 age group. A second peak of about 5 per 1,000 occurs after age 60. The highest carcinoma *in situ* incidence rates are in the 25 to 29 age group. The prevalence of invasive carcinoma is highest in older age groups, rising precipitously after 50. A breakdown in host barriers at the time of menopause has been proposed as explanation for the decreased *in situ* and increased invasive prevalence rates observed in these patients.

Many factors have been associated with cervical disease. Most are related to early sexual activity and multiparity. The incidence is said to be decreased in Jewish women and increased in black women. Socioeconomic status may be the most important predictor inasmuch as the racial disparity is eliminated when

NATURAL HISTORY OF CERVICAL CANCER AND EFFECTIVENESS OF THERAPY

Cervical cancer classically presents with intermenstrual bleeding prompted by coitus or douching. Symptoms invariably occur late in the course of the lesion. Epidemiologic evidence indicates that the natural history of cervical neoplasia should be viewed as a progression from mild dysplasia, through carcinoma *in situ*, to invasive carcinoma. Only a minority of dysplastic lesions progress to carcinoma. It is not clear that carcinoma *in situ* invariably becomes invasive, but epidemiologic data suggest that progression occurs in the vast majority of cases. Both of these premalignant lesions are reliably detected by cytologic techniques.

The duration of the detectable asymptomatic period, as estimated from incidence and prevalence rates, is very long. The mean duration of carcinoma *in situ* varies with age but averages about 10 years. The duration of asymptomatic invasive carcinoma is

5 years for all age groups. It should be emphasized that these are estimated means; the proportion of cervical cancers that become invasive early in their development is not known.

There is no doubt that the earlier the clinical stage of the tumor when detected and treated, the better the prognosis. Survival for carcinoma *in situ* treated with hysterectomy is essentially 100 per cent. But the uncertainty about the natural course of carcinoma *in situ* must be kept in mind. Relative 5-year survival rates for localized and regional invasive carcinoma are about 80 per cent and 40 per cent respectively. The 5-year experience of one screening program demonstrated that 86 per cent of cases detected by cytologic screening were limited to regional invasion, while only 44 per cent of those presenting symptomatically were in this early stage.

SCREENING METHODS AND DIAGNOSTIC TESTS

There are three techniques of cell collection for Papanicolaou staining and cytologic screening of the cervix. The easiest is aspiration from the vaginal pool. More sensitive, but requiring visualization of the cervix with a vaginal speculum, are endocervical swabbing and cervical scraping. The sensitivity of the vaginal aspirate technique has been reported in a range from 62 to 92 per cent in the presence of invasive carcinoma and from 31 to 70 per cent in the presence of carcinoma in situ. The range of reported sensitivities for swabbing is 82 to 92 per cent, for scraping 86 to 100 per cent. There is no consistent difference in detection rates for invasive carcinoma as opposed to carcinoma *in situ* with the swabbing and scraping techniques. The specificity of cytologic diagnosis is very high. In a recent 2-year period, 151 of 25,000 cytologic examinations of the cervix performed at the Massachusetts General Hospital were read as positive. Eighty per cent of these women had uterine cancer. Clearly, more than 99 per cent without disease had negative smears. This high specificity limits the costs associated with false-positive results.

Cytologic smears are not simply positive or negative. Rather, there is a range of findings that reflect various cervical histologies. Doubtful smears may indicate mild or moderate dysplasia or short-term effects of local infection. In such cases, further evaluation and repeat smears should precede referral.

Routine examination of the cervix can be complemented by the use of Schiller's iodine solution. Carcinomatous or dysplastic epithelium does not stain. Such Schiller-negative areas should be biopsied.

Colposcopy is generally not available for routine examination but can play an important role in the evaluation of patients with abnormal cytologic smears or macroscopic abnormalities of the cervix.

CONCLUSIONS AND RECOMMENDATIONS

- The high prevalence, long mean duration of asymptomatic detectable disease, and availability of a highly specific screening test make cervical cancer screening an important task for all primary care providers.
- Known risk factors, including early sexual activity and number of sexual partners, allow selection of high-risk patients and populations.
- Age-specific incidence rates and estimates of preclinical duration indicate that women beyond the usual reproductive age may be at greater risk than generally appreciated.
- Because of the long duration of preinvasive, detectable disease in women of reproductive age, annual screening in the absence of specific risk factors may be unnecessary. Two screens with a short interval (6 months to 1 year) are indicated to reduce the number of false-negative prevalence cases. The interval between subsequent screens can be lengthened for low-risk individuals. The presence of a risk factor, particularly in the menopausal or postmenopausal patient, is an indication for more frequent (i.e., yearly) screening.
- A cytologic smear positive for cancer or severe dysplasia is an indication for referral to a gynecologist for further evaluation, including appropriate biopsies.
- A doubtful smear—suggestive of mild dysplasia—can be further evaluated by the nongynecologist. If a concurrent infection is evident, the smear should be repeated following specific treatment of the infection. If no infection is present, the smear may be repeated after a 3 to 6 month interval. Persistently abnormal smears should be referred for colposcopy or biopsy.

ANNOTATED BIBLIOGRAPHY

Christopherson W.W., *et al.*: Cervix cancer control in Louisville, Kentucky. Cancer, *26*:29, 1976. *(Racial disparity in prevalence explained by socioeconomic variables.)*

Kaiser, R.F., Erickson, C.C., Everett, B.E., *et al.*: Initial effect of community-wide cytological screening on clinical stage of cervical cancer detection in an entire community. J. Natl. Cancer Inst., *25*:863, 1960. *(Reports 5-year experience of early screening program; 86 per cent tumors detected by screening were limited to regional invasion compared to 44 per cent of those presenting symptomatically.)*

Kashgarian, M., and Dunn, J.E.: The duration of intraepithelial and preclinical squamous cell carcinoma of the uterine cervix. Am. J. Epidemiol., *92*:211, 1970. *(Detailed analysis of incidence and prevalence data from Memphis study providing estimates of preclinical duration of disease.)*

Massachusetts Department of Public Health: Papanicolaou testing—Are we screening the wrong women? N. Engl. J. Med., *294*:223, 1976. *(Points out high frequency of screening of young women with low risk.)*

Richart, R.M.: The patient with an abnormal pap smear—Screening techniques and management. N. Engl. J. Med., *302*: 332, 1980. *(Reviews cytologic detection of cervical cancer precursors as well as newer diagnostic and therapeutic approaches utilizing colposcopy and cryotherapy.)*

Richart, R.M., and Vaillant, H.W.: Influence of cell collection techniques upon cytological diagnosis. Cancer, *18*:1474, 1965. *(Reviews sensitivities of endocervical swabbing, cervical scraping and vaginal aspirate techniques.)*

104
Screening for Endometrial Cancer

More than 95 per cent of the cancers of the uterine corpus are adenocarcinomas arising from the endometrium. In the United States, endometrial cancer is a more frequent problem than invasive cervical cancer. Approximately 30,000 cases occur among American women each year. There is some evidence that increases in the incidence of endometrial cancer are parallel to the increased life span among American women, and, more recently, to the increased use of exogenous estrogens among postmenopausal women. Most cases occur in women in whom risk factors are well defined. The tumors often present symptomatically at a time when cure is still possible. Diagnostic tests suitable for indiscriminate screening are not available. It is the responsibility of the primary care provider to be aware of the risk factors and limitations of diagnostic tests, to elicit the pertinent history, and to respond to worrisome symptoms.

EPIDEMIOLOGY AND RISK FACTORS

Advancing age is the single most important risk factor for endometrial cancer. Most tumors occur during the sixth and seventh decades; fewer than 5 per cent occur before age 40. The risk is increased among first-degree relatives of patients with endometrial cancer. Epidemiologic studies have also shown an association with cancer of the breast and cancer of the colon. Case-control studies have also demonstrated a surprisingly high prevalence of obesity and glucose intolerance among patients with endometrial cancer. Between 20 and 80 per cent of patients with tumors were obese, depending on the definition of obesity used in different studies. Up to 40 per cent of patients were found to have diabetes mellitus; this relationship is less clear, partly because of varying definitions of diabetes and the likely correlation with obesity.

Epidemiologic, clinical and experimental data indicating that estrogens, either endogenous or exogenous, play a principal role in the etiology of endometrial carcinoma have been mounting in recent years. The histologic precursor of endometrial cancer is atypical endometrial hyperplasia. Retrospective studies have indicated a progression from cystic hyperplasia through adenomatous hyperplasia to atypical hyperplasia, associated with unopposed estrogen effects. Prospective studies have demonstrated a carcinoma incidence of 10 per cent among patients with atypical endometrial hyperplasia.

A number of clinical syndromes that include

ovarian estrogen excess have been associated with the risk of endometrial cancer. Postmenopausal women with estrogen-secreting tumors have been reported to have a 10 to 24 per cent incidence of endometrial cancer. There is also a high incidence of cancer in patients with polycystic ovary disease; 19 to 25 per cent of young women with endometrial carcinoma have underlying Stein-Leventhal syndrome. It is likely that less well-defined abnormalities of estrogen control explain the association of endometrial cancer with menstrual abnormalities and infertility. Approximately half of all women with endometrial carcinoma and 20 to 30 per cent of married women with endometrial carcinoma are nulliparous.

The principal estrogen in postmenopausal women is estrone, which is peripherally converted from androstenedione produced in the adrenal glands. Peripheral conversion of androstenedione to estrone has been shown to be increased in patients with endometrial cancer, and estrone to estradiol ratios are higher. Peripheral conversion by adipose cells may be the explanatory link between obesity and endometrial cancer.

A number of recent retrospective case-control studies indicate that the use of estrogens postmenopausally substantially increases the risk of endometrial cancer. Rates of endometrial cancer among estrogen users ranged from 4 to 14 times those among control patients in various studies. Several studies have demonstrated dose-response relationship, in that use of estrogen for longer periods of time was associated with greater risk. It has been argued that the association between estrogens and endometrial cancer can be explained in part by a greater likelihood of detection of preexisting tumors in women for whom estrogens are prescribed. Implications of the association for estrogen treatment of menopausal symptoms are discussed in Chapter 114. Recent case-control data suggest a decreased risk among users of combination birth control pills but an increased risk among women exposed to Oracon, a sequential pill containing ethinyl estradiol.

NATURAL HISTORY OF
ENDOMETRIAL CANCER
AND EFFECTIVENESS OF THERAPY

Postmenopausal bleeding, by far the most common symptom associated with endometrial cancer, must always be pursued aggressively. Clinical studies have indicated that, depending on patient selection, cancer is the explanation in from 10 to 70 per cent of women who present with postmenopausal bleeding. In one review of over 400 presentations of bleeding at least 2 years after menopause, 16 per cent of patients had endometrial cancer. The likelihood of malignancy increased with the span of years since menopause.

In a series of over 500 patients from the Mayo Clinic, nearly all presented with postmenopausal bleeding or similar symptoms; only 3 per cent of the tumors were detected in asymptomatic women. In this series, there was little if any correlation between the duration of symptoms and the clinical stage of the tumor at the time of diagnosis. The prognosis for endometrial cancer is generally favorable. In the Mayo series, a 75 per cent 5-year survival rate was reported.

DIAGNOSTIC TESTS

Available data suggest that endometrial cancer almost always presents with early symptoms. There is little evidence that cytopathologic screening can appreciably advance the time of diagnosis in most patients. The diagnosis of endometrial cancer can be made on the basis of a Pap smear of cells aspirated from the vaginal pool or scraped from the cervical os. However, a number of studies have indicated that the sensitivity of the Pap smear in the diagnosis of endometrial cancer is only 70 to 80 per cent. A retrospective review of patients with endometrial cancer who had Pap smears during the year prior to diagnosis found that only 18 per cent had smears that were suggestive of cancer.

Jet wash techniques have been advocated for more direct sampling of the uterine cavity. However, one study of patients without suspected cancer showed that cells extracted with this technique provided a diagnosis in only 3 of 7 cases of adenocarcinoma. None of the tumors that eventually proved to be early and focal were detected by the jet wash method. While cytologic tests may be useful in the diagnostic workup of the patient with symptoms, they cannot be considered useful for screening. Furthermore, a negative test in a symptomatic woman must be followed by endometrial biopsy.

SUMMARY AND CONCLUSIONS

Endometrial carcinoma is a source of substantial morbidity and mortality and has well-defined risk factors. Evidence indicates that endogenous and exogenous estrogen stimulation plays an etiologic role.

While Pap smears potentially advance the diagnosis of cervical cancer, there are no tests as suitable for endometrial cancer screening. A prompt diagnostic workup, including endometrial biopsy, must be initiated by the primary care provider in patients presenting with postmenopausal bleeding.

ANNOTATED BIBLIOGRAPHY

Antunes, C.M.F., Stolley, P.D., Rosenshein, N.B., *et al.*: Endometrial cancer and estrogen use. N. Engl. J. Med., *300*:9, 1979. *(Overall sixfold risk in estrogen users. Increased risk with dose and duration. Stage 0 and 1 tumors are more common in estrogen users.)*

Burke, J.R., Lehman, H.F., and Wolf, F.S.: Inadequacy of Papanicolaou smears in the detection of endometrial cancer. N. Engl. J. Med., *291*:191, 1974. *(Only 18 per cent of Pap smears taken within a year of presentation with endometrial cancer were suggestive of malignancy.)*

Horwitz, R.I., Feinstein, A.R.: Alternative analytic methods for case-control studies of estrogen and endometrial cancer. N. Engl. J. Med., *299*:1089, 1978. *(Points out the potential of bias in case-finding but does not refute increased risk.)*

Jick, H., Walker, A.M., and Rothman, K.J.: The epidemic of endometrial cancer: A commentary. Am. J. Publ. Health, 70:264, 1980. *(Reviews the time series and cross-sectional data supporting the association between estrogen therapy and endometrial cancer and estimates 15,000 cases attributable to estrogens during the period 1971–1975.)*

Knab, D.R.: Estrogen and endometrial carcinoma. Obstet. Gynecol. Surv., *32*:267, 1977. *(Succinct review of clinical and experimental evidence linking estrogen effects with endometrial carcinoma.)*

Lucas, W.E.: Causal relationships between endocrine-metabolic variables in patients with endometrial carcinoma. Obstet. Gynecol. Surv., *29*:507, 1974. *(Exhaustive review with 255 references.)*

Mack, T.M., Pike, M.C., Henderson, B.E., *et al.*: Estrogens and endometrial cancer in a retirement community. N. Engl. J. Med., *294*:1262, 1976. *(Retrospective study indicating risks of approximately 8 times control risks for estrogen users.)*

Malkasian, G.D., McDonald, T.W., and Pratt, J.H.: Carcinoma of the endometrium. Mayo Clin. Proc., *52*:175, 1977. *(Detailed review of 523 cases with 74 per cent 5-year survival rate.)*

Pachecho, J.C., and Kempers, R.D.: Etiology of postmenopausal bleeding. Obstet. Gynecol., *32*:40, 1968. *(Sixteen per cent of 401 women with postmenopausal bleeding had endometrial cancer.)*

Rodrigues, M.A., *et al.*: Evaluation of endometrial jet wash technique in 303 patients in a community hospital. Obstet. Gynecol., *43*:392, 1974. *(Only 3 of 7 cases detected; none of 3 focal tumors detected.)*

Smith, D.C., Prentice, R., Thompson, D.J., and Hermann, W.L.: Association of exogenous estrogen and endometrial carcinoma. N. Engl. J. Med., *293*:1164, 1975. *(Case-control study showing 4.5 times greater risk among exposed women.)*

Weiss, N.S., and Sayvetz, T.A.: Incidence of endomentrial cancer in relation to the use of oral contraceptives. N. Engl. J. Med., *302*:551, 1980. *(Case-control study suggesting decreased endometrial cancer risk among users of combination birth control pills but increased risk among users of Oracon, a particular brand of sequential pills. Accompanying editorial is noteworthy.)*

Weiss, N.S., Szekely, D.R., and Austin, D.F.: Increasing incidence of endometrial cancer in the United States. N. Engl. J. Med., *294*:1259, 1976. *(Cross-sectional data indicating sharp increases in incidence during the 1970s.)*

Wynder, E.L., Escher, G.C., and Mantel, N.: An epidemiological investigation of cancer of the endometrium. Cancer, *19*:489, 1966. *(Extensive retrospective study indicating obesity is a major risk factor.)*

Ziel, H.K., and Finkle, W.D.: Increased risk of endometrial carcinoma among users of conjugated estrogens. N. Engl. J. Med., *293*:1167, 1975. *(Case-control study showing risk increasing with duration of exposure.)*

105
Vaginal Cancer
and Diethylstilbestrol

Vaginal cancer is a rare disease, accounting for approximately 1 per cent of gynecologic malignancies. More than 90 per cent of vaginal cancers are squamous cell tumors. Elderly women are at greatest risk, and because of the extensive lymphatic drainage of the vagina, the 5-year survival rate is only 20 to 25 per cent.

Of greater concern to the primary care provider is adenocarcinoma, or clear-cell carcinoma of the vagina, which occurs in young women who were exposed to diethylstilbestrol or other synthetic estrogens *in utero*. While these tumors are quite rare, the population at risk is large. Increasing public awareness and concern bring many patients to their doctors with questions regarding diethylstilbestrol exposure. The primary physician must carefully follow the literature on the natural history of this malignancy if he is to appropriately counsel and evaluate these patients.

DIETHYLSTILBESTROL AND
VAGINAL CANCER

Diethylstilbestrol is a synthetic estrogen first produced in 1938. After early studies indicated it was helpful in preventing spontaneous abortion, it and other synthetic estrogens were used extensively from the 1940s until 1971 in pregnant women at risk for miscarriage. It has been estimated that between 100,000 and 160,000 women born between 1960 and 1970 were exposed to diethylstilbestrol or similar drugs *in utero*. Because these agents were used more extensively in the 40s and 50s, well over 1 million women are estimated to have been exposed.

In 1970, a cluster of cases of the then very rare adenocarcinoma of the vagina, occurring in daughters who had been exposed to DES *in utero*, was reported from Massachusetts General Hospital. Since that time, the association has been confirmed, and several hundred cases of clear-cell carcinoma have been recorded and investigated. A history of DES exposure has been elicited in approximately two-thirds of all cases of malignancy.

A subsequent prospective study of 110 exposed women detailed the abnormalities of the cervix and vagina that can be found in women at risk, in addition to clear-cell carcinoma. Vaginal adenosis, the presence of glandular epithelium in the vagina, was found in 35 per cent of exposed women, but in only 1 per cent of matched controls. Cervical erosion was present in 84 per cent of exposed women and in only 38 per cent of controls. Gross structural abnormalities of the cervix were found in 22 per cent of exposed women, but were not found among controls. No cases of carcinoma were identified in this study. The cumulative incidence of carcinoma in exposed daughters is not known; estimates of from 1 per thousand to 1 per 10,000 have been made. All abnormalities of the vagina and cervix identified to date occur more commonly in women who were exposed early *in utero*, particularly before 18 weeks of gestation.

While tumors have been identified in preteenage patients as young as 8, more than 90 per cent of tumors have been found in daughters 14 or older. The majority of tumors occur between ages 14 and 20, suggesting that the period of greatest risk occurs when the abnormal vaginal or cervical epithelium is stimulated by ovarian hormones with the onset of puberty. It is too early to say with certainty whether the decreased incidence after age 20 indicates a true decrease in risk with age or is a result of the current age distribution of the cohort at risk.

SYMPTOMS AND NATURAL HISTORY OF
VAGINAL CANCER AND
EFFECTIVENESS OF THERAPY

The natural history of clear-cell carcinoma is still unfolding. Most cases present with abnormal vaginal bleeding or discharge, but because of increasing public and professional awareness, an increasing percentage of cases are detected in the asymptomatic stage. Adenosis has been found in proximity to adenocarcinoma in over 95 per cent of cases, and is therefore considered a malignant precursor by some. Transitions from adenosis to carcinoma have not, however, been documented.

Limited follow-up information indicates that clear-cell carcinoma is an aggressive tumor. Metastases have been found at the time of surgery in 17 per cent of cases of Stage 1 disease and in the majority of cases of Stage 2 disease. Short-term follow-up of registry cases of clear-cell carcinoma has indicated that recurrence, death, or both occur in approximately 25 per cent of patients.

DIAGNOSTIC TESTS

Although the discovery of abnormal cytology has led to the detection of some cases of clear-cell carcinoma, the Pap smear has been shown to have a relatively low sensitivity (80 per cent) for detecting this lesion. This may be explained by the relatively high degree of differentiation of the neoplastic cells, which may resemble endocervical cells. The cells may also be obscured by a heavy polymorphonuclear infiltration. The initial examination of a woman exposed in utero to diethylstilbestrol or similar drugs must therefore include, in addition to direct inspection of the vagina and cervix and cytologic sampling, careful Schiller's iodine staining and biopsies of areas that appear red or fail to stain with the iodine solution. Colposcopy is a complementary procedure. It is particularly useful in patients with abnormal iodine staining or cytology. Colposcopy should be performed by an experienced gynecologist.

CONCLUSIONS AND RECOMMENDATIONS

- As many as 1 million women are at risk for abnormalities of the genital tract, including clear-cell adenocarcinoma, because of *in utero* exposure to diethylstilbestrol or other synthetic estrogens.
- Risk of malignancy among exposed women is low. Nevertheless, because of the significant morbidity and mortality associated with these tumors, careful case-finding and evaluation are indicated. Since routine screening procedures such as the Pap smear are inadequate, patients at risk must be identified by careful history-taking if they are to receive proper evaluation and counseling.
- It is recommended that exposed daughters with symptoms such as vaginal discharge or bleeding be promptly examined regardless of age. Asymptomatic daughters with a history of exposure should have an initial evaluation at age 14 with subsequent yearly examinations.
- More frequent examinations are advised when extensive epithelial changes are present. When possible, such examinations should be performed by a gynecologist experienced in the use of the colposcope.

ANNOTATED BIBLIOGRAPHY

Heinonen, O.P.: Diethylstilbestrol in pregnancy: Frequency of exposure and usage pattern. Cancer, *31*:573, 1973. *(Drug utilization data for 1960s indicated that 100,000 to 160,000 women born in the U.S. during that decade were exposed in utero.)*

Herbst, A.L., Kurman, R.J., Scully, R.E., and Poskanzer, D.C.: Clear-cell adenocarcinoma of the genital tract in young females. N. Engl. J. Med., *287*:1259, 1972. *(Registry report of 91 cases 2 years after the initial report of 7 clustered cases in* Cancer *in 1970.)*

Herbst, A.L., Poskanzer, D.C., Robboy, S.J., *et al.*: Prenatal exposure to stilbestrol: A prospective comparison of exposed female offspring with unexposed controls. N. Engl. J. Med., *292*:332, 1975. *(Prospective examination of 110 exposed and 82 unexposed females. No cancers were found, but adenosis and other abnormalities were common among exposed individuals.)*

Herbst, A.L., Scully, R.E., and Robboy, S.J.: Effects of maternal DES ingestion on the female genital tract. Hosp. Pract. October, 1975. *(General review with update of registry cases.)*

106
Evaluation of Abnormal Vaginal Bleeding

Vaginal bleeding that occurs at an inappropriate time or in an excessive amount may be a sign of important pathology or simply a manifestation of a functional disorder. In postmenopausal women, cancer is the principle concern, accounting for about 25 per cent of cases in this age group. A number of confusing terms have been used to describe the timing, duration and amount of abnormal bleeding, including polymenorrhea (frequent but regular episodes of uterine bleeding), menorrhagia (bleeding normal in timing but excessive in amount and duration), metrorrhagia (excessive, prolonged bleeding occurring at irregular intervals), and epimenorrhea or intermenstrual bleeding (occurring between otherwise normal menstrual periods).

The primary physician needs to distinguish the patient with dysfunctional bleeding from one likely to have pelvic pathology and to decide when referral for a D&C or other diagnostic procedure is indicated. The task is particularly important and often difficult in the perimenopausal woman, because the alteration in menstrual activity coincides with the time that the incidence of malignancy increases.

PATHOPHYSIOLOGY AND CLINICAL PRESENTATION

Dysfunctional bleeding is defined as abnormal bleeding in the absence of tumor, inflammation or pregnancy. The pathophysiology varies with the age of the patient. In teenagers, immaturity of the hypothalamic-pituitary-gonadal axis is often responsible. In women of reproductive age, emotional or physical stress may alter hypothalamic-pituitary function and disturb the menstrual cycle. Abnormal bleeding may also result from ovarian dysfunction with inadequate progesterone production due to alterations in LH-FSH secretion, which can be triggered by stress (see Chapter 107). In the perimenopausal woman, bleeding accompanies anovulation due to onset of senile ovarian failure.

Unruptured ovarian follicles persist, and functioning corpora lutea are absent. The endometrium shows hyperplasia due to unopposed estrogen effect; there is little if any secretory pattern because of the lack of progesterone. Ovulation does not occur, and bleeding results when progesterone production returns or excessive proliferation results in sloughing of the overstimulated endometrium. This condition results in irregularity of the menstrual interval, periods of amenorrhea, and episodes of very heavy and prolonged bleeding when the heavily built-up endometrium finally sheds.

Anatomic lesions of the uterus, tubes and ovaries can result in abnormal vaginal bleeding. In general, ovulation continues in such cases, and the normal menstrual intervals are preserved, but there is intermenstrual bleeding or excessive menstrual blood loss. *Uterine fibroids* are the most common cause and are estimated to occur in 30 per cent of women over the age of 35; they account for about one third of cases. Only those fibroids that are submucosal in location and involve the uterine cavity lead to bleeding. Since they are so common, they may coexist with another cause of abnormal vaginal bleeding. Periods are often very heavy. *Carcinoma of the cervix* is among the most important sources of abnormal bleeding, though it accounts for only about 3 per cent of cases. Bleeding is often postcoital, typically intermenstrual and described as slight spotting. It results from surface ulceration which may occur in early stages of the disease. *Cervical polyps* and *cervical erosions* due to cervicitis present similarly, with slight spotting noted intermenstrually, especially after coitus. *Adenocarcinoma of the endometrium* is an important cause of bleeding in the postmenopausal woman, but almost 20 per cent of cases are detected in menstruating women, though very rarely before 40. Heavier than normal periods, as well as intermenstrual blood loss, are noted. Initially, the intermenstrual problem is reported as a watery discharge containing small amounts of blood. *Ovarian tumors,* whether benign or malignant, rarely result in abnormal bleeding, unless they are endocrinologically active.

Retained products of gestation represent a very common cause of abnormal uterine bleeding after abortion; blood loss is often heavy. *Ectopic pregnan-*

cy is characterized by delay of the regular period, followed by spotting, often in conjunction with unilateral pelvic pain. Intraperitoneal hemorrhage results if there is tubal rupture, but this occurs in less than 5 per cent of cases. A careful menstrual and contraceptive history is most useful.

Pelvic inflammatory disease may alter the normal pattern of menstrual bleeding by disturbing ovarian function, as well as affecting the endometrial surface. *Intrauterine devices* also alter the endometrial surface and can be similarly responsible for heavy menstrual bleeding or intermenstrual bleeding.

Bleeding may be associated with *hypothyroidism* or *hyperthyroidism;* these can produce abnormally heavy periods. *Oral contraceptives* can cause intermenstrual spotting, so-called breakthrough bleeding. *Bleeding diatheses* or *iron deficiency* may present as abnormally heavy periods.

DIFFERENTIAL DIAGNOSIS

Abnormal vaginal bleeding can be broadly divided into anatomic, dysfunctional, inflammatory, endocrinologic and hematologic etiologies with vaginal, uterine, tubal and ovarian sources (see Table 106–1).

Table 106–1.   Important Causes of Abnormal Vaginal Bleeding

Anatomic Lesions
1. Uterine fibroids
2. Cervical erosions
3. Cervical polyps
4. Retained products of gestation
5. Ectopic pregnancy
6. Carcinoma of the endometrium
7. Carcinoma of the cervix
8. Ovarian neoplasms

Dysfunctional Bleeding
1. Immaturity or senescence of the hypothalamic-pituitary-ovarian axis
2. Inadequate luteal phase
3. Ovarian senescence
4. Endometriosis

Inflammation
1. Pelvic inflammatory disease
2. Intrauterine devices

Endocrine Disturbances
1. Hyperthyroidism
2. Hypothyroidism
3. Oral contraceptive use

Hematologic Disturbances
1. Bleeding diatheses
2. Iron deficiency
3. Anticoagulation therapy

WORKUP

History. One should first attempt to establish whether any vestige of menstrual regularity remains since hematologic and anatomic lesions (with the exception of pregnancy) usually do not interfere with ovulation. Dysfunctional bleeding of the anovulatory type is suggested by complete irregularity of menstrual periods and months of amenorrhea. Although it is useful to assess the severity of bleeding (for example, by inquiring into the number of pads used), such information is more helpful for management than for diagnosis. More important is obtaining information on the patient's normal menstrual cycle, its duration, frequency and intensity, and how the current bleeding pattern compares to it. The presence of postcoital bleeding, trauma, IUD, hormone or drug use, recent abortion, unprotected intercourse, breast engorgement, morning sickness, emotional stress, weight loss, iron deficiency anemia, symptoms of hypothyroidism, easy bruising, abdominal pain or dyspareunia can be useful for determining etiology. Shoulder pain representing diaphragmatic irritation from abdominal bleeding may be reported.

Physical Examination. Assessment of vital signs should include a check for postural drop in pressure, suggesting significant loss of intravascular volume. Pallor, skin changes indicative of hypothyroidism, petechiae or purpura need to be noted. A thorough speculum and bimanual pelvic examination is essential, taking particular care to note any cervical erosions, uterine or adnexal masses, or focal tenderness.

Laboratory Studies. A Pap smear of the cervix is mandatory for proper assessment of cervical lesions. Vaginal cytologic sampling is especially important in older women, because endometrial cancer is a concern. Acetic acid may need to be added to cytology preservative if the smear sample is bloody.

In patients aged 12 to 58, pregnancy is always a possibility. Urine should be tested for the presence of human chorionic gonadotropin (HCG); a negative result within 6 to 7 weeks of the last menstrual period does not rule out a pregnancy. A complete blood count will help assess the severity of blood loss, and a peripheral smear may show signs of iron deficiency. Evaluation for a bleeding diathesis is indicated in the presence of petechiae or purpura and should include a platelet count, bleeding time, prothrombin time, partial thromboplastin time, and perhaps fibrin or split products. A TSH and free T_4 will detect hypothyroidism (see Chapter 100). A cervical culture for gonorrhea as well as for other organisms is needed in the patient with pain on motion of the cervix and adnexal tenderness (see Chapter 113); an elevated sedimentation rate supports a suspicion of pelvic inflammatory disease. When a pelvic mass is detected on pelvic examination, an ultrasound examination can help in determining whether the lesion is solid or cystic.

INDICATIONS FOR REFERRAL

Any patient with abnormal vaginal bleeding who has a mass lesion, an abnormal Pap test, or a high risk for carcinoma of the cervix or endometrium (see Chapters 103 to 105) should be referred to a gynecologist. The consultation is especially important for any postmenopausal woman who experiences the new onset of staining or bleeding. Perimenopausal and postmenopausal patients will usually require a D&C to ensure the absence of malignancy. In one retrospective series, 23 per cent of women with postmenopausal bleeding were found to have endometrial carcinoma. Immediate hospital admission and gynecologic consultation are essential if ectopic pregnancy is a possibility, because life-threatening hemorrhage is a real, albeit slight, risk. The same applies in cases of recent abortion, because placenta tissue may be retained. Bleeding in pregnancy is a definite indication for an emergency obstetric consultation. Nonpregnant women who are not bleeding heavily can be referred on an ambulatory basis.

SYMPTOMATIC MANAGEMENT AND PATIENT EDUCATION

Symptomatic management of dysfunctional bleeding can be accomplished by the primary care physician. Dysfunctional bleeding can be stopped in most patients by administration of progestational agents. *Ethinyl estradiol* (Estinyl) 0.05 mg. once daily, or up to three times daily, can be administered to control bleeding, followed by *medroxyprogesterone* (Provera), 10 mg. daily for 7 days, then discontinued for one week to await bleeding. A period of observation for the return of normal cycles should follow. If bleeding recurs and precipitating factors such as drugs or emotional stress have been ruled out, maintenancy therapy may be employed. In patients who do not desire pregnancy, estrogen-progestin combination pills may be used. Patients who would like to conceive should be referred. In young patients with anovulatory dysfunctional bleeding, oral contraceptives may regularize periods and control blood loss, but will not alter the underlying cause.

Correction of any iron deficiency (see Chapter 83) or hypothyroidism (see Chapter 100) should be carried out, and any pelvic infection treated (see Chapter 113).

When anovulatory bleeding is diagnosed, it is important for the patient to know that reproductive capacity is not lost, that the condition is usually self-limited, and that the possibility of malignancy is low under the age of 40. Directing attention to any contributing situational stresses may prove beneficial. Patients experiencing breakthrough bleeding on low-dose estrogen oral contraceptives need to be queried to be sure they are strictly adhering to their regimen (see Chapter 115). If they are taking the medication on schedule, switching to another preparation with a slightly greater estrogen dose is indicated.

The perimenopausal patient who is being referred to the gynecologist usually ought to be told that further assessment for the possibility of malignancy is necessary. When discussed openly, the concerns which most patients already harbor can be addressed and often lessened, since the majority of cases are not likely to be cancerous.

ANNOTATED BIBLIOGRAPHY

Aksel, S., and Jones, G.S.: Etiology and treatment of dysfunctional uterine bleeding. Obstet Gynecol., *44*:1, 1974. (*A study to determine specific FSH and LH patterns associated with dysfunctional uterine bleeding.*)

Isaacs, J.H., and Ross, F.H.: Cytologic evaluation of the endometrium in women with postmenopausal bleeding. Am. J. Obstet Gynecol., *131*:410, 1978. (*A retrospective series of 143 women with postmenopausal bleeding found endometrial carcinoma in 23 per cent. A prospective study in 69 showed good correlation of endometrial cytology with curettage results, but 1 out of 9 carcinomas was missed.*)

Quick, A.M.: Menstruation in hereditary bleeding disorders. Obstet. Gynecol., *28*:37, 1966. (*An excellent discussion of the role of hematologic pathology in abnormal menstrual bleeding.*)

Reyniak, J.V.: Dysfunctional uterine bleeding. Reprod. Med., *17*:293, 1976. (*A thorough review of the problem.*)

Scommegna, A., and Dmowski, W.P.: Dysfunctional uterine bleeding. Clin. Obstet. Gynecol., *16*:221, 1973. (*Another comprehensive review.*)

Shane, J.M., Naftolin, F., and Newmark, S.R.: Gynecologic endocrine emergencies. JAMA, *231*:393, 1975. (*A succinct review of gynecologic endocrine emergencies that cause uterine bleeding.*)

107
Evaluation of Secondary Amenorrhea

Amenorrhea is defined as the absence of menstruation in a woman of reproductive age. In the United States, the mean age for menarche is 13.3 years (range 11 to 17); the mean age for menopause is 49 (range 35 to 55). Primary amenorrhea is defined as failure of menstruation to occur by age 17. Secondary amenorrhea is defined as cessation of established menses for 6 or more months. In an epidemiologic study of an unselected population, the incidence of secondary amenorrhea was 3.3 per cent.

The primary physician is frequently consulted by the otherwise asymptomatic woman who has missed a period or two. Recent discontinuation of oral contraceptives and fear of pregnancy are commonly encountered. One needs to be able to recognize the common causes of secondary amenorrhea, realize when simple counseling is sufficient, and know when to initiate a more extensive workup, such as gonadotropin assays and tomography of the sella.

PATHOPHYSIOLOGY AND CLINICAL PRESENTATION

Amenorrhea reflects an interruption in the regulation of menstruation. In a normal menstrual cycle, FSH stimulates development of follicles and production of estradiol, which causes the endometrial lining to increase in width and the glands to elongate. At midcycle, there is an FSH-LH surge triggered by high estrogen levels and a small increase in serum progesterone. Ovulation occurs, and estradiol and progesterone are produced by the corpus luteum. Under the influence of progesterone, the endometrial glands become secretory. In the late luteal phase, estradiol and progesterone decline, the stroma becomes edematous, and the blood vessels necrose, resulting in menstrual bleeding.

In secondary amenorrhea, there may be inadequate gonadotropic activity due to hypothalamic or pituitary disease, ovarian failure, local disease of the uterus with normal endocrine function, obstruction of the cervix, or androgen excess.

In the majority of women with secondary amenorrhea, FSH and estrogen stimulation are normal, but cyclic LH secretion is absent. Alterations in the hypothalamic-pituitary axis can be triggered by emotional stress, concurrent illness, sudden weight loss, drugs, or any other significant physical stress. This so-called *functional amenorrhea* occurs in such situations as starting school or a new job, severe illness, anxiety over pregnancy, crash dieting, strenuous athletic training, or use of phenothiazines, reserpine or birth control pills. Periods usually return within a few months. Loss of cyclic LH production may also cause mild hirsutism and acne due to stimulation of ovarian androstenedione, testosterone and estrogen. Prolonged stress may eventually lead to loss of LH release. The amenorrhea noted after oral contraceptive use rarely lasts more than 6 months unless there is a history of a previous menstrual disorder. The incidence of postpill amenorrhea lasting more than 6 months is less than 1 per cent.

Pituitary tumors may cause amenorrhea by destroying normal glandular tissue or by stimulating secretion of prolactin. Slow-growing *chromophobe adenomas* may present with amenorrhea, due to decline in LH and FSH production. Amenorrhea can occur prior to changes in the sella turcica or the onset of clinical hypothyroidism, since TSH secretion may continue for a while longer. Headache and visual field loss are late signs of an expanding mass lesion. Some chromophobe adenomas (estimates run as high as 70 per cent) are associated with excess prolactin levels. Recent reports show that previously undetected *microadenomas* can sometimes be found by computed axial tomographic study of patients with secondary amenorrhea and hyperprolactinemia. About 30 per cent of patients with hyperprolactinemic secondary amenorrhea turn out to have radiologically detectable tumors. Many patients with elevated prolactin levels do not have galactorrhea (see Chapter 108).

Polycystic ovarian disease (Stein-Leventhal syndrome) is characterized by amenorrhea, infertility, hirsutism and obesity in conjunction with bilaterally enlarged, polycystic ovaries. Persistent LH secretion is believed to be a major factor. Infertility (found in about 75 per cent of cases), is a common symptom, followed by hirsutism (70 per cent) and amenorrhea (50 per cent).

Bilateral *ovarian tumors* rarely destroy enough ovarian tissue to cause amenorrhea, but granulosa-cell tumors, which produce excess estrogen, and arrhenoblastomas, which synthesize excess androgen, may be responsible for amenorrhea. *Radiation injury* and *cancer chemotherapy* are iatrogenic sources of ovarian failure.

Endometrial scarring from radiation therapy, septic abortion or overly vigorous curettage can produce adhesions which obliterate the uterine cavity (Asherman's syndrome). Similarly, cervical trauma can result in scarring and in obstruction of menstrual flow.

An important endocrine source of amenorrhea is *uncontrolled diabetes mellitus*. When control is adequate, periods are normal, but flagrantly poor control manifested by polyuria, polydipsia, and polyphagia can be complicated by amenorrhea. Marked *hypo-* and *hyperthyroidism* are accompanied by amenorrhea in many instances; other thyroid symptoms are usually evident and often dominate the clinical presentation. Mild hypothyroidism may lead to hyperprolactinemia and amenorrhea. *Cushing's syndrome* is another endocrinologic cause of suppressed periods; symptoms of cortisol excess are usually obvious by the time amenorrhea is present.

DIFFERENTIAL DIAGNOSIS

The causes of secondary amenorrhea can be grouped in an anatomic-pathophysiologic fashion. Common and important etiologies are shown in Figure 107–1. The most frequent etiology, excluding pregnancy, is "functional," reflecting concurrent emotional or physical stress or drug use. In one epidemiologic study, the most important factor associated with development of secondary amenorrhea was age: most cases were found in women under 25 or over 39. In addition, secondary amenorrhea was more frequent in smokers and in divorced or single women.

The true incidence of functional amenorrhea is unknown, because many patients do not come to medical attention, but it certainly represents the vast majority of cases. Pituitary tumors are rare, but are important to detect.

WORKUP (see Fig. 107–1)

Evaluation ought to begin by first ascertaining if the patient is pregnant. A simple *HCG precipitation slide test* performed on a first morning voided urine is more than 90 per cent sensitive when performed 6 weeks after the last menstrual period. If the test is negative and suspicion persists, it can be repeated in

a week, when the HCG concentration will have risen, or serum can be drawn immediately for the more sensitive β-subunit determination.

Once the pregnancy issue is settled, evaluation for other etiologies can proceed. Among the less common causes of amenorrhea, but of greatest consequence to long-term survival, are occult neoplasms of the sellar region. Unlike ovarian or adrenal tumors, these may present with few symptoms other than amenorrhea, making diagnosis difficult unless a high index of suspicion is maintained. However, embarking on an elaborate workup in every patient with amenorrhea is bound to be wasteful, because the incidence of pituitary tumors is so low. High-risk patients who deserve detailed endocrinologic and radiologic study need to be identified.

History. A menstrual history that includes age of onset, character of normal cycles, timing of missed periods, and any prior pregnancies or abortions should be obtained. Detailed inquiry into any emotional problems, changes in eating habits, dieting and drug use is required. The patient should be asked about concurrent stress factors, including recent changes in school, job, family or social relationships. History of sexual activity, contraceptive use and symptoms of pregnancy should be pursued. The patient also needs to be asked about headaches, breast discharge, change in body hair pattern, and symptoms of thyroid or adrenal disease.

Physical examination should include assessment of weight, secondary sex characteristics, and skin; any signs of thyroid or adrenal disease ought to be noted. The breasts are checked for evidence of galactorrhea, masses, or darkening of areola (as seen in pregnancy). On pelvic examination, it is important to check for any clitoromegaly, evidence of estrogenization of vaginal mucosa, appearance of the cervix, patency of the canal, and size of the uterus and ovaries. Rectopelvic examination will help differentiate culde-sac masses from feces or a retroflexed uterus.

When history and physical examination are unremarkable and pregnancy has been ruled out, one needs to decide whether further evaluation is indicated at the present time. The nonpregnant woman who has missed one or two periods, has a normal physical examination and is involved in a stressful situation such as the first year of college or boarding school, a new job or a new city can be observed for 6 months before further workup is planned. If periods have not returned by 6 months and there is no obvious emotional stress to account for the problem, further assessment is indicated.

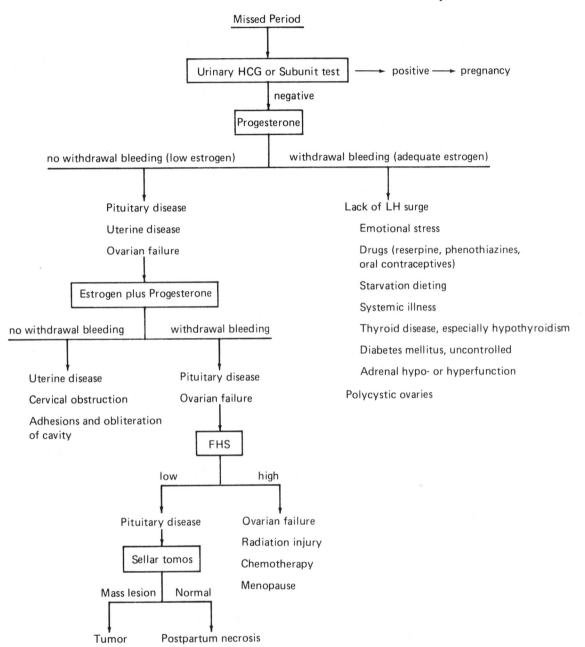

Fig. 107–1.   Evaluation and differential diagnosis of secondary ammenorrhea.

Laboratory studies. The first step of a more detailed assessment (see Fig. 107–1) is to determine if there is sufficient estrogen effect. If there is, it indicates that amenorrhea is due to a disturbance of cyclic LH secretion and progesterone production. Estrogen effect can be assayed by the administration of *exogenous progesterone,* which will result in withdrawal bleeding if estrogen secretion has been adequate. To test the response to progesterone, medroxyprogesterone (Provera) can be administered orally, 10 mg. per day for 5 days, and withdrawal bleeding awaited. Another way to assess estrogen effect is to note the pattern made by *cervical mucus* on a glass slide; the mucus from a patient with normal estrogen levels has a fernlike pattern.

Patients in whom withdrawal bleeding occurs have adequate estrogen, suggesting that the problem involves a lack of LH surge or is due to polycystic disease (if in conjunction with hirsutism, obesity and infertility). The vast majority will have a "functional" type of amenorrhea due to temporarily disturbed LH secretion of hypothalamic origin. Assessment for polycystic ovary disease can be noninvasively done by ultrasound, though persistently elevated *LH levels* are very suggestive of the diagnosis, if the patient is obese, hirsute or infertile. Laparoscopy can be reserved for difficult cases. Patients with normal estrogen effect do not require testing for Cushing's syndrome unless there is clinical evidence of excess cortisol. The same is true for diabetes and thyroid disease, although occult hypothyroidism may trigger an increase in prolactin, which interrupts menses. Thus a TSH is probably worth ordering, though hyperprolactinemia is usually accompanied by low estrogen levels.

Failure of the progesterone to induce bleeding implies inadequate endogenous estrogen production or target organ failure. These patients require a more extensive evaluation for the possibility of pituitary disease, uterine pathology, or inadequate ovarian function.

If bleeding follows administration of estrogen plus progesterone, the problem is either at the hypothalamic-pituitary level and an evaluation for tumor is required, or the difficulty resides with the ovaries. Measurement of *FSH level* will distinguish between these; a four- to fivefold elevation in FSH points to ovarian, low FSH to pituitary disease.

Serum prolactin levels have helped to identify patients likely to have tumors; one third of patients with elevated levels have been found to have mass lesions. However, many of the "prolactinomas" are small; *tomography* and, sometimes, computerized axial tomagraphy are necessary for their detection. The importance of detecting these "microadenomas" derives from the fact that they may enlarge dramatically with pregnancy and stay enlarged, leading to possible compression of adjacent structures. On conventional tomograms of the sella turcica, small prolactinomas are symmetrical and give a double contour to the sellar floor. Thus, in the patient with amenorrhea that persists for 6 to 12 months, one might obtain a serum prolactin level; if it is elevated in the absence of hypothyroidism or recent phenothiazine or oral contraceptive use (known stimuli to prolactin secretion), an aggressive search for pituitary tumor should be undertaken.

INDICATIONS FOR REFERRAL

Patients found to have ovarian failure, suspicion of Stein-Leventhal syndrome, or uterine scarring should be sent to the gynecologist for further evaluation. Virilization deserves consultation with the gynecologist and endocrinologist, though serum testosterone, androstenedione, and urinary 17-ketosteroid levels can be obtained prior to referral. Evaluation for a pituitary neoplasm should be done in conjunction with the endocrinologist and neuroradiologist. In any patient in whom amenorrhea of unclear etiology has persisted for 12 months, the opinion of a subspecialist may be reassuring to both patient and primary physician.

SYMPTOMATIC THERAPY

Since functional amenorrhea is a harmless condition, there is no medical need to reestablish menstrual cycles by prescribing estrogen-progesterone combinations. However, some women request medication to induce a period because they are uncomfortable living with the uncertainty of waiting for resumption of normal flow.

Even though the spontaneous recovery rate for women with functional amenorrhea is quite high, in some patients it may be palliative to provide psychological reassurance by administering a trial of a progestogen to induce menstrual shedding. Progesterone should not be administered more frequently than every other month to allow for observation of the return of spontaneous menses. A typical dose is 10 mg. of medroxyprogesterone for the first 5 days of every other month.

PATIENT EDUCATION

The first priority is to inform the patient who presents with one or two missed periods as to whether or not she is pregnant. Sometimes this essential communication is forgotten. In addition, the primary physician can reassure the patient with functional amenorrhea that menstrual bleeding is not essential for health and that periods usually return within a few months, often soon after resolution of a stressful situation. Patients whose amenorrhea followed use of oral contraceptives can be reassured that they have not been rendered infertile and that normal ovulatory periods resume in over 99 per cent of patients by 6 months. If conception is not desired, the need for mechanical contraception should be stressed, because the incidence of spontaneous ovulation is high in functional amenorrhea.

ANNOTATED BIBLIOGRAPHY

Boyar, R., Kapen, S., Weitzman, E., et al.: Pituitary microadenoma and hyperprolactinemia. N. Engl. J. Med., *294*:263, 1976. *(Secondary amenorrhea with hyperprolactinemia and no galactorrhea. Microadenomas found on polytomograms.)*

Farber, M.: Evaluation of secondary amenorrhea. Clin. Obstet. Gynecol., *20*:805, 1977. *(A succinct review emphasizing the central role of the progestin withdrawal test in a cost-effective evaluation.)*

Fries, H., et al.: Epidemiology of secondary amenorrhea. II. A retrospective evaluation of etiology with special regard to psychogenic factors and weight loss. Am. J. Obstet. Gynecol., *118*:473, 1974. *(A comprehensive discussion of the epidemiology of secondary amenorrhea related to weight loss and stressful life events.)*

Jacobs, J.S.: Prolactin and amenorrhea. N. Engl. J. Med., *295*:954, 1976. *(Discusses significance of prolactin evaluation in assessment of amenorrhea.)*

McDonough, P.G.: Amenorrhea—Etiologic approach to diagnosis. Fertil. Steril., *30*:1, 1978. *(A comprehensive review using hypergonadotrophic, hypogonadotrophic, and androgen excess as the physiologic organization of the differential diagnosis.)*

Nakano, R., Hashiba, and N. Kotsuji, F.: A schematic approach to the workup of amenorrhea. Fertil. Steril., *28*:229, 1977. *(A good description of sophisticated endocrine tests used in the precise determination of amenorrhea.)*

Pettersson, F., Fries, H., and Nillius, S.J.: Epidemiology of secondary amenorrhea. I. Incidence and prevalence rates. Am. J. Obstet. Gynecol., *117*:80, 1973. *(A sample of 2000 Swedish women with a 1-year incidence of 3.3 per cent and a prevalence of 4.4 per cent. A relationship to oral contraceptives was found in 16 per cent of the women with amenorrhea.)*

Shearman, R., and Fraser, I.: Impact of new diagnositic methods on the differential diagnosis and treatment of secondary amenorrhea. Lancet, *1*:1195, 1977. *(A prospective series of 90 women who had at least 12 months of secondary amenorrhea; 39 per cent had hyperprolactinemia; 11 per cent had pituitary tumors, and most had galactorrhea or hyperprolactinemia.)*

Shearman, R.P.: Prolonged secondary amenorrhea after oral contraceptive therapy. Lancet, *2*:64, 1971. *(A review of the syndrome of postpill amenorrhea.)*

108
Evaluation of Abnormal Breast Discharge

Discharge from the breast is an abnormal finding except in late pregnancy and the postpartum period. Discharges may be serous, bloody, or opalescent. When a bloody or serous discharge appears, the task is to exclude carcinoma; when galactorrhea is the presenting problem, the possibility of an occult pituitary neoplasm must be evaluated.

PATHOPHYSIOLOGY AND CLINICAL PRESENTATION

Nonmilky unilateral breast discharges reflect local inflammatory or neoplastic lesions. The pathophysiology of inflammatory and neoplastic discharges is straightforward, involving glandular irritation and the production of clear or bloody material. The neoplasms are most often benign. Adenocarcinoma occurs in approximately 5 per cent of all patients with breast discharges, but in 26 per cent of those with bloody discharge. Bloody discharge due to carcinoma may present in the absence of a breast mass.

The pathophysiology of *galactorrhea* is not well understood; it has only a limited relationship to hyperprolactinemia. In the common, idiopathic form of galactorrhea, menses are normal and 85 per cent of such patients have normal prolactin levels. The cause of galactorrhea is believed related to local breast factors after the capacity for lactation has been induced previously by childbirth or another stimulus. Galactorrhea in conjunction with *amenorrhea* is often associated with high prolactin levels, but only 20 per cent of patients with hyperprolactinemia have galactorrhea. Galactorrhea occurs when high levels of prolactin act on a breast primed by estrogen and progesterone, accounting for its occurrence just after pregnancy or use of oral contraceptives. Prolactin secretion may increase as a result of an autonomously functioning prolactinoma, or because of agents acting on the hypothalamus; for example, thyroid-releasing hormone (TRH) may stimulate prolactin, accounting for the association of galactorrhea with hypothyroidism.

The importance of galactorrhea is its relationship to *hyperprolactinemia* and the association of hyperprolactinemia with pituitary adenomas. In one study of 235 patients with galactorrhea, all those with prolactin values above 300 ng. per ml. had pituitary neoplasms; 57 per cent of those with values above 100 ng. per ml. had tumors. In the same series, 6 women with prolactin levels in the normal range of 1 to 20 ng. per ml. were found to have adenomas, but 4 had acromegaly and 1 had had prior radiotherapy, so only 1 patient without acromegaly and with a normal serum prolactin had an untreated tumor.

Galactorrhea may be first noted as an isolated finding by the patient or discovered during the physical examination. Amenorrhea may or may not be concurrent. Occasionally, the patient is discovered to have galactorrhea during an infertility workup. Less frequently, patients present with other symptoms, such as headache or visual symptoms associated with pituitary adenomas.

DIFFERENTIAL DIAGNOSIS

Nonopalescent breast discharges are caused by local intramammary lesions. Benign lesions predominate; in one series, fibroadenosis, ductal papilloma, papillomatosis and papillary cystadenoma accounted for over two-thirds of cases. Less common benign disease include ductal ectasia, squamous metaplasia, fat necrosis, breast abscesses, eczema of the nipple, and mastitis. About 5 per cent are cancers.

The differential diagnosis of galactorrhea includes idiopathic cases, pituitary tumors, drugs, and hypothyroidism. The largest single group of patients (32 per cent in one series) have the idiopathic variety, with normal periods and normal prolactin levels. The hypothalamic-pituitary causes of galactorrhea include prolactin-producing pituitary adenomas, the empty sella syndrome, and, less commonly, craniopharyngiomas or pinealomas. About one-third of pa-

tients with galactorrhea and amenorrhea are found to have neoplasms. Persistent galactorrhea after childbirth accounts for less than 10 per cent of cases. Drugs associated with galactorrhea include oral contraceptives, tranquilizers (phenothiazines, benzodiazepines, haloperidol), and, less commonly, reserpine, methyldopa, isoniazid, and imipramine. Primary hypothyroidism is a definite cause. Galactorrhea has also been associated with heroine addiction.

Various local factors (e.g., chest trauma or breast manipulation) as well as central lesions (e.g., head trauma, sarcoidosis) have been noted in association with galactorrhea.

WORKUP

Serous or Bloody Discharge. In evaluating nongalactorrheic discharge, one needs to inquire about breast masses, previous breast cancer, family history of breast cancer, any prior discharge, breast infections, or biopsies. Careful inspection and palpation of the breasts are obviously essential, as is examination of axillary nodes. Skin lesions, such as Paget's disease of the nipple or herpes zoster, should be noted. Fluid should be expressed and examined for clarity, purulence, and blood. The discharge should be tested for occult blood and sent for cytologic examination.

The patient with a nonbloody, cytologically negative discharge and no breast lumps can be followed expectantly and need not be subjected to further workup at the present time. Alternatively, a local excisional biopsy can be considered. Since carcinoma is a possibility in patients with a bloody discharge, they should undergo mammography and be referred to a surgeon for an opinion regarding local excision or simple mastectomy.

Galactorrhea. The workup for galactorrhea should include questioning about recent pregnancy, abortion, current presence or absence of normal menstrual periods, symptoms of hypothyroidism, and presence of headache or visual complaints. A careful review of drug use, particularly oral contraceptives and major tranquilizers, needs to be pursued. Physical examination ought to include a careful examination of the breast, although no increased risk of breast cancer has been found in patients with galactorrhea. Confrontation testing of the visual fields and fundoscopic examination are important, though usually normal. Any signs of hypothyroidism (see Chapter 100) should be noted, and confirmed by ordering a TSH and free T_4.

The development of prolactin assays and the occasional association of galactorrhea with high prolactin levels and pituitary tumors have made prolactin testing a very important adjunct to assessment; however, prolactin levels may be affected by stress, time of day, sleep or breast stimulation. Accuracy is enhanced by placing a catheter in the patient's vein and having the patient rest in a recumbent position for an hour before a morning sample is drawn. The patient with galactorrhea and amenorrhea is at increased risk for a pituitary neoplasm and should be prolactin tested.

Radiographic examination of the sella turcica should be obtained in any patient with a markedly elevated prolactin level or symptoms and signs suggestive of pituitary adenoma. Formal visual field evaluation by an ophthalmologist or optometrist should be performed in patients with abnormal sella turcica films.

From a practical standpoint, regular menses and a normal prolactin level in a patient with galactorrhea make the likelihood of a clinically important pituitary tumor remote. Patients in whom the likelihood of tumor is low can be followed carefully with periodic determinations of prolactin, usually at 1-year intervals; if prolactin levels become elevated, tomograms of the sella can be ordered.

SYMPTOMATIC MANAGEMENT

Symptomatic management of galactorrhea depends on the degree of concern shown by the patient. In patients who are not bothered by the discharge, no treatment is indicated except for explanation, follow-up, and discontinuation of drugs associated with the production of galactorrhea. In patients with idiopathic galactorrhea who are bothered by the discharge, the most effective treatment is the use of ergot derivatives; their dopaminergic effects lower prolactin secretion, may lessen galactorrhea, and often restore regular menses.

PATIENT EDUCATION

Patients with breast discharges are worried about cancer. Open discussion of their concerns is basic to alleviating excessive fears; the chances of a neoplasm can be reviewed. Fear that may be engendered by the possibility of a pituitary adenoma can be lessened by explaining the slow growth and good prognosis associated with the majority of prolactinomas. The patient with galactorrhea and amenorrhea should be informed that numerous options for induction of fertility are available and that these may be pursued according to the patient's wishes. By providing accurate information, moral support, and close follow-up, the primary physician can prevent a great deal of unnecessary suffering.

ANNOTATED BIBLIOGRAPHY

Adler, R.A.: The evaluation of galactorrhea. Am. J. Obstet. Gynecol., *127*:569, 1977. *(A useful diagnostic classification.)*

Atkins, H., and Wolff, B.: Discharges from the nipple. Br. J. Surg., *51*:602, 1964. *(A review of 203 cases from the Breast Clinic at Guys Hospital; 171 cases without a lump had histologic examination with 71 cases of fibroadenosis, 43 of direct papilloma, 21 of papillary cyst adenomas, and only 14 carcinomas. A treatment plan is proposed.)*

Boyd, A.E., Reichlin, S., and Turksoy, R.N.: Galactorrhea-amenorrhea syndrome: Diagnosis and therapy. Ann. Intern. Med., *87*:165, 1977. *(High basal prolactin levels [150 mg./ml.] that increase by 100 mg./ml. after TRH or chlorpromazine are suggestive of tumor.)*

Frantz, A.G.: Prolactin. N. Eng. J. Med., *298*:201, 1978. *(A well-synthesized review; 17 refs.)*

Gambrell, R.D., Greenblatt, R.B., and Mahesh, V.B.: Postpill and pillrelated amenorrhea-galactorrhea. Am. J. Obstet. Gynecol., *110*:833, 1971. *(A careful study of 10 women with postpill amenorrhea-galactorrhea; 5 had previous amenorrhea. It began while on contraceptives in 3, and after in 3; 4 were identified by physician examinations.)*

Gomez, F., Reyes, F.I., and Faiman, C.: Nonpuerperal galactorrhea and hyperprolactinemia. Clinical findings, endocrine features and therapeutic responses in 56 cases. Am. J. Med., *62*:648, 1977. *(A superb review emphasizing that many cases are without precise diagnosis; prolactin suppression tests were of no value and prolonged observation remains essential. Pituitary adenomas were found in 17, myxedema 2, phenothiazine 6; 27 were considered dysfunctional.)*

Hooper, J.H., Welsh, V.C. and Shackleford, R.T.: Abnormal lactation associated with tranquilizing drug therapy. JAMA, *178*:506, 1961. *(An incidence of abnormal lactation of 26 per cent was found in 100 women receiving tranquilizers; the effect was dose-dependent.)*

Kleinberg, D.L., Noel, G.L., and Frantz, A.A.: Galactorrhea: A study of 235 cases, including 48 pituitary tumors. N. Engl. J. Med., *296*:589, 1977. *(A comprehensive review finding a 2 per cent incidence of pituitary tumors overall and 34 per cent in connection with amenorrhea. The largest*

group, 32 per cent, had idiopathic galactorrhea without amenorrhea. Ergot derivatives are an effective treatment.)

Reichlin, S. (editorial): The prolactinoma problem. N. Eng. J. Med., *300*:313, 1979. *(A succinct statement on the implication of discovering approaches to treating small prolactin-secreting pituitary adenomas.)*

109
Evaluation of Vulvar Pruritus

Vulvar itching in young women is annoying, but rarely a sign of serious illness; in older women it may be a manifestation of malignancy. A specific cause can usually be identified, making etiologic treatment possible. The primary physician needs to be aware of the common vulvar irritants, inflammatory conditions and infestations as well as the appearance of early malignancy so that use of nonspecific therapies and delay in detection of carcinoma are avoided.

PATHOPHYSIOLOGY AND CLINICAL PRESENTATIONS

In the genital area only the vulvar and perineal skin have sensory receptors which trigger the sensation of itching when irritated. The mucosa of the vagina and cervix are not innervated in such a manner. Of the many etiologies of vulvar pruritus, squamous *carcinoma of the vulva* is the most ominous. The typical patient is elderly; 70 per cent of cases appear in women over 60 years of age; however, the condition may appear at any age, and recent data suggest an increasing incidence of carcinoma *in situ* among younger women. Squamous cell carcinoma of the vulva may present with single or multiple papules or macules, which can be confluent or discrete. Spread is to inguinal and deep pelvic nodes. Occasionally, a patient with carcinoma complains of a lump or an ulcerated lesion. Itching may be intense, sometimes in conjunction with a slightly bloody discharge. Delay in presentation is common; often the patient gives a history of unsuccessful trials of topical agents for symptomatic relief from itching. Epidemiologically, there is an association with early menopause, obesity, diabetes and nulliparity.

Premalignant skin changes, referred to as *vulvar dystrophies*, present as thickened white lesions; formerly, such lesions were included under the term "leukoplakia." When there is no atypia, the risk of cancer is nil. Sometimes there is scaling, erythema or a thin pale wrinkled appearance, as in *lichen sclerosus*, which may contain atypical cells. *Paget's disease* of the vulva is a diffuse scaling process involving the anal region as well; in 5 per cent of cases, there is an underlying adenocarcinoma.

Atrophic vaginitis may produce considerable itching. The mucosa is red and thin; sometimes a mild discharge is present. It occurs postmenopausally from estrogen lack and is seen in women who have undergone oophorectomy as well as in normal menopause (see Chapter 114).

Infectious forms of vaginitis are often very itchy, such as those due to *Candida* and *Trichomonas*. Characteristic vaginal discharges are present (see Chapter 112). Infestations with mites or lice are very uncomfortable. *Scabies* produces papular lesions and itching which may occur anywhere on the body; involvement of the skin between the fingers is very characteristic but not always present. *Pediculosis* is confined to areas covered by hair, since eggs are deposited on the hair shafts (see Chapter 187).

Irritations caused by scratching, maceration and chemical agents are common. Deodorants, soaps, douching agents, bubble baths and contraceptive foams may incite allergic reactions or chemical irritations, leading to itching. Some patients habitually scratch themselves, but often the precipitant is inadequate hygiene; the warm moist environment and chafing fosters maceration of skin in conjunction with the itching and scratching. Cutaneous candidiasis may arise in such an environment, especially when the patient is pregnant or diabetic. Pantyhose exacerbate the problem, as does urinary incontinence. Women who shave their pubic hair are often bothered by pruritus.

DIFFERENTIAL DIAGNOSIS

In young women, vaginitis, pediculosis, scabies, chemical irritants, poor hygiene, use of pantyhose, and allergic reactions are the major etiologies of vaginal itching. The same etiologies apply to older women, but atrophic vaginitis and vulvar carcinoma also become major considerations. Premalignant conditions include lichen sclerosus and Paget's disease. Any condition capable of causing pruritus may present with vulvar itching. Primary cutaneous candidiasis is common among obese diabetic women.

WORKUP

It is important to inquire about vaginal discharge, maceration, skin rash, urinary incontinence, vulvar lesions and other sites of itching. Possible irritants and allergens need to be identified, such as creams, soaps, bubble baths, vaginal deodorants, douches, and contraceptive foams. The sexual history or presence of genital itching in partners or roommate may suggest infection or infestation. Information related to the duration of the problem and responses to prior treatments can be useful. Presence of an ulceration or nodule which has persisted or grown should be ascertained.

The vulva and perineal skin is inspected for macules, papules, scaling, erythema, ulcerations, pigmented lesions, hypopigmentation, excoriation, rash, lice, and mites. A close look at the hair shaft may reveal lice eggs (nits), which are pathognomonic of the infestation (see Chapter 187). A speculum examination helps to identify any vaginitis or discharge (see Chapter 112). Inguinal nodes should be palpated. A smear of the discharge for identification of an organism and a urinalysis for glycosuria are the major laboratory studies needed. Any suspicious lesions should be referred for biopsy; lesions can be stained with toluidine blue to direct selection of biopsy sites.

SYMPTOMATIC MANAGEMENT, PATIENT EDUCATION, AND INDICATIONS FOR REFERRAL

The management of vulvar pruritus is most likely to be successful when a specific etiology can be identified. Self-treatments and potentially irritating soaps or creams ought to be stopped. Incontinent patients will benefit from washing and using protective pastes such as zinc oxide. Biopsy-proven lichen sclerosus without atypia may respond to 2 per cent testosterone propionate cream applied two or three times a day for a period of 6 months. Hyperplastic dystrophy without atypia often responds to topical corticosteroid therapy within 6 weeks. Treatments of vaginitis and mite or lice infestations are detailed in Chapters 112 and 187. Atrophic vaginitis may require a topical estrogen cream (see Chapter 114).

When poor hygiene or excessive moisture are suspected to be contributing to the problem, the patient should be instructed to avoid tight garments such as pantyhose and to use absorbent white cotton underwear.

Occasionally, an antihistamine sedative may be used at night to relieve itching and break the itch-scratch cycle. In the absence of infection or other specific etiology, hydrocortisone cream or lotion might be tried. While vaginitis is treated with a specific agent, application of topical hydrocortisone may facilitate symptomatic relief. Persistence of any suspicious lesion requires referral for consideration of biopsy.

ANNOTATED BIBLIOGRAPHY

Friedrich, E.G., Jr.: Lichen sclerosus. J. Reprod. Med., *17*:147, 1976. *(Topical testosterone may be an effective treatment.)*

Friedrich, E.G., Jr.: Vulvar pruritus—A symptom, not a disease. Postgrad. Med., *61*:164, 1977. *(An excellent review.)*

International Society for Study of Vulvar Disease. Committee on Terminology: New nomenclature for vulvar disease. Obstet. Gynecol., *47*:122, 1976. *(The introduction of "dystrophy" to substitute for a confusing collection of terms.)*

Kaufman, R.H.: Hyperplastic dystrophy. J. Reprod. Med., *17*:137, 1976. *(The risk of malignancy is low and is present only in cases that show atypia.)*

Woodruff, J.D., Julian, C., Puray, T., et al.: The contemporary challenge of carcinoma in situ of the vulva. Am. J. Obstet. Gynecol., *115*:677, 1972. *(Emphasizes need for early diagnosis.)*

110
Medical Evaluation of Dyspareunia and Other Female Sexual Dysfunctions
ANN B. BARNES, M.D.

DYSPAREUNIA

Dyspareunia, or painful intercourse, is probably more common than physicians realize because patients may not volunteer the complaint. It often requires an aware and sympathetic clinician to uncover the problem. Pain on intercourse may be the presentation of pelvic disease or a symptom that disrupts a marriage. The primary physician is often in the best position to evaluate the causes and manage the problem.

PATHOPHYSIOLOGY AND CLINICAL PRESENTATION

Several pathogenic mechanisms may be responsible for painful intercourse. They include inflammatory lesions, failure of lubrication, anatomic problems and psychological conflicts. Pain can arise from friction against inflamed tissue or by jarring of deeper inflamed parametrial structures. Failure of normal vaginal lubrication may produce pain or spasm. Physical impediments to penile penetration of the vagina may be due to surgery, inflammation or anatomic variants. The psychological mechanisms of dyspareunia reflect a variety of conflicts, fears and hostility (see Chapter 217).

In premenopausal women, inadequate lubrication because of too little foreplay is among the most frequent causes of dyspareunia. In postmenopausal patients, atrophic vaginitis is an important factor. Scant production of vaginal secretions may also reflect fears, misunderstandings, marital conflicts and hostilities. Concern about venereal disease and cancer are other common underlying issues which can inhibit normal lubrication.

Dyspareunia may be due to anatomic difference between partners, especially when the woman's vagina is functionally or anatomically small. A tight or thick hymenal ring, marked vaginal constriction, or partial fusion of the labia can cause pain on intercourse.

Irritation of the vulva caused by tight-fitting clothes, lack of hygiene, or infection is found in patients complaining of *pain on intromission*. Fungal vulvovaginitis and bacterial infection of the vagina, cervix, and Bartholin's gland duct are common. A cyst of the Bartholin's gland duct occurs when mechanical irritation and the attendant inflammatory reaction obstruct the ductal lumen. Viral vulvitis from herpes vaginalis is usually so painful that intercourse is not attempted. Condylomata can be painful and may bleed, but usually do not inhibit intercourse.

Deep dyspareunia may occur with endometriosis, ovarian cysts, adhesions, and pelvic inflammatory disease. These sources of pain on intercourse cause difficulty when penetration is deep. Penile thrusting moves the entire uterus, with resultant pulling on the peritoneum. Acute or defervescing pelvic inflammatory disease or endometritis will produce pain even on gentle motion.

A thin vulvar surface and vaginal mucosa are less resilient and less resistant to trauma. These vaginal changes take place in women who are anorexic, breast-feeding, or menopausal, or who have had pelvic irradiation.

Vaginismus, defined as involuntary spasm of the perineal muscles induced by any attempt at physical penetration, is an important though uncommon cause of dyspareunia.

DIFFERENTIAL DIAGNOSIS

The causes of dyspareunia can be listed according to whether there is pain on intromission or on deep penetration (Table 110-1).

WORKUP

One needs to determine whether dyspareunia occurred with the first effort at intercourse or has developed recently secondary to organic change or a situational problem. The patient should be asked whether pain occurs before penetration, on penetration or only after deep penetration. It is important to establish whether the patient can insert a tampon without pain; if she can, mechanical obstruction is unlikely. A history of previous surgery, pelvic inflammatory disease or radiation may suggest the etiology. Failure to localize the site of coital pain suggests psychogenic dyspareunia. A history of sexual fears, time spent on foreplay and feelings toward the partner should be sensitively obtained (see Chapter 217). Interviewing the husband or sexual partner is essential to an adequate evaluation. The duration of dyspareunia should be determined, because symptoms which have existed for years may not resolve even after a medical condition is identified and corrected.

The most important part of the workup is pelvic examination. The physician should inspect for signs of vulvovaginitis, atrophic vaginitis, narrowed introitus, cervicitis, and congenital abnormalities. Observation of involuntary spasm on attempted examination suggests vaginismus. Palpation may identify a uterine mass, a retroverted uterus or tenderness. The cervix should be manipulated to see if pain is produced. Examination for loss of pelvic support, rectocele or cystocele is needed. A smear should be obtained for cervical cytology to detect underlying malignancy.

A complete blood count, sedimentation rate, and cervical culture are indicated when there is evidence on physical examination suggesting pelvic inflammatory disease (see Chapter 113). Pelvic ultrasound may be indicated to help define a suspected pelvic mass. Referral to a gynecologist for laparoscopy is indicated when endometriosis, adhesions, or an adnexal mass is under consideration.

SYMPTOMATIC MANAGEMENT, PATIENT EDUCATION, AND INDICATIONS FOR REFERRAL

The patient without organic pathology who is troubled by inadequate lubrication should be sympathetically reassured that she is healthy and provided advice, which may include insisting on more prolonged foreplay and use of a water-soluble lubricant jelly (e.g., Lubafax). Contraceptive creams should not be used for lubrication because they often cause dehydration and may worsen soreness. Oral-genital foreplay, trying different positions for coitus and guiding the man's penis for insertion are other suggestions which can be made. The *postmenopausal* woman with an atrophic vaginal mucosa can be given estrogen cream to use topically on an intermittent basis (see Chapter 114).

Table 110–1. Important Causes of Dyspareunia

PAIN GREATEST ON INTROMISSION	PAIN GREATEST ON DEEP PENETRATION
Inadequate lubrication	Pelvic inflammatory disease
Size discrepancy in partners	Ovarian cyst
Incompletely ruptured hymen	Endometriosis
Bartholin's gland cyst	Pelvic adhesions
Stricture	Relaxation of pelvic support
Inadequate episiotomy	
Vaginitis	
Atrophy of vaginal and vulvar tissue	
Vaginismus	

If there is an underlying vaginal or pelvic infection, it should be treated and the patient advised to refrain temporarily from intercourse (see Chatpers 112 and 113). A cyst of the Bartholin's gland duct may spontaneously drain following frequent warm soaks in the bath tub, which sometimes relieves the obstruction, marsupialization by a gynecologist may be required to provide adequate drainage if the cyst is badly inflamed and infected.

There is no cure for herpes vaginalis; most symptomatic measures are of limited help. The patient must wait for the lesions to heal on their own before resuming intercourse.

Patients bothered by pain on deep penetration may be more comfortable lying on one side during coitus so that deep penetration is limited.

Retained suture material in episiotomy scars, vulvar islands of adenosis (ectopic columnar epithelium) or nerve endings previously damaged by herpetic infection may require local excision for relief of pain.

The patient with a narrow introitus should be referred to a gynecologist for a trial of vaginal dilators. Vaginismus may be managed by education, relaxation and Kegel exercises, all of which are usually best accomplished by an experienced therapist or sex therapy clinic.

Failure to succeed in identifying or relieving dyspareunia should prompt referral to the gynecologist. This ought to be done only after a thorough evaluation has been performed, the sexual history elicited, any infection treated, advice on sexual technique provided, and lubricants have been tried. Referral to a psychiatrist or sex therapist, involving both partners, might also be considered. Nevertheless, constant education and reassurance as to the lack of physical danger associated with the symptom are important when there is no evidence of underlying disease. The patient's fears and concerns must be sensitively explored and specifically addressed, as must any marital discord (see Chapter 217).

EXCITEMENT AND ORGASMIC PHASE DYSFUNCTIONS

Causes of female sexual dysfunction beyond those resulting in dyspareunia have only recently been explored in systematic fashion. Data are still sketchy but are beginning to accumulate. Psychogenic etiologies still predominate.

Excitement phase problems beyond inadequate lubrication are manifested by poor libido. Drug-induced decrease in sexual desire has been identified and is similar to that seen in men. Antihypertensive agents which cross the blood-brain barrier, (e.g., reserpine and methyldopa) sometimes diminish libido. Oral contraceptives, particularly the sequential variety (which are no longer marketed), have depressive and libido-reducing side effects in about 5 to 10 per cent of women who use them. Antidepressants, minor tranquilizers, alcohol, phenothiazines, hypnotics and opiates have been linked to reduction in libido, though it is unclear if it is the underlying emotional problem rather than the drug that is more at fault. Libido is a very sensitive indicator of general physical health, and any intercurrent illness will blunt it. The third trimester of pregnancy often produces a diminution in desire. There is no evidence that estrogen deficiency has an impact on libido, but androgen deficiency does. Loss of androgen synthesizing capacity (e.g., by hypophysectomy or adrenalectomy) can lead to losses of desire and capacity for orgasm.

Orgasmic dysfunction from medical causes is seen in patients who previously functioned normally. In one study, loss of orgasmic capacity among diabetic women was found to have a 35 per cent prevalence. Excitement phase functions were normal, and the severity of the problem correlated with duration of the diabetes. As with excitement phase problems, any illness can interfere with this phase of sexual activity. Usually the problem is global when illness is present, and all sexual functioning is reduced. Correlations between individual disease states and isolated orgasmic dysfunction remain to be further elucidated.

An increasingly common problem is the use of *cytotoxic chemotherapy* in young women with malignancies. There may be a marked loss of libido, lack of lubrication, hypoestrogenism from ovarian failure

and inhibition, as well as hot flashes. The depression which accompanies confronting a chronic, malignant disease, combined with the fatigue which follows surgery and chemotherapy, further distresses patients and impairs sexual functioning. Marital problems may ensue. Patient and partner need to be informed of these side effects of therapy prior to its use, and be supported through therapy. For some women, these side effects are sufficient reason to decline or discontinue such medication. Other women may experience few such side effects and need to be encouraged to sustain contraceptive practices to avoid harm to a developing fetus.

ANNOTATED BIBLIOGRAPHY

Chapman, R.M., Sutcliffe, S.B., and Malpas, J.S.: Cytotoxic-induced ovarian failure in women with Hodgkin's disease I and II. JAMA, *242*:1877, 1979. *(Study of sexual function in 41 women.)*

Fordney, D.S.: Dyspareunia and vaginismus. Clin. Obstet. Gynecol., *21*:205, 1978. *(A comprehensive review emphasizing behavioral therapy and the role of sex clinics; 36 refs.)*

Huffman, J.W.: Office gynecology: Relieving dyspareunia. Postgrad. Med., *59*:223, 1976. *(A useful overview.)*

Kolodny, R.: Sexual dysfunction in diabetic females. Diabetes, *20*:557, 1971. *(Isolated orgasmic phase dysfunction identified in 35 per cent.)*

Lamont, J.A.: Vaginismus. Am. J. Obstet. Gynecol., *131*:632, 1978. *(A review of the presentation and treatment of 80 patients with vaginismus.)*

Solberg, D., Butler, J., and Wagner, N.: Sexual behavior in pregnancy. N. Engl. J. Med., *288*:1098, 1973. *(Third-trimester is associated with reduced libido.)*

Story, N.: Sexual dysfunction resulting from drug side effects. J. Sex. Res., *10*:132, 1974. *(Antihypertensive agents which cross the blood-brain barrier are an important cause of reduced libido.)*

Sutcliffe, S.B.: Cytotoxic chemotherapy and gonadal function in patients with Hodgkin's disease. Facts and thoughts. JAMA, *242*:1898, 1979. *(Comments on treatment of side effects of chemotherapy.)*

111
Approach to the Patient with Pelvic Pain

Pelvic pain is a major source of concern and morbidity in women. Dysmenorrhea or painful periods affect approximately half of menstruating women at some time, and an estimated 10 per cent are incapacitated by the problem, with much time lost from work and school. Acute episodes of pelvic pain are also common and may represent potentially serious pathology. The primary physician should be able to distinguish pain of a functional nature from that due to infection or an anatomic lesion, and know when referral to the gynecologist or urgent hospital admission is indicated. Moreover, one should be able to provide the young woman bothered by dysmenorrhea with rational and effective therapy in conjunction with psychological support.

PATHOPHYSIOLOGY AND CLINICAL PRESENTATION

Acute Pain. Pelvic pain of acute onset may result from pelvic inflammatory disease, ectopic pregnancy, torsion of the tube or ovary, rupture of an ovarian cyst, or extrapelvic pathology such as acute appendicitis or ureteral stone. *Pelvic inflammatory disease* (PID) usually causes little pain until infection has spread from the cervix via lymphatics into the parmetria and fallopian tubes. The process may not occur for weeks or even months after initial contact with an infected partner. The consequent acute salpingitis is characteristically bilateral, though one side may be more involved than the other, and peritoneal signs may follow if pus escapes from the tube and soils the overlying peritoneum. The gonococcus was once considered the predominant offending organism, but more careful bacteriologic investigation based on culdocentesis or laparoscopic sampling of fallopian tubes has revealed other organisms which can produce the infection. It is estimated that gonorrhea accounts for a third to a half of pelvic inflammatory disease; other agents commonly implicated include alpha strep, *E.coli, Staphylococcus aureus,* and anaerobic organisms such as *Bacteroides.* The roles of chlamydia, T-strain mycoplasma, and cytomegalovirus are less well defined (see Chapter 113).

There is a striking association between menstrual periods and onset of gonococcal PID, suggesting that spread from the cervix may occur during menstruation. Prior gonorrhea appears to increase the likelihood of nongonococcal PID, possibly by causing tubal damage. The recurrent nature of PID may be due to fallopian tube damage that impairs bacterial clearance. Pelvic inflammatory disease can be provoked by abortion, endometrial biopsy, hysterosalpingograms, D & C, and hysterectomy. The use of an intrauterine device (IUD) increases the risk of PID, particularly in nulliparous women.

Ectopic pregnancy is a much feared cause of acute pelvic pain, since catastrophic hemorrhage may ensue from tubal rupture. In most cases, the period is delayed by 1 to 2 weeks, followed by recurrent spotting. Severe hemorrhage occurs in less than 5 per cent of cases, causing sudden severe pain and hypotension. There may be mild, unilateral tenderness in those cases without bleeding. Patients with previous PID are at greater risk for ectopic pregnancy.

Torsion of the tube with or without ovarian involvement is seen mostly in young women, many of whom have otherwise normal adnexa. Severe, acute unilateral pain and distention are found without an elevation of white count, fever, or increased sedimentation rate, unless complicated by ischemic necrosis.

Ovarian cysts may spontaneously rupture or twist on their pedicles. Rupture can be associated with marked blood loss, thereby presenting in a fashion similar to that of a ruptured ectopic pregnancy. More commonly, only small amounts of fluid or blood are released, causing milder, often recurrent, discomfort. Torsion of the pedicle can lead to ischemic gangrene of a cyst and present as acute unilateral pelvic pain with local peritoneal signs, fever and leukocytosis. Sometimes the twisting reverses itself spontaneously and only mild intermittent symptoms result.

Chronic Pain. Conditions predisposing to recurrent or chronic pelvic pain are generally less ominous than those responsible for acute pain. Common etiologies include primary dysmenorrhea, endometriosis, adenomyosis, chronic pelvic inflammatory disease, intrauterine devices, ovarian cysts and fibroadenomas.

Pain occurring in conjunction with menstruation is termed *dysmenorrhea* and is defined as *primary* when onset is shortly after menarche and unaccompanied by recognized pelvic pathology. Primary dysmenorrhea beginning months or even a few years after menarche is presumably linked to the onset of ovulatory periods. The condition is believed to result from exaggerated uterine contraction secondary to excess prostaglandin synthesis by the endometrium. Psychogenic factors are thought by some to play a role, perhaps in lowering the threshold for pain. The patient typically complains of crampy or aching pelvic pain, sometimes accompanied by nausea, vomiting and diarrhea. Onset coincides with the signs of menstrual bleeding, and pain can last from several hours to a few days. The natural history of the condition is one of gradual resolution with advancing age, but episodes can occur until menopause. Occasionally, patients experience a remission following childbirth, but there are no studies documenting the frequent claim that childbirth in itself resolves the problem.

The onset of dysmenorrhea after the age of 25 suggests an underlying anatomic lesion. Such episodes of *secondary dysmenorrhea* frequently begin several days before menstruation and may worsen or diminish with the onset of bleeding. Major causes of secondary dysmenorrhea include endometriosis, pelvic inflammatory disease, and IUD use.

Endometriosis is seen mostly in women between the ages of 25 and 45, many of whom are nulliparous; mean age at time of diagnosis is 37. The condition is due to the presence of functioning ectopic endometrial tissue, located in such places as the ovaries, uterosacral ligaments, cul de sac and peritoneum. The origin of the ectopic tissue is unclear. Pain can begin days or even a week before menstruation, tends to subside with bleeding, and is usually bilateral, deep-seated or aching, with radiation to the rectum or perineal region. There is often a history of infertility, dyspareunia, or menorrhagia.

A retroverted and fixed uterus or nodular uterosacral ligaments are sometimes detectable on physical examination. Symptoms due to endometriosis depend on actively functioning endometrial tissue, but bear no relationship to the amount of endometrial tissue present. The condition resolves with menopause, but often hysterectomy is resorted to.

Adenomyosis is related to endometriosis in that there is ectopic endometrial tissue, but it is localized to the myometrium and occurs mostly in older women. Incidence is greatest in women 41 to 50. The condition can cause menorrhagia, dysmenorrhea and an enlarged, sometimes tender, uterus. Pain is referred to the back and rectum as the uterus enlarges. Endometrial carcinoma is found with slightly increased frequency in patients with adenomyosis.

Chronic pelvic inflammatory disease is another source of secondary dysmenorrhea with exacerbation of pain occurring around the time of menstruation. A history of previous venereal disease, dyspareunia, menstrual irregularity, backache, rectal pressure, or pelvic pain with fever is often obtained. The physical examination typically reveals tender, thickened adnexal organs; bilateral involvement is characteristic, though one side may predominate.

Intrauterine devices are an important source of secondary dysmenorrhea and heavy bleeding. The rate of removal because of bleeding and pain ranges from 4 to 15 per cent. The crampy menstrual pain can occur in previously normal patients who never experienced dysmenorrhea; parity has little impact, but bleeding seems to be worse in women whose periods were scanty before IUD insertion.

Benign neoplasms, predominantly dermoid cysts, cystadenomas, and uterine fibroids may produce a chronic aching localized to one side of the pelvis. The pain may be intermittent, secondary to periodic leakage of irritant contents, or, occasionally, chronic. Chronic intermittent discomfort which is worse at the time of ovulation or in the latter half of the cycle is sometimes a feature of benign ovarian lesions. The majority of benign cystic or solid ovarian tumors are painless unless complicated by torsion or rupture, which can produce severe acute abdominal pain. Pain is a rather late feature of cervical, uterine, ovarian or tubal malignancy.

Strictly speaking, *mittleschmerz* or intermenstrual pain is not a form of dysmenorrhea since it occurs in midcycle at the time of ovulation. It is more common on the right side than the left and may be accompanied by bleeding. There is some evidence that the ovary is the source of the blood loss. The pain, believed due to distention of the ovarian capsule, is harmless but annoying and a source of concern.

In the large number of patients who have significant pelvic complaints but in whom no disease is found on repeated examinations, including laparoscopy, a diagnostic classification of *enigmatic pelvic pain* has often been utilized. This syndrome has been characterized as occurring in premenopausal women who have usually borne children. The pain is described as dull; it is localized to the suprapubic area or one or both of the iliac fossae, with frequent referral to the medial aspect of the thighs. Discomfort is usually worse before menstruation, and deep dyspareunia is often reported. Discharge and menorrhagia are sometimes noted; gastrointestional symptoms are rare.

DIFFERENTIAL DIAGNOSIS

The causes of pelvic pain can be organized into acute, chronic and recurrent categories, with the latter group separated by their relationship to the menstrual period (see Table 111-1). Uterine hypoplasia and retroverted uterus are no longer considered causes of dysmenorrhea.

WORKUP

For the patient with acute pain, the first task is to assess the need for immediate hospitalization, because some etiologies are potential medical emergencies. A rectal temperature and a check for postural changes in blood pressure or pulse indicative of significant volume depletion are essential. The abdomen is examined for evidence of peritonitis. Speculum examination is performed for detection of vaginal discharge, bleeding, and any cervical pathology. Bimanual palpation should establish that the pain is pelvic in origin, help to further localize the problem, and identify any masses or distorted anatomy. Exquisite pain on motion of the cervix is a classic finding in

---

Table 111-1.   Important Causes of Pelvic Pain

Acute Pain
  1. Pelvic inflammatory disease
  2. Ectopic pregnancy with rupture
  3. Twisted fallopian tube, ovary or ovarian cyst
  4. Ruptured ovarian cyst
  5. Extrapelvic disease (e.g., appendicitis)
Recurrent Pain with Menstruation
  1. Primary dysmenorrhea
  2. Endometriosis
  3. Adenomyosis
  4. Chronic pelvic inflammatory disease
  5. Intrauterine devices
Recurrent Pain Unrelated to Menstruation
  1. Mittleschmerz
  2. Leaking ovarian cysts
Chronic Pain
  1. Psychogenic pain
  2. Malignancy
  3. Benign neoplasms
  4. Enigmatic pelvic pain

---

acute PID, but the sign is indicative only of generalized pelvic irritation and not pathognomonic for PID. Rectovaginal examination should not be overlooked, because gastrointestinal pathology or a cul de sac mass may be discovered.

The necessary laboratory studies for acute pelvic pain are few, but should be obtained promptly. A complete blood count (CBC), differential, sedimentation rate, urinalysis, and pregnancy test in any woman of reproductive age are of greatest utility; however, obtaining a negative urine HCG test during the first 6 weeks after the last menstrual period does not rule out the diagnosis of ectopic pregnancy.

Any patient with high fever, postural signs or peritoneal signs should be sent directly to the hospital, even before laboratory results are available or detailed history elicited. However, even if the situation is urgent, a few historical facts can help establish the diagnosis. Inquiry is needed into any delay in menstrual period, dyspareunia, IUD use, shaking chills, abnormal vaginal discharge or bleeding, recent abortion, and location and spread of pain. Development of generalized severe pain is a worrisome symptom indicating possible peritoneal involvement, especially in conjunction with a rigid abdomen and absent bowel sounds. Unilateral pain suggests a local tubal or ovarian problem, whereas bilateral involvement is more indicative of PID or another cause of diffuse pelvic irritation. Gastrointestinal and urinary symptoms such as constipation, nausea, vomiting, diarrhea, flank pain, and dysuria need to be asked about in order to avoid mistaking appendicitis, acute pyelonephritis or ureteral stone for a pelvic etiology.

If the pain is chronic or recurrent, a more detailed history should be obtained during the office visit. The relationship of the pain to the menstrual cycle is of central importance. Radiation of the pain may give a clue to its origin. Pain due to cervical, uterine or vaginal pathology is often referred to the low back or buttock, while that which is tubal or ovarian in origin is generally localized to one side and referred to the medial aspect of the thigh. Menstrual and obstetrical history should be elicited in detail. Any emotionally stressful situations should be elucidated. It is essential to find out what the patient understands about menstruation and identify any gaps in her knowledge. A detailed pelvic examination needs to be carried out, looking in particular for adnexal thickening, cervical discharge, uterine masses, fixation of any structures, ovarian masses, and focal tenderness.

Laboratory studies beyond a CBC, SED rate, and urinalysis contribute little to the evaluation unless a mass is felt, in which case ultrasound may help define fibroids and distinguish solid from cystic masses. Laparoscopy or D & C may become necessary to establish a diagnosis.

SYMPTOMATIC MANAGEMENT AND PATIENT EDUCATION

The management of the young woman with *primary dysmenorrhea* requires patience and restraint in use of pain medication. Women may be severely handicapped by menstrual cramping and resort to a variety of over-the-counter medicines for relief of pain. If these do not work, there may be a request for stronger medication. Potentially addictive analgesics have little place in initial management.

The woman with primary dysmenorrhea should first be told that her examination is normal and that other gynecologic problems and infertility are unlikely. Taking time to clear up misconceptions and answer questions about menstruation can be very productive. It is sometimes comforting to explain that many women experience relief as they grow older, but it should be pointed out that there is no controlled evidence to support the notion that childbirth resolves the problem. Warm baths and mild analgesics such as aspirin can provide many patients with some symptomatic relief.

Drug therapy programs are designed to inhibit prostaglandins or have a direct relaxant effect on the uterus. Aspirin in doses of two or three tablets four times a day may provide some pain relief; the drug is a prostaglandin synthetase inhibitor. Patients who have found aspirin ineffective should be treated with more potent prostaglandin inhibitors. Indomethacin, 25 mg. b.i.d., and other nonsteroidal anti-inflammatory drugs, such as ibuprofen, naproxen, and flufenamic acid, have proven to be effective in clinical trials. Studies utilizing vitamin B_6 alone and with magnesium are in progress, based on empirical success in uncontrolled studies.

The beta-2 adrenergic agent terbutaline has been found to reduce the frequency and amplitude of uterine contractions. It may be worth a trial, but side effects of tremor, palpitations and flushes sometimes limit its use. When medication, particularly prostaglandin synthetase inhibitors, is prescribed, the patient should be instructed to begin the drug a day or two before she expects her period. If she is uncertain about the timing of menses, a basal body temperature chart will help to identify ovulation; drug therapy is then best begun 13 days following ovulation.

Since primary dysmenorrhea occurs with ovulation, it can also be treated with oral contraceptives, which will suppress ovulation and relieve cramps in 80 to 90 per cent of patients. Progestins may also inhibit ovulation but are not as effective clinically in alleviating symptoms, perhaps because of their prostaglandin-stimulating effect. Occasionally, a teenager will complain of menstrual pain as an excuse to obtain oral contraceptives.

Pain due to IUD use may be sufficient grounds for removal. Therapy for most causes of secondary dysmenorrhea require gynecologic referral, but PID ought to be treated by the primary physician (see Chapter 113).

INDICATIONS FOR REFERRAL

Patients with a mass lesion detected on physical examination should be referred, though a pelvic ultrasound study may be worth obtaining prior to the visit to the gynecologist. Suspicion of chronic pelvic inflammatory disease, endometriosis, adenomyosis, ovarian cyst, or any other condition that might be better assessed by laparoscopy should lead to consultation with the gynecologist, who may be able to provide reassurance to both patient and primary physician as well as to determine if further assessment is necessary. Surgical therapy for primary dysmenorrhea (involving dilatation of the fibromuscular tissue at the level of the internal os, presacral neurectomy, or uterosacral ligament resection) is worth considering only in severe cases if all other forms of treatment have failed and the patient is severely incapacitated by her symptoms. Hysterectomy is a last resort for patients with secondary amenorrhea who have already fulfilled their reproductive potential.

ANNOTATED BIBLIOGRAPHY

Abraham, G.E.: Primary dysmenorrhea. Clin. Obstet. Gynecol., *21*:139, 1978. *(A good review of physiology, and includes a discussion of the use of vitamin B_6 and magnesium as therapy for dysmenorrhea.)*

Akerlund, M., Anderson, K.E., Ingemarsson, I.: Effects of terbutaline on myometrial activity, uterine blood flow, and lower abdominal pain in women with primary dysmenorrhoea. Br. J. Obstet. Gynecol., *83*:673, 1976. *(Argues that increased uterine pressures are associated with dysmenorrhea, and that this could be abolished with a selective beta-2 receptor stimulant, such as terbutaline.)*

Beard, R.W., Belsey, E.M., Lierberman, B.A., and

Wilkinson, J.C.: Pelvic pain in women. Am. J. Obstet. Gynecol., *128*:566, 1977. *(A study comparing 18 patients with pain and normal laparoscopy and a group with documented pathology; a higher incidence of necrotic qualities was found in patients with pain and no evident pathology.)*

Editorial: A new line of dysmenorrhoea. Br. Med. J., *1*:461, 1975. *(A short article introducing the concept that dysmenorrhea is due to local prostaglandin excess and may be abolished by the use of prostaglandin inhibitors, such as indomethacin.)*

Editorial: Enigmatic pelvic pain. Br. Med. J., *2*:1041, 1978. *(A review of the difficult problems of managing pelvic pain in the absence of detectable pathology.)*

Editorial: Primary dysmenorrhoea. Br. Med. J., *1*:65, 1977. *(A terse discussion of the therapies that have been tried to relieve dysmenorrhea.)*

Filler, W.W., and Hall, W.C.: Dysmenorrhea and its therapy: A uterine contractility study. Am. J. Obstet. Gynecol., *106*:1, 1970. *(Suggests that women with dysmenorrhea have raised uterine tonicity and irregular uterine contractions.)*

Halbert, D.R., Demers, L.M., and Jones, D.E.D.: Dysmenorrhea and prostaglandins. Obstet. Gynecol. Surg., *31*:77, 1976. *(A review of the literature indicating that prostaglandin concentrations were raised in some, but not all patients with primary dysmenorrhea.)*

Swartz, A., Linder, H.R., Naor, S.: Primary dysmenorrhea: Alleviation by an inhibitor of prostaglandin synthesis and action. Obstet. Gynecol., *44*:709, 1974. *(A double-blind study showing the effectiveness of a prostaglandin synthetase inhibitor, flufenamic acid, in controlling dysmenorrhea.)*

Trobough, G.E.: Pelvic pain and the IUD. J. Reprod. Med., *20*:167, 1977. *(A thorough review of the role of IUDs in producing pelvic pain; 36 refs.)*

Ylikorkala, O., and Dawood, M.Y.: New concepts in dysmenorrhea. Am. J. Obstet. Gynecol., *130*:833, 1978. *(A solid and comprehensive review on which rational therapy can be designed; 119 refs.)*

112

Approach to the Patient with Abnormal Vaginal Discharge

Abnormal vaginal discharge is among the most frequent gynecologic complaints the primary physician is asked to evaluate. Some degree of discharge is normal, but complaints of dysuria, offensive odor, staining, itching or accompanying rash point to a pathologic etiology. Uncomplicated vaginal discharge rarely presages serious illness, but can be an irritating and recurrent problem for the patient. The primary physician should be able to identify the cause of the discharge by its appearance and simple laboratory tests as well as detect venereal transmission and underlying disease. Management of vaginitis requires proper choice of antimicrobial agents. Patient education is necessary to reduce recurrences.

PATHOPHYSIOLOGY AND CLINICAL PRESENTATION

The normal vaginal discharge consists of desquamated vaginal epithelial cells, lactic acid, and secretions from cervical glands. An abnormal discharge may result from infection with bacteria, yeasts or parasites. Atrophy secondary to estrogen deficiency produces a mucosa more vulnerable to injury. Inflammation produces desquamation of cells and stimulates glandular secretion from the cervical area. Other pathogenic factors, such as foreign bodies, trauma, recent surgery, alteration of the normal vaginal flora by antibiotic use, and chemical irritants, may disrupt or inflame the vaginal mucosa, increasing the amount of discharge. Rarely, neoplastic change produces an increase in discharge.

The clinical presentation of vaginitis involves a discharge that is notable because of its amount, color or odor. Clinical presentation depends in part on the underlying etiologic agent.

Trichomoniasis is reported in 3 to 15 percent of asymptomatic women seen in private practice and in up to 50 to 75 per cent of prostitutes. The prevalence among women attending gynecology clinics is approximately 15 to 20 per cent. Sexual transmission of trichomoniasis is well established; peak incidence occurs in woman between the ages of 16 and 35. The most prominent symptom is pruritus; it is the sole complaint in 25 per cent of patients; another 50 per cent may seek treatment for pruritus and discharge, while 25 per cent are symptom-free. Vulvar edema may result and give rise to dyspareunia. Dysuria accompanies infection in approximately one-fifth of cases. Physical examination generally reveals erythema, edema, and occasionally characteristic petechial hemorrhages or frank excoriations of the external genitalia. Vaginal discharge may be copious and is usually yellow to green, frothy, and foul-smelling.

Vulvovaginal candidiasis is very common. Yeast is often recovered as a commensal organism. In one private practice study, the incidence of candidiasis was 8.5 per cent, and of these individuals, 25 per cent were asymptomatic. The most common complaint is vulvar pruritus in association with a meager discharge. Symptoms are usually rather rapid in onset, occurring shortly before menstruation when the pH of the vagina falls. On physical examination, erythema, edema and excoriation are often prominent; sometimes there are pustules apparent on the skin. The discharge is typically thick, white, somewhat adherent, and often described as resembling cottage cheese.

Nonspecific vaginitis was a term previously used to denote vaginal inflammation and discharge occurring in the absence of *Trichomonas, Candida* or Gonorrhea. The term is probably a misnomer, because recent careful studies have identified *Hemophilus vaginalis* as the causative organism, either alone or as suggested by other recent studies in association with anaerobic organisms such as *Bacteroides*. On wet-mount one often sees short motile rods and "clue cells" (vaginal epithelial cells covered by small gram-negative rods).

The clinical picture is usually of infection that is milder than that due to *Trichomonas* or *Candida*. The discharge is slight to moderate, less irritating and less likely to be pruritic or burning. Patients may complain of an unpleasant odor that is described as fishy in quality. There is typically little evidence of vaginal irritation, though minimal redness occurs in approximately 20 per cent of affected women.

Gonococcal infection, atrophic vaginitis and herpes simplex infection may also cause vaginal discharge (see Chapters 113, 114, and 184).

DIFFERENTIAL DIAGNOSIS

The major cause of an abnormal vaginal discharge is inflammation due to vaginal infection. Common infectious causes include *Candida, Trichomonas,* and *Hemophilus vaginalis*. Occasionally, discharge results from gonorrheal cervicitis, herpes genitalis or macerated condyloma acuminatum.

If an infectious etiology is not identified, irritants and foreign bodies must be considered. The most common irritants are IUDs, condoms, spermicidal foams, creams, deodorants, sprays, soaps and excessive douching. Foreign bodies include tampons, sexual implements and laminaria. Discharge may be increased postoperatively after an episiotomy, hysterectomy, conization, or cauterization. Cervicitis may be produced by infection, erosion or eversion. Postmenopausal women with estrogen deficiency may have senile or atrophic vaginitis causing abnormal discharge and increased susceptibility to infection. Neoplasms of the vulva, vagina or upper genital tract as well as cervical polyps and uterine fibroids may produce excessive discharge.

A large number of cases are misattributed to nonspecific vaginitis; a number of women who complain of excess discharge merely have physiologic midcycle cervical mucus production or an increased perception of the normal mucosal discharge.

WORKUP (see Table 112-1)

History should determine the onset of the discharge, its appearance, amount, associated symptoms and smell. Need for a pad or tampon is a clue to excessive discharge. History of exposure to venereal disease needs to be considered. The relationship of the discharge to coitus, pregnancy, pessaries, surgery, or oral contraceptives should be noted. Inquiry should be made into associated symptoms such as dysuria, pruritus, pain, dyspareunia, and skin rash. Known allergies need to be reviewed in conjunction with use of douches, bubble baths, soaps or genital deodorants. Symptoms suggestive of diabetes and the recent or current use of antibiotics or corticosteroids need to be considered in a search for alterations in vaginal flora or host defenses. Any self-treatment is worth careful inquiry.

Physical examination should include external inspection for erythema, trauma, edema, excoriation, maceration, condyloma, and rash. Speculum examination, includes looking for foreign bodies, discharge, cervicitis, and prolapse. The discharge should be noted for color, odor and consistency. A white cheesy discharge is characteristic of *Candida*; a green and frothy one is associated with *Trichomonas*; and a thin gray discharge is associated with bacterial infection. With the speculum in place, the walls of the va-

Table 112-1. Causes of Vaginal Discharge

AGENT	PREDISPOSING FACTORS	SYMPTOMS	pH	TRANSMISSION	DIAGNOSIS
Trichomonas	Sexually active Frequent douching	Malodorous discharge, itching, dysuria and dyspareunia	Vulvar irritation, gray to green malodorous discharge, vaginal inflammation with petechiae pH 4.5-6.0	1. Venereal with reservoir in male urethra 2. Families 3. Autogenous reinfection	1. Wet-mount with motile flagellated parasite and many polys 2. Occasionally appears in Pap smears
Candida	Pregnancy, recent broad-spectrum antibiotics, diabetes mellitus, oral contraceptives and corticosteroids	Musty odor, white discharge, dyspareunia, postcoital burning, pain with washing or sitting	Vulvar erythema, possibly pustules or excoriation, gray-white cheesy, curdlike discharge pH 4.0-4.7	1. Usually endogenous with predisposing factors 2. Possible venereal 3. Infection from GI tract	1. KOH stain shows hyphae and buds 2. Culture on Nickerson medium
"Nonspecific" vaginitis— Hemophilus vaginalis and anaerobes	Sexually active Estrogens	Malodorous thin discharge, occasionally itchy but may be asymptomatic	Turbid thin pasty discharge adheres to vaginal walls, rarely pools in posterior fornix pH 5.0-5.5	1. Local factors 2. Venereal from asymptomatic males 3. Families	1. Wet-mount—clue cells (bacilli within epithelial cells) 2. Vaginal culture
Gonococcal	Sexually active History of VD Multiple partners	Discharge— profuse often foul-smelling; fever, pain, dyspareunia, frequently dysuria, itching	Green purulent cervical discharge, fever, cervical and pelvic tenderness, adnexal mass	1. Venereal	1. Gram-negative intracellular diplococci 2. Culture on Thayer-Martin medium
Herpes vaginalis	Sexually active Prior infection Multiple partners	Pain, dysuria, urinary retention dyspareunia, itch, fever	Mild discharge, blisters on vulva, vesicular lesions on vagina and cervix, fever, inguinal adenopathy, sometimes secondary bacterial infection with profuse discharge	1. Venereal 2. Close contact with infected person	1. Multinuclear giant cells on scraping 2. Rise in convalescent serum antibody titers
Atrophic vaginitis	Postmenopause Surgical castrate	Itching, burning, dysuria, dyspareunia secondary to dryness, bleeding	Vulvar, urethral inflammation, pale, thin vaginal mucosa	1. Endogenous involutional process	1. Minimal estrogen effect on mucosa measured by maturation index 2. Low serum estradiol and high FSH

gina and the cervix are examined to detect any cervicitis in conjunction with vaginitis. The characteristics of the various causes of vaginitis are presented in Table 112–1. A pale thin mucosa in postmenopausal women is consistent with atrophic vaginitis. Inspection of the cervix also includes a check for polyps, erosion or eversion. Bimanual palpation needs to be performed for cervical tenderness and uterine or adnexal masses.

Laboratory studies. Microscopic examination of the discharge is essential to diagnosis. Adding a drop of *10 per cent KOH* to a sample of the discharge dissolves most cellular material and aids in identifying the filamentous hyphae and budding forms characteristic of *Candida*. Microscopic examination with 10 per cent KOH has a 40 to 80 per cent sensitivity. *Gram stain* is even more sensitive. A *wet-mount* with a drop of normal saline on a slide of the freshly placed discharge can be prepared to help identify *Candida*, motile flagellated *Trichomonas*, and *Hemophilus*. The sensitivity of wet mount examination for detection of *Trichomonas* is about 25 per cent, while for culture, sensitivity is 90 per cent. In the diagnosis of *Hemophilus* infection, wet-mount examination for "clue" cells, (bacilli within epithelial cells) can be helpful. Investigators have found clue cells present in 44 per cent patients with *Hemophilus* as compared with 18 per cent of those without, making it a somewhat useful but not pathognomonic finding.

The discharge should be *cultured* for gonococci (see Chapter 113) as well as for other bacterial forms when a diagnosis is not established by wet mount and clinical examination, especially if antibiotic therapy is being contemplated.

Vaginal pH may be determined with litmus paper and can be of some help in making a diagnosis, but considerable overlap exists among various etiologies.

A few general laboratory studies are often helpful. A *CBC* and *sedimentation rate* are indicated if pain is present and pelvic inflammatory disease possible. *Urinalysis* should be obtained to check for pyuria and bactiuria, especially if there is concurrent dysuria. Fasting and 2-hour postprandial *blood sugars* are indicated when *Candida* recurs. A *Pap smear* should be done, recognizing that it may be abnormal in the presence of inflammation. In patients who are certain to return for follow-up, it may be reasonable to defer the Pap test until the vaginitis has been treated.

SYMPTOMATIC MANAGEMENT

Trichomonas vaginalis. Asymptomatic vaginal or urethral colonization with this parasite is common, and probably does not require therapy. Many cases respond to douching with 1 tablespoon vinegar per pint of water. If vaginal discharge or symptoms of dysuria or urinary frequency are marked, metronidazole (Flagyl) is the treatment of choice, though some controversy surrounds its use due to carcinogenicity noted in animal studies. This drug is probably most effective if administered orally in a dose of 250 mg. three times a day for 10 days, but single-dose treatment with 2.0 gm. by mouth may suffice. Some authorities advocate simultaneous treatment of male sexual partners; others treat the male only if the female relapses. Treatment of the male partner is most effective when there is a single sexual partner. It may be optimal to culture the male and restrict treatment to those in whom a *Trichomonas* infection

has been documented by culture. Because of the disulfiramlike effects of metronidazole, patients should be instructed to avoid alcohol intake while taking the drug.

Alternatives to metronidazole, such as nitroimidazole drugs, share the risks of metronidazole therapy. A topical agent known as furazolidone, sometimes in combination with nifuroxime (Tricufuron), is available; symptomatic relief is achieved in 80 per cent, but microscopic cure occurs in a smaller percentage of cases than those treated with systemic medication.

Candida albicans vaginitis. Underlying causes such as use of antibiotics, oral contraceptives, or corticosteroids or presence of diabetes or pregnancy need to be identified and attended to first. Therapy must be directed at the etiology when possible as well as at the organism. Nystatin vaginal suppositories used twice a day for 14 days have been the mainstay of treatment for *Candida*. Nystatin is promoted in combination form with other antibacterial agents or corticosteroids; these should rarely be used because they are associated with an increased incidence of adverse reactions and greater cost. The introduction of clotrimazole (Lotrimin) and miconazole nitrate 2 per cent (Monistat) has provided alternate approaches to topical treatment of candidiasis. The course of treatment can be shorter than with nystatin; numerous clinical studies have shown that a 7-day course of clotramizole achieves clinical and mycologic cure in 77 to 95 per cent of affected patients. When clotramizole was compared to miconazole, it was slightly but not significantly more effective; however, cure is achieved with little or no adverse reaction and in a shorter time.

Oral therapy for candidiasis should be considered in recurrent or inveterate candidiasis when reinfection from the gastrointestinal tract is possible. An oral course of nystatin, 500,000 units three times a day for 10 to 14 days, is indicated to remove the intestinal source of reinfection.

Symptomatic relief from the discomfort of the infection can sometimes be obtained by using witch hazel compresses or cool water and hastened by cautious application of hydrocortisone cream to the vulva. The patient should avoid irritant soaps, pantyhose, and hot baths, and should substitute cotton for nylon underwear. Sometimes prolonged therapy, treatment of consorts, eradication of intestinal sources and prophylactic measures may not totally eradicate infection, especially when host defenses are compromised. After treatment, plain yogurt or lactobacillus capsules may be placed in the vagina to restore the normal flora.

"Nonspecific" vaginitis—Hemophilus vaginalis.
It used to be common practice to treat "nonspecific" vaginitis with sulfonamide vaginal creams. Results were frequently disappointing and controlled studies often found that placebo therapy provided similar results. This is not surprising in view of the fact that *Hemophilus vaginalis* has been identified as the causative organism. A recent study comparing metronidazole with sulfonamide treatment for this type of vaginitis showed that metronidazole 500 mg. twice daily for 7 days was far superior. Ampicillin 250 mg. four times daily for 10 days or a similar dose of tetracycline is a reasonable alternative therapy. The effectiveness of metronidazole treatment must be balanced against the potential risks of carcinogenesis. Metronidazole should be used as seldom as possible and only in the lowest effective dose for the shortest possible time. Male partners are often treated as well in cases with multiple recurrences.

Gonorrhea. See Chapter 113.

Herpes genitalis (see Chapters 134 and 184). There is no cure. The goal of treatment is to achieve some degree of symptomatic relief. Rest, warm baths and adequate analgesia should be prescribed. The astringent effects of tea bags may provide some palliation of the painful mucosal erosion. Moral support is essential to the management of this incurable, frequently recurrent viral infection. Since herpes may contribute to the development of cervical neoplasia, regular yearly Pap smear examinations are advisable.

Atrophic vaginitis. The objective is to treat any superimposed infection to restore normal mucosal integrity and elasticity of the vagina. This is best achieved by topical use of estrogen.

PATIENT EDUCATION

Patients need to be informed that most asymptomatic vaginal discharges are self-limited and of little consequence. They should be advised to avoid douches, irritant soaps, bubble baths, and genital deodorants as well as nylon panties, prolonged pantyhose use and wet bathing suits. A period of several days of abstention from sexual intercourse can be advised to observe whether this has an ameliorative effect on symptoms. Because results are often slow, the patient should be reassured that cure is usually achieved, but that occasionally considerable time is necessary. Patients who complain of unpleasant vaginal odors in the absence of discharge usually improve with restoration of good hygiene. Referral to a gynecologist should be made when the symptoms persist. Discharges due to cervicitis, postsurgical, or neoplasia also require referral to a gynecologist.

ANNOTATED BIBLIOGRAPHY

Davis, B.A.: Vaginal moniliasis in private practice. Obstet. Gynecol., *34*:40, 1969. *(A review of 1001 consecutive patients, revealing an 8.5 per cent incidence of* Candida *that was asymptomatic in 25 per cent. Pregnancy, oral contraceptives, antibiotics, and steroids increase the incidence.)*

Kaufman, R.H.: The origin and diagnosis of "nonspecific vaginitis." N. Engl. J. Med., *303*:637, 1980. *(Argues that evidence now supports* Hemophilus vaginalis *as the organism responsible for "nonspecific" vaginitis.)*

Palmer, A.: Vaginitis. Practitioner, *214*:666, 1975. *(An excellent review of anatomy, physiology, and the causes of vaginal discharge.)*

Pheifer, T.A., Forsyth, P.S., Durfee, M.A., et al.: Nonspecific vaginitis: Role of *Hemophilus vaginalis* and treatment with metronidazole. N. Engl. J. Med., *298*:1429, 1978. *(Corynebacterium vaginale [Hemophilis vaginalis]* was isolated from 94 per cent (17/18) of symptomatic patients compared with 1/18 normal controls. Sulfonamide was found ineffective, while metronidazole was effective in 80/81 patients with nonspecific vaginitis.)

Rein, M.F., and Chapel, T.A.: Trichomoniasis, candidiasis and the minor venereal diseases. Clin. Obstet. Gynecol., *18*:73, 1975. *(A thorough review of the clinical characteristics and sensitivity of diagnostic approaches to the major causes of vaginitis; 54 refs.)*

Spiegel, C.A., et al.: Anaerobic bacteria in nonspecific vaginitis. N. Engl. J. Med., *303*:601, 1980. *(Reports that certain anaerobes act with* H. vaginalis *as causes of nonspecific vaginitis.)*

Zuspan, F.E.: Management of patient with vaginal infections. J. Reprod. Med., *9*:1, 1972. *(An invitational symposium, the opinions of a number of experts are offered in this article.)*

113

Approach to the Patient with Gonorrhea

HARVEY B. SIMON, M.D.

At present there continues to be a dramatic increase in the incidence of venereal disease. A number of rather dissimilar disorders are transmitted by direct sexual contact. The great majority of patients with venereal disease present to an ambulatory care facility, and should be diagnosed and treated in this setting. At the same time, the physician must be alert to serious systemic complications requiring hospitalization. In addition, patient education is critical to prevent inadequate treatment and recurrent infections. Finally, the responsibility of the physician must extend beyond the diagnosis and treatment of an individual patient to the identification and treatment of sexual contacts who may otherwise harbor and further disseminate these infections.

The epidemic nature of venereal disease in the United States today is particularly evident in the case of the most prevalent of these infections, gonorrhea. The number of reported cases of gonorrhea has more than doubled in the past 10 years, and exceeded one million for the first time in 1976. Because of the underreporting of venereal diseases, it can be safely estimated that at least three million cases of gonorrhea now occur annually in the U.S.

PATHOPHYSIOLOGY AND CLINICAL PRESENTATION

The clinical features of gonorrhea differ greatly in the male and female. In the male, clinical symptoms usually follow sexual exposure within 2 to 10 days. The risk that a male will acquire gonorrhea following a single exposure to an infected partner is approximately 35 per cent. Absence of symptoms does not indicate absence of infection. Indeed, it has recently been recognized that up to 10 per cent of infected males are asymptomatic carriers of the gonococcus and are fully capable of transmitting the disease. In the male, gonorrhea is principally an infection of the anterior urethra, and hence the major symptom is purulent urethral discharge, often accompanied by urinary frequency and dysuria. Although spread of infection to the prostate or epididymis is uncommon in the antibiotic era, gonococci occasionally gain entry into the bloodstream to produce disseminated infection.

In the female, the cervix is the favored site of gonococcal infection. However, up to 80 per cent of women with gonococcal infection are asymptomatic and must be identified through epidemiologic case-finding. When symptoms do occur, cervical discharge is most common. While the vagina itself is usually spared, the gonococcal infection may spread downward from the cervix to produce urethritis, presenting as dysuria and frequency. Infection of Bartholin glands presents as labial swelling and pain, and rectal infection presents as anorectal discomfort. If, on the other hand, gonococcal infection spreads upward from the cervix, more serious processes may develop. Such upward spread is particularly likely at the time of menstruation and can produce a variety of syndromes. Gonococcal endometritis can cause pelvic pain and abnormal vaginal bleeding, while salpingitis characteristically leads to fever, chills, leukocytosis and a tender adnexal mass. Both systemic and pelvic signs and symptoms are even more pronounced in frank pelvic peritonitis, and further intraperitoneal spread may produce gonococcal perihepatitis with right upper quadrant pain and tenderness.

As a result of changing sexual practices, primary extragenital infections are being encountered more frequently. Gonococcal infection of the pharynx is usually asymptomatic, but can present as an acute exudative pharyngitis, with fever and cervical lymphadenopathy. Gonococcal proctitis is also most often asymptomatic, but can present as proctitis with anorectal discomfort, tenesmus, or rectal bleeding and discharge.

While gonococcal infection invariably begins with the direct infection of a mucosal surface during sexual activity, these organisms may then gain access to the bloodstream to produce bacteremia and systemic spread of infection. This is most common in women, especially at the time of menstruation, but occurs in males as well. Symptoms of the primary gonococcal infection may be absent, making the diagnosis more difficult. Perhaps the most common manifestation of bacteremic gonococcal infection is the "dermatitis-arthritis syndrome." Patients have fever, chills and other constitutional symptoms. Skin lesions are an important clue to diagnosis; these are typically pustular, hemorrhagic or papular, are few in number, and tend to be most common on the distal extremities. Tenosynovitis, especially involving the extensor surfaces of hands and feet, and migratory polyarthritis are typically seen. During the early stage of systemic infection, blood cultures are often positive, but joint cultures are characteristically negative. Later in the course of untreated patients, however, gonococci can produce frank septic arthritis; these patients have less fever, no skin lesions, and negative blood cultures, but more impressive joint swelling and pain, often with purulent synovial fluid in which gonococci can be demonstrated by Gram stain or culture. In rare instances, gonococci can produce osteomyelitis or even life-threatening bacterial meningitis or endocarditis.

DIFFERENTIAL DIAGNOSIS

The major differential diagnosis involving gonococcal cervicitis is vaginitis caused by other bacteria, *Trichomonas* or *Candida*. While the differential diagnosis of gonococcal salpingitis and peritonitis mainly includes nongonococcal pelvic inflammatory disease (PID), it must be remembered that other conditions, including appendicitis, ectopic pregnancy, hemorrhagic ovarian cysts, and endometriosis can produce similar clinical findings, but may require urgent therapy very different from the treatment of PID. In the male, nongonococcal urethritis enters the differential diagnosis. Gonococcal infection needs to be considered among the causes of pharyngitis and proctitis.

WORKUP

The diagnosis of gonorrhea requires a high index of suspicion and a careful sexual history. Physical examination in men with urethritis is usually normal except for purulent urethral discharge. In asymptomatic women, the physical examination is normal, but cervicitis may produce cervical inflammation, discharge, and marked cervical tenderness. Adnexal tenderness and fullness are signs of salpingitis, and may be unilateral or bilateral in women with gonor-

rhea. Tubal abscesses may be suspected because of a palpable mass, and rebound tenderness is a sign of pelvic peritonitis.

Pelvic inflammatory disease due to organisms other than the gonococcus may present similarly. Clinical features favoring the gonococcus include purulent cervical discharge, onset early in the menstrual cycle, no previous history of PID, and exposure to a male with urethritis.

A properly made *Gram stain* of the urethral discharge is a highly reliable diagnostic tool in the male. The smear is made by carefully inserting a swab into the anterior urethra and then rolling the swab on a glass slide, which is air-dried, fixed and Gram-stained in the usual manner. If typical bean-shaped gram-negative diplococci are seen within polymorphonuclear leukocytes, the diagnosis is almost certain; diplococci in extracellular locations are suggestive but not diagnostic. The absence of organisms makes the diagnosis of gonorrhea in a male with urethral discharge quite unlikely. Unfortunately, in the female, the Gram stain of a cervical discharge is much less helpful, with up to 40 per cent false-negatives and some false-positives due to nonpathogenic vaginal *Neisseria*.

In both sexes, *cultures* confirming the diagnosis of gonorrhea are mandatory. *Neisseria gonorrhoeae* is a very fragile and fastidious organism which requires special handling in the lab. The gonococcus is readily killed by drying, so all cultures must be plated promptly. Ideally, this should be done by the physician at the time of examination by streaking the swab across the surface of the culture medium in a Z-shaped pattern. Special culture media must be used. While chocolate agar has been the traditional medium used, a modified Thayer-Martin medium is preferred for specimens obtained from genital, anal or pharyngeal sites because the addition of antibiotics to this medium suppresses the growth of nonpathogenic *Neisseria* species and other bacteria. The culture medium should be at room temperature at the time of inoculation. Because the gonococcus requires a high CO_2 concentration to grow, cultures should be promptly incubated in a candle jar or CO_2 incubator. When this is not possible, the cultures should be planted on modified Thayer-Martin medium in bottles with a 10% CO_2 atmosphere. These bottles should be kept capped until the moment of inoculation and should be held in an upright position when open to prevent the loss of CO_2, which is heavier than air.

In the male, cultures of the anterior urethra suffice unless homosexual contacts are suspected, in which case cultures of the anal canal and pharynx are also indicated. In the female, the endocervix should be cultured by inserting a swab into the cervical os through a speculum which has been lubricated only with water. In all women, rectal cultures are indicated because rectal infection can result simply from direct spread of infection from the genital tract. When pharyngitis is suspected, throat culture is mandatory. When acute arthritis is present, joint fluid should be obtained by arthrocentesis and should be evaluated with cell counts, sugar and protein determinations, Gram stain and culture.

PRINCIPLES OF MANAGEMENT

The therapy of gonorrhea has undergone dramatic changes over the past 35 years. During this time, there has been a steady increase in the penicillin resistance of the gonococcus, so that the currently recommended doses of penicillin are 30 times greater than the initial regimen used with success in 1943. Until recently, this penicillin resistance was just a matter of degree, since it was based on chromosomal mutations decreasing the permeability of the cell wall to penicillin and other antibiotics. While simply increasing the dose of penicillin used against these organisms was very successful, a new problem was recognized in 1975, when gonococcal strains were isolated which resist the effects of even massive doses of penicillin because they produce penicillinase. At present, these organisms have produced only isolated cases of human infection, but if they become more prevalent, the current therapeutic schedules will need major revisions. As of 1979, however, penicillin remains the drug of choice for gonorrhea.

For *uncomplicated urethritis* or *cervicitis,* or for the treatment of asymptomatic individuals exposed to know gonorrhea, either of two regimens may be used: intramuscular procaine penicillin plus probenecid, which reduces renal penicillin excretion, or oral ampicillin plus probenecid. Oral tetracycline or intramuscular spectinomycin is recommended for patients allergic to penicillin.

Patients with *rectal gonorrhea* usually respond to the same regimens used for uncomplicated genital tract infections. Treatment of gonococcal pharyngitis may be more difficult; the basic penicillin or tetracycline schedules should be tried initially, but spectinomycin is ineffective, and treatment failures may require more intensive therapy.

In all patients with gonorrhea, it is mandatory to test for cure by follow-up urethral, cervical and anal cultures 1 to 2 weeks after completion of therapy. Organisms isolated from patients who are treatment failures should be submitted for testing to determine whether they are penicillinase-producing. Patients who are not cured following initial penicillin or tetracycline treatment should be retreated with 2 gm. spectinomycin intramuscularly.

Patients with *disseminated gonococcal infections* require more intensive therapy. In the arthritis-dermatitis syndrome, initial therapy with intravenous aqueous penicillin G for 3 days, followed by oral ampicillin, is ideal. If hospitalization is impractical, the patient reliable, the diagnosis clear-cut, and the case mild, outpatient treatment with ampicillin alone is acceptable. Tetracycline is the drug of choice for penicillin-allergic patients unless they are pregnant. Gonococcal osteomyelitis, meningitis or endocarditis require more intensive and prolonged parenteral antibiotic therapy.

Women with *pelvic inflammatory disease* require special consideration. In mild cases, treatment is the same as for uncomplicated disease. These patients must be closely followed to ensure compliance and efficacy. However, hospitalization should be strongly considered, especially if the diagnosis is not completely certain and surgical emergencies are possible. In addition, pregnant patients, women suspected of having pelvic abscesses or frank peritonitis, very toxic patients, and those who do not respond to outpatient therapy should be hospitalized and treated with intravenous penicillin or tetracycline. Patients who are both pregnant and penicillin-allergic present a difficult problem. Cephalosporins are usually effective, but may cause allergic reactions. Erythromycin is safe, but appears less effective. Spectinomycin is effective, but safety for the fetus has not been established.

Unless cervical Gram stains and cultures are positive for gonococci, it is impossible to clinically differentiate gonococcal from nongonococcal pelvic inflammatory disease. Clinical features favoring the gonococcus include purulent cervical discharge, onset early in the menstrual cycle, no previous history of PID, and exposure to a male with urethritis. All patients with PID should be treated at least with a regimen effective for gonococci. Nongonococcal PID is usually caused by multiple organisms, including bacteroides, enteric gram-negative bacilli and streptococci. Therefore, if nongonococcal PID seems likely, or if patients fail to respond to therapy for the gonococcus, antibiotic programs effective against these other organisms should be considered.

All patients with gonorrhea should have serological tests for syphilis. Seronegative patients treated with procaine penicillin do not need follow-up serologies because this regimen is effective for incubating syphilis; however, patients receiving ampicillin, tetracycline or spectinomycin should have follow-up serologies in 3 months. All cases of gonorrhea should be reported to the appropriate local health department. Because many patients with gonorrhea are asymptomatic, vigorous case-finding represents the only present hope for controlling this epidemic.

THERAPEUTIC RECOMMENDATIONS

Uncomplicated gonorrhea in men or women, or asymptomatic individuals exposed to known gonorrhea

- Procaine penicillin G, 4.8 million units divided into two intramuscular injections at the same visit, together with 1 gm. probenecid by mouth, *or*
- Ampicillin 3.5 gm. by mouth, or amoxicillin 3.0 gm. by mouth, in a single dose, together with 1 gm. probenecid by mouth, *or*
- Tetracycline 500 mg. by mouth four times a day for 5 days (total, 10 gm.). Tetracycline is contraindicated in pregnancy. All tetracyclines are ineffective in single-dose therapy; other tetracyclines are no more effective than tetracycline hydrochloride.

All of these regimens are very effective. Single-dose treatment is preferred in potentially unreliable patients. The procaine penicillin regimen is preferred in men with anogenital infection. Ampicillin (in a single dose) and spectinomycin are not effective for gonococcal pharyngitis. Tetracycline may eliminate coexisting chlamydial infection and result in fewer cases of postgonococcal urethritis. Spectinomycin is the treatment of choice for treatment failures and for infection with penicillinase-producing gonococci. On rare occasions, a penicillinase-producing gonococcus is also spectinomycin-resistant; patients infected with these organisms may be treated with cefoxitin 2.0 gm. in a single intramuscular injection, together with 1.0 gm. probenecid by mouth.

Outpatient treatment of gonococcal pelvic inflammatory disease

- Penicillin G, 4.8 million units divided into two intramuscular doses at the first visit, plus 1 gm. probenecid by mouth, followed by ampicillin 500 mg. four times a day for 10 days, *or*
- Ampicillin, 3.5 gm. orally, or amoxicillin, 3.0 gm. orally, plus 1 gm. probenecid orally, followed by

ampicillin or amoxicillin 500 mg. four times a day for 10 days, *or*
- Tetracycline 500 mg. four times a day for 10 days.

Hospitalized patient with gonococcal PID

- Penicillin G, crystalline, 20 million units intravenously each day until improvement is apparent, followed by ampicillin 500 mg. orally four times a day to complete 10 days.
- Alternatively, tetracycline 500 mg. intravenously four times a day until improvement is shown, then 500 mg. orally four times a day to complete 10 days. Tetracycline is contraindicated in pregnancy.

Gonococcal bacteremia and arthritis

- Penicillin G, crystalline, 10 million units intravenously daily until improvement begins, followed by ampicillin 500 mg. orally four times a day to complete 7 days, *or*
- Ampicillin 3.5 gm. orally plus 1 gm. probenecid orally, followed by ampicillin 500 mg. orally four times a day for at least 7 days, *or*
- Tetracycline 500 mg. four times a day for 7 days. Tetracycline is contraindicated in pregnancy, *or*
- Erythromycin, 500 mg. intravenously every 6 hours for at least 3 days, followed by 500 mg. erythromycin orally four times a day to complete 7 days of therapy.

ANNOTATED BIBLIOGRAPHY

Gonorrhea

Blankenship, R.M., and Holmes, R.K.: Treatment of disseminated gonococcal infection. N. Engl. J. Med., *290*:267, 1974. *(A study of short-term intravenous antibiotic therapy of disseminated gonorrhea. Although standard recommendations still suggest oral ampicillin following 3 days of intravenous penicillin, this study suggests that the 3 days of IV treatment will suffice in most patients.)*

Handsfield, H.H., Lipman, T.O., Harnisch, J.P., *et al.*: Asymptomatic gonorrhea in men. N. Engl. J. Med., *290*:117, 1974. *(An important study showing that asymptomatic males can be prolonged urethral carriers of* N. gonorrhoeae *and may be an important reservoir of infection. All sexual contacts of patients with gonorrhea should be cultured, whether male or female and whether symptomatic or not.)*

Holmes, K.K., Counts, G.W., and Beaty, H.N.: Disseminated gonococcal infection. Ann. Intern.

Med., *74*:979, 1971. *(A useful clinical review of the gonococcal "dermatitis-arthritis" syndrome.)*

Jaffe, H.W., Biddle, J.W., Thornsberry, C., *et al.*: National gonorrhea therapy monitoring study: *In vitro* antibiotic susceptibility and its correlation with treatment results. N. Engl. J. Med., *294*:5, 1976. *(A nationwide multicenter study of antibiotic susceptibility of gonococci providing the rationale for current therapeutic recommendations.)*

Klein, E.J., Fisher, L.S., Chow, A.W., *et al.*: Anorectal gonococcal infection. Ann. Intern. Med., *86*:340, 1977. *(A clinical review of rectal infections in women and homosexual males.)*

Lightfoot, R.W., and Gotschlich, E.C.: Gonococcal disease. Am. J. Med., *56*:347, 1974. *(A review stressing the basic microbiologic aspects of the gonococcus.)*

McCormack, W.M.: Treatment of gonorrhea—Is penicillin passé? N. Engl. J. Med., *296*:934, 1977. *(A lucid summary of the basic mechanisms, epidemiologic patterns, and therapeutic complications of antibiotic-resistant gonococci.)*

Wiesner, P.J., Tronca, E., Bonin, P., *et al.*: Clinical spectrum of pharyngeal gonococcal infection. N. Engl. J. Med., *288*:181, 1973. *(A clinical study of gonococcal pharyngitis.)*

Pelvic Inflammatory Disease

Cunningham, F.G., Hauth, J.C., Strong, J.D., *et al.*: Evaluation of tetracycline or penicillin and ampicillin for treatment of acute pelvic inflammatory disease. N. Engl. J. Med., *296*:1380, 1977. *(A study of 197 women showed that both regimens were effective. Notably, pelvic abscess developed ten times more often in nongonococcal PID.)*

Eschenbach, D.A., Buchanan, T.M., Pollock, H.M., *et al.*: Polymicrobial etiology of acute pelvic inflammatory disease. N. Engl. J. Med., *293*:166, 1975. *(An excellent study of the microbiology of acute pelvic inflammatory disease.)*

Eschenbach, D.A., Harnisch, J.P., and Holmes, K.K.: Pathogenesis of acute pelvic inflammatory disease: Role of contraception and other risk factors, Am. J. Obstet. Gynecol., *128*:838, 1977. *(An excellent review of the increased risk of PID in patients with IUDs, particularly in nulliparous women.)*

114
Approach to the Menopausal Woman

Menopause is a difficult stage for women in our society because of the emphasis on youth. Although many of the emotional and physical changes blamed on menopause are actually more general manifestations of aging and not tied to decreased estrogen levels, the cessation of menstruation has major symbolic significance and, as a result, many symptoms and complaints are attributed to it. The naive hope that taking exogenous estrogen would protect the user from normal aging, coronary disease, and other conditions has for the most part proven ill-founded. Moreover, a disturbing association between estrogen therapy and increased risk of endometrial cancer has appeared in addition to previously recognized cardiovascular complications.

If one uses the generally accepted definition of menopause as a full year without menstrual flow in a previously menstruating woman, then the incidence of menopause is 10 per cent by age 38, 20 per cent by age 43, 50 per cent by 48, 90 per cent by 54 and 100 per cent by age 58. In addition, the prevalence of surgically induced menopause is estimated to be 25 to 30 per cent of women in their mid-50s.

The primary physician can do a great deal to help women pass through this potentially trying stage with confidence and dignity. It is important to provide relief from disabling symptoms, such as severe hot flashes, while avoiding unnecessary exposure to estrogen therapy and its attendant risks.

PHYSIOLOGY AND CLINICAL PRESENTATION

The essential cause of menopause is decreased estrogen production by the aging ovaries, resulting in cessation of menses and rise in gonadotropins. Some estrogen production continues, but its source is primarily peripheral conversion of delta-4-androstene-dione. The diagnosis of menopause is confirmed by a marked increase in the gonadotropins; maximum levels of FSH and LH occur within 1 to 2 years of onset and remain high for 10 to 15 years. The physiologic events are identical in surgically induced menopause, but the time course is shorter, with FSH and LH rising to high levels within 20 to 30 days. Approximately 25 per cent of women do not experience any symptoms, perhaps because of non-ovarian sources of estrogen production.

Hot flashes, believed to be related to rate of estrogen withdrawal and resultant vasomotor instability, are among the most specific of menopausal symptoms. An uncomfortably warm sensation radiates upward from the chest to neck and face and lasts seconds to a few minutes before subsiding. Eating, exertion, emotional upset and alcohol are known precipitants. As many as 20 episodes per day occur; in most patients, the condition lasts for 2 to 3 years but may continue for 6 years or more. Prevalence of severe, disabling hot flashes ranges from 10 to 35 per cent of menopausal women. No link between emotional makeup and symptoms has been demonstrated, though it is clear that the flashes can be very distracting and cause considerable misery and upset.

Other clinical manifestations of estrogen decline include atrophy of the vaginal mucosa and vulvar epithelium. The vagina becomes smaller and less compliant; lubrication decreases. Women may present with complaints of itching, discharge, bleeding or painful intercourse. The uterus becomes smaller, but this causes no symptoms. The urethra becomes atrophic, and perineal bacteria colonize the area, increasing the risk of urethritis and dysuria.

There is no evidence that estrogen decline is the cause of an increased incidence of cardiovascular disease in menopausal women, nor do estrogens protect against such problems or ameliorate risk factors such as hyperlipidemia. In fact, hypertriglyceridemia and increased risk of angina have been noted. Osteoporosis is probably a concomitant of aging and not a specific manifestation of menopause, because the process has been documented to begin years before menopause or any fall in estrogen levels. However, osteoporosis can be minimized by supplying estrogen on a prophylactic basis (see Chapter 152).

Various functional and psychological symptoms such as headache, nervousness and depression, which frequently occur during the climacteric, are more a reflection of the emotional stress attending this difficult stage of life than a result of a change in hormonal milieu. Some women report feeling better emotionally on estrogen therapy, but this probably represents a placebo effect. No specific psychiatric problems have been found to be linked specifically to menopause.

The cosmetic changes associated with aging have been attributed by some to a decrease in estrogens, but clinical evidence is to the contrary. Breast atrophy, loss of skin turgor, and redistribution of fat to the abdomen and thighs have not been shown to be influenced by estrogen therapy and most likely are part of the more general process of aging.

PRINCIPLES OF MANAGEMENT

The objectives are to alleviate any disabling symptoms that result from estrogen deficiency and to provide support for the host of emotional and functional problems likely to occur in the context of aging.

The most difficult decision is whether to employ *systemic estrogen therapy*. Epidemiologic data are accumulating which point to increased risks of cardiovascular disease and endometrial carcinoma associated with estrogen use in menopausal patients. For example, the Framingham study revealed twice the incidence of angina in menopausal women using estrogen than in those who did not, although rates for myocardial infarction were similar. The incidence of endometrial carcinoma has been found in case control studies to parallel estrogen use and to be 4.5 to 13.9 times that of non-users. The risk is independent of other known factors; it declines with cessation of causative therapy. Although no increased risk of breast carcinoma has been found, estrogen does stimulate tumor growth in some patients (see Chapter 118). Other adverse effects of estrogen include fluid retention, blood pressure increase, gallstones, glucose intolerance, and headaches; recurrent uterine bleeding often takes place. There does not appear to be an increased risk of thromboembolism in those on estrogen replacement, but caution is appropriate in patients with known peripheral vascular disease.

With such a list of potentially serious adverse effects to contend with, one must exert considerable care in selecting patients for estrogen therapy to ensure that expected benefits will outweigh the substantial risks involved with its use. At the present time, very severe, *incapacitating hot flashes* seem to be the only definite and widely agreed upon indication for prescribing estrogen to menopausal women. Although *osteoporosis* can be minimized by prophylactic use of estrogen, it is not clear whether the risk of compression fractures can be substantially reduced. Once osteoporosis occurs, it cannot be reversed by any form of therapy; it is only the rate of further bone resorption that can be slowed. Whether to embark on a course of estrogen treatment depends on the perceived risk of severe osteoporosis (see Chapter 152).

Topical estrogen will restore turgor to the vaginal mucosa. Some systemic absorption takes place; its effect is uncertain and the risks of adverse effects must still be considered present, though probably to a lesser degree. The impact of topical estrogen therapy on incidence of endometrial carcinoma is unknown; due to the proximity of the uterus, it is possible that substantial local effects may occur. Thus, topical estrogen cream should be prescribed only for women with severe symptoms definitively attributable to *atrophic vaginitis* and unresponsive to simpler measures such as use of a water-soluble vaginal lubricant.

Estrogen is no more effective than placebo for the relief of headache, palpitations, irritability, decreased libido and minor psychiatric symptoms.

Since adverse effects of estrogen are a function of dose and duration of therapy, the lowest effective dose should be used, and therapy should be cycled to prevent uninterrupted stimulation of the endometrium. The need for continued treatment ought to be periodically reevaluated. Any unexplained vaginal staining or bleeding should initiate an evaluation for underlying pelvic malignancy. Actually, one of the unquantified risks of replacement therapy is the increase in frequency of endometrial biopsies and D&C procedures.

Most of the problems encountered by menopausal women can be handled safely without resorting to replacement therapy. For example, painful coitus due to vaginal atrophy can be prevented by use of a water-soluble lubricant. Muscle tone, appearance, and sense of well-being can be improved by a carefully tailored program of gentle exercises, including walking or swimming. Multiple bodily complaints such as fatigue, headache, arthralgias, etc., should be investigated systematically. If an underlying depression is discovered, specific treatment should be undertaken (see Chapter 215). Patients troubled by preexisting emotional and/or physical problems are probably going to have more difficulty as they grow older, necessitating continuation and enhancement of treatment as they pass such important milestones of aging as menopause.

PATIENT EDUCATION

Since the emphasis in our society is on youth and vitality, the physician has an important supportive role to play in helping the menopausal woman to adjust psychologically and maintain her sense of self-worth and well-being. Discussion of the physiologic consequences of menopause and their clinical manifestations can give the patient a rational basis for understanding her own symptoms and properly attributing them. This might save many anxious phone calls and office visits. One can take advantage of this milestone to interest the patient in a program of regular exercise, attainment of ideal weight and cessation of any self-destructive habits such as smoking. The woman needs to know that any incapacitating symptoms due to estrogen lack can be controlled and that they are self-limited. During the perimenopausal period, women should be reminded to use contraception because ovulation and unwanted pregnancy may occur. Reassurance that capacity for normal sexual activity will continue after menopause is often tremendously comforting. Lack of need for special vitamin supplements should be pointed out, since the lay press heavily encourages their use and this unnecessary expense can be considerable.

If estrogen therapy is being considered, the patient must share in the decision with full awareness of the potential risks and benefits. Patients on estrogen therapy must be reminded to stop the estrogen for 7 days each month and not to increase the dose on their own. The need for regular follow-up and prompt reporting of any abnormal vaginal bleeding, breast masses, leg swelling, etc., needs to be emphasized.

THERAPEUTIC RECOMMENDATIONS

- Estrogen therapy should be reserved for incapacitating symptoms. The decision to treat with estrogens should be made jointly by the physician and patient.
- If prescribed, systemic estrogen should be used in the minimal effective dose (usually the equivalent of 0.625 mg. of conjugated estrogens daily), for as short a time as possible; rarely more than 1 or 2 years. The need for continued treatment should constantly be reevaluated. When estrogens are used for hot flashes, it is suggested that discontinuation be attempted during winter months.
- Therapy should be cyclical, 21 days on, 7 days off, to prevent uninterrupted stimulation of the endometrium. Some authorities advise adding a progestin (e.g., medroxyprogesterone acetate [Provera], 10 mg.) during the last 5 days of the estrogen cycle in order to reduce endometrial buildup.
- The development of osteoporosis may be lessened by the administration of high doses of estrogen

(1.25 mg. per day of conjugated estrogens), but permanent therapy is never indicated. Estrogen therapy cannot replace lost bone, so it is not a therapy for established osteoporosis. Patient selection for prophylactic therapy needs to be individualized and carefully considered (see Chapter 152).

- Severe atrophic vaginitis with dysuria or dyspareunia will respond to topical estrogen which should be given for no more than 3 weeks at a time; topical therapy applied as little as once or twice a week may be effective. Systemic absorption occurs, but its effect is uncertain. Milder cases, with painful coitus only, can be treated with a water-soluble lubricant (e.g., Lubafax).

- Medical surveillance of patients on estrogen is mandatory. Blood pressure measurement, breast and pelvic examination, and Pap smear should be done every 6 months. When a woman requires estrogen for more than a year, a referral to a gynecologist should be made for consideration of endometrial biopsy, which is advocated by some clinicians.

- Uterine fibroids, hypertension, diabetes and hypertriglyceridemia are relative contraindications to estrogen use and demand careful monitoring. A history of myocardial infarction, pulmonary embolism, thrombophlebitis or malignancy of breasts or uterus generally precludes treatment with exogenous estrogens.

ANNOTATED BIBLIOGRAPHY

Ballinger, C.G.: Psychiatric morbidity and the menopause: Clinical features. Br. Med. J., *1*:1183, 1976. *(A description of psychiatric symptoms during the menopause.)*

Boston Collaborative Drug Surveillance Program: Surgically confirmed gallbladder disease, venous thromboembolism and breast tumors in relation to postmenopausal estrogen therapy. N. Engl. J. Med., *290*:15, 1974. *(Postmenopausal estrogen therapy increases risk of gallstones, but not of thromboembolism or breast tumor.)*

Coope, J., Thompson, J.M., and Poller, L.: Effects of "natural oestrogen" replacement therapy on menopausal symptoms and blood clotting. Br. Med. J., *4*:139, 1975. *(Thromboembolic disease is not increased by estrogen therapy.)*

Detre, T., Hayashi, T.T., and Arches, D.F.: Management of the menopause. Ann. Intern. Med., *88*:373, 1978. *(An excellent current review.)*

Gordon, T., Kannel, W.B., Hjortland, M.L., *et al.*: Menopause and coronary heart disease. The Framingham Study. Ann. Intern. Med., *89*:157, 1978. *(The dramatic rise in coronary heart disease associated with menopause is documented with a doubled risk in postmenopausal women on hormones.)*

Grodin, J.M., Siiteri, P.K., and MacDonald, P.C.: Source of estrogen production in postmenopausal women. J. Clin. Endocrinol. Metab., *36*:207, 1973. *(Documents peripheral conversion of androstenedione to estrogen in the adrenals of postmenopausal women.)*

Hoover, R., Gray, L.A., Sr., Cole, P., *et al.*: Menopausal estrogens and breast cancer. N. Engl. J. Med., *295*:401, 1976. *(No increased risk of breast cancer.)*

Jick, H., Watkins, R.N., Hunter, J.R., *et al.*: Replacement estrogens and endometrial cancer. N. Engl. J. Med., *300*:218, 1979. *(Long-term estrogen users in a large Seattle group practice showed an annual risk of 1 to 3 per cent for users and a risk less than one-tenth as great for nonusers. A reduced incidence of endometrial cancer paralleled the downward trend in the use of replacement estrogens.)*

Lindsay, R., Hart, D.M., Aitken, J.M., *et al.*: Long-term prevention of postmenopausal osteoporosis by oestrogen: Evidence for an increased bone mass after delayed onset of oestrogen treatment. Lancet, *1*:1038, 1976. *(Suggests a benefit from estrogen use.)*

Molitch, M.E., *et al.*: Massive hyperlipemia during estrogen therapy. JAMA, *227*:522, 1974. *(A case report reminding clinicians of the risk of increased triglycerides.)*

Rechner, R.E.: Benign breast disease in women on estrogen therapy: A pathologic study. Cancer, *29*:273, 1972. *(The incidence of breast disease is not increased.)*

Rosenberg, L., Armstrong, B., Jick, H.: Myocardial infarction and estrogen therapy in postmenopausal women. N. Engl. J. Med., *294*:1256, 1976. *(No increase in risk of myocardial infarction.)*

Smith, D.C., Prentice, R., Thompson, D., *et al.*: Association of exogenous estrogen and endometrial carcinoma. N. Engl. J. Med., *293*:1164, 1975. *(Among the first reports of the association of endometrial cancer with estrogen use.)*

von Eiff, A.W.: Blood pressure and estrogen. Estrogens in the postmenopause. Front. Horm. Res.,

3:177, 1975. *(Reversible hypertension in 18 per cent of women on estrogen replacement.)*

Wenz, A.C.: Psychiatric morbidity and menopause (editorial*). Ann. Intern. Med., 84:331, 1976. (Psychiatric symptoms are not a function of estrogen deficiency.)*

Ziel, H.K., and Finkle, W.D.: Increased risk of endometrial carcinomas among users of conjugated estrogens. N. Engl. J. Med., *293*:1167, 1975. *(Another early report of the association of estrogen and endometrial cancer.)*

115

Approach to Fertility Control
ANN B. BARNES, M.D.

The ideal contraceptive is perfectly safe, effective, inexpensive, acceptable, and available. None exists. The efficacy of individual contraceptive agents is expressed in several ways. *Theoretical effectiveness* refers to the ability of the medication, device or procedure to prevent pregnancy if applied under ideal conditions. *Use effectiveness* combines theoretical effectiveness with inherent patient-related lapses in application. *Extended use effectiveness* adds the dimension of time. All are important aspects of evaluation of approaches to fertility control.

The primary physician should be knowledgeable about the effectiveness, difficulties, and adverse effects of available contraceptive methods in order to help the patient or couple intelligently select one which suits them best.

NATURAL METHODS

Natural methods of birth control do not meet the demands of most sexually active individuals in industrialized societies. Faithfully practiced *rhythm,* with daily basal body temperature recording, usually results in one pregnancy every 2 years or at least one more child than planned by the couple by their late thirties. Rhythm practiced by abstinence according to menstrual dates is less effective. Rhythm controlled by following the cervical mucus cycle is confounded by infections, dietary changes, douching habits, oral medications, patient understanding of her anatomy, and availability of testing materials. One needs to understand reproductive anatomy and physiology and to have privacy in order to conduct such tests. These ingredients are unavailable to many Americans. The *amenorrhea of lactation* is useful, but the duration of ovarian inactivity in an individual is hard to predict or follow. *Withdrawal* is probably the most commonly used natural contraceptive tech-

nique. Unfortunately, sperm migration from the female perineum occasionally occurs, as does some discharging of semen prior to ejaculation.

BARRIER CONTRACEPTIVES

Condoms have extended use effectiveness. Pregnancies may occur in 3 per 100 couples per year using condoms, which means that properly used, this method is 97 percent effective. For a few cents more than the cheapest devices, high-quality thin condoms are available, use of which is accompanied by very little loss of sensation. The condom is inexpensive and widely available. It requires no medical intervention or prescription. Failure by means of rupture is rare, but easily recognized.

Diaphragms are synthetic rubber barriers mounted on covered rims which deny access of sperm and penis to the anterior vaginal wall and cervical os. There are three widely used rims: all flex, coil spring and flat spring. These have minor differences in characteristics and provide alternatives for fitting a variety of women. The largest diaphragm which will cover the cervix and anterior vagina from the pubis symphysis to the posterior fornix, without uncomfortably stretching the rest of the vagina, should be selected. The diaphragm should not be so big that the penis could get between the pubic symphysis and its rim, nor so small that it is beyond the reach of the exploring finger. The vagina has no bony limitations and will continue to stretch with sexual activity, so that size checks are warranted in the first year and at 2- to 3-year intervals thereafter. Parturition will also alter the size of the vagina. Only massive weight changes of 25 per cent of body weight or more require refitting of diaphragms, despite popular belief.

Diaphragms with a small amount of spermicidal cream or jelly, properly used, are 97 per cent effective; that is, similarly to condoms, 3 pregnancies per 100 fertile women per year would be expected. The cream facilitates insertion but need not be used in the large amounts recommended by the manufacturers, as it is unpleasantly messy. The diaphragm is worn for 6 hours after the last coital event, since this is the length of time during which sperm motility persists. It may be worn for longer periods of time, but like all vaginal contraceptives, will then become associated with an unpleasant odor. It may also be worn while the patient is swimming or during menstruation.

The diaphragm must be fitted to the individual woman by a physician, nurse, or trained technician. The cost of the diaphragm is reasonable, but manufacturers advocate massive use of creams, which adds to the expense. The patient must have some understanding of her anatomy and not be concerned about exploring her reproductive organs. Some adolescents reject the diaphragm as representing premeditated sexual intercourse, which they find less acceptable than spontaneous events. Women in their twenties seldom voice such a complaint. Some women cannot be adequately fitted with a diaphragm for anatomical reasons. The cervix may not protrude into the vagina adequately (absent pars vaginalis). The cervix may be displaced posteriorly by retroversion or extreme anteversion.

Spermicidal creams and *jellies* may have a high theoretical effectiveness, but lesser use effectiveness. Most contain nonoxyl-9 as the spermicidal agent. The physical nature of the creams and jellies and difficulty in their application often result in inadequately smearing the cervical os, so that sperm invasion is not prevented. Both men and women complain of the dehydrating effect of spermicidal agents and may report burning sensations. *Foams* have better physical properties allowing more adequate smearing of the cervical os; however, foams are effective only for short periods of time, and reapplications are necessary. This increases their cost. They also contain nonoxyl-9 and will cause irritation. Although failure rates as high as 50 per cent have been reported in some studies, others claim a 97 per cent success rate, with only 3 pregnancies per 100 fertile women per year. *Encapsulated foams* compared to foams applied through applicators are far less successful because the capsule may not be inserted deeply enough into the vagina or may not disintegrate at the appropriate interval to adequately smear the cervical os. Foams have the advantage of being readily accessible in both supermarkets and drug stores, and do not require medical instruction or prescription.

Cervical caps are individually molded to a par-

ticular cervix and are difficult to apply repeatedly. Their use requires an extensive amount of physician and nurse teaching, and they are more costly than diaphragms. For these reasons, they have found little general application.

Under development are hydrophilic foam-impregnated disposable *urethane sponges,* which once inserted into the vagina, expand to cover the cervix adequately and provide large amounts of nonoxyl-9. It is hoped that these will be inexpensive and readily available without a prescription.

INTRAUTERINE DEVICES (IUDs)

The idea of inserting materials into the uterine cavity to prevent nidation and fetal development is ancient. The precise mechanism of action of intrauterine contraception is unknown. What appears to be important is the area of surface contact. IUDs may be constructed out of a variety of inert substances. Copper enhances their effectiveness. Modern technology has provided many inexpensive plastic models. At present, the Lippes loop and Safe-T-Coil seem to have pregnancy rates similar to those of properly used condoms and diaphragms—i.e., 3 per 100 women per year. Their expulsion rates are 19 per 100 women, and occasionally it is necessary to remove them because of bleeding or pain, at a rate of about 11 per 100 women per year. The copper 7 has a similar failure rate and slightly lower expulsion, bleeding and pain rates. The copper devices are particularly useful in nulliparous women, but are often too small for parous women. The cost of the IUD is variable; most are rather inexpensive. There are additional charges for insertion. At the present time, copper devices may be worn for 3 years, and the other varieties for longer periods.

Inserting anything through the internal cervical os evokes pain similar to that of cervical dilatation during labor. Frequently a vasovagal response may occur, or the women may simply complain of feeling sick to her stomach. Attention must be paid to the orientation of the uterus so that the device is inserted into the uterine cavity and not out the endocervical canal into the peritoneal cavity.

The string used for insertion and retrieval is made of slippery monofilament. This may act as a conduit between the never sterile vagina and the usually sterile endometrial cavity. The risk of subsequent sepsis is enhanced. The risk of laparoscopy-verified pelvic inflammatory disease in nulligravid sexually active women with IUDs has been found to be seven times greater than that for similar women who were not using an IUD. For parous women, the risk was only three times greater. Whether this difference between nulliparous and parous women is a result of prior delivery or the limitations on sexual activity and multiple partners imposed by childbearing is not clear. The problem with increasing the risk of pelvic inflammatory disease in young sexually active women is that if inadequately treated, such disease may lead to infertility. At present, tubal damage from infection is the least well-treated cause of infertility. For rape victims, IUDs have been inserted when morning-after pills containing estrogen are contraindicated. Prophylactic antibiotics must be considered as well.

ORAL CONTRACEPTIVES

Morning-after pill. Large doses of estrogen (50 mg. of diethylstilbestrol daily for 5 days or ethinyl estradiol 0.5 mg. twice a day for 5 days) will result in withdrawal bleeding, denying the conceptus an environment for nidation. Such doses usually cause nausea, and antiemetic medication is needed. Provided that nidation has not already occurred, this therapy may work. However, failures are reported.

Combination pill. Combinations of synthetic estrogens and progesterones have been found to have use effectiveness rates that exceed most estimates of effectiveness of condoms, diaphragms and IUDs. Although some claim the failure rates may be as high as 5 to 10 per cent, others say only one pregnancy per 100 users per year will occur. The combination pill appears to prevent cyclic FSH and LH release, which are required for ovulation. At the present time, combination pills consist of ethinyl estradiol and norethindrone, mestranol and norethynodrel, ethinyl estradiol and norgestrel, or mestranol and ethynodiol diacetate. In various combinations, packets are made up for taking the pills from the fifth day of the menstrual cycle for the subsequent 21 days; some packets have placebos so that one pill is taken daily.

More than two dozen combination oral contraceptive pills are available in the United States. In general, it is most useful to renew any prescription with which a patient is satisfied, as long as the patient has no new symptoms or habits which warrant discontinuation of any oral contraceptive.

Since risk of cardiovascular problems seems to

Table 115–1.   Effects of Synthetic Progestins*

ESTROGENIC	ANDROGENIC
Norethynodrel	Norgestrel
Ethnodiol	Norethindrone
All others have none	Norethindrone acetate
	Ethnodiol
	Norethynodrel (has none)

In order of decreasing potency.

increase as estrogen doses rise above 50 ug/day, it is best to begin with a pill containing 50 ug of either mestranol or ethinyl estradiol. The lowest possible progestin dose will help minimize bothersome side effects such as increased appetite, steady weight gain, acne, and depression. Patients who have a history of symptoms suggesting hyperresponsiveness to endogenous estrogens (premenstrual breast engorgement and soreness, cyclic weight gain, heavy periods) may benefit from a preparation containing a progestin with minimal estrogenic effect, and perhaps some antiestrogenic or androgenic qualities. Similarly, a patient bothered by acne or hirsutism should not be given a preparation with an androgenic progestin (see Table 115–1). Other side effects such as nausea seem related to estrogen content.

Low-dose or "minidose" oral contraceptives were developed to minimize adverse effects of estrogens by decreasing the dose below 50 μg. The preparations need to be taken religiously to be maximally effective and may cause breakthrough bleeding or even amenorrhea. As a result, they are not prescribed for first-time users unless concern about estrogen-related side effects is significant. There is no available evidence that the rate of cardiovascular complications is lower with these agents.

It is helpful to become familiar with four or five combination pills and their minor differences, rather than using the most recently marketed combinations. Providing the patient with full, understandable information at the initiation of therapy will ward off many anxious phone calls. In particular, if one or two pills are missed, they can be made up by doubling the dose for the next one or two days, but barrier contraception is recommended for the remainder of the cycle. If three or more consecutive pills are missed, the pills should be stopped altogether, allowing withdrawal bleeding to occur, and then started 1 week after the last pill was taken. However, failure to take oral contraceptives regularly is an indication for trying another form of birth control.

Patients require follow-up care yearly, checking

for headaches, hypertension, breast masses, cervical abnormalities, phlebitis, and signs of cardiovascular or cerebrovascular disease.

Physicians are generally unaware of the high discontinuation rate among oral contraceptive users. Factors involved include the patient's perceptions of need and attitudes about taking medications that affect the sex organs. Oral contraceptives may cost several dollars a month and require a medical prescription, important barriers for adolescents. Despite these factors and known side effects, birth control pills continue to be the most used, safest birth control method for most women under 30. The pill's relative safety is most apparent in countries where the risk of dying in childbirth is high.

Adverse effects. The major hazards of oral contraceptives are cardiovascular. The relative risks of cardiovascular events in users as compared to nonusers are reported to be 4 to 11 times greater for thromboembolism, 4 to 9.5 times greater for thrombotic stroke, 2 times greater for hemorrhagic stroke, and 2 to 12 times greater for myocardial infarction. Mortality from myocardial infarction rises sixfold in women over 40 who are smokers. Overall excess death rate annually has been estimated to be 20 per 100,000, with risk concentrated in women over 35, especially if they smoke cigarettes and have used oral contraceptives for 5 years or more. Division of data at 35 years of age is arbitrary, and it would be prudent to assume that risk gradually increases with age.

Any population of women provided with oral contraception will show a rise in mean blood pressure in about 3 months. Prospective studies have found that the incidence of *hypertension* increases two- to sixfold in users as compared to nonusers. Patients with hypertension are at increased risk and should not use oral contraceptives. It is wise to check blood pressure before renewing a patient's prescription. The progesterone in the birth control pill, like the progesterone in the secretory phase of the menstrual cycle, increases aldosterone secretion, and estrogen increases renin substrate.

There is a twofold increase in the risk of *gallbladder disease* in users as compared to nonusers, due to increased cholesterol saturation of bile. The frequency of gallstones appears to rise after 2 years' usage and to reach a plateau after 4 to 5 years' usage. This risk must be balanced against the increased risk of gallbladder disease associated with multiparity. Another hepatobiliary problem is development of highly vascular *hepatic adenomas,* which can rupture spontaneously, resulting in serious hemorrhage, isolated cases have appeared in the literature. In cases, most patients were using the pill more than 5 years. The actual risk is unknown. Finally, estrogen use has been associated with *cholestatic jaundice,* but oral contraceptive use does not worsen cases of mild viral hepatitis and need not be discontinued unless cholestasis or hepatocellular injury is severe.

At present, there is no evidence of increased risk of *cancer* from use of oral contraceptives by premenopausal women. However, the growth of certain cancers may be stimulated by estrogens; these include carcinoma of the breast (see Chapter 118), cervix and endometrium (see Chapter 137). Most studies have shown a diminished incidence of fibroadenomas and benign fibrocystic disease of the breast in pill users.

There appears to be an increased risk of *congenital malformations* with inadvertent exposure of the fetus to birth control pills in early pregnancy, but this is a subject of continued dispute. Masculinization of the fetus was reported with earlier pill preparations.

Metabolic and *endocrinologic effects* are numerous. Thyroid-binding globin levels increase, which in turn raises the serum thyroxine level. Glucose tolerance falls as circulating growth hormone rises and peripheral resistance to insulin occurs. Triglyceride levels increase, sometimes dramatically, with the concurrent boost in lipoprotein production.

A few miscellaneous effects are worth noting. Birth control pills increase the frequency of *migraine headache* in patients with prior migraine attacks. Anecdotal reports of *exacerbation of lupus erythematosus* appear in the obstetric literature. Sensitivity to sunlight and chloasma (mask of pregnancy) are seen in some users and fade with discontinuation.

A number of gynecologic conditions are affected by use of these agents; effects may be beneficial or detrimental. Patients with menstrual irregularities prior to oral contraceptive use will have regular pill-induced periods while taking the medication. Upon discontinuation of the pills, some will revert to their previous irregularity. Rarely, *amenorrhea* due to ovarian suppression will persist for several months, even a year (see Chapter 107). Usually, menses return promptly, and fertility rates in the first 3 months of discontinuation are increased. Occasionally, a patient will notice nipple discharge (nonpuerperal lactation) with oral contraceptives. The mechanism is not clear.

Table 115–2.   Contraindications of Oral Contraceptives

Absolute Contraindications
1. Thromboembolic disorders, cardiovascular disease, thrombophlebitis, or a past history of these conditions or other conditions which predispose to them
2. Markedly impaired liver function from severe hepatitis, alcoholism, etc.
3. Known or suspected estrogen-dependent neoplasm (cancers of the breast, endometrium, etc.)
4. Undiagnosed genital bleeding
5. Known or suspected pregnancy

Relative Contraindications
1. Migraine headache
2. Hypertension
3. Familial hyperlipidemia
4. Epilepsy
5. Uterine leiomyoma
6. History of idiopathic obstructive jaundice of pregnancy
7. Smoking one-half pack or more per day
8. Diabetes mellitus
9. Severe heart disease
10. Patient unreliability

Many patients with *dysmenorrhea* find marked relief with oral contraceptives. If the dysmenorrhea is associated with endometriosis, the response is variable, with many patients complaining of exacerbation of symptoms rather than relief.

With these side effects in mind, absolute and relative contraindications can be listed (Table 115–2). Patients exposed to diethylstilbestrol have used birth control pills with no evidence to date of either beneficial or deleterious effects.

ABORTION

Studies by Planned Parenthood have not found that a substantial number of American women rely on abortion as the sole method of birth control, nor has any trend to such a reliance been noted. Rather, abortion is used as a backup when other methods fail. Frequently, the necessity for an abortion initiates effective contraceptive use, particularly in those under 20 years of age. No adverse effect of first trimester induced abortion on future childbearing has been demonstrated. The effect of second trimester abortions in rupturing cervical tissue is controversial. Rarely, an anomalous cervix may become incompetent, requiring cerclage if the patient wishes to carry future pregnancies to term.

OVERALL RISKS

Used alone by women 30 and under, condoms, diaphragms, IUDs, birth control pills and first trimester abortion have a mortality risk of 1 to 2 per 100,000, significantly lower than the 12 per 100,000 delivery-related risk rate. After age 30, the risk of birth control pills rises, especially in smokers, but is still less than the morbidity and complications of childbearing without fertility control. The lowest level of mortality is achieved by a combination of contraception with access to early abortion.

STERILIZATION

In 1965, one third of the married couples in the United States used oral contraception, sterilization or IUDs. By 1975, almost three quarters used one of these methods. Sterilization is now the most frequently used method of contraception among couples married for a decade or more, as well as among couples who have had all the children they want.

Vasectomy is the simplest and safest means of sterilization. Only a few surgical instruments and local anesthesia are required. The procedure may be done in a clinic, doctor's office, ambulatory surgical day care unit, or hospital. The procedure does not lead to impotence; rather, men with problems associated with impotence may blame vasectomy. It takes about 90 days of average ejaculatory activity to completely empty the spermatic cord and accessory glands of residual sperm. Thus, the vasectomy subject should have a postoperative semen analysis before he is considered sterile. Alternate methods of birth control should be used in the interim. Circulating antibodies to sperm may be induced by foreign proteins as well as by sperm. The effect of elevated sperm antibodies on a man's health is not clear, but has been the subject of much concern. Despite the concern, vasectomy still appears safe and effective, and is the least expensive form of permanent sterilization. Recanalization when ends of the vas are tied too closely together may account for failures. Reanastomosis may be carried out with microsurgical techniques; however, only about one third of patients undergoing reanastomosis father live-born children.

The causes of diminished fertility are multifactorial and include damage to nerves adjacent to the vas, the age of the patient, the age of the partner, and motivation for the initial procedure and for reanastomosis.

Procedures on the fallopian tubes. In 1975, 2 per cent of women 25 to 34 years of age underwent tubal sterilization. Surgical division of the fallopian tubes after delivery is easily accomplished, either with normal vaginal delivery or with cesarean section. The procedure adds 1 to 2 days to the patient's hospitalization. Procedures which leave the two ends of the fallopian tubes in close proximity (Pomeroy technique, in which a suture ties a knuckle of tube and the apex of the knuckle is excised) may have a failure rate of 2 per cent. Other methods which leave the two severed ends well separated have less than 1 per cent failure rates. When there is concern for the survival of the newborn, postpartum sterilization is contraindicated.

Vaginal tubal ligation is usually not done postpartum through the vagina because of the increased vascularity and the risk of sepsis. A skilled obstetrician-gynecologist can do interval sterilizations under local anesthesia, usually in a day care or hospital facility. However, leiomyoma, endometriosis, or previous infection may obstruct the approach to the tube.

The *minilaparotomy* involves a small abdominal incision of 1 to 2 inches done under local anesthesia through the peritoneum. Each fallopian tube is identified, ligated and divided. The incision is closed with resorbable sutures, and a bandage is applied. The patient is able to go home within a few hours.

These methods have the advantage of simplicity and require commonly used instruments. They have been taught to surgical technicians in third world countries. Such procedures may be unsuitable in an obese or anxious patient. In fact, other methods are more commonly used in the United States.

Laparoscopy requires expensive special instrumentation and an experienced gynecologist or surgeon. Although it can be done under local anesthesia, general endotracheal anesthesia is more commonly used. A preparatory D&C is usually done (as many patients consider themselves sterile at the time the appointment is made) in anticipation of, rather than after, laparoscopy. A fiberoptic endoscope is inserted through a subumbilical incision, and a second instrument accompanies the endoscope or is inserted through the pelvic incision. The tubes are cauterized or both cauterized and divided. Alternatively, plastic rings or clips are used to occlude them. Cauterization has the lowest failure rate; however, clips are advocated as being less likely to cause damage to bowel. In fact, complications and failures with clips are often remedied by cauterization. Furthermore, the half-life of the plastic materials used for occlusion has not been clearly defined, and very little 5-year data are available.

In experienced hands, laparoscopy is highly effective with minimal risk in a healthy woman. Most insurance carriers will pay for such procedures, though some require a euphemistic indication such as "recurrent situational anxiety." Laparoscopy may be accomplished on a 1-day basis, although most hospitals do not offer day care facilities. The patient may be expected to continue her normal menstrual life and menopause. Anastomosis of severed fallopian tubes is accomplished by careful surgical procedures with or without optical magnification. However, as with vasectomy, the rate of achieving patency is higher than that of live births. Motivating factors, patient age, concurrent disease, or attitudes of the partner as well as surgical technical details account for the low fertility rate.

In general, tubal sterilization should be considered irreversible. The procedure is indicated when the patient requests it. Many requests for anastomosis of divided tubes come when the procedure is initially advocated by a physician or partner. A woman of 23 with three children may be firm in her desire for sterilization, whereas a woman of 34 with five children may be unwilling to consider it. On the average, women are 28 to 30 years old at the time of tubal sterilization; 88 per cent are married, 6 per cent have never been married.

The federal government will not reimburse for sterilization done at the time of abortion, because the combined procedure has been found to be more hazardous than either done separately. The rare instance in which this does not hold true is the patient in whom the risk of anesthesia is unduly high, such as a woman with myasthenia gravis. There is no federal reimbursement for sterilization of minors or mentally incompetent patients. Though awkward in individual cases, on the whole, such regulations have been necessary to prevent widespread abuse of easily accomplished, low-risk surgical procedures done without due respect for the patient's understanding or desires. In addition the government will not pay for hysterectomies done solely for the purpose of sterilization. The public acceptability of sterilization is suggested by government reports of women interviewed in 1970 and reinterviewed in 1975; one half had changed their method of birth control, and most of these changed to sterilization.

PRINCIPLES OF MANAGEMENT

The choice of birth control is best viewed in terms of the patient's age and family expectations. *Unmarried adolescents and women in their early twenties* may use oral contraceptives with a high degree of safety and acceptability. Contraindications are infrequent in this age group, and the cost, in general, is not beyond their reach. Diaphragms may be as effective, but often are less acceptable. Condoms and foam are adequate as long as they are always available. Their use depends on motivation, which can be lacking at times. IUDs are effective, but the risk of pelvic sepsis that may affect future childbearing is a concern.

For sexually active *26- to 35-year-olds,* birth control pills, diaphragms and condoms may be equally effective, and choice is simply a matter of preference. IUDs may be a reasonable choice for women aware of the risk of pelvic inflammatory disease and willing to seek help promptly at the first sign of infection. IUDs are often quite acceptable in parous women and may be ideal for child-spacing. The smoker should be asked to stop if she wants to use oral contraceptives. Many patients in this age group have completed their families and request sterilization. Nulliparous women in this age group who desire sterilization present a problem to many health care providers. If the patient is not well known to the clinic or physician, one can suggest she practice contraception for a year, then undergo sterilization if she still wants to. When such advice is given, perhaps half the patients return for the procedure. The others go elsewhere or change their minds.

For *women over 35,* the risk of birth control pills makes them a less desirable choice than the other methods discussed. *The woman over 40* is not a candidate for oral contraception. Moreover, she may have a leiomyoma, making IUD insertion difficult. Though she is near the menopause, sterilization often relieves recurrent anxiety associated with risk of pregnancy. An ECG and chest x-ray are important preoperative procedures in such women undergoing general endotracheal anesthesia.

PATIENT EDUCATION

There are few areas in primary care where patient education is so important to decision-making. Diagrammatic and written material is available from most commercial distributors of contraceptive products, Planned Parenthood, many women's advocate organizations, the American College of Obstetrics and Gynecology, and the American Medical Association. It is most important that information be clearly written in the patient's native language, and that the patient be given an opportunity to ask questions and demonstrate her understanding.

The need to offer sympathetic and nonjudgmental counseling cannot be overemphasized. It is the physician's task to help the patient select the form birth control which is safest, most effective and personally acceptable. (See individual sections for relevant patient education issues.)

INDICATIONS FOR REFERRAL

Patients may need or request referral for counseling on emotional responses to sexual activity and contraceptive techniques. Referral to a social worker, sex therapist or psychiatrist with an interest in the area may be useful, but thorough discussion between the primary physician and patient usually suffices.

When a surgical procedure is being considered, the patient should meet with the gynecologist to discuss the issue in more detail. Referrals of medically uncomplicated patients may be made by phone. For patients with known medical problems, a careful prior history and physical examination and written referral to the specialist are helpful, so that the risks of the various procedures may be carefully discussed and therapy individualized. Patients who seem unable to use any form of birth control offered may also be referred to any of the above-named specialists, in the hope that an alternate approach will enhance motivation.

ANNOTATED BIBLIOGRAPHY

Barnes, A.B., Cohen, E., Stoeckle, J.D., and McGuire, M.T.: Therapeutic abortion: Medical and social sequels. Ann. Intern. Med., *75*:881, 1971. *(Summarizes impact on the patient from medical and social perspectives.)*

Boston Women's Health Book Collective: Our Bodies, Ourselves. New York: Simon & Schuster, 1976. *(A useful volume for many Americans, but may be too opinionated and difficult for patients with educational disadvantages.)*

Chapel, T.A., and Burns, R.E.: Oral contraceptives and exacerbation of lupus erythematosus. Am. J. Obstet. Gynecol, *110*:366, 1971. *(A case report of worsening SLE.)*

Collaborative Group for the Study of Stroke in Young Women: Oral contraception and increased risk of cerebral ischemia or thrombosis. N. Engl. J. Med., *288*:871, 1973. *(The incidence of thrombotic stroke showed a ninefold increase among women using oral contraceptives; hemorrhagic stroke showed less dramatic, but still significant, increase.)*

Ecklman, D.A., Benger, G.S., and Keith, L.: Intrauterine Devices and Their Complications. Boston: G. K. Hall, 1979. *(Careful evaluation of current literature; clear and complete.)*

Edmondson, H.A., Henderson, B., and Benton, B.: Liver cell adenomas associated with use of oral contraceptives. New Engl. J. Med., *294*:470, 1976. *(A study of 42 women with matched controls showed a dramatic rise in incidence of liver adenomas, correlated with prolonged use of pills which are more likely to contain mestranol as the synthetic estrogen.)*

Hatcher, R.A., Stewart, G.K., Stewart, F., *et al.:* Contraceptive Technology (ed. 9), 1978–1979. New York: Halsted Press, 1979. *(This volume is usually updated every 2 years; a useful handbook.)*

Hennekens, C.H., and MacMahon, B.: Oral contraceptives and myocardial infarction. N. Engl. J. Med., *296*:1166, 1977. *(Editorial reviewing current data suggesting increased risk of cardiovascular disease among women of various age groups using oral contraception. Stresses caution in such use among older women and the need for more data on younger women.)*

Kaminsky, H. (ed.): Proceedings of the First National Conference on the Safety of Fertility Control. Int. J. Gynecol. Obstet., *15*(2), 1977. *(This volume includes many excellent articles, such as the one by Tietze on statistical information about contraception.)*

Kopit, S., and Barnes, A.B.: Patients' response to tubal division. JAMA, *236*:2761, 1976. *(Of 197 patients who underwent tubal division, 93.5 per cent said they would make the same choice again. Those who were regretful could not be readily identified by any preoperative characteristic such as age, parity, or marital status.)*

Lancet, October 8, 1978. *(This issue contains reports of Vessey and the Oxford Family Planning Area as well as of the Royal College of General Practice studies, letters from the President of the Royal College of Obstetrics and Gynaecology and the President of the Royal College of General Practice, providing useful clinical commentary.)*

Langer, A., Devanesam, M., Pelosi, M., *et al.:* Choice of an oral contraceptive. Am. J. Obstet. Gynecol., *126*:153, 1976. *(Discussion of the biochemistry and pharmacology of available types of oral contraceptives, with review of their physiological effects and contraindications.)*

Potter, R.G.: Length of observation seen as a factor affecting contraceptive failure. Milbank Memor. Fund Q., *38*:140, 1960. *(Failure rates increased with time of observation.)*

Rosenberg, L., Armstrong, B., and Jick, H.: Myocardial infarction and estrogen therapy in postmenopausal women. N. Engl. J. Med., *294*:1256, 1976. *(Study from the Boston Collaborative Drug Surveillance Program indicating no statistically significant association between regular use of estrogen and nonfatal myocardial infarction.)*

Rosenfield, A.: Oral and intrauterine contraception: A 1978 risk assessment. Am. J. Obstet. Gynecol., *132*:92, 1978. *(Review of risks and benefits involved with these methods of contraception; 92 refs.)*

Ten-Year Progress Report of the Center for Population Research. Office of Research Reporting, NICHD, Building 31, Room 2A-34, National Institutes of Health, Bethesda, MD 20014. *(Excellent source of fertility and population statistics.)*

Tyson, J.E., and Felig, P.: Medical aspects of diabetes in pregnancy and the diabetogenic effects of oral contraceptives. Med. Clin. North Amer., *55*:947, 1971. *(Peripheral insulin resistance and glucose intolerance occur.)*

Westrom, L., Bergstrom, L.P., and Mandh, P.A.: The risk of pelvic inflammatory disease in women using intrauterine contraceptive devices as compared to nonusers. Lancet, 2:221, 1976. *(Risk of PID was seven times greater than for similar women not using IUDs.)*

World Health Organization: WHO study finds natu-

ral family planning to be "relatively ineffective" even with careful teaching. Fam. Plan. Perspect., *11*:40, 1979. *(Natural methods reported to have a high failure rate.)*

116
Approach to the Infertile Couple
ANN B. BARNES, M.D.

Fertility rates are affected by socioeconomic circumstances, disease patterns, war, and use of contraceptive techniques; they vary from place to place. Fertility may be measured by the census of live-born children in a population, but the variations do not inversely reflect infertility. Epidemiologic data on involuntary infertility are inadequate. Social scientists' data on samples of populations lack medical documentation. Data from infertility clinics lack documentation of the patient selection process and the population from which the patients are drawn. Estimates of infertility in populations of industrialized nations vary from 5 per cent to a high of 22 per cent.

The primary physician is often the first to be consulted by the couple unable to conceive. Although the usual request is to find or rule out a medical cause for the problem, there is also a need to identify any psychological or socioeconomic barriers to conception. Treatment is frequently carried out by individuals specializing in infertility, but the primary care physician should become proficient in performing the initial assessment and knowing when referral is indicated. Principal tasks include providing accurate advice and uncovering treatable etiologies.

PATHOPHYSIOLOGY AND CLINICAL PRESENTATION

Any disorder involving the male or female reproductive system may interfere with function to a degree sufficient to cause infertility.

Men. Inability to sustain an erection is a major contributor to the problem (see Chapters 128 and 217). *Varicoceles* are found in up to 40 per cent of males in infertility clinic populations. Theories suggest that venous distentions interfere with the normal cooling mechanism in the testes and result in disturbance of spermatogenesis. Oligospermia or azospermia may be temporary or permanent. Genetic disor-

ders and damage from bacterial or viral *infections* (e.g., postpubertal mumps) are often irreversible, whereas psychogenic factors, *depression,* and situational *stress* can cause transient declines in spermatogenesis. Nevertheless, the number of sperm thought to be required for fertilization continues to drop, as investigators continue to identify pregnancies intiated by men with sperm counts below 5 to 10 million. The ability of *sperm* to penetrate the zona pellucida of the ova, as well as the biochemical, immunologic and bacterial nature of the *semen,* is presently under investigation. *Anatomic anomalies* such as proximal location of the urinary meatus may lead to the deposition of sperm and semen too far from the cervical os.

Women. *Ovulatory disorders* are among the most frequent causes of failure to conceive. Any of the many causes of amenorrhea (see Chapter 107) may be responsible. A few deserve elaboration. Polycystic ovaries accompanied by low estrogen production with or without hirsutism, virilism, or obesity will produce severe difficulties, including infertility; when this condition is associated with moderate to high estrogen levels, infertility may be less of a problem. Inadequate follicular development with consequently inadequate corpus luteum formation is estimated to occur with 4 per cent of all ovulations and is claimed to occur in as many as 20 per cent of infertile women. Endometriosis is found in 8 to 15 per cent of infertility clinic populations. The person with testicular feminization (testosterone insensitivity) is typically attractive in appearance and has well developed breasts, but lacks pubic and axillary hair, ovaries, and a competent uterus.

Tubal disorders closely follow ovulatory difficulties as sources of infertility. Pelvic inflammatory disease, particularly nongonococcal in origin, is the most serious problem. A prospective study of 415 patients with pelvic inflammatory disease confirmed by laparoscopy and followed with repeat laparoscopy revealed that of those with a single episode of salpingitis, 12.1 per cent had tubal occlusion; of those with two infections, 35 per cent had occlusion; and of those with three or more, 75 per cent, had occluded tubes. Other pelvic infections, abdominal infections, and surgery in childhood (e.g., appendectomy) may lead to tubal adhesions. Infections associated with IUDs are a problem. Postpartum infection has an unusually frequent association with tubal occlusion. Infections following induced abortion, particularly if inadequately treated (e.g., with inappropriately low doses of antibiotics), unrecognized, or not brought to medical attention may lead to infertility. Unfortunately, oil-based radiopaque dyes used for uterotubograms (hysterosalpingograms) in some countries have also been associated with adhesions. Uncommon causes in the United States are pelvic trauma from vehicular accidents, ulcerative colitis, regional ileitis, tuberculosis, and schistosomiasis. In general, processes that cause adhesions as opposed to tubal epithelial damage seem to have a better prognosis.

Uterine problems play a less frequent role in infertility. Congenital anomalies, such as absence or duplication of the uterine fundus, often present as repeated pregnancy wastage. Complete duplication of cervix and uterus tends to diminish fertility, but less so than anomalies causing distortion of a single uterine cavity. Septate and deeply arcuate uteri may be more useful after hysteroscopic or operative repair. Urinary tract anomalies are estimated to occur with 25 per cent of congenitally abnormal uteri. They are found more frequently in the completely duplicated situation or when one side of the mullerian duct is missing. Leiomyoma uteri may distort or obstruct the uterine cavity. Resection and re-resection have been surprisingly successful. The forgotten IUD is occasionally a cause of infertility. The role of uterine glycosaminoglycan to stimulate conversion of sperm proacrosin to acrosin, a step necessary for sperm penetration of the zona pellucida, is an area of current investigation.

Cervical factors are attributed to as many as 20 per cent of the female infertile population. Cervical incompetence may account for repeated abortion or later trimester pregnancy losses. The incompetence can result from inadequate innervation, disturbances in synthesis or breakdown of prostaglandin, or defects in muscle and collagen fibers. Incompetence of the cervix may also compromise its role in resisting the entry of infectious agents into the sterile uterine cavity. The role of cervical mucus is little understood. Its physical characteristics in cystic fibrosis seem an obvious factor; the importance of cervical mucus antibodies and proteins as a sole cause of infertility is difficult to prove, yet it is the focus of much speculation.

Occasionally, the *vagina* is implicated as the cause of infertility. An intact or nearly intact hymen, a septum, or a constricting ring in the upper vagina can limit access to the cervix. Total absence of the vagina is only rarely associated with sufficient development of the cervix and uterus to allow fertility at all. As a site of infection, the vagina may prove to be an important cause of pregnancy wastage. Trichomonas, *Candida albicans,* chlamydia, mycoplasma, *Hemophilus vaginalis,* streptococci, and gonococci are all associated with cervical and vaginal discharge (see Chapter 112); their role in vaginally related obstructions to conception is not clear, though their role in pregnancy wastage is established. When these organisms lead to pelvic inflammatory disease, they become more clearly accountable for infertility.

Viral infections of the *vulva* and *labia,* particularly herpes vaginalis and condyloma accuminatum (see Chapters 112, 184, 186) are usually only temporary impediments to fertility. Vulvar surgery *per se* need not cause infertility. Similarly, paralysis or hemipelvectomy may or may not be blamed for infertility; much of the impediment derives from the social and emotional impact of these conditions.

Both Partners. *Interpersonal problems* are an important etiologic factor. The desire for children may not be shared, equally by both partners. This may be overt, with one partner seeking medical assistance to persuade the other. More often, it is covert. There may be anxiety over how family responsibilities will interfere with career development, or one partner may not want to lose the economic and social freedom of a childless couple. Sometimes one partner may be concerned about sharing the other's affection with a child. Some may feel inadequate or unwilling to assume parental duties. Such concerns can lead to sexual inactivity or frigidity. Transient situational problems arise. The young professional person may be under considerable job pressure; travel may interfere with optimal moments for insemination. Acknowledged or unrecognized homosexual preference may also interfere with fertility.

CLINICAL COURSE

The prognosis of infertility can be estimated from experiences reported by infertility clinics. In one study, 24 per cent of couples achieved pregnancy within 3 months of clinic registration. Another study showed that most conceptions occurred within 1 to 2 years, though the number continued to rise for 4 to 5 years after registration. There appears to be no difference in prognosis between couples with primary or secondary infertility. Recent evidence suggests that the prognosis for recurrent abortion is better than the approximately 20 per cent live birth rate previously estimated. Patients with ovulatory problems do reasonably well; those with tubal problems have more difficulty. In some series, pregnancy following tubal surgery occurred in 10 per cent of patients, whereas following minimal procedures, 79 per cent of couples achieved a live birth. Anastomosis of surgically divided vas deferens or fallopian tubes by a specialist is highly successful in achieving patency, but overall, only about one third of such procedures are followed by a live birth. Couples whose infertility involves multiple factors do less well than those in whom only one factor is present.

DIFFERENTIAL DIAGNOSIS

Male factors account for 30 to 40 per cent of cases. (See Chapter 128). Among female factors, ovulatory disturbances account for 40 per cent, tubal disorders for 10 to 30 per cent, cervical factors for 20 per cent and uterine factors for 8 per cent. Table 116–1 lists some of the most important etiologies.

WORKUP

Healthy couples who plan to discontinue barrier or oral contraceptive methods require no workup, since conception usually follows within a short period of time. Women who had ovulatory problems prior to use of birth control pills may conceive as readily. The same is true for patients discontinuing IUDs. Cautiously optimistic reassurance can be given with advice to check back in 1 year if difficulty occurs.

The primary physician need not hesitate to initiate an infertility workup, because infertility investigations frequently meet with early success and the physician already has knowledge of the patient's socioeconomic and psychological status. The investigation often provides opportunities for patients to consider the interaction between their life-styles, life expectations, and interpersonal relationships.

After a couple has tried to conceive for a year, i.e., during 12 consecutive menstrual cycles uninterrupted by intentional contraception or unintentional factors such as travel or illness of a partner, a *post-*

Table 116-1.   Important Etiologies of Infertility

MALE FACTORS	FEMALE FACTORS
1. Impotence	A. Ovulatory
2. Postpubertal mumps	1. Genetic disorders
3. Varicoceles	2. Hypothalamic dysfunction
4. Hypospadias	
5. Cancer chemotherapy	3. Pituitary insufficiency
6. Prostatitis	4. Inactive or polycystic ovaries
7. Genetic disorders	
8. Pituitary insufficiency	5. Endometriosis
9. Hypothyroidism	B. Tubal
10. Radiation	1. Infection, PID
11. Inadequate spermatogenesis	2. Adhesions
	3. Postsurgery
12. Seminal fluid inadequacies	C. Uterine
	1. Congenital malformations
13. Excess heat	2. Fibroids (repeated abortion)
	D. Cervical and Vaginal
	1. Poor mucus quality from infection, trauma, or estrogen deficiencies
	2. Anatomic abnormalities
	E. Vulvar
	1. Infections

coital examination of the woman is a useful way to initiate the infertility evaluation. The woman is asked to come for her appointment within 6 hours of coitus in the midcycle or second half of the menstrual cycle. If her partner is unable to respond on demand, the appointment is simply rescheduled. Repeated failure may provide a clue to presence of difficulties involving the marital relationship, social circumstances, or a partner's physical well-being. Postcoital tests provide an opportunity for a complete history and physical examination, with particular inquiry into history, age at menarche, and pregnancy history. Inquiry into any surgery or deliveries should be made; if any biopsies were done, pathology reports need to be obtained. The history and physical examination should include a search for evidence of a concomitant medical problem, such as thyroid disease (rarely a cause when it is not clinically obvious), diabetes mellitus, long-standing renal disease, or use of anti-hypertensive medications. A careful pelvic examination is essential, taking special note of any palpable adnexal, ovarian, or tubal mass or thickening of the uterosacral ligaments. During the pelvic examination the patient's response to the procedure may provide an opportunity to inquire into her feelings about sexual intercourse as well as to observe anatomic impediments.

A specimen should be obtained from the cervical

os, placed on a glass slide, and observed under high power. Five or more motile sperm found in the specimen confirms her partner's competence. Most physicians also look at a sample from the vaginal vaults, particularly if the cervix is directed away from the dependent parts of the vagina, as is seen in uterine retroversion. A negative post-coital test means very little and can occur even though the man is fertile. However, a repeated failure does justify a request for an examination of the partner (See Chapter 128), and sometimes an analysis of the semen is revealing. However, *semen analysis* is presently an inadequate way of defining causes of infertility. The volume of semen, the number of sperm, their shape and mobility may be recorded, but correlation of count with fertility is often poor.

If the patient complains of amenorrhea or oligomenorrhea, a *maturation index* may be obtained. In this procedure, the vaginal wall is scraped, the scrapings are applied to two separate microscopic slides, and the slides are submitted in preservative for cytologic examination. A low maturation index shows few mature superficial squamous cells and suggests a lack of estrogen stimulation. A high maturation index shows that 20 to 50 per cent of the superficial squamous cells are mature, and represents evidence that estrogen is present in amounts sufficient to mature the vagina, although the amounts may still be inadequate for production of withdrawal bleeding from the endometrium.

To establish ovulatory capacity, *serum progesterone* can be drawn on days 21 to 23 of the cycle, when the level should be 2 to 4 times its baseline. Endometrial biopsy may also be useful, but is more expensive, more painful, and may remove the long-awaited pregnancy. *Temperature charts* can also be used to identify ovulatory cycles; each morning the patient records oral temperature, using a special thermometer graduated in tenths (not two-tenths) of degrees Fahrenheit. Since this procedure is a constant daily reminder of one's infertility, it may be more depressing than helpful.

If the serum progesterone is low or the menstrual periods are so infrequent that it is impractical to obtain a progesterone level, one should assess pituitary function by ordering *serum prolactin, FSH,* and *LH* determinations. The findings of an elevated serum prolactin is an indication for skull tomograms to define the sella turcica in search of a pituitary tumor or empty sella syndrome (see Chapter 107). A normal prolactin usually rules out these rare problems. Elevations of lutenizing hormone and follicle stimulating hormone suggest ovarian failure. Ovarian failure,

whether caused by genetic factors, disease, or treatment such as cancer chemotherapy or radiation, is presently untreatable.

If the FSH alone is elevated beyond the normal range for the ovulatory woman, the patient should be referred to an endocrinologist or gynecologist interested in endocrinology for further investigation; there may still be some chance of pregnancy.

If there is an isolated LH elevation, the test should be repeated with careful attention to the day of the menstrual cycle to exclude the ovulatory peak. With the repeat LH, the serum free and total testosterones and androstenedione should be ordered; increased levels of these in the context of persistently high LH suggest polycystic ovary syndrome.

A *pelvic ultrasound* study can be a useful preliminary step in identification of a pelvic mass, particularly in distinguishing a cystic lesion from a solid one. If after the initial history, physical examination, postcoital test, and serum progesterone, it is evident that tubal or uterine factors are most likely to be causing infertility, a *uterotubogram* (hysterosalpingogram) may be helpful if a uterine anomaly seems likely. However, in the presence of recent or even long past pelvic inflammatory disease, it may cause a recrudescence adding to the infertility problem.

Intravenous pyelogram is sometimes used in selecting patients for uterotubograms, but the identification of an absent kidney or duplicated urinary structure does not automatically mean that there must be mullerian duct anomalies in an infertile woman and need for a uterotubogram. There should be positive evidence on physical examination or a history of pregnancy wastage.

Laparoscopy is presently one of the more useful procedures in investigation of infertile women. Adhesions are most commonly found. Endometriosis, an unpalpable fibroid, or polycystic ovaries may also be discovered. Often tubal patency and position may be confirmed more accurately than by radiologic investigation. Not to be forgotten is the importance of negative findings.

INDICATIONS FOR REFERRAL

Any anatomic lesions in the male or female require referral to the urologist or gynecologist respectively. Referrals of women should be made to an interested gynecologist, rather than to a general surgeon, because most of the latter are not adequately trained in female infertility.

In general, if any marital, social, or personal problems have arisen such that pregnancy is not desired as soon as possible, gynecological referral should be delayed until circumstances change. At times, these problems are the cause of infertility and may deserve psychiatric evaluation. When referral is indicated, patients should be encouraged to ask questions and voice their concerns to the specialist. If a working relationship is not developed, the primary physician may be helpful in finding an alternative. Patients with prolonged infertility (3 to 4 years) become discouraged and will seek alternate opinions. Here, the primary physician can help by inquiring into the expertise of the subsequent specialists. It is particularly important in the referral for tubal repair to select a gynecologist skilled in the procedure, since success rates vary considerably and results are often discouraging. Yet, it is unusual for a women with tubal occlusion to refuse surgery; even with the slimmest chance of success, most women still will choose surgical repair.

PATIENT EDUCATION AND COUNSELING

Whenever a test comes out normal, it is important to reassure the woman about her normality, particularly if she harbors guilt or fear about an episode of infidelity, a previous abortion, or an out-of-wedlock pregnancy.

The investigation of infertility provides an opportunity to educate patients about normal human reproduction. This area is still omitted from many school curricula, and is inadequately covered in others. Education for both partners about the menstrual cycles, frequency of coitus, and male and female sexual attitudes and responses may provide the cure.

Infertility studies may be the necessary impetus for encouraging the chronically ill to follow medical regimens attentively. Infertility may also lead to reconsideration and redesign of drug regimens for other problems (e.g., antihypertensive agents and cancer chemotherapy drugs may interfere with conception; see Chapters 21 and 88 respectively).

The couple that is still unsuccessful after a year of trying can be given some reassurance as they begin to undergo evaluation. Nearly one-quarter of such couples achieve pregnancy within 3 months, while one-half do so within the year.

Infertility resulting from lack of privacy due to the presence of a child or in-laws needs to be approached with careful and understanding explanation, perhaps in conjunction with a family member, clergy, or mental health professional. A home visit by the visiting nurse may sometimes be helpful in delineating the problem and suggesting solutions. Despite the patient's frequent efforts to medicalize social problems, there may be no medical solution; instead, attention may need to be directed to the home environment.

ANNOTATED BIBLIOGRAPHY

Cook, I. D.: The natural history and major causes of infertility. *In* Diczfalusy, A. (ed.): The WHO Symposium on Advances in Fertility Regulation. Copenhagen: Scriptor, 1977. *(A hard to obtain but most useful overview of the problem.)*

Diugnan, N. M., Jordan, J. A., Couglan, B. M., and Logan-Edwards, R.: One thousand consecutive cases of diagnostic laparoscopy. J. Obstet. Gynecol. Brit. Cwlth., 79:1016, 1972. *(There are many series on laparoscopy, but this is one of the most useful. The role of ovarian biopsy, however, is not supported by most other authors.)*

Gorry, G. A., Pauker, S. G., and Swartz, W. B.: Diagnostic importance of the normal finding. N. Engl. J. Med., 298:486, 1978. *(Emphasizes the value to the patient of a normal finding.)*

Malone, L. J., and Ingersoll, F. M.: Myomectomy in infertility. *In* Berman, S. J., and Kistner, R. W. (eds.): Progress in Infertility, ed. 2. Boston: Little, Brown, 1975. *(Good discussion of the efficacy of the procedure on improving fertility.)*

Masters, W. H., and Johnson, V. E.: Human Sexual Response. Boston: Little, Brown, 1966. *(The classic modern work on the physiology and pathophysiology of sexual activity.)*

Southam, A. L., and Buxton, C. L.: Factors influencing reproductive potential. Fertil. Steril., 6:25, 1957. *(This paper provides a background on which to measure current infertility clinic reports.)*

Tietze, C., Gutmacher, A. F., and Rubin, S.: Time required for conception in 1727 planned pregnancies. Fertil. Steril., 1:338, 1950. *(An early, careful study. The first author continues to be the most useful statistician reporting in the area of fertility and contraception.)*

U. S. Department of Commerce: Statistical Abstracts, 1978. *(A volume available yearly from the U. S. government containing summary tables of vital statistics on many subjects.)*

Westrom, L.: Effect of acute pelvic inflammatory disease on fertility. Am. J. Obstet. Gynecol., *121*:707, 1975. *(A total of 415 women treated for PID reviewed after 9.5 years; 88 [21.2 per cent] were involuntarily childless. Tubal occlusion was more common after nongonococcal disease than after gonorrheal salpingitis.)*

117

Approach to the Woman with an Unwanted Pregnancy

ANN B. BARNES, M.D.

"It is natural to man to die, as to be born: and to a little infant, perhaps, the one is as painful as the other."
Francis Bacon, *Of Death* (1612)

INCIDENCE

There were 3,168,000 live births and approximately one million legal induced abortions in the United States in 1976. The national abortion-to-live-birth ratio rose between 1975 and 1976 by 15 per cent, from 272 abortions per thousand live births to 312. Increasingly, women obtain abortions in their home states—90 per cent did so in 1976. About one third of the women who obtained abortions were under 19, one third were 20 to 24, and one third were over 25 years of age.

Presently, about one-half of all pregnancies in women under 19 end in abortion. This group, particularly those under 15, is the only part of the population in which fertility is increasing. Planned Parenthood estimates that about 200,000 unwanted births occurred in this age group in 1976. It is in this age group that sex education and information are most needed. About one-third of pregnancies in women 20 to 29 and nearly half of pregnancies in women over 30, end in induced abortion. At the time of abortion, 75 per cent of women are unwed. Eighty-nine per cent of abortions are done before 12 weeks gestation, most by suction curettage. The trend toward decreases in abortion-related deaths continued in 1976, when 1 per 100,000 (26 women) died, compared to 3.4 per 100,000 in 1975. Maternal mortality dropped from 12.8 to 12.3 per 100,000 in the same period. The percentage of abortions done after 12 weeks continues to drop. Although the number of repeated abortions increased, there was no evidence from a Planned Parenthood study that women were substituting abortion for conventional contraception.

In considering the risk of achieving pregnancy, wanted or unwanted, Tietze estimated the risk of pregnancy after a single coital act to be between 1 in 25 and 1 in 50. He used Kinsey's estimates of coital frequency of 3.7 times per week for 16- to 20-year-olds, 3 times for 21- to 25-year-olds, 2.6 for 26- to 30-year-olds, 2.3 for 31- to 35-year-olds, and 2.0 for 36- to 40-year-olds. Using a different approach, others have estimated that sexually active, fertile women have a 30 per cent chance of becoming pregnant during each cycle.

The woman who suspects an unwanted pregnancy often calls upon her primary physician soon after a period is missed to have the diagnosis confirmed. In order to provide assistance, the physician needs to know the resources available in the community for abortions, prenatal care, placement, and the indications and risks of various abortion methods, as well as the woman's emotional makeup and social situation. An unwanted pregnancy, especially in the younger patient, is a reflection of the need for patient education in reproductive matters, which should be carried out at the time of the medical encounter to prevent recurrences.

CLINICAL PRESENTATIONS

The presentations of women with unwanted pregnancies are as varied as all human experience. However, certain patterns occur which reflect stress points as well as socioeconomic pressures that touch each individual similarly. A pregnancy may reassure a woman of her unique ability and her potential continuity. The decision to abort is usually a practical one. Few women "want" an abortion. Few perceive a risk; the risk of dying in childbirth is not a deterrent to sexual relations or pregnancy. Indeed, it is hard to tell the sick cardiac patient that she is not capable of carrying a pregnancy to term and that for her safety the pregnancy should be aborted. No woman, no matter how ill, likes to be told she "can't be a woman."

A number of presentations are particularly important because of their psychosocial circumstances and ramifications for prevention of future pregnancy.

In both rural and urban areas, *incest* persists to a greater extent than most professional people assume. It may occur between father and daughter, but frequently involves a mother's boyfriend or second husband and a child. Brother and sister pregnancies also occur. Often the mother is so offended by the implications of the incest that she will never appear with the pregnant youngster. The pregnant youngster is confused, scared, and may be unaware of what is going on. Usually it is beyond a physician's capability to change the social situation from which such a pregnancy arose, but encouraging the patient to have an IUD inserted at or after the procedure or prescribing birth control pills may prevent a future pregnancy even if the social setting cannot be improved.

Adolescent women are no different from young men in their perception of risks. "Oh, it will never happen to me," or "I can do it once and it will be OK." Other teenagers feel unwanted or unloved and see a pregnancy as providing a companion who will want them and love them. The impracticality of this dream may be stressed, and usually parental permission for abortion is promptly forthcoming. Such young women are likely to become pregnant repeatedly, as medical intervention can seldom affect the surrounding circumstances.

Other young women are angry at their parents and see a pregnancy as a way of getting even or "really hurting" them. They may not be eager for any abortion that is arranged by their parents, and often are not enthusiastic participants in prenatal care either. That the fate of the unborn might be similar to their own sometimes sways their decisions as to whether to continue the pregnancy.

The 15-year-old unmarried couple who come together are charming in their innocent trust, but may be masking substantial personal problems.

Most second trimester abortions are done on teenagers. The number decreases each year, but because the complications of the procedure increase with the passing weeks of gestation, this remains an important problem. At first, there may be a problem of denial, but denial is usually hard to sustain after two missed periods. Then there is the problem of how to get help. Many teenagers are uninformed on such matters and often turn to their uninformed peers. Perhaps an older sister, a friend, or an older brother will be able to provide information. Alternately, a suspicious mother will drag her daughter to the doctor. Such patients provide monosyllabic histories and may even mumble or not answer inquiries at all.

The *older teenager* or 20-year-old often presents early with an unwanted pregnancy, and simply wants to "get it over with." Such patients are often able to accept office curettage (menstrual extraction) with little difficulty and minimal or no anesthesia. Contraception is usually accepted with alacrity.

The 20-year-old who presents in the second trimester often signals marked ambivalence. Counseling, including an opportunity for her to express her mixed feelings, is expecially necessary.

The *rape victim* may be repulsed at the thought of a baby inside her from such a horrible experience. She may present near or after 12 weeks, and may not be able to cooperate in either the pelvic examination or other care.

Women in their *thirties* and *forties* seek abortion with the same air of practicality as younger women, but are often touched with a tinge of remorse that there may not be many more opportunities for motherhood ahead. This attitude is as common in unmarried as in married women. Others come for abortion forced by the economic reality of childbearing. Often the husband has made the economic decision and the pregnant woman accepts it as the best course, but is far from eager. At this time, such women are not receptive to the suggestion of permanent sterilization.

Patients undergoing amniocentesis for genetic counseling do so on the assumption that they would accept induced abortion, which usually would occur between 20 and 24 weeks gestation, often after they have experienced fetal movement (quickening). The feeling of being a failure and unable to have a normal child will add to the normal hormonally-induced depression that follows any pregnancy termination and requires supportive care. Sometimes there is a touch of anger with the sadness, and the primary physician will be asked to arbitrate the advice of the genetic counselor and the obstetrician.

One of the saddest situations involves the *previously infertile woman* when she comes to have taken away that which she wanted most for as much as

5 or 10 years because of a preconceived idea of what a normal family should be, economic problems, or change of attitude of an aging spouse.

Patients who present for *repeat abortions* tend to generate feelings of frustration in health care personnel. They may return because they made the same mistake again, or because they tried a different form of birth control that was not properly explained or has failed. Other women need to reassure themselves of their fertility; in such cases, no form of birth control will work. A few lack motivation for any self-help. Others may be prostitutes, earning cash for a drug or alcohol habit. Others are severely ill mental patients. There is little evidence that the pregnancy affects the course of the mental illness or that the mental illness will affect the outcome of the pregnancy, except insofar as their illness affects their socioeconomic status and ability to physically care for themselves.

PRINCIPLES OF MANAGEMENT

One must first confirm the diagnosis of pregnancy. A first morning voided urine is collected about 40 days from the last menstrual cycle (LMP) or 10 days after the first missed period and saved in a clean container. Usually the specimen will contain sufficient human chorionic gonadotropin (HCG) for a positive slide test. It is important to practice the test several times before utilizing it, in order to ensure that the test is done correctly. A positive or negative pregnancy test of this nature does not by itself prove or disprove a pregnancy, but rather must be interpreted in conjunction with the patient's signs and symptoms. The patient may complain of some nausea; often breast tenderness is the first clue the patient can recount. It is particularly important to repeat the test or obtain the more expensive determination of the serum beta subunit of HCG if the patient thinks she is pregnant and urinary pregnancy tests are repeatedly negative. In general, if a woman thinks she's pregnant, she should be considered so until proven otherwise.

The earlier that an abortion is performed, the less the risk of complications. However, the risk increases each week of pregnancy, and approaches the risk of term delivery after the thirteenth week; nevertheless, there may be some time to resolve conflicts, make practical economic arrangements, or find the most appropriate resource within the community. Though most abortions are done in the state in which the pa-

the patient resides, availability of services is inconsistent, and some patients may have to travel long distances to unfamiliar surroundings. Planned Parenthood and the National Organization for Women usually have a list of referral centers and local resources. Local medical societies are less often helpful, although the district offices of the American College of Obstetrics and Gynecology are usually well informed.

It takes about 1,000 operative procedures, many under local anesthesia, to provide enough experience for an individual physician to develop skill commensurate with the national average complication rate. Thus, referring the patient to an experienced facility may be wiser than asking an associate who only occasionally does abortions to help out. However, Planned Parenthood or a direct call may clarify whether a new physician has just started or a waiting list is too long for a particular patient's needs.

Local and general anesthesia have the same rate of complications. Local anesthesia is associated with febrile and convulsive morbidity; general anesthesia with hemorrhage, cervical injury, and uterine perforation. General anesthesia usually costs more, but can still be used on a one-day ambulatory basis. Patients with venereal disease are particularly at risk for febrile complications. Patients should be tested for blood type, and immune globulin (RhoGAM or mini-RhoGAM) should be given to Rh-negative women (15 percent of the population). The postabortion period is also a good time for rubella immunization. The cervix may not prevent introduction of bacterial infection into the sterile uterine cavity for about 2 weeks following abortion, consequently, abstinence from coitus should be advised for this period. Longer periods of abstinence are usually unacceptable to the patient. All abortion facilities encounter patients who have coitus with a partner eager to console immediately following an abortion.

If products of conception are retained, bleeding and fever usually do not occur for about 3 days; then cramping pain, a tender uterus, and temperature elevation, possibly with an elevated white count and sedimentation rate, will be found. Repeat curettage with oral, or possibly intravenous, antibiotics, is indicated. Passage of fetal parts may spontaneously resolve the problem; however, this is not dependable.

Uterine perforation is usually recognized at operation. If it is not, it may lead to peritonitis, hemorrhage, or even prolapse of bowel through the uterus and cervix with obstructive symptoms. If a perforation is recognized at operation, bed rest, careful monitoring, and intravenous or liquid diet will often resolve the hazard, averting the need for exploratory surgery.

First trimester abortions are done with cervical dilatation over 8 to 12 hours with *laminaria* insertion or with dilators after anesthesia is administered. Following dilatation, *suction curettage* is carried out. Evidence is accumulating which suggests the slower laminaria dilatation may diminish the frequency of cervical malfunction in future pregnancies.

After 12 weeks, the fetal parts no longer can be removed with ease through a cervix dilated with standard dilators. Loss of blood may be excessive and the procedure incomplete. Second trimester abortion usually requires dilatation by insertion of several *dilateria* (laminaria japonica [Japanese seaweed] gas-sterilized). These are hydrophilic, swell on absorption of water, and gently dilate the cervix to 14 to 18 mm. in diameter. However, dilateria connect the never-sterile vagina with the sterile endometrial cavity and its contents. Furthermore, the uterine contents are removed from the normal maternal defenses to infection. Usually the abortion relieves this risk of sepsis, but some women get infections and, thus, some abortions are covered by prophylactic intravenous or oral antibiotics. Coverage should be directed against bowel flora. The abortion is carried out within 12 to 14 hours after laminaria insertion, usually with large *suction* instruments. At present, data from the Center for Disease Control indicate that this is the safest method of abortion up to 20 weeks. It is unusual for abortions to be done between 20 and 24 weeks. Legal intervention is required after 24 weeks.

Other methods in use for second trimester abortions include the installation of 40 mg. of *prostaglandin* E_2 alpha into the amniotic cavity, which produces uterine contractions and risk of cervical rupture if not accompanied by use of vigorous laminaria or oxytocin infusion for cervical softening. If oxytocin is given for cervical softening or to facilitate prostaglandin and hypertonic saline therapy, the volume of fluid should be watched to avoid water intoxication. Patients must be hospitalized for this procedure. The products of conception are usually viable when delivered. For this reason, some institutions combine 40 cc. of 23.9% saline with the prostaglandin.

Installation into the amniotic cavity of up to 200 cc. of 23.9% *saline* through the abdominal wall with a 20 or 22 gauge spinal needle, 3½ inches long, will usually lead to prompt demise of the products of conception followed in 14 to 36 hours with erratic labor and passage of the products of conception. As with prostaglandin, suction curettage subsequent to the passage of the products of conception is frequently required. Urea has been used in place of saline, but is expensive. The desire to avoid saline arises out of the known changes in coagulation factors, which rarely result in clinical disseminated intravascular coagulation or hemorrhage. Also, hypertonic saline is lethal to the mother if injected into her bloodstream; first, she will taste salt, and then will feel chest pain or pressure from pulmonary hypertension before losing consciousness due to brain damage. The procedure should be halted at the first taste of salt, and 5% dextrose and water should be infused to dilute the salt.

A combination of laminaria dilatation and hypertonic saline or prostaglandin is currently in use for 16–20 week abortion. Prostaglandin E_2 vaginal suppositories are being used with increasing frequency, as is intramuscular insertion of prostaglandin analogs.

Hysterotomy has the highest complication rate and appears unjustified at the present time. Furthermore, because the uterus is small, the uterine incision traverses the fundus, putting the patient at risk for rupture in subsequent pregnancy.

Laparoscopic sterilization at the time of induced abortion has been shown to be more hazardous than either procedure performed separately. The federal government will not pay for the two procedures simultaneously in Medicaid recipients, nor in federally funded insurance plans. This is probably wise except in those rare instances where the risk of using anesthesia twice is greater than the risk of the combined procedure, as in a patient with myasthenia gravis, multiple sclerosis, or severe heart disease.

Abortions may be done in conjunction with dental extractions, orthopedic surgery, biliary or GI surgery, or procedures on the lungs or endocrine organs. Some cardiac surgeons, neurosurgeons, and orthopedic surgeons are concerned about possible sepsis and will wish to use antibiotics prophylactically.

Despite the hazards listed above, legal abortions are safer than normal deliveries. Abortions in the hands of the inexperienced physician or outside the legal channels of care are a serious risk. With financial discrimination against certain segments of the population, it is not surprising to hear of *"criminal abortions"* again. The major problems are sepsis and hemorrhage. The signs of complications usually appear within 3 days, but usually the patient does not present for treatment until 7 to 10 days after "criminal" abortion. The history is usually not forthcoming, or the patient says she fell down the stairs and started to bleed. A complete physical examination is required. The punched-out, clean, clear ulcers of potassium permanganate tablets on opposing vaginal mucosal surfaces are a familiar indication of illicit attempts at self-abortion. Complete blood count, differential and blood cultures are essential; intravenous colloid or blood products are often needed. An upright KUB x-ray may indicate free air in cases of uterine perforation or suggest gas gangrene if coathangers or unsterile metal probes were used.

PATIENT EDUCATION

Individualized instruction on reproductive processes and contraception can be effective when given at the time the patient presents for abortion, at the abortion, and following the procedure. About one half of patients who undergo therapeutic abortion return for follow-up. However, unwed women who have a delivery and place the child for adoption frequently do not return for their postpartum checkups, and they have an 80 per cent risk of returning with another unwanted pregnancy within 2 years. On the other hand, 80 per cent of abortion patients are found to be using contraception appropriately after the procedure. The number of abortions arising out of lack of awareness of contraceptive needs or methods emphasizes the need for public education as well as informing the individual.

Patients are frequently concerned about the effect of abortion on future childbearing. This is an area of great controversy, but, at the present time in the United States, it would appear that one, and even two, therapeutic abortions do not statistically alter one's chances of normal childbearing. It should be kept in mind that about 20 per cent of all human pregnancies end in spontaneous abortion, discarding 95 per cent of the chromosomally abnormal fetuses. Thus, the patient should be reassured that a spontaneous abortion may have no relationship to an earlier induced abortion. There may be individual situations in which the therapeutic abortion has weakened the cervix so that it will prematurely open in a subsequent pregnancy, but it has been hard to document a cause-and-effect relationship or to predict which individuals are at risk for such an outcome. Fortunately, the numbers are small and not statistically significant.

The positive impact that understanding and support by the primary physician can have during this trying period should not be ignored or underestimated. Availability to answer questions and help work out the practicalities of the situation can foster a strong doctor-patient alliance which later can be used therapeutically to prevent recurrence and minimize the trauma of the unwanted pregnancy. An appointment to return for discussion after the abortion may be much appreciated.

INDICATIONS FOR REFERRAL

- If a physician, nurse, or nurse clinician has personal objections to abortion, the patient should be referred if she requests pregnancy termination.
- It is unusual for women undergoing pregnancy termination, even teenagers, and incest and rape victims, to require referral for mental health care. The primary physician, or associated social worker, often can provide appropriate opportunity for discussion of the psychosocial ramifications.
- If the primary physician or health unit has insufficient time or resources for counseling, most abortion clinics can provide patients with psychological support.
- Planned Parenthood, or local women's groups, may have listings of support groups that can be particularly useful in the face of individual harassment by "Right to Life" advocates found in some areas.

At the present time, federal regulations limit access to abortion for women on welfare and those with federal insurance, including those in the armed services. Yet, it has been shown that the hazard of childbearing is worse for women who have not completed high school or are of a lower socioeconomic status. Further, state, federal, and prepaid health plan restrictions on abortion run the danger of fostering a return to "criminal abortions" and their high risks of morbidity and mortality.

ANNOTATED BIBLIOGRAPHY

Alan Guttmacher Institute: Family Planning Perspectives, *11*(1), Jan./Feb., 1979. *(An ultimate source of current research and opinion.)*

Boston Women's Health Book Collective: Our Bodies, Ourselves. New York: Simon & Schuster, 1976. *(Consumer writers; useful alternate resource to professional publications.)*

Center for Disease Control: Abortion Surveillance 1977, issued August 1979. HEW Publication No.

(CDC) 78–8205. *(A source which will be continually updated to provide current information.)*

Tietze, C.: Probability of pregnancy resulting from a single unprotected coitus. Fertil. Steril., *11*:485, 1960. *(The risk is 2 to 4 per cent.)*

American College of Obstetricians and Gynecologists, Chicago, Illinois: Pertinent *Technical Bulletins. (Current practice guidelines recommended in the United States by a specialty organization.)*

118

Management of Breast Cancer
JACOB J. LOKICH, M.D.

Breast cancer is not only the most common malignancy of women in the United States today, but it is also among the most responsive to therapy; many of the therapeutic modalities can be managed by the primary care physician. Unfortunately, in spite of the expanded therapeutic armamentarium for breast cancer, survival and potential for cure of these lesions remain relatively unchanged.

There is much controversy over the best means of treating primary, curable breast cancer. The primary care physician needs to explain to the patient the options for therapy, and guide the initial evaluation; he may take part in administration of chemotherapy as well as monitoring the patient. Local therapy may be supplemented by the use of adjuvant hormonal or chemotherapy, but at present adjuvant therapy is thought to improve chances of survival only in premenopausal patients.

The management of advanced disease requires an understanding of hormone responsiveness and chemotherapeutic regimens. These may be administered in the office setting with careful monitoring. Combination therapy and sequential systemic therapy are being actively explored.

CLINICAL COURSE

The course of breast cancer is determined for the most part by the stage of tumor at presentation and the adequacy of treatment. Seventy per cent of patients with a tumor less than 5 cm. in size and confined to the breast can expect to live 10 years. With lymph node involvement, rate of survival decreases, according to the number of nodes involved, with a 10-year survival rate of 10 to 20 per cent for patients with involvement of regional lymph nodes.

In addition to stage of tumor and tumor size, prognosis is determined by the pathologic grade of tumor and the presence or absence of estrogen receptor protein (ERP) within the tumor specimen. The clinical course of breast cancer is unique because metastatic lesions may develop after a long period of freedom from disease, even after as many as 20 years. Thus, 5 years without evidence of spread does not indicate cure.

Breast cancer may metastisize to almost any site in the body, but five general categories have been distinguished by Smalley and coworkers, which are correlated with predictable response to therapy and prognosis (Table 118–1). It is evident that even in patients with metastatic disease, median survival may exceed 3 years, and there does not have to be significant change in quality of life when palliative radiation and chemohormone therapy are used throughout that period. Today more than 50 per cent of patients with metastatic breast cancer may respond to therapy but only a small portion (perhaps less than 10%) show complete regression. The median duration of, response is not more than 12 to 18 months.

PRINCIPLES OF MANAGEMENT

The therapeutic options for those women diagnosed by an incisional or excisional biopsy have expanded in recent years, accompanied by greater *pa-*

Table 118–1.   Patterns of Recurrence and Survival in Breast Cancer

PATTERN	INCIDENCE %	MEDIAN TIME (MONTHS) RELAPSE	SURVIVAL
Multiple metastases	19	9	4
Pulmonary	12	36	18
Bone	26	15	29+
Effusions*	16	39	44
Skin and subcutaneous†	26	15	27+

*+ Minor skin nodules
†+ Minor bone metastases

tient participation in choice of therapy. It is no longer justified to perform a biopsy and immediate mastectomy under the same anesthesia. Patients should be fully informed of the diagnosis, promptly staged, and advised of the therapeutic options.

Staging procedures should be performed only in patients in whom adjuvant chemotherapy is being considered, because alternative therapies are applicable in the presence of metastatic disease. Staging procedures at the time of primary surgery or radiation therapy should include a chest x-ray and liver function tests. The other major site of metastases, the skeletal system, should be evaluated when the patient has symptomatic pain or the disease is pathologic stage II (spread to local nodes). Pathologic evidence of spread to nodes is needed (rather than relying on simple clinical assessment for nodal involvement), because 25 per cent of palpable lymph nodes are histologically negative; in contrast, nonpalpable nodes are positive in 40 per cent of patients. It is only in pathologic stage II patients or in patients with primary tumors of more than 3 cm. in diameter that the expense of routine bone evaluation is justified. If there is clinical indication for bone evaluation, both radionuclide scan and standard metastatic series should be obtained. Liver scan should be obtained only in patients with hepatomegaly or an elevated serum alkaline phosphatase.

Treatment of Localized Disease. There are two major therapeutic options: total mastectomy and radiation therapy with partial mastectomy. The effectiveness and morbidity of each procedure must be discussed with the patient so that an informed decision can be reached.

Complete mastectomy (total or modified radical) involves removal of all breast tissue and axillary lymph nodes. Ten-year follow-up studies have shown that the procedure provides "cure" of localized disease. Removal of the entire breast also precludes the risk of a second primary tumor in the same breast and helps to establish whether there are any other foci of tumor at the time of initial treatment. Finally, with total mastectomy, the extent of tumor in the lymph nodes can be readily determined.

Radiation therapy with partial mastectomy involves removal of a section of breast; this is not a "lumpectomy." Local recurrence rates appear to be comparable to, if not better than, those achieved by surgery alone. The 10-year survival rate has not been determined, since follow-up has not exceeded 5 years.

However, the five-year survival rate is similar to that for total mastectomy.

The primary care physician can help the patient to reach a decision by avoiding the terms "radical," "simple," and "lumpectomy." The patient must balance the cosmetic advantage of partial mastectomy and radiation therapy with the established effectiveness of surgery.

Adjuvant chemotherapy for breast cancer is presently undergoing extensive clinical trails throughout the United States and abroad. There are now preliminary data that indicate that for the *premenopausal patient* with *positive lymph nodes,* adjuvant chemotherapy of 12 months duration may extend the disease-free interval as well as improve chances for survival. The adjuvant chemotherapy programs used in clinical trials are CMF (cyclophosphamide, methotrexate, and 5-fluorouracil) and triple-drug regimens of adriamycin with and without BCG (bacillus Calmette Guerin) immune therapy. The adriamycin programs are designated primarily for patients with a high risk of relapse (4 or more positive nodes). Immune therapy is used at present only in clinical trials.

Patients with negative nodes and those with positive nodes who are menopausal or postmenopausal have so far not improved survival with adjuvant chemotherapy. Nonetheless, ongoing clinical trials may yet identify an impact of this therapy. Patients with regional breast cancer or cancer confined to the breast and regional lymph nodes should be considered for clinical trials but should not routinely receive chemotherapy outside the aegis of a research protocol.

Monitoring patients after definitive local therapy is contingent, at least in part, on whether or not adjuvant chemotherapy is also being used. In general, adjuvant chemotherapy is administered on a monthly basis, and, therefore, patients are seen monthly. Patients may be monitored more definitively with an extensive examination at 3-month intervals for the first year, at 4-month intervals for the second year, and thereafter at 6-month intervals.

Monitoring should include a complete history and physical examination as well as a precise evaluation of the other breast. At annual intervals for the first 5 years, a mammogram may be obtained; the test need not be more frequent than every 2 years if there are clinical examinations every 6 months. Follow-up examination of the bones should be undertaken only in patients who develop symptoms of bone pain. The crucial concern in monitoring patients with breast cancer is the increased risk of a second primary tumor, which may also be curable. The identification of early metastatic disease is inconsequential, because systemic therapy should be used only in patients with either rapidly growing tumor or symptomatic disease.

Treatment of Advanced Disease. Advanced disease includes not only distant metastases in bone, lung, or liver but also extensive regional tumor, the so-called "neglected" primary tumors of the breast. Patients with *extensive regional tumor* have a surprisingly favorable prognosis; the prolonged time of survival already achieved indicates that the malignancy is relatively low-grade. Many of these tumors are responsive to hormonal management as well as local radiation therapy. The concomitant use of these two therapies may be associated with a long or protracted life expectancy.

Stage III breast cancer (inoperable local disease confined to the skin, breast, or lymph nodes) may be treated in the following sequence: (1) biopsy for histologic confirmation and ERP assay; (2) systemic therapy, either hormone or chemotherapy, to determine the effectiveness of the systemic treatment and to reduce the bulk of tumor; (3) local therapy, which may be either mastectomy followed by radiation therapy or radiation therapy alone. The median length of survival after effective treatment is 18 to 24 months.

The management of *advanced metastatic breast carcinoma* is determined in part by sites of metastases and age (menopausal status). The decision to treat and the timing of therapy are dependent upon the presence or absence of symptoms and/or the growth rate of the tumor. There are three categories of therapy for advanced breast cancer: hormone therapy, chemotherapy, and combination therapy.

The decision to employ *hormone therapy* and prediction of response are based upon site of disease, age, and presence of ERP. *ERP positivity* indicates that a response to hormonal therapy may be expected

in 50 to 60 per cent of patients. It must be emphasized that the presence of estrogen receptors does not indicate which hormone treatment may be effective, and, in fact, either estrogen withdrawal by ablation or estrogen supplements by exogenous hormone may be effective. Less than 5 per cent of ERP-negative patients achieve a response. Therefore, unless the menopausal status and site of disease strongly suggest a high likelihood of response, ERP-negative patients are almost never treated with hormone management.

The sites of disease most often associated with hormone response are pulmonary nodules, pleural effusions, osseous lesions, and cutaneous disease. There is a very remote likelihood of response to hormonal manipulation in patients with hepatic metastases, lymphangitic pulmonary involvement, brain metastases, or skin lesions *en cuirasse*.

Hormone management is also a function of age (see Table 118–2). The least responsive group is *perimenopausal*. From the time of menopause to five years afterward, the response to ablation or estrogen supplements is meager. These patients have been treated with androgens, with a response rate of 20 per cent or less. Androgen therapy is associated with significant side effects of masculinization and is, therefore, used rather sparingly. In *premenopausal* patients, tumor develops in a setting of estrogen abundance; consequently *ablative procedures* are almost invariably used; oophorectomy is associated with a response in 40 to 50 per cent of patients. The response may last for 6 to 12 months, and upon relapse, adrenalectomy is usually performed. In *postmenopausal* patients, the tumor develops in an estrogen-depleted environment; therefore, *estrogen* is the first hormonal manipulation to be employed. A response may be achieved in 40 to 50 per cent of patients, but in 20 per cent of patients, tumor growth may be exacerbated. Postmenopausal patients who worsen on hormone therapy may undergo combined

Table 118–2.   Hormonal Regimens in Management of Advanced Breast Cancer

HORMONE	DOSE/SCHEDULE	PATIENT POPULATION	RESPONSE RATE (%)
Estrogen*			
Diethylstilbestrol (DES)	15 mg./day	Postmenopausal	40–50
Ethinyl estradiol (Estinyl)	3 mg./day		
Progesterone			
Megestiol acetate (Megace)	40 mg. four times a day	Postmenopausal	20
Androgens			
Testosterone propionate	100 mg. IM 3 times week	Perimenopausal	15
Antiestrogens			
Tamoxifen	10 mg. twice daily	All groups	35

*Exacerbates 20% of patients

adrenalectomy and oophorectomy; response occurs in 75 per cent. Thus, the response of selected patients to hormonal ablation is not necessarily age-dependent.

Following an initial response to hormonal therapy, a relapse usually occurs, but a subsequent secondary response is not uncommon. Patients initially treated with estrogen may, upon relapse, be managed with estrogen withdrawal and sustain a second response. Later they may be reinduced with maximal doses of estrogen or with an alternative hormone preparation, such as progesterone or androgens. For the most part, such secondary responses are short-lived and are not of the quality of the initial response. It is important to recognize that the effect of hormonal therapy on tumor bulk may not be observed for 1 or 2 months, even though the agent may begin working immediately. Relief of bone pain is much more rapidly achieved.

Hormonal therapy occasionally results in exacerbation of bone pain or tumor growth. The mechanism is not known; in a small percentage of these patients, the opposite hormonal maneuver (i.e., ablation or supplementation) may induce an antitumor effect. In some institutions, patients are monitored in the hospital for a 10-day period to determine whether tumor stimulation occurs. This is particularly useful in patients with multiple bone lesions, because serious hypercalcemia may occur occultly. The hypercalcemia is preceded by hypercalciuria, which is an indication of stimulatory effect by the hormone. In patients without bone lesions, urine calcium monitoring is of little value. Exacerbation has been reported predominantly with estrogen therapy, but it has occurred in association with the use of progesterone and androgens and adrenalectomy.

Tamoxifen, a new hormonal agent, is a competitive inhibitor of endogenous estrogen. The agent, binds to estrogen receptors on the cell surface. An antitumor effect may be achieved by the agent in tumors whose growth is promoted by endogenous estrogen. Since estrogens are derived not only from the ovary but also from the adrenal gland, the tamoxifen therapy may be an alternative to adrenalectomy. Comparative studies on the effectiveness of tamoxifen and adrenalectomy are in progress. At present, it appears that tamoxifen, which has a very low level of toxicity, has a response rate comparable to other forms of hormone therapy.

The utilization of *cytotoxic agents* for chemotherapy of breast cancer has been expanded since Cooper introduced multiple-agent therapy in 1969. Single-agent therapy is rarely used today in the management of breast cancer, since response rates and durations of remissions are dramatically improved by use of multiple-drug regimens. Unlike hormonal therapy, the chemotherapeutic regimens are associated with a substantial increment in adverse effects. The major adverse effect for women is alopecia, which compounds the cosmetic insult of mastectomy and the loss of femininity associated with hormonal

Table 118–3.   Chemotherapeutic Regimens in Management of Advanced Breast Cancer

REGIMEN	DOSE	ROUTE	SCHEDULE	RESPONSE RATE (%)
CMF*				30-60
Cyclophosphamide	100 mg.	Oral	For 10 days, every 28 days	
Methotrexate	30 mg./m.²	Intravenous	Day 1 and 8	
Fluorouracil	300 mg./m.²	Intravenous	Day 1 and 8	
C-A†				40-80
Cyclophosphamide	500 mg./m.²	Intravenous	Every 3 weeks	
	or			
	100 mg.	Oral	Day 3-6	
Doxorubicin	50 mg./m.²	Intravenous	Every 3 weeks	
A-V				40
Doxorubicin	60 mg./m.²	Intravenous	Every 3 weeks	
Vincristine	1.5 mg./m.²	Intravenous	Every 3 weeks	
CAF				40-60
Cyclophosphamide	100 mg.	Oral	For 10 days	
Adriamycin	50 mg./m.²	Intravenous	Days 1 and 8	
Fluorouracil	500 mg./m.²	Intravenous	Days 1 and 8	
CMFVP				40-80
(Cooper regimen)	Variable	Variable	Variable	

*Low-dose regimen

†In all doxorubicin regimens, the doxorubicin is discontinued beyond 450 mg./m.² cumulative dose

ablation. Myelosuppression and gastrointestinal toxicity are the other major ill effects of these drugs (see Chapter 88).

The chemotherapeutic regimens most commonly used to manage advanced breast cancer are listed in Table 118–3. *CMF* (Cytoxan, methotrexate, 5-fluorouracil) may be used in high- or low-dose regimens. Response rates are comparable; the primary difference is the frequency of visits needed for treatment. The high-dose schedule requires twice monthly visits, the associated alopecia and acute gastrointestinal upset are still substantial.

The regimen that uses *cytoxan* and *adriamycin* imposes uniform alopecia, which is total; treatment is administered every 3 weeks. The response rate may be somewhat higher than with CMF, but for the most part the duration of response is comparable. The maximum cumulative dose for adriamycin, which is a cardiotoxic drug, is 450 mg./m.^{2}. Not uncommonly, patients may be managed by an initial induction with CMF and, upon relapse, can be treated with adriamycin in combination with vincristine. The response rate in such patients is about 20 per cent; when adriamycin and vincristine are used as the first regimen, the response rate approaches 40 per cent.

When one chemotherapy regimen fails, it is important that the secondary regimen not incorporate any of the previous drugs, because the tumor usually has established resistance to them; they will only limit the doses of the other drugs that can be used within the multiple-drug regimen. In patients who fail to respond to the regimens outlined in Table 118–3, either primarily or secondarily after a response, subsequent conventional chemotherapy is generally ineffective, and experimental drugs may be tried.

The combination of hormone manipulation (either addition or ablation) and multiple-drug chemotherapy has been advocated on the basis of a possible synergistic interaction. It has been suggested that the hormone-sensitive clone of malignant cells may be independent of the cytotoxic-sensitive cell. In spite of this rationale, there have been relatively few studies that have demonstrated a synergistic effect from the combination of hormones and chemotherapy management.

Chemotherapy should be considered after hormonal manipulations have failed. However, the likelihood of response to chemotherapy is decreased when the tumor has been demonstrated to be resistant to other kinds of treatment. In addition to tumor resistance, most tumor burden is increased, thereby decreasing the likelihood of response.

Breast cancer is exquisitely responsive to *radiation therapy*. One of the most common patterns of recurrence that requires palliation is that of metastatic bone lesions and local cutaneous recurrence. The latter may develop in small subcutaneous implants, and these may coalesce to form a tumor en cuirasse with secondary obstruction to dermal lymphatics and enormous lymphedema. The pain and incapacity from this complication of breast cancer is significant and may be avoided by local radiation therapy at a time when tumor on the chest wall is minimal.

Metastatic bone lesions are present in more than 60 per cent of patients with breast cancer; the lytic lesions in particular are generally associated with pain. Local radiation therapy at relatively low doses of 2,000 to 3,500 rads may abort the pain, although persistent structural defects as a consequence of cortical erosion may necessitate orthopedic support and even internal fixation for weight-bearing bone structures.

Another important role for radiation therapy in the palliation of metastatic breast cancer is in patients who develop metastatic brain lesions, which may occur in over 10 per cent of patients with breast cancer. The radiation sensitivity and responsiveness of the tumor make this form of therapy an excellent treatment modality for brain metastases. An extended period of survival can be achieved.

PATIENT EDUCATION

See Principles of Management and Chapters 87 and 90.

ANNOTATED BIBLIOGRAPHY

Baker, L.H., Vaughn, C.B., Al-Sarraf, M., Reed, M.L., and Vaitkewicius, V.K.: Evaluation of combination vs. sequential cytotoxic chemotherapy in the treatment of advanced breast cancer. Cancer 33:513, 1974. *(Multiple drug vs. sequential single drug cytotoxic chemotherapy is compared. The results are similar for patients receiving sequential vs. simultaneous combination therapy. In particular, survival was not different.)*

Bonadonna, G., Brusamolino, E., Valagussa, P., *et al.*: Combination chemotherapy as an adjuvant treatment in operable breast cancer. N. Engl. J. Med., *294*:405, 1976. *(This article represents the* initial definitive presentation which acted as a confirmation of the success of early adjuvant trials in breast cancer and served as a forerunner for subsequent trials.)

Brunner, K.W., Sonntag, R.W., Alberto, P., et al.: Combined chemo- and hormonal therapy in advanced breast cancer. Cancer, *39*:2923, 1977. *(A recent randomized trial comparing hormone and chemotherapy in combination with one another. The hormone therapy was variable but consistent with standard choices based on menopausal status. The combination of hormone and chemotherapeutic approaches was consistently superior in response rates and survival, suggesting that the tumor may have chemotherapy sensitive clones as well as hormone-sensitive lines which are therefore individually attacked by this therapeutic modality.)*

Canellos, G.P., DeVita, V.T., Gold, G.L., et al.: Combination chemotherapy for advanced breast cancer: Response and effect on survival. Ann. Intern. Med., *84*:389, 1976. *(The expanded American experience with the three-drug regimen known as CMF; summarizes those prognostic determinants which predict response and survival.)*

Haskell, C.M., Sparks, F.C., Graze, P.R., and Korenman, S.G.: Systemic therapy for metastatic breast cancer. Ann. Intern. Med., *86*:68, 1977. *(The UCLA conference reviews adjuvant therapy as well as hormone therapy for advanced disease and emphasizes the role of estrogen receptor protein and other clinical factors in predicting response. The singular experience at UCLA and the use of immune therapy is also presented.)*

Kennedy, B.J.: Hormonal therapies in breast cancer. Semin. Oncol., *1*:119, 1974. *(This article develops the rationale and the practical use of primary and secondary endocrine therapy in the management of breast cancer; by a leading authority.)*

Legha, S.S., Davis, H.L. and Muggia, F.M.: Hormonal therapy of breast cancer: New approaches and concepts. Ann. Intern. Med., *88*:69, 1978. *(A good review of hormonal treatments; it includes discussion of estrogen receptor antagonists.)*

Levene, M.B., Harris, J.R., and Hellman, S.: Treatment of carcinoma of the breast by radiation therapy. Cancer, *39*:2840, 1977. *(The initial definitive experience of the Joint Center for Radiation Therapy; more than 150 patients with primary breast cancer were treated by radiation therapy. Results are reviewed emphasizing the ability to control disease locally and maintain a satisfactory cosmetic result. The issue of long-term control and survival is not addressed because of the short follow-up.)*

McGuire, W.L., Horwitz, K.B., Zara, D.T., et al.: Hormones in breast cancer. Metabolism, *27*:487, 1978. *(A detailed review of hormone receptor proteins and their implications for therapy.)*

Priestman, T., Baum, M., Jones, V., and Forbes, J.: Comparative trial of endocrine versus cytotoxic treatment in advanced breast cancer. Br. Med. J., *1*:1248, 1977. *(An unusual prospective randomized trial comparing chemotherapy of a cytotoxic nature with endocrine therapy in advanced breast cancer, and suggesting that cytotoxic therapy is more than twice as effective in terms of inducing response and also in terms of improving survival.)*

Stoll, B.A.: Hormonal management of advanced breast cancer. Br. Med. J., *2*:293, 1969. *(This article represents a definitive treatise by the world authority on the use of hormones; supplements the book publications by the same author.)*

Yonemoto, R.H., Tan, M.S.C., Byron, R.L., et al.: Randomized sequential hormonal therapy vs. adrenalectomy for metastatic breast carcinoma. Cancer, *39*:547, 1977. *(This study compares hormone ablation and, specifically, adrenalectomy with sequential exogenous hormones in more than 200 patients. Although the response rate to adrenalectomy was generally superior to other forms of hormone therapy not significantly changed by adrenalectomy, overall survival was unchanged.)*

9

Genitourinary Problems

119
Screening for Syphilis
HARVEY B. SIMON, M.D.

Syphilis, like tuberculosis, has become dramatically less prevalent since the introduction of effective antibiotic therapy in the 1940s. As a result, manifestations of the disease have become less familiar to practitioners. If a patient is not identified and treated during the primary or secondary stages of the disease, the infection becomes latent and is identifiable only by means of laboratory tests until late, often irreversible, clinical manifestations appear. The prevention of destructive cardiovascular and neurologic lesions by means of appropriate screening for latent syphilis is an important task for the primary physician. Because false-positive results are common and are potentially traumatic for the patient, it is critical that the sensitivities and specificities of the various serologic tests be understood.

EPIDEMIOLOGY AND RISK FACTORS

With the exception of infection in utero or, very rarely, by means of blood transfusion, syphilis is exclusively transmitted sexually by direct contact with infectious lesions. It follows that risk increases with sexual activity. Since syphilis is readily treated with antibiotics, it is less common in populations with access to medical care. The reported incidence of syphilis among nonwhites in the United States is 20 times that among whites. Rates are highest in urban areas. It must be remembered, however, when comparing incidence rates in different populations, that case reporting has been shown to be more complete in public clinics than among private practitioners. The age-specific incidence rates parallel those of gonorrhea, with the peak incidence for both diseases occurring between ages 20 and 25. A diagnosis of gonorrhea, nongonorrheal urethritis, or another sexually transmitted disease should be considered a risk factor for syphilis. Presumably because they tend to have multiple sexual contacts, homosexuals are at particularly high risk. In the United States, nearly 40 per cent of all males with primary, secondary, or early latent syphilis reported being either homosexual or bisexual.

The importance of an accurate sexual history in determining risk of syphilis is obvious. Patients with early syphilis report an average of three recent sexual contacts. The probability that a known contact will develope syphilis has been shown to be approximately 50 per cent.

NATURAL HISTORY OF SYPHILIS AND EFFECTIVENESS OF THERAPY

Treponema pallidum enters the bloodstream within a few hours after innoculation through intact mucous membranes or abraded skin. A primary lesion occurs at the site of the innoculation between 10 and 90 days after contact. This incubation period de-

486

pends on the size of the innoculum, but is usually less than 3 weeks. The painless chancre usually resolves within 4 to 6 weeks, ending the *primary stage*. The *secondary stage* is usually heralded by a maculopapular rash that appears approximately 6 weeks after the primary lesion has healed. When the rash subsides, after 2 to 6 weeks, the untreated patient enters the *latent stage* (arbitrarily divided into *early latent* for the first 2 years and *late latent* thereafter).

Because anorectal or vaginal chancres are not likely to be brought to medical attention, primary syphilis is usually not diagnosed among homosexual men or among women. In 1974, while more than 40 per cent of syphilis cases were detected in the primary stage among heterosexual males, only 23 per cent and 11 per cent respectively were detected in the primary stage among homosexual males and among females.

Natural history studies from Oslo and Tuskegee indicate that approximately one third of untreated syphilitics will develop clinically manifest tertiary disease and that autopsy evidence of cardiovascular syphilis can be found in more than one half. In the retrospective Oslo study, 10 per cent of patients had clinically evident cardiovascular syphilis, 7 per cent neurosyphilis, and 16 per cent gummatous disease. The incidence of cardiovascular syphilis was higher and that of neurosyphilis was lower in the prospective Tuskegee study.

Factors that influence the progression to clinical tertiary disease are incompletely understood. Congenital syphilis or disease contracted before age 15 does not predispose to cardiovascular tertiary disease. In general, late complications seem more likely to occur among untreated men than women.

The antibiotic regimens recommended in Chapter 134 are highly effective in eradicating early syphilis. If response to therapy is appropriately monitored by following the quantitative VDRL titer, the risk of late complications is virtually eliminated. Antibiotic treatment of late syphilis has less predictable results. Improvement among patients with general paresis has been reported in 40 to 80 per cent of cases. Not surprisingly, structural cardiovascular changes caused by syphilis are not reversed by antibiotic treatment.

SCREENING AND DIAGNOSTIC TESTS

Serological tests for syphilis depend on reactions to either a nonspecific reaginic antibody or to a specific antitreponemal antibody. The former tests include the sensitive and easily automated rapid plasma reagin test (RPR) and the quantitative VDRL flocculation test. While these tests are virtually 100 per cent sensitive during the secondary stage of syphilis, their sensitivity is only 70 per cent during primary, latent or late disease. Their specificity is approximately 70 per cent during all stages. Acute false-positive reactions, which revert to negative within 6 months, may follow acute infections or vaccinations. Chronic false-positive reactions can be expected among patients with autoimmune disease, as well as among drug addicts and the elderly. Approximately 15 per cent of patients with systemic lupus erythematosus (SLE), 25 per cent of drug addicts, and 10 per cent of people over 70 have false-positive reactions. The more expensive antitreponemal tests are both more sensitive and specific. The most commonly used is the fluorescent treponemal antibody absorption test (FTA-ABS). It has a sensitivity of 85 per cent in primary disease, 100 per cent in secondary disease and 98 per cent in latent or late disease. While it is highly specific, false-positives do occur, but the results are generally interpreted as borderline. Such equivocal results are more likely during pregnancy or in patients with SLE. The treponema pallidum immobilization test (TPI) is less sensitive than the FTA-ABS but essentially 100 per cent specific for past or present treponemal infection. The diagnosis of syphilis is discussed further in Chapter 134.

CONCLUSIONS AND RECOMMENDATIONS

- Syphilis is now a relatively uncommon disease. Nevertheless, screening for latent disease is simple, and the late manifestations of syphilis are entirely preventable if treatment is instituted early.
- Many patients have been screened routinely at the time of marriage, during prenatal care, prior to giving blood or on hospital admission. Frequent screening is unnecessary, but the nonreactivity of sexually active individuals, particularly those with multiple sex partners, should be documented at approximately 5-year intervals. Special indications for screening include contact or infection with other sexually transmitted diseases and pregnancy.
- Nontreponemal tests such as the RPR or VDRL are appropriate for screening because of their sensitivity and simplicity. FTA-ABS and other treponemal tests should be reserved for confirming a diagnosis suspected on the basis of clinical presentation or positive nontreponemal tests.

ANNOTATED BIBLIOGRAPHY

Brown W.J.: Status and control of syphilis in the United States. J. Infect. Dis., *124*:428, 1971. *(A somewhat dated but useful quantitative review of syphilis epidemiology in the United States.)*

Clark E.G., and Danbold, N.: The Oslo study of the natural course of untreated syphilis. Med. Clin. North Am., *48*:613, 1964. *(A restudy of case material of untreated syphilis collected 1891–1910.)*

Jaffe, H.W.: The laboratory diagnosis of syphilis. Ann. Intern. Med., *83*:846, 1975. *(A more recent review of diagnostic tests including discussion of the RPR.)*

Rockwell, D.H., Yobs, A.R., Moore, M.B., Jr.: The Tuskegee study of untreated syphilis. Arch. Intern. Med., *114*:792, 1964. *(Report of a prospective study of untreated syphilis in 412 black males in its 30th year. Notable for the ethical questions raised as well as the natural history of syphilis.)*

Sparling, P.F.: Diagnosis and treatment of syphilis. N. Engl. J. Med., *284*:642, 1971. *(An extensive review of both diagnostic tests and treatment schedules.)*

120
Screening for Asymptomatic Bacteriuria and Urinary Tract Infection

When urinary tract infection is associated with symptoms, the early resolution of these symptoms and the resulting reassurance of the patient is justification enough for treatment that involves little risk. However, efforts to detect and treat asymptomatic bacteriuria are based on the assumption that treatment reduces the likelihood of subsequent morbidity due to symptomatic infection, sepsis or chronic renal disease. The risk of such complications depends on the clinical situation, including the age and sex of the patient. For some, risk is well defined, and treatment is indicated; for others, the most significant morbidity may be related to the side effects of inappropriate treatment. It is therefore critical that the physician appreciate the different implications of bacteriuria in different settings.

EPIDEMIOLOGY AND RISK FACTORS

The prevalence of bacteriuria depends on age and sex. Among neonates, positive cultures are found in about 1 per cent of both males and females. During school-age years, the prevalence among boys is as low as 0.03 per cent, compared with 1 to 2 per cent among girls. Prevalence among females increases by 1 per cent of the population per decade; throughout childbearing age, the prevalence is 2 to 4 per cent, and by age 50, it has reached 5 to 10 per cent. Geriatric males are almost as likely to have bacteriuria as females because of the high incidence of prostate and other urologic disease and subsequent instrumentation in this group. Prevalence in these older age groups reaches 15 per cent.

The greater susceptibility of younger women and girls can be explained anatomically, in that a short urethra allows easier access to the bladder, facilitating colonization by perineal organisms. Risk increases with local trauma associated with sexual activity and the relaxation of pelvic supporting structures with age. Anatomic changes may also explain the slightly higher prevalence of bacteriuria (2 to 4 per cent) among pregnant women. Alternatively, since users of birth control pills have a similarly increased risk, this prevalence may reflect estrogen-mediated dilatation of the urethra.

It must be kept in mind that prevalence figures indicate the extent of bacteriuria at a single point in time. Since risk factors are shared by many and bacteriuria frequently resolves spontaneously as well as after therapy, the cumulative prevalence of bacteriuria is higher. By age 30, approximately 25 per cent of women have experienced symptoms consistent with urinary tract infection.

Structural abnormalities, including obstruction of the urethra or ureters, significant vesicourethral reflux, neurologic lesions and foreign bodies are important additional risk factors for bacteriuria.

NATURAL HISTORY OF ASYMPTOMATIC BACTERIURIA, AND EFFECTIVENESS OF THERAPY

Asymptomatic and symptomatic urinary tract infections have the same epidemiologic correlates. Asymptomatic infections can become symptomatic; bacteriuria can persist after symptoms have resolved. Ninety per cent of women with bacteriuria have had symptoms some time in the past, nearly 70 per cent within the preceding year. While both asymptomatic and symptomatic infections can resolve spontaneously, the urine is more likely to become sterile after treatment. Approximately 80 per cent of women with bacteriuria have sterile urine after appropriate antibiotic treatment. However, follow-up studies indicate that only 55 per cent of those treated will have sterile urine at the end of 1 year. Sterile urine spontaneously developed in fully 36 per cent of untreated bacteriuric women during the same period. Significantly, women who had recurrences of infection after treatment were more likely to have associated symptoms than those who had persistent or relapsing bacteriuria. Symptomatic infection recurs within 3 years in 40 per cent of women.

Special risks are associated with bacteriuria during pregnancy. Among women with bacteriuria identified early during pregnancy, there is a 40 per cent incidence of acute pyelonephritis without prophylactic treatment. Bacteriuria is also associated with higher incidences of premature delivery, perinatal infant mortality and preeclampsia.

The importance of chronic or recurrent bacteriuria in the etiology of chronic renal failure has been de-emphasized as diverse noninfectious etiologies for the pathologic findings of interstitial nephritis have been recognized. Patients with bacteriuria are more likely to be hypertensive. They are also more likely to have identifiable abnormalities on IVP, including small kidneys, delayed excretion, caliceal dilatation and blunting, ureteral reflux, stones and other obstructive lesions. However, chronic renal failure rarely occurs as a complication of urinary tract infection in the absence of structural abnormalities. Evidence indicates that such abnormalities predispose patients both to chronic renal failure and recurrent infection. Definitive studies that address this important question have not yet been performed.

In addition to symptomatic urinary tract infection and chronic renal disease, the clinician must also be concerned with the possibility that chronic asymptomatic infection is a potential source of disseminated infection, such as endocarditis. This danger is particularly likely in the male patient with prostate disease and infection who requires instrumentation. Bacteremia has been documented in as many as 50 per cent of males whose urine is infected at the time of the procedure; it is relatively rare when the urine is sterile.

SCREENING AND DIAGNOSTIC TESTS

Asymptomatic bacteriuria is a laboratory diagnosis that requires careful definition. Because voided urine is easily contaminated by urethral and (in women) perineal flora during micturition, cultures of clean voided urine must be cultured quantitatively. The probability of infection in a patient whose specimen contains 10^5 col./ml. is nearly 100 per cent for males but only 80 per cent for females. Two such positive cultures in a female increase the probability of infection to 95 per cent. False-negative findings are more likely if the patient is undergoing vigorous diuresis, if the urine is unusually acid (pH 5.5) or if the specimen was inadvertently contaminated with antibacterial detergents. Spurious positive cultures are more frequent, due to unclean collection technique, contaminated collection equipment or failure to promptly culture the urine.

A single culture of urine collected on urethral catheterization with $\geq 10^5$ col./ml. has a predictive value of infection of 95 per cent. Catheterization should be limited to patients requiring relief of obstruction or those who absolutely cannot cooperate with collection techniques. The risk of introducing infection during catheterization may be as high as 5 per cent. The risk of inducing bacteremia in men with an infected urinary tract approaches 50 per cent. When suprapubic percutaneous bladder aspiration is used in young children or to resolve confusing problems in the adult, infection can be presumed if any bacterial growth other than that of skin contaminants occurs.

Nonquantitative approaches to diagnosis include microscopic examination for bacteria and clinical tests of bacterial activity such as the reduction of nitrate to nitrite. These and the less specific signs of urinary tract inflammation such as pyuria, hematuria, and proteinuria may be helpful in making a presumptive diagnosis in the symptomatic patient. They may also indicate the need for urine culture when incidental abnormalities are detected in the asymptomatic patient. Confirmation of infection with quantitative culture technology should always precede a therapeutic decision in the absence of symptoms.

CONCLUSIONS AND RECOMMENDATIONS

- Bacteriuria, both symptomatic and asymptomatic, is a common phenomenon with well-defined risk factors.
- Treatment is moderately effective in the short run, but because of high rates of spontaneous recurrence and resolution, the likelihood that bacteriuria will be noted with longer follow-up is not significantly influenced by short-term therapy.
- Symptomatic infections are generally not prevented by treatment of asymptomatic bacteriuria in nonpregnant women.
- While there is an association between bacteriuria and renal abnormalities, there is no evidence that this is an etiologic relationship. Furthermore, there is no evidence that treatment of infection in the absence of urinary tract abnormalities will prevent progressive renal disease.
- Screening for asymptomatic bacteriuria is recommended only in selected high-risk populations including: (1) pregnant women; (2) elderly males with clinical prostatism or other urologic abnormalities, particularly before and after required instrumentation; (3) all patients recently catheterized; (4) patients with known renal calculi or other structural abnormalities of the urinary tract.

ANNOTATED BIBLIOGRAPHY

Asscher, A.W., Sossman, M. *et al.*: The clinical significance of asymptomatic bacteriuria in the nonpregnant woman. J. Infect. Dis., *120*:17, 1969. *(Controlled trial of treatment of asymptomatic bacteriuria. Concludes that screening for bacteriuria in nonpregnant women is unlikely to be of value.)*

Freedman, L.R., Seki, M., and Phair, J.P.: The natural history and outcome of antibiotic treatment of urinary tract infections in women. Yale J. Biol. Med., *37*:245, 1965. *(Short-term follow-up cultures overestimate benefits of treatment.)*

Gower, P.E., Haswell, B., Sidaway, M.E., and deWardener, H.E.: Follow-up of 164 patients with bacteriuria of pregnancy. Lancet, *1*:990, 1968. *(Fewer than 20 per cent of those not treated in this study incurred pyelonephritis.)*

Kass, E.H., and Zinner, S.H.: Bacteriuria and renal disease. J. Infect. Dis., *120*:27, 1969. *(Exhaustive review of the links between bacteriuria and renal disease. Authors conclude that a causal relationship has been demonstrated in cases of pyelonephritis in pregnancy and bacteremia postcatheterization but not in progressive renal disease among adults.)*

Takahashi, M., and Loveland, D.B.: Bacteriuria and oral contraceptives. JAMA, *227*:762, 1974. *(Fifty per cent higher prevalence among oral contraceptive users.)*

121

Screening for Prostatic Cancer
JOHN D. GOODSON, M.D.

Prostatic carcinoma is perhaps the most common malignancy among men in the United States. The lifetime probability that a man will incur clinical prostatic cancer is between 5 and 6 per cent, but the probability of death due to prostatic cnacer is approximately 2 per cent. Even the patient with clinically evident disease is more likely to die of something else. Pathologic studies indicate that occult prostatic cancer is even more prevalent than these figures suggest.

The physician faces a great deal of uncertainity in making clinical decisions about prostatic cancer. The tumors are exceedingly common and have the potential to cause significant morbidity and mortality. They also have a variable, often indolent course and a higher prevalence in those whose health is often more limited by coincident diseases. The clinician should be aware of the unpredictable natural history of the disease and the limitations of therapy when considering the use of screening tests for prostatic cancer.

EPIDEMIOLOGY AND RISK FACTORS

The incidence of prostatic carcinoma increases with age. Reports of age-specific prevalence range from 5 to 15 per cent during the sixth decade, 10 to 30 per cent during the seventh decade, and 20 to 50 per cent or higher after age 70. Such prevalence estimates have increased over the years as detailed histologic study of glands removed at surgery has become more common. Clinical detection of prostatic cancer is highest in whites of Northern European origin and American blacks. A history of prostatitis does not seem to be a risk factor, but benign prostatic hypertrophy may predispose the patient to malignant disease. There is no clear etiologic relationship to environmental factors, socioeconomic status, fertility, or endogenous androgen level. Regional variations in the prevalence of prostatic cancer reflect either differences in unidentified environmental factors or variation in case detection methods.

NATURAL HISTORY OF PROSTATIC CANCER AND EFFECTIVENESS OF THERAPY

Unfortunately, the biologic behavior of prostatic carcinoma varies widely, making individual cases unpredictable. In most of the reported cases of prostatic cancer, the patient presents with symptoms of urinary tract outflow obstruction such as hesitancy, frequency, nocturia and loss of stream volume and force. In up to 20 per cent of cases, presentation includes signs or symptoms of early metastasis such as bone pain.

Approximately 50 per cent of isolated prostatic nodules found on routine rectal examination in the asymptomatic patient are subsequently proven to be malignant. Such presentations account for 10 per cent of all prostatic cancers. Another 10 per cent of cases are discovered incidentally during microscopic examination of glandular tissue after removal for reasons other than suspected malignancy.

The clinical course after diagnosis is remarkably variable and depends on the degree of histologic differentiation of the tumor more than the extent of disease. Most incidentally discovered tumors have well-differentiated isolated malignant foci. Even without treatment, survival in these patients is the same as that in age-matched controls. A minority of latent tumors have diffuse poorly differentiated histology. Prognosis in these cases is nearly as poor as in those

with metastases at presentation. The mean duration of the asymptomatic stage of prostatic cancer has been estimated to be between 10 and 30 years, but it is apparent that a substantial number of cases with poorly differentiated tumors are on the short end of the distribution. It is also clear that tumors can run a very aggressive course after they become clinically manifest. In some older series, the median survival from diagnosis to death in untreated patients was less than 2 years.

This variability in natural history makes assessment of the efficacy of therapeutic interventions difficult. Some have argued that early and aggressive intervention with surgical extirpation of involved tissue and radiation therapy to involved areas may prolong survival in patients in whom the tumor is isolated to the gland or is locally metastatic. However, no form of intervention applied to asymptomatic patients, either with latent carcinoma or carcinoma found on biopsy of a suspected malignant nodule, has been shown to improve survival. With older patients, most oncologists withhold treatment until symptoms of obstruction or metastasis develop. More aggressive therapy is reserved for patients without serious comorbid conditions.

SCREENING AND DIAGNOSTIC TESTS

Careful digital examination of the rectum is the only practical screening technique for prostatic carcinoma. The finding of a hard (similar in consistency to the tip of the nose), stony, and asymmetric prostate is highly suggestive of malignancy. Fixation to adjacent tissue and a loss of the lateral prostatic sulcus suggests local metastasis. The isolated prostatic nodule, though possibly an indication of localized disease, is a nonspecific finding. It occurs in up to 5 per cent of men over 50 years of age and 10 per cent of men over 70. Approximately 50 per cent of such nodules are prostatic cancers.

While acid phosphatase is found in normal hyperthrophied or malignant prostatic tissue, measurement of serum levels is not a sensitive test for early disease. Elevated levels are found in 80 per cent of individuals with bony metastasis, but in only 5 to 15 per cent of those with localized disease. Measurement of acid phosphatase levels has a reported specificity of greater than 90 per cent. The physician should be aware, however, that transient elevations of less than 24 hours' duration can occur following prostatic massage of the hypertrophied nonmalignant gland. A recently introduced radioimmunoassay for prostatic acid phosphatase has an increased sensitivity for early disease.

CONCLUSIONS AND RECOMMENDATIONS

- Routine yearly rectal examination is recommended for the detection of asymptomatic prostatic nodules. Stool obtained should be tested for the presence of occult blood as a screen for early colorectal cancer.
- Prostatic nodules in younger patients should be referred for biopsy. Nodules in elderly patients or those with comorbid conditions should be followed at 6-month intervals and biopsied only if there is an increase in size or symptoms of outflow obstruction or bone pain appear.
- While radioimmunoassay or counterimmunoelectrophoretic techniques for determining acid phosphatase levels may allow more sensitive detection of early disease, routine screening is not recommended on the basis of currently available data regarding benefits of early detection. Routine chemical determination of acid phosphatase is not sensitive enough to detect early disease.

ANNOTATED BIBLIOGRAPHY

Armenian, H.K., Lilienfield, A.M., Diamond, E.L., and Bross, I.D.: Relation between benign prostatic hyperplasia and cancer of the prostate. Lancet, 2:115, 1974. *(Retrospective analysis of patients with BPH showed a 5.1 relative risk for prostatic cancer versus age-matched controls.)*

Blackard, C.E., Millinger, G.T., and Gleason, D.F.: Treatment of Stage I carcinoma of the prostate: A preliminary report. J. Urol., *016*:729, 1971. *(No difference in survival of patients with localized carcinoma treated surgically or hormonally, or with no therapy at all.)*

Guinan, P., Bush, I., Ray, V., et al.: The accuracy of the rectal examination in the diagnosis of prostate carcinoma. N. Engl. J. Med., *303*:499, 1980. *(Finds the rectal examination to be the most efficient test with a sensitivity of 69% and specificity of 89%. Accompanying article cautions about limits of RIA acid phosphatase screening.)*

Heaney, J.A., Chang, H.C., Daley, J.J., and Prout, G.R.: Prognosis of clinically undiagnosed prostatic carcinoma and the influence of hormonal therapy. J. Urol., *118*:283, 1977. *(Survival among patients with incidentally found moderate or poorly differentiated carcinoma was significantly reduced. Survival in patients with well-differentiated carcinoma was unchanged.)*

Hudson, P.B., and Stout, A.P: Prostatic cancer. N.Y. State J. Med., *351*, 1966. *(Fifty-two per cent of prostatic nodules were malignant.)*

Hutchison, G.B.: Epidemiology of prostatic carcinoma. Semin. Oncol., *3*:151, 1976. *(Excellent review of epidemiologic data.)*

Klein, L.A.: Prostatic carcinoma. N. Engl. J. Med., *300*:824, 1979. *(An excellent review. A detailed approach to each stage of prostatic malignancy is outlined.)*

Rullis, I., Shaeffer, J.A., and Lilien, O.M.: Incidence of prostatic carcinoma in the elderly. Urology, *6*:295, 1975. *(Two thirds of males over 80 had prostatic cancer.)*

122
Screening for Cancers of the Lower Urinary Tract

Lower urinary tract cancers include tumors of the renal pelves, ureters, bladder and urethra. These lesions can logically be considered together because of similar cell types—more than 95 per cent consist of transitional cells, squamous cells or a combination of the two—and because of common epidemiologic correlates.

Cancer of the lower urinary tract is viewed by many primary physicians as a relatively benign tumor that principally affects the elderly. Nevertheless, approximately 30,000 new cases occur each year in the United States; 10,000 deaths per year can be attributed to bladder cancer. The lifetime probability of incurring cancer of the bladder is approximately 2 per cent for white males and 1 per cent for white females.

Risk factors, including a strong association with occupational exposure, have been well defined. A weaker association with tobacco use has more recently been demonstrated. Screening tests are available. Although there is still insufficient understanding of the natural history of bladder cancer to allow specific screening recommendations, the physician must understand the epidemiology of these tumors as well as the potential costs and benefits of various screening practices.

EPIDEMIOLOGY AND RISK FACTORS

Cancer of the lower urinary tract is a tumor of older age groups; in the United States, the mean age at the time of diagnosis is 68 years. The incidence increases at a constant rate during adult life, varying from 1 per 100,000 per year at age 20 to 200 per 100,000 per year at age 80 for white males. Females have approximately one-third the risk of males. In the United States, whites are twice as likely to have bladder tumors as nonwhites. Urban dwellers, too, have consistently been shown to have a higher incidence of lower urinary tract tumors when compared to people who live in rural or suburban areas.

The most notable risk factor for development of lower urinary tract cancers is occupational exposure to aromatic amines, first noted in England in 1895. Subsequently, dyestuff workers were shown to have a ten to fiftyfold increased risk of bladder carcinoma. Compounds most closely associated with bladder carcinogenesis include 2-naphthylamine and benzidine. Recent case-control studies indicate excess risk among men who worked with dyestuffs, rubber, leather, or painting or other organic chemicals. It has been estimated that these occupational exposures are responsible for 18 per cent of bladder cancer cases. As little as two years' exposure may be sufficient to increase risk, but the time between exposure and subsequent cancer may be as long as 45 years.

Smoking has been implicated as a risk factor for bladder cancer in many studies, most of which indicate that smokers have a twofold increase in risk compared to nonsmokers. Other suggested risk factors include pelvic irradiation, which was used in the past for dysfunctional bleeding, heavy coffee consumption, and abuse of phenacetin-containing analgesics.

NATURAL HISTORY OF LOWER URINARY TRACT CANCERS AND EFFECTIVENESS OF THERAPY

The natural history of lower urinary tract tumors is not well defined. Prognosis at the time of diagnosis depends on both clinical stage, defined by depth of penetration and extent of metastases, and histologic grade of the tumor. There is often close correlation between depth of penetration and histologic grade. Urothelial tumors are grossly subdivided into papilloma, papillary carcinoma, and transitional cell carcinoma. These gross morphologic distinctions have histologic counterparts that are highly predictive of 5-year survival. Grade 1 papillary carcinoma (papilloma) has a 5-year cure or clinical control rate of approximately 95 per cent. Grade 2 papillary carcinoma (papillary carcinoma) has a 5-year survival rate of only 25 per cent. The outlook for Grade 3 papillary and infiltrating carcinoma (transitional cell carcinoma) is worse. Prognosis for patients with squamous carcinoma is also very poor, unless the tumor is well differentiated. Clinical staging systems that distinguish between levels of tumor penetration of the bladder have also been shown to have good prognostic value. Overall, about 50 per cent of patients with treated bladder cancer survive for 5 years. However, multiple synchronous and asynchronous tumors are the rule in lower urinary tract cancer, contributing to morbidity and eventual mortality.

Hematuria is the most common presentation of lower urinary tract cancer. Other symptoms suggestive of cystitis may also occur. While it has been claimed that 75 per cent of tumors promptly diagnosed after a first episode of hematuria are localized, little data on this subject are available. The likelihood that screening tests, including urinalysis and urinary cytology, would significantly advance the time of diagnosis is likewise unproven. A progression from urothelial atypia to sessile carcinoma *in situ* or papilloma to higher grade malignancy has been postulated. Studies of the natural history of urothelial carcinoma *in situ* indicate that the majority of lesions progress to more malignant forms. While early lesions are much less likely to be detected cytologically, 3.7 per cent of detected tumors were *in situ* in one study. The usual synchronous and asynchronous multiplicity of such tumors makes it difficult to assess the benefits of early detection.

SCREENING TESTS

Urinary cytology is the most specific screening test for lower urinary tract cancers. Reports of the sensitivity of cytology in detecting bladder carcinoma vary from 50 to 90 per cent. Studies have consistently demonstrated that sensitivity increases with the grade of malignancy. While invasive transitional cell carcinoma can regularly be detected with 90 per cent or greater sensitivity, sensitivity rates for papillomas and papillary carcinomas range from 0 to 50 per cent.

Studies of cytologic screening of high-risk populations have been conducted. In one such study, screening of 285 exposed workers produced positive results in 31, 10 of whom had the diagnosis of cancer confirmed at cystoscopy. Within 4 years, 11 additional tumors developed among the 21 cytology-positive, cystoscopy-negative patients. Cystoscopy was also performed in the 254 workers with negative cytologic findings; only 1 case of bladder cancer was diagnosed on that examination. In general, the specificity of urinary cytology depends on the skill of the cytologist. False-positive rates as low as 1 per cent and as high as 20 per cent have been reported.

The value of other urinary sediment abnormalities, particularly hematuria, has not been well defined. In one study of cytologic detection, hematuria was absent in 50 per cent of true-positive cytologic diagnoses.

Cystoscopy and radiographic procedures cannot be considered screening tools. They should be reserved for patients who present with symptoms suggestive of urinary cancer or who have positive cytologies. Frequent follow-up cystoscopies are also a part of the postoperative care of the patient with bladder cancer.

CONCLUSIONS AND RECOMMENDATIONS

- Lower urinary tract cancer is associated with significant morbidity and mortality.
- Risks of occupational exposure to dyestuffs, rubber, leather and leather products, and paint and organic chemicals have been well defined. Smoking is associated with a smaller, but significant, increase in risk.
- Urinary cytology is an imperfect but useful screening test for high-risk groups.
- There is no evidence that screening significantly advances the time of diagnosis in an individual case or that early treatment influences the outcome. Nevertheless, because of the relatively high speci-

ficity and lack of morbidity associated with cytologic screening, identification of patients at high risk due to occupational exposure, with subsequent yearly cytologic screening, is indicated. Screening of asymptomatic smokers without risk of occupational exposure is not recommended.

ANNOTATED BIBLIOGRAPHY

Cole, P.: Coffee-drinking and cancer of the lower urinary tract. Lancet, *1*:1335, 1971. *(Further case-control data identifying association between coffee-drinking and cancer of the lower urinary tract, particularly among women.)*

Cole, P., Hoover, R., and Friedell, G.H.: Occupation and cancer of the lower urinary tract. Cancer, *29*:1250, 1972. *(Case-control study identifying excess risk among 5 occupation categories: dyestuffs, rubber, leather and leather products, paint and organic chemicals. There was no identifiable risk in those who worked with nonorganic chemicals, petroleum or printing.).*

Cole, P., Monson, R.R., Haning H., and Friedell, G.H.: Smoking and cancer of the lower urinary tract. N. Engl. J. Med., *284*:129, 1971. *(Case-control data indicating that smokers have a two-fold risk of developing bladder cancer.)*

Foot, N.C., Papanicolaou, G.N., Holmquist, N.D., and Seybolt, J.F.: Exfoliative cytology of urinary sediments (a review of 2,829 cases). Cancer, *11*:127, 1958. *(Sensitivity of 62 per cent in detecting tumors of renal pelves, bladder or ureters, 8 per cent in renal tumors, and 15 per cent in prostatic tumors. High specificity.)*

Jewett, H.J.: Cancer of the bladder. Diagnosing and staging. Cancer, *32*:1072, 1973. *(Good, brief review of presenting symptoms and staging.)*

King, H., and Bailar, J.C.: Epidemiology of urinary bladder cancer: a review of selected literature. J. Chron. Dis., *19*:735, 1966. *(Extensive review with 134 references.)*

Melamed, M.R., Koss, L.G., Ricci, A., and Whitmore, W.F.: Cytohistological observations on developing carcinomas of the urinary bladder in men. Cancer, *13*:67, 1960. *(Documents cytologic identification of latent bladder cancer in patients with occupational exposure.)*

Tweeddale, D.N.: *Urinary Cytology.* Boston: Little, Brown, 1977. *(Detailed text with chapters on pathology of urinary tract tumors and clinical value of cytology that are useful for the generalist.)*

123
Evaluation of Hematuria
LESLIE S.-T. FANG, M.D.

Practically every disease of the genitourinary tract may at some time produce hematuria. However, since hematuria is often the only symptom of genitourinary neoplasia, its presence demands a thorough investigation to ascertain the underlying etiologic factors. The primary physician may encounter a patient complaining of gross hematuria or may find microscopic hematuria on routine examination of the urine. One needs to be able to initiate an effective workup and decide when referral for urologic evaluation or renal biopsy is necessary.

PATHOPHYSIOLOGY AND CLINICAL PRESENTATION

Normally, fewer than 1000 red blood cells are excreted in the urine each minute. If the rate of excretion is 3000 to 4000 red blood cells per minute, 2 to 3 red blood cells will be seen under the high power field and microscopic hematuria can be detected. If the rate of excretion exceeds 1 million red blood cells per minute, macroscopic or gross hematuria will result.

Intrinsic lesions of the genitourinary tract involving the kidneys, ureters, bladder, prostate or urethra can all produce hematuria. Hematuria can also result from intrinsic periurethral problems, systemic diseases, and use of certain drugs.

Symptoms associated with hematuria may provide important clues to etiology. Renal colic is usually secondary to renal calculi, but may occasionally be associated with the passage of clots. Frequency, dysuria, urgency and suprapubic pain often indicate inflammatory lesions of the lower urinary tract. Dull flank pain with fever and chills suggest pyelonephritis (see Chapter 129). Occasionally, systemic or multisystemic complaints such as fever, rash or joint pains indicate an underlying systemic disease. However, not uncommonly, hematuria may occur without any associated symptoms, yet the majority of cases have a definable cause. When a thorough workup fails to reveal an etiology, the patient is said to have "essential hematuria." Renal biopsy of such patients

often shows minimal glomerular or interstitial disease. Long-term prognosis is excellent.

In view of the high incidence of structural lesions associated with hematuria, a thorough workup to establish the etiology is necessary regardless of the mode of presentation.

DIFFERENTIAL DIAGNOSIS

Intrinsic genitourinary lesions involving the kidneys, ureters, bladder, prostate and urethra can all produce hematuria. The diagnoses in 1000 cases of gross hematuria and 500 cases of microscopic hematuria are tabulated in Tables 123–1 and 123–2. Gross hematuria was most commonly associated with inflammatory lesions and neoplasms; in this series, infection accounted for 34 per cent and neoplasms accounted for 31 per cent of the final diagnoses of patients presenting with gross hematuria. Benign prostatic hypertrophy accounted for another 12.5 per cent of the diagnoses. Microscopic hematuria was most commonly associated with infection and benign prostatic hypertrophy, the former being the final diagnosis in 28 per cent of the patients.

Rarely, *periureteral inflammatory lesions* in the appendix, colon or pelvic structures can produce microscopic hematuria.

On occasion a *systemic illness* such as lupus erythematosus, bacterial endocarditis, or rheumatic fever is the source of hematuria. *Blood dyscrasias,* such as hemophilia, sickle cell disease, polycythemia vera and leukemia, and *hemorrhagic disorders,* such as thrombocytopenic purpura and various coagulation defects, can be responsible for red cells in the urine.

Drugs such as anticoagulants, salicylates, methanamine preparations, and sulfonamides have been known to cause hematuria. However, hematuria in a patient on anticoagulants requires thorough evaluation because an underlying urologic lesion is often found.

If a thorough workup fails to reveal an etiology, the patient is said to have *essential hematuria.*

Table 123-1.   Diagnosis in 1000 Cases of Gross Hematuria*

DIAGNOSIS	PATIENT(%)
Kidneys	15.0
Tumor	3.5
Infection	3.0
Calculus	2.7
Trauma	2.0
Obstruction	1.5
Others	2.3
Ureters	6.5
Calculus	5.3
Tumor	0.7
Others	0.5
Bladder	39.5
Infection	22.0
Tumor	14.9
Others	2.6
Prostate	23.6
Benign hyperplasia	12.5
Infection	9.0
Tumor	2.1
Urethra	4.3
Stricture	1.7
Calculus	1.3
Others	1.3
Essential Hematuria	8.5

*Lee, L.W., *et al.*: JAMA, *153*:782, 1953.

Table 123-2.   Diagnosis in 500 Cases of Asymptomatic Microscopic Hematuria*

DIAGNOSIS	PATIENT(%)
Kidneys	6.2
Calculus	3.4
Cyst	1.2
Hydronephrosis	0.6
Tumor	0.4
Others	0.6
Ureters	0.8
Calculus	0.4
Ureterocoele	0.4
Bladder	8.6
Infection	6.6
Tumor	1.8
Others	0.2
Prostate	23.6
Benign hyperplasia	23.6
Urethra	23.4
Infection	21.2
Calculus	1.8
Others	0.4
Essential Hematuria	44.0

*Greene, L.F., *et al.*: JAMA, *161*:610, 1956.

WORKUP

The history is of paramount importance in narrowing the scope of the workup. History of trauma ought to direct attention to possible renal, ureteral, or urethral injury. Massive hematuria is usually associated with bladder neoplasm, benign prostatic hypertrophy or trauma. Passage of large bulky clots implicates the bladder as the source, while long shoestring-shaped clots suggest a ureteral origin. Past history of analgesic excess makes analgesic nephropathy a possibility. A prior history of nephritis requires consideration of chronic nephritis as the etiology of the hematuria. Family history of renal diseases may suggest polycystic kidney disease or hereditary nephritis.

Physical examination should include note of any fever, hypertension, rash, purpura, petechiae, friction rub, heart murmur or joint swelling. Presence of hypertension suggests renal parenchymal disease. The abdomen has to be carefully examined for enlargement of one or both kidneys, liver, or spleen. A thorough prostatic examination in the male and a pelvic examination in the female are essential.

Laboratory studies must include a careful examination of the *urinary sediment*. Presence of white cells and bacteria would favor a diagnosis of cystitis. White cell casts imply the presence of pyelonephritis or interstitial nephritis. Red cell casts strongly suggest glomerulonephritis. A urine specimen should be sent for routine *culture*. Culture for urine acid-fast bacillus needs to be obtained if sterile pyuria and hematuria persist.

A *three-glass test* (see Chapter 133) should be done to attempt to identify the site of the bleeding. Initial hematuria is usually associated with anterior urethral lesions such as stenosis and urethritis. Terminal hematuria usually arises from a lesion in the posterior urethra, bladder neck or trigone. Total hematuria is associated with lesions at the level of the bladder or above.

Renal function should be checked to rule out renal parenchymal lesions. *Twenty-four-hour urine* collection for creatinine and protein determination should be done to assess renal function and quantitatively assess degree of proteinuria. Heavy proteinuria (greater than 2 gm. per 24 hours) is usually associated with glomerular lesions (see Chapter 124). In the presence of renal colic, the urine should routinely be strained to detect the presence of calculi or papillae. Urine specimens should also be sent for cytology in patients over age 40 with hematuria, because they are at increased risk for a neoplasm.

Flat plate and upright films of the abdomen are obtained and carefully examined to ascertain renal size and detect the presence of calcifications.

If these tests fail to define the origin of the

hematuria, an *intravenous pyelogram* with *nephroto-mograms* should be done. Renal and ureteral abnormalities can accurately be defined. A postvoid film should be obtained to assess the amount of postvoid residual urine in order to estimate the degree of bladder neck obstruction. *Ultrasonography* is useful to differentiate a solid mass from a cystic lesion if the differentiation cannot be made on nephrotomograms. *Renal angiography* is reserved for evaluation of possible renal trauma, suspicious renal masses, and possible arteriovenous malformations.

If there is clinical evidence of glomerular disease (red cell casts, heavy proteinuria), *immunologic studies* should be performed and a renal biopsy considered. The immunologic tests of diagnostic use include ANA, LE prep, anti-DNA antibodies and complement levels for the diagnosis of systemic lupus erythematosus; ASLO titer, antistreptokinase, antihyaluronidase, and complement levels for the diagnosis of poststreptococcal glomerulonephritis; and immunoelectrophoresis for the diagnosis of multiple myeloma.

INDICATIONS FOR REFERRAL

If a distinct lesion is still not defined or there is suspicion of a bladder lesion, it is necessary to proceed to *cystoscopy*. The procedure is particularly useful during periods of active bleeding. Careful examination of the ureteral orifices for bleeding and biopsy of suspicious lesions are essential.

Referral to the nephrologist should be considered if renal biopsy is necessary for the establishment of a diagnosis that will affect the selection of therapy. Renal biopsies should be reserved for patients with clinical evidence of glomerular disease. Rarely, renal biopsies may be indicated if the preceding studies have not led to a diagnosis.

PATIENT EDUCATION

It is essential to impress upon the patient the necessity of a complete evaluation of hematuria. The high incidence of potentially curable neoplasms in patients over the age of 40 makes thorough investigation in this group mandatory.

ANNOTATED BIBLIOGRAPHY

Chen, B.T., Ooi, B.S., Tan, K.K., *et al.*: Causes of recurrent hematuria. Q.J. Med., *41*:141, 1972. *(Series of 82 patients.)*

Greene, L.F., O'Shaughnessy, E.J., Jr., and Hendricks, E.D.: Study of 500 patients with asymptomatic microhematuria. JAMA, *161*:610, 1956. *(Diagnoses in 500 cases of microscopic hematuria.)*

Koehler, P.R., and Kyaw, M.M.: Hematuria. Symp. Radiol. Intern. Med., *59*:201, 1975. *(Radiologic evaluation of patients with hematuria.)*

Kudish, H.G.: Determining the cause of hematuria. Postgrad. Med., *58*:(6):118, 1975. *(Good overview of etiologies and diagnostic considerations.)*

Lee, L.W., Davis, E., *et al.*: Gross urinary hemorrhage: A symptom, not a disease. JAMA, *153*,782, 1953. *(Diagnosis in 1000 cases of gross hematuria.)*

124

Evaluation of Proteinuria
LESLIE S.-T. FANG, M.D.

Normal individuals excrete less than 150 mg. of urinary protein each day; the mean is 40 to 50 mg. Excretion in excess of 150 mg. per 24 hours is classified as clinically significant proteinuria. Causes range from benign forms, such as exercise and orthostatic proteinurias, to glomerulonephritis with rapidly deteriorating renal function. Office evaluation is frequently prompted by an incidental finding of proteinuria on routine urinalysis. The objective of the outpatient workup is to establish the presence of significant proteinuria, search noninvasively for treatable underlying conditions, and select patients who need referral for renal biopsy.

PATHOPHYSIOLOGY AND CLINICAL PRESENTATION

Small amounts of protein (2 to 8 mg. per 100 ml.) are normally found in the urine of healthy individuals, but at a concentration below that detectable by routine methods. Two thirds of this protein is low molecular weight globulin of serum origin, the remainder albumin and nonserum protein.

Significant proteinuria can occur by a number of mechanisms:

1. Increased glomerular permeability;
2. Increased production of abnormal proteins small enough to pass freely through the glomerulus (e.g., Bence Jones protein);
3. Decreased tubular reabsorption (e.g., due to interstitial nephritis);
4. Lower urinary tract disease;
5. Fever, heavy exertion congestive failure, postural changes, and surgical trauma, all believed related to changes in renal blood flow.

Proteinuria can present as an isolated asymptomatic finding on urinalysis, as edema of unknown etiology, or as part of the clinical picture in a patient with known renal or systemic disease. Cases in which less than 2 gm. of protein are excreted daily are more likely to be asymptomatic.

Heavy proteinuria results in progressive decline in the serum albumin level and plasma oncotic pressure and can lead to formation of edema. When more than 3.5 gm. of protein are excreted per day and the serum albumin falls to less than 3.0 mg. per 100 ml., nephrotic syndrome is said to be present. Cholesterol is often increased in these patients, and lipiduria is common. Clinically, the edema usually begins in the medial aspect of the ankles, but on occasion there is only periorbital puffiness.

Other presenting symptoms reflect associated renal dysfunction or underlying systemic diseases.

DIFFERENTIAL DIAGNOSIS

Asymptomatic proteinuria. Proteinuria without other abnormalities in an asymptomatic patient can be transient or persistent. *Transient proteinuria* can occur in association with exercise, orthostatic changes, lower urinary tract diseases and, occasionally fever or congestive failure. *Persistent proteinuria* occurs in patients with mild glomerular and tubular pathology.

Symptomatic proteinuria. Heavy proteinuria resulting in nephrotic syndrome is usually the result of glomerular disease (Table 124–1), but can occur with severe tubular injury.

Intrinsic glomerular diseases account for 75 per cent of the conditions causing nephrotic syndrome. In adults, membranous glomerulonephritis is the most common histologic abnormality seen on biopsies of patients with nephrotic syndrome.

Nephrotic syndrome may be associated with systemic illnesses that can produce glomerular pathology (Table 124–2). Among these illnesses, diabetes mellitus, systemic lupus erythematosus and amyloidosis are the most commonly encountered.

Rarely, marked proteinuria may be seen in tubular disorders (Table 124–3).

Table 124–1.   Glomerular Diseases Causing Nephrotic Syndrome

1. Membranous glomerulonephritis
2. Minimal change disease
3. Focal and proliferative glomerulonephritis
4. Membranoproliferative glomerulonephritis

Table 124–2.   Systemic Diseases Causing Nephrotic Syndrome

Common causes of nephrotic syndrome
1. Diabetes mellitus
2. Systemic lupus erythematosus
3. Amyloidosis
Less common causes of nephrotic syndrome
1. Infection (subacute bacterial endocarditis, shunt infection, malaria, syphilis, hepatitis, schistosomiasis)
2. Toxins (heroin, mercury, bismuth, gold, penicillamine)
Uncommon causes of nephrotic syndrome
1. Allergens (bee stings, serum sickness)
2. Mechanical causes (constrictive pericarditis, renal vein thrombosis, obstruction of inferior vena cava)
3. Malignancy (Hodgkin's disease, lymphoma and other tumors)
4. Pregnancy
5. Congenital (Fabry's disease, nail-patella syndrome, Alport's disease)

Table 124–3.   Tubular Disorders Associated with Proteinuria

1. Analgesic abuse
2. Pyelonephritis
3. Fanconi's syndrome
4. Cadmium and mercury poisoning
5. Balkan's nephropathy
6. Lowe's syndrome
7. Hepatolenticular degeneration

WORKUP

Most workups begin with a *dipstick* check of a random urine sample. The test is specific for albumin and can detect concentrations in excess of 30 mg. per 100 ml. A negative test does not rule out significant proteinuria, since excretion may be intermittent or composed of protein other than albumin. Also, false-negatives can occur if dilute specimens are used. Therefore, note of the specific gravity should be made along with the test results. False-positive dipstick reactions can be seen in patients receiving large doses of cephalosporins.

A *24-hour urine collection* is the only satisfactory quantitative method for determination of significant proteinuria. Adequacy of collection can be judged by simultaneous determination of total creatinine. Depending on muscle mass, the total 24-hour urine creatinine should be 15 to 24 mg. per kg.

Once significant proteinuria is established, the evaluation is tailored to whether the patient is asymptomatic or symptomatic. In *asymptomatic proteinuria,* several urinalyses should be performed to determine if the proteinuria is transient or persistent. Transient orthostatic or exercise-induced proteinuria is benign and may occur in the absence of underlying disease, usually in young adults. In such cases, invasive procedures and extensive workups should be avoided. Persistent asymptomatic proteinuria, on the other hand, is associated with a high incidence of renal pathology and warrants the same investigation as in patients with symptomatic proteinuria.

In *symptomatic proteinuria,* history should be reviewed for known renal disease, streptococcal infections, drug allergies, toxin exposure, diabetes, hypertension, analgesic intake (especially phenacetin-containing compounds), urinary tract infections, and family history of renal disease. Erect and supine blood pressure should be measured, and the patient checked for skin rash, retinopathy, adenopathy, tricuspid valve disease, congestive heart failure, constrictive pericarditis, abdominal masses or organomegaly, periorbital, sacral and ankle edema, prostatic enlargement, and signs of joint inflammation.

Once the presence of significant proteinuria has been established, the history taken, and the physical examination performed, certain laboratory studies can be very helpful; the following should be obtained in most patients:

- *Urinalysis with examination of the sediment* is the single most important test and should be done on a freshly collected specimen. Red cell casts indicate glomerulonephritis (though the absence of erythrocytes on one sample does not rule out glomerulonephritis). White cell casts are found in pyelonephritis and interstitial nephritis. Oval fat bodies are due to lipiduria in patients with nephrotic syndrome. A negative or weakly positive dipstick test combined with a positive sulfosalicylic test for protein suggests the presence of myeloma protein in the urine, since the dipstick is specific for albumin only.

- *Creatinine clearance* is best for determination of renal function and approximates glomerular filtration rate. A serum creatinine and a 24-hour urine collection for urinary creatinine are simultaneously obtained. Random BUN or creatinine levels are less accurate than a clearance determination, but are useful for following the patient once the creatinine clearance is known.

- *KUB* can be used to judge kidney size, which may help to elucidate etiology (e.g., small, shrunken kidneys suggest significant, chronic, bilateral disease). *Intravenous pyelogram* is essential for the diagnosis of chronic pyelonephritis and is an excellent way to judge kidney size. It gives an estimate of individual kidney function, based on how well the contrast material is concentrated and excreted. When creatinine clearance is reduced by over 75 per cent, the kidneys may not sufficiently concentrate contrast media for visualization. The incidence of contrast-media-induced acute renal failure is higher in diabetics, in patients with multiple myeloma, and in patients with renal insufficiency; *renal ultrasound studies* may be more appropriate in these patients.

- *Complete blood count* will identify any anemia due to severe subacute or chronic renal insufficiency. It is also present at some point in all cases of myeloma.

- *Serum albumin* level correlates inversely with the severity of proteinuria.

- *Protein selectivity index* is useful for diagnosis and therapy in patients with nephrotic syndrome. Proteinuria is considered selective when urine contains large amounts of proteins of low molecular weight. A high degree of selectivity in patients with nephrotic syndrome suggests minimal change disease, which is responsive to corticosteroids.

In most instances, these tests should be done on all patients with significant proteinuria. More specific investigations for individual conditions are indicated only when clinical or laboratory data suggest a particular underlying condition. The workup of proteinuria can be done sequentially; a wasteful "pan scan" should not be ordered initially.

INDICATIONS FOR REFERRAL

At times, the diagnosis may remain unclear, even after extensive laboratory testing. In such instances, a referral for renal biopsy is indicated if the result will have important therapeutic and/or prognostic implications. Most causes of glomerulonephritis do not respond to therapy; thus, biopsy is of academic interest only. However, at times it will be impossible to rule out the treatable forms of glomerulonephritis, such as minimal change disease and, perhaps, idiopathic membranous nephropathy. When faced with this situation, the primary physician should obtain the consultation of a nephrologist to help decide the usefulness of a biopsy.

PRINCIPLES OF MANAGEMENT AND PATIENT EDUCATION

Asymptomatic Proteinuria. Transient proteinuria may not be associated with underlying renal disease and is by and large benign. Patients should be reassured, and therapy is not warranted. Persistent proteinuria is often associated with renal pathology; however, idiopathic proteinuria as an isolated finding without other associated abnormalities has been found to have an excellent prognosis in two prospective studies with 5 to 18 years follow-up. These patients should be carefully followed and referred to a nephrologist for biopsy if the situation changes.

Symptomatic Proteinuria. In proteinuria associated with systemic diseases such as multiple myeloma, diabetes, or systemic lupus erythematosus, treatment should be directed toward the underlying diseases (see Chapters 98 and 139). In proteinuria secondary to renal disease, therapy is dependent upon the renal pathology defined by biopsy.

In patients with nephrotic syndrome, general measures that can provide symptomatic relief include a high-protein diet, sodium restriction and the judicious use of diuretics. Specific therapeutic interventions that have been of benefit include the use of corticosteroids and immunosuppressive agents in children and adults with minimal change disease. Recent studies have also shown alternate-day steroids to be of some benefit in nephrotic syndrome secondary to membranous glomerulonephritis. The literature should be followed for developments in this area, for the issue is not yet settled.

ANNOTATED BIBLIOGRAPHY

Becker, E.L.: Proteinuria in renal diseases. Bull N.Y. Acad. Med., 46:830, 1970. *(General and basic review of proteinuria.)*

Heinemann, H.O., Maack, T.M, and Sherman, R.L.: Proteinuria. Am. J. Med., 56:71, 1974. *(A good discussion of the pathogenesis of proteinuria.)*

Robinson, R.R.: Idiopathic proteinuria. Ann Intern. Med. 71:1019, 1969. *(Short review of idiopathic benign proteinuria.)*

Robinson, R.R.: Orthostatic proteinuria: Definition and prognosis. Kidney, 4(3): 1, 1971. *(Review of pathogenesis and prognosis of orthostatic proteinuria.)*

Smith, F.G., Stanley, T.M., and McIntosh, R.M.: The nephrotic syndrome: Current concepts. Ann. Intern. Med., 76:463, 1972. *(Detailed definition of nephrotic syndrome and the renal pathologic conditions that can result in nephrotic syndrome.)*

125
Evaluation of Lower Urinary Tract Dysfunction
JOHN D. GOODSON, M.D.

Patients with lower urinary tract dysfunction present with complaints of hesitancy, dribbling, frequency, loss of stream volume and force, incontinence or urgency. The primary physician must collect sufficient data to ensure that renal function is not jeopardized and that there is not a serious underlying condition which requires treatment. Having done this, the physician and the patient can then decide whether the symptoms justify the risk and expense of a more detailed and invasive evaluation.

PATHOPHYSIOLOGY AND CLINICAL PRESENTATION

The maintenance of urinary continence depends on the integrated function of the bladder, urethra, pelvic floor and nervous system. In the normal individual, the detrusor muscle of the bladder wall is under dual sympathetic and parasympathetic control. Sympathetic activity combines the beta adrenergic effect of detrusor relaxation with the alpha adrenergic effect of bladder neck contraction to accomplish bladder filling. Parasympathetic activity produces contraction of the detrusor and, together with voluntary relaxation of the external sphincters of the pelvic floor, results in voiding. The urethra is mechanically oriented to the bladder so as to facilitate continence; complete bladder emptying depends on unimpeded flow.

The process of voiding usually begins with a sensation of bladder fullness mediated by sensory nerves in the bladder wall. Detrusor contraction is initiated via a parasympathetic reflex arc. Voluntary relaxation of the pelvic external sphincter allows the bladder to empty.

The process can be disturbed at many levels. If the destrusor muscle fails to generate sufficient contractile force, the bladder will not empty completely. The patient will complain of frequent urination and poor stream force. Likewise, irritation of the detrusor from either an acute or a chronic inflammatory process can cause muscular overactivity or reduced bladder capacity.

An abnormal urethrovesical angle or a weakened pelvic musculature will allow excessive urinary flow and may produce stress incontinence and dribbling. Any intrinsic or extrinsic impediment to flow through the urethra will lead to loss of stream force, hesitancy, and incomplete bladder emptying. The patient will void frequently in small amounts. Eventually, persistent urethral obstruction results in chronic distention of the bladder, leading to detrusor failure and the inability to urinate.

Interruption of the autonomic reflex arc produces a hypotonic autonomous bladder, while damage to the spinal cord above the arc usually leads to bladder spasticity. With both, the patient will void small amounts frequently, and stream force will be diminished.

Anticholinergic drugs and tranquilizers with anticholinergic properties can interfere with bladder contraction by inhibiting cholinergic transmission. Symptoms can develop rapidly when such medications are used in patients with preexisting lower urinary tract dysfunction.

Lower tract dysfunction can be psychogenic in origin or reflect impaired cortical function. There is frequency of urination or even incontinence, but dribbling and hesitancy are usually absent.

Many patients have multiple coexisting deficits. Each lesion requires separate identification.

DIFFERENTIAL DIAGNOSIS

The differential diagnosis of lower urinary tract dysfunction can be organized along functional and anatomic lines (Table 125–1). Various *bladder abnormalities* can produce lower urinary tract complaints. Trigonitis often accompanies cystitis and is the most common cause of urinary frequency. Chronic interstitial cystitis is a condition with reduced bladder capacity and found almost exclusively in women. A small bladder can also develop following pelvic irradiation, pelvic surgery or tuberculous cystitis. Chronic outflow obstruction can produce bladder herniation and formation of diverticula that prevent complete emptying. Any extrinsic or intrinsic mass can impinge on the bladder and reduce its holding capacity.

Urethral obstruction can arise from both intrinsic and extrinsic factors. Strictures of the urethra occasionally develop following gonococcal urethritis, urethral trauma, and pelvic irradiation. Rarely, a stone or a tumor will cause partial obstruction. Congenital valves of the urethra usually produce symptoms in childhood, whereas prostatic median bars produce symptoms in adulthood. Extrinsic urethral compression is seen in males with prostatic enlargement. Symptoms of urethral irritation and obstruction in the absence of an identifiable cause are attributed to so-called prostatosis in the male and urethral syndrome in the female.

Pelvic floor incompetence resulting from a difficult vaginal delivery or direct perineal injury causes a loss of the normal urethrovesical angle and external sphincter strength. In some cases, the formation of a cystocele further impairs control.

Neurologic abnormalities can be divided into those that affect the cord above the reflex arc, those that affect the reflex arc *per se,* those that develop following the administration of drugs, and those affecting the cerebral cortex. Interruption of the cord above the sacral segments is rarely complete in pa-

Table 125-1.   Causes of Lower Urinary Tract Dysfunction

I.   Bladder abnormalities
    A. Intrinsic
        1. Infection (trigonitis)
        2. Chronic interstitial cystitis
        3. Postradiation fibrosis
        4. Bladder diverticula
        5. Detrusor failure
        6. Postoperative
    B. Extrinsic
        1. Pelvic or abdominal mass
II. Urethral obstruction
    A. Instrinsic
        1. Stricture (postradiation, infection, trauma)
        2. Stone
        3. Tumor
        4. Congenital lesion (valves, median bar)
    B. Extrinsic
        1. Prostatic enlargement (infection, benign prostatic hypertrophy, cancer, granulomatous prostatitis)
        2. Pelvic abscess
        3. Prostatosis
III. Pelvic floor incompetence
        1. Muscular relaxation (postpartum, post-traumatic)
        2. Cystocele
        3. Denervation
IV. Neurologic abnormalities
    A. Cord-related problems
        1. Congenital lesions (meningomyelocele)
        2. Infection (transverse myelitis)
        3. Demyelinating diseases (multiple sclerosis)
        4. Vascular insufficiency
        5. Disc herniation
        6. Tumors (intrinsic, extrinsic)
    B. Reflex arc dysfunction
        1. Infection (herpes, tabes dorsalis, arachnoiditis)
        2. Congenital lesions (meningomyelocele)
        3. Demyelinating diseases (multiple sclerosis)
        4. Diabetes
        5. Tumors (cord, pelvic)
        6. Trauma
    C. Cortical dysfunction
        1. Normopressure hydrocephalus
        2. Dementia
        3. Oversedation
        4. Encephalitis
    D. Drugs
        1. Anticholinergics
        2. Major tranquilizers
        3. Antidepressants
V.   Psychogenic factors
        1. Anxiety
        2. Psychosis

tients seen in general clinical practice. Partial abnormalities develop with diabetes, multiple sclerosis, tabes dorsalis, and intrinsic or extrinsic cord compression from tumor or disc herniation. Such abnormalities are frequently associated with some form of reflex arc dysfunction as well. Occasionally, isolated arc dysfunction is seen, due to herpes infections, diabetes, or multiple sclerosis. Drugs with anticholinergic properties often cause trouble with voiding. Impaired cortical function may cause difficulty with voluntary relaxation of the external sphincter. *Psychogenic etiologies* include anxiety and psychosis.

Other causes of frequency unrelated to lower urinary tract dysfunction are those which produce a diuresis, such as diabetes insipidus, poorly controlled diabetes mellitus, diuretic use, and excessive fluid intake.

WORKUP

The evaluation of the patient with hesitancy, dribbling, frequency, or loss of stream volume and force requires assessment of each component involved in maintaining urinary continence.

History and Physical Examination. Much can be determined by history and physical examination alone.

Bladder. Frequency associated with dysuria and fever suggests a urinary tract infection (see Chapter 129). Frequent small voidings are consistent with a small bladder; bladder contraction or extrinsic compression should be suspected. However similar complaints can also arise from a large, distended bladder in which voiding is essentially spillage off the top. To distinguish between the two, the lower abdomen should be noted for distention and the suprapubic area percussed and palpated for evidence of an enlarged bladder. Straight catheterization for residual urine following voiding is safe and frequently diagnostic.

Urethra. Obstruction produces loss of stream force initially and bladder distention secondarily. The patient should be carefully questioned about antecedent gonococcal urethritis, urethral instrumentation, or radiation. In the male, rectal examination is essential, palpating the prostate to get some idea of size, though size alone does not reliably correlate with the degree of obstruction especially if median lobe enlargement is responsible for symptoms.

Pelvic floor. Incompetence is most often seen in multiparous women and can be assessed with the patient in the lithotomy position by observing pelvic motion during coughing and the Valsalva maneuver. Pelvic muscle denervation will be suggested by a history of trauma or coexisting neuropathy.

Nervous system. Abnormalities above the autonomic reflex arc produce frequent, small voidings. Such patients should be screened for a history of cord trauma, multiple sclerosis, syphilis, and vascular insufficiency. Aside from certain metabolic disorders, conditions that directly affect the cord are generally associated with other neurologic deficits; these should be searched for by a careful neurologic examination in order to determine the specific level of the lesion. The autonomic arc can be assessed on physical examination by checking the bulbocavernosus reflex. Normally, squeezing the clitoris or glans penis will cause anal sphincter contraction. An absent reflex suggests interruption. Since control of the anal sphincter is similar to that of the bladder, the examiner can estimate the functional competence of both systems by checking anal tone on rectal examination and by noting the patient's ability to contract the sphincter voluntarily. In certain situations, such as poliomyelitis, the sensory component of the arc is preserved and the patient will complain of painful distention, but will be unable to generate bladder contraction.

Regardless of the suspected etiology, all patients should be asked about prescription and nonprescription medications which affect autonomic function, such as tricyclic antidepressants, major tranquilizers, and anticholinergics and an effort should be made to determine amounts and patterns of fluid consumption.

Laboratory evaluation should include a two-hour postprandial blood sugar as a screen for diabetes, a serologic test for syphilis, BUN, creatinine, and urinalysis. The presence of pyuria suggests inflammation within the urinary tract. Hematuria raises the possibility of neoplasm or some other lesion in the bladder, urethra, or prostate (see Chapter 123). A morning urine osmolality after overnight fluid deprivation should be obtained if diabetes insipidus is suspected; normal persons are able to concentrate their urine to over 700 milliosmoles per liter.

Straight catherization following voiding is a simple office technique for assessing the residual urine volume. A residual volume of greater than 50 cc. is abnormal.

The *cystometrogram* (CMG) is a valuable aid in determining the functional characteristics of suspected neurogenic abnormalities. Normal individuals sense bladder filling between 100 and 200 cc., have a nonurgent desire to void at 250 to 350 cc., and experience detrusor contraction at 400 to 550 cc. A spastic bladder will demonstrate a small capacity and recurrent uninhibited contractions (see Fig. 125–1, line B). An atonic bladder will demonstrate a large volume and little contractile force (Fig. 125–1, line C).

Urine flow rates provide the clinician with information helpful for initially assessing outflow obstruction and for monitoring patients during follow-up.

Radiologic studies are important for defining anatomic defects. The *intravenous pyelogram (IVP)* is particularly useful when outflow tract obstruction is suspected. The test allows an estimate of the post-void residual bladder volume and identifies any de-

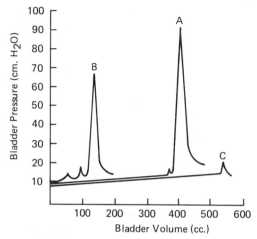

Fig. 125-1. Cystometrogram findings. (A) Normal pressure-volume relationship; (B) the uninhibited neurogenic bladder; (C) the atonic bladder.

trusor hypertrophy, bladder diverticula, or intravesicular prostate enlargement. The *voiding cystourethrogram (VCUG)* can identify specific areas of urethral obstruction, such as might occur as a result of stricture formation.

INDICATIONS FOR REFERRAL

Consultation with a neurologist is necessary when a demyelinating disease, an intrinsic cord lesion, or extrinsic cord compression is suspected, especially if myelography is being considered. Patients with urethral obstruction or a bladder lesion should be referred to the urologist for further assessment with cystoscopy or more detailed flow studies.

SYMPTOMATIC MANAGEMENT AND PATIENT EDUCATION

While evaluation is in progress, the patient should be instructed to avoid situations or medications which might place stress upon the lower urinary tract. Fluid overload following excessive coffee, tea or alcohol consumption or unnecessary diuretic or methylxanthine use should be avoided. Anticholinergics, antidepressants and tranquilizers should be used cautiously, if at all. Infections can exacerbate the clinical severity of any abnormality; the patient should be alerted to contact the physician if dysuria, fever or flank pain develops.

Definitive treatment of specific lower urinary tract abnormalities requires an etiologic diagnosis (see Chapters 131 and 136). However, many patients will have an unrevealing initial evaluation and can be followed conservatively as long as they are able to tolerate their symptoms and have no evidence of deterioration in renal or bladder function or evidence of malignancy (e.g., hematuria or a prostatic nodule).

ANNOTATED BIBLIOGRAPHY

Badenoch, A.W.: Chronic interstitial cystitis. Br. J. Urol. *43*:718, 1971. *(Short clinical review of an unusual syndrome. Primary symptoms are frequency and suprapubic pain relieved by voiding.)*

Castro, J.E., and Griffiths, H.L.J.: The assessment of benign prostatic hypertrophy. J. R. Coll. Surg. Edinb., *17*:194, 1972. *(Technique for calculation of urethral calibre based on flow rates and bladder pressure.)*

Culp, D.A.: Benign prostatic hypertrophy. Urol. Clin. North Am., *2*:29, 1975. *(Clinical review with a discussion of the differential diagnosis.)*

Khanna, O.P.: Disorders of micturition. Urology, *8*:316, 1976. *(Excellent review of bladder neuropharmacology and various treatment modalities.)*

Meares, E.M.: Bacterial prostatitis *vs* "prostatosis." JAMA, *224*: 1372, 1973. *("Prostatosis" produces symptoms of outflow obstruction without evidence of infection. Treatment is palliative.)*

Messing, E.M., and Stamey, T.A.: Interstitial cystitis. Urology, *12*:381, 1978. *(The diagnosis of interstitial cystitis should be considered in women with persistent lower urinary tract symptoms and negative cultures and urine cytologies. Diagnosis and treatment are discussed.)*

O'Dea, M.J., Hunting, D.B., and Greene, L.F.: Nonspecific granulomatous prostatitis. J. Urol., *118*:58, 1977. *(An unusual cause of outflow obstruction in males which must be differentiated from carcinoma. Natural history is toward gradual resolution.)*

Wein, A.J., Raezor, D.M., and Benson, G.S.: Management of neurogenic bladder dysfunction in the adult. Urology, *8*:432, 1976. *(Review of the surgical and nonsurgical options in the treatment of the neurogenic bladder.)*

126
Evaluation of Penile Discharge
JOHN D. GOODSON, M.D.

Urethral discharge in the male can range from a relatively trivial moistening of the penile meatus to copious purulent fluid associated with severe dysuria and secondary urinary retention. The number of known causes is limited, and the most important responsibility of the primary physician is to distinguish gonococcal from nongonococcal etiologies in order that appropriate therapy can be initiated and complications avoided.

PATHOPHYSIOLOGY AND CLINICAL PRESENTATION

Numerous bacterial and nonbacterial organisms can invade the mucosal lining of the male urethra. Slightly less than half the urethritis seen in urban venereal disease clinics is due to gonococcal infection. The patient with *gonococcal urethritis* usually presents with a 2- to 4-day history of dysuria and penile discharge. The discharge is thick and purulent; on Gram stain, polymorphonuclear leukocytes and gram-negative intracellular diplococci are the characteristic findings. Systemic gonococcemia develops in approximately 3 per cent of patients.

In contrast, patients with *nongonococcal urethritis* (NGU) present with symptoms of longer duration, occasionally 3 to 4 weeks. The discharge is mucoid and frequently scant. On Gram stain, polymorphonuclear leukocytes and pleomorphic extracellular gram-negative and gram-positive organisms are seen. Only 20 per cent of ambiguous Gram stains (rare extracellular gram-negative diplococci) will be shown by subsequent culture to represent gonococcal infection.

Nongonococcal urethritis can develop from infection by a number of organisms with a low level of tissue invasiveness and unusual cultural requirements. *Chlamydia trachomatis* is responsible for 40 to 60 per cent of these cases and has been isolated from asymptomatic female consorts. The role of *Ureaplasma urealyticum* or T-strain *mycoplasma* is still debated since their prevalence in asymptomatic individuals is high. *Trichomonas vaginalis* and *Candida albicans* are both occasional causes of urethritis.

Reiter's syndrome is a relatively common connective tissue disorder of unknown etiology characterized by conjunctivitis or iritis, acute symmetrical polyarthritis, circinate balanitis, keratodermia blennorrhagica, mucosal ulcerations and urethritis. One or a combination of symptoms may be present at any one time (see Chapter 139). Many of these patients present with a mucoid or purulent penile discharge, mild dysuria and few eye, joint or skin complaints. The histocompatibility antigen HLA-B27 is found in up to 96 per cent of these patients (10 per cent of controls). Whether this histocompatibility antigen correlates with a predisposition to viral, bacterial or other infections that subsequently lead to the symptom complex is still unknown.

Trauma and *acute prostatitis* can also produce a discharge. A bloody discharge suggests lower genitourinary tract *neoplasm*.

DIFFERENTIAL DIAGNOSIS

The differential diagnosis of urethral discharge can be divided into infectious and noninfectious causes (Table 126–1). The known infectious causes are *Neisseria gonorrhoeae*, *Chlamydia trachomatis*, *Candida albicans* and *Trichomonas vaginalis*. The noninfectious causes are Reiter's syndrome, trauma, and malignancy of the lower urinary tract.

Table 126–1. Causes of Urethral Discharge in Males

Infectious causes
  1. *Neisseria gonorrhoeae*
  2. *Chlamydia trachomatis*
  3. *Candida albicans*
  4. *Trichomonas vaginalis*
  5. *Ureaplasma urealyticum*
Noninfectious causes
  1. Reiter's syndrome
  2. Trauma
  3. Cancer of lower genitourinary tract

WORKUP

History. The duration and character of the discharge can be informative. A spontaneous purulent discharge usually indicates gonococcal infection; a scant mucoid discharge points toward a nongonococcal etiology. Inquiry should be made concerning symptoms of localized gonorrheal infection (pharyngitis, proctitis), of systemic gonococcemia (arthritis, punctate skin lesions, sepsis), or Reiter's syndrome (polyarthritis, dermatitis, conjunctivitis).

A careful search for sexual contacts who have gonorrhea is important in the historical evaluation of all patients with a penile discharge; however, both female and homosexual male consorts can be asymptomatic.

Physical examination should be checked for systemic signs of gonococcemia and Reiter's syndrome. Fever, punctate, centrally hemorrhagic, necrotic skin lesions, tenosynovitis, and polyarthritis, suggest gonococcemia. Reiter's syndrome can be manifest by any combination of conjunctivitis, iritis, mucosal ulceration (oral or meatal), circinate balanitis (ulceration and erythema on the penile glans), keratoderma blennorrhagica (pustular or hyperkeratotic lesions on the soles of the feet), and acute symmetrical polyarthritis (knees, ankles, heels and sacroiliac joints), in addition to urethritis.

Laboratory studies. Since the clinical presentation of patients with gonococcal and nongonococcal urethritis often overlaps, all patients with penile discharge must be carefully evaluated to exclude gonococcal infection. The Gram stain and culture of the urethral discharge are essential to accurate diagnosis. The finding of Gram-negative intracellular diplococci is highly predictive of gonococcal urethritis with greater than 95 per cent specificity, while mixed Gram-negative and Gram-positive pleomorphic extracellular organisms are suggestive of a nongonococcal etiology. A "wet" saline preparation and a KOH preparation should be done in ambiguous cases to screen for the presence of *Trichomonas* and *Candida,* respectively. All patients should have a gonorrhea culture and serology for syphilis regardless of Gram stain results. When cultures and Gram stains are not diagnostic and a therapeutic trial of treatment for nongonococcal urethritis is unsuccessful, or when there is a reasonable suspicion of Reiter's syndrome, the patient can be checked for the presence of HLA-B27 histocompatibility antigen.

Undiagnosed or bloody discharge warrants cytologic examination of the discharge and urine for neoplastic cells and referral to a urologist for possible cystoscopy.

PATIENT EDUCATION

Patients with gonococcal urethritis and NGU must be told that the successful treatment of the disease depends on the eradication of the infecting organism in all sexual partners. Both partners must be screened regardless of complaints and treated in the same fashion as the symptomatic patient. The exception to this general rule is that there is no evidence to support the treatment of the homosexual partner of the male with NGU.

Treated patients should be strongly encouraged to return for follow-up culture and to seek medical attention immediately if symptoms should return.

There are no firm data concerning abstinence from intercourse during the treatment period, but it seems reasonable to suggest 2 to 5 days of treatment before resumption of sexual activity.

SYMPTOMATIC MANAGEMENT

Treatment must be etiologic to be effective (see Chapters 132, 134).

ANNOTATED BIBLIOGRAPHY

Arnett, F.C., McClusky, O.E., Schacter, B.Z., and Lordon, R.E.: Incomplete Reiter's syndrome: Discriminating features and HLA-B27 in diagnosis. Ann. Intern. Med., *84:*8, 1976. *(Description of 13 patients who presented primarily with oligoarticular, asymmetric arthritis. The diagnosis of Reiter's syndrome was suspected due to the presence of HLA-B27 in 12.)*

Holmes, K.K., Hansfield, H.H., Wang, S.P., et al.: Etiology of nongonococcal urethritis. N. Engl. J. Med., *292:*1198, 1975. *(Culture data from males with NGU definitely identified Chlamydia trachomatis in 42 per cent. No other organism was statistically more frequent in NGU patients when compared to controls. Chlamydia was also isolated in female partners of symptomatic males.)*

Jacobs, N.J., and Kraus, S.J.: Gonococcal and nongonococcal urethritis in men. Ann. Intern. Med., *82:*7, 1975. *(Ninety-eight per cent of specimens which were definitely positive for gonococcus on*

Gram stain were culture-positive. Ninety-seven per cent that were definitely negative were culture-negative. Twenty-one per cent of stains that were equivocal were gonococcal culture-positive.)

Kaufman, R.E., and Wiesner, P.J.: Nonspecific urethritis. N. Engl. J. Med., *291*:1175, 1974. *(Short clinical review.)*

McCormack, W.M., Braun, P., Lee, Y.H., *et al.*: The genital *Mycoplasma.* N. Engl. J. Med., *288*:78, 1973. *(Balanced review of the role of T mycoplasma in NGU.)*

Morris, R., Metzger, A.L., Bluestone, R., and Teraski, P.I.: HLA-B27—A clue to the diagnosis and pathogenesis of Reiter's syndrome. N. Engl. J. Med., *290*:554, 1974. *(Ninety-six per cent of patients with Reiter's syndrome were HLA-B27 positive.)*

Schacter, J.: Chlamydial infections. N. Engl. J. Med., *298*:428; 490; 540, 1978. *(Excellent review of the role of chlamydial organisms in genitourinary infection.)*

Weinberger, H.W., Ropes, M., Kulka, J.P., and Bauer, W.: Reiter's syndrome, clinical and pathologic observations. Medicine, *41*:35, 1962. *(Excellent clinical review.)*

127

Evaluation of Scrotal Pain, Masses and Swelling

A mass, generalized enlargement or acute pain involving the scrotum may be noted by the patient or discovered incidentally on physical examination. Patients with scrotal complaints are often concerned about loss of sexual function and the possibility of cancer. The primary physician needs to be able to promptly recognize torsion and epididymitis and differentiate benign masses from those suggestive of malignancy, which require referral for urologic evaluation.

PATHOPHYSIOLOGY AND CLINICAL PRESENTATION

Almost all *testicular neoplasms* are malignant and of germ cell origin. The metastatic lesion may be histologically different from the primary lesion; on occasion, extensive metastasis occurs with little evidence of the primary tumor. Fortunately, these tumors are not common, accounting for less than 1 per cent of all deaths from neoplasms in men; however, they are the third most frequently found tumor in men between ages 20 to 34, having an estimated incidence of 2 to 3 per 100,000 men. Incidence is increased in those with an undescended testicle and remains high even if orchiopexy is performed or the testicle is removed; the risk seems to be genetically determined.

Typically the tumor presents as a hard, heavy, firm, nontender mass that does not transilluminate, but sometimes the lesion is smooth or even resilient in nature, leading to confusion with benign etiologies even though it blocks transmission of light. Metastasis may result in a palpable left supraclavicular node or epigastric mass. A few of these malignancies produce chorionic gonadotropin or estrogen, leading to gynecomastia. Others may be painful if there is hemorrhage into the tumor.

Nontesticular, intrascrotal malignancies are usually firm and do not transilluminate.

Testicular torsion presents with acute pain and a firm tender mass in a young patient. The intense pain may be associated with nausea and vomiting and may be confused with an abdominal process. The condition is most prevalent among adolescent boys and becomes much less common in adulthood. There may be no history of antecedent trauma.

Trauma produces acute testicular pain and swelling similar to torsion or infection. It does not predispose to cancer.

Mumps orchitis is usually seen 7 to 10 days after parotitis and is most often unilateral in association with fever, swelling, pain and tenderness. On occasion parotitis is absent.

Cystic masses containing fluid or sperm often develop spontaneously. They are slow-growing, usually painless, and may be large and fluctuant. *Hydroceles* are cystic accumulations of clear or straw-colored fluid within the tunica vaginalis or processus vaginalis. *Spermatoceles* are intrascrotal cysts containing sperm which derive from the small tubules of the epididymis. The space between the testicle and tunica vaginalis may also fill with fluid secondary to impaired drainage or inflammation.

In *epididymitis,* which often occurs secondary to prostatic infection and sometimes in association with carcinoma of the testes, the epididymis is cordlike, tender, swollen and palpably distinct from the testicle.

Varicoceles arise from incompetent venous valves. They occur on the left in 97 per cent of cases, because the left spermatic vein empties directly into the renal vein, resulting in transmission of considerable hydrostatic pressure into the scrotum when the valves are incompetent and the patient stands. Varicoceles have a "bag of worms" appearance and are usually nontender; they decrease in size when the patient is recumbent.

Inguinal hernias can lead to scrotal enlargement as bowel tracks through the inguinal canal and pushes down into scrotum.

DIFFERENTIAL DIAGNOSIS

The differential diagnosis of a soft painlessly enlarged scrotum includes hydrocele, spermatocele, nonincarcerated bowel herniating into the sac, and nonincarcerated generalized edema. Painful scrotal swelling is caused by epididymitis, orchitis, torsion of the cord, trauma, or, less commonly, hemorrhage into tumor. A firm, hard, nontender nodule or a smooth one that cannot be transilluminated represents carcinoma till proven otherwise.

WORKUP

History. It is important to determine whether or not the lesion is painful, how long it has been present and whether there has been any change, recent trauma, inguinal hernia, prostatitis, or mumps. Age may be helpful in diagnosis; for example, epididymitis is much more common in older patients than is torsion, which occurs in the 15 to 40 age group. A complaint of heaviness usually means tumor, hydrocele or epididymitis. It is important for therapeutic purposes to establish whether infertility has been a problem, as may occur with come varicoceles. (see Chapter 115).

Physical examination. The scrotum must be carefully inspected and palpated. Inspection should include note of any erythema, masses, hernias, or varices. To palpate the scrotal contents properly, one should stand to one side and use both hands, one to support the testicle and the other to feel and identify each structure. The head of the epididymis is usually situated above the testis; the body and tail run posteriorly and are separately palpable.

One should try to assess if a lesion is cystic or solid, testicular or nontesticular. Transillumination with a penlight in a darkened room is needed to help determine whether the lesion is cystic or solid. Cystic lesions allow transmission of light in most instances, although a bloody exudate may not. A mass that appears extratesticular and cystic is most likely benign and either a spermatocele, a cyst of the epididymis, or hydrocele. If it is hard, does not transilluminate, or is reported to be steadily growing, tumor must be considered and urological evaluation is necessary even if the mass appears to be extratesticular. In patients suspected of having testicular tumors, the breasts should be checked for gynecomastia, the abdomen for masses and the supraclavicular lymph nodes for enlargement. Inguinal adenopathy does not suggest testicular tumor because the testicular lymphatics drain into the para-aortic nodes. Scrotal nontesticular lymphatics drain into the inguinal nodes.

Laboratory studies. A urinalysis is helpful in all cases for detection of pyuria or bacteriuria suggestive of an infectious process. Semen analysis should be performed only when infertility is a concurrent complaint. A right-sided varicocele or suddenly appearing left-sided varicocele requires further evaluation because of the possibility of venous obstruction or renal carcinoma; in such cases an intravenous pyelogram is indicated.

Summary. An acutely painful, swollen scrotum requires urgent assessment because if torsion of the testes is present, permanent damage may occur within hours. Acute epididymitis and torsion are the two main causes. Epididymitis is suggested by its occurrence most often in men over age 40, a more gradual onset in the context of urinary tract symptoms, a tender boggy prostate gland, a tender cordlike epididymal mass, or a urinalysis revealing pyuria and bacteriuria. The finding of a firm tender mass of acute onset in a young patient must be considered torsion till proven otherwise. Urgent urologic consultation is necessary to determine whether or not the scrotum should be explored. Sometimes it can be very difficult to distinguish torsion from epididymitis on clinical grounds, and surgical exploration is mandatory.

PATIENT EDUCATION AND SYMPTOMATIC MANAGEMENT

The patient with a nontender cystic, clearly extratesticular mass can be reassured that the lesion is not a cancer. Concern about fertility sometimes arises. Fertility is compromised only occasionally in a patient with a varicocele. The reassurance can be most comforting.

Most hydroceles and cystic lesions do not require therapy, but the patient should be instructed to return if the enlargement becomes uncomfortable or interferes with intercourse. The patient should understand that surgery is an option that will not threaten virility or fertility. Patients may want a hydrocele removed for cosmetic reasons or relief of discomfort. Aspiration of a hydrocele is to be avoided. Patients with inguinal hernias that are at risk of causing strangulation of bowel should be advised to have them repaired (see Chapter 63).

INDICATIONS FOR REFERRAL

Referral to a urologist should be swift in cases of torsion, because surgical exploration must not be delayed if a viable testicle is to be preserved. Patients in whom tumor is suspected also need prompt surgical evaluation, because early disease is almost 100 per cent curable. Any mass that cannot be confidently defined as cystic and as separate from the testicle should be subjected to a urologist's examination. A patient with varicocele should be referred if it does not deflate when he lies down, is painful, or is associated with infertility. Referral to a general surgeon is needed for the patient with a poorly reducible hernia.

ANNOTATED BIBLIOGRAPHY

Beccia, D.J., Krane, R.J., and Olsson, C.A.: Clinical management of nontesticular intrascrotal tumors. J. Urol., *116*:476, 1976. *(Even extratesticular masses may be malignant.)*

Essenhigh, D.M.: Scrotal swelling. Practitioner, *212*:216, 1974. *(A succinct review of scrotal lesions organized around the anatomy.)*

Gott, L.J.: Common scrotal pathology. Am. Fam. Physician, *15*:165, 1977. *(A good discussion of the diagnosis and management of common scrotal lesions.)*

Rous, S.N.: Intrascrotal problems. In Urology in Primary Care. St. Louis: C.V. Mosby, 1976, p. 131. *(A discussion of scrotal lesions, focusing on the need to explore suspected torsion within a few hours.)*

128

Medical Evaluation of Male Sexual Dysfunction
ERIC J. SACKNOFF, M.D.

Approximately 10 per cent of medical outpatients are experiencing sexual dysfunction at any one time. In recent years, the primary physician has taken a more active role in evaluation and management of sexual problems as a result of advances in understanding of sexual pathophysiology and increases in the number of patients openly complaining of sexual difficulties. One is frequently called upon to distinguish organic from psychogenic etiologies and to initiate corrective measures. The workup of any sexual problem requires thorough investigation from both physical and psychological perspectives (see Chapter 217).

NORMAL AND PATHOLOGIC PHYSIOLOGY AND CLINICAL PRESENTATIONS

Normal responses to erotic stimuli may be organized into three categories: (1) a general response mediated by the autonomic nervous system resulting in increases in pulse rate and blood pressure and a diminution of auditory and visual senses; (2) an erectile response; and (3) ejaculation.

The erectile response may occur from one of two erectile centers in the body: the psychic (or cortical) erectile center and the reflex (or spinal) erectile center. Visual, auditory or olfactory sensations will produce erection by stimulating the psychic erectile center located in the cerebral cortex. Tactile stimulation of the penis produces afferent impulses carried by the internal pudendal nerve, which synapses in the reflex erectile center (sacral cord segments, 2, 3 and 4), and from there efferent impulses pass over the pelvic nerves (nervi erigentes) to the parasympathetic plexuses. These impulses produce dilation of the arterioles of the corpora and closure of the arteriovenous shunts, leading to development of an erection. The shunts permit arterial bypass of the corpora in the flaccid state.

Continued stimulation of the glans results in a summation of stimuli, triggering ejaculation. First there is elevation and closure of the internal vesical sphincter, followed by expulsion of secretions from the prostate, vas deferens and seminal vesicles. The presence of ejaculatory fluid in the posterior urethra promotes still another reflex via the pudendal nerve, which causes rhythmic contraction of the striated perineal musculature and expulsion of the semen through the urethra.

Orgasm consists of all the coordinated sensations resulting from the sequence of events described above. The ejaculatory response appears to be a function of the sympathetic nervous system and is entirely separate from the mechanism of erection, which is dependent on the parasympathetic nervous system. Erection may occur in the quadriplegic with a cervical fracture or dislocation of the spinal cord, because the reflex center below the lesion is still intact, though the psychic center above has been isolated. This explains why neurologic lesions of the lower spinal cord involving the reflex erectile center, especially those of the sacral cord, can result in organic impotence.

It is not clinically useful to label all problems related to male sexual function as "impotence." Rather, each dysfunction should be classified according to the specific impairment of sexual physiology involved. Male sexual dysfunctions can be divided into disorders of erection and ejaculation. *Impotence* denotes the inability to obtain or maintain an erection. *Premature, retarded* or *retrograde ejaculation* describes difficulties with the orgasmic phase of sexual activity. When there is a prior history of normal sexual functioning, the disorder is termed "secondary"; if satisfactory erection and ejaculation have never been achieved, it is labeled "primary."

It is important to recognize that most normal men have occasional episodes of erectile failure, especially at times of stress, fatigue or distraction. Only when the rate of failure to achieve successful coital connection approaches 25 per cent of opportunities is it proper to invoke the clinical diagnosis of impotence.

Lesions in any part of the sexual apparatus, its blood supply or innervation may produce a problem in sexual function. Among the most tragic of lesions are traumatic *spinal cord injuries* resulting in paraplegia. Fortunately, capacities for erection and even ejaculation are often preserved; however, erections are totally abolished when there is complete local destruction of spinal segments S_2 to S_4 or their roots. Some degree of reflex erection can usually occur in all other cord injuries above this level. The higher the location of the lesion, the better the chances of a good erection. About 60 per cent of paraplegics regain penile erections 1 to 24 months after injury. The percentage of erections is higher if the injury is above T_{11}, lower if below. Ejaculation is rare when the lower thoracic and upper lumbar segments (approximately to L_3) of the cord are so extensively damaged that the nearby sympathetic components are destroyed. Sexual sensation is abolished with transection anywhere above the sacral level. Following tactile stimulation, a paraplegic must look to confirm that reflex erection has occurred. Ejaculation can only be documented by feeling wetness with the fingers. Orgasm must be identified by feeling for perineal muscle contractions. Herniated intervertebral discs and metastatic cancer of the vertebral column, especially between T_{10} and L_5, which cause local swelling and destruction of spinal cord tissue, may produce a similar clinical picture.

A second group of common lesions involves the autonomic fibers of peripheral nerves, with diabetes and surgical procedures most often responsible. One out of four young men with *diabetes* is believed to develop impotence, and another 10 per cent have some impairment in potency. The forerunner of erectile impotence in the diabetic is most often retrograde ejaculation. The presence of dry orgasm or milky postcoital urine augurs that potency may be extinguished within a year. There are substantial indications that diabetic impotence is due to peripheral neuropathy affecting the parasympathetic pelvic plexuses, nervi erigentes, etc. Few observers implicate premature arteriosclerosis or secondary hypogonadism (see Chapter 98).

Surgical procedures often leave the patient with sexual dysfunction following transection of autonomic fibers. In simple prostatectomy, whether transurethral, suprapubic or retropubic, erectile impotence is only occasional and is a function of age, prior potency, extent of surgical dissection and psychological expectations. However, over 80 per cent of patients undergoing simple prostatectomy, regardless of the type of procedure performed, will develop some degree of retrograde ejaculation due to surgical destruction of the internal sphincter mechanism at the bladder neck. The surgically destroyed or the neurologically incompetent internal sphincter allows retrograde flow of seminal fluid into the bladder, producing a dry emission. Normal ejaculation will not occur under these circumstances, because the external sphincter tightens to retain urine. Simple perineal prostatectomy has a much higher incidence of impotence due to unavoidable direct dissection of parasympathetic fibers along the posterior capsule. Open perineal biopsy and posterior urethral reconstruction can result in impotence; transperineal or transrectal needle biopsy of the prostate does not. Radical prostate, bladder or colorectal surgery can produce impotence due to surgical damage to the pelvic autonomic nerves, notably the nervi erigentes as they course through the perirectal, retroperitoneal tissues. Following radical retroperitoneal lymph node dissection for testicular tumors, young men may develop ejaculatory failure due to bilateral resection of the para-aortic sympathetic ganglia, but rarely erectile impotence. Bilateral sympathectomy of lumbar ganglia at L_1 will inhibit ejaculatory capacity, but not orgasmic sensation, in over half of cases.

Prostatic disease plays a variable role as a source of sexual difficulty. Prostatitis may cause painful ejaculations and even hematospermia. Premature ejaculation and postcoital fatigue occur, but impotence is not characteristic. Benign prostatic hypertrophy does not interfere with sexual functioning. Impotence may be the first sign bringing the patient with cancer of the prostate to the physician. Advancing centrifugal growth of neoplastic tissue in the posterior lobe of the prostate may induce local swelling and destruction of the parasympathetic fibers that run along the posterolateral aspect of the prostate. Compulsive vesiculoprostatitis represents a chronic congestive syndrome of gradual onset which may appear to result in progressive weakening of the quality of erection, although complete erectile impotence is not a primary part of the syndrome. The condition often occurs with habitual self-inhibited masturbation in an adult, lifelong limitation of sexual activities to heavy petting, chronic coitus interruptus with a sexually inert partner, or habitually hastened acts fraught with anxiety related to threatened interruptions. Other symptoms of this psychosomatic syndrome may include sacroiliac ache, irritating sensations in the glans penis, urinary urgency and frequency, minor weakness of the urinary stream, overflow prostatorrhea (especially after straining), and sometimes hematospermia.

Very obvious performance problems ensue from *penile* or *urethral damage.* Pelvic fractures, resulting from crush injuries in which the posterior urethra is ruptured, cause impotence in 25 to 30 per cent of cases. Nonperformance may result from painful intromission associated with Peyronie's disease, balanitis, acute gonorrhea, herpes genitalis, or phimosis. Hypospadias with a downward chordee of the shaft can preclude intercourse. With *priapism,* erection may be only partial and insufficient for intercourse because irreversible fibrosis of the corpus cavernosum has occurred. A large hernia or hydrocele may mechanically interfere with coitus, although potency should be intact.

Many *drugs* can interfere with sexual function by affecting autonomic transmission or libido. Drug effects are often unpredictable and may vary from patient to patient and with dosage and duration; they are usually reversible by reducing or discontinuing the medication. Antihypertensives are frequently to blame (see Chapter 21). Ganglionic blocking agents may inhibit parasympathetic activity from the sacral segments of the cord or sympathetic activity from the sympathetic chain. Parasympathetic inhibitors produce impotence, while sympathetic inhibitors result in faulty ejaculation. Psychotropic agents may also be responsible for unpredictable forms of sexual dysfunction. The phenothiazines suppress central sympathetic activity; they are capable of producing such side effects as decreased libido, impaired ejaculation, erectile impotence and retrograde ejaculation. The anticholinergic effects of tricyclic antidepressants may interfere with erection. Large doses of alcohol can acutely depress the sexual reflexes to the point of abolishing them. The chronic alcoholic is usually impotent because of either the direct toxic effect of the alcohol or the high blood level of circulating estrogens seen in alcoholic liver disease. Exogenous estrogen therapy may have a similar effect of diminishing the libido.

Drug abuse involving barbiturates, heroin, morphine or methadone can result in major disturbances of sexual potency; most are reversible. Marijuana, amyl nitrite, hashish and lysergic acid diethylamide may heighten the perception of the sexual experience, but do not specifically increase or decrease potency. Amphetamines, in moderate users, may increase libido and delay orgasm, thus prolonging the sexual act; however, impotence often occurs with chronic, heavy use. Cocaine increases sexual excitability in males and females, but side reactions including a flight of ideas may interfere with sustained sexual performance. Episodes of painful priapism may develop in chronic users.

Impaired potency and reduced libido are often features of *endocrinopathies*. Addison's disease tends to lead to loss of libido and to impotence. Cushing's syndrome, except when due to adrenal carcinoma, impairs libido and potency after an intitial period (weeks or months) of marked increase. Untreated hypothyroidism may diminish libido; in severe cases, a degree of impotence exists. Acromegaly leads to early potency impairment and premature extinction of function; decline in function is frequently preceded by a hyperlibidinal period. Hypogonadism, whether due to chromosomal, pituitary or testicular disorders, involves nondevelopment or regression of the secondary male sex characteristics along with feeble libido and waning potency.

Vascular insufficiency is becoming a more widely recognized source of impotence in older men. Unexplained, progressive weakening of erection can be the first symptom of aortoiliac vascular disease (see Chapter 17). Impairment of blood flow due to atheromatous narrowing occurs at or near the bifurcation of the abdominal aorta and the iliac arteries immediately distal. Almost 40 per cent of men with stenosis and nearly 75 per cent those with occlusion develop impotence. Some of the younger men can initiate erection, but are unable to maintain it. Symptoms of claudication in association with impotence, aortic or femoral bruits, and diminished peripheral pulses describe the Leriche syndrome.

Table 128–1.   Organic Causes of Sexual Dysfunction*

CAUSE	PERCENTAGE OF PATIENTS (N=77)
Diabetes mellitus	41.5
Vascular insufficiency	16.8
Peyronie's disease	15.5
Hypogonadism	12.9
Postsurgical impotence	10.3
Neurologic disease	9.0
Trauma	7.7
Medications	3.8
Priapism	2.5
Excessive alcohol abuse	1.2

* Montague, *et al.*: Urology, *14*(6):545, 1979.

lowed a variety of surgical procedures. Sexual dysfunction secondary to various neurologic diseases occurred in 9 per cent.

The high percentage of organic causes of sexual dysfunction in this series most probably reflects the selection bias for patients with organic disorders at a tertiary referral center composed of urologists, vascular surgeons and psychiatrists. In a typical primary care practice, however, functional causes of sexual dysfunction account for 75 to 90 per cent of the cases.

However, the widespread use of drugs affecting the autonomic nervous system makes pharmacologic agents an epidemiologically important source of impotence and ejaculatory disturbances. Table 128–2 provides a listing of some of the more important etiologies of secondary impotence and ejaculatory disturbances.

DIFFERENTIAL DIAGNOSIS

In the vast majority of patients with a prior history of normal function, impotence has an emotional basis (see Chapter 217).

In a recent review of 165 men with sexual dysfunction seen at the Cleveland Clinic, 51 per cent were found to have functional disorders, 47 per cent had organic disorders, and 2 per cent had incomplete evaluations (see Table 128–1). Peak incidence of sexual dysfunction occurred between the ages of 50 and 59. Of those suffering from organic sexual dysfunction, diabetes mellitus accounted for 41.5 per cent. In 16.8 per cent, sexual dysfunction was due to vascular insufficiency. Those with Peyronie's disease (15.5%) could not penetrate due to marked chordee or inability to achieve sufficient erection. In 12.9 per cent, hypogonadism, due to low levels of serum testosterone, was a factor. In 10.3 per cent, impotence fol-

WORKUP

History can be instrumental in evaluating sexual dysfunction, particularly in separating psychogenic from organic causes. Since an intact nervous system, blood supply and sexual apparatus are necessary to achieve an erection, any occurrence of erection and ejaculation even if rare, strongly suggests that the problem is emotional rather than organic. The absence of an erection does not rule out a psychogenic cause, but often one is able to elicit from patients with a psychogenic etiology a story of an occasional erection (particularly on awakening from sleep). Even if an emotional etiology is suspected, every patient needs to be questioned thoroughly in a search for evidence of an underlying medical problem contributing to or causing the sexual dysfunction. Of primary importance are a history or symptoms of di-

Table 128-2. Important Organic Causes of Secondary Sexual Dysfunction

CAUSE	EFFECT		
	Decreased Libido	Impotence	Ejaculatory Failure
Drugs			
Alcohol	+	+	+
Amphetamines		+	
Antidepressants		+	
Barbiturates		+	
Clonidine		+	
Cocaine		Priapism with chronic abuse	
Guanethidine	+		+ (Retrograde)
Methadone		+	
Phenothiazines	+	+	+
Cord Lesions			
Well above T$_{11}$	Sensation abolished		+/−
Below T$_{11}$	Sensation abolished	+	+
Peripheral Autonomic Neuropathy			
Diabetes		+	+ (Retrograde)
Surgical Procedures			
Simple prostatectomy (all approaches)		Occasional	+ (Retrograde)
Perineal prostatectomy		+	
Open perineal biopsy		+	
Radical prostatectomy, bladder or rectal surgery		+	
Radical retroperitoneal node dissection			+
Bilateral sympathectomy			+
Prostatic Disease			
Benign prostatic hypertrophy		No effect on function	
Cancer of the prostate		+	
Vesiculoprostatitis		+/−	
Prostatitis			Painful
Penile and Urethral Lesions			
Pelvic fractures		+	+
Hypospadias			+
Priapism			+
Phimosis, herpes, balanitis		Painful intromission	
Peyronie's disease		Painful intromission	
Hernia or hydrocele		Interferes with coitus	
Endocrine Diseases			
Addison's disease	+	+	
Cushing's syndrome	+	+	
Hypothyrodism	+	+/−	
Acromegaly		+	
Hypogonadism	+	+	
Vascular Disease			
Aortoiliac insufficiency		+	

abetes, antihypertensive or tranquilizer use, prostate surgery, alcohol abuse, claudication, urethral discharge and concurrent neurologic deficits. Detailed description of the specific difficulty with sexual performance is needed to determine whether erection, ejaculation or both are affected.

Physical examination can provide helpful clues to etiology. For example, postural fall in blood pressure may be a sign of autonomic insufficiency, and characteristic skin changes may alert one to the pres-ence of thyroid disease, Addison's disease or Cushing's syndrome. The flaccid penis ought to be inspected for tumor, inflammation, or phimosis of the foreskin and the hard plaques of Peyronie's disease along the dorsolateral aspect of the shaft. If possible, assessment of the erect penis should be attempted, especially if disease of the shaft is suspected, so that precise information on degree of chordee or erectile weakness can be obtained. Testicles and prostate are checked for masses, nodules and tenderness. Intrascrotal pathology such as varicocele, hydrocele or inguinal hernia may mechanically interfere with performance and can be readily detected by a careful examination (see Chapter 127).

The aorta and femoral arteries need to be palpated and auscultated for signs of bruits and other occlusive disease when there is a history of claudication (see Chapter 17). Neurologic assessment includes testing for pain sensation in the genital and perianal areas and a check of the bulbocavernosus reflex. This reflex is achieved when the anal sphincter contracts around the examining finger upon squeezing the glans. A positive response indicates that $S_{2,3,4}$ are intact. Other aspects of neurological function also deserve thorough testing, looking for cortical, brain stem, cord or peripheral deficits.

Laboratory studies are rarely cost-effective in themselves, but may confirm a clinical suspicion. Probably the most important is a 2-hour postprandial glucose test to detect diabetes. Since neurogenic bladder dysfunction is associated with diabetic impotence, a cystometrogram and postvoid residual measurement may be of help when diabetes is confirmed. In retrograde ejaculation, examination of a postintercourse urine will find it filled with sperm. Doppler flow study is indicated in suspected aortoiliac disease (see Chapter 17). Nocturnal penile tumescence study is useful for detecting erectile capacity.

permanent loss of function. Impotence secondary to aortoiliac disease is correctable with skilled bypass graft surgery. Most endocrine imbalances can be corrected. Even castration does not necessarily lead to sexual impotence; replacement androgen therapy is often successful in maintaining function. Coitus after routine prostatectomy is usually possible 4 to 6 weeks after surgery. Ability to perform may return following removal of a significant hydrocele or repair of an inguinal hernia. Even cord lesions due to tumor may be sufficiently reduced by irradiation or decompression surgery to help the patient regain some function, at least temporarily.

In patients with learned inhibitions and interpersonal problems, sex counseling and therapy can be extremely helpful. A graduated series of encounters is prescribed, beginning with simple, mutual pleasures and progressing toward intercourse in a non-threatening setting designed to diminish performance anxiety and encourage personal experience. Masters and Johnson report a success rate of 60 per cent in men with primary impotence (no history of successful penetration), and of 75 per cent in men with secondary impotence. Referral to a psychotherapist may be necessary when sexual problems stem from specific interpersonal reactions, such as repressed rage, guilt feelings, unconscious incestuous feelings, or marital issues (see Chapter 217).

SYMPTOMATIC MANAGEMENT AND INDICATIONS FOR REFERRAL

When impotence results from drug use, dose reduction or discontinuation of the medication is the treatment of choice. More complicated approaches are needed when impotence is more permanent, e.g., due to previous surgery or diabetes; in such instances, the patient should be referred to a urologist for evaluation for penile prosthetic surgery. In selected patients with Peyronie's disease, the urologist may be able to perform resection of the hard plaque and replacement with a dermal skin graft from the abdomen, a procedure which has met with considerable success. Relief from the acute discomfort of a boggy, mushy prostate can often be accomplished by repeated prostatic massage. This manual decongestant therapy often provides good temporary results, but a permanent cure is unlikely. In patients with retrograde ejaculation, recovery of live spermatozoa from the bladder may be feasible if the couple wishes to attempt artificial insemination.

Fortunately, a number of organic etiologies are reversible. Most infections can be cleared without

ANNOTATED BIBLIOGRAPHY

Abelson, D.: Diagnostic value of the penile pulse and blood pressure. A Doppler study of impotence in diabetics. J. Urol., *113*:636, 1975. *(This paper provides early research data on penile circulation in diabetics who report sexual impotence.)*

Cass, A.S., and Godec, C.J.: Urethral injury due to external trauma. Urology, *11*(6):607, 1978. *(This short paper provides statistical reference to the degree of impotence following urethral injury due to external major trauma.)*

Frosch, W.A.: Psychogenic causes of impotence. Med. Asp. Hu. Sexual., *12*:57, 1978. *(This article differentiates psychogenic from organic causes of impotence and provides an easy method for obtaining information from the history.)*

Karacan, I.: Advances in the diagnosis of erectile impotence. Med. Asp. Hu. Sexual. *12*(5):85, 1978. *(This excellent article summarizes the use of nocturnal penile tumescence studies.)*

Karafin, L., and Kendall, R.A.: Psychosomatic problems in urology. *In* Urology. Hagerstown, Md:

Harper & Row, 1977, Chapter 29. *(This chapter provides a broad review of the sexual problems seen in a typical urologic practice.)*

Levine, S.B.: Marital sexual dysfunction: Introductory concepts. Ann. Intern. Med., *84*:448, 1976. *(This paper, written by a psychiatrist, clearly outlines the emotional forces contributing to marital sexual dysfunction.)*

Machleder, H.I.: Sexual dysfunction in aorto-iliac occlusive disease. Med. Asp. Hu. Sexual., *17*:125, May, 1978. *(This paper outlines the various vascular diseases and their relationship to sexual dysfunction.)*

Masters, W.H., and Johnson, V.E.: Human Sexual Inadequacy. Boston: Little, Brown, 1970. *(This excellent complete textbook provides a thorough description of cases in all categories of sexual inadequacy. It is less technical than their first book, Human Sexual Response.)*

Montague, D.K., James, R.E. Jr., DeWolfe, V.G., and Martin, L.M.: Diagnostic evaluation, classification, and treatment of men with sexual dysfunction. Urology, *14*(6):545, 1979. *(A review.)*

Oliven, J.F.: Clinical Sexuality: A Manual for the Physician and the Professions, ed. 3. Philadelphia: J. B. Lippincott, 1974. *(This textbook is a superb manual which covers all phases of sexuality. It is well organized and provides a wealth of clinical, psychiatric and therapeutic information.)*

Prout, G.R., Jr.: Succinct description of the pathophysiology of retrograde ejaculation. Med. Asp. Hu. Sexual., *12*(6):131, 1978. *(This brief discussion clearly describes a common condition following simple prostatectomy.)*

Sacknoff, E.J., and Dretler, S.P.: Urologic emergencies. *In* E.W. Wilkins, A. Moncure, and J. Dineen, Textbook of Emergency Medicine. Baltimore: Williams & Wilkins, 1978; Chapter 22.) *(One portion of this chapter describes sexual impotence associated with urethral rupture due to pelvic fracture. Subsequent impotence should be considered when deciding between early or delayed operative repair of posterior urethral rupture.)*

129
Approach to the Woman With Urinary Tract Infection
LESLIE S.-T. FANG, M.D.

Among adult women, urinary tract infection is the most common of all bacterial infections. Between 20 and 30 per cent of women will have a urinary tract infection in their lifetime, and 40 per cent of women with one infection will have a recurrence. Thus, urinary tract infections represent a significant source of morbidity among women. For the primary physician, evaluation should be directed at the detection of any anatomic abnormalities that may predispose the patient to recurrent infections; therapy should be aimed at the eradication of infection to minimize morbidity.

PATHOPHYSIOLOGY AND CLINICAL PRESENTATION

Current evidence suggests that most episodes of urinary tract infection in adult women are secondary to ascending infection. Bacteria reach the bladder through the urethra and may then ascend to the kidneys through the ureters. Hematogenous spread has rarely been implicated in the pathogenesis of urinary tract infections.

Bacteria that commonly cause urinary tract infection are found in the periurethral area in up to 20 per cent of adult women. This colonization of the vaginal introitus has been shown to be the essential first step in the production of bacteriuria and plays an important role in recurrent urinary tract infections. Entry of bacteria into the bladder through the relatively short female urethra can occur spontaneously, but urethral trauma such as that associated with sexual intercourse has also been incriminated. Serial determinations of urine bacterial counts before and after sexual intercourse demonstrated significant increases following 30 per cent of the intercourse episodes. Transient bacteriuria therefore occurs frequently in the sexually active female.

The establishment of a bladder infection depends upon a number of factors: the virulence of the bacteria introduced; the number of organisms introduced;

and most important, a lapse in the normal host defense mechanisms. A number of host defense mechanisms normally act together to decrease the likelihood of infection. Normal voiding eliminates some organisms. Certain chemical properties of the urine are antibacterial; urine with a high urea concentration, low pH and high osmolarity supports bacterial growth poorly. The most important host defense mechanism resides in the ability of the bladder mucosal surface to phagocytose bacteria coming into contact with it. Abnormalities in these host defense mechanisms will result in recurrent and complicated urinary tract infections.

In approximately 30 per cent of cases of sustained bladder infection, further extension of the infection through the ureters into the kidneys can occur. The presence of reflux will increase the chance that infection will ascend. Once infected urine gains access to the renal pelvis, it can enter the renal parenchyma via the ducts of Bellini at the papillary tips, and then spread outward along the collecting ducts, leading to parenchymal infection.

Urinary tract infections are associated with a number of clinical syndromes. *Symptomatic abacteriuria* or *acute urethral syndrome* occurs in about 10 to 15 per cent of patients who present with dysuria, frequency, urgency, and suprapubic or flank pain. They are found to have insignificant bacterial growth on urine cultures, and urinalyses are usually unimpressive, with few white cells and no bacteriuria. The etiologic agent responsible for the syndrome has not been identified, but *Chlamydia*, viruses, L-form bacteria, and gonococci have all been implicated.

Symptomatic bacteriuria in the form of cystitis or pyelonephritis is the most common of the clinical syndromes. Cystitis has traditionally been thought to present primarily as frequency, urgency, dysuria and bacteriuria. Pyelonephritis, on the other hand, is generally believed to be associated with fever, flank pain and systemic symptoms such as nausea and vomiting. Unfortunately, numerous investigations have shown that the ability to differentiate between bladder and kidney infection on clinical grounds alone is quite limited. Studies using bilateral ureteral catheterization to directly localize the site of infection have demonstrated that many patients with upper tract infection present with symptoms supposedly characteristic of lower tract infection. Moreover, patients whose infection is limited to the bladder may occasionally have fever, flank pain and systemic symptoms usually associated with pyelonephritis. Thus the traditional clinical clues are at best imprecise for identifying the site of infection; it is probably more appropriate to regard all patients with symptomatic bacteriuria as a group and rely upon other means to localize the problem to the upper or lower urinary tract.

Recurrent infections are responsible for the group of patients who present with repeated episodes of symptomatic bacteriuria. Two basic patterns of recurrences are recognized: *relapse,* in which the original organism is suppressed by antimicrobial therapy and then reappears when the antibiotic is stopped; and *reinfection,* in which the original organism is eradicated by antimicrobial therapy, and the recurrence is due to the introduction of a new bacterial strain. Approximately 80 per cent of recurrences are due to reinfection. Ureteral catheterization studies have demonstrated that the majority of reinfections occur in patients in whom infection is restricted to the bladder, whereas the majority of relapses occur in patients with renal parenchymal infection.

Groups frequently bothered by recurrent infections include (1) sexually active women, who report a temporal relationship of urinary symptoms to intercourse, (2) patients with compromised host defenses due to underlying systemic illness or residual urine in the bladder, and (3) patients with upper tract infections.

DIFFERENTIAL DIAGNOSIS

The differential diagnosis of symptoms referable to the urinary tract is limited. If dysuria is present, patients with vaginal infections or urethritis may occasionally be mistakenly thought to have urinary tract infection. History of vaginal discharge, or evidence of discharge on pelvic examination, together with a urinalysis, will usually resolve the issue.

Patients with renal calculi or embolic renal infarcts may present with flank pain and hematuria mimicking pyelonephritis. Again, examination of the urine and urine culture will rapidly settle the ambiguity, since in such cases, cultures are sterile and no bacteria are seen on Gram stain.

WORKUP

The pace and the order of the various tests included in the workup of urinary tract infections are largely dictated by the patient's clinical presentation.

In *acutely ill patients* presenting with fever, flank pain and systemic symptoms, the most important consideration is the possibility of an obstructive lesion. Infection behind an obstruction constitutes a medical and urologic emergency requiring prompt therapeutic intervention. Patients should be asked about diabetes, sickle-cell anemia, or history of excessive analgesic abuse, because people with these problems are at higher risk of papillary necrosis and subsequent obstruction by a sloughed papilla. Likewise, history of past renal calculi should be of some concern in an acutely ill patient; such patients should have early urologic evaluations to rule out the possibility of obstruction.

The physical examination needs to include a temperature determination, check for tenderness in the costovertebral angles and suprapubic area, and careful pelvic examination to rule out vaginal and cervical infections.

The laboratory workup begins with a careful urinalysis and Gram stain of the unspun urine. In patients with a convincing history of dysuria, frequency, urgency and suprapubic pain, but with benign urinalysis with few white cells and no bacteria, acute urethral syndrome should be suspected; a negative urine culture supports the diagnosis. In most patients, urinary tract infection is confirmed by the presence of pyuria, hematuria and bacteriuria on Gram stain of the unspun urine. Presence of one organism under high power field examination represents clinically significant bacteriuria (10^5 organisms/cc).

The localization of the site of infection is important to appropriate management. The ability to differentiate between upper and lower tract infection on clinical grounds is limited. The urinalysis is helpful only in the rare instance when white cell casts are present in a patient suspected of having upper tract infection. The only direct method of localization of the site of infection is bilateral ureteral catheterization, a method which is generally considered too invasive for general application.

Numerous indirect methods of localization have been devised, but most are of limited value because they lack sensitivity and specificity. The most promising of the indirect techniques is the demonstration of antibody coating of bacteria in the urine. Immunofluorescence studies have shown that bacteria originating from the kidneys are coated with antibodies, while bacteria associated with lower urinary tract infections are usually antibody-negative. There has been at least 95 per cent correlation with the results obtained by direct methods of localization. Unfortunately, the assay is primarily a research tool at present and is not generally available.

Numerous investigations have suggested that the response to therapy is dependent upon the site of the infection; therefore, some clues to the site can be obtained by following clinical responses. For example, lower tract infections, as defined by the absence of antibody coating of bacteria in the urine, have been found to respond to a single dose of 3.5 gm. of amoxicillin as well as to the conventional 10 to 14 days of therapy. Upper tract infections, on the other hand, have a high relapse rate.

Currently, the clinical response to therapy probably provides the most convenient means of delineating therapeutic guidelines for outpatient management of urinary tract infections. In this schema, patients should have a follow-up culture 2 weeks after the termination of therapy. Patients in whom infection persists despite an appropriate course of antibiotics should be investigated for obstruction, renal parenchymal involvement, and postvoid residual urine.

When one is confronted with a patient with recurrent infections, questions of radiologic and urologic evaluations are invariably raised. Such studies are probably not necessary for every patient with recurrent infections. Recent studies examining the role of intravenous pyelography in patients with recurrent infections have demonstrated that urography is a rather low-yield procedure in terms of influencing subsequent therapeutic modalities. Radiographic and urologic evaluations should therefore be reserved for patients in whom anatomic abnormalities are suspected. Currently, patients who fail to respond to appropriate antimicrobial therapy and those with relapsing infections should undergo intravenous pyelography. If evidence of reflux is suggested by intravenous pyelography, a voiding cystourethrogram should be done to document the degree of reflux. Urologic evaluation is indicated when urethral meatal stenosis is strongly suspected.

PRINCIPLES OF THERAPY

Therapy should be dictated in part by the clinical presentation. Acutely ill patients presenting with fever, chills, flank pain, nausea and vomiting should be hospitalized and started on parenteral antibiotics. In patients with gram-negative rods on urine Gram stain, an antibiotic with adequate coverage of Enterobacteriaceae (such as ampicillin) should be used initially until the sensitivity of the causative organism is ascertained. In patients with suspected gram-negative bacteremia from a genitourinary source, aminoglycosides may be more appropriate. Gram-positive cocci seen on urine Gram stain often prove to be enterococci, which are also sensitive to ampicillin. Failure to respond to antibiotics to which the presenting organisms are sensitive should raise the possibility of anatomic abnormalities, and the patient should undergo a radiologic evaluation.

Patients presenting with mild to moderate symptoms can usually be managed as outpatients. If acute urethral syndrome is documented, symptomatic therapy with fluids and urinary analgesics such as phenazopyridine (pyridium) is usually adequate. Some clinicians recommend a short course of tetracycline to both sexual partners, especially if significant pyuria is present and symptoms last longer than 4 days. Recurrences of symptoms are common in patients with acute urethral syndrome.

Patients with mild to moderate symptoms and gram-negative rods on urine Gram stain should be started on either a sulfonamide or a penicillin derivative, which will cover over 90 per cent of Enterobacteriaceae found in the community. Many clinicians believe that the therapy of infection ought to be tailored to the site of infection. Lower tract infections respond to a short course of antibiotics, including single oral dose regimens, as well as to 10- to 14-day courses. Upper tract infections, on the other hand, are characterized by frequent relapses and should be treated for longer periods (4 weeks) with the appropriate antibiotic. Since clinical clues often cannot accurately distinguish between upper and lower tract infections, follow-up urinalyses and cultures are essential to judge the efficacy of therapy.

In patients with recurrent infections, the clinical setting is again of importance in selecting the appropriate form of therapy. In sexually active women with recurrent reinfection, single nocturnal doses of ampicillin, nitrofurantoin and trimethoprim-sulfamethoxazole have been found to be effective in minimizing the frequency and severity of the infection. In older patients with bladder distention, postvoid residual urine, and recurrent reinfection, prophylactic therapy with trimethoprim-sulfamethoxazole has been beneficial. In patients with defined anatomic abnormalities such as significant reflux or nephrolithiasis, surgical correction, when appropriate, should be undertaken to decrease the severity of recurrent infections.

INDICATIONS FOR REFERRAL OR ADMISSION

Hospitalization is indicated in patients with severe symptoms such as rigors, high fever, flank pain, nausea and vomiting. Patients with suspected obstruction and those unable to maintain oral intake also require hospitalization. Referral to a urologist is indicated if a surgically correctable anatomic abnormality is detected or suspected.

PATIENT EDUCATION

Certain general measures are important in minimizing the possibility of recurrent infection. The patients should be instructed about increasing fluid intake during symptomatic periods and maintaining urine flow around the clock. Patients with urinary tract infections temporally related to sexual intercourse would probably benefit from voiding after intercourse. They should also be convinced of the importance of the follow-up visits for repeat urinalysis and culture.

ANNOTATED BIBLIOGRAPHY

Fang, L.S.T., Rubin, N.E., and Rubin, R.H.: Localization and antibiotic management of urinary tract infection. Ann. Rev. Med., *30*:225, 1979. *(Discussion of the importance of localization of site of infection in the management of patients with urinary tract infections.)*

Jones, S.M., Smith, J.W., and Sanford, J.P.: Localization of urinary tract infections by detection of antibody-coated bacteria in urine sediment. N. Engl. J. Med., *290*:591, 1974. *(Indicating the high degree of sensitivity and specificity of the technique.)*

Sanford, J.P.: Urinary tract symptoms and infections. Ann. Rev. Med., *26*: 485, 1976. *(Excellent review of clinical syndromes and therapeutic approach.)*

Stamey, T.A., Grovan, D.E., and Palmer, J.M.: The localization and treatment of urinary tract infections: The role of bactericidal urine levels as opposed to serum levels. Medicine, *44*:1, 1965. *(Early delineation of importance of localization.)*

Stamm, W.E., *et al.*: Causes of the acute urethral syndrome in women. N. Engl. J. Med., *303*:409, 1980. *(Those women with pyuria usually had an organism recovered from the bladder, though the colony count was less than 10^5 per ml.; few women without pyuria had infection.)*

Turck, M.: Localization of the site of recurrent urinary tract infectons in women. Urol. Clin. North A., *2*:433, 1975. *(Differentiation of relapses and reinfection and the importance of using clinical responses to help in localization of site of infection.)*

130
Approach to the Patient with Nephrolithiasis
LESLIE S.-T. FANG, M.D.

Nephrolithiasis is a significant medical problem incurring substantial morbidity and cost. One autopsy series estimated the prevalence as 1.12 per cent. In most industrialized countries, 1 to 3 per cent of the population may be expected to have a calculus at some time. The annual frequency of hospitalization for nephrolithiasis is estimated at 1 per 1000 population. In the outpatient setting, the primary physician may encounter patients with a history of renal calculi, asymptomatic nephrolithiasis, or acute colic. One needs to identify the nature of the stone and any precipitating factors, prevent further stone formation, and know when referral for surgical intervention is needed.

PATHOPHYSIOLOGY AND CLINICAL PRESENTATION

Two major groups of factors are important in the pathogenesis of stones: (1) changes which increase the urinary concentration of stone constituents and (2) physiochemical changes.

Increase in concentration can occur with reductions in urinary volume or increases in excretion of calcium, oxalate, uric acid, cystine or xanthine.

CALCIUM-CONTAINING STONES. The majority of calcium-containing stones contain calcium oxalate; hypercalciuric and hyperoxaluric states promote their formation.

Hypercalciuric states can be categorized into three groups: increased absorption of dietary calcium, increased resorption of calcium from bone, and presence of a renal calcium leak. Combinations of these factors can be at play in certain clinical settings. *Hyperoxaluria* is less common than is hypercalciuria. It may result from increased absorption of dietary oxalate, as occurs in small bowel disease, from increased endogenous production of oxalate due to a genetic deficiency in enzymes in the glyoxalate pathway or a deficiency of pyridoxine, an important cofactor in glyoxalate metabolism, or rarely, from

markedly increased ingestion of oxalate or one of its precursors.

MAGNESIUM AMMONIUM PHOSPHATE STONES (STRUVITE). Struvite formation occurs in an alkaline environment and is almost invariably associated with urinary tract infection due to a urea-splitting organism.

URIC ACID STONES. Hyperuricosuric states are seen in patients with primary and secondary gout. Occasionally, persistently acid urine promotes uric acid stone formation even in the absence of increased urinary uric acid concentration. In myeloproliferative disorders and during chemotherapy, significant hyperuricosuria can occur, and uric acid stone can form if adequate urine flow and alkalinization are not maintained.

CYSTINE STONES. Cystine stones are found exclusively in patients with cystinuria who have an inherited disorder in which renal and gastrointestinal transport of cystine, ornithine, lysine and arginine is abnormal.

XANTHINE STONES. These occur in xanthinuria, an extremely rare genetic disorder of purine metabolism associated with a deficiency of xanthine oxidase. Rarely, xanthine stones may be seen in patients taking xanthine oxidase inhibitors for treatment of uric acid disorders.

Physicochemical factors that have been identified as important in stone formation include changes in urinary pH and urinary concentrations of magnesium, citrate, organic matrix and pyrophosphate. Alkaline pH favors struvite formation, and acidic pH facilitates formation of uric acid and xanthine stones.

High urinary concentrations of magnesium, citrate, pyrophosphate and certain anions are potent inhibitors of stone formation. Deficiencies in one or more of these inhibitors have been identified in some patients with recurrent stones.

Three major theories have been advanced to explain stone formation and growth. The matrix-nucleation theory suggests that some matrix substances form an initial nucleus for subsequent stone growth by precipitation. The precipitation-crystallization theory suggests that when the urinary crystalloids are present in a supersaturated state, precipitation and subsequent growth occur. The inhibitor-absence theory postulates that the deficiency of one or more of numerous agents known to retard stone formation leads to nephrolithiasis. Evidence for and against each of these theories has been collected; multiple factors may be involved in any given patient.

Clinical presentation is usually renal colic of varying severity presenting as unilateral flank pain, back and loin pain with radiation into the groin and testicle. The presenation may be mistaken for pyelonephritis and occasionally abdominal and pelvic processes, but the initial workup should rapidly lead to the correct diagnosis.

Occasionally, asymptomatic calcareous calculi are detected on abdominal x-rays taken for other reasons.

In the United States, about two thirds of all renal calculi are composed of either calcium oxalate or calcium oxalate mixed with calcium phosphate (Table 130–1). Struvite or magnesium ammonium phosphate stones occur almost exclusively in patients with urinary tract infections due to urea-splitters, and contitute about 15 per cent of stones analyzed. Stones of pure uric acid account for another 8 per cent. Other stones occur infrequently and are composed of cystine, xanthine and salicates.

Natural history of stone formation is still not clearly delineated. The likelihood of recurrence of calcium stones with time was examined propectively in one study of patients who formed single stones. An exceedingly high incidence of recurrence was found, with a mean time to recurrence of 6.78 years. With time, cumulative recurrence approached 100 percent. Recurrence seemed to take place early in half of the patients, but could take up to 20 years. On the other hand, other studies have found a more benign course.

In one, a group of 101 patients was followed for an extended period (mean 7 years); additional stone formation was observed in only a third. These differences undoubtedly reflect heterogeneity among patients in the respective referral groups. In any case, the incidence of recurrence is high enough to justify evaluation and consideration of preventive treatment.

DIFFERENTIAL DIAGNOSIS

The disease states associated with nephrolithiasis are best categorized according to the type of stones formed. In many instances, stone formation is a manifestation of a systemic disease (see Table 130–2).

WORKUP

In the evaluation of the patient with recurrent nephrolithiasis, knowledge of the stone composition is essential to rational management. Obtaining the stone for analysis is the single most important study; therefore, urine should be strained for stones when renal colic is present. Ideally, studies of the stone should include the use of quantitative chemical analyses in addition to crystallographic examination.

History. When there is no stone available for analysis, certain aspects of the clinical history can be helpful in the evaluation. The age of the patient at onset of nephrolithiasis should be obtained because metabolic disorders such as hyperoxaluria, cystinuria, xanthinuria and renal tubular acidosis are often associated with stones at an early age; idiopathic calcareous nephrolithiasis and primary hyperparathyroidism commonly occur after age 30. The sex of the patient can also be helpful, because idiopathic nephrolithiasis is more common in males, whereas primary hyperparathyroidism is more common in fe-

Table 130–1.   Types of Renal Calculi*

CRYSTAL NAME	CHEMICAL NAME	FREQUENCY (%)
Whewellite	Calcium oxalate monohydrate ⎫	
Weddelite	Calcium oxalate dihydrate ⎬	33
Apatite, pure	Calcium phosphate ⎭	4
Mixed	Calcium oxalate and phosphate	34
Brushite	Calcium phosphate	2
Struvite	Magnesium ammonium phosphate	15
Uric acid	Uric acid	8
Cystine	Cystine	3

* Prien, E. L.: Urol. Clin. North Am., *1*:229, 1974.

Table 130–2.   Important Conditions Associated with Nephrolithiasis

I. Calcium stones
  A. Increased gastrointestinal calcium absorption
    1. Primary hyperparathyroidism
    2. Sarcoidosis
    3. Vitamin D excess
    4. Milk-alkali syndrome
    5. Idiopathic nephrolithiasis
  B. Increased bone calcium resorption
    1. Primary hyperparathyroidism
    2. Neoplastic disorders
    3. Immobilization
    4. Distal renal tubular acidosis
  C. Renal calcium leak
    1. Idiopathic hypercalciuria
  D. Hyperoxaluria
    1. Small bowel disease
    2. Enzymatic deficiency
    3. Pyridoxine deficiency
    4. Increased ingestion
II. Magnesium ammonium phosphate stones
  A. Alkaline environment
    1. Urinary tract infection due to urea-splitting organism
III. Uric acid stones
  A. Increased uric acid production
    1. Primary gout
    2. Secondary gout (myeloproliferative disorder, chemotherapy)
IV. Cystine stones
  A. Inherited disorder of amino acid transport
V. Xanthine stones
  A. Xanthine oxidase deficiency
  B. Use of xanthine oxidase inhibitor

males. A past history of stones is invaluable if their composition has been previously determined. Any prior history of systemic illnesses (such as sarcoidosis or cancer) and any prior urinary tract infections should be noted. Family history of nephrolithiasis may suggest a hereditary metabolic disorder. Careful dietary history should also be taken to rule out excessive oxalate or calcium intake. It is important to check for use of drugs that would promote calcium or uric acid excretion.

Physical examination is not particularly revealing in most cases, but should be checked for evidence of a systemic disease, such as sarcoidosis (lymphadenopathy, organomegaly) or breast cancer.

Laboratory evaluation should include a urinalysis for determination of pH and an examination of urinary sediment for crystals. An alkaline pH suggests infection with urea-splitting organisms and struvite formation. Inability to acidify the urine pH below 5.3 despite systemic acidosis suggests renal tubular acidosis. Serum ought to be obtained for determinations of calcium, uric acid, BUN, and creatinine and a 24-hour urine collected for creatinine, calcium, uric acid and oxalate.

Repeated determinations of fasting serum calcium and phosphorus are necessary if primary hyperparathyroidism is suspected. Serum albumin should also be determined, since 40 to 45 per cent of the serum calcium is protein-bound. If the serum calcium is elevated and hyperparathyroidism is suspected clinically, confirmation of the diagnosis can be made by obtaining a simultaneous PTH determination, which should reveal an inappropriately elevated level (see Chapter 94). If the clinical presentation suggests a rare cause of nephrolithiasis, such as cystinuria or xanthinuria, special 24-hour collections of urine should be sent for study.

Roentgenographic evaluation includes a KUB and an intravenous pyelogram. The flat plate radiograph of the abdomen can provide an estimate of renal size and is important in detecting the presence of small radiopaque stones. Staghorn calculi usually denote magnesium ammonium phosphate or cystine stones. The latter usually have a more laminated appearance. Intravenous pyelogram provides better details of any renal abnormalities that may be present, as well as the level of the obstruction caused by the renal calculus.

The laboratory evaluation permits identification of stones and hyperexcretory states and therefore allows rational therapy.

PRINCIPLES OF MANAGEMENT

Because of the high incidence of stone formation and its attendant morbidity, preventive therapy is indicated in all patients with nephrolithiasis.

In general, maintenance of dilute urine by means of vigorous fluid therapy around the clock is beneficial in all forms of nephrolithiasis. Specific therapy should be tailored to the type of stones involved.

Calcium-containing stones. Primary hyperparathyroidism should be corrected surgically when feasible (see Chap. 94). Vitamin D excess and milk-alkali syndrome are readily correctable by cessation of intake. Steroids have been found to be effective in patients with sarcoidosis (see Chap. 48).

Patients with *hypercalciuria* require limitation of dietary calcium, including careful avoidance of dairy products. Thiazides decrease urinary calcium excretion; and hydrochlorothiazide, 50 mg. given twice a day, has been found to be effective. Primary hyperparathyroidism has to be ruled out prior to the use of thiazides in order to avoid hypercalcemia. Phosphates (in the form of neutral phosphate or cellulose phosphate) have been used to decrease absorption of calcium and have been found to be effective in decreasing stone formation. Diarrhea and extraskeletal calcifications are the major side effects of phosphate therapy.

Patients with *Hyperoxaluria* need to have their intake of dietary oxalate limited. Tea, rhubarb, and many green leafy vegetables should be avoided. Dietary calcium, on the other hand, should not be restricted, since calcium has been shown to cause increases in urinary excretion of oxalate. In the rare patient with pyridoxine deficiency, replacement would improve the hyperoxaluric state.

Studies in those patients with *no identifiable metabolic disorder,* have demonstrated drastic reduction in new stone formation when given allopurinol and a thiazide. In one study, *30* such patients formed 6 stones, as compared to a predicted 31.8 stones, during a 1- to 7- year follow-up period. The use of allopurinol is based on the supposition that so-

dium hydrogen urate crystals are reasonable heterogeneous nuclei for calcium oxalate crystal growth.

Magnesium ammonium phosphate stones. These are often very large and may have to be removed surgically. Acidification of the urine with ascorbic acid, along with appropriate antibiotic treatment to eradicate any urinary tract infection, is essential for the prevention of recurrences of struvite.

Uric acid stones. Maintenance of copious urine flow, allopurinol therapy, and alkalinization of the urine are the mainstays of therapy. The solubility of uric acid is a hundred times higher at pH 7 than at pH 4.5, and every attempt should be made to maintain an alkaline urine by giving 100 to 150 mEq of bicarbonate per 24 hours in divided doses. In patients with myeloproliferative disorders undergoing chemotherapy, prophylactic uses of allopurinol, saline diuresis and alkalinization should eliminate the incidence of uric acid stone formation.

Cystine stones. Copius urine flow and maintenance of urinary pH above 7.5 are important in preventing and dissolving cystine stones. D-penicillamine has also been shown to be effective, but significant side effects may be encountered.

Xanthine stones. Limitation of dietary purines, maintenance of urine flow, and maintenance of very high urine pH (greater than 7.6) minimize difficulties. Prophylactic alkalinization and forced diuresis should be employed in patients with myeloproliferative disorders on xanthine oxidase inhibitors.

In addition to the therapeutic interventions outlined, several other less well-evaluated modes of therapy have been advocated. Administration of magnesium oxide may improve the solubility of urinary oxalate. It has been suggested that methylene blue is an effective inhibitor of calcium oxalate stone formation.

INDICATIONS FOR ADMISSION

In a patient with renal colic, the needs for hospitalization and other intervention are dictated by the clinical presentation. Patients with mild symptoms can be managed as outpatients with oral analgesics, and instructed to maintain a high fluid intake and urine output around-the-clock. These patients should be told to strain the urine in order to retrieve calculi for stone analysis.

Patients with severe pain, nausea, and vomiting need hospitalization for intravenous hydration and pain control. In these patients, KUB and intravenous pyelogram are indicated to localize and determine the extent of the obstruction. In the majority of cases, stones will pass spontaneously. Patients with severe symptoms and persistent obstruction beyond 3 to 4 days should be referred for urologic evaluation.

Patients presenting with fever, chills, and symptoms of renal colic require hospitalization and prompt intervention. If the presence of an infection behind an obstructed ureter is indeed confirmed, antibiotic coverage and surgical decompression are mandatory.

PATIENT EDUCATION

Meticulous care must be taken in giving dietary instructions. Lists of foods high in calcium or oxalate should be provided to help guide the patient's choices. Instructions should also be given to help patients divide their fluid intake evenly to maintain a dilute urine at all times. Patients who need to alkalinize their urine ought to be instructed in how to measure urinary pH with litmus test tapes. Long periods of immobilization should be avoided, and appropriate fluid intake should be prescribed if such situations are anticipated.

ANNOTATED BIBLIOGRAPHY

Coe, F.L.: Treated and untreated recurrent calcium nephrolithiasis in patients with idiopathic hypercalciuria, hyperuricosuria or no metabolic disorder. Ann. Intern. Med., *87*:404, 1977. *(Study demonstrating efficacy of thiazide and allopurinol in patients with recurrent nephrolithiasis.)*

Coe, F.L., Keck, J., and Norton, E.R.: The natural history of calcium urolithiasis. JAMA, *238*:1519, 1973. *(Retrospective study indicating that calcium urolithiasis is a recurrent disease incurring significant morbidity.)*

Smith, L.H.: Medical evaluation of urolithiasis: Etiologic aspects and diagnostic evaluation. Urol. Clin. North Am. *1*(2):241, 1974. *(Discussion of the importance of adequate medical history, laboratory data and stone analysis in the evaluation of stone disease.)*

Thomas, W.C., Jr.: Medical aspects of renal calculous disease. Treatment and prophylaxis. Urol. Clin. North Am. *1*(2):261, 1974. *(Discussion of therapeutic programs directed to alter urine in such a way that it becomes undersaturated with respect to the offending crystalloid.)*

Williams, H.E.: Nephrolithiasis. N. Engl. J. Med., *290*:33, 1974. *(Excellent review of pathogenesis and treatment of renal calculi.)*

131
Management of Benign Prostatic Hypertrophy
JOHN D. GOODSON, M.D.

Benign prostatic hypertrophy (BPH) is a nearly ubiquitous condition in aging American males and is a frequent cause of urinary tract outflow obstruction. The primary physician must distinguish BPH from the other causes of outflow obstruction (see Chapter 125), determine its severity, and design a therapeutic approach which will provide symptomatic relief, preserve renal function, and prevent infection.

PATHOPHYSIOLOGY

Benign prostatic hypertrophy arises from nodular hyperplasia of prostatic stromal, epithelial and muscular elements. Growth is primarily centered in the periurethral glandular tissue, but frequently the lateral lobes show significant enlargement. The etiology of age-related prostatic hyperplasia is still unknown, though it is reasonably well established that androgenic changes at a cellular level are a major factor. Unfortunately, it is not known which specific hormonal manipulations would be most efficacious in reversing or slowing the process.

Regardless of the lobe(s) involved, BPH is manifest clinically by urinary tract outflow obstruction or infection. As the gland enlarges, urine flow through the urethra diminishes and bladder muscular hypertrophy ensues. Nonetheless, bladder emptying is usually incomplete. The resulting residual urine predisposes to infection. Numerous saccules or bladder herniations form between the thickened overlapping muscular bands that compose the detrusor. These diverticula are incompletely emptied with voiding, further predisposing to infection. Ureteral dilatation is common in advanced cases of chronic retention due to increased bladder pressure. Hydronephrosis and renal deterioration may follow shortly thereafter.

When the detrusor is no longer able to generate sufficient pressure to overcome urethral obstruction, bladder failure occurs, and urinary retention develops. If there is a large fluid load or the contractile function of the bladder is otherwise impaired by anticholinergic or sympathomimetic drugs, the patient may be unable to void (see Chapter 125).

The hyperthrophied prostate is highly vascularized and predisposed to bleeding; painless hematuria is not uncommon.

The complications of chronic retention caused by BPH include hydronephrosis, loss of renal concentrating ability, diminished hydrogen ion excretion, and renal failure. As noted, residual urine volumes, which predispose to infection and overflow incontinence, also develop.

CLINICAL PRESENTATION AND COURSE

Patients with clinically significant urethral obstruction due to BPH generally present with symptoms of hesitancy, loss of stream force, frequency, nocturia, double voiding and dribbling. It is most common for patients to have a waxing and waning symptomatic course with very gradual deterioration over several years. Sometimes, urinary tract infection is the first indication of outlet obstruction. Hematuria may be an early symptom of BPH, but neoplasm must always be excluded (see Chapter 123).

Unfortunately, the rectal examination of the prostate is of little help in assessing the degree of obstruction due to gland enlargement, though it does provide a reasonable estimate of overall gland volume. Normally, one can readily feel over the top of the gland; this becomes more difficult as the gland enlarges. The inability to palpate the distal margins of the gland generally indicates massive enlargement (over three times normal size).

BPH in the elderly can have protean manifestations. It may cause so-called *silent prostatism,* which can produce a lower abdominal mass due to bladder enlargement; confusion; anorexia; a palpable kidney; anemia; a bleeding diathesis, secondary to hydrone-phrosis and uremia; altered medication requirements, as a consequence of diminished renal clearance; and incontinence, related to overflow.

PRINCIPLES OF MANAGEMENT

Assessment. In cases of urinary outflow obstruction from BPH, the clinician must determine the extent to which the patient is bothered by his symptoms. For some, frequency and nocturia significantly interfere with a restful night of sleep, while for others they are a minor inconvenience. It is generally best to see the patient repeatedly over a 3- to 6-month period in order to get a general sense of how his symptoms are progressing before making any major therapeutic decisions.

A BUN, creatinine, complete blood count and urinalysis should be obtained on all patients in order to assess renal function. Observation of the patient while he is voiding may be helpful. Straight catheterization after voiding is a simple office procedure that can give a direct assessment of bladder emptying; more than 50 to 100 cc. of residual urine is abnormal.

In most patients, an intravenous pyelogram (IVP) should also be obtained to assess upper and lower tract function. With obstructing prostatic enlargement, excretory films frequently demonstrate bladder wall trabeculations and a significant intravesicular prostatic component. The postvoiding film shows a residual urine volume. A voiding cystourethrogram (VCUG) gives a better portrayal of bladder wall diverticula, trabeculations and residual urine volume. A cystometrogram (CMG) should be added to the evaluation in order to screen for a coincident abnormality of bladder function. Flow studies are helpful in the initial management and ongoing monitoring of patients (see Chapter 125).

Treatment. Many patients with symptomatic BPH can be managed conservatively. Repeated *prostatic massage* (3 to 4 times over a 2-week period) and *frequent intercourse* are felt to reduce obstruction. Any prostatic infection should be treated (see Chapter 133).

The patient should be told to void frequently and to avoid beverages that are likely to produce a diuresis (coffee, tea, alcohol), particularly before bed. Diuretics should be taken early in the day, in order to avoid nocturnal bladder distention. Drugs, such as anticholinergics, mild tranquilizers, and antidepressants, that can exacerbate the symptoms of bladder outflow obstruction should be used only with great care.

Surgical therapy is indicated in patients with deterioration of bladder or renal function as evidenced by large postvoid residuals, hydronephrosis on IVP, repeated urinary tract infections, or increasing BUN and creatinine. It is more difficult to assess the subjective inconvenience BPH causes the individual patient. Clearly, there are some men who are greatly troubled by outflow obstruction but who have little demonstrable deterioration in bladder or renal function. The identification of patients in whom surgery would be helpful depends on the careful clinical assessment by the primary physician and an experienced consulting surgeon.

Transurethral resection of the prostate (TURP) is a procedure associated with low morbidity and is useful in patients with small glands or in older, debilitated patients. A *retropubic* or a *suprapubic prostatectomy* may be required if the gland is substantially enlarged. All of these operations have a low mortality rate (less than 5 per cent). Most patients are able to maintain sexual potency regardless of the surgical approach used, though temporary dysfunction may occur (see Chapter 128). Incontinence is unusual, except following radical surgical procedures.

If, for reasons of age or concomitant disease, a patient is considered inoperable, chronic Foley or suprapubic *catheter drainage* may be necessary. Recently, *antiandrogens* have been used with some success to shrink hypertrophied prostatic tissue, but these drugs must still be considered experimental.

It must be remembered that most prostatic operations leave a substantial amount of prostatic tissue in place, and postoperative patients must be subsequently screened for the development of malignancy (see Chapter 121). Furthermore, since residual prostatic tissue will continue to hypertrophy, renal function must be monitored in all patients so that any return of obstructive symptoms will be detected.

MANAGEMENT RECOMMENDATIONS

- All patients should have a baseline BUN, creatinine, complete blood count and urinalysis.
- An IVP is necessary to assess upper tract function and the clinical severity of obstruction. A CMG should be done to assess bladder muscle function.

- Patients should be followed initially, unless there is risk of sepsis or deterioration in renal function. Fluid loads and drugs which affect bladder function must be avoided. Infection should be treated appropriately.
- Surgical consultation should be obtained early, though the decision to operate is contingent on symptomatology, bladder and renal function, and risk of infection.

ANNOTATED BIBLIOGRAPHY

Blandy, J.P.: Benign prostatic enlargement. Br. Med. J., *1*:31, 1971. *(Short clinical review.)*

Castro, J.E., and Griffiths, H.L.J.: The assessment of patients with benign prostatic hypertrophy. J. R. Coll. Surg. Edin., *17*:190, 1972. *(No correlation was found between gland size or symptoms and calculated urethal area.)*

Castro, J.E., Griffiths, H.L.J., and Edwards, D.E.: A double-blind, controlled, clinical trial of spironolactone for benign prostatic hypertrophy. Br. J. Surg., *58*:485, 1971. *(Seventy-six per cent of patients treated with placebo had symptomatic improvement at 6 months, illustrating the subjectivity of symptoms.)*

Culp, D.A.: Benign prostatic hypertrophy. Urol. Clin. North Am., *2*:29, 1975. *(Clinical review with a discussion of the differential diagnosis.)*

Finestone, A.J., and Rosenthal, R.S.: Silent prostatism. Geriatrics, *26*:89, 1971. *(Seven cases illustrating the protean presentations of BPH in the elderly.)*

Finkle, A.L., and Prian, D.V.: Sexual potency in elderly men before and after prostatectomy. JAMA, *196*:125, 1966. *(Eighty-four per cent of patients who were potent preoperatively maintained potency after prostatectomy [TURP, perineal, suprapubic]. The highest level of impotency occurred with the perineal approach.)*

Geller, J.: Medical treatment of benign prostatic hypertrophy. In J.E. Castro (ed.): The Treatment of Prostatic Hypertrophy and Neoplasia. Lancaster, England: Medical and Technical Publishing Co., Ltd., 1974. *(Good review of current hormonal theories of BPH.)*

132

Management of Nongonococcal Urethritis
JOHN D. GOODSON, M.D.

Nongonococcal urethritis (NGU) is a venereal disease which rivals gonorrhea in terms of frequency in the male. It can occur as an isolated infection or may follow gonococcal urethritis within a period of 1 to 3 weeks. In about half the patients, infection with *Chlamydia trachomatis* appears responsible for NGU; in the remainder, the etiology is often uncertain, although T-strain mycoplasma (*Ureaplasma*) may account for some of these infections, and Reiters syndrome for others. Management of urethritis involves distinguishing gonococcal from nongonococcal etiologies and instituting prompt antibiotic therapy.

CLINICAL PRESENTATIONS AND COURSE

Nongonococcal urethritis (NGU) often presents differently from gonococcal disease, but Gram stain and culture of the discharge are needed to rule out gonorrhea. Patients with gonococcal infection generally have a short symptomatic period (2 to 4 days) and a purulent discharge that on Gram stain demonstrates polymorphonuclear leukocytes (PMNs) and intracellular gram-negative diplococci. The finding on Gram stain of intracellular gram-negative diplococci is over 95 per cent specific for gonorrhea. Patients with NGU typically have a longer symptomatic period and a scant, watery discharge. The Gram stain in patients with NGU usually demonstrates a few PMNs and mixed organisms. Patients originally treated for gonococcal urethritis who have persistent symptoms following therapy and who are found to have negative follow-up cultures for gonococci are likely to have NGU. NGU is a disease of males; a female counterpart to NGU has not been identified.

Reiter's syndrome is characterized by various combinations of conjunctivitis, iritis, acute asymmetrical polyarthritis (see Chapter 139), circinate balanitis, keratodermia blennorrhagica, mucosal ulcerations and urethritis. Many patients present first with urethritis, though involvement of other organ systems is frequently found or appears with in a few weeks.

Nongonococcal urethritis tends to produce a low level of symptomatology and may wax and wane over several weeks. Spontaneous resolution can occur. Prostatitis, epididymitis and urethral stricture formation have been reported in untreated or poorly treated infections, but these complications are very rare. Most patients with Reiter's syndrome experience a self-limited illness, though in a minority a chronic or recurrent illness with arthritis develops (see Chapter 138).

PRINCIPLES OF MANAGEMENT AND THERAPEUTIC RECOMMENDATIONS

Every patient with symptoms of urethritis should have a Gram stain of a urethral specimen, and the specimen should be cultured for gonococci (see Chapter 113). If there is a spontaneous discharge, this material can be used. Otherwise, a sterile swab should be inserted into the penile meatus. Alternatively, the urethral fraction of clean-voided urine, the VB_1 specimen (see Chapter 133), can be obtained and centrifuged, and the pellet Gram-stained and cultured.

If no definite gram-negative intracellular diplococci are seen on Gram stain, the diagnosis of NGU should tentatively be made. The final diagnosis depends on a negative gonococcal culture. It is not necessary to culture for *Chlamydia* or *Ureaplasma*. These patients should be treated with *tetracycline* 250 mg. four times a day orally for 14 to 21 days. Those allergic to tetracycline should receive erythromycin 250 mg. four times a day orally for 14 to 21 days. Sulfisoxazole (500 mg. four times a day for 10 to 14 days) can be used, but has a lower response rate.

Although a female counterpart to NGU has not been identified, some authorities recommend that the female sexual partner be treated the same as the male patient. Treatment of the male homosexual partner of the patient with NGU does not seem to be necessary.

Persistent symptoms of NGU after treatment should prompt a repeat course of therapy of longer duration and a careful search for possible reinfection.

The patient who has been adequately treated twice and in whom reinfection has been excluded should be watched for the development of Reiter's syndrome. The treatment for Reiter's syndrome is palliative, involving anti-inflammatory agents such as aspirin or indomethacin for arthritic complaints. Conjunctivities and mucocutaneous symptoms are self-limited and usually require no systemic treatment.

If gram-negative intracellular diplococci are seen on Gram stain, the diagnosis of gonococcal urethritis can be made with reasonable certainty. The culture will provide confirmation. These patients should receive either 4.8 million units of penicillin G injected in two sites at the same visit along with 1 gm. of probenecid orally, or ampicillin 3.5 gm. orally with 1 gm. of probenecid. Those allergic to penicillin should receive either tetracycline 1.5 gm. orally followed by 500 mg. four times a day for 4 days, or spectinomycin 2.0 gm. intramuscularly (see Chapter 113).

Patients with nongonococcal urethritis should be examined carefully for other venereal diseases (herpes infection, venereal warts, lice, syphilis). A serologic test for syphilis is indicated (see Chapters 119 and 134).

ANNOTATED BIBLIOGRAPHY

Bowie, W.R., Wang, S.P., Alexander, E.R., et al.: Etiology of nongonococcal urethritis. J. Clin. Invest. 59: 735, 1977. (Evidence for Ureaplasma role in NGU in those with negative cultures for Chlamydia.)

Holmes, K.K., Handsfield, H.H., Wang, S.P., et al.: Etiology of nongonococcal urethritis. N. Engl. J. Med., 292:1198, 1975. (Forty-two per cent of NGU patients were Chlamydia culture positive. Careful screen for other infectious agents was unproductive.)

Jacobs, N.J., and Kraus, S.J.: Gonococcal and nongonococcal urethritis in man. Ann. Intern. Med. 82:7, 1975. (Of 400 men with urethritis, 54 per cent had NGU and 46 per cent had gonorrhea. Ninety-eight per cent of specimens that were definitely positive for gonococcus on Gram stain were culture positive. Ninety-seven per cent that were definitely negative were culture negative. Twenty-one per cent that were equivocal were gonococcal culture positive.)

Kaufman, R.E., and Wiesner, P.J.: Nonspecific urethritis. N. Engl. J. Med., 291: 1175, 1974. (Short clinical review.)

King, A.: Nonspecific urethritis. Med. Clin. North, Am. 56:1193, 1972. (Ninety per cent of nongonococcal urethritis were "nonspecific.")

McCormack, W.M., Braun, P., Lee, Y.H., et al.: The genital mycoplasma. N. Engl. J. Med., 288:78, 1973. (Balanced review of the role of T mycoplasma in NGU.)

Schacter, J.: Chlamydial infections. N. Engl. J. Med., 298:428, 490, 540, 1978. (Excellent review of role of chlamydial organisms in genitourinary infection.)

Weinberger, H.W., Ropes, M., Kulka, J.P., and Bauer, W.: Reiter's syndrome, clinical and pathologic observations. Medicine, 41:35, 1962. (Excellent review of clinical findings.)

133

Management of Acute and Chronic Prostatitis

JOHN D. GOODSON, M.D.

Chronic prostatitis is a common infection that can cause persistent and annoying symptoms, while acute prostatitis is less common but potentially much more serious. Both conditions require accurate recognition and treatment by the primary physician; prompt initiation of therapy is especially important for acute prostatitis.

CLINICAL PRESENTATION AND COURSE

Acute prostatitis. The condition is readily identified by the onset of diminished urine flow, perineal pain, dysuria and fever. On gentle rectal examination, the gland is enlarged, exquisitely tender and boggy. Abdominal examination occasionally reveals striking bladder distention. Some patients may appear toxic at the time of presentation.

Chronic prostatitis. In older men, the symptoms are generally those of bladder outflow obstruction. Patients complain of frequency, dribbling, loss of stream volume and force, double voiding, hesitancy and urgency. Younger men more often complain of dribbling and intermittent pain in the perineum or testicles. Some patients present initially with hematuria, hematospermia or painful ejaculations. In most cases, rectal examination reveals an enlarged prostate with a variable amount of asymmetry, bogginess and tenderness. Untreated or incompletely treated chronic prostatitis is characterized by recurrent symptomatic exacerbations, though these may be separated by long asymptomatic intervals.

Infection of the gland must be differentiated from other conditions such as benign prostatic hypertrophy (BPH) (see Chapter 131), prostatic carcinoma (see Chapter 137), and "prostatosis," all of which can produce a similar symptom complex (see Chapter 125).

Both acute and chronic prostatitis can cause urinary tract and systemic complications. The acutely infected gland may lead to renal parenchymal infection or bacteremia. Rarely, acute infection will progress to a well-defined abscess of the gland. Chronic infection can produce small prostatic stones which may serve as a nidus for further inflammation and recurrent symptomatic bouts of infection.

PRINCIPLES OF MANAGEMENT

Acute prostatitis accompanied by severe pain, high fever, and marked leukocytosis requires hospitalization. Antibiotics must be given intravenously to achieve high tissue levels of the drug. Such patients must be examined rectally for the presence of a fluctuant prostatic mass suggestive of an abscess, which may necessitate surgical drainage. Less toxic patients can be treated as outpatients with oral medication.

Chronic prostatitis is difficult to eradicate. Success in these cases has been achieved with long-term trimethoprim-sulfamethoxazole treatment, but the cure rate after one course of therapy is less than 50 per cent. The low cure rate achieved with antibiotics in chronic prostatitis requires that therapeutic goals be adjusted to the patient's age.

When a cure is not achieved in younger patients, antibiotic therapy is directed toward suppression of prostatic inflammation and prevention of upper tract

infection or obstruction. Transurethral prostatic resection or total prostatectomy provides a surgical alternative when repeated courses of antibiotics fail. Both operations are associated with significant morbidity, including possible impotence or sterility, and should be reserved for older patients. Recurrent infection associated with prostatic stones is an indication for removal of the gland.

Careful adherence to culture technique is necessary to confirm the diagnosis and essential to identification of the responsible organism. *E. coli* and other enteric bacteria are the predominant pathogens, though numerous other bacteria have been cultured. Viruses, *Chlamydia, Mycoplasma* and parasites are occasionally implicated. Tuberculous prostatitis is an unusual complication of disseminated mycobacterial disease.

Urines representing urethral, bladder, and post-prostatic-massage specimens (labeled VB_1, VB_2, and VB_3) are collected (see Appendix at end of this chapter) in addition to any prostatic secretions which can be expressed as a result of massage. Vigorous massage should be avoided in patients with severe acute prostatitis, because of the risk of inducing bacteremia. Gram stain of the expressed prostatic secretions (EPS) or the spun VB_3 specimen will often demonstrate organisms; cultures of the EPS and VB_3 should show significant growth (greater than 5,000 colonies/ml.), while the VB_1 and VB_2 should be sterile. Direct culture of the prostate via the rectum or the urethra has not proved reliable. Culture for *Chlamydia* and *Mycoplasma* requires special techniques and should be reserved for difficult or protracted infection.

Curative antibiotic therapy is indicated by the elimination of bacteria from prostatic fluid. Since the gland's secretions are normally acidic (pH 6.5–7.4), the most efficacious drugs are those which readily penetrate membranes (lipid-soluble) and are ionically trapped (basic). Trimethoprim and erythromycin have these characteristics. Animal studies have demonstrated good prostatic fluid levels for both. With chronic infection, the prostatic fluid becomes alkaline, a situation that tends to reduce trimethoprim concentrations. As a result, some men are not cured even by prolonged courses of antibiotic therapy. Trimethoprim is more effective than erythromycin against gram-negative bacteria and consequently is preferred. The combination of trimethoprim and sulfamethoxazole, a sulfa drug with a similar half-life, acts synergistically on a wide range of gram-negative and gram-positive infections, with the notable exception of enterococci. Ampicillin and most other antibiotics enter the acutely inflamed prostate, but penetration of the chronically infected gland is uncertain. Minocycline penetrates the prostate reasonably well.

The EPS and VB_3 should be inspected and cultured following the treatment period to determine the efficacy of therapy. A BUN and creatinine should be obtained at the initial visit and periodically thereafter depending on the chronicity and severity of symptoms. An intravenous pyelogram is indicated when there is evidence of renal deterioration or symptoms of persistent outflow obstruction.

THERAPEUTIC RECOMMENDATIONS AND PATIENT EDUCATION

- *Acute prostatitis* requires appropriate Gram stains, cultures of EPS and VB_3, and immediate treatment. Patients with high fever, leukocytosis, and severe perineal pain need intravenous antibiotics, antipyretics, and analgesics; hospitalization is indicated. In the presence of marked outflow obstruction, suprapubic bladder decompression may be necessary. A fluctuant prostatic mass suggestive of an abscess requires surgical drainage. Until culture and sensitivity data are available, treatment of the toxic patient is directed toward gram-negative bacteria, utilizing parenteral ampicillin or gentamicin.
- For the nontoxic patient, the combination of 160 mg. trimethoprim and 800 mg. sulfamethoxazole twice a day orally is preferred. Ampicillin, 500 m.g. four times a day, tetracycline at the same dose, or minocycline, 100 mg. twice a day, would be a reasonable alternative in sulfa-allergic individuals. Treatment should be continued for 10 to 14 days.
- *Chronic prostatitis* requires a prolonged antibiotic course; 160 mg. trimethoprim and 800 mg. sulfamethoxazole orally twice daily for 6 weeks is recommended. After treatment, the patient should be followed closely for return of infection. A second antibiotic course of up to 12 weeks' duration may be necessary in refractory infections. If these measures fail to control infection, a brief course of an aminoglycide antibiotic should be considered.
- Patients should be warned of the chronic and relapsing nature of the disease and alerted to the early signs of infection in the upper urinary tract. They can also be reassured that isolated prostatitis does not cause infertility or impotence.
- *Local measures* reduce symptoms in both acute and chronic infections. Sitz baths two to three times a day for 20 minutes can relieve perineal

pain. The patient with a partial obstruction should be told to void while in a warm water bath with pelvic muscles relaxed. Prostatic massage will relieve gland congestion in chronic cases and can be repeated every 1 to 2 weeks. Massage of the acutely infected gland is contraindicated since it can produce bacteremia. Stool softeners, antipyretics, analgesics and bed rest are all helpful. The patient should avoid alcohol, coffee, tea or other beverages which might produce rapid bladder expansion. The physician should discontinue or reduce in dose, if possible, anticholinergics, sedatives, and antidepressants, all of which can impair bladder function.

ANNOTATED BIBLIOGRAPHY

Drach, G.W.: Problems in diagnosis of bacterial prostatitis: Gram-negative, Gram-positive and mixed infections. J. Urol., *111*:630, 1974. *(Careful culture documentation of infection in 105 patients with prostatitis. Gram-positive organisms were found most frequently* [Staphylococcus aureus *and* Streptococcus] *but were felt to represent a more benign disease for which antibiotic suppression was not recommended. Gram-negative isolates were felt to increase the risk of urinary tract infection and suppression was recommended.)*

Fair, W.R., Crane, D.B., Schiller, N., and Heston, W.D.W.: J. Urol., *121*:437, 1979. *(Prostatic fluid from men with chronic infection was found to have a mean pH of 8.32* [basic]. *This may explain why some men are not cured by trimethoprim and sulfamethoxazole since the trimethoprim would be ionically excluded.)*

Hensle, T.W., Prout, G.R., Jr., and Griffin, P.: Minocycline diffusion into benign prostatic hypertrophy. J. Urol., *118*:609, 1977. *(Minocycline penetrates well into noninfected prostate.)*

Meares, E.M., Jr.: Infected stones of the prostate gland. Urology, *4*:560, 1974. *(Prostatic stones are found in 13.8 per cent of men. Most are asymptomatic, but where recurrent infection is demonstrated, the gland and stones must be removed.)*

Meares, E.M.,. Jr.: Prostatitis. Urol. Clin. North Am., *2*:3, 1975. *(An excellent review.)*

Meares, E.M., Jr.: Long-term therapy of chronic bacterial prostatitis with trimethoprim-sulfamethoxazole. Can. Med. Assoc. J., *112*:225, 1975. *(Twelve weeks of combination treatment produced an initially good response in 74 per cent. Only 31 per cent remained cured for a 3-month follow-up period.)*

O'Dea, M.J., Moore, S.B., and Greene, L.F.: Tuberculous prostatitis. Urology, *11*:483, 1978. *(Tuberculosis may present in the prostate. Multiple biopsies are necessary to make the diagnosis.)*

Pfan, A. and Sacks, T.: Chronic bacterial prostatitis: New therapeutic aspects. Br. J. Urol., *48*:245, 1976. *(Chronic prostatitis refractory to trimethoprim and sulfamethoxazole was successfully treated with kanamycin, an antibiotic more readily trapped in the alkaline fluid of the infected gland.)*

Smart, C.J., and Jenkins, J.D.: The role of transurethral prostatectomy in chronic prostatitis. Br. J. Urol., *45*:654, 1973. *(Good results in treating chronic infection, but up to three operations may be required to remove all infected tissue. Recommended TURP for patients in whom sterility is not an issue.)*

Sporer, A., and Auerbach, O.: Tuberculosis of the prostate. Urology, *11*:362, 1978. *(Tuberculosis of the prostate results from hematogenous dissemination of disease and is a frequent site of genitourinary involvement.)*

Stamey, T.A.: Urinary Infections. Baltimore: Williams & Wilkins, 1972. *(Excellent chapter on male urinary tract infections.)*

Stamey, T.A., Meares, E.M., Jr., and Winningham, D.G.: Chronic bacterial prostatitis and the diffusion of drugs into the prostatic fluid. J. Urol., *103*:187, 1970. *(Discussion of the ideal drug for prostatic infection and the concept of ion trapping.)*

Schwartz, H.: Prostatitis. Prog. Clin. Biol. Res., *6*:1365, 1976. *(An argument is made for the equivalence of the major broad-spectrum antibiotics in the treatment of prostatitis.)*

APPENDIX:
URINE AND PROSTATIC FLUID COLLECTIONS

The appropriate diagnosis and management of infections involving the urinary tract depend on the correct identification of the responsible pathogen. The clinician must ensure the collection of urine specimens with a minimal amount of contamination. Careful patient instruction, adequate hydration and assistance where necessary are essential to obtaining accurate, useful results.

Standard Clean-Voided Specimen

The *female patient* is told to straddle or squat over the toilet and to spread the labia with the nondominant hand. This position is maintained throughout collection. With the other hand the vulva is swabbed front to back with three sterile gauze pads soaked in sterile water or with a sponge soaked in a mild nonhexachlorophene soap. A small amount of urine is then passed. This is a urethral specimen and can be saved if bacterial or protozoan urethritis is suspected. More urine is voided and collected in a sterile cup. Alternatively, the patient can be told to slide the cup into a freely flowing stream to collect a true midstream specimen. The adequacy of collection can be confirmed by examining for epithelial cells; their presence indicates vulvar or urethral contamination.

With an elderly patient, the assistance of a family member or a nurse may be needed. When repeated contamination is suspected, straight catherization of the bladder can be done with relatively little risk. Suprapubic bladder aspiration with a large bore spinal needle after careful preparation of the skin should be reserved for cases of urethral obstruction when the bladder is distended on physical examination.

Specimen collection in the *male* varies with the clinical situation. When cystitis is suspected, the patient retracts the foreskin and cleans the glans penis with three gauze pads or soap sponges. A small amount of urine is voided into the toilet and then a midstream specimen is collected. When urethritis or prostatitis is suspected, voided bladder specimens are indicated.

Voided Bladder Specimens (Fig. 133–1)

The patient retracts the foreskin and cleans the glans penis. The first 10 cc. is collected and labeled VB_1 (voided bladder one) and represents a urethral specimen, useful in cases of suspected urethritis (see Chapters 126 and 132). A midstream specimen is collected in the standard fashion. This specimen is labeled VB_2. The bladder must not be completely emptied. While the patient maintains foreskin retraction with one hand, the physician massages the prostate with continuous strokes. The resulting prostatic fluid

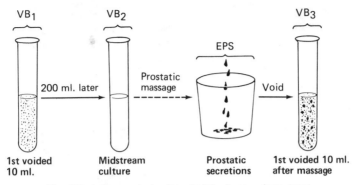

Fig. 133-1. Segmented cultured of the lower urinary tract in the male. (Adapted from Meares, E.M., and Stamey, T.: Bacteriologic localization patterns in bacterial prostatitis and urethritis. Invest. Urol., 5:492-518, 1968)

is collected in a sterile container labeled EPS (expressed prostatic secretion) and can be used for culture and Gram or acid-fast stain. If no fluid is obtained, the patient is instructed to milk the penis, starting from the base and moving toward the tip. Finally, if there is still no fluid, the patient is told to void another 10 cc. into a sterile container. This specimen is labeled VB_3 and represents roughly a 100:1 dilution of prostatic fluid; it can be cultured or spun and stained. Vigorous prostatic massage can produce a transient bacteremia and should be avoided if acute prostatitis is suspected; if the patient has chronic prostatitis and known valvular heart disease, endocarditis prophylaxis may be necessary (see Chapter 11).

The EPS and VB_3 can be inspected under the microscope for the presence of fat globules, leukocytes and organisms. A Gram stain should be prepared and examined, since it may aid in identifying the responsible organism. With prostatic infections, growth will occur in VB_3 and EPS, but not in VB_1 and VB_2. When there is bacterial growth in both VB_2 and VB_3 samples, a prostatic infection may be masked by a bladder infection. In this situation, antibiotics which sterilize the bladder contents but do not penetrate the prostate (such as penicillin G, 500 mg. four times a day orally, or macrodantoin, 100 mg. three times a day orally) may be given for 2 to 3 days before specimen collection. With prostatic infection, the EPS and VB_3 will still grow organisms.

Urethral catheterization of the male is rarely required for culture and should be reserved for the symptomatic relief of marked outflow obstruction.

BIBLIOGRAPHY

Meares, E.M., and Stamey, T.: Bacteriologic localization patterns in bacterial prostatitis and urethritis. Invest. Urol., 5:492, 1968.

134

Management of Syphilis and Other Venereal Diseases
HARVEY B. SIMON, M.D.

Syphilis

In 1943, the dramatic efficacy of penicillin treatment was established, and for the next 15 years the incidence of new cases of syphilis declined steadily to a low of about 6000 in 1957. Although *Treponema pallidum,* the spirochete which causes syphilis, has not developed resistance to penicillin, the incidence of syphilis has increased progressively in the last 20 years, largely due to a change in sexual mores, with many new cases occurring in adolescents, young adults and homosexuals.

PATHOPHYSIOLOGY AND CLINICAL PRESENTATION

Man is the only natural reservoir of *T. pallidum.* Except for transplacental transmission, virtually all cases are acquired by sexual contact with persons having active infectious lesions. *T. pallidum* readily penetrates abraded skin and intact mucous membranes to multiply locally and disseminate through the lymphatics and bloodstream.

The course of syphilis can be divided into primary, secondary, latent and tertiary phases. The lesion of *primary syphilis* is the chancre, which occurs at the site of inoculation about 3 weeks after exposure. The chancre is usually located on the genitalia, but depending on sexual practices, it can occur in the anal canal, on oral mucosa, hands, or even more unusual locations. The lesion begins as a small papule which enlarges and undergoes superficial necrosis to produce an ulcer with a clean base and sharp margins. The chancre is typically painless, and patients are free of constitutional symptoms, though regional nodes may be enlarged. The chancre is teeming with spirochetes and is highly infectious.

Even without therapy, the chancre will heal completely in 2 to 6 weeks. However, about 2 months after the primary infection, the features of secondary syphilis may appear. *Secondary syphilis* is a systemic disease. A flulike syndrome is common, as is generalized lymphadenopathy. The most characteristic feature of secondary syphilis is a generalized skin eruption. Lesions may be macular, papular or papulosquamous, but tend to be symmetric and uniform in size; typically, the palms and soles are involved. Mucous patches and split papules often occur on the mucous membranes. Secondary syphilis can involve many other organs; clinical manifestations may include aseptic meningitis, hepatitis, nephritis or uveitis. Patients with secondary syphilis are contagious.

As in primary syphilis, the manifestations of secondary syphilis resolve spontaneously even without therapy, although up to 25 per cent of patients exhibit a brief relapse of secondary lesions. Untreated patients without active lesions are considered to have *latent syphilis.* About two-thirds of these individuals remain entirely asymptomatic, but in the remaining one-third, the lesions of tertiary syphilis develop, usually 10 to 40 years after primary infection. The major forms of *tertiary syphilis* include: (1) cardiovascular, with aneurysmal dilatation of the ascending aorta and aortic insufficiency; (2) neurosyphilis, which may be asymptomatic or present as general

paresis with disorders of intellect and personality, or as tabes dorsalis, with ataxic gait, impaired pain and temperature sensation, autonomic dysfunction and hypoactive reflexes; (3) gummas, which are isolated, slowly progressive destructive granulomatous lesions of skin, bone, liver or other organs.

Congenital syphilis occurs as a result of transplacental transmission of spirochetes during the second or third trimester of pregnancy. Fetal loss is about 60 per cent, and up to half of surviving infants have stigmata which can result in serious permanent handicaps. Congenital syphilis can be prevented by prompt treatment of maternal infection.

DIAGNOSIS

Treponema pallidum cannot be cultured in the laboratory, but the diagnosis of syphilis can be made by direct visualization of treponemas from the chancre; however, this is a specialized technique which requires dark field or fluorescent microscopy and very experienced observers. As a result, the diagnosis usually depends on clinical features and serological testing. The most widely used serological tests for syphilis use a lipoidal extract of mammalian tissues for the antigen. Examples include the VDRL, Hinton and RPR tests. These are excellent screening tests, but the false-positive rate is as high as 20 per cent, often as the result of unrelated infections or inflammatory diseases which produce hyperglobulinemia. More specific serological tests use treponemal antigens and can be used to distinguish true-positive from false-positive results. The best of these treponemal tests is the FTA-Abs (see Chapter 113).

PRINCIPLES OF MANAGEMENT AND THERAPEUTIC RECOMMENDATIONS

The results of treatment of early syphilis are excellent. *Treponema pallidum* is very sensitive to *penicillin.* Because the organism multiplies slowly, the goal is to attain relatively low, but long-lasting, antibiotic levels. Present Public Health Service recommendations include:
- Early syphilis (incubating, primary, secondary, early latent stages): 2.4 million units of benzathine penicillin intramuscularly at a single session. Alternatively, one may give 600,000 units of procaine penicillin intramuscularly daily for 8 days. Penicillin-allergic patients may receive tetracycline or

erythromycin 500 mg. by mouth four times a day for 15 days. Tetracycline is contraindicated in pregnancy.

• Syphilis of greater than 1 year's duration (latent or tertiary stages): benzathine penicillin 2.4 million units intramuscularly for 3 consecutive weeks. Alternatively, patients may receive 600,000 units of procaine penicillin intramuscularly daily for 15 days. Some authorities suggest substantially higher doses of penicillin for neurosyphilis. Penicillin-allergic patients should receive tetracycline or erythromycin 500 mg. by mouth four times a day for 30 days.

Immunity to syphilis is incomplete and reinfection may occur, especially in patients treated with penicillin within a year of infection. Follow-up of patients is essential. Equally important is the reporting of cases to appropriate public health authorities, so that investigation of contacts can be carried out.

Other Venereal Diseases

HERPES GENITALIS

In addition to syphilis, gonorrhea (see Chapter 113) and nongonococcal urethritis (see Chapter 132), many other infections can be transmitted by sexual contact. The most common of these are viral infections. *Herpes genitalis* is caused by sexual transmission of *herpes simplex* virus, Type II. After a short incubation period averaging 2 to 10 days, vesicular lesions develop on the genitalia; these are penile lesions in the male; in the female they may affect the external genitalia or the vagina and cervix. The lesions ulcerate early, and although they may be asymptomatic, pain is sometimes severe, and regional lymphadenopathy and fever may be prominent. In most patients, herpes genitalis is self-limited, but the disease can pursue a relapsing course which is all the more frustrating because no form of treatment is of demonstrated efficacy (see Chapter 184). Herpetic infection during pregnancy is particularly worrisome, since neonatal herpes can be a devastating disease.

CONDYLOMATA ACUMINATA

Another viral disease which appears to be sexually transmitted is condylomata acuminata, or venereal warts. These typically present as painless papillomatous lesions of the moist mucocutaneous regions of the genitalia. Generally, venereal warts should be treated with careful topical application of 20 per cent podophyllin solution, but large lesions may require electrocoagulation or excision (see Chapter 186).

Other Viral Infections

Although other viral infections, including cytomegalovirus and hepatitis, can be transmitted sexually (see Chapters 52 and 70), their major impact is not on the genital tract, and the great majority of cases are transmitted nonsexually.

SCABIES AND PUBIC LICE

It should be noted that cutaneous infestations with mites or pubic lice commonly result from intimate contact. Patients present with pruritus of the pubic region. The diagnosis of pubic lice or "crabs" is made by seeing the organism either with the naked eye or with a magnifying lens. Scabies, which is caused by mites, produces papules and burrows which may be scraped and examined microscopically in wet mounts to visualize the organism. Topical lotions, such as 1 per cent gamma benzene hexachloride (Kwell) are effective treatments. Bedding and clothing should be laundered (see Chapter 187).

VAGINITIS (see Chapter 112)

Although not strictly speaking a venereal disease, vaginitis may be perpetuated by sexual contact and may therefore require simultaneous treatment of male sexual partners. This is particularly true of trichomonal vaginitis, caused by the protozoan *Trichomonas vaginalis*. The diagnosis is made by direct microscopic examination of a wet mount of the vaginal discharge. *Hemophilus vaginalis* is another organism which has been implicated (see Chapter 112).

CHANCROID AND GRANULOMA INGUINALE

The gram-negative bacillus *Hemophilus ducrey,* causes chancroid, which presents as dirty, shaggy, painful genital ulcers often accompanied by regional adenopathy. Sulfonamides or tetracyclines are recommended for treatment.

Painless, slowly progressive genital ulcers are

characteristic of granuloma inguinale, caused by the gram-negative bacterium *Donovania granulomatis.* Tetracycline or erythromycin is the treatment of choice. Both chancroid and granuloma inguinale are rare in temperate climates.

LYMPHOGRANULOMA VENEREUM

A microorganism belonging to the *Chlamydia* group of obligate intracellular parasites is the cause of lymphogranuloma venereum. In this disease, the primary genital lesion is a small, painless papule which heals spontaneously and often escapes notice. The major impact of the disease is on the regional lymphatics. Inguinal nodes enlarge and may suppurate to produce chronic draining sinuses. Scarring and lymphatic obstruction may result. Rectal fibrosis and strictures are late residua. Sulfonamides, tetracycline, and erythromycin are effective treatments.

ANNOTATED BIBLIOGRAPHY

Orkin, M., and Maibach, H.I.: This scabies pandemic. N. Engl. J. Med., *298*:496, 1978. *(A detailed review of the clinical features of scabies.)*

Pheifer, T.A., Forsyth, P.S., Durfee, M.A., *et al.*: Nonspecific vaginitis: role of *Haemophilus vaginalis* and treatment with metronidazole. N. Engl. J. Med., *298*:1429, 1978. *(A provocative reappraisal of the common problem of nonspecific vaginitis. Haemophilis vaginalis was the etiologic agent in most patients. Traditional therapy with sulfonamide vaginal cream and orally administered doxycycline and ampicillin was ineffective. Oral metronidazole therapy was effective, but its efficacy must be weighed against its possible toxicity.)*

Rein, M.F., and Chapel, T.A.: Trichomoniasis, candidiasis, and the minor venereal diseases. Clin. Obstet. Gynecol., *18*:73, 1975. *(An overview of miscellaneous sexually transmitted diseases.)*

Sparling, P.F.: Diagnosis and treatment of syphilis. N. Engl. J. Med., *284*:642, 1971. *(An excellent review of the serologic diagnosis and antibiotic management of syphilis.)*

135
Management of Chronic Renal Failure
LESLIE S.–T. FANG, M.D.

Although diverse diseases can lead to chronic renal failure, the clinical manifestations and functional derangements are remarkably constant. Hemodialysis and transplantation have increased the capacity to prolong survival and function, but the primary physician continues to have a very important role, being responsible for initial conservative management of the patient with decreasing renal function. The objectives are to prevent or minimize the complications of uremia in order to forestall the need for dialysis, monitor the disease, and judge when referral to the nephrologist is indicated for consideration of dialysis or transplantation.

PATHOPHYSIOLOGY AND CLINICAL PRESENTATION

Chronic renal faulure can result from glomerular, vascular or tubular disease. Congenital anomalies, infection, metabolic diseases, obstructive urology, or collagen vascular disease can all lead to renal insufficiency. Independent of underlying disease, the major clinical manifestations of chronic renal failure result from disturbances in electrolyte and fluid balance, elimination of metabolic wastes and other toxins, erythropoietin production, and blood pressure control. Considerable controversy exists about the contribution of urea or other toxins to the production of many of the symptoms associated with chronic renal failure.

Fluid and electrolyte problems. These include hyperkalemia, volume overload, hypocalcemia, hyperphosphatemia and metabolic acidosis. With moderate renal insufficiency, concentration is impaired, so that patients drink and excrete more water than normal to handle the same solute load; this results in polydipsia, polyuria and nocturia. The ability to dilute urine is compromised with further renal impairment, producing isosthenuria and obligate fluid intake. As renal function continues to decline, olguria supervenes. The situation is similar with sodium; moderate renal failure produces mild *salt wasting.* In the later stages, sodium excretion becomes limited, *salt retention* develops, and edema supervenes.

Potassium excretion is usually preserved until late in the course, when potassium retention occurs as oliguria develops and the ability of the distal tubule to secrete potassium is compromised.

Decreased renal function produces phosphate retention, secondary hypocalcemia and consequently *secondary hyperparathyroidism.* Decreased intestinal calcium absorption secondary to impaired hydroxylation of vitamin D also contributes to hypocalcemia.

Acidosis results from the compromised kidneys' inability to excrete urinary ammonium and, with further impairment, titratable acid. Acidosis also results from loss of bicarbonate reabsorption and hydrogen ion secretion. Loss of bicarbonate due to diarrhea may also contribute to acidosis.

Endocrine functions. Impairment of the kidneys' endocrine function contributes to anemia, hypertension, and congestive failure, which may further compromise renal function. *Decreased erythropoietin* results in a mild to moderate normochromic normocytic anemia. (Anemia also comes as a consequence of increased hemolysis and bleeding, aggravated by impaired platelet adhesiveness.) *Increased renin levels* may occur, causing modest hypertension and fluid retention.

Clinical presentation. Early in renal failure, anorexia, lassitude, fatigability and weakness are prominent symptoms. As failure worsens, the patient may complain of pruritus, nausea, vomiting, constipation or diarrhea. Shortness of breath may occur secondary to cardiomyopathy and fluid overload.

Edema, hypertension and pericarditis are common late in the course. Neurologic manifestations include drowsiness, lethargy, peripheral myopathy, seizures and, terminally, coma.

Course. The course of renal failure is punctuated by periods of rapid deterioration, often precipitated by dehydration or infection. The rate of progression depends on the underlylng renal disease and the efficacy of conservative therapy. The rate of progression from moderate renal insufficiency appears to be more rapid for patients with diabetic nephropathy or severe hypertension and to be slower for patients with polycystic kidneys. However, progress to death or dialysis in patients with advanced renal failure appears to be reasonably predictable, with a mean survival of 100 to 150 days.

PRINCIPLES OF MANAGEMENT

Conservative management of renal failure can prolong survival and preserve function outside the hospital. Principles of management involve compensating for the excretory, regulatory, and endocrine functions of the kidney. The goals of therapy are to reduce symptoms, slow progression of the underlying disease and avoid preventable complications.

Protein intake. The excretory function of the kidneys involves removal of nitrogenous waste, uric acid and drugs. The cornerstone of therapy is to *reduce protein intake* to prevent worsening of azotemia. Restriction to 0.5 gm. of protein per kg. per day usually allows sufficient amounts for daily requirements while lessening progression of renal failure. By utilizing a diet high in essential amino acids, some investigators have been able to restrict proteins to 0.3 gm. per kg. per day. Essential amino acids appear to be the most effectively utilized source of nitrogen and can lead to the lowest rate of urea nitrogen development. Alpha keto analogues of essential amino acids have been purported to spare nitrogen even more than essential amino acids, but are quite costly and unpalatable.

Fluids and electrolytes. Judicious fluid and electrolyte management is exceedingly important because patients with chronic renal failure have difficulty adjusting to variations of either excessive intake or rigid restriction of salt and fluids. Prior to the late stages of renal failure, *salt and fluid intake* must be adequate to match the excess losses which occur as tubular function begins to deteriorate. Restriction of intake can actually accelerate renal damage by causing decreased extracellular volume and reduced renal perfusion. Concentrating ability can be measured by determining the specific gravity of a first morning urine specimen, and sodium requirements can be estimated by testing a 24-hour urine collection for sodium excretion. In the later stages, as excretion of sodium and water becomes limited, cautious sodium and fluid restrictions become necessary.

Since *potassium excretion* is preserved until late in the course of renal failure, there is no need to restrict its intake until oliguria sets in. However, prior to the onset of oliguria, it is prudent to avoid use of potassium-sparing diuretics and indefinite potassium supplementation. Moreover, since acidosis worsens hyperkalemia, it should be corrected promptly. On the other hand, severe hypokalemia can itself cause tubular damage; therefore, serum potassium should be monitored regularly and low levels corrected.

Hypocalcemia and *secondary hyperparathyroidism* are best countered by reducing the elevations in phosphate which result from decreased renal excretion of the anion. The principle of therapy is to lower serum phosphate by reducing dietary sources, inhibiting absorption through administration of aluminium hydroxide antacids, and maintaining adequate calcium levels by pharmacologic doses of vitamin D and exogenous calcium. This will reduce the prevalence of secondary hyperparathyroidism and the consequent metabolic bone disease. *Hyperuricemia* can be controlled by drugs that interfere with the production of uric acid such as allopurinol.

Correction of *acidosis* becomes desirable when the serum bicarbonate falls below 15. Any external acid loads, such as aspirin, excess protein intake or infection, should be removed. Sodium bicarbonate is given as long as the sodium load can be tolerated. The goal is to titrate the serum bicarbonate level back to the 16 to 20 range.

Hematologic problems. Anemia in the patient with chronic renal failure may be severe enough to cause symptoms. Androgens have been shown to stimulate red cell production and can be used successfully in some patients. Others may require repeated transfusions. Repeated transfusions carry the risk of hepatitis and may result in sensitization of leukocyte HLA antigens, which may complicate the ease with which a cadaver donor may be found for

renal transplantation. On the other hand, evidence is accumulating to suggest that transfusions prior to transplantation enhance subsequent graft survival. In some centers, prospective transplant candidates are being purposefully transfused prior to transplantation.

Patients with chronic renal failure should be cautioned to avoid antiplatelet drugs. Abnormalities in *platelet function* can be aggravated by drugs such as aspirin. These abnormalities can be corrected by dialysis.

Cardiovascular complications. These are frequent as renal failure advances. The goal of *hypertension* treatment is to decrease pressure without reducing renal perfusion. The preferred antihypertensive agents are hydralazine, alpha-methyldopa and propranolol. Diuretics and ganglionic blockers may compromise glomerular filtration.

The onset of *congestive heart failure* poses a very difficult problem, especially late in the course of the disease when the ability to excrete sodium may be very limited. Salt restriction and a trial of a loop diuretic (e.g., furosemide) may be tried but are often insufficient. Digitalization must be done with care, since renal excretion of digoxin is compromised (see Chapter 27). Dialysis may be the only recourse in patients with refractory fluid overload.

Neuromuscular difficulties. Lethargy, inability to concentrate, and asterixis improve with protein restriction. However, *peripheral neuropathies* often progress in spite of comprehensive conservative therapy. *Muscle cramping* and tetany respond to correction of hypocalcemia.

Itching, hiccups and nausea. These symptoms are not life-threatening, but certainly contribute to the patient's misery and require attention. Pruritus can be quite stubborn, but topical agents for symptomatic relief help. Prochlorperazine is effective in lessening hiccups and nausea.

Adjustment of medications. Doses of drugs that are excreted renally or are nephrotoxic must be adjusted; this is one of the most crucial aspects of chronic renal failure management. Digoxin and aminoglycoside antibiotics are important examples of agents to be used with extreme care in the uremic patient.

Of chief importance is early detection and correction of any condition which may further compromise renal function. Urinary tract infection and gastrointestinal bleeding are among the most common problems that can cause acute decompensation, in addition to those mentioned earlier, i.e., hypertension, congestive heart failure, dehydration, and severe anemia.

PATIENT EDUCATION AND SUPPORT

Successful therapy and good morale are strongly dependent upon a well developed doctor-patient relationship. The patient must be educated about chronic renal failure and the rationale behind therapy, because compliance is central to successful conservative management, especially if the treatment program requires dietary restrictions. Renal failure is a serious chronic disease, often precipitating depression, denial, anger and noncompliance. The physician's patience, understanding, support and interest are powerful but sometimes underutilized elements of the treatment program.

It is important to adapt the treatment program to the patient's psychological style. In general, the patient should have a sense of control over his life by knowing the logic and purpose behind each therapy. Treatment alternatives must be presented honestly, completely and optimistically. It is necessary to include the family in discussions about diet, medications, prognosis and therapeutic options. Psychosocial management should aim at minimizing dependence and social isolation.

INDICATIONS FOR REFERRAL AND ADMISSION

Patients can generally be managed as outpatients, but referral to a nephrologist should be made when hemodialysis or transplantation warrants consideration. Usually, vascular access needs to be constructed about 3 to 4 months prior to the start of hemodialysis to permit maturation of the fistula and allow revision of vascular accesses when needed. When transplantation is anticipated, HLA typing of patient and family should be carried out to identify suitable donors.

Hospitalization may also be required for control of fluid overload, hypertension, hyperkalemia or infection. In general, the multiplicity of possible metabolic disturbances in the patient with chronic renal insufficiency demands careful follow-up and constant adjustments of the treatment program.

MANAGEMENT RECOMMENDATIONS

Protein and Calories

- 0.5 gm./kg. per day of high-quality protein when the patient is symptomatic or acidotic, 0.5–0.75 gm./kg. per day when the BUN is greater than 75 but the patient is asymptomatic.
- Maintain calorie intake at 40 to 50 cal./kg. per day.

Fluids

- With mild to moderate renal insufficiency, fluid restriction is not necessary unless there is concomitant hypertension or congestive heart failure.
- Restrict fluids only in the presence of oliguria. Intake should equal urine output and insensible losses.

Sodium

- With mild to moderate renal insufficiency, salt restriction is not necessary.
- In patients with hypertension or congestive heart failure, salt restriction to 4 gm. of sodium daily may be necessary.
- Restrict sodium in the presence of oliguria or CHF.

Potassium

- In hypokalemia, administer potassium supplements in low doses and check levels frequently. Do not maintain indefinite KCl supplementation.
- Avoid aldosterone-inhibiting diuretics in patients with moderate renal insufficiency.
- Monitor potassium frequently in oliguric patients. Treat levels greater than 6 mEq/liter and admit if ECG changes accompany levels greater than 6.5 mEq/liter. Mild chronic hyperkalemia is best treated with the use of exchange resins such as sodium polystyrene sulfonate (Kayexalate), given by mouth or instilled as an enema in sorbitol. Kayexalate exchanges sodium ion for potassium ion; therefore be alert to possible sodium and volume overload.

Calcium and Phosphate

- Correct hyperphosphatemia with phosphate-binding antacids, usually 30 ml. of aluminum hydroxide gel three times a day before meals.
- Hypocalcemia despite normalization of serum phosphate requires calcium supplements and/or vitamin D in pharmacologic doses.

Acidosis

- Treat when bicarbonate is less than 15 or symptoms attributable to acidosis.
- Remove external acid load.
- Treat acidosis with sodium bicarbonate, 600 mg. twice daily initially, and titrate bicarbonate to the 16–20 range. Follow serum potassium and calcium levels during treatment of acidosis since both may fall.

Anemia

- Transfuse for high output failure or angina. Avoid unnecessary blood work and injections.
- Avoid antiplatelet drugs.
- Oral ferrous sulfate, 325 mg. per day, should be given to patients with iron deficiency.
- Weekly injections of nandrolone decanoate, 100 mg., can be administered to male patients.

Congestive Heart Failure

- Treat with restriction of salt.
- Add furosemide if congestive failure persists.
- Digoxin can be used, but frequent monitoring of digoxen levels is needed.

Itching, Hiccups and Nausea

- Treat uremic complications by controlling the dietary protein intake.
- Prochlorperazine 5–10 mg. p.o. four times daily may be effective for nausea.
- Itching may respond to menthol and phenol lotions or cholestyramine; recently, ultraviolet light has been used successfully.

Dialysis and Transplantation

- The conservative management outlined is directed toward the prolongation of the symptom-free period. When dietary therapy becomes intolerable or is no longer effective, dialysis or transplantation must be considered. Referral to a nephrologist is mandatory at this point. The primary physician should continue to participate in the important decisions about dialysis and transplantation.

ANNOTATED BIBLIOGRAPHY

Baehler, R.W., and Galla, H.J.: Conservative management of chronic renal failure. Geriatrics, September 1976, p. 46. (*A good review.*)

Bennett, W.M., Singer, I., Golper, C.J.; et al.: Guidelines for drug therapy in renal failure. Ann. Intern. Med., *86*:754, 1977. (*Excellent review of drug therapy in patients with renal insufficiency.*)

Feldman, H.A., and Singer, I.: Endocrinology and metabolism in uremia and dialysis: A clinical review. Medicine, *54*:345, 1975. (*Excellent discussion of metabolic conplications of uremia.*)

Giordano, C.: Role of diet in renal disease. Hosp. Pract., November 1977, p. 113. (*A review of nitrogen metabolism, emphasizing reutilization of endogenous nitrogen with advice on dietary management of uremia.*)

Hendler, E.D., Goffinet, J.A., et al.: A controlled study of androgen therapy in anemia of patients on maintenance hemodialysis. N. Engl. J. Med., *291*, 1046, 1974. (*A controlled crossover study demonstrating benefit of androgen therapy.*)

Schwartz, W.B., and Kassirer, J.P.: Medical management of chronic renal failure. Am. J. Med., *44*:786, 1968. (*A symposium that remains a classic reference on the subject.*)

136

Management of the Incontinent Patient

JOHN D. GOODSON, M.D.

Incontinence in the adult patient can result from metabolic, neurologic, or structural abnormalities. Intermittent urine loss is an inconvenience or embarrassment; constant incontinence can predispose to local skin breakdown and serious infection. The primary physician must be attuned to the personal needs of the individual patient, aware of the long-term risks of severe incontinence, and able to use drugs which improve bladder function. Urologic consultation may be necessary.

PATHOPHYSIOLOGY

The detrusor muscle of the bladder is normally under simultaneous sympathetic and parasympathetic control. During the filling phase, sympathetic tone predominates. The detrusor relaxes under beta adrenergic influence. During voluntary emptying, parasympathetic stimulation produces detrusor contraction; at the same time sympathetic tone decreases, the external sphincter of the pelvic floor relaxes, and abdominal muscles tighten. Normally the urethra is oriented to the bladder so as to facilitate continence.

Abnormalities of lower urinary tract function occur at many levels (see Chapter 125 and Table 125–1). Those lesions which affect the reflex arc generally produce a distended, hypotonic bladder and, as a result, voiding consists primarily of uncontrolled spillage. Diabetes, pernicious anemia complicated by subacute combined degeneration, multiple sclerosis, and isolated peripheral neuropathies are the most frequent etiologies. Viral and bacterial infections of the spinal cord, nerve roots or peripheral nerves can have similar effects.

Severe outflow obstruction, such as occurs with progressive benign prostatic hypertrophy (BPH) or chronic prostatitis, can lead to bladder atony if the detrusor muscle fails.

Structural abnormalities of the pelvic floor affect the internal and external sphincters and impair normal voluntary control mechanisms. As a result, the patient is unable to store urine between voidings. Pelvic relaxation and cystocele formation from previous vaginal delivery or perineal surgery are common causes of such incontinence in women. In men, damage to the external sphincter from prostatic surgery can impair control.

Any condition which irritates the bladder, especially the trigonal region, will interfere with the internal sphincter. In some patients, a urinary tract infection may be sufficient to produce partial loss of bladder control.

Finally, urinary continence depends on intact frontal lobe function. Patients with cortical degenerative diseases or normopressure hydrocephalus (NPH) may be unaware of their own voiding patterns, and therefore will be functionally incontinent.

CLINICAL PRESENTATION AND COURSE

The clinical presentation of the incontinent patient can vary from occasional inadvertent voiding associated with coughing or straining to constant urine leakage. In some patients, incontinence develops slowly, while in others the onset is abrupt. The symptom complex and its onset can be helpful in identifying the cause in individual cases.

Structural abnormalities are common; they are suggested by a history of perineal trauma or surgery. In female patients, perineal operations or repeated vaginal deliveries are frequent antecedent events. Such patients become symptomatic over an extended period of time and will usually give a history of worsening stress incontinence. Male patients may report rapidly developing symptoms following prostatic surgery.

The patient with an abnormality in the reflex arc may be more difficult to identify. In the extreme case, he will complain of abdominal fullness and discomfort due to an enlarged bladder. In most cases, however, the arc is only partially impaired. There may or may not be historical evidence to suggest a systemic disease such as diabetes, pernicious anemia, tabes dorsalis, or a toxic neuropathy. Careful examination will be necessary (see Chapter 125).

The patient with incontinence due to self-neglect will generally present with frontal lobe findings. Normopressure hydrocephalus (NPH) will also be associated with dementia and gait instability (see Chapter 157). The family will frequently give a history of progressive deterioration of mental competence and attention span.

Regardless of the suspected abnormality, rapid deterioration of continence must suggest the possibility of a urinary tract infection (UTI). In some patients, especially the elderly, the classic UTI symptom complex of dysuria, urgency, and frequency may be lacking.

MANAGEMENT RECOMMENDATIONS

- All patients should be carefully screened for diabetes (see Chapter 91), tabes dorsalis (see Chapter 119) pernicious anemia (see Chapter 77), toxic neuropathies and urinary tract infection (see Chapter 120).
- Regardless of whether the primary abnormality is sphincter incompetence or bladder atony, fluid loads, coffee, tea and alcohol should be avoided. The physician should limit the use of diuretics, scheduling them to be given in the morning, and the use of anticholinergics or anticholinergic-like drugs (tranquilizers, antidepressants and antipsychotics), if possible.

- Patients with bladder atony should be told to void frequently. The use of the Credé maneuver (low abdominal pressure applied externally during voiding) will facilitate bladder emptying.
- Patients with mild pelvic floor weakness should be instructed to exercise the perineal muscles involved with stream termination. Males should be told to contract the anal sphincter in a regular daily exercise pattern. Females should be instructed to do the same with the vaginal sphincter. Some women show improvement of the urethrovesicular angle with the use of a vaginal tampon and regain urinary control. In some men, postoperative incontinence is difficult to treat, and occasionally a penile clamp is required.
- The cholinergic agonist bethanechol (Urecholine) can be used to improve detrusor contractility in patients with mild bladder atony that is not due to outflow obstruction. A dose of 10 to 50 mg. orally four times a day is titrated to the patient's needs. The adrenergic agonist phenylephrine given orally in a dose of 20 to 40 mg. per day can be used to improve bladder neck tone and restore control of urination in the presence of weakened pelvic musculature and following surgical instrumentation of the urethra. Repeated cystometrograms are necessary for monitoring the effects of these drugs.
- Surgical intervention should be considered if there is urethral obstruction. Pelvic reconstructive procedures should be considered in women with severe stress incontinence. Urologic consultation is necessary in evaluating these patients.
- The patient and family should be taught the need for local hygiene, particularly elderly patients in whom surgery is impractical and pharmacologic intervention is too dangerous. The use of diapers and frequent bathing should be encouraged. Macerated skin must be gently cleansed and kept dry with frequent turning and hot lamps.

ANNOTATED BIBLIOGRAPHY

Khanna, O.P.: Disorders of micturition. Urology 8:316, 1976. *(Excellent review of bladder neuropharmacology and various treatment modalities.)*

Turner-Warwick, R., and Whiteside, C.G.: Clinical urodynamics. Urol. Clin. North Am., 6:1, 1979. *(The entire issue is devoted to the subject of urodynamics.)*

Wein, A.J., Raezer, D.M., and Benson, G.S.: Management of neurogenic bladder dysfunction in the adult. Urology 8:432, 1976. *(Short review of the approach to the patient with a neurogenic bladder.)*

137

Management of Genitourinary Cancers

JACOB J. LOKICH, M.D.

Cancers of the genitourinary tract are comparable in incidence to those of the gastrointestinal (GI) tract, with approximately 175,000 cases annually. Unlike GI malignancies, a number of these tumors are slow-growing, readily detectable in the early stages, and responsive to radiation or chemotherapy or curable by surgery. A less favorable characteristic of these malignancies is their ability to obstruct the urinary tract, producing infection and renal failure.

The genitourinary cancers may be separated into three categories: genital carcinomas in men, genital carcinomas in women, and pure urinary carcinomas, the last including carcinomas of the kidney and bladder. Carcinomas of the ureter, urethra, and accessory organs are rare and therefore relatively inconsequential.

The tumors of the genitourinary tract are often localized and managed singularly by surgery or by radiation therapy. The primary care physician, however, has an important role in early diagnosis and in therapeutic management of advanced disease, particularly those tumors that are responsive to drug management such as prostatic and testicular carcinomas.

Carcinoma of the Prostate

EPIDEMIOLOGY

Malignancy in the prostate gland is age-related, and it is estimated that by the age of 80 more than 50 per cent of men may have an adenocarcinoma within the prostate gland. Prostatic cancer has, therefore, been thought to represent a degenerative process as much as a neoplastic one. The condition is often approached therapeutically as an incidental development, since mortality in the elderly is frequently secondary to another disease. In fact, however, the morbidity and mortality rates from prostatic cancer are substantial, and every case warrants a meticulous clinical approach to therapy.

CLINICAL PRESENTATION AND COURSE

Malignancy in the prostate gland often presents as urethral obstruction; occasionally, the clinical picture of acute renal failure may be observed. Bone is the most common site of metastases. Osteoblastic metastases predominate, and, unlike those from breast cancer, prostatic metastases are commonly painful. Bone pain is the overwhelmingly prevalent cause of morbidity from prostate cancer.

Two rare clinical disorders associated with prostatic cancer represent unique complications. Cushing's syndrome has been reported in cases of prostate cancer, related to the production of adrenocorticotropic hormone (ACTH) by the tumor with secondary adrenal hyperplasia. In patients who undergo adrenalectomy to control progressive disease, incidental adrenal adenomas have been described. Such patients may be among those having Cushing's syndrome associated with prostatic cancer; mechanism is unknown.

A second clinical disorder associated with prostate cancer is bronchogenic carcinoma. In patients with underlying prostate cancer who subsequently develop pulmonary lesions, the most likely cause of the lesion is a second primary tumor originating from the lung, considering the rarity of pulmonary metastases from prostate cancer and the 15 per cent frequency of bronchogenic carcinoma in patients with prostate cancer.

PRINCIPLES OF MANAGEMENT

Extension of the tumor beyond the capsule of the prostate gland mandates a systemic approach to therapy, but localized tumor (Stages A and B) may be managed either by *local surgery* or by *radiation therapy* to the pelvis. Both methods of treatment are associated with a substantial incidence of impotence, and this feature may be of critical importance to the patient.

Local palliation and relief of pain from bone lesions are achieved promptly with radiation therapy, but the mainstay of therapy is a systemic hormonal treatment. Since the late 1940s and the studies of Charles Huggins, hormonal therapy has been a standard form of treatment for metastatic prostate cancer. Orchiectomy has produced significant tumor regression, as measured by relief of pain from bony metastases or reduction in the size of the primary tumor.

Hormone therapy for prostate cancer involves a variety of options, ranging from orchiectomy to use of estrogens and antiandrogen medications. Androgens stimulate the tumor, and the removal of the primary source of androgens by orchiectomy removes most endogenous hormone production, although it

Table 137-1. Exogenous Hormone Therapy for Prostatic Cancer

HORMONE	DOSE SCHEDULE	COMMENT
Antiandrogens		
Cyproterone	Investigational	Unavailable at present
Flutamide	Investigational	
Chlormadimone	Investigational	
Estrogens		
Diethylstilbestrol	1-5 mg. daily	Response in 75% of patients
Ethinyl estradiol (Estinyl)	1 mg. daily	Response in 75% of patients
Diethylstilbestrol diphosphate (Stilphostrol)		Intravenous preparation
Miscellaneous		
Estramustine	Investigational	Investigational, combined estrogen and alkylating drug
Progesterone	Variable	Unevaluated
Tamoxifen	10 mg. twice daily	Limited effectiveness

does not affect the secondary source, the adrenal glands. In fact, adrenalectomy and hypophysectomy have been used as tertiary therapeutic measures. Before such ablative surgery is resorted to, hormonal preparations should be administered (Table 137–1).

Hormone therapy should be reserved for patients who do not respond to orchiectomy or who refuse the procedure; hormones should not be used concomitantly with orchiectomy. The principal class of hormones used has been estrogens, which function as competitive inhibitors or blockers of circulating androgens, presumably competing for androgen receptor sites on the tumor cell. The effect of diethylstilbestrol or ethinyl estradiol is comparable to orchiectomy in inducing tumor regression. However, a primary complication of estrogen therapy, particularly high doses given to the elderly, has been secondary vascular thrombosis, both arterial and venous. This complication may develop as a consequence of a drug-induced hypercoagulable state compounded by the presence of malignancy and advanced age. In this clinical setting, the concomitant use of either salicylates or coumarin anticoagulation may be employed. An intravenous diethylstilbestrol preparation, Stilphostrol, is available and was initially thought to have important clinical advantages, but it is associated with substantial nausea and vomiting. Estrogens may also cause marked gynecomastia, which may be prevented in patients on estrogen therapy by radiation to the breast. All men who undergo estrogen therapy should receive prophylactic, single-dose breast irradiation.

An alternative hormonal approach employs *antiandrogens,* such as flutamide, which are peripheral inhibitors of the androgen effect. Although they also produce impotence, they do not induce either the hypercoagulable state or the debilitating gynecomastia associated with estrogen therapy. The other hormone preparations listed in Table 137–1 are either of limited effectiveness or unavailable for general use.

MONITORING THERAPY

Acid phosphatase elevations have been associated with prostate cancer and, rarely, with Gaucher's disease. A specific acid phosphatase fraction unique to prostate cancer has recently been identified. However, an elevated serum level of the enzyme can be found in only 50 per cent of patients with metastatic prostate cancer, and the quantitative level is not directly related to the host tumor burden. Nonetheless, *serum acid phosphatase* is a useful monitor of the ef-

fectiveness of treatment and may be employed in conjunction with serial measurements of plasma carcinoembryonic antigen. Still, any specific correlation with the antitumor effect should incorporate additional objective and subjective parameters of tumor response.

Testicular Cancer
EPIDEMIOLOGY

Testicular cancer is the most common malignancy in men between the ages of 20 and 30.

CLINICAL PRESENTATION AND COURSE

Both seminomas and nonseminomatous germinal tumors commonly present as painless testicular masses in young men (see Chapter 127). These are rapidly growing tumors that spread by the lymphatics and blood.

PRINCIPLES OF MANAGEMENT

Testicular tumors grow rapidly. Seminomas are exquisitely responsive to *radiation therapy* and cured in more than 90 per cent of cases. Germ-cell tumors that have extended beyond the testicle have a cure rate of less than 50 per cent. *Chemotherapy* is often effective and may improve survival.

A solid, nontransilluminating, painless testicular mass in a young man should be presumed to represent a primary testicular carcinoma and needs to be treated by *testicle removal* through an inguinal canal approach (as opposed to a transscrotal operative procedure).

Staging includes chest film and lung tomograms, lymphangiogram, and assays for alpha-fetoprotein and human chorionic gonadotropin. If there is no evidence of metastatic disease, an ipsilateral complete *lymphadenectomy* and a contralateral partial lymphadenectomy to the level of the aortic bifurcation are mandatory. Retrograde ejaculation commonly develops after the lymphadenectomy, and in some instances it may not be fully reversible. In addition to these staging procedures, a blind supraclavicular exploration and biopsy of scalene nodes may be performed to ensure that there are no microscopic or occult metastases.

For patients with a tumor identified in the retroperitoneal lymph nodes or in visceral sites (most commonly in the lungs), multiple-agent chemotherapy is employed. An important breakthrough in the management of testicular cancer has been made in the last 5 years. Even patients with metastatic disease have a chance for cure as a consequence of the development of a new drug, *cis-platinum,* used in conjunction with vinblastine and bleomycin in a three-drug combination program. This regimen has produced remission and cure in some cases.

Ovarian Cancer
CLINICAL PRESENTATION

Carcinoma of the ovary is an occult tumor, with more than 40 per cent of patients presenting with advanced local, extrapelvic, or intra-abdominal disease. The occult location of the tumor in the pelvis and the cystic nature of these neoplasms may allow for enormous tumor growth before any clinical signs or symptoms develop.

PRINCIPLES OF THERAPY

Therapeutic options in ovarian cancer are substantial and include surgery, radiation therapy, and chemotherapy. The tumor is exquisitely responsive. *Surgery* for ovarian cancer often necessitates "debulking" or tumor removal. Omentectomy as well as total abdominal hysterectomy and bilateral salpingo-oophorectomy are performed, in addition to the reduction of tumor masses throughout the abdominal cavity. This is believed to lessen the host tumor burden and increase the effectiveness of ancillary or adjunctive therapeutic modalities, such as radiation or chemotherapy.

Radiation therapy to the pelvis or to the abdomen (for patients with disease that extends beyond the pelvis) has been advocated as a routine adjunct to surgery and as a palliative procedure. The impact on survival has not been established. The rationale for abdominal and pelvic irradiation is based on the fact that ovarian tumors not infrequently cause recurrent ascites and bowel obstruction, leading to progressive inanition as a consequence of malabsorption and protein sequestration in the abdominal space. Other forms of radiation therapy (e.g., those using ^{32}P or ^{198}Au) have been employed with some success, both as an adjuvant therapy in patients with ascites and as a primary therapeutic modality.

The *alkylating drugs* have been the mainstay of systemic therapy for ovarian cancer. The simplest regimen uses one drug, such as melphalan or phenylalanine mustard. When alkylating drugs are employed in intermittent courses—monthly or every 6 weeks—30 per cent of patients with extensive abdominal tumor respond, and a substantial proportion of patients achieve a complete response for an extended period of time. Recently, the combination of an alkylating drug with doxorubicin (Adriamycin) or cis-platinum has achieved response in up to 80 per cent of patients. The effect on survival of combination chemotherapy regimens, compared to that of single-agent regimens, has yet to be established. The achievement of more substantial regression of disease, confirmed by "second-look" operations, suggests that multiple-modality and multiple-drug therapies should be the standard approach to ovarian cancer.

Carcinoma of the Uterus
CLINICAL PRESENTATION

Endometrial cancer and cancer of the uterine cervix are frequently detected early as a consequence of routine Pap screening or early vaginal bleeding (see Chapter 106).

PRINCIPLES OF THERAPY

The management of these tumors is almost exclusively the responsibility of the gynecologic surgeon and rarely involves the primary care physician. Nonetheless, in some patients with tumors of the uterus, the disease recurs or metastasizes, necessitating palliative management. The use of progesterone for endometrial cancer has been advocated, although the data in the literature are predominantly anecdotal. Responses are achieved for the most part in patients with pulmonary nodules and not in patients who have pelvic extension of the tumor or who have received prior radiation therapy. More than 50 per cent of patients have responded to chemotherapy using cyclophosphamide (Cytoxan) and doxorubicin (Adriamycin). This combination regimen should be considered the standard form of treatment for patients who do not have a co-morbid problem, such as heart disease, that precludes the use of either the alkylating drugs or doxorubicin.

Cancers of the uterine cervix are epidermoid or squamous in origin, as opposed to the glandular carcinomas of the endometrium, and are not hormonally responsive. Radiation therapy can often cure localized disease. For patients who relapse, bleomycin is used in combination with vincristine and mitomycin C or methotrexate. Methotrexate has been associated with renal impairment; since many of the patients with recurrent cervical cancer develop ureteral obstruction, the use of methotrexate may be precluded.

Renal Cell Carcinoma (Hypernephroma)
CLINICAL PRESENTATION AND COURSE

Renal cell carcinoma is notorious for its many confusing presentations. It may cause fever of unknown origin, occult hematuria; or be the source of excess erythropoetin, parathormone-like substance, renin, or prostaglandin. In addition, an unusual syndrome of hepatic dysfunction has been described which regresses with removal of the primary tumor and occurs in the absence of liver metastases.

The natural history of the tumor is unique. It has been associated with spontaneous regression as well as long intervals before the appearance of metastases, which may be curable when solitary and to the lung. Moreover, there are reports that metastatic disease may show regression when the primary is removed although this latter issue is rare and controversial.

PRINCIPLES OF THERAPY

When tumor is confined to the kidney, cure is commonplace; when it extends beyond Gerota's capsule, the prognosis is quite poor. A major proportion of patients with hypernephroma present with or develop metastases in the presence of the primary tumor; management of the primary and secondary lesions is problematic. Some authorities suggest that removal of the primary tumor may be associated with regression of metastases, although a total of only 45 to 50 cases have been reported in the literature. Large series have failed to demonstrate that removal of the primary tumor in the presence of metastases significantly affects survival or regression of metastases. Therefore, the primary tumor should be removed only if there is local pain or hemorrhage. Metastases in the lung, bone, or brain are more specifically managed by drug or radiation therapy.

Systemic therapy for renal cell carcinoma has not identified any active chemotherapeutic drugs. Two important reviews have suggested that vinblastine and, possibly, doxorubicin in combination with a nitrosourea may have a modicum of activity, but other

published data are lacking. Hormone therapy, and particularly progesterone and androgens, has been associated with responses in about 20 per cent of patients, although the responses are not necessarily associated with prolonged survival.

Bladder Cancer
EPIDEMIOLOGY

Patients at increased risk of bladder cancer include heavy smokers, those exposed to naphthalene from industrial contact, and patients who have used cyclophosphamide. There are no long-term epidemiological data at present on the relation between saccharin and bladder cancer, although animal studies suggest an association. The issue remains controversial.

CLINICAL PRESENTATION

Tumors of the bladder are usually detected early in association with gross or microscopic hematuria (see Chapter 123). Specific monitoring of patients at high risk for bladder cancer with urinary cytology is advocated (see Chapter 122).

PRINCIPLES OF THERAPY

The tumor is often curable with local surgery or radiation therapy. Metastatic bladder cancer uncommonly extends beyond the pelvis, but, with metastases to the lung, the use of systemic chemotherapy must be considered. The development of regimens that employ cis-platinum in conjunction with cyclophosphamide and doxorubicin have achieved substantial regression in patients with metastatic disease. For local recurrence of tumor resistant to radiation, chemotherapy may be introduced into the bladder.

ANNOTATED BIBLIOGRAPHY

Bagshaw, M.A., Ray, G.R., Pistenma, D.A., Castellino, R.A., and Meares, E.M., Jr.: External beam radiation therapy of primary carcinoma of the prostate. Cancer, *36*:723, 1975. *(A summary of the use of radiation therapy for carcinoma of the prostate employing high-dose extended field therapy in the Stanford University tradition. In* the total population of more than 400 patients the efficacy of radiation therapy appears comparable to surgery.)

Blackard, C.: The Veterans Administration Cooperative Urological Research Group Studies of carcinoma of the prostate: A review. Cancer Chemo. Rep., *59*:225, 1975. *(A summary of the impact of estrogen therapy on prostate cancer in more than 3,000 patients and a analysis of the effect of estrogen in inducing cardiovascular deaths. The controversial original publication by the VA study group is clarified.)*

Carter, S.K., and Wasserman, T.H.: The chemotherapy of urologic cancer. Cancer, *36*:729, 1975. *(A comprehensive analysis of single agents and ongoing national programs employing chemotherpy for cancers of the prostate, bladder and kidney as well as the testes.)*

Einhorn, L.H., and Donohue, J.: Cis-diamminedichloroplatinum, vinblastine, and bleomycin combination chemotherapy in disseminated testicular cancer. Ann. Intern. Med., *87*:293, 1977. *(The original publication of the three-drug regimen is reported for disseminated testicular cancer with an 85 per cent disease-free status.)*

Huggins, C., and Hodges, C.V.: The effect of castration, of estrogen and of androgen injection on serum phosphatases in metastatic carcinoma of the prostate. Cancer Res., March 22, 1941. *(This classic article presents the first awareness of the* influence of hormones on prostate cancer and served as a basis for the Nobel Prize for Charles Huggins.)

Lokich, J.J., Harrison, J.H.; Renal cell carcinoma: Natural history and chemotherapeutic experience. J. Urol., *114*:371, 1975. *(A review of the natural history of renal cell carcinoma at a single institution and the experience with hormone therapy and chemotherapy. The association of paraneoplastic syndromes, splenomegaly, bilaterality of tumors, and delayed appearance of metastases is indicated. The lack of response to systemic forms of treatment is emphasized)*

Staubitz, W.J., Early, K.S., Magoss, I.V., and Murphy, G.P.: Surgical treatment of nonseminomatous germinal testes tumors. Cancer *32*:1206, 1973. *(Surgical approach to testicular cancer is reviewed in general as well as specifically citing an experience in more than 70 patients. This work and that of Skinner [J. Urol., 106:84, 1971] serve as the basis for the surgical approach.)*

Tobias, J.S., and Griffiths, C.T.: Management of ovarian carcinoma: Current concepts and future prospects. N. Engl. J. Med., *294*:818, 1976. *(An updated review of the approach to ovarian cancer in two parts incorporating surgery, chemotherapy, and radiotherapy and an analysis of the concept of second-look operations and debulking.)*

10

Musculoskeletal Problems

138
Evaluation of Acute Monoarticular Arthritis

The patient with acute monoarticular arthritis must be diagnosed promptly because of the possibility of an infectious etiology and its potential for rapid joint destruction. Proper recognition of noninfectious causes is also of importance because a number of these conditions are readily treatable.

PATHOPHYSIOLOGY AND CLINICAL PRESENTATION

The major pathogenic mechanisms of acute monoarticular arthritis are bloodborne infection, nonsuppurative immunologically mediated inflammation, crystal-induced inflammation, and trauma. Regardless of etiology, joint manifestations are similar. The joint is painful, tender and swollen; it may be warm and erythematous as well.

Septic arthritis derives predominantly from hematogenous seeding of the synovium. Once in a while, direct extension from a site of trauma or from osteomyelitis is encountered. Among previously healthy patients, *disseminated gonorrhea* is the most frequent etiology of joint infection. Dissemination occurs in about 1 to 3 per cent of individuals with gonorrhea (see Chapter130). Over 80 per cent of individuals with disseminated gonococcal infection

develop arthritis. Women account for two-thirds of cases; pregnancy and menstruation increase the risk of dissemination. Initially, there is a bacteremic stage with fever, polyarthralgias, minimal joint effusion, necrotic skin lesions, positive blood cultures and sterile joint fluid. This phase of the illness is followed in about 5 days by a septic joint stage, with monoarticular or occasionally polyarticular pain, marked joint swelling, effusion, and resolution of skin lesions. During the septic joint stage, gonococci can be recovered from the joint in about 50 per cent of patients. The bacteremic stage occurs within 3 days of onset of symptoms, and septic arthritis within 8 days.

Acute nongonococcal septic arthritis occurs in patients with altered host defenses (diabetes, cirrhosis, immunoproliferative disease, immunosuppressive therapy) or damaged joints (trauma, rheumatoid arthritis). Gram-positive organisms account for most nongonococcal infections, with *Staph. aureus* being the leading cause. Gram-negative organisms may be responsible for infections in very debilitated, chronically ill patients. Gram-negative infection is most likely to occur in an inpatient setting. Onset is typically acute (except in patients with rheumatoid arthritis). Fever, chills and joint complaints are prominent. If the patient is very debilitated or immunosuppressed, fever may be indolent. The larger joints are most likely to become involved. In a series of 59 patients with nongonococcal joint infection, 75 per cent presented with knee infection; the remainder of cases involved the shoulders, wrists, elbows, hips or ankles.

Articular destruction can be rapid. Within 10 days of nongonococcal infection, radiographic evidence of cartilage and bone damage may appear. Joint injury from gonococcal arthritis is less precipitous.

Acute gout is among the most common causes of acute monoarticular arthritis. Uric acid crystals in the joint fluid incite a brisk inflammatory response after their ingestion by polymorphonuclear leukocytes. The condition predominates among middle-aged and elderly men. Onset is rapid, peaking within 12 to 24 hours. The great toe is the classic site, but ankles, wrists, knees and olecranon bursae are other important locations. A dusky, reddened skin often develops over the inflamed joint, and can extend beyond it. Crystals of uric acid are found in the joint fluid; they are needlelike and negatively birefringent when viewed under the polarizing microscope. The serum uric acid may be normal at the time of an attack. Tophi, hypertriglyceridemia, hypertension, mild diabetes and obesity are associated findings in some patients (see Chapter 149).

Pseudogout resembles gout pathophysiologically, though clinical features differ. The condition results from crystals of calcium pyrophosphate inducing joint inflammation. Chondrocalcinosis is usually present. About 4 to 5 per cent of elderly patients with degenerative joint disease demonstrate calcium pyrophosphate deposition in the fibrocartilage. Most are asymptomatic, but on occasion an acute arthritis flares in the knee, wrist or shoulder. Men and women are affected with equal frequency. Under the polarizing microscope, the crystals show weakly positive birefringence and a blunted appearance. X-rays may reveal calcium deposition in the joint space, indicative of chondrocalcinosis. Ten per cent of patients with chondrocalcinosis have an underlying endocrinologic disease such as hyperparathyroidism, hemochromatosis, myxedema or diabetes.

Rheumatoid arthritis is associated with an increased incidence of septic arthritis, but may by itself give rise to an acutely inflamed joint. Occasionally the disease starts out as an acute monoarticular problem. There are no unique features to the acute arthritis, unless some pre-existing rheumatoid manifestations are present, such as subcutaneous nodules, morning stiffness, ulnar deviation, or symmetrical metacarpophalangeal and proximal interphalangeal joint involvement (see Chapter 139).

Reiter's syndrome most often causes an acute asymmetrical polyarthritis, but in the early stages one joint may predominate. Knees, ankles, metatarsophalangeal joints and proximal interphalangeal joints are typical sites of the arthritis; sacroiliac and spinal involvement can also occur. Conjunctivitis, urethritis, balanitis or keratoderma blennorrhagicum of the soles may precede the arthritis or appear later (see Chapter 126). Young males are primarily affected; about 75 per cent are HLA-B27 positive.

Ankylosing spondylitis is another disease of young men which can cause acute monoarticular inflammation; however, spinal involvement manifested by low back pain and stiffness is usually the initial presentation. Arthritis of the hip, knee or shoulder eventually develops in about 25 per cent, and on rare occasions may precede back symptoms and present as an acute monoarticular arthritis. Over 90 per cent of white patients are HLA-B27 positive; in contrast, only 50 per cent of blacks show B27 positivity.

The acute arthritis of *inflammatory bowel disease* resembles ankylosing spondylitis in its spinal manifestations, but peripheral joint involvement is more common. Onset of arthritis is typically acute, usually in a single joint of the leg, followed in a few days by arthritis in other joints. Knees and ankles are most frequently affected; proximal interphalangeal, elbow, shoulder and wrist joints may also become inflamed. Arthritis is seen in patients between the ages of 25 and 45, at least 6 months or more after an attack of colitis. It is uncommon for the arthritis to precede gastrointestinal symptoms. Patients with systemic manifestations of the disease (uveitis, erythema nodosum, mucosal ulcers) are more likely to suffer from arthritis (see Chapter 65).

Psoriatic arthritis appears in several forms and affects about 7 per cent of patients with psoriasis. The most frequent variety produces acute swelling and pain of one to three interphalangeal digits ("sausage" fingers); the flexor tendon sheath becomes inflamed, as well. Psoriatic skin lesions precede onset by months to years in most cases; rarely, the arthritis predates or coincides with the development of skin changes. Nail pitting is characteristic. Women outnumber men by a small percentage, and age of onset is similar to that of rheumatoid arthritis, with which it may be confused.

Trauma can produce an acute effusion, often due to hemarthrosis. On occasion a hairline fracture of the subchondral bone will be noted. Since traumatic effusions resolve spontaneously within 10 to 14 days, persistence of pain and swelling indicates another etiology. Trauma to periarticular soft tissue may also cause acute swelling and pain referable to the joint.

DIFFERENTIAL DIAGNOSIS

The differential diagnosis of acute pain and swelling in a single joint includes infections, crystal-induced arthropathy and trauma. The gonococcus is the leading infectious agent, followed in frequency by gram-positive organisms (staphylococci, steptococci and pneumococci), and in compromised hosts by gram-negative coliforms, *Salmonella* and *Pseudomonas*. Gout and pseudogout are the important crystal-induced etiologies.

Several polyarticular diseases may initially present with one acutely inflamed joint or with symptoms that are greatest in a single joint. These mono-articular presentations of polyarticular disease are seen in rheumatoid arthritis, Reiter's syndrome, ankylosing spondylitis, psoriatic arthritis and the arthritis of inflammatory bowel disease.

Joint pain may occur as a result of inflammation of soft tissue or vessels adjacent to the joint, as in cellulitis or thrombophlebitis. Traumatic or inflammatory processes in the adjacent periarticular structures include tendinitis, peritendinitis, ligamentous strain and bursitis.

WORKUP

History. The first objective is to establish whether or not the joint is infected. Although examination of the joint fluid is the single most important diagnostic test, history may provide useful information regarding the likelihood of an infectious etiology as well as a source of infection. Abrupt onset in conjunction with fever and chills points to a septic etiology, as does a history of skin lesions, vaginal or urethral discharge, gonorrhea exposure, diabetes, concurrent rheumatoid arthritis, immunosuppression, or previous trauma. Occurrence of acute trauma is suggestive of periarticular injury or hemarthrosis. A history of previous attacks suggests gout or pseudogout. Location is of some help diagnostically. Inflammation in the big toe points to gout, especially in an elderly male; but in diabetics, extension of osteomyelitis into the joint must be ruled out. Large joints, particularly the knees, are the most common sites of

nongonococcal septic arthritis. Associated back pain raises the possibility of one of the spondyloarthropathies. The patient's age can be an important clue. Pseudogout is most common in older patients, unless there is an underlying endocrinopathy causing chondrocalcinosis. Disseminated gonococcal infection is more common among sexually active young people. Reiter's syndrome and ankylosing spondylitis are also diseases of young people.

Physical examination should include a recording of the rectal temperature. Almost all patients with septic arthritis will be febrile. Low-grade fever may also be noted in gout and rheumatoid arthritis, but a high fever suggests infection. Inspection of the skin should include a search for necrotic skin lesions on the extremities (indicative of disseminated gonorrhea), tophi, rheumatoid nodules, pitting of the nails and other psoriatic manifestations, erythema nodosum, the hyperkeratotic blisters of keratoderma blennorrhagicum, and circinate balanitis. The eyes are examined for conjunctivitis and iritis, the mouth for mucosal ulceration and the heart for murmurs; aortic insufficiency is found in some of the spondyloarthropathies.

All joints must be carefully examined to be certain that the problem is limited to one joint; inspection may reveal more than one inflamed area. It is important to be sure that the joint and not a periarticular structure is the site of the problem. Sometimes this distinction is impossible to make, but preservation of range of motion despite pain in the area reduces the likelihood of joint involvement. The probability of a periarticular process is increased by finding tenderness and swelling centered about a soft tissue structure, rather than over the joint space. The spine should be examined carefully for restriction of motion and tenderness, indicative of spondylitis. The genitalia need to be checked for any discharge which must be cultured for gonorrhea.

Laboratory studies. Aspirating and examining *joint fluid* is the single most important diagnostic procedure in the evaluation of acute monoarticular arthritis. A turbid appearance to the fluid points to an inflammatory etiology, blood suggests trauma, and a straw-colored fluid is seen with degenerative disease and minor trauma. The fluid should be Gram stained; in about 60 per cent of cases, the Gram stain will reveal the causative organism. It is most important to immediately culture the joint fluid onto proper media (including Thayer-Martin plates for detection of gonococci). Smears of the joint fluid may show organisms in the absence of a positive culture if antibiotics have already been taken. A repeat tap of the joint will improve the diagnostic yield of Gram stain and culture if the first arthrocentesis is negative.

Other studies to be performed on the joint fluid include a white cell count and differential, mucin clot assessment, glucose determination and polarizing microscope examination for crystals. With the exceptions of Gram stain, culture, and examination for crystals, no single test result is diagnostic. The white cell count, differential, glucose and mucin clot are helpful when considered together. A white count greater than 100,000 with 95 per cent or more polymorphonuclear cells and a glucose below 25 is strongly suggestive of infection. However, gonococcal arthritis often does not cause a sharp fall in glucose while rheumatoid arthritis can; a white count in the 50,000 range does not rule out a septic joint. The mucin clot is friable in all inflammatory effusions.

Two *blood cultures* should be obtained when an infectious etiology is suspected. *CBC, sedimentation rate, rheumatoid factor* and *serum uric acid* are often ordered, but usually are of only marginal utility compared to examination of the joint fluid. The same is true for x-ray studies in the early stage of acute joint inflammation, since most films reveal only soft tissue swelling, regardless of etiology. About 10 to 14 days later, narrowing of the joint margin and subchondral bone erosion may be noted in a septic joint, but not within the first week. In acute cases, x-ray findings are present in patients with chondrocalcinosis or fracture. In chondrocalcinosis there is calcification along the joint margin.

A few other studies may occasionally contribute to evaluation. An *HLA-B27 determination* can be helpful when there is a question of Reiter's syndrome or ankylosing spondylitis. A *biopsy* of the synovium should be considered in the setting of a chronic undiagnosed monoarticular arthritis, because tumor (e.g., pigmented villonodular synovitis) and chronic infection (e.g., tuberculosis) need to be ruled out.

SYMPTOMATIC MANAGEMENT

Until a diagnosis is established, the patient may feel better with rest, immobility of the joint, and warm packs. Use of anti-inflammatory agents should be postponed for at least 12 hours to allow for repeat arthrocentesis if the first one is nondiagnostic. If pain is unbearable and a diagnosis is not yet established, an analgesic without anti-inflammatory effects (e.g., codeine) may be used. After a second negative arth-

rocentesis, it is reasonable to institute anti-inflammatory therapy empirically in the absence of a specific diagnosis as long as gout and infection have been ruled out. Aspirin is safe for initial use. More definitive therapy must be based on an etiologic diagnosis (see Chapters 113, 147, 149).

INDICATIONS FOR REFERRAL AND ADMISSION

Septic arthritis requires hospital admission, treatment with intravenous antibiotics, and consultation with an infectious disease specialist. Cases of monoarticular arthritis which remain undiagnosed should be reviewed with a rheumatologist.

ANNOTATED BIBLIOGRAPHY

Bilka, P.J.: Physical examination of the arthritic patient. Bull. Rheum. Dis., *20*:596, 1970. *(An excellent discussion of the usefulness of physical examination.)*

Edeiken, J.: Arthritis: The roles of the primary care physician and the radiologist. JAMA, *232*:1364, 1975. *(Differentiates between those conditions which have mainly clinical findings from those with specific roentgenographic manifestations.)*

Fries, J.F., and Mitchell, D.M.: Joint pain or arthritis. JAMA, *235*:199, 1976. *(An excellent flow chart based article emphasizing judicious use of the laboratory.)*

Gelman, M.I., and Ward, J.R.: Septic Arthrits: A complication of rheumatoid arthritis. Radiology, *122*:17, 1977. *(Points out the problem of detecting superimposed infection and suggests radiologic criteria to help in identification.)*

Goldenberg, D.L., and Cohen, A.S.: Acute infectious arthritis: A review of patients with nongonococcal joint infections (with emphasis on therapy and prognosis). Am. J. Med., *60*:369, 1976. *(A review of clinical and laboratory data in 59 patients. Many had Gram-negative infections.)*

Hansfield, H.H., Wiesner P.J., and Holmes, K.K: Treatment of gonococcal arthritis-dermatitis syndrome. Ann. Intern. Med., *84*:661, 1976. *(High-dose I.V. penicillin G or oral ampicillin alone was effective.)*

Holmes, K., Counts, G., and Beaty, H.: Disseminated gonococcal infection. Ann. Intern. Med.,

74:979, 1971. *(Arthritis occurred in 38 of 42 patients with disseminated disease. Classic paper describing the syndrome, with 141 refs.)*

McCarty, D. J.: A basic guide to arthrocentesis. Hosp. Med., *77*: November 1968. *(A clear, well-illustrated guide to this important procedure.)*

Mitchell, W.S., Brooke P.M., Stevenson R.D., et al.:

Septic arthritis in patients with rheumatoid disease. J. Rheumatol, *3*:124, 1976. *(Thorough discussion of pathophysiology and diagnosis.)*

Newman, J.H.: Review of septic arthritis throughout the antibiotic era. Ann. Rheum. Dis., *35*:198, 1976. *(Little change in incidence or distribution of organisms. Poor prognosis is due to delay.)*

139

Evaluation of Polyarticular Arthritis

DANIEL E. SINGER, M.D.

The differential diagnosis of polyarticular complaints comprises a bewildering array of diseases. Nonetheless, the primary care physician can chart a simple, logical course that will minimize diagnostic error and maximize patient benefit. The initial evaluation should focus on answering the following basic questions:

1. Are the patient's complaints truly articular?
2. Is the arthritis inflammatory or degenerative?
3. Is the problem local or systemic?
4. How sick is the patient?

PATHOPHYSIOLOGY AND CLINICAL PRESENTATION

Polyarthritis can result from a degenerative or an inflammatory process. Noninflammatory forms of arthritis are, in most cases, the result of breakdown in joint cartilage and secondary mechanical disruption of the joint, i.e., degenerative arthritis. This may be a primary process or may be associated with an underlying disease, such as hemochromatosis. Uncommon mechanisims of nondegenerative noninflammatory joint injury include hemarthrosis, joint infarction, leukemic infiltration, and myxedematous changes.

Inflammatory arthritis results from the aggregation of inflammatory cells and their products in the joint space and synovium. Infection, gout, pseudogout, and the immunologically mediated diseases—rheumatoid arthritis, lupus, the spondyloarthropathies—all produce an inflammatory type of arthritis.

The typical features of the more common inflammatory arthropathies are given in Table 139–1.

DIFFERENTIAL DIAGNOSIS

Polyarticular disease may be inflammatory (see Table 139–1) or noninflammatory in origin. Osteoarthritis (OA) accounts for almost all noninflammatory cases, but hemophilia, sickle cell disease, leukemia and myxedema may be responsible in rare instances.

Table 139–1. Common Inflammatory Polyarthritides

1. **Rheumatoid arthritis.** Female predominant subacute symmetrical polyarthritis often involving PIPs, MCPs, wrists. AM stiffness is characteristic. Rheumatoid factor positivity is found in approximately 75% of cases and is associated with nodules and more aggressive articular and extra-articular disease.

2. **Systemic lupus erythematosus.** Usually occurs in young women, with high prevalence in blacks. Characterized by symmetrical polyarthralgias or nondeforming arthritis, with malar rash, pleuritis, leukopenia, immune thrombocytopenia, hemolytic anemia, glomerulonephritis. ANA is positive in nearly all cases. Renal disease and cerebritis are most life-threatening.

3. **Scleroderma.** Sclerodactyly and more general skin tightening, Raynaud's phenomenon, impaired esophageal motility, lung, heart, and renal involvement with malignant hypertension predominate. Articular symptoms are mild. ANA is often positive with a speckled pattern.

4. **Psoriatic arthritis.** Peripheral form is characteristically asymmetrical, oligoarticular involving DIP joints, and may be very erosive. Spondylitic form can mimic ankylosing spondylitis but the extent of disease is less; HLA-B27 positivity is associated with the spondylitic form.

5. **Reiter's syndrome.** Primarily a disease of young men, defined by arthritis, nongonococcal urethritis, and conjunctivitis, although the latter two features may be fleeting and not simultaneous. It may follow bowel infections, e.g., *Salmonella, Shigella.* Joints involved are often asymmetrical, lower extremity. Heel pain with plantar fasciitis and calcaneal periostitis is distinctive. Mild spondylitis and HLA-B27 positivity are common.

6. **Ankylosing spondylitis.** Again primarily a disease of young men. Inflammation of the joints and fibrous tissue of the spine with subsequent calcification and ossification produces the typical sacroiliitis and fused spine. Back pain, abnormal Shober's test and reduced chest expansion result. Uveitis, HLA-B27 are highly associated.

7. **Polyarticular gout.** Often, there is a past history of transient mono- or oligoarthritis; serum uric acid is usually but not necessarily elevated. Diagnosed by identifying urate crystals in synovial fluid (see Chapter 149).

8. **Pseudogout.** Calcium pyrophosphate crystal deposition disease: rarely polyarticular, patient often elderly, knee characteristically involved, cartilage calcification seen on x-ray; diagnosis made by identifying calcium pyrophosphate crystals in synovial fluid.

9. **Gonococcal arthritis.** Migratory polyarthritis and tendinitis that may lead to a frank infected joint and vesicular-pustular skin lesions. Diagnosis is made by culture of organism from cervix, urethra, or rectum as well as blood, skin, or synovial fluid (see Chapter 113).

10. **Acute hepatitis B arthritis.** Acute polyarthritis with urticarial skin lesions; occurs in preicteric phase and wanes as icteric phase develops. Diagnosed by laboratory evidence of hepatitis and hepatitis B antigen positivity (see Chapter 70).

WORKUP

Use of "official" criteria in diagnosing rheumatic disease. Diagnosis in the rheumatic diseases often depends on a pattern of clinical findings rather than on some specific pathologic abnormality. As a result, criteria have been proposed to help objectify the diagnosis of rheumatoid arthritis (RA), systemic lupus erythematosus (SLE), and other related conditions. These criteria capture the essential features of the diseases and are necessary for epidemiologic and therapeutic studies. However, they should be applied cautiously to any given patient.

The American Rheumatism Association (ARA) criteria for RA stress chronicity (greater than 6 weeks), presence of symmetrical polyarthritis, positive rheumatoid factor, skin nodules, and consistent x-ray changes. Clearly, the patient who has RA at week 7 has had RA during weeks 1 through 6. Similarly, a symmetrical disease or even monoarticular arthritis can be due to RA. Thus, the diagnostic criteria are not perfectly sensitive, especially in the early phases of the disease. Nor are they highly specific; numerous other diseases can meet ARA criteria for RA. To increase specificity, the ARA has listed 20 conditions (including gout, SLE, scleroderma, and infections) whose presence invalidates the use of the criteria to diagnose RA.

The basic message for the clinician is that chronic inflammatory polyarthritis is often RA, but if there are atypical features (e.g., lack of symmetry or lack of rheumatoid factor positivity) one should be sure no other cause is present.

The diagnosis of SLE poses similar problems. The so-called preliminary criteria for SLE are a list of 14 clinical features, of which 4 must be present for diagnosis. These include nondeforming polyarthritis or arthralgias, characteristic skin changes, evidence of serositis, hemolytic anemia, thrombocytopenia, and proteinuria. A study comparing these criteria against the diagnoses of experienced rheumatologists in cases of arthritis indicated that the hematologic manifestations, pleuritis, pericarditis, photosensitivity, and Raynaud's phenomenon correlated highly with the clinicians' diagnoses. In addition, the presence of a high titer ANA (a test which came into common use after the criteria were published) in conjunction with arthritis or any of the other clinical findings was highly predictive of SLE. The study emphasizes that for the individual patient, the diagnosis of SLE must be entertained when *any* of the clinical characteristics of the disease is associated with a positive ANA.

Workup Strategy

The initial assessment of the patient who presents with polyarticular joint complaints should determine whether the complaints are truly articular, whether the underlying disease is inflammatory or not, whether it is systemic or focal, and whether vital organ function or joint integrity is endangered.

The answers to these questions can be provided by a careful history and physical examination supplemented by a complete blood count and erythrocyte sedimentation rate (see Table 139-2). Synovial fluid analysis is very helpful if an accessible effusion is

Table 139–2. Distinguishing Inflammatory from NonInflammatory Articular Disease

	NONINFLAMMATORY	INFLAMMATORY
History	MCP and carpal joints rarely involved	MCPs and carpals often involved
	Little AM stiffness and much relief of pain with rest	AM stiffness is the hallmark; symptoms persist even without mechanical stress
	Few systemic effects	Patient often systemically ill, fatigued
	Little relief with anti-inflammatory medications	Clear-cut benefit from aspirin
Physical examination	MCP and carpal joints rarely involved	MCPs and carpals often involved
	Joints rarely warm red or swollen. Often merely bony enlargement	Synovitis is the central feature
	Extra-articular findings rare*	Extra-articular disease is common
Laboratory tests	CBC is normal	Anemia and/or other abnormalities often present
	ESR<30	ESR>40
	RF and ANA usually negative	RF and or ANA may be positive

* Throughout this chapter, noninflammatory arthritis has implied primary OA. This is usually the case. However, there are other diseases producing OA-like arthritis or a mildly inflammatory arthritis. These illnesses may have severe extra-articular manifestations. An example is the degenerative arthritis associated with hemochromatosis.

present. The rest of the laboratory tests that are available for rheumatologic diagnosis are best used to modify one's initial impression, and rarely are helpful when used as a general rheumatologic screening procedure.

History. Patients complain of pain, stiffness, and loss of function—generally in that order. The physician should attempt to identify the anatomic basis of the symptoms by asking the patient to specify exactly where the pain is located, what aggravates it, and what functional loss has occurred. For the most part, joint symptoms are well localized and bear a logical relationship to the use of the joint. Hand involvement will reduce grip strength. Shoulder involvement prevents hair combing. Hip disease is characterized by difficulty in rising from a seated position, and in putting on shoes and stockings. Cervical spine involvement makes back-parking difficult. Neuropathic pain (see Chapter 155), bone pain, and myalgias are often

confused with arthritis by the patient. These difficulties rarely have a specifically articular location, and do not produce typical articular loss of function. For example, a common neuropathic mimic of arthritis of the hands is the carpal tunnel syndrome. Here, poorly described pains in the hand may be associated with loss of grip strength. However, paresthesias, a sense of the hands being "ballooned" in size, aggravation of symptoms by sleep or driving, together with physical findings characteristic of median nerve entrapment will reveal the diagnosis.

After obtaining a specific description of the patient's complaints, one should ask in detail about other joints not mentioned. Complaints that initially appear to be monoarticular may turn out to be polyarticular on further questioning. The *distribution* of involved joints can be relatively specific for certain diagnoses. Thus, symmetrical enlargement with pain and limitation of motion of the proximal interphalangeal joints (PIPs) and distal phalangeal joints (DIPs), without metacarpophalangeal (MCP) or wrist involvement and without an AM stiffness pattern, suggests osteoarthritis. As a general rule, involvement of MCPs, wrists, or elbows implies inflammatory disease and should strongly discourage a diagnosis of osteoarthritis, unless some clear predisposing antecedent trauma has occurred, e.g., old fractures or a history of working a jack-hammer. The distribution of joint involvement in rheumatoid arthritis is characteristically symmetrical and often includes the interphalangeal (IP), MCP, carpal, or metatarsophalangeal (MTP) joints. Temperomandibular (TM) joint arthritis is relatively specific for RA. Asymmetrical DIP disease characterizes the peripheral form of psoriatic arthritis. Bilateral heel pain suggests Reiter's syndrome and the other spondyloarthropathies. Overall, the pattern of joints involved best helps to distinguish OA from the inflammatory arthritides. Within the set of inflammatory arthritides, joint distribution suggests initial diagnostic possibilities.

Concurrent with establishing the distribution of involved joints, one should determine the *temporal pattern* of the disease. A chronic, subacute, additive process occurs in many cases of RA. Sudden, explosive, symmetrical polyarthritis, while found with RA, strongly suggests "serum sickness" diseases, e.g., early hepatitis B infection or delayed penicillin allergy. Desultory arthralgias, arthritis, or tenosynovitis involving first one joint and then a second, after the first's symptoms are receding, typify gonococcal disease (see Chapter 113). A similar migratory pattern is noted in rheumatic fever. In establishing the temporal pattern, the physician should probe into the distant past as well. Has the patient ever had any other episodes of arthritis in the past? Gout may present as polyarthritis but more often, one uncovers a prior episode of podagra or other lower extremity monoarthritis (see chapter 149). Young adult men with ankylosing spondylitis often give a history of unexplained mono- or oligoarthritis occurring in their teens.

A few questions are particularly helpful in deciphering the patient's articular complaints. First, are the involved joints stiff as well as painful, and if so are they stiffer after rest or after activity? Inflammatory arthritis, in particular RA, is characterized by maximal stiffness after inactivity, so-called "AM stiffness." This stiffness persists for one or more hours. In contrast, osteoarthritis is characterized by maximal symptoms with use. If there is some stiffness with rest in OA, it passes quickly with activity. Second, have anti-inflammatory agents helped? RA patients reach for their aspirin as soon as they awaken, and they clearly feel worse if they miss a dose. The response in OA patients is much less dramatic. Third, has the patient noted joint redness, warmth, and/or swelling? The value of this question depends on the detail and believability of the patient's response. A well-described "hot joint," as opposed to diffuse hand or foot swelling, probably indicates true inflammation, whether or not the current examination suggests arthritis. A negative response coupled with a negative examination suggests a noninflammatory and perhaps nonarticular etiology.

After determining the temporal and spatial pattern of the patient's illness, the physician should assess its *severity*. First, are there symptoms at night? Joint pain awakening the patient at night indicates a severe problem. Bone and neurologic pain may also occur at night. Second, what desired activities has the patient discontinued because of arthritis? The answer to this question depends on several factors, including the patient's premorbid level of activity, his attitudes toward work and pain, as well as the biologic severity of the disease. However, the answer reveals the overall impact of the illness and the urgency of the patient's complaint. Third, how systemically ill is the patient? Marked daily fatigue, the need for afternoon naps, weight loss, fever—all suggest active systemic illness.

Inflammatory arthritides are often associated with disease in other organ systems. Thus, a detailed review of systems is mandatory. In particular, one should ask about the new onset of Raynaud's phenomenon (a marker of scleroderma, SLE, and RA),

the presence of nasopharyngeal ulcers, rashes, hair loss, fever or illness with sun exposure, or a history of pleuritis or pericarditis (all indicators of SLE). Chronically scratchy eyes or dry mouth suggests Sjögren's syndrome. A history of chronic or bloody diarrhea suggests inflammatory bowel disease. (see Chapter 65). Dysuria, conjunctivitis, and balanitis are found in Reiter's syndrome (see Chapter 126). Details about past or present psoriasis or unusual skin lesions (e.g., erythema nodosum) will also aid diagnosis. Questions about family history are pertinent to the spondyloarthropathies, gout, and Heberden's nodes. In addition, it is critical to know what other medical problems the patient has had, what his medications are, and whether he uses alcohol or other drugs heavily.

The physician should appreciate the influence of *age, sex,* and *race*. The probabilities of different forms of arthritis vary with these determinants. SLE and RA for example, are female predominant, while ankylosing spondylitis is male predominant. Onset of rheumatic fever or ankylosing spondylitis is nearly always before age 40. Peak incidence for SLE occurs in the premenopausal period, although later onset is not rare. The incidence of RA is less dependent on age, with new onset occurring in the elderly as well as in the young. Gout in women is mainly a postmenopausal disease; in men, it occurs at all adult ages. One point regarding race is worth noting. Despite the archetypal picture of a red butterfly rash on a Caucasian face, SLE is particularly common among black women, one study citing a prevalence of 1 in 250.

Physical examination. The physical examination is basically a continuation of the same approach, documenting the pattern and type of joint involvement and the nature of any extra-articular disease. The myriad of extra-articular manifestations of arthritic diseases makes a detailed general physical examination mandatory. Certain aspects deserve emphasis. First of all, one should carefully palpate around the elbows, the Achilles tendons, and the pinnae searching for nodules and tophi. When pathologically confirmed, nodules and tophi are specific indicators of RA and gout, respectively. The nails should be examined for clubbing, which is associated with pulmonary osteoarthropathy and inflammatory bowel disease (see Chapter 41), and pitting, characteristic of psoriasis. In fact, nail pitting adjacent to erosive DIP arthritis can justify the diagnosis of psoriatic arthritis in the absence of any skin psoriasis. Fingertip atrophy with healed or active ulcers suggests severe

Raynaud's syndrome, and should prompt a search for the calcinosis, subungual telangiectasias, and skin tightening of scleroderma. Other skin findings of value include the malar eruption of SLE, urticarial lesions of hepatitis B infection, the vesicular/pustular erption of gonococcal infection (see Chapter 113), the nodules and palpable purpura of the vasculitides (see Chapter 168) and erythema nodosum. This last skin finding is often associated with painful periarticular inflammation about the ankles as well as with true arthritis and should prompt a chest x-ray looking for evidence of sarcoidosis. Erythema nodosum is also a finding in inflammatory bowel disease, and may be part of Behçet's syndrome. There are many other skin findings with the rheumatic diseases, attesting to the common parallel involvement of skin and synovium.

The eyes should be examined for conjunctivitis and iritis (see Chapter 191), suggestive of Reiter's syndrome and spondylitis, and fundoscopic changes such as hemorrhages, exudates, and ischemic lesions consistent with systemic lupus and vasculitis. "Cotton-wool" exudates are the most common eye lesion in SLE. The oral and nasal mucosa should be examined for ulcers which when painful suggest SLE or Behçet's syndrome, and when painless suggest Reiter's syndrome. Thyroid evaluation may reveal hypothyroidism which can produce numerous musculoskeletal problems. Pleural or pericardial rubs are found in RA and SLE. Heart murmurs characterize rheumatic fever and SBE; mitral valve murmurs sometimes occur in SLE, and aortic regurgitant murmurs in the spondyloarthropathies. Splenomegaly is found in a variety of rheumatic diseases, including RA and SLE.

A detailed examination of the joints is very valuable in distinguishing periarticular from true articular disease, inflammatory from noninflammatory arthritis, and in objectively documenting which joints are abnormal. In general, the joint examination should assess the presence of tenderness, erythema, warmth, effusion, bony enlargement and mechanical abnormalities—e.g., limitation of motion, instability, subluxation, and tendon injury. An informative examination of the joints need take only a few minutes.

The primary physician is often faced with the problem of stiffness or pain in the hand. A valuable screening test for the presence of a joint or tendon abnormality is that of "curling." The patient is asked to extend the MCP joints and then maximally flex the PIP and DIP joints. This is quite different from making a fist where the MCPs are flexed as well. Curling is normal when a patient can bring his fingertips into apposition with his palm. Any limitation of motion in the PIP or DIP joints will interfere with curling. In addition, any inflammation along the entire length of the dorsal extensor tendons will also produce abnormal curling. As a sensitive but nonspecific test, curling is most useful in ruling *out* hand joint disease.

Another test that is useful but rarely performed by the general physician is Shober's test. Any patient with back pain or an arthritis pattern that suggests spondyloarthropathy should have this assessment of lumbar mobility. A mark is made on the patient's skin above the fifth lumbar vertebra and another mark 10 cm. above the first while the patient is standing upright. The patient is then asked to bend forward maximally. With normal lumbar flexion, the two marks should now be at least 15 cm. apart. Shober's test is a nonspecific screening procedure. Any form of lumbar spine disease and even simple lumbar paraspinous muscle spasm may reduce lumbar flexion. However, when coupled with evidence of spine disease elsewhere—e.g., abnormal chest expansion—an abnormal Shober test can suggest ankylosing spondylitis. Similarly, an abnormal test in a patient complaining of hip or knee arthritis raises the probability of spondyloarthropathy.

Some forms of periarticular disease require particular attention. Bursitis and tendinitis commonly mimic arthritis. Subacromial bursitis and bicipital tendinitis can be confused with shoulder joint disease (see Chapter 142); lateral epicondylitis (tennis elbow) and olecranon bursitis for elbow joint disease (see Chapter 145); trochanteric bursitis (see Chapter 143) and anserine bursitis (see Chapter 144) for hip and knee disease respectively. Familiarity with these entities is essential to proper diagnosis and therapy.

Another important type of periarticular disease is that manifested by "frozen" joints and flexion contractures. Severe limitation of motion of a joint may occur with an intrinsically normal joint. Disuse due to neurologic disease or periarticular pain may lead to tightening of periarticular fibrous tissue and secondary contractures. The clinical presentation may be mistaken for arthritis, but normal joint x-rays and lack of indicators of inflammatory arthritis, plus an awareness of a predisposing illness, will lead to the correct diagnosis.

Laboratory studies. A large number of laboratory tests, both simple and esoteric, are used in the evaluation of arthritic complaints. However, diagnostic hypotheses should be developed primarily from a detailed and directed history and physical examination. Diagnostic confusion that persists at the end of the physical examination is rarely resolved by laboratory results. The primary physician needs to know the indications and limitations of available studies.

SYNOVIAL FLUID ANALYSIS If a synovial effusion is present in a patient whose diagnosis is still undetermined, it should be tapped. A white blood cell (WBC) count of greater than 3000 per mm^3 should be considered inflammatory; less than 1000 suggests OA or a mechanical derangement. A count between 1000 and 3000 is ambiguous. The presence of urate or calcium pyrophosphate crystals is diagnostic of gout and pseudogout respectively (see Chapter 138). Similarly, the diagnosis of joint infection is made by Gram stain and positive cultures of joint fluid (see Chapter 138). Often, one obtains a synovial fluid WBC count of 5-20,000, without crystals, bacteria or other distinctive attributes. All that one can conclude at that point is that the patient has inflammatory arthritis, type unspecified.

ERYTHROCYTE SEDIMENTATION RATE. The erythrocyte sedimentation rate (ESR) is useful as a screen for inflammatory disease and for monitoring therapy. In one study of patients with OA and RA, more than 90 per cent of those diagnosed as having RA had an ESR greater than 30 (Westergren) while only 10 per cent of those with OA had such a rapid ESR. These are crude figures and will vary with age and type of clinical presentation, as will the relative prevalence of OA and RA. The point of clinical usefulness is that a high ESR (e.g., > 40 mm./hr.) suggests inflammatory disease. An ESR should be obtained on all arthritis patients.

RHEUMATOID FACTOR. Nearly all patients with polyarthritis are tested for rheumatoid factor (RF). The exact relationship of RF and RA is a matter of great speculation. It is clear that one can have RA and be RF negative, or conversely, one can be RF positive and not have arthritis. In general, 70 to 80 per cent of all patients meeting ARA criteria for RA are RF positive. This, of course, means that almost 30 per cent of RA patients are seronegative. Moreover, 5 to 15 per cent (increasing with age) of so-called normals are RF positive. The higher the titer of RF, the more likely the diagnosis of RA. RF negativity does not rule out RA nor does RF positivity rule it in. RF can also be positive in other connective tissue diseases and in chronic infections, e.g., SBE. The RF test is most helpful in confirming the diagnosis of RA when one's probability of RA was high prior to the test.

ANTINUCLEAR ANTIBODY (ANA). The ANA is very sensitive but not very specific. More than 95 per cent of patients diagnosed as having SLE are ANA positive. Consequently, one is fairly safe in concluding that a patient who is ANA negative does not have SLE. However, the ANA may be positive in drug-induced lupus, RA, scleroderma, and chronic hepatitis among other illnesses, and may be positive in normals. Recent research has focused on the presence of antibodies to more homogeneous nuclear components. At the present time, it seems that antibodies to native DNA and to the so-called Sm antigen are more specific indicators of SLE than the ANA test.

HLA TYPING. Over the past decade, much research has been devoted to the association between rheumatologic disease and HLA types. The most dramatic example of this is the relationship between HLA-B27 and ankylosing spondylitis. While 5 per cent of the general population is B27 positive, 95 per cent of patients with ankylosing spondylitis are B27 positive. Since the prevalence of ankylosing spondylitis is less than 1 per cent of males, most B27 positive males will *not* have spondylitis (see Chapter 2). Therefore, HLA typing for B27 positivity is a sensitive but nonspecific test for spondylitis. A high percentage of patients with inflammatory spondylitis associated with Reiter's syndrome, inflammatory bowel disease, and psoriasis are also B27 positive. In cases of seronegative (i.e., RF negative) inflammatory arthritis, particularly with evidence of spine involvement, B27 positivity strongly supports the diagnosis of inflammatory spondyloarthropathy. As with the RF and ANA tests, B27 testing is useful only if one has a strong suspicion of the diagnosis prior to the test. The test should not be ordered indiscriminately for all cases of back pain.

URIC ACID LEVEL. Serum uric acid levels are obtained in most arthritis patients and too often serve as the primary basis for a diagnosis of gout. Definitive diagnosis requires observing urate crystals in the synovial fluid (see Chapter 138). A normal serum uric acid does not rule out the diagnosis of gout nor does an elevated level rule it in.

X-RAYS. The question of appropriate x-rays is often raised. In osteoarthritis, joint x-rays are abnormal by the time the patient becomes symptomatic. However, the converse is not true. Degenerative changes are commonly found in asymptomatic joints. In new onset inflammatory arthritis, the x-ray may show only soft tissue swelling. As such, it serves more as a baseline examination than as a diagnostic test. In oligoarticular disease, the few involved joints should be x-rayed. In polyarticular disease, if no one joint is outstandingly worrisome, films of both hands and wrists assess the most joints for the least radiation. In cases of suspected spondyloarthropathy, films of the sacroiliac joints may provide definite evidence of sacroiliitis.

INDICATIONS FOR ADMISSION AND REFERRAL

The diagnosis of polyarticular arthritis may remain uncertain for a long period of time. For the most part, arthritis is not life threatening. Short-term risk to the patient is posed primarily by extra-articular disease. *The physician must assure himself that no active infection or vasculitis is present and that the patient's eyes, lungs, heart, kidneys and other vital organs are not endangered.* Thus assured, he may approach the problems of diagnosis and therapy at a more relaxed pace on an outpatient basis; otherwise, hospitalization is needed.

Any patient with inflammatory polyarthritis who is systemically ill or who has vital organ involvement should be seen by the rheumatologist as soon as possible. When a patient with less serious illness remains undiagnosed after completion of the initial workup, referral to a rheumatologist may be appropriate. Patients with clear-cut osteoarthritis require referral only when severity warrants consideration of surgical therapy (see Chapter 148). In cases of RA, early consultation with a rheumatologist may be helpful in the design of a total therapeutic program (see Chapter 147).

SYMPTOMATIC THERAPY

Provided that acute gout and infection have been ruled out and pending results of the remainder of the initial evaluation, the patient bothered by symptoms of joint inflammation may be given aspirin at a dose of about twelve 325-mg. tablets per day, or one of the newer nonsteroidal anti-inflammatory agents (see Chapter 147).

ANNOTATED BIBLIOGRAPHY

American Rheumatism Association: Primer on the Rheumatic Diseases, ed. 7. New York: The Arthritis Foundation, 1973. *(This brief text covers nearly all rheumatic diseases, and contains, in its appendices, the detailed "ARA criteria" for RA, SLE. A new edition should soon be available.)*

Anderson, R.J.: The diagnosis and management of rheumatoid synovitis. Ortho. Clin. North Am. 6: 629, 1975. *(An excellent, logical article outlining the main points of diagnostic and therapeutic concern in RA.)*

Brewerton, D.A., *et al.*: Ankylosing spondylitis and HL-A 27. Lancet, *1*:904, 1973. *(One of the earliest reports of the association of ankylosing spondylitis and what is now known as HLA-B27.)*

Calin, A.: HLA-B27: To type or not to type? Ann. Intern. Med., *92*:208, 1980. *(A critical assessment of the use of B27 typing in clinical practice.)*

Fessel, W.J.: SLE in the community. Arch. Intern. Med., *134*:1027, 1974 *(This is the report where the claim of a prevalence of 1/250 black women is made.)*

Harler, N.M., Franck, W.A., Bress N.M., and Robinson, D.R.: Acute polyarticular gout. Am. J. Med., *56*:715, 1974. *(A study of this uncommon presentation of a very common disease.)*

Katz, W.A. (ed.): Rheumatic Diseases. Philadelphia: J. B. Lippincott, 1977. *(This text emphasizes the clinical problem rather than the disease. The first quarter of the text deals with the approach to given articular complaints, e.g., elbow problems, shoulder problems. Subsequently, individual disease entities are considered.)*

Lawrence, J.S.: Rheumatism in Populations. London: W. Heinemann, 1977. *(This is a text devoted to the epidemiology of arthritis, based heavily on British studies.)*

McCarty, D.J. (ed.): Arthritis and Allied Conditions, ed. 9. Philadelphia: Lea and Febiger, 1979. *(The current dominant American reference textbook of rheumatology.)*

Polley, H.F., and Hunder, G.G.: Rheumatologic Interviewing and Physical Examination of the Joints. Philadelphia: W.B. Saunders, 1978. *(A wonderfully useful short text on the physical examination of the joints. Excellent photographs and drawings.)*

Trimble, R.B., *et al.*: Preliminary criteria for the classification of SLE. Arthritis Rheum. *17*:184, 1974. *(This short paper analyzes the usefulness of the typical "criteria" approach to rheumatologic diagnosis, specifically in distinguishing SLE from RA.)*

140
Evaluation of Back Pain
ROBERT J. BOYD, M.D.

Back pain is common and can be disabling. When a patient presents with back pain, serious underlying problems must be considered, because early recognition of tumor, infection, disc herniation and vertebral compression fracture is essential to effective management and avoidance of permanent injury. After the description of lumbar disc herniation by Mixter and Barr in 1933, it became increasingly apparent that disc disease is frequently responsible for recurring mild low back discomfort and episodes of severe back pain with sciatica. Most back pain is due to musculoligamentous strain, degenerative disc disease, or facette arthritis, and will respond to symptomatic treatment. Occasionally, back pain may be due to problems originating outside the spinal axis. The frequency of back pain requires that the primary physician be skilled in its assessment and conservative management and knowledgeable about the indications for myelography and surgery.

PATHOPHYSIOLOGY AND CLINICAL PRESENTATION

The patient with *low back musculoligamentous strain* presents after a specific episode of bending, twisting, or lifting. The strain is usually severe and is associated with a feeling of something giving way in the lower back; the onset of pain in the lower lumbar area is immediate. There may be tearing of muscle fibers or distal ligamentous attachments of the paraspinal muscles, usually at the iliac crest or lower lumbar/upper sacral region. Resultant bleeding and spasm cause local swelling and marked tenderness at the site of injury. Pain radiates across the low back, often to the buttock and upper thigh posteriorly; radiation of pain into the lower leg is rare.

In *lumbar disc herniation*, there is often a several-year history of recurring mild mid–low back pain related to minor back strain, with symptoms clearing spontaneously within a few days. Attacks occur with increasing frequency and severity at intervals of several months to several years. Eventually, pain may radiate in the distribution of a lower lumbar nerve root, and bed rest may be needed in increasing

amounts before symptoms resolve. Numbness, paresthesias and weakness often develop in the areas supplied by the irritated nerve root.

The pathophysiology of disc disease is not completely understood. It is felt that lower lumbar disc degeneration and attritional changes are due to the concentration of stress at the lumbosacral level. Stresses result from the enormous longitudinal and sheer forces that are a consequence of upright posture and are aggravated by bending strain. The disc annulus may become injured, inflamed and weakened, leading to localized back pain. Pain receptors in the longitudinal ligaments probably mediate the recurring attacks of local back pain. Eventually, the disc may become so weakened that it bulges posteriorly during relatively minor stress; compression and irritation of a lumbar nerve root result, and radicular symptoms develop. The clinical syndrome of back and leg pain in the distribution of a specific lumbar root is due to compression of an inflamed and sensitive root.

Disc herniation at the L_{4-5} or L_5 -S_1 level accounts for 95 per cent of disc ruptures, with the L_5 and S_1 nerve roots affected, respectively. With S_1 root irritation, pain, numbness and paresthesias involve the buttock, posterior thigh, calf, lateral aspect of the ankle and foot, and lateral toes. Calf atrophy and a diminished or absent ankle jerk can occur as well as plantar flexion weakness. With L_5 root compression, pain radiates to the dorsum of the foot and great toe, and the only neurologic deficits may be extensor weakness of the great toe and numbness of the L_5 area on the dorsum of the foot at the base of the great toe (Fig. 140–1). In the rarer instance of high lumbar disc herniation, pain radiates to the anterior thigh, and the knee jerk may be diminished or absent. Quadriceps atrophy and weakness may be found, and reverse straight leg raising often reproduces the back and anterior thigh pain.

With lower lumbar disc herniations, there is often lumbar paraspinal muscle spasm that limits lumbar motions. There may be a list away from the side of the disc herniation, so-called sciatic scoliosis, and frequently there is tenderness of the lower lumbar spine and sciatic notch. Straight leg raising on the affected side is limited by back and leg pain which increases on ankle dorsiflexion at the extreme of straight leg raising.

Vertebral compression fracture in normal bone requires severe flexion-compression force and is acutely painful. Spontaneous vertebral body collapse, or pathologic fracture, is most commonly seen in elderly patients with severe osteoporosis (see Chapter 152), in patients on long-term steroids (see Chapter 101), and in cancer patients with lytic bony metastases. Usually there is a history of sudden back pain brought on by a minor stress. The discomfort is noted at the level of fracture, with local radiation across the back and around the trunk, but rarely into the lower extremities. The fracture is more likely to be in the middle or lower levels of the dorsal spine, which helps differentiate the problem from lumbar disc herniations, 95 per cent of which occur at the L_4 or L_5 disc level.

The most common spinal tumor is *metastatic carcinoma*, which often presents with waist level or midback pain of insidious onset, gradually increasing in severity and aggravated by activity. Typically, the pain is not relieved by lying down, and night pain is frequent. The disc spaces are spared; disc space height is usually maintained, although collapse of the vertebral body due to destruction and weakening of bone is common. A history of previous malignancy and insidious increase in midback pain that is not relieved by lying down is highly suspicious of metastatic tumor. Breast, lung, prostate, gastrointestinal and genitourinary neoplasms frequently metastasize to the spine. Purely lytic lesions, which are often due to renal or thyroid carcinoma, are seen occasionally. *Myeloma* is the most common primary bone tumor involving the spine. Early in its course, the tumor may be difficult to differentiate from compression fracture due to osteoporosis.

Vertebral osteomyelitis is rare and involves the disc space as well as the vertebral bodies. It is usually hematogenous in origin but may occasionally follow a spinal procedure, such as lumbar puncture, myelography, discography, or disc surgery. Dull continuous back pain is the usual presentation, often in conjunction with low-grade fever and spasm over the paraspinous muscles. Tenderness to percussion over the involved vertebrae is common. A compression fracture or an *epidural abscess* may develop and result in root pain, weakness, and even paraplegia. The progression from spinal ache to paraplegia may be rapid, occurring over the course of a few days.

Ankylosing spondylitis usually occurs in young men; morning back stiffness is a prominent feature. Diminished chest expansion is the earliest physical finding. Occasionally there is a previous history of inflammatory bowel disease. The mechanism of the disease is unknown; spinal x-rays may be normal in its early phases. Initial radiologic changes occur in the sacroiliac joints and include narrowing of the joint space and reactive sclerosis; eventually obliteration of the space and fusion of the joint may occur. Over 90 per cent of patients are HLA-B27 positive (see Chapter 139).

Spondylolisthesis denotes forward subluxation of a vertebral body. In adults, the condition results from degenerative changes and arthritis of the facet joints, usually at L_{4-5} or L_5-S_1, with forward slippage of 10 to 20 percent of the vertebral body diameter. About 70 per cent of patients with spondylolisthesis have chronic low back pain; sciatica is infrequent. The pain is due to strain imposed on the ligaments and intervertebral joints.

Intraspinal tumors may present like herniated discs. However, marked progression of neurologic deficits despite adequate conservative therapy may be a clue to the existence of a tumor inside the spinal canal.

Extraspinal tumors may eventually cause root impingement and simulate sciatica due to disc disease. Tumors of the retroperitoneum, pelvis and large bowel may extend to the roots. This is a very late development; metastases may occur earlier.

Depression may present with chronic low back pain. Often there is a history of previous back problems or onset at the time of a minor injury. Mild muscle spasm might be noted on physical examination; characteristically, the intensity of complaints and the degree of disability are much greater than the minor limitations found on examination. Multiple somatic symptoms are common (see Chapter 215). Many of these patients appear refractory to therapy, often unwilling to take an active role in their own treatment. Some even seem to derive a sense of legitimacy and self-worth from their suffering (see Chapter 218).

Malingering implies conscious deception for the sake of obtaining gain from being ill. Inconsistencies in symptoms and physical findings typify the malingerer. These often can be brought out by distracting the patient.

DIFFERENTIAL DIAGNOSIS

The differential diagnosis of back pain can be considered in terms of whether or not there is root pain. Conditions that produce root injury include lumbar disc herniation, late osteomyelitis, epidural abscess, compression fracture, intraspinal tumor, extraspinal neoplasms, and, occasionally, spondylolisthesis. Musculoligamentous strain, ankylosing spondylitis, most cases of spondylolisthesis, depression, and the very early phases of spinal osteomyelitis and epidural abscess usually cause back pain without root involvement. Occasionally a retroperitoneal neoplasm may be the source of difficulty.

WORKUP

History. In addition to elucidating mode of onset, location, radiation, aggravating and alleviating factors, and course of illness, one needs to inquire about fever, numbness, weakness, root pain, and recent injury. Previous therapy for back problems, recent lumbar puncture, concurrent illness, and chronic corticosteroid use also should be looked into. A discussion of emotional and social stresses is indicated when symptoms persist in the absence of obvious structural pathology. It is important to check for somatic symptoms of depression (see Chapter 215).

Physical examination. The back should be examined with the patient unclothed, observing the back while the patient is standing for symmetry, muscle bulk, posture and spinal curves. Spinal motions are assessed; flexibility is of greatest importance. One needs to look for muscle spasm and spinal segments that do not move freely. Description of what limits back motion is more important than estimating degrees of motion, which is imprecise at best. The spine is palpated for focal tenderness suggestive of tumor, infection, fracture and disc herniation. Tiptoe and heel walking tests gross motor function of ankle plantar flexors (L_5-S_1 disc, S_1 root) and dorsiflexors (L_{4-5} disc, L_5 root) respectively. With the patient sitting, the knee jerks (L_{3-4}) and ankle jerks (S_1) are tested. With the patient supine, strength of the long toe extensor (L_5 root), cutaneous sensation, and straight leg raising are evaluated. The L_5 autonomous area of sensation is on the dorsum of the foot at the base of the great toe, S_1 autonomous sensory area is along the lateral border of the foot and the fifth toe (see Fig. 140–1). Thigh and calf circumferences are measured looking for evidence of atrophy, and lower extremity joint motions are tested. Abdomen, rectum, groin, pelvic visceral and genitalia are examined, and peripheral pulses palpated. Femoral nerve sensitivity is usually present with higher lumbar ($L_{2,3,4}$) root irritation. The prone position allows palpation of the back and buttocks. Lower lumbar spine and sciatic notch sensitivity usually are found with lower lumbar disc problems.

Straight leg raising (SLR) is an important com-

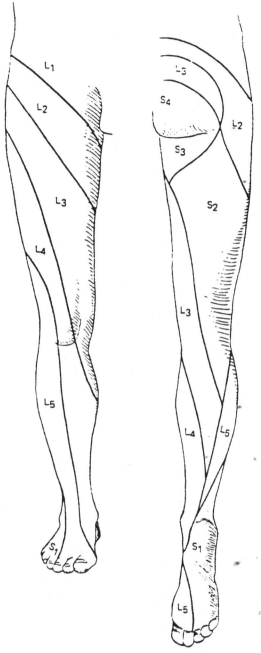

Fig 140–1. Lower extremity dermatomes. (Finneson, B. E.: *Low Back Pain.* Philadelphia: J. B. Lippincott. 1973)

ponent of the assessment for disc disease. The maneuver is a sensitive test of disc herniation. SLR stretches the lower nerve roots; in the presence of disc herniation the additional root stretching causes impingement and pain. SLR is positive when back or root pain is reported upon passively lifting the straightened leg with the patient supine. This should not be confused with hamstring muscle tightness, which can also cause discomfort on straight leg raising. Maximal L_5 and S_1 root movement occurs at 60–80° of SLR, whereas there is much less L_4 and minimal L_2 or L_3 movement. Thus a positive SLR is of maximal use in locating an L_5-S_1 or $L_{4.5}$ disc, but its absence does not rule out herniation higher up.

Performing SLR on the opposite side also causes root movement. In the presence of a severely herniated disc, root pain may occur, especially with an L_5-S_1 disc. It is felt that a positive contralateral SLR test is specific for large disc herniation, suggesting an extruded disc fragment, though there may be a large percentage of false-negative results.

If severe pain is reported on elevation and resistance occurs, yet the leg can be raised another 20° or 30° when the patient is distracted, the test is "negative" and other causes of the pain should be sought, such as hamstring muscle tightness. Dorsiflexion of the ankle at the extreme of SLR may exacerbate the pain of disc herniation on SLR testing and is particularly useful when the SLR test is equivocal.

Laboratory studies. For the majority of patients with back pain, a careful history and physical usually suffice for diagnosis. Nevertheless, x-rays of the spine are usually obtained in order to rule out a serious unexpected bony abnormality such as lytic lesions. Although routine x-rays are common practice, the cost-effectiveness of ordering back films on every patient is an unresolved question. X-rays are often low in yield of diagnostic information; for example, in the patient with low back pain, the finding of normal disc spaces does not rule out the diagnosis of disc herniation. Moreover, a narrowed disc space does not distinguish between disc rupture and asymptomatic degeneration. The presence of osteophytes extending from the vertebral bodies indicates only long-existing disc degeneration and attempts at repair. Often lumbosacral films are more useful for reassuring the patient than for making a diagnosis. X-rays are also of little use in early osteomyelitis, because there are few radiographic abnormalities in the first week to 10 days, except for slight disc space narrowing; vertebral end-plate destruction and reactive bone formation develop later.

There are a number of situations in which spinal films are particularly useful for diagnosis. Suspected ankylosing spondylitis is an indication for radiographs of the spine and sacroiliac joints. Syndesmophytes and obliteration of the sacroiliac joints are characteristic x-ray findings. A positive test for *HLA-B27* helps to confirm the diagnosis when there is some uncertainty, but the test is not indicated unless there is a high index of suspicion. When back pain is localized to the high lumbar or thoracic region, spinal films should be ordered, because compression fracture or metastatic bone disease may be present.

Bone scan is indicated for suspected metastatic disease of the spine and early osteomyelitis. An elevated sedimentation rate and increased uptake on technetium bone scan further suggest the diagnosis of osteomyelitis. Gallium scan and computerized axial tomography of the spine may be helpful in defining soft tissue involvement or abscess formation.

Immunoelectrophoresis (IEP) of serum and urine will diagnose most cases of myeloma. Crudely screening for myeloma with a CBC, erythrocyte sedimentation rate (ESR), and serum globulin level is probably sufficient when clinical suspicion is not high. The diagnosis must be suspected when back pain is accompanied by unexplained anemia and very high ESR. Nevertheless, such findings are quite nonspecific and may also be due to a chronic inflammatory process.

Myelography is indicated when there are progressive neurologic deficits, such as loss of sphincter control or severe numbness and weakness of the lower extremities. The temptation to perform myelography in the patient with chronic refractory pain is strong, but the test should be reserved for patients with objective findings that are amenable to surgery or radiation therapy. *Electromyography* may be needed to document peripheral nerve deficits and help select patients who require myelography.

INDICATIONS FOR REFERRAL

Patients with progressive neurologic deficits require prompt neurologic and surgical consultations. The same is true for individuals with acute vertebral collapse, particularly to assess stability of the fracture. Suspicion of osteomyelitis or epidural abscess is an indication for immediate hospitalization and infectious disease consultation; treatment must be early to be effective.

If a patient with refractory pain does not respond to conservative measures, referral to an orthopedist or neurosurgeon with a particular interest in back problems can be helpful. Even if the patient has no neurologic deficits and is thus not a surgical candidate, the referral can serve to reassure such a person that a surgically correctable lesion is not being overlooked, and that the efforts of the primary physician are appropriate.

SYMPTOMATIC MANAGEMENT AND PATIENT EDUCATION

Acute back pain. Acute musculoligamentous strain, degenerative disc disease, and herniated lumbar disc with or without sciatica can usually be managed by bed rest; approximately 98 per cent of patients respond favorably. The patient may be severely incapacitated by pain at rest as well as with movement. The acute discomfort usually persists for at least several days. Symptomatic measures consist of local heat or warm baths and use of mild analgesics. An oral narcotic analgesic such as codeine, 30 to 60 mg., or meperidine, 50 mg., is sometimes required every 4 hours for several days to achieve relief of severe acute pain. Most so-called muscle relaxants are actually minor tranquilizers; they have little direct effect on muscles but can be of help to the patient who cannot sleep. The patient should be advised to find the most comfortable position in bed; lying supine with pillows behind the knees and a low pillow for the head usually suffices. Lying on one's side with the hips and knees flexed is sometimes quite comfortable; lying prone is usually not.

The patient should be allowed up only to go to the bathroom, and rest should be continued until there is no discomfort in bed. Then, activity can be resumed gradually, beginning with getting up for meals and progressing to walking and sitting as tolerated. The patient should be prepared to return to bed promptly if significant pain recurs. Bed rest may be needed for as long as 2 to 3 weeks.

If pain remains severe and intractable after 3 weeks of strict bed rest, or if an important neurologic deficit develops, such as foot drop, gastroc-soleus or quadriceps weakness, or incontinence, hospitalization is indicated for enforced bed rest, myelography, and consideration of surgery.

A reasonable program of back care should be discussed when recovery from acute symptoms allows gradual mobilization and resumption of normal activities. The patient must understand that pain is a normal protective response to injury or inflammation; discomfort should be used as a guideline to determine the pace of increasing activity. However, minor discomfort, stiffness, soreness, or mild aching should not interfere with progressive mobilization.

If symptoms recur or marked pain develops in re-lation to a specific activity or level of activity, the patient should temporarily limit himself for several days. If pain increases within 24 hours of performing a new or greater level of activity, the activity should be halved each day until a tolerable level is reached, and then gradually increased. The patient can be encouraged to progress as rapidly as symptoms permit.

Although acute symptoms will subside with rest, proper back care should become a way of life for the patient. The patient ought to be advised to avoid activities which cause pain as well as such potentially injurious actions as repetitive bending, heavy lifting (over 10 to 20 pounds) or shoveling snow. The patient must understand the limited goals of exercise, which are to restore and maintain the flexibility and strength of the back so that good posture can be attained and chances of recurrent injury minimized. Instruction sheets are often useful (see Figs. 140–2 and 140–3) to supplement instruction in the office. Mild daily exercise and more vigorous exercise 2 to 3 times a week are also encouraged. Walking briskly for 20 minutes once or twice a day, supplemented by swimming twice weekly for up to 30 minutes, fulfills such an exercise requirement; stationary bicycling or jogging can be substituted for swimming.

Chronic back pain. Patients with chronic refractory back pain and no clear anatomic deficits pose one of the most difficult long-term management problems encountered in primary care practice. Many of these patients do not take an active role in their own treatment and frustrate the efforts of physicians while continuing to complain of discomfort. Although there are no simple solutions to the management of such individuals, some important objectives can be achieved: identification and treatment of underlying psychopathology; avoidance of inappropriate tests, addictive medications and unnecessary surgery; and preservation of the individual's capacity to function independently.

When a careful and thorough assessment fails to identify significant musculoskeletal pathology or neurologic deficits, diagnostic and therapeutic attention must be directed to the possibility of an occult depression or character disorder. Discovery of an underlying depression should be followed by consideration of tricyclic therapy (see Chapter 215). Recognition of a character disorder can lessen the frustration associated with trying to "cure" the patient. Therapeutic efforts are best directed at helping the patient to find ways other than suffering to achieve a sense of self-worth. Attempting to remove a person's one source of personal value (albeit maladaptive) is

How to get along with your back

Sitting: Use a hard chair and put your spine up against it; try and keep one or both knees higher than your hips. A small stool is helpful here. For short rest periods, a contour chair offers excellent support.

Standing: Try to stand with your lower back flat. When you work standing up, use a footrest to help relieve swayback. Never lean forward without bending your knees. Ladies take note: shoes with moderate heels strain the back less than those with high heels. Avoid platform shoes.

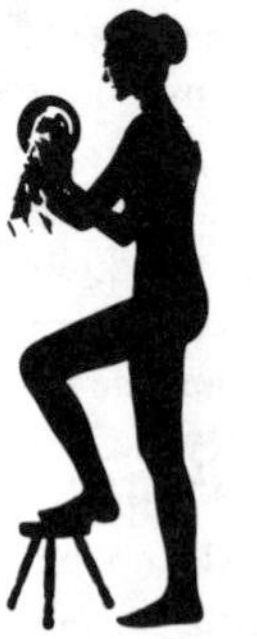

Sleeping: Sleep on a firm mattress; put a bedboard (¾" plywood) under a soft mattress. Do not sleep on your stomach. If you sleep on your back, put a pillow under your knees. If you sleep on your side keep your legs bent at the knees and at the hips.

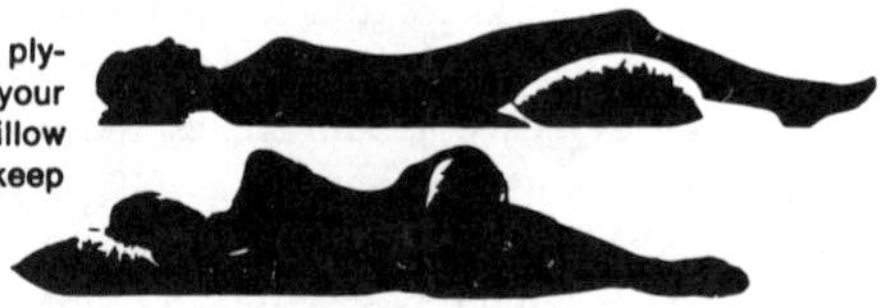

Driving: Get a hard seat for your automobile and sit close enough to the wheel while driving so that your legs are not fully extended when you work the pedals.

Lifting: Make sure you lift properly. Bend your knees and use your leg muscles to lift. Avoid sudden movements. Keep the load close to your body, and try not to lift anything heavy higher than your waist.

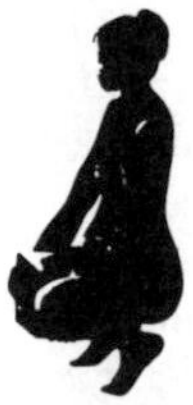

Working: Don't overwork yourself. If you can, change from one job to another before you feel fatigued. If you work at a desk all day, get up and move around whenever you get the chance.

Exercise: Get regular exercise (walking, swimming, etc.) once your backache is gone. But start slowly to give your muscles a chance to warm up and loosen before attempting anything strenuous.

See your doctor: If your back acts up, see your doctor; don't wait until your condition gets severe.

Fig. 140–2. Sample instruction sheet describing care of the back. (McNeil Laboratories, Fort Washington, PA)

Exercises for low back pain

General Information:

Don't overdo exercising, especially in the beginning. Start by trying the movements slowly and carefully. Don't be alarmed if the exercises cause some mild discomfort which lasts a few minutes. But if pain is more than mild and lasts more than 15 or 20 minutes, *stop* and do no further exercises until you see your doctor.

Do the exercises on a hard surface covered with a thin mat or heavy blanket. Put a pillow under your neck if it makes you more comfortable. Always start your exercises slowly—and in the order marked—to allow muscles to loosen up gradually. Heat treatments just before you start can help relax tight muscles. Follow the instructions carefully; it will be well worth the effort.

Do exercises marked (**X**)

in numerical order

for _____ minutes

_____ times a day.

Take the medication

prescribed for you

_____ times daily

for_____ .

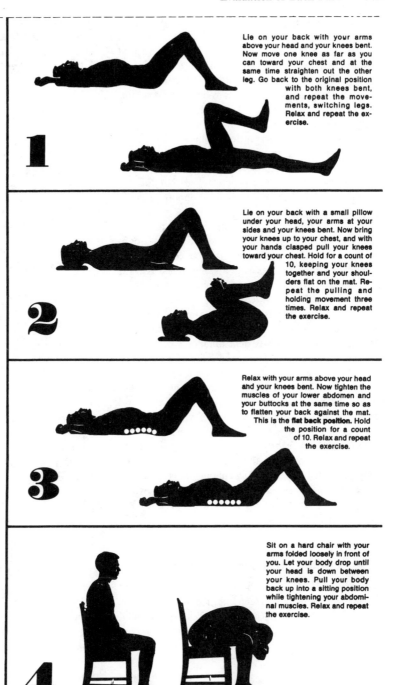

1 Lie on your back with your arms above your head and your knees bent. Now move one knee as far as you can toward your chest and at the same time straighten out the other leg. Go back to the original position with both knees bent, and repeat the movements, switching legs. Relax and repeat the exercise.

2 Lie on your back with a small pillow under your head, your arms at your sides and your knees bent. Now bring your knees up to your chest, and with your hands clasped pull your knees toward your chest. Hold for a count of 10, keeping your knees together and your shoulders flat on the mat. Repeat the pulling and holding movement three times. Relax and repeat the exercise.

3 Relax with your arms above your head and your knees bent. Now tighten the muscles of your lower abdomen and your buttocks at the same time so as to flatten your back against the mat. This is the **flat back position**. Hold the position for a count of 10. Relax and repeat the exercise.

4 Sit on a hard chair with your arms folded loosely in front of you. Let your body drop until your head is down between your knees. Pull your body back up into a sitting position while tightening your abdominal muscles. Relax and repeat the exercise.

Fig. 140–3.   Sample instruction sheet describing exercises for low back pain (McNeil Laboratories, Fort Washington, PA)

bound to be sabotaged by the patient, unless there is something to replace it (see Chapter 218).

Patients with chronic refractory back pain are at considerable risk for invasive testing (e.g., myelography) and surgery, even though they may lack symptoms and signs that are considered proper indications for such procedures. The primary physician needs to protect these patients from unnecessary and potentially harmful interventions. One way to accomplish this objective is to arrange a consultation for the patient with an orthopedic surgeon or a neurosurgeon experienced in back problems, so that the patient does not feel the need to go "shopping around" for a surgeon.

Avoiding repeated use of narcotics for pain control is another important and difficult aspect of managing these patients. There may be repeated demands for strong analgesic agents, but unless there is an acute and reversible etiology for pain, the use of narcotics should be limited if at all possible. Many patients with chronic back pain may initially be unwilling to participate in their own treatment. Establishing a strong doctor–patient alliance (see Chapter 1) and attending to emotional difficulties may be necessary before the patient can be actively engaged in a program of self-help. Then advice which emphasizes good posture, proper body mechanics, postural exercises, and a general program of physical conditioning may be received more enthusiastically. Arranging regularly scheduled visits at intervals agreed upon by both physician and patient can help provide support and forestall many phone calls and unscheduled office appearances. Even though symptoms may not disappear, it is often possible to keep the patient functioning independently.

ANNOTATED BIBLIOGRAPHY

Ahstrom, J. (ed.): Low back pain assessment and management. In Current Practice in Orthopaedic Surgery, Vol. 8. St. Louis: C. V. Mosby, 1979, Chap 1. *(A detailed discussion of current concepts of assessment and management of low back pain.)*

American Medical Association: Skeletal muscle relaxants. *In* AMA Drug Evaluations, ed. 3. Littleton, Mass.: PSG Publishing Company, 1977, p. 1023. *(There is no evidence at the present time that sedative agents used as muscle relaxants have a direct muscle-relaxant effect; rather, the reduction in muscle tone may be dependent on their centrally acting sedative effects.)*

Baker, A.S., Ojemann, R.G., Swartz, M.N., et al.: Spinal epidural abscess. N. Eng. J. Med., 293:463, 1975. *(In a series of 39 patients, the typical progression was from spinal ache to root pain, followed by weakness and paralysis. Osteomyelitis was the cause in 38 per cent and bacteremia in 26 per cent.)*

Bickerstaff, E.R.: Neurological Examination and Clinical Practice, ed. 3. Oxford: Blackwell Scientific Publications, 1975. *(A good text for additional information regarding details of the neurological examination, including straight leg raising.)*

Howorth, B.: Examination and Diagnosis of the Spine and Extremities. Springfield, Ill.: Charles C Thomas, 1962. *(A detailed discussion of the technique of back examination is included in this text.)*

Larrienere, R.P.T.: Procedures for treatment by physical therapy. In The Low Back Patient. Masson Publishers, U.S.A., 1979. *(A recent brief text outlining current concepts of physical therapy procedures and back care advice; well illustrated.)*

Rothman, R., and Simeone, F. (eds.): The Spine. Philadelphia: W. B. Saunders, 1975. *(An excellent and comprehensive textbook with in-depth discussion of low back problems including specific indications for surgical treatment.)*

Ruge, D., and Wiltse, L. L. (eds): Spinal Disorders: Diagnosis and Treatment. Philadelphia: Lea & Febiger, 1977. *(This text includes a good discussion of spondylolisthesis and mechanical back problems.)*

141
Evaluation of Neck Pain
ROBERT J. BOYD, M.D.

The primary physician is often faced with the patient who complains of a stiff neck; most of the time the problem is musculoskeletal in origin. Although the majority of musculoskeletal etiologies are not serious, they can result in considerable discomfort. One should be able to provide symptomatic relief to the person with a minor neck problem, and identify the patient with a serious complication of cervical spine disease, such as root compression or cord injury that requires surgical attention.

PATHOPHYSIOLOGY AND CLINICAL PRESENTATION

Severe *neck strain* is one of the most frequent causes of neck pain and usually results from a specific injury. Tearing of muscle fibers can cause bleeding, swelling, severe muscle spasm and pain. Symptoms increase gradually over several hours, often becoming most severe the day following the acute event. The anterior or posterior ligaments of the cervical spine may be disrupted. When the injury is not complicated by root or spinal cord compression, there are no neurologic deficits.

Neck pain from *cervical paraspinal muscle spasm* is usually secondary to neck strain or prolonged, unconscious muscle contraction associated with emotional stress. The problem is usually self-limited, though it may recur. Muscles spasm also occurs with cervical arthritis and cervical disc disease.

Trauma or degenerative changes in the intervertebral discs or joint facettes can be a source of neck pain and result in ankylosis or subluxation of the cervical spine, termed *cervical spondylosis*. Immobility and consolidation of the joint may ensue. Usually the process is localized to the lower cervical levels, such as C_{4-5}, C_{5-6}, or C_{6-7}. Degenerative changes and spurring at the cervical disc spaces are prominent. The condition presents as recurring neck stiffness and mild aching discomfort, with progressive limitation of neck motion over months to years. Lateral rotation and lateral flexion of the neck toward the painful side are limited; pain is precipitated or increased by such motions.

Cervical disc degeneration can lead to narrowing of the neural foramina, causing *root impingement* and pain. Pain radiates in the distribution of the affected nerve root, and there may be associated paresthesias, numbness and weakness. The C_5, C_6 and C_7 nerve roots are most often affected. C_5 root compression results in the development of pain, paresthesias and numbness in the anterosuperior shoulder and anterolateral aspect of the upper arm and forearm; decreased biceps jerk and weakness of elbow flexion are found on examination. Compression of the C_6 nerve root produces symptoms in the dorsoradial aspect of the forearm and thumb, while C_7 impingement is denoted by altered sensation in the middle of the hand. The brachioradialis tendon reflex is affected by conditions altering C_5 and C_6, and the triceps jerk by injury to the C_7 and C_8 roots.

Whiplash is a lay term used to denote neck injury from an automobile accident. Typically, there is sudden hyperextension of the neck followed by flexion, resulting in musculoligamentous strain. Neurological deficits are rare unless there is an accompanying cervical spine fracture leading to root or cord compression. The problem of neck pain is often complicated by concurrent legal proceedings.

DIFFERENTIAL DIAGNOSIS

The musculoskeletal causes of neck pain include muscle strain, muscle spasm, cervical spondylosis, and cervical root compression. Lymphadenopathy (see Chapter 8), angina pectoris (see Chapter 14), and meningitis are important etiologies of cervical pain which may be mistaken for a musculosketal one.

WORKUP

History. Inquiry should focus on elucidating precipitating events, aggravating and alleviating factors (particularly specific neck movements), area of maximal tenderness, radiation of pain, presence of numbness or weakness in the extremities, course, past history of similar problems, and previous therapeutic efforts. One also needs to consider symptoms suggestive of coronary artery disease (see Chapter 14) or meningeal irritation.

Physical examination must include full visualization of the neck, thorax, and upper extremities. Neck motions are assessed, including flexion-extension, left and right lateral flexion, and left and right rotation. Palpation must be carefully done to identify the point of local tenderness, which gives the best indication of the structure involved. The upper extremities should also be carefully examined, including evaluation of tendon reflexes, strength, sensation, range of motion, and pulses. Every patient with fever and neck pain needs to be tested for meningeal signs.

Laboratory studies. Cervical spine x-rays are mandatory when there is root pain or a neurologic deficit, and should include AP, lateral, oblique and flexion-extension views in all cases to check for fracture, subluxation, narrowing of foramina and soft tissue abnormalities. An electrocardiogram is needed when chest pain radiates into the neck and jaw, or the patient with isolated neck pain has risk factors for coronary disease.

SYMPTOMATIC MANAGEMENT

Neck pain due to minor muscle ligament strain is usually self-limited when aggravating activities are avoided. Heat and gentle massage may ease muscle spasm. There is no good evidence that injecting anesthetic into the tender body of a muscle in spasm speeds resolution of the problem. Injection may actually injure the muscle. Occasionally, a soft cervical collar is needed if symptoms persist. The collar should be worn for several days to a few weeks, and used at all times until pain clears. Once pain lessens, the collar can be worn at times when added support may be helpful, such as at night or when riding in a motor vehicle. So-called muscle relaxants are of limited value; they act predominantly by sedating the patient. Cervical traction is indicated for severe, chronic, or recurrent neck pain due to cervical spondylosis or disc herniation associated with radiculitis. Sitting cervical traction is employed at home for 20 to 30 minutes, 2 to 4 times a day, using 6 to 10 pounds of weight. The cervical traction apparatus needs to be carefully aligned, pulling slightly forward at an angle of about 20° to follow the natural line in the neck. Mild analgesics such as aspirin, acetaminophen or propoxyphene, plus a mild tranquilizer such as chlordiazepoxide, may be helpful, as well.

INDICATIONS FOR ADMISSION AND REFERRAL

If pain is intractable to conservative measures, if there is significant weakness in the upper extremity, or if there is evidence of cord pressure or long tract signs, neurosurgical or orthopedic referral is indicated. Surgery may be necessary when signs of cord injury are present, unless further cervical traction in hospital results in rapid improvement. Presence of meningeal signs is an obvious indication for urgent hospitalization.

ANNOTATED BIBLIOGRAPHY

American Medical Association: Skeletal muscle relaxants. *In* AMA Drug Evaluations, ed. 3. Littleton, Mass.: PSG Publishing Company, 1977, p. 1023. *(There is no evidence at the present time that sedative agents used as muscle relaxants have a direct muscle-relaxant effect; rather, the reduction in muscle tone may be dependent on their centrally acting sedative effects.)*

Bailey, R.W. (ed.): The Cervical Spine. Philadelphia: Lee & Febiger, 1974. *(A good discussion of cervical spine problems emphasizing degenerative processes and trauma.)*

Miller, M., Gehweiler, J., Martinez, S., et al.: Significant new observations on cervical spine. Am. J. Roentgenol., *130*:659, 1978. *(An excellent recent article on x-ray abnormalities and cervical spine trauma.)*

Penning, L.: Normal movements of the cervical spine. Am. J. Roentgenol., *130*:317, 1978. *(An in-depth discussion of cervical spine biomechanics.)*

White, A., and Panjabi, J.: Basic kinematics of the human spine—Review of past and current knowledge. Spine, *3*:12, 1978. *(Review of kinetics, authoritative and current.)*

142
Evaluation of Shoulder Pain
ROBERT J. BOYD, M.D.

Shoulder pain is among the more common musculoskeletal complaints seen in office practice. Acute shoulder pain will usually precipitate a visit to the physician when symptoms interfere with daily activity. Ninety per cent of nontraumatic shoulder pain is due to tendinitis. Besides being capable of identifying an etiology, the primary physician needs to know how and when to utilize physical therapy, joint injection, and anti-inflammatory agents. Referral to an orthopedist should be reserved for refractory cases.

PATHOPHYSIOLOGY AND CLINICAL PRESENTATION

Injury or degenerative change in the rotator cuff, bicipital tendon, or acromioclavicular joint can produce pain localized to the shoulder joint. Characteristically, there is focal tenderness and aggravation of pain on shoulder movement. Patients report difficulty dressing, combing their hair or reaching up. Degenerative disease of the glenohumeral joint is uncommon; symptoms include mild stiffness, crepitus, and low-grade aching discomfort related to vigorous or sustained use. Pain originating in or about the shoulder may be referred to the upper arm or radiate to the neck, elbow or forearm; it does not follow a specific cervical root distribution. Although pain originating in the neck may radiate to the shoulder, it is brought on by neck motion rather than by shoulder movement and is usually not affected by shoulder position. However, there may be poorly localized sensitivity to touch extending into the shoulder, vaguely simulating shoulder pathology (see Chapter 141).

Rotator cuff disease. The tendons of the cuff are subjected to considerable mechanical stress. Degenerative and attritional changes take place over time in the tendons and lead to structural weakening. Tendinitis and tears may ensue. Calcific deposits develop as degenerating tendon fibers become pulverized and collections of calcium salts form. These deposits may contribute to local mechanical irritation by causing a bulge in the tendon and decreasing the clearances under the acromion and coraco-acromial ligament. Fibrous scarring with limitation of motion often occurs as part of the repair mechanism.

Calcific tendinitis is frequent and commonly affects the supraspinatus tendon. Usually there is no major precipitating event. It can cause acute or chronic pain; initially the pain is localized to the vicinity of the greater tuberosity and acromion process. Pain is worsened by abduction and elevation of the shoulder joint. X-rays may demonstrate calcium deposits in the tendon.

Bursitis is rarely a primary condition; usually it is secondary to calcific tendinitis. The subdeltoid bursa lies just above the supraspinatus tendon. The acutely inflamed and bulging tendon may irritate the overlying bursa. In addition, calcium deposits in the tendon may evacuate into the subbursal space or rupture into the bursa; when such material ruptures into the bursa, pain and tenderness may be felt in the upper third of the humerus.

Rupture. A weakened rotator cuff may rupture spontaneously as a result of minimal trauma. Patients with tears often present with surprisingly little pain. Local sensitivity is maximal over the greater tuberosity and rotator cuff (see Fig. 142–1). Active abduction of the shoulder and rotation are markedly limited while passive range of motion is full.

In *adhesive capsulitis* or *frozen shoulder syndrome*, pain and tenderness are located diffusely about the anterior and posterior regions of the shoulder joint capsule. Active as well as passive motions of the glenohumeral joint are limited. Diffuse pain gradually increases about the shoulder, and glenohumeral motion slowly decreases over several weeks. The condition is often refractory to most forms of treatment.

Biceps tendinitis of the shoulder is less common than rotator cuff tendinitis, and often follows a forward flexion strain. Elbow flexion against resistance will usually reproduce the pain, which is over the anterior aspect of the shoulder and upper arm. Characteristically, there is tenderness localized to the area about the long head of the biceps, in the bicipital

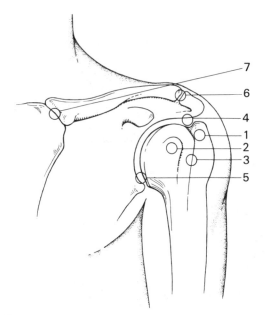

Fig. 142–1. Trigger points. Palpable "trigger points" during the examination reveal the site of the pathology, corroborate the history, and indicate the type of therapy. *1,* The greater tuberosity and the site of supraspinatus tendon insertion. *2,* Lesser tuberosity, site of subscapularis muscle insertion. *3,* Bicipital groove in which glides the bicipital tendon. *4,* Site of the subdeltoid bursa. *5,* Glenohumeral joint space. *6,* Acromioclavicular joint. *7,* Sternoclavicular joint. (Redrawn from Cailliet, R.: *Shoulder Pain.* Philadelphia: F. A. Davis, 1966)

groove over the proximal anterior margin of the humerus (see Fig. 142–1).

Infection. The shoulder joint may become contaminated by an improperly performed injection and present with marked swelling, redness and fever.

Dislocation. Dislocation usually results from trauma to the shoulder while it is hyperextended. Dislocations are most often anterior and characterized by loss of the shoulder's rounded appearance. There is prominence of the acromion, limitation of movement by pain, and displacement of the humerus away from the trunk. X-rays of the shoulder confirm diagnosis; axillary and tangential views must be obtained for full assessment because routine AP and lateral films may miss posterior dislocations.

Rheumatoid disease. Rheumatoid arthritis involving the shoulder is characteristically bilateral, with morning stiffness (see Chapter 147).

Acromioclavicular degenerative lesions. Degenerative changes are seen in patients who do heavy labor or engage in contact sports. Pain is localized to the acromioclavicular joint and nonradiating; tender-

ness is maximal over the joint. Shrugging the shoulder causes pain.

NONMUSCULOSKELETAL CONDITIONS. *Shoulder-hand syndrome* (also referred to as reflex sympathetic dystrophy) follows myocardial infarction, stroke, trauma and a host of other events. The characteristic features are persistent burning, "causalgic" pain, diffuse tenderness, immobilization of the shoulder and vasomotor changes in the hands. *Gallbladder disease* is suggested by pain at the tip of the scapula in conjunction with concurrent upper abdominal pain and tenderness. With *diaphragmatic irritation*, pain may be referred to the trapezius area running from the shoulder to the lateral aspect of the neck.

DIFFERENTIAL DIAGNOSIS

Shoulder pain can be divided into intrinsic and referred causes. Among the former are supraspinatus tendinitis, rotator cuff degeneration and tear, adhesive capsulitis or frozen shoulder, bicipital tendinitis, traumatic dislocations, rheumatoid arthritis and degenerative joint disease. Tendinitis accounts for over 90 per cent of nontraumatic cases of shoulder pain. Referred pain is seen with cervical root compression (see Chapter 141), spinal cord tumor, brachial plexus injury, angina (see Chapter 14), gallbladder disease, and diaphragmatic irritation (see Chapter 53).

WORKUP

History. One should inquire about previous trauma or an inciting event, location and radiation of pain, specific limitations of movement, associated neurologic deficits, aggravating and alleviating factors, previous history of shoulder problems, and therapies utilized. It is important to be sure there are no symptoms suggestive of angina, gallbladder disease or diaphragmatic irritation. An occupational history is occasionally revealing, especially if the patient has engaged in heavy labor or sports.

Physical examination. The shoulder is observed for any distortion of the normal surface anatomy, which is indicative of a dislocation or a severe inflammatory process. Next, the patient is asked to move the shoulder through a full range of motion, including internal and external rotation, abduction and elevation. This is followed by testing passive movement of the shoulder. The scapula is stabilized while glenohumeral joint motion is tested (Fig. 142–2). The shoulder is then palpated for "trigger points" to

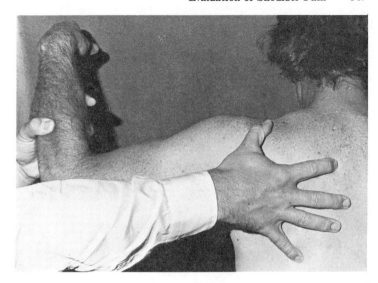

Fig. 142-2. Stabilization of the scapula while testing glenohumeral joint motion. (Katz, W. A.: *Rheumatic Diseases*. Philadelphia: J. B. Lippincott, 1977)

help reveal the site of pathology (Fig. 142-1). These include the greater tuberosity, site of the subscapularis insertion; bicipital groove, along which the bicipital tendon glides; the subdeltoid bursa, which is often inflamed in supraspinatus tendinitis; the glenohumeral joint space, and the acromioclavicular joint, an often overlooked site of degenerative disease and dislocation. The supraclavicular region is examined for tenderness, seen with brachial plexus injury. Careful neurologic and vascular examinations of the limbs are needed for detection of numbness, weakness, or vascular occlusion.

Neck, chest, heart and abdominal examinations are necessary in searching for sources of referred pain. Cervical disease is often mistaken for a shoulder problem. Cervical root compression is readily distinguished from intrinsic shoulder disease by the elicitation and reproduction of pain on neck motion to the side of complaint. Brachial plexus injury causing shoulder pain is associated with tenderness on deep pressure over the neurovascular bundle and scalene muscles of the supraclavicular fossa. Pain due to myocardial ischemia usually originates in the precordial region, but may present as shoulder or neck pain radiating into the arm. Relief with rest or nitroglycerin supports the diagnosis.

Laboratory studies. Most laboratory tests are only confirmatory; the history and physical examination suffice in the vast majority of cases. However, shoulder films are important when dislocation of the glenohumeral or acromioclavicular joint is suspected; tangential and axillary views of the shoulder must be obtained, because dislocation may be missed on standard AP and lateral films. Calcium deposits along the course of a tendon may be seen on shoulder x-rays of the patient with tendinitis. Cervical spine films are needed when neck motion reproduces the shoulder pain or root compression symptoms are noted (see Chapter 141).

When infection is suspected in the joint or joint capsule, aspiration, Gram stain and culture are urgent so that definitive therapy can be initiated without delay (see Chapter 138). When a peripheral nerve deficit is discovered on neurologic examination, electromyography may help to better characterize the lesion. The need for an electrocardiogram, gallbladder study, chest fluoroscopy, or radionuclide scan is dictated by the presence and nature of referred pain and associated physical findings.

INDICATIONS FOR REFERRAL

Glenohumeral and acromioclavicular dislocations and rotator cuff tears should be referred to an orthopedist for therapy as soon as the diagnosis is made or suspected. Most other causes of shoulder pain can be managed initially by the primary physician.

SYMPTOMATIC THERAPY

Tendinitis of the rotator cuff. This condition usually responds well to rest and anti-inflammatory agents followed by progressive exercises designed to

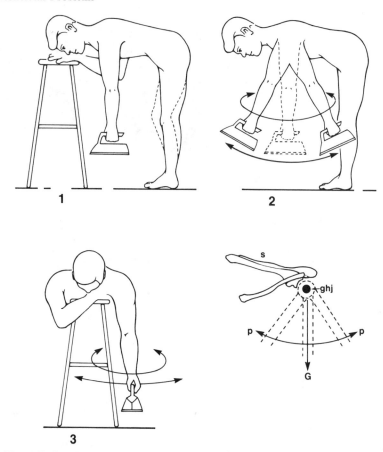

Fig. 142–3. Active pendular glenohumeral exercise (so-called Codman exercises). *1*, The posture to be assumed to permit the arm to "dangle" freely, with or without a weight. *2*, The arm moves in forward-and-back sagittal plane, in forward and backward flexion. Circular motion in the clockwise and counterclockwise direction is also done in ever-increasing large circles. *3*, The front view of the exercise showing lateral pendular movement actually in the coronal plane. The lower right diagram shows the effect of gravity, *G*, upon the glenohumeral joint, *ghj*, with an immobile scapula, *s*. The *p*-to-*p* arc is the pendular movement. (Redrawn from Cailliet, R.: *Shoulder Pain*. Philadelphia: F. A. Davis, 1966)

help the patient regain and preserve full range of motion. During the first few days of acute tendinitis, one can apply ice packs for 20-minute periods to reduce pain and swelling. A sling can be used to help rest the shoulder. Oral anti-inflammatory agents frequently contribute to the patient's comfort. A prompt and dramatic response is often obtained with phenylbutazone, 100 mg. 3 times daily; however, indomethacin, 25 to 50 mg. 3 times daily, is almost as effective and considerably safer, because, unlike phenylbutazone, it is not associated with agranulocytosis.

If shoulder pain does not respond to a course of systemic anti-inflammatory medication, and tenderness is well localized to the greater tuberosity/rota-

tor cuff area anterolaterally just under the margin of the acromion, local injection of a corticosteroid can be attempted. The point of maximum tenderness must be carefully found and marked, and 1 to 2 cc. of a local anesthetic (e.g., 2% lidocaine) injected into this area. If pain is substantially relieved by the local anesthetic, 40 mg. methylprednisolone (Depo-Medrol) or an equivalent steroid can be injected into the same area. Within several hours, the anesthetic will wear off and shoulder pain may again flare for 2 to 3 days, then gradually resolve.

Immobilization should not be prolonged beyond 4 to 7 days, because fibrosis and restriction of movement may develop. To prevent permanent limitation,

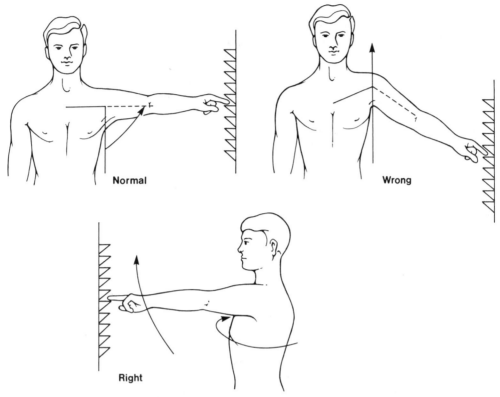

Normal

Wrong

Right

Fig. 142–4. Correct and incorrect use of "wall climbing" exercise. The wall climbing exercise frequently is done improperly. The normal arm climbs with normal scapulohumeral rhythm. When there is a pericapsulitis, the wall climb in abduction is done with "shrugging" of the scapula and accomplishes nothing. The wall climb should be started facing the wall and gradually turning the body until the patient is at a right angle to the wall. (Redrawn from Cailliet, R.: *Shoulder Pain.* Philadelphia: F. A. Davis, 1966)

the patient is taught active range of motion exercises to be performed at home as soon as the pain has sufficiently subsided. Pendulum exercises are prescribed for the early phases of recovery, even though mild pain may persist, to stretch the joint capsule and increase range of motion without furthering injury. It is essential that the patient not actively abduct or elevate the shoulder. The patient bends forward at the waist, dangles the arm, often with the help of a weight, and swings the arm in forward-and-back, side-to-side and ever-increasing circular motions. The head is rested upon the other hand and the elbow kept straight (Fig. 142–3).

Further exercises, such as "wall-climbing," shoulder shrugging and others (Fig. 142–4) are employed as pain further subsides and range of motion increases. It is important to recognize that some "pulling" discomfort will be felt during these exercises, since they are designed to stretch the capsule and increase range of motion. In fact, if no stretching is

felt, chances are the exercise is not being done correctly. Jerky extreme movements must be avoided, because these leave residual pain and worsen injury. Exercises should be performed 3 or 4 times daily for about 5 minutes each time.

Aspirin may be a helpful adjunct to exercise by providing some anti-inflammatory effect as well as analgesia. Narcotics should be avoided if possible. Oral steroids are not indicated for acute episodes since they take days to become fully effective, and the acute condition is usually self-limited.

Forward flexion of the shoulder should be substituted for abduction and the patient advised to make a habit of putting the involved arm into dress; shirt- and coat-sleeve first. If there is a large deposit of calcium in the shoulder and disabling chronic discomfort or frequent acute recurrences of pain develop, surgical excision of the calcific deposit, partial acromionectomy and division of the coracoacromial ligaments may be needed.

Frozen shoulder. Treatment is difficult. Although the problem is partially self-limited, in that pain subsides and some motion returns eventually, the recovery may not be complete and limitation of movement may remain. The treatment program is similar to that for acute tendinitis with a few important differences. The patient with a frozen shoulder is often tense, passive and dependent. A low threshold for pain is common. Thus, attention must be given to the patient's personality and environment as well as to the shoulder in order to achieve results. Use of a minor tranquilizer may help to lessen anxiety and enable these individuals to take the active role necessary to regain function. Discussion and resolution of family and job stresses are helpful for the same reasons.

Medication for pain should be limited to non-narcotic anti-inflammatory agents. A short course of oral corticosteroid therapy—for no more than 5 to 10 days, to avoid adrenal suppression—may have impressive effects in stubborn cases. One starts with 20 to 40 mg. of prednisone per day, tapering rapidly over the 5- to 10-day course of therapy.

Active exercises are the most valuable therapeutic modality, but may be difficult to start in the passive, tense, fearful patient. The patient can start with pendulum exercises and progress as in therapy for tendinitis. It may be necessary to assist the patient initially, demonstrating that there is no harm in moving and stretching the joint and capsule. Once range of motion is increased, overhead stretching, such as hanging from a chinning bar, is excellent; reaching for the ceiling or door frame above the head and slightly behind the body is also very beneficial. There is no evidence that shoulder manipulations or local steroid injections are of any value.

Biceps tendinitis management. Management is similar to that described for rotator tendinitis: anti-inflammatory medication, pendulum exercises and limitation of other shoulder motions initially. Occasionally, local cortisone injection into the area of tenderness is helpful; it can be done by carefully and precisely identifying the area of pain. Rarely, surgical division and reattachment of the long head of the biceps is necessary.

PATIENT EDUCATION

The patient must be made to realize that thorough recovery from tendinitis requires active participation in the treatment program. Many individuals seek only relief from pain and expect oral or injectable medication to suffice. They must be told that repeated pain and limitation of function are bound to ensue if the exercise program is not taken seriously.

ANNOTATED BIBLIOGRAPHY

Bateman, J.E.: The Shoulder and Neck. Philadelphia: W.B. Saunders, 1972. *(A good standard textbook for further reference.)*

Calliet, R.: Shoulder Pain. Philadelphia: F.A. Davis, 1973. *(A clearly written and well-illustrated monograph that provides in-depth discussion of tendinitis.)*

Cave, E., Burke, J., and Boyd, R.: Trauma Management. Chicago: Year Book Medical Publishers, 1974. *(In particular, Chapter 17 provides an excellent discussion of shoulder girdle injuries, including shoulder dislocations, for further reference.)*

143
Evaluation of Hip Pain
ROBERT J. BOYD, M.D.

Hip pain can be a major source of misery for the patient and family. The joint is essential to locomotion and weight-bearing and is frequently subject to trauma and chronic mechanical stress. Assessment of hip pain requires determinations of severity and disability as well as etiology, because surgery is now a practical therapeutic option for disabled patients refractory to conservative measures.

PATHOPHYSIOLOGY AND
CLINICAL PRESENTATION

The hip is supplied by the obturator, sciatic, and femoral nerves. Pain originating in or around the hip can be felt in the groin or buttock, with radiation to the distal thigh and anteromedial aspect of the knee. Occasionally, pain from the hip may be felt only in the thigh and knee. Pain occurs in the distribution of the L_2 and L_3 roots, and rarely is referred to the lower leg or foot. Conversely, pain due to a problem outside the hip may be referred to the hip if the lesion irritates the femoral, sciatic or obturator nerve, or nerve roots. Extra-hip problems include herniation of high lumbar discs, retroperitoneal or pelvic tumor, and femoral hernia; aortoiliac insufficiency may also present with hip and buttock pain (see Chapter 17).

Hip pain may be focal or diffuse, depending on the extent to which the joint and surrounding structures are involved in the pathologic process. For example, bursitis is characterized by focal pain and tenderness over the site of the bursa; synovitis is more diffuse, involving the entire joint capsule. Stiffness, limitation of motion, limp, and crepitus are frequent accompaniments of pain. Swelling is usually not evident and is difficult to detect, since the joint is buried deeply in soft tissues.

The major mechanisms of hip disease include cartilaginous degeneration, synovial inflammation, tendinitis and consequent bursitis, fracture and ischemia.

Osteoarthritis. The hip is a major site of degenerative joint disease (see Chapter 148); the elderly are most affected. Onset is often insidious, beginning with minor aching or stiffness that may be unilateral or bilateral. Symptoms are characteristically exacerbated by prolonged standing, walking or stair-climbing. Stiffness is present on getting up after long periods of sitting. The hip begins to loosen up on first moving about, but worsens with continued activity. As osteoarthritis gradually progresses, it results in decreasing hip motion, increasing stiffness, and increasing pain. A limp may develop as joint architecture is disrupted and weight-bearing becomes painful. The course of the disease is usually marked by spontaneous exacerbations and remissions.

On physical examination, the patient with substantial disease characteristically holds the leg in flexion, external rotation and adduction. There may be an antalgic gait, positive Trendelenburg sign (buttock falls when standing on opposite foot) indicative of abductor weakness, and limitation of hip motion, with or without crepitus. Pain, muscle spasm and guarding occur when the examiner attempts to take the hip through the full range of motion. There may be buttock atrophy involving the gluteus maximus posteriorly and the gluteus medius more laterally. With severe degenerative arthritis of the hip, there may be a marked flexion deformity and pain in the hip joint even at rest.

Rheumatoid arthritis. The hips are rarely affected in rheumatoid disease until other joints have become involved. Pain is characteristically bilateral and associated with morning stiffness, which lessens with activity. During flares of the disease, the hip joint is tender to palpation, and capsular fullness and thickening may be felt if effusion or chronic synovitis are present. Flexion contractures occur in advanced cases (see Chapter 147).

Ankylosing spondylitis. The disease is unique among the spondyloarthropathies in that the hip is sometimes affected. Concurrent sacroiliac and spinal involvement is usually present and in itself may cause pain radiating into the hip or buttock (see Chapters 138 and 139).

Hip fracture is most prevalent in the elderly, who are subject to frequent falls and osteoporosis. The femoral neck and intertrochanteric region are common fracture sites. There may be loss of normal surface architecture, acute joint deformity, severe pain, guarding and restriction of flexion and external rotation. Active straight-leg raising is impaired. X-rays are diagnostic.

Septic arthritis. Joint infection in the hip most often follows hematogenous seeding (see Chapter 138). Since the joint is deep-seated, the ordinary signs of infection may not be readily evident. Fever, hip or knee pain (due to pain referral) and inability to bear weight are early symptoms. The thigh is often held in flexion, and a bulging, tender joint capsule may be palpable.

Idiopathic avascular necrosis. Aseptic necrosis of the femoral head is believed due to ischemia. The condition is most often seen in patients on chronic corticosteroid therapy. Alcoholics, patients with hemoglobinopathies, and those who work under conditions of increased atmosphere pressure are also at risk. Patients report gradual onset of focal pain and limitation of movement. X-rays are diagnostic; they show wedge-shaped areas of increased density and segmental collapse of the femoral head.

Bursitis. Inflammation of the bursa occurs as a consequence of trauma or spread of an inflammatory process. There is focal pain with tenderness over the bursa. *Trochanteric bursitis* is felt on the lateral aspect of the hip, posterior to the trochanter. Symptoms are increased by direct pressure or hip flexion and internal rotation. Pain may worsen at night and radiate down the leg to the knee. *Iliopectineal bursitis* causes pain on flexion and tenderness localized to the lateral border of Scarpa's triangle. *Ischiogluteal bursitis* presents with buttock pain that is worse on prolonged sitting, occurs at night, and occasionally radiates down the leg posteriorly, simulating sciatica.

Polymyalgia rheumatica. This is a disease of the elderly, characterized by bilateral aching of the hips, thighs, and shoulders in conjunction with a very high sedimentation rate (see Chapter 150). Passive range of joint motion is usually preserved.

Pigmented villonodular synovitis. This uncommon granulomatous disease of the synovium presents with slowly progressive pain and limitation of movement. X-rays show large cystic areas about the hip joint, distinguishing the condition from degenerative joint disease.

Referred pain. Any pelvic, abdominal or retroperitoneal process irritating the obturator muscle can cause pain referred to the hip and worsened by internal rotation of the hip joint.

DIFFERENTIAL DIAGNOSIS

Hip pain is usually due to degenerative joint disease. Other causes include joint infection, avascular necrosis of the femoral head, bursitis, polymyalgia rheumatica, rheumatoid arthritis, and, rarely, ankylosing spondylitis and villonodular synovitis. Pain may be referred to the hip from lumbar or pelvic problem such as high lumbar disc herniation, retroperitoneal tumor or abscess, or obturator or femoral hernia. Aortoiliac insufficiency may present with hip and buttock pain.

WORKUP

History. One should ascertain the onset, location, and radiation of the pain as well as inciting and alleviating factors, and the presence of numbness or weakness. It is particularly important to inquire directly about trauma, involvement of other joints, morning stiffness, relationship of pain to activity, response to rest, steroid or alcohol use, and current infection or fever. There are a few pitfalls regarding history; for example, stiffness by itself is a nonspecific finding, because it may occur with degenerative disease as well as with rheumatoid involvement of the hip. The response to continued activity may be of more help; stiffness usually worsens in degenerative disease and lessens in rheumatoid arthritis. Bilateral cramping hip and buttock pain that comes on with walking and is relieved by rest may actually be a sign of vascular insufficiency rather than of joint disease.

Physical examination. The hip should be looked at for deformities such as flexion or adduction contractures that are seen with rheumatoid disease, and for fixed external rotation, suggesting a fracture of the femoral neck. Gait is also important to check. The hip is then put through the full range of passive motion to detect crepitus, limitation of movement, flexion contracture, muscle spasm or guarding. Normal range of hip flexion-extension is $-20°$ to $90°$ with the knee straight and $0°$ to $120°$ with the knee flexed. Normal adduction-abduction is $-20°$ to $90°$; normal internal-external rotation is $-50°$ to $+50°$. Among the earliest limitations of movement in hip disease is internal rotation with the hip hyperextended. Palpation of the joint and individual bursae for focal tenderness and swelling is important for detecting a localized inflammatory process.

Circumference measurements should be made of the thigh at a fixed distance from a bony reference point such as the tibial tubercle of the knee, the anterior superior iliac spine, or the midpatella. Atrophy is suggestive of intrinsic hip disease. Femoral pulses need to be palpated for diminution and auscultated for bruits. Pelvic and rectal examinations are helpful in searching for tumors which may cause referred pain. The back should be examined for evidence of L_{1-2} or L_{2-3} disc herniation (see Chapter 140). Neurologic assessment of the lower extremities is needed to test for weakness, sensory loss and reflexes.

Laboratory studies. Hip x-rays are essential to the assessment of hip pain. They may be diagnostic of degenerative joint disease, rheumatoid arthritis, avascular necrosis, or fracture. Weight-bearing films help one judge the severity of degenerative hip disease by disclosing the extent of joint space narrowing. Sacroiliac and spine films are needed if ankylosing spondylitis is under consideration (see Chapter 139). Other laboratory studies worth ordering are few in number. A CBC, sedimentation rate and rheumatoid factor are useful if an inflammatory process is being considered (see Chapter 139). If a septic joint is suspected, aspiration for Gram stain and culture is urgent (see Chapter 138).

SYMPTOMATIC THERAPY AND INDICATIONS FOR REFERRAL

Degenerative disease. Simple treatment measures for relief of an acute exacerbation include bed rest, aspirin, limitation of sitting, and crutch or cane support. Once acute symptoms lessen, the patient can begin a program that includes avoidance of activities that specifically aggravate pain, rest periods of one hour twice daily with local heat to the hip, daily mild exercise of walking short distances as tolerated, aspirin or acetaminophen regularly, cane support, weight reduction in the obese, and specific daily range of motion and strengthening exercises, preferably outlined by a physical therapist. Acute exacerbations of hip pain can often be managed effectively by a few weeks of bed rest and several weeks' use of a partial weight-bearing crutch. If conservative measures fail to control symptoms, and the patient is active, surgery may be needed. Since results of hip reconstructive procedures are now quite good and the procedure has relatively low risk, referral for consideration of surgery need not be delayed indefinitely if symptoms are disabling and not well controlled by conservative measures. The need for reconstructive surgery must be a joint decision of patient, primary physician and orthopedic surgeon.

Bursitis. Anti-inflammatory medication should be tried, e.g., indomethacin, 25 mg. three times daily for 1 to 2 weeks. If pain does not respond and if tenderness is well localized to a bursa, a local steroid injection can be given, using 2 cc. of 2% lidocaine (Xylocaine) followed by 40 mg. methylprednisolone (Depo-Medrol) in 1 cc. injected into the tender area. Primary physicians who are unfamiliar with the technique of injecting a hip bursa should refer the patient to an orthopedist or rheumatologist. *Polymyalgia rheumatica* responds to low-dose steroids (see Chapter 150), and *rheumatoid arthritis* to nonsteroidal anti-inflammatory agents (see Chapter 147).

Hip fracture and *septic arthritis* are indications for immediate hospitalization.

ANNOTATED BIBLIOGRAPHY

Beckenbaugh, R., and Ilstrup, D.: Total hip arthroplasty—Review of 333 cases with long follow-up. J. Bone Joint Surg., *60*(A):306, 1978. *(A carefully studied series of total hip replacement patients.)*

144

Evaluation of Knee Pain
ROBERT J. BOYD, M.D.

The knee joint is frequently the site of trauma, degenerative disease, and rheumatologic conditions. Disability can be considerable because of inability to bear weight. The primary physician is called upon most often for minor acute injuries or chronic knee pain that limits mobility. Occasionally, an acute monoarticular arthritis is encountered. The popularity of jogging and especially long-distance running has markedly increased the prevalence of acute and recurrent knee complaints.

PATHOPHYSIOLOGY AND CLINICAL PRESENTATION

Degenerative disease, trauma-induced soft tissue derangements, and inflammatory processes are the predominant mechanisms of knee pain in the adult. The pain is characteristically worsened by weight-bearing and may radiate into the anterior thigh, posterior calf or pretibial region. An inflamed joint capsule produces diffuse pain; bursitis causes more focal discomfort; a tear in the meniscus may result in pain along the joint line. Locking of the joint suggests a loose body or torn meniscus. Hip disease occasionally presents as knee pain (see Chapter 143).

Degenerative disease. Changes often originate in the medial joint compartment and patellofemoral joint, related in part to mechanical stresses. The entire joint may be painful, but often the discomfort is localized to the anterior and medial portions of the knee. Prolonged standing or walking may precipitate or worsen symptoms. Mild stiffness is common on first arising in the morning and on getting up after a long period of sitting; it initially improves on moving about, but worsens with continued activity. Symptoms gradually progress, but may take many years to become disabling. Considerable degenerative change and joint destruction can occur before serious knee pain develops. Small effusions may appear after prolonged weight-bearing, but few other signs or symptoms of inflammation occur.

Rheumatoid disease. Rheumatoid arthritis commonly affects the knees. Pain, swelling and morning stiffness are characteristic. Symmetrical polyarticular involvement is the rule, with joints in the hands, feet, ankles and wrists often affected. Symptoms wax and wane; the course is chronic (see Chapter 147). Other rheumatoid diseases can produce a similar picture (see Chapter 139).

Acute monoarticular arthritis. The knee is a frequent site of septic arthritis, gout, pseudogout, early rheumatoid arthritis, rheumatic fever, palindromic rheumatism and disseminated gonorrhea. Usually there is the acute onset of unilateral swelling, pain, and generalized tenderness (see Chapter 138). Motion is limited and muscle spasm prominent.

Knee sprain. Ligamentous injury caused by excessive joint strain is extremely frequent. Sprain injuries range from minor tears of a few fibers to complete tears of entire ligaments resulting in loss of joint stability. Mild sprains produce tenderness and local swelling without joint effusion or loss of joint stability. In moderate sprains, there is pain on stressing the joint, voluntary restriction of movement, some joint instability and swelling due to an effusion. Severe sprains involve total loss of integrity and immediate swelling, marked joint instability, severe pain and a large effusion. The collateral and cruciate ligaments are frequently injured in contact sports; ligamentous injuries are uncommon in joggers.

Degeneration or tear of a meniscus. An acute tear occurs as a result of excessive weight-bearing, twisting, or valgus or varus stress, and may be associated with partial or complete disruption of collateral or cruciate ligaments. There is usually a history of acute trauma and immediate swelling due to tissue disruption and bleeding. Joint locking may occur. If swelling does not develop until the next day, damage is likely to be confined to the meniscus and not involve the ligament; such swelling is due to a reactive joint effusion. Chronic internal derangements caused by degeneration or tear of the meniscus produce recurrent pain, swelling, and a knee that gives way, catches, or locks.

Chondromalacia patellae. Degeneration of the posterior patellar cartilage is the cause of this condition. Dessication, thinning, fissure formation and ultimately erosion of the cartilage occur. Mechanical factors are suspected, though unproven. Chondromalacia is the most common cause of knee pain in joggers. The patient presents with retropatellar aching that is worsened by standing up, climbing stairs or any other form of bent-knee strain. There may be stiffness after inactivity, but there is usually no locking or giving way to the knee. Pain can be elicited by applying pressure against the patella with the knee actively extended. X-rays are normal until late stages, when the posterior surface of the patella becomes irregular and marginal osteophytes develop.

Baker's cyst. Rupture of one of these popliteal fossa cysts can cause acute inflammation with pain, swelling and limitation of knee flexion. The inflammation may extend down into the calf and simulate thrombophlebitis. Baker's cysts usually communicate with the knee joint space and most commonly occur in patients with osteoarthritis or rheumatoid disease. An unruptured cyst causes only mild aching and stiffness. Trauma may initiate a rupture.

Prepatellar bursitis results from repeated trauma—hence, the name "housemaid's knee." Swelling, tenderness and occasionally erythema over the prepatellar bursae are present. Bursitis of the suprapatellar and infrapatellar bursae have similar presentations, with findings localized to the bursal site.

Villonodular synovitis is a granulomatous inflammatory condition of the synovium which lines the joints, bursae and tendon sheaths. Etiology is unknown. It affects young adults, predominantly men, and presents with unilateral pain, persistent swelling, intermittent knee locking and, occasionally, a palpable mass. Diagnosis requires arthroscopy or surgical exploration.

DIFFERENTIAL DIAGNOSIS

The list of conditions which can cause knee pain is extensive and includes those that cause polyarticular disease as well as those that are confined to the

Table 144–1. Differential Diagnosis of Knee Pain

KNEE INVOLVEMENT							
ASYMMETRICAL				SYMMETRICAL			
ONE KNEE ONLY		ONE KNEE PLUS OTHER JOINTS		KNEES ONLY		SYMMETRICAL POLYARTHRITIS	
Acute	*Chronic*	*Acute*	*Chronic*	*Acute*	*Chronic*	*Acute*	*Chronic*
Sprain	Osteoarthritis	See Chap. 139		Rheumatoid arthritis	Osteoarthritis	See Chap. 139	
Strain	Baker's cyst			Juvenile RA	Chondromalacia patellae		
Acute gout	Chronic gout			Early phase of other rheumatoid diseases	Bursitis		
Meniscus tear	Chrondromalacia patellae			Trauma	Rheumatoid arthritis		
Early rheumatoid disease	Bursitis				Juvenile RA		
Gonococcal arthritis	Meniscal injuries				Chronic gout		
Septic arthritis					Neuropathic joints		
Reiter's syndrome					Hemophilia		
Bursitis							
Pseudogout							
Pallindromic rheumatism							
Ruptured Baker's cyst							
Hemophilia							
Sickle cell disease							
Cassion's disease							
Rheumatic fever							

Adapted from Katz, W. A.: *Rheumatic Diseases.* Philadelphia: J. B. Lippincott. 1977.

knee. A clinically useful classification system is to group etiologies according to whether they are acute or chronic, symmetrical or asymmetrical, and monoarticular or polyarticular (see Table 144–1).

WORKUP

History. Besides ascertaining the pain's quality, location, alleviating and aggravating factors, and associated symptoms such as swelling, redness and warmth, it is necessary to determine if the problem is acute or chronic, symmetrical or asymmetrical, and mono- or polyarticular. By combining a careful description of the problem with a characterization of its pattern and chronicity, one can quickly focus the evaluation onto a relatively limited set of conditions having similar clinical presentations (see Table 144–1).

ACUTE UNILATERAL KNEE PAIN. One should inquire about trauma, jogging, locking, swelling, pain on climbing stairs, concurrent fever, purulent vaginal or urethral discharge, rash, recent strep infection or sore throat, heart murmur, morning stiffness, and urethritis or conjunctivitis (see Chapter 138). Any prior history of gout, sickle cell disease or hemophilia should be checked for. When swelling is localized, it is important to determine the exact site, since it may be a clue to bursitis or a Baker's cyst.

CHRONIC UNILATERAL KNEE PAIN. Questioning ought to cover previous or recurrent trauma, pain in association with prolonged walking, standing or climbing stairs, knee locking, crepitus, focal swelling and recurrent acute episodes or exacerbations.

ACUTE OR CHRONIC UNILATERAL KNEE PAIN WITH CONCURRENT ASYMMETRICAL INVOLVEMENT OF OTHER JOINTS. See Chapter 139.

ACUTE BILATERAL KNEE PAIN. The focus of inquiry should be on the symptoms of rheumatoid disease (see Chapters 139 and 147) and recent trauma.

CHRONIC BILATERAL KNEE PAIN. The questioning can be similar to that for chronic unilateral disease, but there should also be consideration of rheumatoid symptoms (see Chapter 139).

ACUTE OR CHRONIC BILATERAL KNEE PAIN WITH CONCURRENT SYMMETRICAL INVOLVEMENT OF OTHER JOINTS. See Chapter 139.

Physical examination. A complete physical examination must be performed because many systemic illnesses can present with knee pain. Skin and integument are examined for rash, clubbing, psoriatic changes, rheumatoid nodules, pallor, alopecia, and tophi; conjunctivae for erythema and petechiae; oral cavity for aphthous ulcers; lymph nodes for enlargement; chest for signs of consolidation and effusion, heart for murmurs and rubs; abdomen for organomegaly and tenderness; pelvis for vaginal discharge and adnexal tenderness; urethral for discharge and penis for balanitis. This is in addition to a thorough check of all joints and complete neurologic testing.

Examination of the knee should begin with a careful inspection for distortion of normal contours and irregular bony prominences at the joint margin.

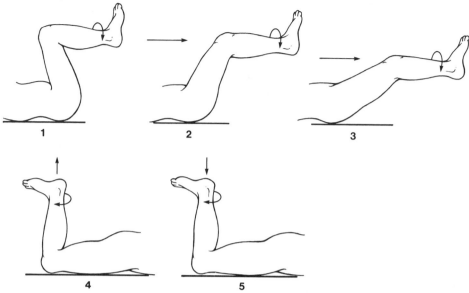

Fig. 144–1. Meniscus signs (examination). *1, 2, 3, McMurray test.* The patient is supine with knee flexed, heel touching the buttocks at the start. The leg is internally rotated for lateral meniscus testing or externally rotated for medial meniscus testing. Then the knee is fully extended. A painful click occurs if there is a meniscus lesion. The test is more meaningful in the first phase of knee extension. Full extension limitation does not indicate an anterior meniscus lesion. *4, 5, Apley test.* The patient is prone. Leg is internally or externally rotated with simultaneous traction. Pain indicates a capsular or ligamentous lesion. Rotation with downward pressure that causes pain indicates meniscus lesion. (Redrawn from Cailliet, R.: *Knee Pain and Disability.* Philadelphia: F. A. Davis, 1973)

It is important to check for muscle atrophy. Measurements of knee, calf, and thigh circumferences can help quantitate the loss of muscle mass. Presence of an effusion needs to be determined; this is done by noting an increased knee circumference at midpatella and feeling for a distended fluctuant capsule with a fluid wave and ballotable patella. The joint line should be palpated for localized joint line tenderness suggestive of a meniscal tear. The McMurray and Apley tests are performed for suspected meniscal injury (see Fig. 144–1). The bursal regions should be assessed for focal tenderness and swelling indicative of bursitis.

Range of motion needs to be determined. The knees normally extend symmetrically 180°, and may hyperextend an additional 5° or 10°. Knee flexion is also symmetrical and limited to 135° to 170° by posterior soft tissue contact or by the heel striking the buttock. Collateral and cruciate ligaments should be examined for stability. Collateral ligaments are tested by applying mediolateral valgus-varus strain with the knee in full extension and in 15° to 20° of flexion. Cruciate stability is determined by anterior-posterior displacement of the upper tibia on the fixed lower femur with the knee in extension and in 90° of flexion (Fig. 144–2).

Laboratory studies. There is no set of "routine" laboratory studies for assessment of knee pain. When there is trauma, x-rays are needed to rule out fracture, and stress films are indicated to determine joint stability. Knee films are also indicated for suspected degenerative or rheumatoid disease. Weight-bearing films best demonstrate degree of joint obliteration. Acute monoarticular effusions require prompt arthrocentesis for Gram stain and cultures to rule out a septic process (see Chapter 138). Joint fluid is sent for determinations of the white cell count, differential, and glucose, and is examined for crystals. Rheumatoid factor, sedimentation rate, antinuclear antibodies, uric acid, ASLO titer and HLA-B27 may be useful in evaluation of selected mono- and polyarticular problems (see Chapters 138 and 139).

SYMPTOMATIC THERAPY AND INDICATIONS FOR REFERRAL

Acute pain often responds to restriction of weight-bearing activities; only absolutely necessary walking is allowed, and kneeling, squatting and stair-climbing are forbidden. Isometric quadriceps and hamstring exercises help prevent thigh weakness and

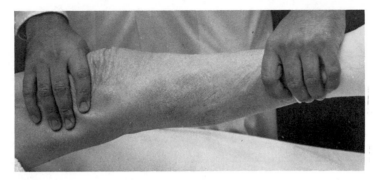

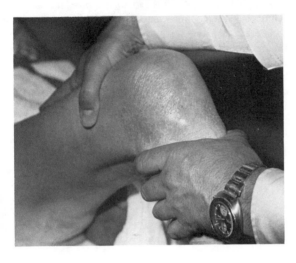

Fig. 144-2. *(top)* Testing for lateral instability of the knee by fixating the lower femur with one hand and forcibly abducting and adducting the joint while grasping the leg. *(bottom)* "Drawer sign" performed by drawing the upper tibia back and forth upon the fixated femur. (Katz, W. A.: *Rheumatic Diseases.* Philadelphia: J. B. Lippincott, 1977)

atrophy. Aspirin may be quite helpful symptomatically when used in pharmacologic doses of 2 to 4 gm. per day. If the problem is one of acute severe injury and pain, especially if the knee gives way or locks and there is a question of joint instability or internal derangement, prompt orthopedic referral is essential. Arthroscopy may be needed.

ANNOTATED BIBLIOGRAPHY

Helfet, A.J.: Disorders of the Knee. Philadelphia: J.B. Lippincott, 1974. *(A good standard orthopedic text, including detailed discussion of the orthopedic aspects of knee problems.)*

Jackson, R.W., and Dandy, D.J.: Arthroscopy of the Knee. New York: Grune & Stratton, 1976. *(Detailed description of arthroscopic technique as a guide to assessing knee problems.)*

Jones, R.E., Smith, E.C., and Reisch, J.S.: Effects of medial meniscectomy in patients older than 40 years. J. Bone Joint Surg. 60(A):783, 1978. *(Following meniscectomy for degenerative tears, there is a high ,incidence of osteoarthritis, and current feeling is that retention of as much of the meniscus as possible is important to protect the compartment from further articular cartilage stress and degeneration.)*

Laskin, R.S. (ed.): Symposium on disorders of the knee joint. Orthop. Clin. North Am., 10(1):1, 1979. *(A discussion of problems affecting the knee joint.)*

Royer, H.R. (ed.): Sports injuries. Orthop. Clin. North Am., 1(3):1, 1978. *(Further reference on management and assessment of athletic injuries.)*

Smillie, I.S.: Injuries of the Knee Joint, ed. 4. New York: Churchill Livingstone, 1975. *(A classic text discussing traumatic knee problems in depth.)*

Watanabe, M.: Present state of arthroscopy. Int. Orthop., 2:101, 1978. *(Further information regarding use of arthroscopy in evaluating and managing knee problems.)*

145

Approach to Minor Orthopedic Problems of the Elbow, Ankle, and Foot
ROBERT J. BOYD, M.D.

Most minor orthopedic problems seen in the office that involve the elbow, ankle or foot are due to trauma. The frequency of such problems has increased with the growth in popularity of jogging and racquet sports. The primary physician should be able to diagnose the more common problems, initiate conservative therapy, and decide when orthopedic referral is necessary.

ELBOW

Tennis elbow. A frequent injury among players of racquet sports is lateral epicondylitis or "tennis elbow." It is usually self-limited. Symptoms occur on wrist extension and strong grasp, and subside on simple avoidance of aggravating activities. There is associated tenderness well-localized to the proximal attachment of the common extensor tendon at or near the lateral epicondyle (Fig. 145–1). It may take several weeks for pain to clear. Any painful activity is best avoided, including racquet sports, shaking hands, forceful use of the arm in hammering or unscrewing jars, or using a screwdriver. There is no certain way to prevent recurrences of epicondylitis related to playing tennis, but proper stroking of shots with a firm wrist and proper elbow positioning may be helpful. Elbow bands are often tried but usually are of limited value; however, sometimes they allow play when mild pain is present.

If symptoms do not clear promptly, systemic anti-inflammatory medication (e.g., indomethacin, 25 mg. three times daily for 1 week) should be tried. Local steroid injection may eventually be needed,

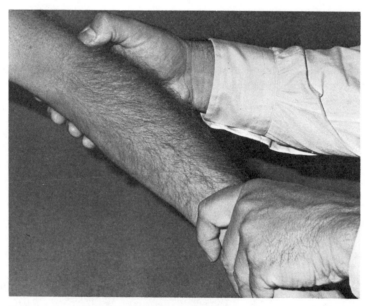

Fig. 145–1. Technique of palpating the lateral epicondyle to elicit "point" tenderness typical of "tennis elbow." (Katz, W. A.: *Rheumatic Diseases.* Philadelphia: J. B. Lippincott, 1977)

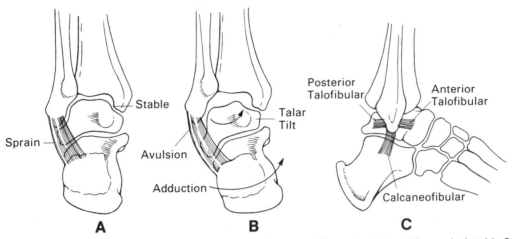

Fig. 145-2.   Lateral ligamentous sprain and avulsion. The lateral ligaments of the ankle are depicted in C. The anterior talofibular and the calcaneofibular ligaments are the ligaments most frequently involved in inversion injuries. A is the simple sprain in which the ligaments remain intact and the talus remains stable within the mortice. B depicts avulsion of the lateral ligaments, and the talus becomes unstable and tilts within the mortice when the calcaneus is adducted. (Redrawn from Cailliet, R.: *Foot and Ankle Pain.* Philadelphia: F. A. Davis, 1968)

though results may not be very dramatic. The area of well-localized tenderness is carefully identified and injected with 1 cc. of 2% lidocaine (Xylocaine) followed by injection of 40 mg. of methlyprednisolone (Depo-Medrol).

Olecranon bursitis usually follows direct bruising or irritation in response to protective sponge pad, ace bandage, and systemic anti-inflammatory agents. Occasionally aspiration of the bursa and installation of steroid is needed.

ANKLE

Ankle sprain. A sprain is the most common ankle injury. Lesions range from minor ligamentous damage to complete tear or avulsion of the bony attachment, fracture and dislocation. A *strain* does not involve loss of joint stability or tearing of ligaments, whereas a sprain does. Sprain occurs when stress is applied while the ankle is in an unstable position, causing the ligaments to overstretch. During plantar flexion the joint is least stable and most susceptible to eversion or inversion forces. Such stresses are encountered during running or walking over uneven surfaces. Evaluation is facilitated by early presentation, because the event producing injury is likely to be remembered and swelling is confined to the site of injury.

An *inversion injury* is the most common type of sprain, causing damage to the lateral ligaments. There is often a history of inversion during plantar flexion; a snap or tear may have been heard or felt. Passive inversion of the ankle produces pain. Swelling invariably occurs, usually anterior to the lateral malleolus at the onset; ecchymoses are common. Simple strain does not result in joint instability, whereas with a sprain, the joint loses stability and the talus tilts when the calcaneus is adducted (see Fig. 145-2). This produces a talomalleolar gap on the lateral aspect of the ankle. If swelling or pain interferes with evaluation, an x-ray assessment after nerve block may be needed to determine joint instability. X-rays are taken with the ankle fully inverted. The degree of talar tilt is diagnostic.

Control of swelling is the first and immediate priority of management, because effusion and hemorrhage further stretch and distend the joint and predispose to adhesions. An elastic bandage, ice water and elevation are often helpful in controlling edema. The ankle should be placed in ice water for 15 to 20 minutes and then elevated. An ice pack may substitute for immersion. Cold application is repeated every few hours. X-rays can be done after taping, ice water and elevation.

A strain or minor sprain can be managed by repeated ice packs, followed within 48 hours by hot soaks. The elastic bandage is used for 1 to 2 weeks to control swelling and provide stability. Partial weight-bearing is accomplished by utilizing a crutch until

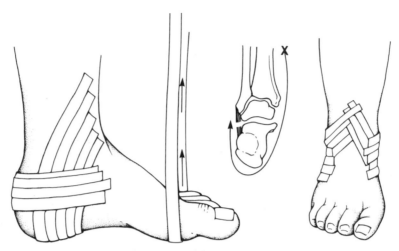

Fig. 145-3. Taping a sprained ankle. The purpose of taping an ankle is to prevent further stretching of the injured ligaments until healing has occurred. The ankle must be inverted or everted to place the strained ligament at rest. The center figure depicts an avulsed lateral ligament. The tape here begins from inside and the runs under the foot to finish on the outer leg holding the heel *everted*. The horizontal strips minimize rotation of the forefoot. (Redrawn from Cailliet, R.: *Foot and Ankle Pain.* Philadelphia: F. A. Davis, 1968)

pain subsides. Nonweight-bearing exercises are started within 2 to 3 days of injury; these include active plantar flexion, dorsiflexion, toe flexion, inversion and eversion.

Once pain subsides and swelling resolves, full weight-bearing can be resumed. Running should be postponed another 1 to 3 weeks depending on severity of injury. With mild ligamentous laxity of the ankle and repeated minor sprains, proper taping to support the lateral structures is indicated for athletic activity that involves contact, running, or jumping, particularly on uneven ground. Tape strips are applied from the medial aspect to the lateral aspect of the ankle (Fig. 145-3) to hold the heel and ankle in eversion and provide support. Exercises to strengthen the ankle evertors and high-laced leather supportive shoes may also be helpful.

Ankle sprain is a serious injury; if ligaments are torn and result in marked ankle instability (determined by examination under anesthesia or stress x-rays) surgical repair or at least cast immobilization for 4 to 8 weeks will be needed. Serious sprain requires prompt orthopedic referral to maximize chances of healing and restoration of joint stability.

An *eversion injury* often causes bony damage and may result in tearing of the deltoid and inferior tibiofibular ligaments. Orthopedic referral is necessary.

FOOT

Bunions. Bunions result from chronic trauma due to shoes that are too narrow. The trauma induces reactive inflammation in the underlying medial bursa of the first metatarsophalangeal (MTP) joint. Pain can usually be controlled by use of properly fitted, adequately wide shoes. Injecting the inflamed bursa with a steroid preparation may give symptomatic relief in refractory cases; otherwise, orthopedic referral for consideration of surgical treatment is indicated.

Hammertoes. This deformity is caused by hyperextension of the MTP joint and flexion contracture of the proximal interphalangeal (PIP) joint. A painful callus forms over the tip of the toe and dorsal aspect of the PIP joint. Spacious, well-padded shoes will often relieve the painful calluses. Surgical consultation is needed if properly fitting shoes do not provide relief.

Metatarsalgia. This condition is characterized by pain in the sole of the forefoot across the metatarsal heads. It is often difficult to explain, and usually requires orthopedic analysis and use of carefully designed and fitted pads for support.

Neuroma. Excessively narrow, high-heeled shoes may result in medial-lateral compression of the fore-feet, with irritation and pressure on the branches of the digital nerves as they course between the second and third or third and fourth metatarsal heads. On examination, there is maximum tenderness between the metatarsal heads. Hypertrophy and fibrosis of the nerve results in neuroma formation. Recurrent, often disabling neuritic pain, numbness, and paresthesias may occur after standing or walking. Simple longitudinal arch supports and wide shoes with low or medium heels will usually reduce compression and relieve symptoms, but on occasion surgical excision of the neuroma is needed if these measures fail.

Plantar fasciitis. Pain in the vicinity of the heel is most commonly a result of plantar fasciitis. It occurs in patients who have done a great deal of walking, standing or running, particularly if unaccustomed to such activity. In joggers it is caused by a tight gastrocnemius-soleus complex that limits ankle dorsiflexion. Pain is felt under the heel, not over it, and may radiate into the sole. Point tenderness is found at the proximal portion of the arch near the plantar medial aspect of the calcaneus. X-rays are not particularly helpful, because many asymptomatic patients have calcaneal spurs, which are probably incidental findings. Raising the heel ¼ inch reduces the tension on the plantar fascia. If a calcaneal spur is causing symptoms, a doughnut-shaped sponge pad can be placed under the heel inside the shoe to alleviate pressure on the painful area. In refractory cases, a corticosteroid and local anesthetic can be injected into the site of the pain. Prevention includes use of jogging shoes with a sturdy arch support, heel lifts, and stiff shank to help minimize stress on the plantar fascia; gastrocnemius stretching exercises before running are also important (see Chapter 10).

Achilles tendinitis. The Achilles tendon is a common site of injury, especially among joggers. Hypertrophy of the gastrocnemius and soleus muscles can cause loss of flexibility in the musculotendinous unit and lead to injury when there is overuse. The best treatment is prevention, accomplished by gastrocnemius stretching exercises before and after running (see Chapter 10).

Heel pad degeneration. With aging, the pad loses its shock-absorbing quality, and pain results. Pain is felt directly on the calcaneal pad. A sponge and elevation of the heel may alleviate the discomfort. Pain is self-limited, though direct injection of anesthetic may be needed in severe cases.

Peripheral vascular insufficiency (see Chapter 17) *and peripheral neuropathies* (see Chapter 155) are important causes of foot pain and should be kept in mind. Conversely, patients with diminished sensation, such as diabetics, must be examined diligently for ulcerations and skin infections of the feet; if allowed to go undetected and untreated, these may lead to osteomyelitis and amputation.

ANNOTATED BIBLIOGRAPHY

Inman, V.T.: Surgery of the Foot. St. Louis: C.V. Mosby, 1973. *(A detailed discussion of operative procedures for foot problems.)*

Klenerman, L.: The Foot and Its Disorders. Oxford: Blackwell Scientific Publications, 1976. *(Further reference for common foot problems.)*

O'Donoghue, E.H.: The treatment of Injuries to Athletes, ed. 3. Philadelphia: W.B. Saunders, 1976. *(A standard textbook of athletic injuries for further reference.)*

146

Approach to the Patient with Asymptomatic Hyperuricemia

The detection of asymptomatic patients with hyperuricemia has increased markedly with the proliferation of multiphasic screening techniques. Hyperuricemia is defined as a serum uric acid concentration that exceeds the mean by at least 2 standard deviations. The mean, as determined by colorimetric assay (the most commonly used method) is 7.5 mg. per 100 ml. for men and 6.6 mg. per 100 ml. for women. By definition, 2.5 per cent of the population is hyperuricemic; the consequences of being hyperuricemic and the need for lowering the uric acid are subjects of debate. Some have advocated prophylactic therapy in hopes of preventing acute gout, chronic tophaceous gout, stone formation, and renal failure. Others question the cost-effectiveness of such an approach. The primary physician must decide when to treat the asymptomatic patient with an elevated uric acid.

PATHOPHYSIOLOGY AND CLINICAL PRESENTATION

Uric acid is the end product of purine metabolism. In man there is no pathway for further breakdown or uric acid; it must be excreted by the kidneys or the serum level will rise. The pathogenesis of hyperuricemia involves overproduction and underexcretion of urate. It is estimated that one-third of hyperuricemic patients are overproducers, that another third are underexcreters, and that the remainder have a combined deficit.

Overproduction of uric acid is especially marked in patients undergoing treatment for myeloproliferative and lymphoproliferative malignancies and in those with severe psoriasis. Rapid cellular turnover results in production of massive amounts of nucleic acid metabolites that are converted to uric acid. Overproduction may also develop from an increase in *de novo* purine synthesis, as occurs in patients with inborn errors of metabolism. Excessive dietary intake of purine-rich foods is rarely responsible for hyperuricemia, because dietary sources of purine make up only 10 per cent of the uric acid pool.

Underexertion of uric acid occurs if there is an overall decrease in glomerular filtration or a defect in tubular secretion of urate, or if another substance competes with urate for tubular secretion. Thiazides are an important cause of decreased uric acid excretion; low doses of aspirin may also interfere with excretion. Fasting that results in ketosis also seems capable of transiently reducing urate excretion and raising the serum uric acid. Excessive intake of alcohol (greater than 100 gm. per day of ethanol) has been found to produce hyperuricemia and a reduction in excretion. The effect of alcohol was found in one study to be particularly prominent if the patient was fasting at the time of alcohol intake.

Well over 90 per cent of hyperuricemic patients present asymptomatically; many are individuals subjected to multiphasic screening. Half of newly discovered patients in the Framingham study were taking thiazides. Just under 3 per cent of hyperuricemic patients had elevations in uric acid secondary to a concurrent illness such as a myeloproliferative disorder.

NEED FOR THERAPY

The need to treat patients with asymptomatic hyperuricemia continues to be controversial. The publication of review articles with recommendations for managing such patients always generates strong dissenting letters to the editor. The justifications cited for prophylactic therapy are founded on the belief that lowering the uric acid will prevent the development of acute gout, chronic gouty arthritis, gouty nephropathy, and urolithiasis. Because data are inconclusive or conflicting in many instances, the problem of treating the asymptomatic patient remains unresolved. However, recent studies have begun to provide some data that can help guide decision-making.

Acute gout. Two of the three existing population studies on the risk of acute gout in patients with hyperuricemia show that the higher the serum uric acid level, the greater the chance of an attack of acute gout. The incidence of acute gout in the Framingham study was 14 per cent for men with a uric acid between 7.0 and 7.9 mg. per 100 ml., 19 per cent for those with a level between 8.0 and 8.9; and 80 per cent when the level went above 9.0. However, only 10 patients in the entire study population had a serum uric acid above 9.0 mg. per 100 ml. Similar results were obtained in a large community study in Sudbury, Massachusetts. On the other hand, a study of 124 asymptomatic hyperuricemic patients followed in the Kaiser-Permanente system found no relationship between uric acid concentration and development of acute gout.

The costs of preventing attacks of acute gout include the expense of medication and the risk of adverse drug effects. The cost of lifelong prophylactic therapy can reach several thousand dollars, because the mean age at time of detection is 35, and a year's worth of medication can cost well over $100. The prevalence of adverse drug reactions has been reported to be as high as 10 per cent for probenecid and 25 per cent for allopurinol. These costs appear excessive when compared to the safety, efficacy and minimal expense of treating an acute attack of gout with an anti-inflammatory agent. It seems reasonable to wait until an acute attack occurs, rather than to subject the patient to lifelong prophylaxis, especially if the intervals between recurrences of acute gout are measured in years.

Chronic gouty arthritis. The issue of prophylaxis for prevention of chronic gouty arthritis is of only minor importance, because almost all patients with this condition go through a stage of acute gouty attacks before developing chronic joint changes. Thus, asymptomatic patients are at little if any risk for silently falling victim to chronic gouty arthritis.

Impairment of renal function. It is a common assumption that chronic hyperuricemia is potentially harmful to the kidneys and may result in progressive renal damage leading to azotemia. However, recent evidence does not fully support this belief. In a prospective Kaiser-Permanente study comparing 113 patients with asymptomatic hyperuricemia and 193 controls followed for 8 years, there was no significant difference in the incidence of azotemia for the two groups (1.8 per cent versus 2.1 per cent, respectively). The degree of azotemia that developed was always mild (serum creatinines were in the range of 1.3 to 1.7 mg. per 100 ml.).

In the same study, 168 patients with clinical gout were followed for 10 years; similarly, the incidence of azotemia was low and its severity mild. The development of azotemia was unrelated to the degree of control of hyperuricemia. In addition, the investigators studied the records of 1,356 men aged 60 to 69 who were followed for 10 years; there were no deaths from renal failure that were attributable to hyperuricemia. The association between azotemia and hyperuricemia was further assessed by analysis of hyperuricemic patients and matched controls. Excluding those with hypertension, diabetes, and atherosclerosis, there were only 3 cases of azotemia in the hyperuricemia group and none in the matched controls; the difference was not statistically significant. In only 2 cases did hyperuricemia precede azotemia.

The investigators projected from their data that the long-term risk of clinically significant azotemia was minuscule until the uric acid level reached 13.0 mg. per 100 ml. in men and 10.0 mg. per 100 ml. in women. They estimated that only if such levels were sustained for 40 years would the risk of clinically important azotemia become substantial.

The Kaiser study is not the only one to show little evidence for hyperuricemia-induced renal impairment. A 12-year study of 524 gouty patients found no relationship between hyperuricemia and renal function. A 3-year prospective study of hyperuricemic patients with and without renal failure showed no change in renal function when allopurinol was used to normalize the serum urate concentration. A study of hyperuricemic relatives of patients with clinical gout found normal inulin, creatinine, and hippurate clearances.

A frequently quoted study purporting to show a beneficial effect of lowering the serum uric acid level was uncontrolled and involved only 10 patients, of whom all had chronic gout and many had high uric acid excretions. There was no change in serum creatinine during the 23-month mean treatment period of the study. The authors claim that deterioration of renal function was prevented by therapy, but if azotemia is as infrequent and mild as suggested by the Kaiser study, then it is no surprise that there was little change and one can hardly conclude that the effect was due to allopurinol therapy.

One group of hyperuricemic patients *is* at risk for renal failure. These are persons with myeloproliferative or lymphoproliferative disease. They may have a sudden increase in uric acid load after a course of treatment. The resultant hyperuricemia and extreme amount of uric acid excretion may lead to precipitation of uric acid crystals in the renal tubules and cause acute oliguric renal failure. Such patients require prophylaxis with allopurinol before receiving therapy for their proliferative disorder.

In sum, the preponderance of available data argues against the notion that asymptomatic hyperuricemia is associated with a substantial risk of clinically significant renal impairment or that attempts to lower the serum uric acid reduce the risk of azotemia.

Nephrolithiasis. The risk of nephrolithiasis in patients with asymptomatic hyperuricemia was also addressed in the Kaiser study; it was found to be very small. Renal calculi occurred in 3 (2.6 per cent) of 113 hyperuricemic patients and in 2 (1.1 per cent) of 193 controls. In two of the hyperuricemic patients with stones, the stone was composed of calcium. The risk of developing a stone attributable to hyperuricemia was calculated to be less than 1 per cent per year. Among gouty patients, the control of serum uric acid was the same in those who developed stones as in those who did not.

Factors other than hyperuricemia are believed to be important for stone formation. Family history of stone formation is contributory. Two of the three hyperuricemia patients with stones in the Kaiser study had a family history of nephrolithiasis. Urine acidity is a critical factor because the solubility of uric acid falls precipitously as the pH falls from 8.0 to 5.0. The amount of uric acid excreted in the urine per 24 hours has also been suggested as a cause; but careful studies have shown that the level of urinary uric acid is only a weak determinant of stone formation. However, dehydration can precipitate nephrolithiasis (see Chapter 130).

It is interesting to note that urolithiasis is rarely life-threatening. In a study of 1,700 patients with gout, only one patient experienced serious obstructive uropathy.

CONCLUSIONS AND RECOMMENDATIONS

- Asymptomatic hyperuricemia is associated with an increased risk of acute gouty arthritis, but the cost of prophylactic therapy in patients who have never had a single attack of gout greatly exceeds the cost of symptomatically treating an acute attack, should it occur.
- Treatment to prevent chronic tophaceous gout need not be started until clinical evidence of gout develops.
- There is insufficient evidence to justify prophylaxis for prevention of renal impairment unless the pa-

tient has a myeloproliferative or lymphoproliferative disorder and is about to be treated for it. The degree of azotemia that can be attributed to hyperuricemia is mild and clinically insignificant in most other instances.
- The risk of urolithiasis is sufficiently low to justify waiting for the development of a stone before initiating prophylactic therapy, unless the patient has a strong family history of nephrolithiasis.

ANNOTATED BIBLIOGRAPHY

Burger, L.U., and Yu, T.F.: Renal function in gout—An analysis of 524 gouty subjects including long-term follow-up studies. Am. J. Med., *59*:604, 1975. *(Follow-up for 12 years showed that hyperuricemia alone had no deleterious effect on renal function in ambulatory patients with gout.)*

Coe, F.L.: Hyperuricosuric calcium oxalate nephrolithiasis. Kidney Int., *13*:418, 1978. *(An interesting observation that 25 per cent of patients with calcium oxalate stones hyperexcrete uric acid. The mechanism is not known, and allopurinol does not seem to reduce new stone formation.)*

Fessel, J.W.: Renal outcomes of gout and hyperuricemia. Am. J. Med., *67*:74, 1979. *(A carefully done prospective study showing that the risks of renal failure and stone formation are very small and hardly justify prophylactic therapy.)*

Hall, A.P., Berry, P.E., Dawber, T.R., et al.: Epidemiology of gout and hyperuricemia—A long-term population study. Am. J. Med., *42*:27, 1967. *(The Framingham study; 14 per cent of patients with uric acids of 7 to 7.9 mg., 19 per cent with uric serum urates between 8 and 8.9, and 5 out of 6 patients with uric acids over 9 developed gouty attacks.)*

Klinenberg, J.: Hyperuricemia and gout. Med. Clin. North Am., *61*:299, 1977. *(A good review of the significance and treatment of both of these conditions.)*

Liang, M.H., and Fries, J.F.: Asymptomatic hyperuricemia: The case for conservative management. Ann. Intern. Med., *88*:666, 1978. *(A well-developed approach to asymptomatic hyperuricemia.)*

Maclaughlan, M.J., and Rodnan, G.P.: Effects of food, fast, and alcohol on serum uric acid and acute attacks of gout. Am. J. Med., *42*:38, 1967. *(Fasting and consumption of over 100 gm. of al-*

cohol raised urate levels. Acute changes in levels precipitated gouty attacks.)

Paulus, H.E., Coutts, A., Calabro, J.J., *et al.*: Clinical significance of hyperuricemia in routinely screened hospitalized men. JAMA, *211*:277, 1970. *(An early but prophetic paper that argued that an abnormal laboratory finding does not confirm diagnosis or justify therapy.)*

Rastegar, A., and Their, S.O.: The physiologic approach to hyperuricemia. N. Engl. J. Med., *286*:470, 1972. *(An excellent review of the enzymatic defects that lead to increased uric acid.)*

Rosenfeld, J.B.: Effect of long-term allopurinol administration on serial GFR in normotensive and hypertensive hyperuricemic subjects. Adv. Exp. Med. Biol., *41*:581, 1974. *(Normalizing uric acid and following patients for 3 to 4 years produced no beneficial effect on renal function.)*

Yu, T., and Gutman, A.: Uric acid nephrolithiasis in gout: Predisposing factors. Ann. Intern. Med., *67*: 1133, 1967. *(A classic study of 305 gout patients correlating risk of stone formation with uric acid excretion, urine pH, serum urate level and etiology.)*

147
Management of Rheumatoid Arthritis

Management of rheumatoid arthritis (RA) is a challenge because the disease is chronic, relapsing, potentially disabling, and without completely satisfactory methods of treatment. The problem is common. Population surveys indicate that 3 per cent of females and 1 per cent of males have definite or probable RA, based on the diagnostic criteria established by the American Rheumatism Association. Prevalence increases with age, and incidence peaks in the fourth decade. The estimated annual incidence ranges from 0.5 to 3 new cases per thousand per year. The objectives of therapy are to minimize pain and stiffness and preserve range of motion and muscle strength. The primary physician needs to be able to make optimal use of anti-inflammatory agents, know how to design and implement a program of supportive measures, and decide when referral is needed.

PATHOPHYSIOLOGY AND CLINICAL PRESENTATION

RA is a chronic inflammatory condition of unknown etiology, manifested by arthritis of diarthrodial joints in combination with extra-articular lesions and systemic symptoms. Available evidence suggests cellular, humoral, and complement-mediated pathways of immunologic injury. The earliest change is synovial edema and dilatation of small vessels, followed by new capillary formation, synovial proliferation, and infiltration by plasma cells and lymphocytes. Neutrophils migrate into the joint space and are trapped.

A number of mechanisms lead to an inflammatory response. Plasminogen activator, which can trigger the complement system, is produced by the cellular infiltrate. The production of rheumatoid factor by plasma cells and B lymphocytes in the synovium can also activate the complement cascade. Phagocytosis of immune complexes leads to release of lysosomes.

The synovium becomes more hypertrophic, edematous, hypervascular and infiltrated by mononuclear cells. If exuberant granulation tissue (pannus) forms within the inflamed synovium, joint damage may ensue. Pannus is capable of eroding cartilage and bone, typically beginning at the joint margin, then spreading over the entire cartilaginous surface. Lysosomal enzymes released from within the pannus and latent collagenases are believed to contribute to the direct erosive capacity. Often osteopenia is seen in subchondral bone adjacent to the involved joint even before the pannus has denuded the cartilage, and may be due to prostaglandin release from synovial cells.

Initially, an effusion develops, distending the joint capsule. This is followed by damage to the articular surface and weakening of the capsule and periarticular ligaments. Secondary muscle atrophy results and leads to imbalance of opposing muscle groups. The net effect is an unstable, weak, swollen, subluxated joint. The synovium of tendon sheaths and bursae may also be affected by the inflammatory process, which leads to accompanying tenosynovitis and bursitis.

Clinical onset of RA is usually insidious, often beginning with vague *arthralgias, morning stiffness* and *fatigue*. Frank signs of *articular inflammation* (swelling, pain, and warmth) soon follow. The small joints of the hands and feet—the proximal interphalangeals (PIP), metacarpophalangeals (MCP), and metatarsophalangeals (MTP)—are typically among the first to be involved, but knees, ankles, wrists or elbows may also be affected early on. *Tenosynovitis* is common. Initially, the arthritis may be asymmetrical or may even present as a monoarticular arthritis, but symmetrical distribution supervenes in most instances and is characteristic of the disease.

In an occasional patient, RA is preceded by *palindromic rheumatism,* a condition characterized by repeated episodes of transient joint pain, swelling, and redness extending beyond the joint. The condition lasts a few hours to a few days, followed by complete resolution and no permanent joint injury. Fingers, wrists, shoulders and knees are most commonly affected. About 50 per cent of these patients eventually develop typical RA.

Rheumatoid nodules appear in about 25 per cent of patients with rheumatoid arthritis, usually as the disease progresses. These subcutaneous nodules are firm, nontender, and located principally along the extensor surface of the forearm and in the olecranon bursa. The appearance of rheumatoid nodules is an unfavorable prognostic sign, as is persistence of acute disease for more than 1 year, high serum titers of rheumatoid factor, and age under 20 at time of presentation.

Sustained joint inflammation lasting over a year leads to permanent erosion and loss of joint function. At first, the changes are partially reversible, but as cartilage and bone erode, the injury becomes permanent.

Hands and wrists. Characteristic hand deformities include ulnar deviation of the MCP joints, boutonniere deformities of the PIP joints, and swan-neck contractures of the fingers. In the wrists, there is often permanent loss of extension. A boggy, tender, dorsal wrist mass may result from tenosynovitis, and compression of the median nerve can occur. The subsequent *carpal tunnel syndrome* is usually reversible, but nerve damage is permanent by the time wasting of the thenar eminence is obvious.

Feet. Erosion of the metatarsal heads can lead to ventral subluxation. Increased weight-bearing on the inflamed heads and painful callus formation result. Erosive disease may be silent in the MTP joints.

Hips and knees. Involvement of these joints can be a source of much disability, because severe pain on weight-bearing may result. Loss of internal rotation is the first change noted in the hip, followed by flexion contracture. One hip may predominate even though the process is bilateral. In the knee, distention of the suprapatellar pouch by synovial effusion is common. If pressure rises rapidly, there can be herniation of the synovium with formation of a popliteal *Baker's cyst,* which can cause severe pain if it ruptures into the calf. Loss of full knee extension is followed by flexion contractures and gait difficulties.

Other joints. In the *elbow,* extension may be compromised, and olecranon bursitis is often present. *Shoulder* involvement presents as a subacromial or subdeltoid bursitis or as limitation of motion. Erosion of the rotator cuff leads to painful upward subluxation of the humeral head against the acromion. In the *cervical spine,* atlantoaxial subluxation is common, but usually asymptomatic. This development is potentially serious because it can lead to direct compression of the spinal cord or of the blood supply to the brain stem; fortunately, it is a rare event. When the *temperomandibular joint* is affected, there is pain on chewing or biting and difficulty in opening the mouth. *Avascular necrosis of the femoral head* and *vertebral osteoporosis* and collapse are usually a consequence of corticosteroid therapy.

Radiographic manifestations of early disease are soft tissue swelling around the joint and periarticular osteopenia. Relatively uniform narrowing of the joint space occurs as cartilage is destroyed. Periarticular subchondral erosion of bone is noted at the joint margin where pannus has developed. Finally, joint architecture is lost as the joint space is obliterated and erosion of subchondral bone progresses.

Extra-articular manifestations of rheumatoid arthritis develop mostly in patients with high titers of rheumatoid factor and persistent disease, so-called *sero-positive RA.* Pleural effusions with very low glucose concentrations and reduced complement can occur; there may or may not be accompanying pleuritic pain. Interstitial pulmonary changes, pulmonary nodules, and asymptomatic pericardial effusions are detected in some. Keratoconjunctivitis sicca (*Sjögren's syndrome*) has a strong association with RA, being found in up to 15 per cent of patients. Splenomegaly is present in 5 to 10 per cent of those with RA, and lymphadenopathy is not unusual. The combination of RA, splenomegaly and neutropenia (*Felty's syndrome*) is noted in an occasional patient. Neutropenia may be severe, but the arthritis is often quiescent. Vasculitis is believed responsible for a number of systemic manifestations, including fever, mononeuritis multiplex, Raynaud's phenomenon, chronic leg ulcers, mucosal erosions of the gastrointestinal tract, focal ischemia of the digits, and necrotizing mesarteritis. The anemia of chronic disease is seen in a large percent of RA patients.

PROGNOSIS AND COURSE

It is difficult at the outset to predict the course of an individual case, although a high serum titer of rheumatoid factor, extra-articular manifestations and systemic symptoms at the onset of arthritis are unfavorable prognostic signs. Onset before age 30 does not indicate a favorable course. Disease that remains persistently active for over a year is likely to lead to joint deformities and disability. Cases in which there are periods of activity lasting only weeks or a few months followed by spontaneous remission have a better prognosis. In one study, female sex and white race in patients under age 45 were associated with a somewhat less optimistic prognosis.

Most published series on clinical course and prognosis are based on patients who were hospitalized or treated in arthritis centers, thus tending to overrepresent people with severe disease. A study of 200 such people followed for 9 years after discharge found 20.5 per cent without significant disability, 41 per cent moderately disabled, 27 per cent severely crippled, and 11 per cent dependent on others. This does not reflect the prognosis for the majority of rheumatoid arthritics treated exclusively as outpatients, many of whom carry a diagnosis of "probable" RA. Reviews suggest that over 50 per cent of these patients remain fully employed after having disease for 10 to 15 years, with one third having only intermittent low-grade disease, and another third experiencing spontaneous remission.

PRINCIPLES OF MANAGEMENT

The goals are to relieve stiffness and pain, preserve muscle strength and range of motion, and minimize progressive disability and deformity. There is no cure. A number of factors require consideration in design of a management program, including the patient's age, social and occupational responsibilities, emotional makeup, the activity and duration of disease, and results of prior therapies. A balanced, multifaceted approach to therapy is most likely to provide best results, because no single drug or treatment is by itself effective. The basic components of a program must include thorough patient education, adequate rest, proper exercise, and appropriate use of anti-inflammatory agents. Diet plays no role.

Rest can be helpful, but in the patient with mild to moderate disease, complete bed rest is not only unnecessary but potentially harmful. Prolonged rest may lead to flexion contractures, osteoporosis, and muscle atrophy. Only the patient whose acute disease is severe enough to warrant hospitalization should be put to bed, in which case there is some benefit. However, a period of rest during the day can be of considerable benefit to less ill patients with persistently active disease, most of whom are usually bothered by fatigue.

Splinting. Selectively resting individual joints by splinting can help relieve pain and prevent contracture of severely inflamed joints. The principle is to maintain the joint in its physiological position, especially during periods when the joint is stressed. Splinting of the wrist at night is the best example of this form of therapy. The patient with painful tenosynovitis of the wrist can be afforded a decrease in pain and prevention of flexion deformity with its attendant loss of grip. A wrist splint applied at night places the joint in 10° to 15° of extension. A cervical collar worn at night can provide similar relief when the cervical spine is involved. Deformed feet require specially constructed shoes.

Exercise helps to maintain range of motion and muscle strength. Again the goal is to minimize the chances of postinflammatory contractures. Exercises which safely put involved joints through a full range of motion need to be taught to the patient. When pain is too severe for active exercises, isometrics can be performed, and passive exercises can be prescribed and carried out by a physical therapist. Prior application of *heat* or *cold* (either may work) will facilitate the exercise program. Hot baths, paraffin soaks or ice packs are efficacious in loosening stiff joints for many patients. Moist heat is also useful in relieving pain and reducing the length of morning stiffness.

Exercises that utilize important muscle groups are prescribed in order to counteract the development of atrophy, strengthen periarticular tissues, and preserve joint stability. A judicious program of walking can play a similar role. Design and execution of an exercise program can be facilitated by the participation of a physical therapist. To protect the joint from damaging stress, the patient can be instructed in the use of implements which provide a mechanical advantage. Such "joint savers" are available commercially and are most helpful for tasks requiring use of the hands.

Drug therapy. The goals are to provide pain relief and counter joint inflammation. Since most discomfort results from inflammation, a drug that is effective for treatment of RA must have strong anti-inflammatory properties. Although narcotic analgesics without anti-inflammatory effects are sometimes resorted to, their regular use should be avoided since RA requires prolonged treatment, posing the risk of drug dependence.

Aspirin remains the cornerstone of pharmacologic therapy despite the much-promoted introduction of new nonsteroidal anti-inflammatory agents. The drug is clearly the best proven and least expensive agent for treatment of RA. It decreases pain and lessens inflammation, although it has no effect on the course of the illness. The mechanism of action is believed related in part to the inhibition of prostaglandin release. Serum levels of 15 to 20 mg. per 100 ml. are needed in adults under age 60 to effectively suppress the inflammation of rheumatoid arthritis. No standard dose predictably achieves this level, but usually at least 3.6 to 4.8 gm. per day are necessary.

The dose of aspirin can be increased to the point of tinnitus, which is a dependable sign of salicylate toxicity in adults. Temporary mild hearing loss also occurs, especially in the elderly, even at subtoxic doses. The most frequent adverse effects of aspirin are gastrointestinal. In a recent endoscopic study of 82 patients with RA receiving chronic aspirin therapy, 17 per cent had gastric ulcers, 40 per cent had erosions, and 76 per cent had erythema of the gastric mucosa. One-third of patients with gastric ulcers had no symptoms. Frank bleeding occasionally occurs from gastritis or ulceration. Aspirin also inhibits platelet aggregation.

Many forms of aspirin have been introduced with the hope of equaling regular aspirin's efficacy without causing its gastrointestinal side effects. Buffered aspirin does not appear to contain sufficient bicarbonate to prevent aspirin-induced gastric damage. In the endoscopic study cited above, the incidence of gastric ulceration among buffered aspirin users was 31 per cent compared to 23 per cent for patients taking regular aspirin. Those who took enteric-coated aspirin had only a 6 per cent incidence of ulceration ($p < 0.05$). Fasting salicylate levels were equal among all patients in the endoscopic study. However, the bioavailability of enteric-coated aspirin is not well established.

Other salicylates have been promoted. Choline salicylate (Arthropan) is less irritating to the stomach than regular aspirin, but also less effective and much more expensive. Several new salicylate tablets are being marketed, including magnesium salicylate, choline magnesium salicylate and salsalate. There are insufficient data to determine whether these represent any improvement over aspirin.

Ibuprofen (Motrin), *fenoprofen* (Nalfon), and *naproxen* (Naprosyn) represent a class of new nonsteroidal anti-inflammatory agents derived from propionic acid. At maximum doses, these agents have about the same anti-inflammatory effect as 4 to 6 gm. of aspirin. Although the incidence of gastrointestinal bleeding seems to be less with these agents, the data for bleeding are often derived from patients using the agents at submaximal doses. Moreover, fatal hemorrhage has been reported. Gastrointestinal symptoms are the most commonly encountered adverse effects. All of these agents should be used with caution in patients with a history of peptic ulceration. Like aspirin, they may interfere with clotting. In addition, they can cause tinnitus, produce sodium retention, and cost many times more than aspirin.

Use of these agents is best reserved for patients unable to tolerate aspirin; sometimes they may be added to a program of aspirin therapy. Because their cost is high and they are not free of gastrointestinal side effects, they should not be used before a full trial of aspirin has been carried out and salicylate levels in therapeutic range have been documented. Each should be tried at maximum dosage for a 2-week period. If one agent does not work, it is worth trying one of the others, since response seems to be somewhat idiosyncratic. In a double-blind crossover study comparing these 3 drugs, there were groups of patients who preferred a particular agent. Naproxen has the advantage of being effective in twice-daily dosage, but deaths from severe bleeding are more frequent with it than with the other two. These agents have no effect on the course of disease.

Indomethacin has potent anti-inflammatory effects and is a prostaglandin inhibitor. The drug is particularly helpful as a supplement to salicylate therapy; when taken at bedtime it helps to reduce morning stiffness. Indomethacin is not used more frequently in RA because it causes considerable gastrointestinal upset and often clouds the sensorium, especially in elderly patients. *Tolmetin* (Tolectin) is related to indomethacin and has comparable anti-inflammatory effects when used in maximal doses. Patients who derive benefit from indomethacin, but cannot tolerate its side effects, may be given a trial of tolmetin. At recommended doses it has been found to be as effective as 4 gm. of aspirin per day. *Sulindac* (Clinoril) is also chemically related to indomethacin and is heavily promoted by the manufacturer. Like most other nonsteroidal anti-inflammatory agents, it inhibits prostaglandin synthesis; its half-life is 18 hours, making twice-daily dosage feasible. Cost for the daily dose is about the same as that for naproxen, or about 10 times the cost of a daily supply of aspirin. Experience with the drug is limited, but it appears comparable to 2 to 4.8 gm. of aspirin per day. Gastrointestinal side effects are reported in up to 17 per cent. Its role in the management of RA remains to be fully defined.

Gold salts are used in patients with progressive erosive disease in an attempt to stop joint destruction. The agent is unique among drugs used to treat RA in that it has been shown to halt or even partially reverse articular erosion in up to 60 per cent of cases, although its mechanism of action remains unknown. Decrease in inflammatory symptoms is noted in two thirds of patients by the time the cumulative dose reaches 400 to 600 mg. Those who are going to respond do so by the time 1000 mg. have been given. Skin rashes and buccal cavity mucosal ulcers represent minor adverse effects. Serious idiosyncratic reactions include marrow suppression and nephropathy. Consequently, treatment is begun slowly; each dose is preceded by urinalysis and complete blood and platelet counts. Gold is given intramuscularly by weekly injection using gold sodium thiomalate (Myochrysine) or aurothioglucose (Solganal). The former is sometimes associated with an immediate postinjection vasomotor reaction of warmth, erythema and light-headedness.

Toxic reactions are not infrequent; the effects of gold are cumulative. If a skin rash occurs, the agent can be resumed at reduced doses following cessation for a few weeks to be sure a more generalized skin reaction does not set in. The first evidence of marrow suppression or nephropathy requires immediate cessation of therapy. Thrombocytopenia is reversible in early stages. Most patients who respond to gold are treated weekly until the cumulative dose reaches 1 gm.; then administration is cut back to every other week until 1.5 gm. is reached, at which point injections are given once a month. There are no clear indications as to when to stop therapy or how long to continue it.

Penicillamine is another slow-acting drug used in RA patients with erosive disease; the agent may inhibit progression of joint destruction. In one study it retarded bony erosion. However, adverse effects are numerous, potentially serious, and as frequent as with gold. Fatal aplastic anemia, leukopenia, agranulocytosis and thrombocytopenia can occur. Proteinuria is seen in 10 to 15 per cent of patients, and may progress to the nephrotic syndrome. Rashes and autoimmune syndromes such as myasthenia gravis are reported. The drug should be reserved for those who fail to respond to aspirin and gold, and used only after consultation with a rheumatologist. It appears to be as effective as gold.

Hydroxychloroquine can sometimes induce remissions; it is not as potent as gold or penicillamine. At least 4 to 6 weeks are needed before results are detectable. Use of hydroxychloroquine is reserved for chronic cases that lack active joint erosion but are uncontrolled by aspirin. Some rheumatologists recommend using the agent before resorting to gold, though the number is fewer than before. The major toxic effect is visual impairment (even blindness) due to drug accumulation in the retina. Although this complication is rare, its possibility limits dosage to 200 to 400 mg. per day and makes regular ophthalmologic examinations advisable.

Corticosteroids administered as a single *intra-articular injection* of a long-acting preparation may mean the difference between maintenance of daily activity and confinement, especially when a single large weight-bearing joint is inflamed. However, repeated steroid injections into the same joint may hasten its degeneration and increase the risk of infection. *Systemic* corticosteroids have a limited role in treatment because they cause osteoporosis, weaken joints by softening their ligamentous supports, and can produce aseptic necrosis of the femoral head. Moreover, their chronic use results in adrenal suppression and other important complications (see Chapter 101). The only clear-cut indication for systemic steroids is life-threatening extra-articular disease such as vasculitis, pericarditis, or alveolitis. Controversy surrounds systemic steroid use in patients with articular disease only. In extremely difficult situations such as a flare of joint disease that threatens to totally disable the head of a household, some clinicians advocate a small nightly dose of 5 to 7.5 mg. of prednisone to tide the patient over a difficult period.

Disease activity and response to therapy are monitored by reproducible measures such as duration of morning stiffness, sedimentation rate, number of tender swollen joints, strength of grip (measured with a blood pressure cuff), time needed to walk 15 meters, and ring size. The titer of rheumatoid factor does not correlate with disease activity, but does decrease with gold and penicillamine therapy if the patient responds.

The use of *immunosuppressive agents* (*azathioprine* and *cyclophosphamide*) requires the help of the rheumatologist; they are prescribed in extreme situations only.

INDICATIONS FOR
REFERRAL AND ADMISSION

The primary physician can usually provide for the continuous care of most patients with RA, even to the point of administering hydroxychloroquine or gold therapy. However, the occasional case that does not respond to maximal doses of aspirin or the newer nonsteroidal anti-inflammatory agents should be discussed with a rheumatologist before resorting to gold or hydroxychloroquine. Patients refractory to conventional therapy require referral to a rheumatologist for consideration of immunosuppressive therapy or penicillamine, as well as a general review of a patient's overall program.

Referral to a physical or an occupational therapist is basic to design of a good exercise program and should be made for every patient with active disease. Surgical referral is indicated for carpal tunnel syndrome that persists in spite of gold therapy and corticosteroid injection. Trigger finger deformity, tendon rupture with loss of manual dexterity, and refractory dorsal wrist effusions unresponsive after 6 months of therapy are also indications for surgery. Disabling hip or knee destruction with severe impairment of weight-bearing capacity deserves a surgical assessment regarding possible prosthetic joint replacement. Synovectomy may be needed for a single, very refractory joint which cannot be replaced.

When fever, floridly inflamed joints, severe pain, or marked extra-articular disease is present, hospital admission is an obvious requirement.

PATIENT EDUCATION

Patients do best when they know what to expect and can view their illness realistically. Most fear crippling consequences. Without building false hopes, the physician can point out that spontaneous remissions are frequent and that over two-thirds of patients are free of significant disability. Moreover, it should be emphasized that there is much that can be done to minimize discomfort and preserve function. Many patients benefit from being included in the design and implementation of the management plan. By taking into account the patient's life-style and explaining the rationale for exercises, rest and medication, the physician can enlist the active participation of the patient and his family.

Details of drug programs need to be reviewed. For example, some patients scoff at the use of aspirin. Explaining the difference between taking sporadic low doses and near-toxic amounts usually suffices to convince most. The marked difference in cost between aspirin and other agents is also worth discussion. Other patients are concerned about gastrointestinal upset; taking doses with meals, milk or antacids can be suggested.

The benefits achievable with current therapy can be emphasized, yet the patient should be warned not to expect immediate results or complete cure. The physician must be sensitive to possible concomitant depression. Alertness to intercurrent illnesses which can aggravate the underlying disease and to complications which may develop, such as septic arthritis, is important. Patients may consider changing jobs in order to maintain economic viability.

Most important, the patient needs to know that the primary physician understands his situation and is available for support, advice and therapy as the situation arises. A trusting and strong relationship between doctor and patient can sustain many patients and is fundamental to good management of rheumatoid arthritis.

THERAPEUTIC RECOMMENDATIONS

- Aspirin is still the drug of choice. It should be initiated in doses of at least 3 to 6 gm. per day, titrating the therapeutic response against the development of toxicity. Periodically check blood levels and adjust dose to maintain a therapeutic level of 15 to 20 mg. per 100 ml. in patients less than 60 years old.
- Indomethacin, 25 mg. before bed, can supplement aspirin therapy in patients bothered by severe morning stiffness.
- A lack of response or intolerance to aspirin is a reasonable indication for trying one of the newer nonsteroidal anti-inflammatory agents such as ibuprofen (2400 mg. per day), fenoprofen (1800 mg. per day), naproxen (750 mg. per day), or tolmetin (1600 mg. per day). Each should be tried separately for 2 weeks. Occasionally, aspirin and one of these agents can be used together to permit a reduction in dose of aspirin if toxicity is a problem.

- Active erosive disease is an indication for initiating gold therapy. Gold sodium thiomalate (Myochrysine) or aurothioglucose (Solganal) is started with a 10-mg. intramuscular dose, followed by 25 mg. the next week, and 50 mg. weekly until definite improvement is observed or a cumulative dose of 1 gm. of the salt is reached. Urinalysis and blood counts are monitored weekly. If no effect is observed after 20 weeks of therapy, gold therapy should be halted. Otherwise, injections every other week can be continued until 1.5 gm is reached; then 50 ml. per month is the maximal maintenance dosage.
- Patients with stubborn, nonerosive disease can be given hydroxychloroquine (maximum, 400 mg. per day) for at least 8 weeks. Regular retinal examinations are required every 6 months if therapy is continued.
- Drug therapy should be initiated in conjunction with a program of daily range of motion and muscle-strengthening exercises and rest.
- Splinting may be applied, especially at night for the wrists, to support weakened joints and prevent flexion contractures.
- Heat can reduce pain and stiffness and is particularly helpful in the morning before the patient engages in activity.
- Penicillamine may be considered in refractory cases. Immunosuppressive therapy is investigational. For either, consultation with a rheumatologist is required.
- Intra-articular injection of a long-acting corticosteroid is indicated when a single refractory, inflamed joint prevents activity. An injectable suspension, such as triamcinolone acetonide 2.5 mg. to 10 mg. (depending on joint size) and a local anesthetic (e.g., 1 cc. lidocaine) is made up and injected into the joint space.
- Oral prednisone is reserved for only the most desperate situations. Short-term low-dose courses may suffice, such as 5.0 to 7.5 mg. given in the evening.
- Psychological support of the patient is essential, as is thorough instruction regarding treatment program.

ANNOTATED BIBLIOGRAPHY

Cooperating Clinics Committee of the American Rheumatism Association: A controlled trial of gold salt therapy in rheumatoid arthritis. Arthritis Rheum., *16*:353, 1973. (*A controlled trial establishing the efficacy of gold salts.*)

David, J.D., Muss, H.B., and Turner, R.A.: Cytotoxic agents in the treatment of rheumatoid arthritis. South. Med. J., *71*:58, 1978. (*A current review on use of azathioprine and cyclophosphamide.*)

Dingle, J.T.: Articular damage in arthritis and its control. Ann. Intern. Med., *88*:821, 1978. (*A molecular and cellular level discussion of arthritis, focusing on control of catabolic enzyme function and proposing an approach to future therapy.*)

Duthie, J.R.R., *et al.*: Course and prognosis in rheumatoid arthritis. Ann. Rheum. Dis., *23*:193, 1964. (*The course 9 years after discharge of 200 people treated for rheumatoid arthritis in a hospital.*)

Feigenbaum, S.L., Masi, A.T., and Kaplan, S.B.: Prognosis in rheumatoid arthritis. Am. J. Med., *66*:377, 1979. (*Identifies factors in 50 newly diagnosed patients under age 45 which seem to help predict outcome.*)

Fye, K.H.: Conservative management of rheumatoid arthritis. West. J. Med., *129*:121, 1978. (*A good review emphasizing physical therapy and other nonsurgical aspects of care.*)

Hill, H.F.: Treatment of rheumatoid arthritis with penicillamine. Semin. Arthritis Rheum., *6*:361, 1977. (*A good discussion of the use of penicillamine for patients with rheumatoid arthritis.*)

Is all aspirin alike? *Medical Letter, Drug Therapy*, *15*:57, 1974. (*A succinct report on aspirin and its various forms.*)

Kantor, T.G.: Ibuprofen. Ann. Intern. Med., *91*:877, 1979. (*Critical review of this popular nonsteroidal anti-inflammatory agent; 59 refs.*)

Kaye, R.L., and Hammand, A.H.: Understanding of rheumatoid arthritis—Evaluation of a patient education program. JAMA, *239*:2466, (*Evaluation of patient education, demonstrating behavioral changes; patients did not abuse joints as much, got more rest, and used medication more appropriately.*)

Kaye, R.L., and Pemberton, R.B.: Treatment of rheumatoid arthritis: A review including new and experimental anti-inflammatory agents. Arch. Intern. Med., *136*:1023, 1976. (*A good review of the treatment of rheumatoid disease with a rational scheme proposed.*)

Lee, P., Kennedy, A.C., *et al.*: Benefits of hospitalization in rheumatoid arthritis. Q. J. Med., *170*:265, 1974. (*A study of 30 indomethacin-treated patients showed moderate benefit from hospitalization.*)

Lewis, J.R.: Evaluation of ibuprofen, a new anti-rheumatic agent. JAMA, *223*:364, 1975. *(A brief but accurate review of the role of ibuprofen and, by extension, of other anti-inflammatory agents in the treatment of RA.)*

Mills, J.A., Pinals, R.A., Ropes, M.W., *et al.*: Value of bed rest in patients with rheumatoid arthritis. N. Engl. J. Med., *284*:453, 1971. *(Minimal benefit was obtained from enforced rest.)*

Pearson, C.M., *et al.*: Diagnosis and treatment of erosive rheumatoid arthritis and other forms of joint destruction. Ann. Intern. Med., *82*:241, 1975. *(A UCLA clinical case conference which emphasizes both medical and surgical therapy of destructive joint disease. It presents an excellent review of surgical procedures available for the rheumatoid patient.)*

Sigler, J.W., Gluhm, G.B., *et al.*: Gold salts in the treatment of rheumatoid arthritis: A double-blind study. Ann. Intern. Med., *80*:21, 1974. *(This paper reports a 2-year double-blind study in 27 patients, showing objective improvement measured by physical examination, ring size and grip strength, including radiologic evidence of arrest of progression.)*

Silvoso, G.R., Ivey, K.J., Butt, J.H., *et al.*: Incidence of gastric lesions in patients with rheumatic disease on chronic aspirin therapy. Ann. Intern. Med., *91*:517, 1979. *(An endoscopic study showing a high incidence of pathology; one third of patients were asymptomatic. Provides uncontrolled data comparing various aspirin preparations.)*

Werb, Z, Mainardi, C.L., *et al.*: Endogenous activation of latent collagenase by rheumatoid synovial cells. N. Engl. J. Med., *296*:1017, 1977. *(An article that tries to elucidate the mechanism of synovial damage in rheumatoid arthritis, attributing it to activation of latent collagenase.)*

148
Management of Degenerative Joint Disease (Osteoarthritis)

Degenerative joint disease (DJD), the most prevalent arthropathy, is principally a consequence of aging. Prevalence is difficult to estimate; although 50 per cent of adults show degenerative changes on x-ray, no more than 20 per cent are symptomatic. Because the condition is essentially irreversible, the goals of management are to provide relief from pain, minimize further damage to the involved joints, and keep the patient functioning independently.

PATHOPHYSIOLOGY AND CLINICAL PRESENTATION

Degenerative joint disease is characterized by degeneration of articular cartilage and reactive formation of new bone. Unlike rheumatoid arthritis, the synovium plays only a secondary role. What causes the demise of the articular cartilage is incompletely understood. Available evidence suggests a combination of mechanical injury and age-related biochemical change such as an alteration in the glycosaminoglycan class of mucopolysaccharides. This change leads to a decrease in water content of cartilage. Fibrils become less resilient and more readily damaged by trauma; this change may allow penetration of synovial collagenases. It also appears that bone elasticity, which cushions normal trauma, is lost, allowing increased stress to be transmitted directly to the cartilage. Conditions which alter the mechanical relationships of joints—such as trauma, hypermobility, neuropathy, Paget's disease and acromegaly—increase the likelihood that degenerative joint disease will develop.

Fissured hyaline cartilage is incapable of restoration. Eventually, the cartilage frays, shreds and cracks. Underlying bone begins to be remodeled, with thickening of trabeculae; cyst formation is also seen. At the margins of the joint, hypertrophic spurs (osteophytes) eventually develop, followed by buttressing of adjacent cortical bone (osteosclerosis). The joint space narrows in an irregular fashion. There is little synovial reaction unless the degenerative process is very rapid, a piece of cartilage dislodges, or calcium pyrophosphate crystals form and incite an acute inflammatory response (pseudogout).

The patient with DJD typically complains of joint pain that is aggravated by motion and weight-bearing. In addition, there may be stiffness worsened by periods of inactivity. The involved joint can be enlarged due to osteophyte formation, but swelling is usually inconsequential, since soft tissue involvement and effusions are minimal. Examination often reveals crepitus and discomfort on movement of the joint. Occasionally, slight warmth is noted in severely affected weight-bearing joints, but erythema and marked warmth are absent. Limitation of motion, malalignment and bony protuberances from spurs are frequent findings.

The joints most commonly affected include the distal interphalangeal (DIP) joints of the hands, the carpometacarpal joint at the base of the thumb, the hips, the knees, and the cervical and lumbosacral spine.

DIP joints. Disease in these joints is most common in middle-aged and elderly women, and sometimes proves to be quite painful and tender. A low-grade inflammatory response may accompany early rapid mucinous degenerative changes, giving the joint a tender, cystic inflammatory appearance. Later, osteophytes form, giving rise to the characteristic bony protuberances known as *Heberden's nodes.* All inflammatory activity resolves, leaving the joint nontender and with some limitation of motion. Occasionally, a similar process may affect the proximal interphalangeal joints, resulting in *Bouchard's nodes,* which may be mistaken for changes due to rheumatoid arthritis.

Thumbs. The base of the thumb, a site of much physical stress, is quite vulnerable to DJD. There is pain in the region of the thenar eminence and particularly over the carpometacarpal joint. Because the thumb is so important to manual dexterity, the development of arthritis at this site may be quite disabling. Grip becomes impaired and fine movements of apposition are restricted. Osteophytes are palpable and, in rare instances, may encroach upon the flexor tendon sheath, causing tenosynovitis.

Hips. Degenerative hip disease arises in young patients with congenital dislocations or slipped femoral capital epiphyses, and much later from wear and tear in the elderly. Unilateral or asymmetrical distribution is typical. Pain is reported deep in the hip, radiating into the anterior medial thigh, groin, or buttock. The site of radiation may be the only area of discomfort. At first, pain occurs only on weight-bearing, but as DJD progresses, discomfort may become continuous and especially unbearable at night. Sexual intercourse is sometimes compromised. Loss of internal rotation during flexion is the earliest change

and is as reliable as x-ray for diagnosis. The Trendelenburg test (see Chapter 143) is positive.

Knees. DJD of the knee produces pain that is localized to the joint and worsened by weight-bearing. Crepitus is often marked, and range of motion reduced. A very small effusion may be noted. The joint appears enlarged and feels bony. On occasion there maybe very few physical findings, even though pain and x-ray changes are prominent.

Cervical spine. DJD commonly involves the lower cervical spine (see Chapter 141). Although x-ray changes are frequent, most individuals are asymptomatic. Moreover, the correlation between symptoms and x-ray findings is often poor. The patient may complain of pain and stiffness in the neck, but sometimes only pain in the occiput, shoulder, arm, or hand is reported. In a few instances, scapular or upper anterior chest pain is produced. Osteophytes can protrude into the spinal foramina and impinge upon nerve roots, causing pain that radiates into the shoulder, upper arms, hands and fingers (brachial neuralgia). At night, the patient may awaken with paresthesias and numbness is the arms that improve upon getting up and shaking them.

On examination, neck motion is restricted to some extent in all directions and movement reproduces or aggravates symptoms. Reactive muscle spasm and tenderness are often present, and decreased sensation, weakness and diminished reflexes occur when root compression is marked. However, even when symptoms of root compression are reported, neurologic findings may be scant and their absence does not rule out the complication.

Lumbosacral spine. Degenerative changes in the lumbosacral spine involve the intervertebral discs and the apophyseal joints. With aging, the disc nucleus becomes brittle and less elastic. Herniation posteriorly or laterally through a defect in the disc annulus may occur and cause nerve root compression (see Chapter 140). Intervertebral spaces narrow and marginal osteophytes form. The apophyseal joints show typical secondary degenerative changes. The patient reports pain across the lower back with radiation into the buttock and posterior thigh, or down into the lower leg if root compression has occurred (see Chapter 140). Foreward flexion and extension are reduced, but lateral flexion is painless. Focal areas of tenderness are common and often due to spasm of the paraspinous musculature.

Other sites. DJD may involve the great toe at the metatarsophalangeal joint, causing bony enlargement and a valgus deformity. Crepitus and pain in the temporomandibular joint are sometimes seen secondary to bruxism (grinding of the teeth because of anxiety or anger). Pain is reproduced by opening the mouth widely.

Since DJD is not a systemic disease, there are no extra-articular manifestations. Radiographic findings are limited to the joints and include irregular narrowing of the joint space, sclerosis of subchondral bone, bony cysts, marginal osteophytes and buttressing of adjacent bone.

COURSE

Degenerative joint disease is often progressive over months to years; significant disability may ensue, related to pain and restriction of motion. However, clinical remissions do occur, especially in the hands, neck and back. It is important to note that progression is typically limited to a few affected joints and does not become widespread. A study of the natural history of untreated DJD of the knee in 71 patients found it to be especially progressive; the majority of patients ended up with pain at rest. Early onset of symptoms and varus deformity correlated with poor prognosis. Pain at rest and inability to use public transportation occurred over a period of 10 to 18 years. DJD of the hip also follows a relentless course. In most cases of DJD, symptoms in weight-bearing joints are exacerbated by obesity.

PRINCIPLES OF MANAGEMENT

There is no cure for osteoarthritis, but it helps to reduce stress imposed on the joint, maintain normal alignment, and treat pain and muscle spasm. Surgical intervention should be restricted to patients who do not respond to conservative management and are so disabled that they cannot function satisfactorily.

Rest. Some relief can be attained by partially resting the involved joint; this helps to reduce the stress imposed on it. A *cervical collar* can ease neck pain by supporting the spine and resting the paraspinous musculature. It may be necessary to continue use for many weeks, day and night, before significant benefit is achieved. Cervical traction may also help (see Chapter 141). A *corset* or *brace* for the back may be similarly helpful. Limiting the amount of walking a patient does will lessen stress on a weight-bearing joint, but can be counterproductive because stiffness, muscle atrophy and osteoporosis are accelerated, and the patient becomes demoralized from loss of independence and function. However, some relief can be provided without immobilization if the patient uses a walking cane, walker or even forearm crutches. The cane is held on the side opposite the painful joint. Unnecessary strain such as stair climbing should be reduced. Bed rest is essential for relief of back pain (see Chapter 140).

Exercises. Strengthening the supporting muscles may help maintain proper joint alignment. Quadriceps exercises are among the simplest; they can be performed while sitting in a chair by extending the knee and holding the straightened leg horizontal. Isometric and active exercises for the neck improve muscle tone and may sometimes help in cases of painful cervical spine disease. Exercises for the abdominal and parispinous musculature are useful for preventing back problems (see Chapter 140). Gentle walking, cycling and swimming will improve the muscle groups of the hips and knees and provide considerable psychological benefit. There is no evidence that manipulation is of any use. Excessive exercise may only exacerbate pain and cause further disruption of the joint.

Heat. Moist heat can give symptomatic relief from muscle spasm, though it has no effect on the disease itself. Diathermy and ultrasound units are expensive ways to delivering heat to deep-lying tissues. More than 5 or 6 treatments are unnecessary, though some patients derive considerable psychological benefit and a sense of well-being from them.

Drugs. The progression of disease cannot be halted by available drugs, but they can offer symptomatic relief. Anti-inflammatory agents are used. Their effect is probably due as much to their analgesic properties as to their impact on inflammation, because the inflammatory component of DJD is usually minimal. Since DJD is a chronic disease, any drug selected for use should be inexpensive and safe for long-term consumption. Narcotic analgesics should be used sparingly, and only for acute disabling pain. An individual's response to drugs is unpredictable and it may be necessary to try several different agents. Intermittent use of drugs will sometimes suffice.

Because of its low cost, relatively low toxicity, and documented potency, *aspirin* is an excellent first choice. It need not be given in the large doses needed in rheumatoid arthritis to suppress inflammation, but patients usually require up to 2 to 4 gm. per day. Sustained therapy is superior to intermittent use. Acetaminophen is a weak alternative for patients who do not tolerate aspirin, but some patients do find that they are benefited by the drug.

The newer nonsteroidal, anti-inflammatory agents such as *ibuprofen* (Motrin), *naproxen,* and *fenoprofen* may be helpful in patients who fail to obtain sufficient relief with aspirin. *Indomethacin* is usually quite effective for hip pain, especially in early phases of the disease. Unfortunately, its prolonged use is sometimes poorly tolerated in elderly people due to headache, dizziness, nausea, and stomach upset. The efficacy of the new indomethacinlike agents *tolmetin* (Tolectin) and *sulindac* (Clinoril) in DJD is not firmly established, but they seem to be equal to aspirin, though they are 10 or more times as expensive for an equally effective dose. *Phenylbutazone* should not be used chronically due to the risk of marrow suppression. There is no role in DJD for systemic *steroids,* and local injection is rarely indicated.

Antispasmodics are without effect, except for their tranquilizing action. Strong, potentially addicting *analgesics* such as codeine have a limited role, providing temporary relief for severe disabling disease when circumstances make it essential that the patient remain active. Obviously, prolonged use is contraindicated. Propoxyphene (Darvon) is taken by many patients with DJD, but its potential for dependence is considerable—similar to that of codeine—and its analgesic properties are no greater than low doses of aspirin.

INDICATIONS FOR REFERRAL

Physical and occupational therapists can be very helpful to patients with DJD in terms of teaching exercises, giving suggestions on performing the tasks of daily living, and providing psychological support. A referral is indicated for most patients whose DJD interferes with their lives.

Surgical therapy, such as osteotomy, arthroplasty, removal of loose bodies, or joint replacement, deserves consideration in significantly disabled patients. Replacement of hip joints has been particularly successful. The decision to refer for surgery must be made with an understanding of the risks involved and the need to undertake a postoperative exercise program. Surgery should be considered only in patients whose limitation of motion or pain has become so severe that it prevents them from living productively. They must be healthy enough to tolerate surgery and sufficiently motivated to carry out the exercise program needed to ensure full rehabilitation.

PATIENT EDUCATION

Patients need to know that DJD is not reversible; however, they should also be aware that pain can often be lessened and overall functioning preserved. Degenerative disease is not a generalized, systemic illness that produces crippling involvement of most joints. Moreover, those with cervical or lumbosacral disease can be given some hope for a spontaneous remission of severe pain. The need to reduce weight and strengthen supporting muscles should be stressed, as well as the importance of avoiding unnecessarily strenuous activity and addicting analgesics. Surgical options should be discussed with patients who have disabling disease of the hips or knees.

The physician's concern and support are essential to the successful management of any chronic disease, and especially one like DJD, in which the patient's response to the illness has much to do with its effect on his life. Return visits should be scheduled as frequently as needed to provide psychological support. A strong doctor–patient relationship helps many patients to tolerate the disease and remain active.

THERAPEUTIC RECOMMENDATIONS

- Patients with disease of the hips or knees should be instructed to reduce excess weight, exercise regularly to strengthen quadriceps and hip muscles, and avoid excessive stress on these joints (e.g., stair climbing). Gentle walking, swimming or stationary cycling can be prescribed. Isometric exercises and use of a cane or crutches for reduction of weight-bearing are preferred when severe pain limits joint motion. Absolute rest is inadvisable.
- Those with back pain should be instructed to obtain bed rest followed by exercises to strengthen supporting musculature (see Chapter 140). A corset or brace may help.
- Those with cervical pain can be given a soft cervical collar for support. It should be worn at all times, including during the night. Four weeks or more of use may be necessary. Cervical traction is also helpful (see Chapter 141).
- Drug therapy for reduction of pain should be instituted with aspirin, 2 to 4 gm. per day, given on a continuous basis at first. Acetaminophen may be tried in patients who are intolerant to aspirin, but a nonsteroidal anti-inflammatory drug (e.g., ibuprofen 400 mg. four times a day) may be more effective. Indomethacin, 25 to 50 mg. with each meal, may help patients who do not respond to other drugs, particularly those with osteoarthritis of the hip; however, chronic use may be poorly tolerated in the elderly and is associated with risk of gastric irritation. One of the newer indomethacin-like agents may be tried if indomethacin cannot be tolerated.
- In general, use of narcotics should be avoided, because most pain is chronic. However, for an acute

disabling exacerbation, a short course of an agent such as codeine sulfate (30 to 60 mg. every 6 to 8 hours) may reduce pain sufficiently to allow the patient to function.

• Referral for a surgical opinion should be restricted to the well-motivated patient who can tolerate major surgery and has refractory disease of a major weight-bearing joint that significantly interferes with life-style and ability to function satisfactorily.

ANNOTATED BIBLIOGRAPHY

American Medical Association: Skeletal muscle relaxants. *In* AMA Drug Evaluations, ed. 3. Littleton, Mass.: PSG Publishing Company, 1977, p. 1023. *(There is no evidence at the present time that sedative agents used as muscle relaxants have a direct muscle-relaxant effect; rather, the reduction in muscle tone may be dependent on centrally mediated sedative effects.)*

Feinstein, P.A., and Haberman, E.T.: Selecting and preparing patients for total hip replacement. Geriatrics, *32*:91, July, 1977. *(A straightforward guide for the primary physician about total hip replacement.)*

Gainsiracusa, J.E., Donaldson, M.S., et al.: Ibuprofen in osteoarthritis. South. Med. J., *70*:49, 1977. *(A study showing 1800 mg. per day of ibuprofen was as effective as aspirin.)*

Greenfield, S., Solomon, N.E., Brook, R.H., et al.: Development of outcome criterion and standards to assess the quality of care for patients with osteoarthrosis. J. Chron. Dis., *31*:375, 1978. *(An article that reviews the epidemiology of osteoarthritis, emphasizing the difficulty of assessing the efficacy of medical care for people with this disease.)*

Gresham, G.E., and Rathey, U.K.: Osteoarthritis in knees of aged persons: Relationship between roentgenographic and clinical manifestations.

JAMA, *233*:168, 1975. *(A study showing that crepitus, decreased range of motion, pain, bone enlargement and instability are more common in abnormal knees.)*

Hernborg, J.S., and Nilsson, B.E.: The natural course of untreated osteoarthritis of the knee. Clin. Orth., *123*:130, 1977. *(A study of 94 joints in 71 patients showing a generally unfavorable prognosis, with pain developing at rest in the majority of patients.)*

Kellgren, J.H.: Osteoarthritis. Arthritis Rheum., 8:568, 1965. *(A good review.)*

Kellgren, J.H., Lawrence, J.J., and Bier, F.: Genetic factors in generalized osteoarthritis. Ann. Rheum. Dis., *22*:237, 1969. *(The genetic basis of osteoarthritis.)*

Lawrence, J.S., Bremner, J.M., and Bier, F.: Osteoarthrosis prevalence in the population and relationship between symptoms and x-ray changes. Ann. Rheum. Dis., *25*:1, 1966. *(A prevalence of minimal disease in 50 per cent and more significant disease in 20 per cent. Radiographic changes were associated with symptoms in all joints but the lumbar spine.)*

Mankin, H.J.: The reaction of articular cartilage to injury and osteoarthritis. N. Engl. J. Med., *291*:1285, 1974. *(A good review of the biochemistry of cartilaginous change.)*

Mason, D.I., Brooks, P.M., and Buchanen, W.W.: The treatment of osteoarthrosis. Practitioner, *215*:87, 1975. *(A review of treatment of osteoarthritis, with well-reasoned prescribing recommendations.)*

Solomon, L.: Patterns of osteoarthritis of the hip. J. Bone Joint Surg., *58*:176, 1975. *(A detailed clinical and pathologic study of 327 cases of osteoarthritis that revealed normal cartilage failing under normal conditions as well as breakup of articular cartilage due to defective subchondral bone.)*

149
Management of Gout

Gout is among the most common causes of acute monoarticular arthritis. Estimates of prevalence in the United States range from 0.3 per cent to 2.8 per cent of the population; the condition is predominant-

ly a disease of adult men. Inborn errors in purine metabolism and abnormalities in uric acid excretion (see Chapter 146) account for most cases of primary gout. The expanded use of agents that decrease uric acid excretion (e.g., thiazide diuretics) has markedly increased the incidence of secondary gout. In the Framingham study, almost half of new cases were associated with thiazide use.

The primary physician should be able to promptly diagnose and treat acute gout, prevent recurrences, and minimize the chances of complications such as chronic gouty arthritis, nephrolithiasis and renal disease.

PATHOPHYSIOLOGY AND CLINICAL PRESENTATION

Acute gout usually occurs after many years of sustained asymptomatic hyperuricemia. The greater the uric acid concentration, the greater the risk of an acute attack. The mean duration of the asymptomatic period is about 30 years. During this time there may be deposition of urate in synovial lining cells and possibly in cartilage as well. Acute gout develops when uric acid crystals collect in the synovial fluid as a result of precipitation from a supersaturated state or release from the synovium. Trauma, decline in temperature, fall in pH, dehydration, starvation, alcoholic binge, emotional or physical stress, and rapid change in serum uric acid concentration have all been implicated in the process. The pathogenesis of the inflammatory response appears to involve phagocytosis of crystals by leukocytes in the synovial fluid, disruption of lysosomes, release of enzymatic products, activation of the complement and kallikrein systems, and release of leukocyte chemotactic factor.

The typical attack of *acute gouty arthritis* is monoarticular and abrupt in onset, often occurring at night. Symptoms and signs of inflammation become maximal within a few hours of onset and last for a few days to a few weeks. Recovery is complete. The initial attack usually involves a joint of the lower extremity; in about half of patients the first metatarsophalangeal joint is the site of inflammation (podagra). The tarsal joint (located at the instep), ankle, and knee are other common sites of initial attacks. Later episodes may involve a joint of the upper extremity, such as the wrist, elbow or finger; shoulder or hip involvement is rare. Over 80 per cent of attacks occur in the lower extremity; 85 per cent of patients have at least one episode of podagra. About 5 per cent of acute gouty episodes are polyarticular. Some patients are normouricemic at the time of an acute attack.

The joint appears swollen and erythematous; periarticular involvement is also common. There may be a low-grade fever. During resolution, the skin overlying the affected joint often desquamates. The clinical presentation may simulate joint infection (see Chapter 138) or even cellulitis (see Chapter 181).

Interval gout follows the initial attack. There is an asymptomatic period that generally lasts for several years before a second episode of acute gout takes place. The original joint or another joint may be involved in subsequent attacks. Over time, the asymptomatic intervals between acute episodes shorten. In more advanced disease, polyarticular attacks are not uncommon, and resolution may be slower and less complete.

Chronic gouty arthritis (tophaceous gout) takes years to develop. Tophi are noted an average of 10 years after the initial attack of acute gout. The risk of chronic gout is a function of duration and severity of hyperuricemia. Tophi represent sodium urate collections surrounded by foreign body giant cell inflammatory reactions. They can occur in a variety of sites, including the synovium, subchondral bone, olecranon bursa, Achilles tendon, and subcutaneous tissue of the extensor surfaces of the arm. Eventually cartilage erodes, joints become deformed, and chronic arthritis ensues. The joints of the lower extremities and hands are most commonly affected. The process is insidious; the patient notes progressive aching and stiffness. Tumescences may develop over joints of the foot and cause difficulty with wearing shoes. Fortunately the incidence of tophaceous gout has declined markedly with the introduction of effective antihyperuricemic agents. At present, less than 15 per cent of patients with acute gout develop chronic gouty arthritis.

The incidence of *nephrolithiasis* among patients with clinical gout is small. In a prospective study from the Kaiser-Permanente system, the risk of new stone formation in a patient with new onset of gout was less than 1 per cent per year. The probability of stone formation was unrelated to initial serum urate concentration or degree of uric acid control. The mean interval between onset of gout and passage of a stone was 5.5 years. Factors other than serum urate concentration are important to stone formation, and include family history of stone formation, urine pH, hydration status, and possibly the amount of renal uric acid excretion. Stone formation is rarely life-threatening, as demonstrated by one large 7-year study, in which only 1 of 1,700 patients with gout developed obstructive uropathy due to urate lithiasis.

Chronic renal failure is felt to be a potential consequence of hyperuricemia; however, recent data do not fully support this view. Data from the only controlled, long-term, prospective study of the question showed that azotemia was infrequent and, when it did occur, was clinically insignificant during the 10-year follow-up period. Projections based on this data indicate that there is no significant risk of clinically important azotemia until the serum uric acid reaches 13 mg. per 100 ml. in men and 10 mg. per 100 ml. in women *and* is sustained for 40 years. Much of the renal disease in gouty patients is attributable to concurrent hypertension or diabetes, although some investigators wonder whether vascular injury may be crystal-induced.

Acute renal failure can occur from the sudden extreme uric acid load that is produced in the early stages of treatment for lymphoproliferative and myeloproliferative diseases. Uric acid may precipitate in renal tubules and elsewhere in the urinary tract, leading to acute oliguria.

PRINCIPLES OF THERAPY

Acute gouty arthritis. Acute symptoms can be relieved by a number of *anti-inflammatory drugs,* including colchicine, indomethacin, phenylbutazone, and the new nonsteroidal agents such as ibuprofen, naproxen, and fenoprofen.

Without treatment, an acute attack of gout usually resolves within 7 to 10 days, though severe episodes can last for weeks. Initiation of treatment with an anti-inflammatory agent at the very first sign of an acute attack produces a prompt and excellent therapeutic response. Delay of therapy is associated with less dramatic results. Symptomatic treatment is usually continued until symptoms have resolved.

Interval gout. Although prophylactic therapy to prevent acute gouty arthritis is not cost-effective for patients with asymptomatic hyperuricemia (see Chapter 146), it may be worthwhile in patients who have had more than one attack of acute gout, because the intervals between future recurrences are likely to shorten.

Colchicine is highly effective for prophylaxis and is commonly given for 6 to 12 months in conjunction with an agent that lowers the serum uric acid. Initiation of antihyperuricemic therapy without colchicine prophylaxis can precipitate an attack of acute gout. There are no definitive data on the ideal duration of colchicine therapy, but most authorities recommend that it be given for at least 6 months. Cost is minimal; a once-a-day dose suffices. Serious side effects associated with long-term colchicine use are rare, but include agranulocytosis, aplastic anemia and myopathy.

Antihyperuricemic agents are indicated in patients with repeated episodes of acute gout, because the risk of an attack is in part related to the degree of hyperuricemia. *Allopurinol* is currently the agent most widely used to lower the uric acid. It inhibits the enzyme xanthine oxidase and thus blocks the formation of uric acid. The half-life of allopurinol is about 3 hours, but its metabolites are biologically active for up to 30 hours. As a result, the drug can be given once daily. Serum urate levels fall within a week of initiating therapy. Toxic reactions are rare; rash is the most common side effect, and hepatocellular injury occasionally occurs in patients with renal failure. Unfortunately, the drug is expensive. Colchicine is required during the initial phases of therapy. Allopurinol has no effect on acute gouty arthritis.

A *uricosuric agent* is a reasonable alternative to allopurinol therapy as long as the patient does not demonstrate urate nephrolithiasis or hyperexcretion of uric acid (greater than 500 mg. per 24 hours). *Probenecid* and *sulfinpyrazone* are the most commonly used uricosuric drugs. They work by blocking tubular reabsorption of uric acid. These agents are being used with less frequency because of the efficacy of allupurinol; however, they are less expensive than allopurinol. A 24-hour urine specimen must be obtained to be sure that urate excretion is below 500 mg. per 24 hours. If this is the case, a uricosuric drug can be used; otherwise the amount of uric acid excretion that may result from uricosuric therapy could result in crystal deposition and stone formation. At the onset of therapy, the uric acid excretion may reach extraordinary levels; consequently, it is essential that fluid intake be generous (2 to 3 liters per day) to minimize the chances of uric acid precipitation. Alkalinization of the urine to a pH of 6.6 is desirable but difficult to achieve. It can be attempted by administration of large doses of sodium bicarbonate during the day, supplemented by acetazolamide before bed. Potassium citrate may be tried in patients who must restrict their sodium intake, but success is often minimal. Colchicine is needed concurrently with uricosuric treatment to prevent an acute attack of gout.

The uricosuric action of probenecid and sulfinpyrazone is blocked by thiazides and low doses of salicylates; moreover, patients with renal failure do not respond to these drugs.

Dietary factors have received much attention.

There is no need to restrict purine intake because only 10 per cent of circulating purine is derived from dietary sources. However, reduction of excess weight (without fasting) and abstinence from excessive alcohol intake and binge drinking can help prevent future attacks.

Chronic gouty arthritis. Prevention or lessening of chronic tophaceous gout can be achieved by lowering the serum urate level to normal. Allopurinol is the drug of choice for patients with tophaceous gout. Tophi may begin to resolve after several weeks of therapy. Again, colchicine must be given concurrently because mobilization of urate deposits may trigger an acute attack. A uricosuric agent is a reasonable alternative as long as there are no contraindications to its use, such as nephrolithiasis of excess uric acid excretion.

Nephrolithiasis and chronic renal failure. The patient with an established uric acid stone should be given allopurinol and instructed to keep well hydrated (see Chapter 130). Antihyperuricemic therapy for prevention of stone formation is indicated in gouty patients with a history of nephrolithiasis, a family history of kidney stones (see Chapter 146) and, perhaps, extraordinary degrees of uric acid excretion (i.e., greater than 1100 mg. per 24 hours on a routine diet). All patients should be instructed to avoid even temporary dehydration, especially if they live in warm dry climates.

Efforts to prevent chronic renal failure by lowering the serum uric acid level are of questionable utility, though projections based on data from the prospective study cited above suggest that extremely high concentrations of uric acid (13 mg. per 100 ml. in men and 10 mg. per 100 ml. in women) sustained over very prolonged periods (40 years in the analysis) may put the patient at risk for renal failure (see Chapter 146).

PATIENT EDUCATION

The importance of weight control (see Chapter 222), avoidance of excessive ethanol intake (see Chapter 216), and maintenance of good hydration need to be stressed. On the other hand, patients will often find it comforting to know that severe dietary restrictions are unnecessary. Fasting should be prohibited, since it might precipitate an acute episode of gout. Patients must be instructed to take their anti-inflammatory agent at the earliest sign of an attack.

THERAPEUTIC RECOMMENDATIONS

- At the first sign of an attack of acute gouty arthritis, an anti-inflammatory agent such as indomethacin (50 mg. 3 to 4 times daily) should be started; therapy is continued until symptoms resolve, and then tapered over 72 hours. Relief is usually prompt and effective. Delay in initiating therapy is associated with less dramatic results.
- Refractory cases of definite acute gout can be treated with intra-articular or systemic corticosteroids.
- For interval gout, small daily doses of colchicine (0.6 to 1.2 mg. per day) can be given prophylactically when recurrences of acute attacks are becoming increasingly frequent. Antihyperuricemic therapy can be initiated at the same time using allopurinol (300 mg. once daily) or a uricosuric agent (e.g., probenecid 500 mg. 1 or 2 times daily).
- Colchicine should be started at the time of antihyperuricemic therapy and continued for 6 to 12 months to prevent acute gout due to mobilization of urate deposits.
- Antihyperuricemic therapy plus colchicine should help prevent chronic gout and reduce the number of acute gouty attacks.
- If a uricosuric agent is used, therapy should be initiated utilizing small doses (e.g., 500 mg. per day of probenecid) in conjunction with large volumes of fluid (2 to 3 liters per day) to prevent precipitation of uric acid in the urinary tract. Alkalinization of the urine to a pH of 6.6 is desirable during the first week of therapy, but is difficult to achieve; gram doses of sodium bicarbonate are required, supplemented by acetazolamide (250 mg.) before bed.
- For chronic gout, allopurinol is the treatment of choice; colchicine is required during the first 6 to 12 months of therapy.
- Patients need to be instructed to take their anti-inflammatory agent at the first sign of an acute attack. An extra supply should be given for future episodes.
- Gradual reduction to ideal weight, decrease in alcohol intake, and avoidance of dehydration, binge drinking and low-dose aspirin also need to be reviewed with the patient. Fasting should be discouraged, since it might precipitate an attack.
- Patients with clinical gout who require thiazide therapy should receive allopurinol. Asymptomatic patients with mild hyperuricemia on thiazide therapy probably do not need allopurinol (see Chapter 146).

- For gouty patients with urate nephrolithiasis, a strong family history of kidney stones, or marked uric acid excretion (greater than 1100 mg. per 24 hours), allopurinol (300 mg. once daily) and hydration are indicated. Long-term efforts to alkalinize the urine are impractical and need not be attempted.
- The utility of prophylactic therapy for prevention of chronic renal failure is unproven.

ANNOTATED BIBLIOGRAPHY

Burger, L.U., and Yu, T.F.: Renal function in gout—An analysis of 524 gouty subjects including long-term follow-up studies. Am. J. Med., *59*:604, 1975. *(Follow-up for 12 years showed that hyperuricemia alone had no deleterious effect on renal function in ambulatory patients with gout.)*

Fessel, J.W.: Renal outcomes of gout and hyperuricemia. Am. J. Med., *67*:74, 1979. *(A carefully done prospective study showing that the risks of renal failure and stone formation are very small and hardly justify prophylactic therapy.)*

Graham, R., and Scott, J.T.: Clinical survey of 354 patients with gout. Ann. Rheum. Dis., *29*:461, 1976. *(An extensive epidemiologic review.)*

Hall, A.P., Berry, P.E., Dawber, T.R., et al.: Epidemiology of gout and hyperuricemia—A long-term population study. Am. J. Med., *42*:27, 1967. *(The Framingham study; 14 per cent of patients with uric acids of 7 to 7.9 mg., 19 per cent with uric serum urates between 8 and 8.9, and 5 out of 6 patients with uric acids over 9 developed gouty attacks.)*

Maclaughlan, M.J., and Rodnan, G.P.: Effects of food, fast, and alcohol on serum uric acid and acute attacks of gout. Am. J. Med., *42*:38, 1967. *(Fasting and consumption of over 100 gm. of alcohol raised urate levels. Acute changes in levels precipitated gouty attacks.)*

Paulus, H.E., Coutts, A., Calabro, J.J., et al.: Clinical significance of hyperuricemia in routinely screened hospitalized men. JAMA, *211*:277, 1970. *(An early but prophetic paper that argued that an abnormal laboratory finding does not confirm diagnosis or justify therapy.)*

Rastegar, A., and Thier, S.O.: The physiologic approach to hyperuricemia. N. Engl. J. Med., *286*:470, 1972. *(Reviews what is known about enzymatic defects that lead to increased uric acid.)*

Rodnan, G.P., Robin, J.A., et al.: Allopurinol and gouty hyperuricemia: Efficacy of a single daily dose. JAMA, *231*:1143, 1975. *(A study that compared single 300-mg. dose to divided doses, demonstrating that the once-daily dose of allopurinol is adequate.)*

Simkin, P.A.: The pathogenesis of podagra. Ann. Intern. Med., *86*:230, 1977. *(Reviews the current state of understanding of the pathogenesis of gout.)*

Yu, T., and Gutman, A.: Uric acid nephrolithiasis in gout: predisposing factors. Ann. Intern. Med., *67*:1133, 1967. *(A classic study of 305 gouty patients correlating risk of stone formation with uric acid excretion, urine pH, serum urate level and etiology.)*

150

Management of Temporal Arteritis and Polymyalgia Rheumatica

Temporal or giant cell arteritis is a vasculitic disorder of unknown origin that primarily affects people over the age of 60 and rarely occurs before 50. The incidence of temporal arteritis in one population study was 11.7 per 100,000, and its prevalence was 133 per 100,000. In an autopsy study of 389 unselected people, temporal arteritis was found in 1.7 per cent. The importance of temporal arteritis derives from its potential to produce sudden irreversible blindness in approximately one-third of untreated patients.

Temporal arteritis has been reported in 40 per cent of patients with polymyalgia rheumatica (PMR). The exact relationship between the two conditions has yet to be completely elucidated. PMR is characterized by proximal musculoskeletal discomfort and elevated sedimentation rate, often accompanied by fever, malaise and weight loss. It affects patients over 50 and has a 2:1 predominance in females.

The primary physician needs to be alert to the possibility that these diseases may be present, because they can be subtle in presentation and easily dismissed as vague functional complaints. The associated risk of blindness makes recognition and treatment of prime importance. Because polymyalgia rheumatica may be accompanied by temporal arteritis, one needs to decide which patients with PMR require biopsy in search of arteritis.

PATHOPHYSIOLOGY AND CLINICAL PRESENTATION

Temporal arteritis is defined pathologically by histiocytic, lymphocytic and giant cell infiltration of the walls of medium or large arteries. The internal elastic lamina is fragmented in conjunction with proliferation. The inflammatory process occurs predominantly, though not exclusively, in cranial arteries. The condition has many of the characteristics of an autoimmune process, but the precise pathophysiology remains to be elucidated.

The clinical presentations of temporal arteritis reflect direct inflammation of the arterial wall and ischemia secondary to vasculitic narrowing. Headache is reported in 44 to 98 per cent of cases and is an initial symptom in 30 to 45 per cent. The pain is boring or throbbing, often localized to the arteries of the scalp. A tender artery may be noted on combing the hair. Ischemic symptoms such as masseter claudication occur in one-third to one-half of patients. Visual manifestations are due to vasculitis that may involve the ophthalmic or posterior ciliary arteries. Blindness is usually a late symptom, occurring abruptly but frequently preceded by transient visual symptoms. In early studies that included many untreated patients, visual loss occurred in 42 to 50 per cent. Better recognition and prompt treatment has resulted in a drop in frequency of permanent visual loss to 5 to 10 per cent. Constitutional symptoms of fatigue, malaise, anorexia and weight loss occur in the majority of patients. Palpable, tender temporal or occipital arteries are sometimes encountered. A markedly increased erythrocyte sedimentation rate is highly characteristic of the disease. A low-grade anemia of chronic disease is often present as well.

Polymyalgia rheumatica develops gradually over weeks or months. Pain and stiffness of periarticular structures of neck and shoulders is the presentation in two-thirds of cases, with hip and thigh involvement accounting for the other third. Many complain of shoulder and thigh involvement. Morning stiffness and pain with movement are highly characteristic; muscle strength is unimpaired. Synovitis has been documented histologically; muscle biopsies are usually normal or show minor inflammatory infiltrates. Low-grade fever, weight loss and fatigue are commonly present for months before the diagnosis is made.

A PMR patient with headache, tender cranial artery or visual complaints is likely to have temporal arteritis. One study found temporal arteritis in 15 of 33 PMR patients who had such symptoms. However, most patients with symptoms solely of polymyalgia for 6 months do not later incur risk of blindness.

PRINCIPLES OF MANAGEMENT

A critical issue in management is the decision whether to *biopsy* the temporal arteries of patients with PMR. It is known that there is a relationship between PMR and temporal arteritis and that headache and other arteritis symptoms help to identify those who will have positive biopsies. In the defined population studied by the Mayo Clinic, all patients with PMR found to have temporal arteritis had symptoms of arteritis. Though some rheumatologists advocate biopsy of all PMR patients, the data are inconclusive. Some find it difficult to justify the costs associated with biopsying all PMR patients, especially when the need for steroids in asymptomatic patients with positive biopsies is unclear. At the present time, it seems reasonable to defer temporal artery biopsy in those patients with PMR who have no symptoms of temporal arteritis and can be depended on to report any. Should such symptoms arise, biopsy can be promptly performed. The risk to the patient in delaying biopsy until symptoms arise is probably very small, because symptoms almost always precede onset of visual loss.

Temporal artery biopsy has a considerable false-negative rate because the arteritis is often patchy in distribution. When clinical evidence is strong, yet biopsy is negative, treatment can proceed without pathologic confirmation. The false-negative rate can be minimized by obtaining a generous portion of the temporal artery at biopsy. Arteriography is sensitive but nonspecific and unreliable diagnostically, but may be helpful in choosing an area to biopsy, especially if the first attempt was unsuccessful.

The natural history of temporal arteritis is a self-limited one; most cases resolve within 2 years, though there is much individual variation. The disease should be treated initially with substantial daily doses of *prednisone* (40 to 60 mg. per day). Daily therapy is needed; an alternate day schedule does not control the arteritis. The resolution of symptoms is characteristically prompt, and the sedimentation rate falls back to normal levels. The prednisone dose can be titrated against recurrence of symptoms and elevation of the sedimentation rate and should be reduced slowly toward a maintenance dose of 10 to 15 mg. per day. The patient must be carefully watched for recurrence of symptoms and elevation of the sedimentation rate. It is sometimes possible to have the patient completely off steroids within a year. Data suggest that spontaneous remission may occur within 6 months, but in many cases activity persists for 2 to 3 years. Relapses have occurred in up to 20 per cent when treatment was discontinued before 2 years had elapsed. Fortunately in the Mayo Clinic series, blindness did not occur during relapses. Tapering should begin as soon as improvement is evident to minimize the adverse effects of prolonged high-dose steroid therapy (see Chapter 101).

Polymyalgia rheumatica without symptoms of arteritis can be treated with low-dose prednisone, beginning with 10 to 15 mg. per day and tapering as the sedimentation rate falls and symptoms resolve. If improvement does not occur in 1 week, the diagnosis is probably incorrect. Characteristically, the condition responds dramatically to very small steroid doses. These dosages do not protect the patient from the complications of arteritis and require adjustment should vasculitic symptoms occur. However, it is very rare for blindness to occur if the sedimentation rate is normal.

PATIENT EDUCATION

Patients with PMR must be told of the symptoms of arteritis and instructed to report their occurrence immediately. The rationale for daily prednisone therapy needs to be shared with the patient and family to ensure compliance. The usual precautions applicable to anyone on daily prednisone therapy should be reviewed (see Chapter 101).

INDICATIONS FOR REFERRAL

Before steroid therapy is undertaken, consultation with a rheumatologist is indicated if the temporal artery biopsy is negative but the clinical picture strongly suggests the diagnosis of temporal arteritis. Consultation is also indicated in cases of polymyalgia and temporal arteritis which do not respond to steroid therapy.

THERAPEUTIC RECOMMENDATIONS

- Diagnosis of suspected temporal arteritis should be established by confirmatory biopsy, recognizing that a negative biopsy does not rule out the diagnosis.
- At present, there appears to be no justification for performing temporal artery biopsy in patients with PMR who do not have headache or other cranial symptoms suggestive of vasculitis, e.g., tender artery; onset of such symptoms (tongue claudication, visual disturbances, etc.) requires prompt biopsy and high-dose steroid therapy.
- Therapy for temporal arteritis is initiated with 60 mg. of prednisone per day; tapering is started once the sedimentation rate has been substantially reduced and symptomatic control achieved. Daily prednisone therapy is required, usually for 18 to 24 months.
- Tapering can continue over a period of months, arriving at a minimal dose sufficient to keep the sedimentation rate normal and the patient free of symptoms.
- After 18 to 24 months, a cautious attempt at phasing out prednisone therapy can be undertaken; the patient is watched for recurrence of symptoms and rise in sedimentation rate.
- Polymyalgia rheumatica should be treated initially with low-dose prednisone (10 to 15 mg. per day) and slow tapering once symptoms and elevated sedimentation rate have resolved. Therapy is commonly needed for 2 to 4 years.
- The patient needs to be instructed to report at once the onset of any symptoms suggestive of arteritis.

ANNOTATED BIBLIOGRAPHY

Ettlinger, R.E., Hunder, G.G., and Ward, L.E.: Polymyalgia rheumatica and giant cell arteritis. Ann. Rev. Med., *29*:15, 1978. *(A review that tends to favor biopsy in PMR patients.)*

Fauchald, P., Rygvold, O., and Osytese, B.: Temporal arteritis and polymyalgia rheumatica. Ann. Intern. Med., *77*:845, 1972. *(Documents the strong association between the two conditions.)*

Hamilton, C.R., Jr., Shelly, W.M., and Tumulty, P.A.: Giant-cell arteritis: Including temporal arteritis and polymyalgia rheumatica. Medicine (Baltimore), *50*:1, 1971. *(Comprehensive review.)*

Healty, L.A.: Giant cell arteritis (editorial). Ann. Intern. Med., 88:710. 1978. *(A succinct statement encouraging a conservative approach to treating people with polymyalgia.)*

Healty, L.A., and Wilske, K.R.: Manifestations of giant cell arteritis. Med. Clin. North Am., 61:261, 1977. *(Details a wide variety of presentations.)*

Horton, B.T., Magath, T.B., and Brown, G.E.: An undescribed form of arteritis of the temporal vessels. Proc. Staff Meetings Mayo Clin., 7:700, 1932. *(A classic description.)*

Hunder, G.G., Sheps, S.G., Allen, G.L., and Joyce, J.W.: Daily and alternate-day corticosteroid regimens in the treatment of giant cell arteritis. Ann. Intern. Med., 82:613, 1975. *(Alternate-day steroids are not effective.)*

Huston, K.A., Hunder, G.G., Lie, J.T., *et al.*: Temporal arteritis, a 24-year epidemiologic, clinical and pathologic study. Ann. Intern. Med., 88:162, 1978. *(An epidemiologic survey detailing symptoms in an unselected population.)*

Klein, R.G., Hunder, G.G., Stanson, A.W., and Sheps, S.G.: Large artery involvement in giant cell (temporal) arteritis. Ann. Intern. Med., 83:806, 1975. *(Temporal arteritis can be a more generalized condition.)*

Layfer, L.F., Banner, B.F., Huckman, M.S., *et al.*: Temporal arteriography. Arthritis Rheum., 21:780, 1978. *(Arteriography is a highly sensitive but nonspecific test for arteritis.)*

151
Management of Paget's Disease
SAMUEL R. NUSSBAUM, M.D.

Paget's disease of bone, or osteitis deformans, is a focal disorder of unknown etiology characterized by deformity of the bone's external contour and internal structure that results from excessive resorption and rapid new bone formation. The incidence of Paget's disease was reported to be 3.3 per cent in an autopsy series and 0.1 to 4.0 per cent in radiologic studies. The clinical presentation is variable. In the majority of cases, the diagnosis is made when the patient is asymptomatic. An elevated alkaline phosphatase is discovered on multiphasic screening, or x-rays of the pelvis, vertebrae or skull show the hallmark radiolucent (osteolytic) areas with compensatory new bone formation. Symptomatic patients report pain in the back or lower extremities, disturbances of gait, increasing head size, hearing loss and occasionally symptoms related to high output cardiac failure. The primary physician needs to be able to provide symptomatic relief and to know when to utilize agents which suppress osteoclastic activity.

PATHOPHYSIOLOGY AND CLINICAL PRESENTATION

The pathophysiological mechanism of Paget's disease is excessive osteoclastic destruction and resorption of bone followed by unregulated osteoblastic new bone formation. The process culminates in an abnormal pattern of lamellar bone with excessive local vascularity and an increase in fibrous tissue. The resultant bone which is mechanically defective, distorted and enlarged, leads to the cardinal manifestation of Paget's disease: bone pain and pathologic fractures.

The exact mechanism of bone pain in Paget's disease is not understood, and its severity does not always parallel the extent of radiographic involvement. Pain is often exacerbated by weight-bearing, muscular activity, or cold weather, and is often located over lytic areas of bone where active osteoclastic resorption is taking place. Bone pain is most common in the spine, pelvis, skull, femur and tibia.

When the long bones of the lower limbs are affected by Paget's disease, deformity and bowing occur. Often the entire length of the tibia is involved while the fibula is unaffected. Fractures of the long bones, common below the lesser trochanter of the femur and in the upper third of the tibia, result from the mechanical bowing and abnormal bone architecture. The skull is enlarged due to thickening of the calvarium, manifest in the frontal and occipital regions. Hearing loss occurs due to involvement of the ossicles in the middle ear which impinge on the eighth cranial nerve in the temporal bone. Basilar invagination of the skull from its downward pressure on the atlas may cause compression of posterior fossa structures. Vertebral encroachment on the spinal cord or nerve roots may cause compression syndromes, including paraplegia.

High output congestive heart failure may occur in patients with extensive Paget's disease as a result of increased cutaneous blood flow to areas overlying pagetic limb involvement. Calcific periarthritis may mimic the symptoms of ankylosing spondylitis.

Hyperuricemia and gouty arthritis, hypercalciuria and renal calculi, and hypercalcemia precipitated by immobilization can occur. Osteogenic sarcoma is seen in 1 to 5 per cent of patients with Paget's disease, rarely before age 50. Extensive and severe skeletal involvement increases the risk of osteogenic sarcoma, which is heralded by localized pain and bony enlargement and occurs more frequently in the upper extremities and skull.

Laboratory and radiographic evidence reflects the increased osteoblastic and osteoclastic activity of pagetic bone. Serum alkaline phosphatase, produced by osteoblasts, is elevated, as is the urinary hydroxyproline excretion, an index of osteoclastic resorption of bone matrix. A bone scan may show areas of increased technetium uptake before diagnostic changes are visible on standard x-rays.

PRINCIPLES OF THERAPY

Most patients with Paget's disease are asymptomatic and require no specific therapy. Localized mild bone pain can be controlled with analgesics; joint involvement usually responds to anti-inflammatory agents such as salicylates, indomethacin, or any of the new nonsteroidal anti-inflammatory drugs (see Chapter 147). Treatment of Paget's disease with calcitonin, diphosphonate, or mithramycin results in a decrease in osteoclastic resorption and accompanying radiographic and clinical improvement. Although there are no universal criteria for initiation of specific therapy, indications for therapy in Paget's disease include: (1) severe pain in pagetic areas, (2) compression of medulla, cauda equina or auditory nerve with neurologic deficit, (3) high output cardiac failure, (4) hypercalcemia due to immobilization, (5) marked radiographic lytic lesions in long bones and skull representing risk of fracture or brain trauma, (6) multiple fractures, (7) prevention of disfigurement when the skull is extensively involved, (8) recurrent renal calculi due to hypercalciuria, (9) severe hyperuricemia and gout, (10) prophylaxis accompanying extensive orthopedic surgery to reduce vascularity of bone, and (11) prophylaxis when disease is of early onset in an area in which disabling deformity is likely to occur.

Calcitonin, diphosphonate and mithramycin are the principle agents available for specific therapy. They decrease osteoclastic resorption of bone and have been shown to lead to dramatic relief of pain, relief of nerve entrapment syndromes (although auditory acuity does not improve if the ossicles of the middle ear are affected), decrease in cardiac output by a reduction in vascularity of bone and overlying skin, and healing of lytic radiographic lesions.

Salmon calcitonin (Calcimar) must be given parenterally; it is started at 50 to 100 MRC units subcutaneously daily, depending on the severity of disease. Therapy is not only expensive but requires patient education and ability to learn self-injection techniques. With therapy, alkaline phosphatase and urinary hydroxyproline levels return to normal in one third of patients and are decreased in another third; in the balance of cases, decreases are minimal or unsustained, as is symptomatic improvement. Although antibodies against salmon calcitonin develop in approximately 50 per cent of patients, the clinical importance of this phenomenon in leading to relapse is uncertain. Patients who have developed antibodies against salmon calcitonin have had remissions when treated with human calcitonin. Calcitonin dosage may be reduced to 50 MRGU three times weekly when the disease is in remission. Current data suggest that a low dose should be continued indefinitely.

Disodium etidronate (EHDP). Diphosphonate treatment has the advantage of being an oral therapy, but it is also costly. It should not be given at a dose greater than 5 mg. per kg. per day because at higher doses (10 to 20 mg. per kg. per day) it induces a mineralization defect that may lead to increased fracture rates in areas of lytic bone, as well as worsened bone pain. Diphosphonate therapy should be given until a biochemical and clinical remission occurs, then discontinued, with recommencement of therapy at a time of relapse. EHDP should not be used for more than 6 consecutive months. In preliminary studies, combined therapy with calcitonin and diphosphonate has reduced bone turnover to normal in 80 per cent of patients and was not accompanied by mineralization defects or increases in bone pain.

Mithramycin must be administered intravenously. It is given in doses of 15 to 25 mcg. per kg. for 10 days, and suppresses urinary hydroxyproline over several days. Mithramycin should be reserved for dramatic complications of Paget's disease, such as severe high output heart failure or hypercalcemic crisis, because the drug can cause acute though reversible renal, hepatic and hematologic toxicities.

Neurosurgical intervention is necessary in patients with spinal cord or nerve root compression syndromes. Orthopedic procedures such as total hip replacement and tibial or femoral ostectomy may help to restore mobility.

PATIENT EDUCATION AND INDICATIONS FOR REFERRAL

Patients should be instructed to drink at least 2 liters of liquid daily, especially if they are unable to keep active, because immobilization and dehydration can precipitate renal stone formation and hypercalcemia. Prompt neurosurgical consultation is warranted in patients who have evidence of nerve or cord compression. Orthopedic assessment is needed if the patient is severely immobilized by hip pain. Referral to an endocrinologist is needed if conventional medical therapy fails.

THERAPEUTIC RECOMMENDATIONS

- The majority of patients with Paget's disease are asymptomatic; they require no specific therapy but should be seen at yearly intervals for clinical assessment and alkaline phosphatase measurement.
- For relief of mild localized bone or articular pain, analgesics or anti-inflammatory agents can be used.
- Patients with severe bone pain, high output cardiac failure, hypercalcemia, multiple fractures, or risk of fracture, deformity or compression should be given calcitonin, 100 CRF units subcutaneously daily, or EHDP, 5 mg. per kg. per day orally.
- Two baseline measurements of alkaline phosphatase as well as skeletal x-ray survey or bone scan ought to be obtained at the outset of treatment to help later in gauging therapeutic response. Serum alkaline phosphatase correlates well with disease activity; it can be followed at monthly intervals during therapy. Frequent bone scanning is unwarranted.
- When biochemical or clinical remission occurs, EHDP should be discontinued; if calcitonin is being used, it should be reduced to 50 CRF units three times a week.

- Avoidance of dehydration and immobilization is important for prevention of hypercalcemia and kidney stones. At least 2 liters of liquid should be taken daily, especially if the patient is inactive.

ANNOTATED BIBLIOGRAPHY

Bijvoet, O.L.M., Hosking, D.J., Frijlink, W.B., et al.: Treatment of Paget's disease with combined calcitonin and diphosphonate (EHDP). Metabolic Bone Disease and Related Research, 1:25, 1978. (Twenty-five of 30 patients treated with a combination of calcitonin and EHDP obtained complete biochemical remission. Mineralization defects were not seen when EHDP was given with calcitonin.)

Deuxchaisnes, C.N., and Krane, S.M.: Paget's disease of bone: Clinical and metabolic observations. Medicine, 43:233, 1964. (An extensive review of clinical manifestations of Paget's disease with a discussion of calcium balance and metabolic responses to fracture and immobilization.)

Frank, W.A., Bries, N.M., Singer, F.R., et al.: Rheumatic manifestations of Paget's disease of bone. Am. J. Med., 56:592, 1974. (A discussion of the rheumatological symptoms associated with Paget's disease.)

Khairi, M.R.A., Atman, R.D., DeRosa, G.P., et al.: Sodium etidronate in the treatment of Paget's disease of bone. A study of long-term results. Ann. Intern. Med., 87:656, 1977. (Demonstrates therapeutic efficacy of 5 mg./kg. EDHP and complications of higher doses of EHDP.)

Ryan, W.G.: Paget's disease of bone. Ann. Rev. Med., 28:143, 1977. (A succinct review of Paget's disease, emphasizing treatment. There is a comprehensive bibliography.)

Woodhouse, N.J., Crosbie, W.A., and Mohamedally, S.M.: Cardiac output in Paget's disease: Response to long-term salmon calcitonin therapy. Br. Med. J., 4(5998):686, 1975. (A brief report documenting a fall in cardiac output in three patients with Paget's disease treated with salmon calcitonin.)

152
Management of Osteoporosis
SAMUEL R. NUSSBAUM, M.D.

Osteopenia denotes a reduced amount of bone and encompasses both osteoporosis and osteomalacia. *Osteoporosis* refers to a reduction in the mass of bone per unit volume to such an extent that the mechanical support is affected, yet the ratio of mineral phase to organic phase remains normal. *Osteomalacia,* in contrast to osteoporosis, is characterized by a defect in the mineralization of the organic phase of bone.

The significance of osteoporosis can best be appreciated when it is realized that 25 per cent of women over the age of 60 have spinal compression fractures, and 20 per cent of women suffer hip fractures by age 90. In 1968, 700,000 hip fractures in women aged 45 and older were attributed to underlying osteoporosis. New techniques for evaluating decreases in bone mass as well as early therapeutic interventions to prevent reductions in skeletal mass are now available.

PATHOPHYSIOLOGY AND CLINICAL PRESENTATION

The formation and resorption of bone is a continuous process throughout life; under most circumstances the rates of these processes are coupled and equal. Skeletal mass is usually maximal by age 30 and declines after age 40, when the rate of bone resorption is not matched by new bone formation. The rate of decline is more rapid in women than in men, and is maximal within 3 years of menopause; greatest losses take place in the metacarpals, femoral neck and lumbar vertebrae.

In osteoporosis, the rate of bone resorption exceeds that of bone formation. The explanation for the increased rate of bone resorption remains speculative. Estrogens are believed to play a role, because bone resorption is accelerated following menopause, and estrogens seem to inhibit the process. Perhaps women in whom osteoporosis does not develop have larger initial skeletal masses. There is no evidence that aging is associated with increases in parathyroid hormone, nor have epidemiologic studies conclusively demonstrated differences in calcium intake in normal

and osteoporotic women, although fractional intestinal absorption of calcium in elderly persons is decreased.

Conditions other than aging which lead to osteoporosis include Cushing's syndrome, exogenous glucocorticoid administration, chronic heparin therapy, thyrotoxicosis, hypogonadism and hyperparathyroidism. These represent a small percentage of all cases; the vast majority are a consequence of aging.

The progressive decrease in skeletal mass, which may approach 50 per cent, becomes clinically manifest when fractures are sustained spontaneously or after minimal trauma. Fractures most commonly occur in the sacral and lumbar vertebrae, hip, humerus, and wrists. Spinal pain heralds new fractures, and loss of height correlates with collapse of vertebrae. The incidence of new fractures tends to decrease with time, but the clinical course of individual patients and frequency of fractures cannot be predicted.

The characteristic radiographic finding in osteoporosis is loss of horizontal vertebral trabeculae, accentuating the end-plates and resulting in biconcave "codfish" vertebrae. Pseudofractures, when present, are pathognomonic of osteomalacia. Other laboratory features of osteoporosis include normal serum levels of calcium, phosphate, parathyroid hormone, vitamin D, and alkaline phosphatase, though the latter can be elevated in the context of a healing fracture.

PRINCIPLES OF THERAPY

The major goal in management of osteoporosis is to minimize loss of bone mass and risk of fracture. Once a fracture has occurred, symptomatic relief and attempts at halting further osteoporosis are indicated. An important issue is the need for estrogen therapy.

The majority of patients with osteoporosis are postmenopausal women. Women who receive *estrogen therapy* at the time of menopause have a fivefold reduction in the incidence of vertebral crush fractures. Although estrogen treatment of osteoporosis has been advocated for three decades, only recently have sophisticated studies of bone mass confirmed previous clinical observations. When metacarpal mineral content was evaluated after 5 to 7 years of therapy with mestranol or placebo, patients on mestranol had no further loss of bone mass and even slight bone accretion, compared to continued bone loss in the placebo group. Unfortunately, if mestranol was discontinued, bone loss rapidly ensued. A 2-year study comparing calcium carbonate, conjugated estrogens and placebo therapy in 60 postmenopausal women revealed that conjugated estrogens in a dose of 0.625 mg. per day were superior to placebo and $CaCO_3$ in that bone loss as measured by photon absorptiometry was markedly diminished. Calcium therapy was also effective in preventing bone loss, but not to the same extent as estrogen.

The ability of *androgens* such as methandrostenolone to decrease bone resorption is similar to that of estrogens, but masculinizing side effects limit their usefulness in women.

The accumulating evidence that fracture rates and bone loss are decreased in postmenopausal women on estrogen therapy, coupled with knowledge that significant bone loss is not reversible, favors the use of estrogens at the time of menopause to prevent osteoporosis in selected patients.

When osteoporosis is clinically manifested by fractures or when osteopenia appears radiographically, at least 30 to 40 per cent loss of bone mass has occurred, and therapy with estrogen (in women) and supplemental calcium (see below) should be commenced. At this time, there is no universal agreement as to which patients should be considered for prophylactic therapy with estrogens at the time of menopause. Certainly, women with a family history of osteoporosis, who have not been physically active, who relate a history of low calcium intake, who have had multiple pregnancies, or who have a small frame are all predisposed to develop osteoporosis and are candidates for prophylactic therapy. The increased risks of endometrial carcinoma and cardiovascular events in postmenopausal women taking estrogen must be considered (see Chapters 104, 114) before therapy is undertaken.

Calcium and vitamin D. The only therapeutic program which is claimed to *increase* bone formation and skeletal mass is that of calcium 1 gm. daily, vitamin D 50,000 U twice weekly, and fluoride 50 mg. per day. Although biopsies in patients treated with this regimen show increased trabecular bone, concern exists regarding whether this bone is structurally sound. At this time, fluoride remains an investigational drug in the treatment of osteoporosis.

An important component of preventive therapy is ensuring maximal development of skeletal mass. The amount of bone accumulated during growth may be critical to the later appearance of osteoporosis as evidenced by the low incidence of osteoporosis in men and in black women, who have a greater skeletal mass than white women. Adequate bone mass in young people, especially pregnant women in whom consumption of dairy products is minimal, should be insured by calcium and vitamin D supplementation. Patients taking phenobarbital or phenytoin need even greater vitamin D supplementation (see below).

Because calcium therapy has been shown to help prevent bone loss and absorption of calcium decreases with aging, women over 40 should receive daily supplemental calcium, 1 to 2 gm. Larger doses of calcium, particularly in conjunction with vitamin D, may predispose to hypercalcemia and hypercalciuric renal stones.

Fractures. In patients who have sustained vertebral fractures, bed rest and adequate analgesics should be prescribed until the acute pain of the fracture subsides. Ambulation, as tolerated and daily exercise, such as swimming and walking, should be encouraged. Lifting and vigorous physical activity are best avoided. Attention to details, such as proper footwear, canes for support, and an uncluttered home environment may prevent further accidental trauma. Corsets and back braces, if comfortable, may facilitate ambulation in formerly bedridden patients; those who have sustained fractures should then be treated for osteoporosis.

The natural history of osteoporosis and compression fractures is unpredictable in individual patients. Symptomatic improvement cannot be used to measure the response to therapy because of the highly episodic course of the disease, which is characterized by long fracture-free intervals. Noninvasive measurements of bone mass, such as metacarpal measurements or photon absorptiometry, if available, will determine if bone loss has slowed or reversed with therapeutic intervention.

Osteomalacia. In approaching the patient with osteopenia, it is important to exclude osteomalacia. In recently conducted orthopedic studies of hip fractures, 10 to 15 per cent of patients were found to have osteomalacia. The most frequent causes include vitamin D lack, disorders of vitamin D metabolism, gastrointestinal and hepatobiliary disease with malabsorption, systemic acidosis and phosphate depletion related to impaired renal tubular phosphate reabsorption or excess aluminum hydroxide ingestion. A 72-hour fecal fat analysis revealing intestinal malabsorption, urine pH, serum 25-OH vitamin D, phosphate, calcium and bicarbonate determinations often indicate the cause of the mineralization defect. In patients taking phenytoin or phenobarbital, hepatic conversion of vitamin D to the more active metabolite 25-OH vitamin D is impaired; resistance to the actions of vitamin D on bone and gut also occurs. These patients, as well as elderly people (in whom sun exposure is often minimal and consumption of dairy products is often inadequate), have low levels of 25-OH vitamin D and may have elevated parathyroid hormone levels, if vitamin D deficiency is severe.

In the absence of pseudofractures on x-ray, it is not possible to radiologically distinguish osteoporosis from osteomalacia. A bone biopsy that includes sectioning of an undecalcified specimen to allow a search for widened osteoid seams is necessary for definitive diagnosis of osteomalacia. Because it is not feasible to perform bone biopsies on all osteopenic patients, this procedure should be reserved for cases in which uncertainty exists as to whether a significant osteomalacic component is present. In patients who are undergoing surgery for a hip fracture, biopsy should be done at the time of operation, and the pathologist should be alerted that the specimen is not to be decalcified. If the 24-hour urinary calcium is greater than 100 mg., osteomalacia is unlikely.

THERAPEUTIC RECOMMENDATIONS

- Young people, especially pregnant women, should have at least 1 gm. of calcium and 400 U of vitamin D daily.
- Individuals receiving phenytoin or phenobarbital should receive 5000 U daily of vitamin D.
- Postmenopausal women may be treated with 400 U vitamin D daily and elemental calcium to supplement dietary sources to a total of 2 gm. of calcium per day.
- Women who have a family history of osteoporosis, are physically inactive, have had skeletal calcium depletion as a result of previous pregnancies, or have inadequate calcium intake should be considered for estrogen therapy beginning in the *perimenopausal period,* because bone loss is greatest soon after menopause. However, the possible adverse effects of long-term estrogen use must also be weighed (see Chapter 114).
- Asymptomatic *postmenopausal* patients who are found to have radiographic evidence of osteopenia

should receive estrogen therapy, calcium, and vitamin D after assessment of associated risks.
- Estrogen therapy can be employed using conjugated estrogens (Premarin), 0.625 mg. or 1.25 gm. per day, given cyclically for the first 25 days of each month. A National Institute of Aging panel (September 13, 1979) concluded that routine addition of progestins for several days per cycle should not be recommended at present.
- Patients who have sustained fractures as a consequence of osteoporosis can be treated with analgesics and bed rest. When pain subsides, ambulation can begin, followed by mild exercise such as walking or swimming. Avoidance of lifting and other weight-bearing stress is advisable.

ANNOTATED BIBLIOGRAPHY

Horsman, A., Gallagher, J.C., Simpson, M., and Nordin, B.E.C.: Prospective trial of estrogen and calcium in postmenopausal women. Br. Med. J., 2:789, 1977. *(Estrogen treatment prevents and calcium treatment retards postmenopausal bone loss when studied densitometrically and morphometrically, even when instituted an average of 6 years following menopause.)*

Jowsey, J., *et al.*: Effect of continued therapy with sodium fluoride, vitamin D and calcium in osteoporosis. Am. J. Med. *53*:43, 1972. *(Fluoride, in conjunction with vitamin D and calcium, resulted in an increase in new bone formation without microscopic evidence of fluorosis.)*

Lindsay, R., *et al.*: Long-term prevention of postmenopausal osteoporosis by estrogen. Lancet, *1*:1038, May 15, 1976. *(Evidence of increased bone mass even after delayed onset of estrogen therapy—3 to 6 years postmenopause—is presented. This increase in bone mineral content occurs during the first 3 years of estrogen therapy.)*

Quigley, M.M., and Hammond, L.B.: Estrogen-replacement therapy—Help or hazard. N. Engl. J. Med., *301*:646, 1979. *(A brief review of current indications for estrogen replacement therapy in the menopause.)*

Recker, R.R., Saville, R.D., and Heaney, R.P.: Effect of estrogens and calcium carbonate on bone loss in postmenopausal women. Ann. Intern. Med. 87:649, 1977. *(Estrogen and calcium treatment both led to a decrease in bone resorption.*

Estrogen was more effective than calcium by the technique of photon absorptiometry. Authors recommend calcium carbonate supplementation as a preventive measure.)

Thomsom, D.L., and Frame, B.: Involutional osteo- penia: Current concepts. Ann. Intern. Med., *85*:789, 1976. *(A comprehensive review of theo-ries of pathogenesis and a critical evaluation of the limited success of therapeutic regimens. There is an extensive bibliography.)*

11

Neurologic Problems

153
Evaluation of Headache

It has been estimated that headaches generate almost 16 million patient visits in the United States annually and that 6 or 7 per cent of the population suffer headaches that cause loss of time from work or school. Physicians and patients worry about headaches that are persistent, severe, or sudden in onset; tumor is a common concern when the headache persists. However, only the rare patient has a worrisome cause for headache; as a result, it is wasteful to subject all patients to extensive laboratory investigation. The primary physician's most immediate task is to identify on clinical grounds the occasional patient who requires aggressive workup.

PATHOPHYSIOLOGY AND
CLINICAL PRESENTATION

Brain parenchyma is not sensitive to pain, but many intracranial and extracranial structures are. Intracranial sources of pain referable to the head include fibers of the fifth, ninth and tenth cranial nerves, the dural arteries, the arteries of the circle of Willis, the major venous sinuses, and the dura at the base of the skull. Extracranial sites of headache include the skin, fascia, muscles and blood vessels of the scalp, the upper cervical nerve roots, and the muscles of the neck. In general, pain that arises from an intracranial process above the tentorium is perceived in the frontal, temporal or parietal region; pain originating from the posterior fossa and below the occiput is referred to the occiput. However, pain deriving from the posterior half of the sagittal sinus or upper aspect of the transverse sinus in the posterior fossa may be referred to the eye and forehead by way of the first division of the trigeminal nerve. In addition, the spinal tract and nucleus of the fifth cranial nerve plunge down into the area of the upper cervical roots; as a result, head pain may occur when upper cervical injury takes place.

The major mechanisms of headache are traction on pain-sensitive structures, inflammation of vessels and meninges, vascular dilatation, and excessive muscle contraction. A number of mechanisms may be operating simultaneously in a given case; patients frequently report being bothered by more than one type of headache.

Traction headaches. Mass lesions that displace a pain-sensitive structure can produce head pain that is initially intermittent, unilateral, dull, and aching. The discomfort is often relieved by lying down and worsened by straining at stool, cough or bending over. Characteristically the course is progressive, with increase in duration and severity of pain over several months, in conjunction with subtle changes in mental status or development of focal neurologic deficits. The headache may become more generalized if increased intracranial pressure ensues; projectile vomiting is a late complication. Nocturnal awakening is common but not diagnostic.

About one third of patients with *brain tumor* have headache as an early symptom. Initially, the headache may be the sole complaint unaccompanied by focal deficits. However, chronic headache due to a brain tumor usually associated with an abnormality on neurologic examination is uncommon. In a study of 165 patients with chronic headache followed for one year or more and subjected to computerized tomography (CT), there was no headache patient with a normal neurologic examination who had an abnormality on CT, angiography, radionuclide brain scan or skull roentgenogram indicative of tumor. *Brain abscess* may also cause a traction headache, especially in its later stages. Parenteral drug abuse, lung abscess or parameningeal infection can serve as the source of infection. Fever and focal neurologic deficits are often absent. *Chronic subdural hematoma* can also behave in a subtle manner. Head trauma is followed by a symptom-free interval. The injury may be forgotten, but the patient begins to show mental status change and, eventually, focal neurologic deficits.

Inflammatory headaches. Meninges, sinuses or cranial vessels may be involved. Tenderness of the involved structure is characteristic, but is not invariable. *Meningitis* results from hemorrhage or infection reaching the subarachnoid space. Pain is acute in onset, severe, generalized and constant. Symptoms may be particularly intense at the base of the skull, and typically aggravated by forward flexion of the neck. The headache of *giant cell arteritis* (temporal arteritis) is dull, aching or throbbing. Initially it is localized to an involved vessel but can become diffuse; moreover, the inflamed artery may not always be tender or palpable. Patients are elderly and often suffer from polymyalgia rheumatica as well. Sudden blindness is the most serious complication (see Chapter 150).

Vascular headaches. Abnormal vasodilatation produces headaches that are characteristically acute in onset and throbbing. *Migraine* is the most common form of vascular headache and is believed to involve vasoconstriction followed by vasodilatation of extracranial vessels. In addition, there are associated changes in circulating vasoactive agents such as serotonin, norepinephrine, prostaglandins, bradykinin and histamine. Whether these changes are causal or reactive remains to be fully elucidated. Migraine presents in two forms: common and classical; the former can be unilateral or bilateral and is unaccompanied by prodromal symptoms; the latter is unilateral and preceded by transient disturbances in neurologic function (see Chapter 160). Both types are accompanied by nausea and photophobia. The headache is usually throbbing, though it may take a while to reach maximum intensity and become clearly vascular in quality. Symptoms last from a few hours to one or two days. A family history of "sick headaches" is often elicited. Precipitants of migraine include emotional upset, menstruation, and even certain foods in some patients. Headache may occur shortly after or just prior to a period of psychological stress.

Cluster headaches occur mostly in middle-aged men and are characterized by nocturnal episodes of intense unilateral pain localized to the orbit and accompanied by lacrimation, nasal stuffiness, miosis, ptosis, and flushing on the same side as the headache. Headache usually begins a few hours after going to bed, lasts about 1 to 2 hours, and repeats nightly for weeks to months. The headaches usually disappear after a while only to return again several years later. Stress and alcohol are believed to be precipitants, although alcohol is well tolerated between attacks. The exact mechanism of cluster headaches is unknown, but vasoactive substances are believed to have an important role. Although the headache is classified as vascular, it is most often described as steady rather than throbbing.

Systemic infection and *fever* are common causes of cranial vasodilatation and diffuse, throbbing headaches. The headache that frequently accompanies a viral syndrome is typical of this type. Numerous *metabolic disturbances* and *drugs* may lead to vasodilatation and headache. A pounding headache is a prominent symptom of early carbon monoxide poisoning and a common complaint of patients who take nitrates for angina or vasodilators for other conditions.

The mechanism of the occipital headache associated with mild to moderate *hypertension* is unknown. The discomfort is worse in the morning and recedes as the day progresses. This headache resolves with correction of the hypertension and is not to be confused with the muscle contraction and psychogenic headaches which are responsible for most headaches that occur in hypertensive patients.

Muscle contraction headaches. Prolonged and excessive muscle contraction ranks among the leading causes of chronic and recurrent headache. Over 90 per cent of these headaches are bilateral and are often described as a pressure or bandlike sensation about the head. The pain is dull and steady in most instances, worsening as the day progresses and sometimes accompanied by occipital and nuchal soreness. The headache may last days, weeks or even months. Recording of myographic potentials from head and neck muscles reveals vigorous contractions; vasoconstriction can also be detected. The mechanism(s) responsible for excessive muscle contraction have not been fully delineated, but anxiety, depression, and emotional conflicts are common precipitants. These factors may produce migraine headaches in the same patient. Muscle contraction headaches may also occur secondary to muscle strain from cervical spondylosis or temperomandibular joint disease.

Psychogenic headaches. Many psychogenic headaches are of the muscle contraction variety. However, others are unaccompanied by detectable changes in muscle contraction or blood flow; these probably have important symbolic meaning. Depression, conversion reactions, and anxiety are among the causes. Some authorities postulate that such headaches represent somatic expressions of deep-seated conflict, and since the headache serves a psychological function, it may become a way of life for the patient.

Psychogenic headaches are often described in flamboyant terms, without any clear or consistent pattern of timing, location, quality or aggravating or precipitating factors. The pain may last for months or even years. Characteristically the patient uses vivid terms ("feels like an ax," or "lightning," or "something exploding") to depict the pain, yet does so without demonstrating any apparent discomfort. So psychologically engaging is the headache that many of these patients are unaware of their underlying emotional problems.

Postconcussion syndrome (post-traumatic nervous instability) is a complicated state characterized by headache, neck pain, nervousness, emotional lability, crying spells, and inability to concentrate. The symptoms are suggestive of an agitated depression following trauma; the syndrome probably represents a variant of psychogenic headache. The correlation between severity of symptoms and seriousness of the injury is minimal. Often legal proceedings and litigation are pending. Because the headache is sometimes throbbing and reproduced by histamine, some authorities believe it has a vascular component.

Focal pathology. Problems involving the eyes, sinuses, cervical spine, temporomandibular joints or cranial nerves can be important sources of headache. *Eyestrain* is often blamed for headaches, and indeed astigmatism can cause difficulty when the patient must make prolonged use of the eyes for close work. Ocular muscle imbalance is produced as well as sustained contraction of extraocular, frontal and temporal muscles; aching discomfort about the orbit and the frontotemporal regions results. Refraction corrects the problem. *Acute glaucoma* may produce an orbital headache accompanied by cloudy vision (see Chapters 193 and 198).

Sinusitis can lead to pain about the involved sinus and sensitivity of the overlying skin (see Chapter 209). The pain of sinusitis is sometimes described as throbbing in quality and may be worsened by bending over, thus superficially resembling a vascular or traction type of headache. Characteristic is the headache's tendency to begin on awakening, to subside on standing up, only to worsen as the day progresses.

Headache is the most common presenting symptom of *cervical spondylosis.* The pain is often localized to one side of the occiput; it usually starts in the neck and at times may even radiate to the forehead or eye. The discomfort is described as nagging or aching and can frequently be aggravated by neck movement. The mechanism of pain is believed to involve entrapment of upper cervical nerve roots among irritated nuchal ligaments and muscles, as the roots course through toward the occiput.

Disarticulation of the temperomandibular joint results in muscle imbalance that is aggravated by stress. The surrounding muscles of the head and neck go into spasm, causing pain. Discomfort may be described about the jaw, behind the eyes, in the ears, and even down the neck and into the shoulders. Jaw pain, clicking sounds, and difficulty opening the mouth in the morning are reported. On examination there may be jaw muscle tenderness, a palpable condylar head felt on inserting a small finger in the external auditory canal, and perhaps evidence of bruxism on inspection of the teeth.

Tic douloureux (trigeminal neuralgia) is one of the most severe pain syndromes known to man. Paroxysms of lancinating pain occur in middle-aged or elderly patients; these may last only a few seconds but can be excruciating and recurrent. The jaw, gums, lips, or maxillary region may be involved, and a trigger zone is characteristically located in the region (see Chapter 163).

DIFFERENTIAL DIAGNOSIS

The causes of headache can be considered in pathophysiological terms (Table 153–1). Most serious acute headaches are of the inflammatory type, due to meningeal irritation from infection or hemorrhage, giant cell arteritis, or acute purulent sinusitis. Hypertensive encephalopathy and acute glaucoma are important noninflammatory causes of acute headache; however, their associated symptoms usually overshadow the headache and dominate the clini-

Table 153–1. Important Causes of Headache

Traction on Pain-Sensitive Structures

1. Brain tumor
2. Brain abscess
3. Subdural hematoma
4. Cerebral edema (hypertensive encephalopathy)

Inflammation

1. Meningeal inflammation from infection or hemorrhage
2. Giant cell arteritis
3. Sinusitis

Vascular Dilatation

1. Migraine, common and classic varieties
2. Cluster headache
3. Drugs (e.g. vasodilators)
4. Metabolic disturbances (carbon monoxide poisoning, hypoglycemia)
5. Fever

Muscle Contraction—Psychogenic Mechanisms

1. Depression
2. Anxiety
3. Conversion reaction
4. Post-traumatic instability
5. Cervical spine disease
6. Temperomandibular joint disarticulation

Miscellaneous

1. Cranial nerve disease (Trigeminal neuralgia)
2. Eyestrain
3. Acute glaucoma
4. Hypertension (mild to moderate)

cal picture. Less worrisome acute headaches are of the nonmigrainous, vascular variety and include those due to high fever, nitrates, and other vasodilators, carbon monoxide poisoning, hypoglycemia, and drug withdrawal.

Most chronic or recurrent headaches result from vasodilatation, excess muscle contraction, or psychological conflict. The more worrisome chronic headaches are caused by displacement and traction on pain-sensitive intracranial structures; causes include brain tumor, abscess and chronic subdural hematoma. Diseases of the eye, sinus, cervical spine, temperomandibular joint, and cranial nerves must be considered when the etiology of a chronic or recurring headache remains elusive.

More than one type of headache may be present at a given time.

WORKUP

Acute Headache

History should include inquiry into onset, severity, location, and associated symptoms, especially neurologic deficits and fever. A previous history of headaches should also be noted. The patient unaccustomed to having headaches who presents with the sudden onset of the worst headache ever experienced deserves prompt attention, particularly if fever, neck stiffness, ataxia, alteration in mental status, focal neurologic deficit, or visual impairment is reported. Diffuse headache in conjunction with a stiff neck and fever suggest acute meningitis. When acute headache and stiff neck occur in conjunction with ataxia of gait and profuse nausea and vomiting, a midline cerebellar hemorrhage needs to be considered. Cerebellar hemorrhage is uncommon, but early recognition is important because prompt treatment can be lifesaving. Hypertensive encephalopathy may be heralded by diffuse headache, nausea, vomiting, and altered mental status. Acute fever with fronto-orbital headache are suggestive of acute sinusitis. Eye pain and blurred vision raise the possibility of acute glaucoma (see Chapter 193). New onset of headache in an elderly patient requires consideration of temporal arteritis (see Chapter 150).

Acute throbbing headaches are mostly vascular in etiology; the patient needs to be asked about fever, vasodilator use, carbon monoxide exposure, drug withdrawal, and symptoms of hypoglycemia (see Chapter 95).

Physical examination. The blood pressure and temperature should be checked for any elevations, the scalp for cranial artery tenderness; the sinuses for tenderness to percussion. Pupils are noted for loss of reactivity and the corneas for clouding (indicative of acute glaucoma); the disc margins for blunting, the neck for rigidity on anterior flexion, and the neurologic examination for ataxia, alteration of mental status, and focal deficits.

Laboratory studies. Patients with meningeal signs require prompt hospitalization, provided there is no evidence of increased intracranial pressure, a lumbar puncture and examination of the cerebrospinal fluid are indicated to rule out an infectious etiology. If there is concern about raised intracranial pressure, an emergency computerized tomography (CT) study is the test of choice, especially if a treatable lesion such as midline cerebellar hemorrhage is a consideration. Sinus films will identify an opacified area due to sinusitis, and an erythrocyte sedimentation rate should be markedly elevated if temporal arteritis is present. Few laboratory studies are necessary for assessment of a vascular headache, but a serum glucose is needed if hypoglycemia is a genuine concern, and a carboxyhemoglobin level is helpful if carbon monoxide poisoning is suspected.

Chronic and Recurrent Headaches

History. It is important to keep in mind that more than one kind of headache may be present; a full description of each type of head pain must be elicited. The quality of the headache, its location, and course over time are the historical features most helpful for identifying a headache of serious etiology. A dull, steady, recurrent, unilateral headache that occurs in the same area each time and progressively worsens in frequency and severity is suggestive of an intracranial mass lesion. In later stages, the headache may become bilateral and more generalized if intracranial pressure increases. Suspicion of a mass lesion necessitates inquiry into causes of brain abscess and subdural hematoma as well as concern about tumor. It is important to ask about chronic ear or sinus infection that has recently flared, parenteral drug use, and lung infection with abscess formation. Patients with brain abscess need not present with fever or focal neurologic deficits. Recent head trauma and a symptom-free interval between injury and onset of headache are characteristic of subdural hematoma; patients may show only subtle personality changes and be mistakenly thought to have a psychogenic problem.

Most throbbing, recurrent headaches are of vascular origin; migraine accounts for the vast majority. Transient neurologic symptoms preceding the headache, family history of "sick headaches," photophobia, nausea, vomiting, and hemicranial location are indicative of classic migraine. Sometimes the focal neurologic complaints that characterize certain auras may be confused with other causes of transient neurologic disturbances. Diagnosis and differentiation are aided by the subsequent occurrence of headache and complete resolution of symptoms within 24 to 48 hours. When headache is absent, diagnosis can be very difficult, but usually headache does occur and aural symptoms resolve with its onset.

The presentation of common migraine can sometimes cause confusion, because there is no aura, family history is often negative (over 35 per cent of patients report no family history of "sick headaches"), and the headache may be bilateral or shift sides. Nevertheless, the association of a recurrent throbbing headache with nausea and photophobia is quite suggestive; response to ergot further supports the diagnosis.

Headaches that are variable in quality and location, or constant over weeks to months but not relentlessly progressive in severity, are likely to have a muscle contraction or psychogenic etiology. Often there is an underlying depression or anxiety state. It is important to ask about early morning awakening, inability to concentrate, fatigue, low self-esteem, loss of libido, and other somatic symptoms of depression (see Chapter 215) as well as acute and chronic psychosocial problems (see Chapter 214). The patient with a muscle contraction headache may complain of neck soreness, occipital pain, or tightness about the head, typically worsening as the day progresses. When the description of the headache is dramatic, yet given without evidence of much physical distress, suspicion of a psychogenic etiology should be high. It is helpful to check into any recent minor trauma to the head or neck, which may precipitate a post-traumatic syndrome in the patient with an underlying depression. The diagnosis ought to be considered when an agitated patient reports varying types of discomfort that persist in the area of trauma long after evidence of injury. A nonvascular type of headache that lasts for years is also strongly suggestive of a psychogenic or muscle contraction mechanism.

Sometimes a story of headache awakening the patient from sleep is encountered. Although interruption of sleep by headache occurs in many patients with intracranial mass lesions, it is by no means pathognomonic of a traction headache; psychogenic, muscle contraction, and cluster headaches can do the same. If the interruption of sleep takes place on a daily basis at the same time each night for several weeks, the most likely diagnosis is a cluster headache. The presence of ipsilateral tearing and nasal congestion in conjunction with a boring periorbital headache that lasts 2 to 3 hours is further evidence for cluster headache.

A chronic or recurrent frontal or periorbital headache of unclear etiology requires inquiry into symptoms of sinusitis (see Chapter 209), cervical spine disease (see Chapter 141), jaw difficulties, and astigmatism. Patients who get headaches after sustained periods of close-up reading should have their eyes checked for refractive errors, but it is a mistake to blame recurring headaches on eyestrain if headache persists after correction of a refractive error.

An occipital headache that is maximal on awakening in the morning and improves as the day progresses may have a hypertensive etiology, especially if it is not worsening as time goes on. However, an occipital headache that does progress in frequency and severity may be a symptom of a posterior fossa mass; an occipital lobe tumor may be mistaken for migraine because scotomata are sometimes produced which may simulate a migrainous aura.

Physical examination. The temperature and blood pressure should be checked for elevation, the sinuses for focal tenderness, the discs for blurring of the margins, and the visual fields for defects which are suggestive of a mass lesion along the visual pathways. The nasal cavity is examined for a source of discharge and the ears for signs of chronic otitis media (see Chapter 208); both are potential foci for parameningeal infection that could lead to brain abscess. The mouth is tested for a trigger zone indicative of trigeminal neuralgia, the teeth for signs of bruxism, and the temperomandibular joint for limitation of motion and crepitus. With a small finger in each external auditory canal, the examiner can palpate the TM joints as the patient opens and closes the mouth. A prominent condylar head suggests TM joint disease. The neck should be put through a full range of motion, taking note of any limitation of motion and palpating for focal tenderness or zones that reproduce head pain. Patients with muscle contraction headaches often have excessively taut muscles about the shoulders, neck, and occiput. A careful and complete neurologic examination is essential, because the finding of a fixed focal deficit is important evidence of intracranial pathology, especially in a patient with a headache that is progressively worsening.

Laboratory studies. The patient who reports a chronic or recurrent headache that is getting worse with time deserves consideration for computerized tomography (CT), especially if the headache has qualities suggestive of a traction mechanism or if there is an abnormality on neurologic examination. CT is the most sensitive neuroradiologic test for detection of a mass lesion; the false-negative rate is less than 10 per cent and can be further reduced by prior injection of contrast. In a study of 168 ambulatory patients with chronic headache referred for CT, only those with an abnormality on neurologic examination proved to have a clinically important abnormality on CT. All patients with a normal neurologic assessment had normal CT as well as normal skull films,

angiogram or nuclide brain scan. In this study, neuroradiologic investigation was of very low yield in the upper middle-class population that composed the study group, and only served to increase the cost of care, unless one considers the value of a normal test result for the patient. However, an occasional headache patient with a intracranial mass lesion may have a normal neurologic examination; consequently, the patient with a story that is very suggestive of a mass lesion is a reasonable candidate for CT. This is particularly true for the patient with a subdural hematoma, who may not demonstrate a focal deficit until late in the clinical course. Nevertheless, it is essential that there be careful selection of patients for CT in order to avoid overutilization of this expensive resource and excess production of false-positive results (see Chapter 2).

In sum, the efforts taken to perform a careful history and physical examination are well worth the time, for these methods remain the best means available for the accurate diagnosis of headache.

INDICATIONS FOR ADMISSION AND REFERRAL

Any patient with evidence of meningeal irritation, increased intracranial pressure, or malignant hypertension obviously requires prompt hospital admission. Less urgent situations in which an office consultation with a neurologist may be beneficial include episodes of transient neurologic dysfunction suspected of being migrainous, presence of symptoms suggestive of an intracranial mass lesion, and need for further reassurance in a patient with a muscle contraction or psychogenic headache. Dental referral is indicated if temperomandibular joint problems appear responsible for the patient's complaints. Detection of a tender cranial artery in an elderly patient with a high sedimentation rate should be followed by surgical referral for biopsy to definitively diagnose temporal arteritis.

The ophthalmologist needs to be consulted at once if acute glaucoma is felt to be the cause of an acute orbital headache. If prolonged close-up work is resulting in headaches, a referral is in order for a vision check and assessment of the need for refraction.

Patients with psychogenic headache are sometimes reluctant to consider an emotional basis for their symptoms, but a psychiatric consultation for evaluation can often provide better definition of the conflicts that are troubling the patient than is possible in an office visit to a busy primary physician. The diagnostic consultation may also serve as an important learning experience for the patient vis à vis the importance of psychological issues and the role of the psychiatrist in the therapeutic effort. However, it is important that a full medical evaluation be conducted before referral is made; otherwise the patient who believes there is a medical basis for the problem may view the referral as an inappropriate dismissal of his symptoms.

SYMPTOMATIC MANAGEMENT AND PATIENT EDUCATION

Much of the anguish associated with chronic or recurrent headaches is due to concern about etiology. Tumor is a common fear. Although relief of symptoms may be a slow process, it should at least be possible to reduce unnecessary worry. A detailed history, that includes eliciting the patient's concerns, combined with a thorough and careful physical examination and discussion of findings, is essential to providing meaningful reassurance. Occasionally, a very anxious patient will insist on a neuroradiologic procedure (e.g., CT), but medically unnecessary testing can often be avoided if time is taken for careful assessment and explanation.

Muscle contraction headache. Heat and massage may help to ease muscle spasm due to prolonged, sustained muscle contraction. A mild analgesic such as aspirin or acetaminophen may contribute to relief of pain, but many patients who come to physicians with muscle contraction headaches complain that such agents are of little help, and request stronger analgesics. It is important to avoid narcotic use in these patients, because symptoms are likely to be chronic. Most muscle relaxants that are employed for muscle contraction headaches (e.g., chlordiazepoxide, methocarbamol [Robaxin]) have little or no direct action on skeletal muscle; they probably exert a beneficial effect by causing sedation and a lessening of anxiety. Since many of these headaches are a response to environmental or intrapsychic stress, attention should be directed to these important precipitants (see Chapter 214). Many patients find that they tolerate stress better if they carry out a program of regular physical exercise (see Chapter 10). When a cervical spine problem (see Chapter 141) or temperomandibular disease is the source of difficulty, correction of the physical condition causing the muscle imbalance is necessary.

Psychogenic headache. There is no simple treatment for relief of psychogenic headache. Tricyclic antidepressants may help if there is an underlying depression (see Chapter 215), and settlement of pending litigation sometimes leads to a lessening of post-traumatic headache. For the patient in whom headache is a manifestation of a deep-seated conflict, psychotherapy is often necessary. Because the headache may last for months or years, it is important that narcotics and related agents (e.g., propoxyphene), and agents that can be harmful if used in large cumulative doses (e.g., phenacetin) be avoided. A number of popular headache remedies are combination agents that contain phenacetin; cumulative doses of 2 kg. or more have been associated with renal papillary necrosis and interstitial nephritis.

Migraine. See Chapter 154.

ANNOTATED BIBLIOGRAPHY

Brenner, C., Friedman, A.P., Merritt, H.H., and Denny-Brown, D.E.: Post-traumatic headache. J. Neurosurg., *1*:379, 1944. *(A classic paper describing the syndrome.)*

Committee on Classification of Headache: Classification of headache. JAMA, *179*:717, 1962. *(A helpful scheme based on disease mechanisms.)*

Friedman, A.P.: Nature of headache. Headache, *19*:163, 1979. *(A useful summary of the important clinical features of common headaches.)*

Larson, E.B., Omenn, G.S., and Lewis, H.: Diagnostic evaluation of headache: Impact of computerized tomography. JAMA, *243*:359, 1980. *(Neuroradiologic evaluation of headache patients with normal neurologic examinations was expensive and clinically unrewarding.)*

Saper, J.R.: Migraine: I. Classification and pathogenesis. JAMA, *239*:2380, 1978. *(Good review of mechanisms and presentations.)*

White, K.L.: Testimony before the Senate Committee on Labor and Public Welfare, Subcommittee on Health. U.S. Senate, 94th Congress, second session, June 17, 1976. *(Provides statistics on epidemiology of headache and the disability it causes.)*

Wolff, H.G.: Headache and Other Head Pain. New York: Oxford University Press, 1963. *(The classic work on headache; still very useful.)*

154
Evaluation of Dizziness

Dizziness is a common complaint and a troublesome problem that is sometimes hard to evaluate. Patients may complain of a conflicting sense of position, a hallucination of movement, or simple light-headedness. Symptoms can be confusing to the patient and difficult to describe precisely. Dizziness is most often a head sensation, but at times patients use the term when they feel weakness or numbness in the legs or are bothered by gait ataxia. The etiology is rarely a life-threatening process, but symptoms can be very frightening. In a study of 104 consecutive cases, 38 per cent of patients had peripheral vestibular disease, 23 per cent hyperventilation, 13 per cent multiple sensory deficits, 9 per cent psychiatric problems, and 5 per cent cardiovascular or central neurologic illness.

Patients are disturbed by the very disabling nature of the symptom, and physicians worry about an underlying cardiovascular or central nervous system lesion. Most patients are eager for both symptomatic relief and reassurance. In the office evaluation, the objective is to distinguish on clinical grounds between benign and threatening causes, selecting patients with worrisome presentations for laboratory study and radiologic investigation.

PATHOPHYSIOLOGY AND CLINICAL PRESENTATION

Dizziness presents in characteristic ways determined by the underlying pathophysiological process. The major mechanisms are vestibular dysfunction, acutely diminished cerebral perfusion, multiple sensory deficits, metabolic disturbance of the central nervous system, and emotional upset.

Vestibular disease causes vertigo, which is defined as an abnormal sensation of movement. Descriptive terms include "spinning," "weaving," "ground rising and falling," "rocking," "seasickness," "merry-go-round sensation." Nausea, vomiting, and diaphoresis accompany many cases. Severe attacks can throw the patient to the ground. Nystagmus is frequently found on examination or can be induced.

Acutely diminished cerebral perfusion can result in faintness or even loss of consciousness. This form of dizziness is seen in patients with fixed and limited cardiac output, diminished vascular tone, or severe intravascular volume depletion. Symptoms often occur on standing up.

Psychiatric illness is frequently responsible for a light-headed or "foggy" feeling. Hyperventilation accompanying marked anxiety can cause a fall in pCO_2, sudden onset of light-headedness, circumoral paresthesias, and numbness and tingling in the extremities. In less severe instances, the syndrome is not so dramatic; light-headedness, apprehension, mild tremor and sweatiness occur. Depression and psychosis can produce a similar type of "dizziness," the mechanism is unknown but is thought to be related to a confusional state, perhaps complicated by drugs.

Metabolic disturbance of the CNS has a clinical picture similar to that of psychiatric illness. Patients describe their dizziness as a light-headedness. Marked hypoglycemia (see Chapter 95), hypoxia, hyper-and hypocarbia are important etiologies.

Multiple sensory deficits lead to inaccurate visual and positional information. Patients have symptoms when walking or turning and find relief by holding onto someone's hand or a railing. The feeling is sometimes a combination of light-headedness and a sense of abnormal motion. It is found most often in individuals with poor vision, peripheral neuropathy, and cervical spondylosis.

DIFFERENTIAL DIAGNOSIS

Conditions that cause dizziness can be grouped according to pathophysiological mechanism (Table 154–1). Vestibular disease is divided into central and peripheral types. Central lesions are mostly due to basilar artery disease and multiple sclerosis. Peripheral causes include acoustic neuroma, benign positional vertigo, vestibular neuronitis, Meniere's disease and ototoxic drugs.

Cardiac and vascular diseases are a second important group. Faintness on standing may be due to

Table 154–1.   Differential Diagnosis of Dizziness

Vestibular Disease

1. Benign positional vertigo
2. Vestibular neuronitis and ototoxic drugs
3. Meniere's disease
4. Acoustic neuroma and other tumors of the cerebellopontine angle
5. Basilar insufficiency
6. Multiple sclerosis

Cardiac and Vascular Disease

1. Critical aortic stenosis
2. Carotid sinus hypersensitivity
3. Volume depletion and severe anemia
4. Autonomic insufficiency (drugs, diabetes)
5. Diminished vascular reflexes of the elderly

Multiple Sensory Deficits

1. Diabetes mellitus
2. Cataract surgery
3. Some cases of multiple sclerosis
4. Cervical spoudylosis

Psychiatric illness

1. Anxiety
2. Depression
3. Psychosis

Metabolic Disturbances

1. Hypoxia
2. Severe hypoglycemia
3. Hypo- and hypercapnia

similar presentation. Hypoxia, hypoglycemia, hypocarbia and hypercarbia are among the most important.

WORKUP

History. The importance of obtaining the best possible description of what the patient means by "dizziness" cannot be overemphasized, because differential diagnosis depends on it. True vertigo suggests vestibular disease; faintness implies a cardiac, vascular or volume disorder; constant light-headedness may be due to psychogenic or metabolic causes and to multiple sensory deficits when precipitated by walking or turning.

If the patient complains of vertigo, the task is to determine whether the lesion is central or peripheral. Attention to associated clinical findings is essential. The presence of brain stem symptoms and signs (e.g., numbness, weakness, diplopia) rules out a peripheral lesion, but their absence does not rule out a CNS problem, though it does reduce its likelihood. In over three-fourths of cases of vertigo due to basilar artery insufficiency, the vertigo is transient and accompanied by other brain stem symptoms; in the remainder, it is the sole complaint, which makes diagnosis difficult. Episodes are initially in the form of transient ischemic attacks (see Chapter 159). Common associated brain stem findings are dysarthria, facial numbness, hemiparesis and diplopia. Headache may occur between spells. Episodic attacks of vertigo lasting beyond 6 weeks without brain stem signs are not likely to represent basilar disease. Moreover, if vertigo is strictly positional, the cause is not vascular.

There are no characteristic features of vertigo due to central nervous system involvement by multiple sclerosis. Attacks can be sudden, transient, recurrent or persistent. The diagnostic features are evidence of discrete CNS lesions and a course of recurrent dysfunction, with exacerbation after remission. Common sites of sclerotic plaques are the optic nerve, corticospinal tract, posterior columns, cerebellar white matter and medial longitudinal fasciculus, producing visual symptoms, weakness, numbness, ataxia, vertigo, nystagmus and diplopia, respectively.

With peripheral causes of vertigo, timing and precipitating factors help elucidate etiology. If symptoms occur only on change of position and last but a few moments, the diagnosis is benign positional vertigo, a condition mostly affecting people over 60. It may be a recurrent problem. A single bout of severe spontaneous vertigo, sudden in onset, sometimes

critical aortic stenosis, severe volume depletion, the use of antihypertensive drugs, autonomic insufficiency or prolonged confinement to bed. Carotid sinus hypersensitivity results in inappropriate reduction of vascular tone.

Multiple sensory deficits are most common in diabetics and others with poor vision and peripheral neuropathies. Cervical spondylosis disturbs cervical sensory input and contributes to dizziness. The thick lenses used by patients following cataract surgery distort peripheral vision and can confuse their sense of position.

Psychiatric problems are often associated with light-headedness. Patients with anxiety, depression and psychosis report feeling light-headed. At times, tranquilizers and antidepressants are responsible. Metabolic disturbances affecting the CNS have a after a viral illness, is usually vestibular neuronitis. When seen in the context of inner ear infection, it is properly called acute labyrinthitis. Some degree of positional vertigo may remain after the acute illness resolves. Meniere's disease is suggested by acute, recurrent paroxysms of vertigo that are accompanied by tinnitus and temporary hearing loss. Tinnitus, pressure in the ear, and hearing loss are episodic and may precede the other symptoms. Attacks can last for hours to days; residual positional vertigo occurs in 25 per cent of cases.

Acoustic neuromas have a variable presentation and can mimic other etiologies of vertigo. Episodes of vertigo, tinnitus, pressure sensation in the ear, and hearing loss may take place, simulating Meniere's disease. However, hearing loss is slowly progressive in nature rather than episodic or fluctuating. Fatigue and headache occur, possibly due to a vestibulospinal reflex increasing cervical muscle tension. Brain stem symptoms are late findings.

Obtaining a thorough drug history is important. The ototoxic effects of the aminoglycoside antibiotics have been well documented; the diuretic ethacrynic acid also can cause eighth nerve injury, especially in patients with compromised renal function. Potent diuretics may be responsible for severe volume depletion. Vasodilators, phenothiazines, and antihypertensive agents can produce postural light-headedness. Antidepressants and minor tranquilizers cause some patients to feel dizzy.

When the complaint is light-headedness, it is worth asking if standing or turning brings on symptoms. If standing does, antihypertensive, tranquilizer, or antidepressant use should be investigated. During the examination, postural signs, carotid upstroke and cardiac function should be evaluated, especially for signs of hemodynamically significant aortic stenosis. If turning worsens the situation, it is important to evaluate vision and search for other sensory deficits. If light-headedness is a constant sensation, an underlying psychiatric or metabolic disorder is likely. Anxiety and depression are frequent causes.

Physical examination. General appearance can be quite informative. The overly anxious person will appear nervous and may sigh frequently during the interview. Blood pressure and pulse should be taken and noted for changes between readings taken in the supine and standing positions. The skin is examined for pallor and the eyes for nystagmus. (It is important to remember that a few beats of nystagmus on extreme lateral gaze are normal.) The carotid arteries in the neck are checked for bruits (suggestive of cerebrovascular disease) and delay in upstroke (characteristic of severe aortic stenosis). A forceful, sustained left ventricular impulse, single second heart sound, and loud ejection quality murmur on cardiac examination also support a diagnosis of significant aortic stenosis (see Chapters 15 and 28).

A thorough and careful neurologic examination is essential, particularly when the possibility of central vestibular disease is being considered. Most important is examination for a brain stem lesion, which suggests central pathology or extrinsic compression by an acoustic neuroma. Cranial nerves V, VIII, and X can be affected by a large acoustic neuroma pressing at the cerebellopontine angle of the brain stem. Testing of sensory function, peripheral vision, and gait often reveals multiple defects in elderly patients troubled by dizziness.

Provocative maneuvers designed to trigger symptoms and reproduce the patient's complaint can be extremely useful. Hyperventilating for 2 minutes will reproduce the light-headedness that many call "dizziness." Standing quickly from a supine position will cause the susceptible patient to feel faint; turning quickly while walking can cause symptoms in the patient with multiple sensory deficits. Dizziness due to a vestibular disturbance may be tested for by laying the patient down with head extended 45° below the horizontal and turned 45° to one side, then waiting and watching for onset of nystagmus and vertigo. If this vestibular stimulus does not produce symptoms or nystagmus, *caloric testing* can be employed. Each auditory canal is irrigated by syringe for 40 seconds. First, cool water at 30° C. is used, then warm water at 44° C. This test can cause marked symptoms and is needed only if less potent means of vestibular stimulation fail.

Vestibular stimulation in the patient with peripheral dysfunction produces nystagmus after a latent period of 5 to 10 seconds; repeated stimulations produce less nystagmus each time. The nystagmus of peripheral disease does not change direction. In central lesions, there is no latent period and the nystagmus does not fatigue with repeated vestibular stimulation. The nystagmus may be very coarse, vertical, and asymmetric, at times occurring without vertigo; stimulation on one side may produce nystagmus that changes direction.

Maneuvers which alleviate symptoms are also of diagnostic use. Getting up slowly lessens the faint feeling associated with cardiovascular causes; paper bag rebreathing reduces the light, giddy feeling that follows hyperventilation; lying still in one position may halt positional vertigo; touching the examiner's hand helps the patient with sensory deficits. Withholding suspected drugs may be informative.

Laboratory studies. Electronystagmography and audiologic testing are indicated when clinical and provocative data are insufficient to differentiate between central and peripheral causes of vertigo. If acoustic neuroma is suspected, polytomes of the internal auditory canal and audiologic evaluation can be helpful. If basilar transient ischemic attacks are a concern because of transient, isolated vertiginous spells, it is felt by most authorities that it is safer to wait for the appearance of brain stem symptoms than to hastily order angiography or anticoagulation.

SYMPTOMATIC THERAPY AND PATIENT EDUCATION

Dizziness can be controlled in most instances. Therapy is aimed at the underlying pathophysiology. True vertigo responds to avoidance of precipitating positions and movements, use of meclizine 25 mg. t.i.d. and, if nausea and vomiting are not controlled by meclizine alone, prochlorperazine 10 mg. q6h p.r.n.

Cardiovascular faintness requires assuring adequate hydration, standing up slowly, and discontinuing or reducing offending drugs. The patient with critical aortic stenosis should undergo evaluation for surgery (see Chapter 28).

Psychogenic light-headedness may be refractory to symptomatic therapy. For acute hyperventilation, rebreathing into a paper bag is effective. Treatment with an antianxiety agent might help, but it can also cause symptoms. Patients with multiple sensory deficits are aided by use of a walker.

The vast majority of people with dizziness have benign disorders. Symptomatic therapy combined with explanation and reassurance is always comforting. In particular, patients tolerate their problems better when they know that in most instances the symptom can be controlled or will resolve on its own.

INDICATIONS FOR REFERRAL

Neurologic consultation is indicated when there is concern about central vestibular disease or acoustic neuroma.

ANNOTATED BIBLIOGRAPHY

Brachman, D.A., and Hart, C. An approach to the dizzy patient. Neurology, *22*:323, 1972. *(In a series of 104 patients seen in a dizziness clinic, secure diagnoses were reached in 91 per cent, with peripheral vestibular disease, hyperventilation, and multiple sensory deficits making up over two-thirds of cases. Article provides details of diagnostic measures.)*

Fisher, C.M.: Vertigo in cerebrovascular disease. Arch. Otolaryngol., *85*:85, 1967. *(Argues that unaccompanied dizziness is unlikely to be vascular in origin and that it is safe to wait and watch for developments rather than risk anticoagulation or arteriography.)*

Hitselberger, W.E.: Tumors of the cerebellopontine angle in relation to vertigo. Arch. Otolaryngol., *85*:95, 1967. *(In a series of 136 patients with surgically confirmed c-p angle tumors, only 25 per cent had vertigo, only 12 per cent had spontaneous nystagmus, but 92 per cent had decreased response to caloric stimulation. The hearing loss associated with vertigo was progressive, distinguishing this condition from Meniere's disease.)*

Schumacher, G.A.: Demyelinating disease as a cause for vertigo. Arch. Otolaryngol., *85*:93, 1967. *(Makes the important point that nothing in the character of vertigo due to multiple sclerosis is pathognomonic or even characteristic of central origin of vertigo.)*

155

Focal Neurologic Complaints: Evaluation of Nerve Root and Peripheral Nerve Syndromes

AMY A. PRUITT, M.D.

Primary physicians are frequently asked to evaluate complaints of focal numbness, tingling, weakness, pain, or some combination of these. In general, major acute neurologic disease is not at issue during an office visit. Nevertheless, the broad range of outpatient complaints encountered encompasses lesions throughout the nervous system. Disorders of nerve roots and peripheral nerves in the upper and lower extremities are especially common. Several syndromes should be analyzable by the primary physician. Identification and localization of these problems can facilitate thorough neurologic evaluation and accurately segregate those cases which must be referred to a neurologist.

PATHOPHYSIOLOGY AND CLINICAL PRESENTATION

Many peripheral nerves, because of their superficial location, are easily injured mechanically, and others are vulnerable because of specific anatomic variants or because of alterations in anatomy caused by degenerative disease.

Upper Extremity Syndromes

Cervical radiculopathy and myelopathy. Age-related loss of water and elasticity in cervical discs leads to increased stress on vertebral bodies. Osteophytic spurs develop and may encroach on nerve roots (see Chapter 141 and Fig. 155–1). More serious but less common is encroachment on the spinal cord itself by progressive cervical spondylotic changes. Usually a combination of radiculopathy involving the C5, C6, or C7 roots (see Fig. 155–2) and myelopathy is present. The presence of cord compression due to spondylosis is indicated by radicular pain, variable weakness, diminished reflexes and at-

rophy in the arms, with spastic weakness and hyperreflexia in the lower extremities.

It may be difficult to distinguish cervical spondylotic myelopathy from other progressive myelopathies, which include multiple sclerosis, subacute combined degeneration due to vitamin B_{12} deficiency, spinal tumor, syringomyelia, and amyotrophic lateral sclerosis. Suspicion of myelopathy should prompt referral to a neurologist.

Radiologic assessment usually includes cervical spine films. Unfortunately, nearly 50 per cent of patients over age 50 show degenerative cervical spine changes on x-ray, and these do not correlate well with the degree of abnormality found clinically in either radiculopathy or myelopathy. Nevertheless, plain cervical spine films with oblique views to visualize the neural foramina are often informative. If the patient has only radiculopathy, a conservative trial of cervical traction is sometimes helpful (see Chapter 141). If myelopathy is suspected, myelography may be necessary to define the extent of compression, to rule out neoplastic lesions, and to assist the surgeon in a decision about decompressive laminectomy.

Brachial plexus neuritis. A painfully disabling condition, this syndrome develops in many patients after an immunization and presents with severe shoulder and upper arm pain followed by weakness which usually involves the upper roots of the plexus more than the lower ones. Prognosis is ultimately good, but recovery may be prolonged. Clinical examination reveals variable weakness and sensory loss in C5-T1 root distributions (see Fig. 155–2) with diminished deep tendon reflexes. Because of the involvement of many nerve roots, confusion with a cervical disc does not usually arise. Electromyography and nerve conduction studies help to localize the abnormality. Apical lordotic views of the chest should

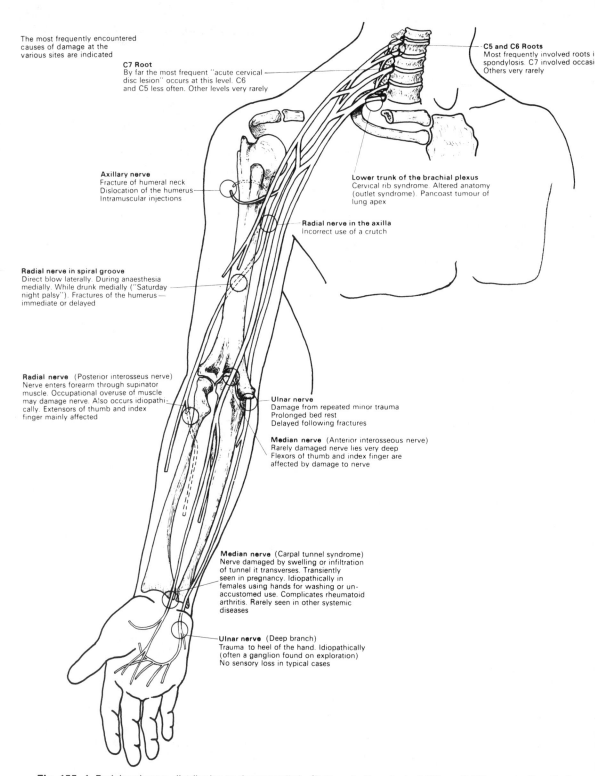

The most frequently encountered causes of damage at the various sites are indicated

C7 Root
By far the most frequent "acute cervical disc lesion" occurs at this level. C6 and C5 less often. Other levels very rarely

C5 and C6 Roots
Most frequently involved roots i spondylosis. C7 involved occasi Others very rarely

Axillary nerve
Fracture of humeral neck
Dislocation of the humerus
Intramuscular injections

Lower trunk of the brachial plexus
Cervical rib syndrome. Altered anatomy (outlet syndrome). Pancoast tumour of lung apex

Radial nerve in the axilla
Incorrect use of a crutch

Radial nerve in spiral groove
Direct blow laterally. During anaesthesia medially. While drunk medially ("Saturday night palsy"). Fractures of the humerus — immediate or delayed

Radial nerve (Posterior interosseus nerve)
Nerve enters forearm through supinator muscle. Occupational overuse of muscle may damage nerve. Also occurs idiopathically. Extensors of thumb and index finger mainly affected

Ulnar nerve
Damage from repeated minor trauma
Prolonged bed rest
Delayed following fractures

Median nerve (Anterior interosseous nerve)
Rarely damaged nerve lies very deep
Flexors of thumb and index finger are affected by damage to nerve

Median nerve (Carpal tunnel syndrome)
Nerve damaged by swelling or infiltration of tunnel it transverses. Transiently seen in pregnancy. Idiopathically in females using hands for washing or unaccustomed use. Complicates rheumatoid arthritis. Rarely seen in other systemic diseases

Ulnar nerve (Deep branch)
Trauma to heel of the hand. Idiopathically (often a ganglion found on exploration) No sensory loss in typical cases

Fig. 155–1. Peripheral nerve distribution to the upper limb. (Patten, J.: Neurological Differential Diagnosis. New York: Springer-Verlag, 1977)

624

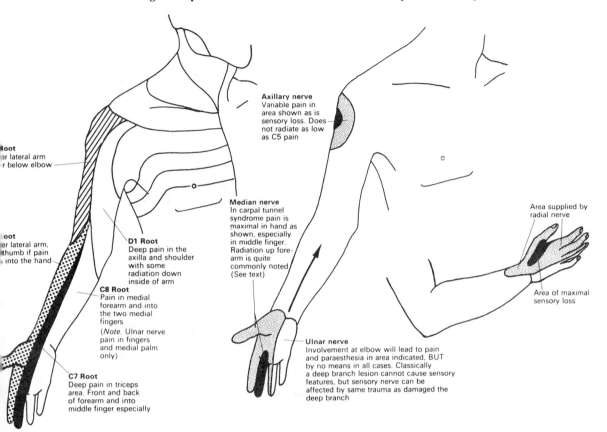

Axillary nerve
Variable pain in area shown as is sensory loss. Does not radiate as low as C5 pain

Median nerve
In carpal tunnel syndrome pain is maximal in hand as shown, especially in middle finger. Radiation up forearm is quite commonly noted (See text)

Area supplied by radial nerve

Area of maximal sensory loss

Root
er lateral arm
r below elbow

oot
er lateral arm,
thumb if pain
 into the hand

D1 Root
Deep pain in the axilla and shoulder with some radiation down inside of arm

C8 Root
Pain in medial forearm and into the two medial fingers
(*Note.* Ulnar nerve pain in fingers and medial palm only)

C7 Root
Deep pain in triceps area. Front and back of forearm and into middle finger especially

Ulnar nerve
Involvement at elbow will lead to pain and paraesthesia in area indicated, BUT by no means in all cases. Classically a deep branch lesion cannot cause sensory features, but sensory nerve can be affected by same trauma as damaged the deep branch

Fig. 155–2. (*Left*) Distribution of root pain and paresthesia. (*Right*) Distribution of peripheral nerve pain and paresthesia. (Patten, J.: Neurological Differential Diagnosis. New York: Springer-Verlag, 1977)

be obtained to rule out the possibility of neoplastic invasion of the plexus from an intrathoracic tumor.

Thoracic outlet syndrome. A cervical rib or bony abnormality of the first rib may lead to pressure on the subclavian artery or brachial plexus as it passes through the thoracic outlet (see Fig. 155–1). Diagnosis is primarily clinical and includes the presence of pain in the arm in certain positions, color changes in the hand, and a pattern of sensory loss and weakness most pronounced in the fourth and fifth fingers. Deep tendon reflexes are usually normal. The differential diagnosis includes Raynaud's phenomenon, ulnar nerve entrapment at the elbow, and compression of the brachial plexus from neoplasm or from fibrosis due to radiation.

Cervical spine films are extremely important to demonstrate cervical ribs or elongated transverse processes of C7. Electromyography may be entirely normal, but will help to exclude a defect at the elbow or a carpal tunnel syndrome. Ultrasonography of the

subclavian artery with the arm held in different positions may help define the extent of compression.

Most surgeons advocate removal of the potentially constricting structures (cervical rib, fascial band to first rib, or first rib). Shoulder exercises to improve posture are often advised first, and orthopedic advice should be sought in each case.

Long thoracic nerve entrapment. This nerve arises from the brachial plexus and innervates the serratus anterior. It is vulnerable to injury in workers who lift or push heavy loads, occurs after direct trauma from heavy backpacks, and may evolve over several months after the injury. The patient notes a change in the appearance of the shoulder, and examination reveals winging of the scapula. Most cases have a good prognosis.

Carpal tunnel syndrome. The median nerve is entrapped at the carpal tunnel (see Fig. 155–1), because of pressure from ligamentous thickening. Most cases are idiopathic, but the disorder may be seen

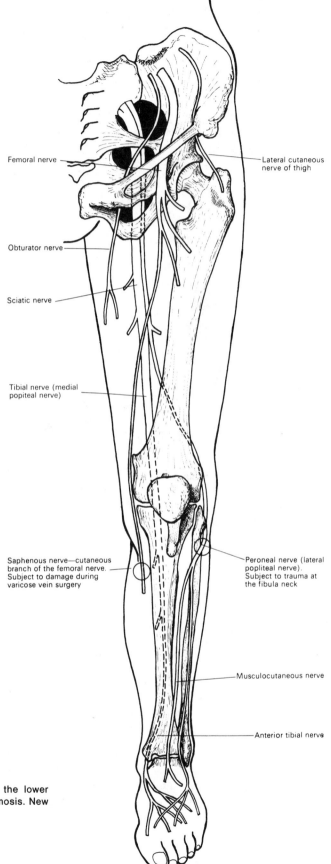

Femoral nerve

Lateral cutaneous nerve of thigh

Obturator nerve

Sciatic nerve

Tibial nerve (medial popiteal nerve)

Saphenous nerve—cutaneous branch of the femoral nerve. Subject to damage during varicose vein surgery

Peroneal nerve (lateral popliteal nerve). Subject to trauma at the fibula neck

Musculocutaneous nerve

Anterior tibial nerve

Fig. 155-3. Peripheral nerve distribution to the lower limb. (Patten, J.: Neurological Differential Diagnosis. New York: Springer-Verlag, 1977)

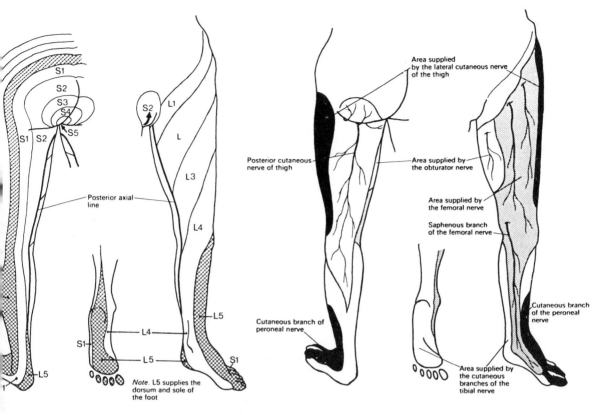

Fig. 155–4. (*Left*) Lumbosacral dermatomes. (*Right*) Lower limb peripheral nerve distribution. (Patten, J.: Neurological Differential Diagnosis. New York: Springer-Verlag, 1977)

with rheumatoid arthritis, pregnancy, acromegaly, hypothyroidism, fractures of the carpal bones, amyloidosis, and myeloma. A combination of pain, paresthesias, and numbness in the median nerve distribution is the earliest complaint, often worse at night (see Fig. 155–2). Later, muscle weakness (particularly of thumb abduction and opposition) occurs, and thenar atrophy may be seen. Importantly, aching pain can be felt as far up as the shoulder and should not distract the examiner's attention from the wrist. Tapping on the wrist may reproduce the pain (Tinel's sign).

Differential diagnosis includes radiculopathy from cervical spine disease, but the exact location of the pain should conform to the median nerve rather than to just one nerve root distribution. Electromyography and nerve conduction studies with motor and sensory conduction latencies of the median nerve provide the most useful data. While some cases respond to conservative therapy (wrist splints, anti-in-

flammatory medications) surgical relief is relatively easy and effective. Failure to respond to surgical therapy should prompt rechecking of the nerve conduction studies, careful re-examination, and consideration of the possibility of coexistant cervical spine disease or of median nerve compression higher in the forearm.

Ulnar nerve entrapment. The most common location of ulnar entrapment is at the elbow (see Fig. 155–1). Causes include fracture deformities, arthritis, faulty positioning of the arm during surgery, or repetitive occupational or recreational trauma (e.g., tennis). Sensation is usually spared in the forearm but there is sensory loss in the fifth finger and half of the fourth (see Fig. 155–2). Wasting of the intrinsic muscles of the hand with weakness of grip occurs later. Nerve conduction studies can accurately localize the site of compression. If there is focal entrapment, repositioning of the nerve or elbow synovectomy may be necessary, but patients with trauma, diabetes, or the so-called "tardy" ulnar palsies (dysfunction developing late after injury) may not improve.

Radial nerve injuries. Compression of the radial nerve most often occurs in the axilla or the upper arm. It may be seen with improperly used crutches, with prolonged pressure during sleep (the Saturday night palsy), or as a result of direct injury. Wrist drop is the prominent feature. Vasomotor or atrophic changes are rarely present, and prognosis is good (recovery within 6 to 8 weeks).

Lower Extremity Syndromes

Lateral femoral cutaneous nerve compression. Also known as meralgia paresthetica, this syndrome involves a nerve formed by branches arising from the second and third lumbar roots. The nerve enters the thigh in close relation to the inguinal ligament, the anterior superior iliac spine, and the sartorius muscle insertion (see Fig. 155–3). It is purely sensory and supplies the anterolateral and lateral aspects of the thigh almost as far as the knee (see Fig. 155–4). Compression causes an extremely unpleasant, characteristic burning pain with increased cutaneous sensitivity. Sitting or lying usually provides relief, but standing or walking exacerbates the pain. The syndrome often occurs in obesity, in pregnancy, or when tight corsets are worn. It is more common in diabetics. Differential diagnosis includes a lesion of the second or third lumbar roots, usually associated with low back pain radiating into the lower leg. Sensory changes in this case will extend further down the leg and more medially, and there is iliopsoas or quadriceps weakness. Weakness and reflex changes do not occur in meralgia paresthetica. The neuropathy tends to regress spontaneously, and weight loss should be encouraged.

Femoral neuropathy. The femoral nerve derives from the second, third, and fourth lumbar roots. Its posterior division is the major innervation to the quadriceps and terminates as the saphenous nerve, which supplies sensation to the medial aspect of the leg as far as the medial malleolus (see Fig. 155–3). Onset of femoral neuropathy is frequently sudden, painful, and followed quickly by wasting and weakness in the quadriceps, loss of knee jerk, and sensory impairment over the anteromedial thigh (see Fig. 155–4). If there is also marked hip flexion weakness, the site of the lesion is usually in the lumbar plexus. Sensory symptoms in the saphenous distribution are uncommon in lesions of the main trunk of the femoral nerve.

Entrapment may occur in the inguinal region and from direct retroperitoneal compression by tumor or hematoma. However, the most common cause is presumed to be nerve infarction, seen usually in diabetics. A combination of thigh pain, weakness, and sensory deficit can be a manifestation of an isolated diabetic femoral neuropathy, although electromyographically, the involvement in such cases is frequently more widespread. While some improvement may occur, the patient is often left quite weak.

Sciatic nerve syndromes. The sciatic nerve arises from the lumbosacral plexus (L4 to S3) and terminates in the common peroneal and tibial nerves (see Fig. 155–3). The tibial nerve supplies gastrocnemius, plantaris, soleus, and popliteus muscles, while its extension into the calf, the posterior tibial nerve, supplies muscles of the calf. All these muscles are involved in plantar flexion. The common peroneal nerve divides into the superficial and deep peroneal nerves. The latter supplies the muscles that dorsiflex the foot and toes. The superficial peroneal nerve innervates the muscles that evert the foot.

Sciatic nerve compression may result from tumors within the pelvis or from prolonged sitting or lying on the buttocks. Gluteal abscesses and misplaced buttock injections have caused sciatic injury. Weakness of the gluteal muscles and pain in the sciatic notch area imply compression within the pelvis. Lesions just beyond the sciatic notch cause weakness in the hamstrings and in all the muscles of the lower leg.

Common peroneal compression usually occurs at the level of the fibular head (see Fig. 155–3) and is seen in cachectic patients following prolonged bed rest, in alcoholics, in diabetics, and in patients placed in tight casts. Injury leads to faulty dorsiflexion and eversion of the foot, producing a characteristic footdrop with a slapping gait. Complete or partial recovery can be expected when paralysis results from transient pressure. Treatment consists of a foot brace and careful avoidance of compressive positions.

Lumbar disc syndromes. Compressive neuropathies of the lower limbs must be distinguished from the very common lumbar disc syndromes. In the lumbar region, the fourth and fifth discs are most frequently affected (i.e., the discs between L4 and L5 vertebral bodies and between L5 and S1 vertebrae). The most common complaint is sudden onset of severe low back pain (see Chapter 140). The inciting event is often trivial, though heavy lifting or an acute twisting motion is sometimes reported. The pain is worsened by bending forward, sneezing, or straining.

The herniated disc can compress one or more nerve roots, but a disc herniation at a particular level generally causes a distinctive picture (see Chapter 140). *L4–5 disc herniation* usually affects the L5 root with pain over sciatic notch, lateral thigh and leg, numbness of web of great toe and lateral leg, weakness of dorsiflexion of the great toe and foot, and no reflex changes (see Fig. 155–4). *L5–S1 disc herniation* catches the S1 root, producing pain down the back of the leg to the heel, numbness in the lateral heel, foot and toe, weakness of plantar flexion, and loss of ankle jerk (see Fig. 155–4). Once the root level is defined, the usual course is a trial of bed rest and analgesia (see Chapter 140) unless there is pronounced weakness, uncontrollable pain, or bladder and bowel dysfunction. In these cases, acute myelography may be necessary to define the extent of disc protrusion and to rule out more unusual causes of lumbar radiculopathy such as a neurofibroma.

WORKUP

Identification of the nerve root or peripheral nerve syndrome and precise localization of the neurologic lesion is possible in the office setting and, in most instances, does not require elaborate knowledge of neuroanatomy or extensive dependence on laboratory studies. Assessment is facilitated by determining (1) whether the problem is peripheral (in a nerve root or peripheral nerve) or central (in the cord or above); (2) whether the problem, if peripheral, is due to a lesion in the peripheral nerve or to nerve root injury; (3) whether there is evidence of cord compression (manifested by signs of myelopathy), particularly with upper extremity syndromes; (4) whether there is evidence (in other extremities) of more widespread peripheral neuropathy (e.g., the diabetic patient with a femoral neuropathy who also has a diffuse peripheral neuropathy); and (5) whether the presence of weakness is due to a muscle or nerve lesion.

The neurologic examination should be organized to address these issues and answer the following questions:

1. Is the lesion upper motor neuron (UMN) or lower motor neuron (LMN)? Fasciculations, flaccidity, and the lack of reflexes indicate a LMN lesion and suggest that the disorder originates at the anterior horn cell or peripheral nerve level. Spasticity and increased reflexes are evidence for a lesion above the

anterior horn cell that supplies the involved musculature. Thus, a cervical disc at the C6 level might decrease the biceps reflex and result in biceps weakness and atrophy, while causing increased reflexes and spasticity below that level.

2. Is the nerve dysfunction confined to one root or dermatome or to one peripheral nerve? A positive answer to this question suggests a compression neuropathy such as a radial, ulnar, or median nerve palsy. Findings of more generalized dysfunction such as diffusely decreased deep tendon reflexes, absent vibration sense at the ankles, and a stocking-glove pattern of sensory loss suggest a more diffuse peripheral neuropathy. Commonly seen forms of peripheral neuropathy include those associated with diabetes mellitus, excess alcohol consumption, toxin and drug exposure, and genetic diseases such as Charcot-Marie-Tooth atrophy. An electromyogram can localize the individual nerve abnormality and can confirm the presence of a generalized neuropathy.

3. Is the weakness due to nerve or to muscle disease? Weakness in conjunction with altered tendon reflexes and sensory loss suggests nerve disease. Primary muscle pathology results in preserved reflexes and normal sensation. Characteristic patterns of muscle weakness occur in the genetically determined muscular dystrophies. The toxic and metabolic myopathies produce largely proximal muscle weakness, in contrast to almost all primary nerve diseases, which affect distal musculature early and preferentially. Serum muscle enzyme elevations are seen in muscle disease, and some muscular disorders are associated with myotonia. The electromyogram coupled with nerve conduction studies can distinguish primary muscle disease from neuropathic processes.

Clinical identification of nerve root and peripheral nerve syndromes is often facilitated by selective use of radiologic, nerve conduction, electromyographic, and serologic studies (as detailed in discussions of each of the important syndromes). However, dependence on laboratory studies for initial assessment is usually not necessary.

INDICATIONS FOR REFERRAL AND ADMISSION

Evidence of acute spinal cord compression is an indication for immediate neurosurgical consultation and hospitalization. The patient with symptoms and signs of a slowly progressive myelopathy requires neurologic consultation, especially if myelography is being considered. A root or peripheral nerve compression syndrome usually needs surgical repair, and the patient with such a problem will need to see the neurosurgeon or orthopedist skilled in its treatment. Nevertheless, before referral, the primary physician should have localized the problem and instituted appropriate initial therapy.

ANNOTATED BIBLIOGRAPHY

Aguayo, A.J., Neuropathy due to compression and entrapment. In Dyck, P.J., *et al. (eds.)*: Peripheral Neuropathy. Philadelphia: W.B. Saunders, 1975, p. 688. *(Detailed discussion of the compression neuropathies.)*

Aids to the Diagnosis of Peripheral Nerve Injuries. ed. 3. London: Her Majesty's Stationery Office, 1976. *(A classic; each muscle test is carefully illustrated and nerve innervation is beautifully diagrammed.)*

Chusid, J.: Correlative Neuroanatomy and Functional Neurology, ed. 18. Los Altos: Lange Medical Publications, 1977. *(Complete with numerous charts and diagrams, this is a succinct discussion of physiologic principles for the purpose of clinical diagnosis.)*

Keim, H.A.: Low back pain. CIBA Clinical Symposia, *25 (3)*: 1973. *(Well-diagrammed discussion of degenerative disc disease with excellent illustration of lumbar disc syndromes.)*

156
Evaluation of Tremor
AMY A. PRUITT, M.D.

Tremor is best defined as a regular oscillation of a body part and must be distinguished from other rapid, involuntary movements. Many patients assume that the development of "shakiness" is a natural concomitant of aging. The physician must determine the significance of a variety of clinically similar tremors that may have widely dissimilar diagnostic, therapeutic, and prognostic implications. Workup involves differentiating the resting tremor of early parkinsonism from essential tremor and differentiating essential tremor from an exaggerated physiologic tremor. As new specific treatments are developed, accurate clinical distinction becomes increasingly valuable. Unfortunately, it may be difficult to differentiate tremors by clinical observation alone, and evaluation requires a working knowledge of simple electrophysiologic and pharmacologic characteristics.

PATHOPHYSIOLOGY AND CLINICAL PRESENTATION

The precise neural mechanisms of tremor remain unknown despite some clinicopathological correlations, such as abolition of the parkinsonian and essential tremors by lesions in the ventrolateral nucleus of the thalamus. Drugs such as L-dopa, which are known to act centrally to increase catecholamines, may worsen essential tremor; this observation has led to the suggestion that beta-adrenergic blockers such as propranolol might exert their therapeutic action by central antagonism of beta-adrenergic receptors.

The patient most frequently reports the insidious onset of "shaking" of a limb. Very likely, he will have ignored the symptom's presence initially, assuming it was due to nervousness or fatigue. However, its steady progression brings him to see the physician. Tremors can be present during maintenance of a posture, at rest, or during an action (intention tremor).

Postural tremors are fine tremors with a frequency of 8 to 12 Hz; they occur normally in everyone during movement and while holding a fixed position. A true "physiologic" tremor is defined as one that does not produce symptoms and is within the above frequency range. It is unaffected by administration of propranolol or alcohol. The movement is usually invisible to the naked eye, but may become exaggerated by anxiety, coffee ingestion, or hyperthyroidism. Drugs, notably lithium and tricyclic antidepressants, may also accentuate this tremor. Amplitude and frequency vary among different people and in the same person at different times.

Intention tremors include those labeled essential (familial) and senile. *Essential tremor* may appear to be a variant or more extreme form of physiologic tremor. However, symptomatic essential tremors are of larger amplitude (hence, visible to the naked eye) and relatively slower frequency than genuine physiologic tremors. Their electromyogram (EMG) characteristically shows synchronous bursts of activity in antagonistic muscle groups. There often is a positive family history and the report of gradual progression; tremor is absent at rest and clearly present in the outstretched arms. It is accentuated by tasks that require precision (e.g., writing, carrying full cups of liquid) and by phenothiazines and haloperidol. It is suppressed by alcohol and propranolol. *Senile tremor* has the same physiological and pharmacological qualities as essential tremor. It is usually first seen in the hands, often remaining there, but sometimes involving the head and legs as well. Essential tremor may begin at any time; senile tremor usually becomes apparent by the sixth or seventh decade.

A more dramatic action tremor is displayed by patients with *cerebellar diseases* and is characterized by progressively increasing amplitude of the tremor as the patient brings the limb toward a target. In younger patients, this is most frequently caused by multiple sclerosis, but similar clinical states may be produced by cerebellar infarction, by degenerative disorders of the spinocerebellar pathways, and by chronic relapsing steroid-sensitive polyneuropathy. This tremor is multiplanar with large, irregular, and relatively slow (2–4 Hz) oscillations. The tremor often is worsened by alcohol. Propranolol has no effect, and no satisfactory therapy is available.

Rest tremors. The most common rest tremor in a relaxed, supported limb is that due to *Parkinson's disease.* It characteristically begins in the fingers and may later involve the arm and the leg. Flexion and extension of the fingers, abduction and adduction of the thumbs, and pronation and supination of the wrist produce the well-known "pill-rolling" movement. Frequently, this is the symptom that brings parkinsonian patients to the physician and may occur well in advance of bradykinesia or postural difficulties characteristic of the full-blown syndrome. It is important, of course, to distinguish this tremor from essential tremor, which demands a different treatment and portends a different prognosis. The parkinsonian tremor is slow (3–8 Hz), and its EMG, quite unlike that of essential tremor, shows alternating discharge in antagonistic muscle groups. This EMG activity is suppressed with voluntary movement.

A few parkinsonian patients may also have a typical action (essential) tremor, and L-dopa therapy may worsen it. Phenothiazines and haloperidol worsen the tremor-at-rest (see Chapter 161).

The definition of tremor as a regular oscillation of a body part serves to distinguish it from other rapid, intermittent movements that bespeak a different neurologic state. For diagnostic, therapeutic, and prognostic purposes, several categories of abnormal involuntary movements should be distinguished from tremor. All of the following involuntary movements (and most true tremors) are greatly reduced or disappear altogether with sleep.

Tics are repetitive, coordinated, usually stereotyped movements that are seen widely in the population and increase in frequency in a given patient in response to stress. They usually involve face or hand muscles, may initially be a conscious mannerism, and usually can be suppressed by voluntary effort. *Hemifacial spasm* is a kind of oscillating movement usually beginning in a middle-aged or elderly person, localized to the facial muscles. It is thought to be due to degenerative lesions of the facial nucleus or peripheral nerve, but the exact mechanism is unknown, and treatment is unsatisfactory.

Asterixis is an irregular, skeletal muscle contraction that results in flapping of the hands, electromyographically coincident with brief pauses at irregular intervals. *Chorea* is an irregular, jerking movement usually involving the fingers and often accompanied by *athetosis,* in which writhing movements of limbs or trunk may be added. *Epilepsy partialis continuens* refers to a focal seizure in which continuous seizure activity may result in a somewhat rhythmic jerking of one body part. Sudden onset of the illness is the most useful distinguishing feature here.

Dyskinesias are rhythmic involuntary movements of the orofacial musculature resulting in tongue protrusion and chewing movements. These are important to recognize because of the frequency with which they occur as early manifestations of the tardive dyskinesia syndrome due to use of phenothiazines and other major tranquilizers.

DIFFERENTIAL DIAGNOSIS

Tremors can be divided clinically into postural, intention and resting types. Most postural tremors are physiologic. Among the intention tremors are the essential, senile and cerebellar varieties. Most resting tremors are due to Parkinson's disease. Tremors must be distinguished from other voluntary movements such as dyskinesias, tics, myoclonus and athetosis.

WORKUP

History. Clinical assessment of tremor is greatly aided by first ascertaining the circumstances under which the tremor occurs. Some tremors are present during maintenance of a posture, some during rest, and others only during an action (the intention tremors). Careful questioning will often identify the type of tremor. Common diagnostic problems include distinguishing the resting tremor of early Parkinson's disease from an essential tremor and an essential tremor from an exaggerated physiologic one. All of these are common and some may, in fact, be present simultaneously in a given patient.

Physical examination is directed primarily at determining whether the tremor is better or worse with activity. The patient should be asked to hold out his hands, to write, to perform rapid alternating movements, and to touch finger to nose repeatedly; the objective is to detect evidence of cerebellar or extrapyramidal disease. The patient should be observed discretely during the history and during other parts of the physical examination, because calling attention to the tremor may worsen it.

Laboratory studies. If there is some question at the end of the examination as to whether the tremor is primarily resting or primarily action, a tremor recording (EMG) may be requested. Many parkinsonian patients will have no other extrapyramidal signs at the time they present with tremor. The EMG can separate the two types, sometimes confirming that both tremors are present simultaneously.

Diagnostic trials. If the diagnosis of essential tremor is entertained, a family history should be sought. This tremor responds to small doses (80 to 120 mg. per day) of propranolol, and the drug may be used in a diagnostic and therapeutic trial, provided there are no medical contraindications. Exaggerated physiologic tremor due to anxiety does not respond substantially to propranolol, although it has been observed that adding diazepam may further reduce essential tremor and, by its antianxiety effect, eliminate exaggerated physiologic tremor as well.

PATIENT EDUCATION AND INDICATIONS FOR REFERRAL

The etiology of the tremor and the fact that it can be controlled should be discussed with the patient. Avoidance of agents that worsen symptoms must be stressed. Patients with intention tremors and cerebellar signs must be referred to a neurologist since demyelinating or hereditary degenerative diseases may be responsible. Disabling tremors refractory to simple therapy may benefit from neurologic consultation.

SYMPTOMATIC MANAGEMENT

1. Essential or familial tremors respond to low, nonbeta-blocking doses of propranolol (80 to 120 mg. per day).
2. Parkinson's tremor should be treated with anticholinergics or L-dopa-containing agents (see Chapter 161).
3. Physiologic tremors are unaffected by propranolol or alcohol but worsened by anxiety, coffee, hyperthyroidism, tricyclics, and lithium. A combination of diazepam and propranolol may lessen severe tremor due to anxiety.

ANNOTATED BIBLIOGRAPHY

Mawdsley, C.: Diseases of the central nervous system: Involuntary movements. Br. Med. J., *4*:572, 1975. *(Overview of abnormal movements with a brief differential.)*

Shahani, B.T., and Young, R.R.: Physiological and pharmacological aids in the differential diagnosis of tremor. J. Neurol. Neurosurg. Psychiatry, *39*:772, 1976. *(Excellent detailed discussion of the EMG in diagnosis of tremor; very readable even without EMG training.)*

Winkler, G.F., and Young, R.R.: Efficacy of chronic propranolol therapy in action tremors of the familiar, senile, or essential varieties. N. Engl. J. Med., *290*:984, 1974. *(The initial clinical trial.)*

157
Evaluation of Dementia
AMY A. PRUITT, M.D.

Dementia is a progressive loss of intellectual ability in which speech, memory, praxis, judgment, and mood may all be altered in varying proportions. There are an estimated 600,000 cases of advanced dementia in the United States, and milder degrees of altered mental status are very common in the elderly (15 per cent of persons over 65 exhibit a degree of intellectual deterioration, according to some estimates). Each patient with dementia deserves careful workup, since as many as 15 per cent may have a condition amenable to therapy. The primary physician should know how to distinguish dementia from other, more specific cortical deficits (aphasia, agnosia, etc.) and should be able to perform an adequate screening examination for potentially reversible disease.

PATHOPHYSIOLOGY AND CLINICAL PRESENTATION

Normal intellectual functioning requires appropriate reception of sensory perceptions, adequate association-making ability, and effective efferent mechanisms to express decisions and responses. Dementia is marked by progressive degrees of inability to adapt to the environment. The patient initially may be noted to have slight impairments in memory, attention, and concentration (often excused or ignored by the family and, at least early in the course, concealed by the patient). Later, he may display impaired judgment on increasingly simple matters, inability to abstract or generalize, and personality change. This last symptom sometimes takes the form of a certain rigidity with perseveration, irritability, or confusion as a result of minor changes in environment. Still later, perception becomes distorted, and the patient is no longer aware of his deficits. Affective disturbances become more prominent, and depression frequently prevails over euphoria or agitation. Finally, the patient may lose interest in personal hygiene and nutrition, and is left helpless and disoriented.

The clinical presentation may be marked by specific signs of neurologic or medical disease (Table 157-1). However, all dementing processes can be distinguished by certain hallmarks. The *pace* of the illness is slowly progressive over a period of months to years; in rare instances the process is more rapid. The *pattern* of the disease is relentless, without stepwise decline or remission. Static, nonprogressive impairment of intellect is more accurately described as "mental retardation."

Table 157-1. Neurologic Diseases Associated with Intellectual Dysfunction

Disease	Physical Signs	Clinical Features
Alzheimer's disease (senile dementia)	Frontal lobe signs	Enlarged ventricles, cortical atrophy by CT scan
Normal pressure hydrocephalus	Gait disorder,* incontinence	Little cortical atrophy by CT scan
Atherosclerotic cerebrovascular disease	Focal deficits*	Episodic dysfunction consistent with strokes
Parkinson's disease	Extrapyramidal signs*	Long-standing disease, extended duration of L-dopa therapy
*Intracranial tumor	Focal signs, papilledema	Subacute evolution, seizures possible
Neurosyphilis	Frontal lobe signs, optic atrophy, Argyll Robertson pupils	Positive VDRL serum/CSF
Huntington's disease	Choreiform movements*	Family history
Creutzfeldt-Jakob disease	Myoclonus,* cerebellar signs, eye movement abnormalities	Subacute course; EEG specific, brain biopsy diagnostic
Multiple sclerosis	Brain stem signs, optic atrophy, spinal cord signs	Usually long-standing disease, episodic illness with remissions
Wilson's disease	Extrapyramidal signs,* hepatic dysfunction, Kayser-Fleischer rings*	Onset in adolescence or young adulthood, psychiatric disorders
Progressive supranuclear palsy	Failure of vertical gaze,* extrapyramidal signs*	Eye movement abnormalities; differentiate from other extrapyramidal disorders

* Invariable; all other physical signs are neither invariably present nor pathognomonic.

DIFFERENTIAL DIAGNOSIS

A useful way of organizing the differential diagnosis of dementia is to divide etiologies into those accompanied by signs and symptoms of medical or neurologic disease. The former includes hypothyroidism, vitamin B_{12} deficiency, thiamine deficiency, progressive multifocal leukoencephalopathy, the dementias associated with neoplastic disease, demen-

tias associated with hemodialysis, and, perhaps inaccurately, "atherosclerotic dementia." This last entity is not a genuine dementia in the sense of progressive loss of all types of intellectual abilities. Instead, it is the end result of recurrent episodic and focal neurologic deficits which should be evident from the history and physical examination. In hypertensive patients, dementia may present in the form of pseudobulbar palsy following repeated lacunar strokes. Hallmarks of this disease are poor emotional control (inappropriate, excessive outbursts of laughing or crying), difficulty with gait, dysarthria, and bilateral signs of corticospinal tract (upper motor neuron) disease.

Neurologic diseases associated with dementia are listed in Table 157–1 and include Alzheimer's disease, normal pressure hydrocephalus, neurosyphilis, Creutzfeldt-Jakob disease (spongiform encephalopathy), Huntington's disease, intracranial tumor, late Parkinson's disease, Wilson's disease, progressive supranuclear palsy, and severe multiple sclerosis. Most of these disorders present with specific, associated neurologic findings. However, Alzheimer's disease and senile dementia, the most common degenerative disorders, do not. They are pathologically and clinically identical except for age of onset (Alzheimer's disease being somewhat arbitrarily reserved for patients with onset at age less than 65.) It has been reported that 4.4 per cent of people over 65 exhibit moderate to severe senile dementia and that about 66 per cent of these fall into the category of idiopathic senile dementia. An additional 10 per cent have a milder form of the disease. The brain is atrophied, the ventricles are enlarged, and evidence of severe vascular disease or infarction is minimal or absent. Neuropathological study reveals neuronal loss, neurofibrillary tangles and senile plaques whose extent does not correlate quantitatively with the degree of dementia. Similar changes are found in the brains of elderly people who are not demented.

Normal pressure hydrocephalus deserves special mention both because of its reversibility and because of a tendency to overdiagnose the entity. The term refers to slow ventricular enlargement without cortical atrophy due to poor cerebrospinal fluid resorption. The brain literally becomes plastered against the skull. Most often, there is no known precipitant, but the condition can occur when there is blockage of CSF resorption due to meningitis or subarachnoid hemorrhage. Dementia, gait disturbance, and incontinence are the classic triad, presumably reflecting disease in areas most affected by ventricular enlargement, namely the frontal lobes and fibers that mediate sphincter and lower extemity function.

Conditions that resemble dementia and are often mistaken for it are schizophrenia, depression, and hysteria. The term delirium should be used to describe an acutely altered mental status often resulting from drug ingestion or withdrawal, fever, hy-

poxia, hypercapnia, encephalitis, hyperthyroidism, or metabolic abnormality.

WORKUP

The goal of the workup is to distinguish dementia from other causes of intellectual impairment, such as metabolic disorders and psychiatric illness, and to identify the etiology of the dementia.

History. Detailed questioning should define the temporal course of the illness, ascertaining whether the process is, indeed, chronic and progressive and determining occurrence of past, focal neurologic insults. Specific inquiry is needed into previous gastric surgery (B_{12} deficiency), neck surgery (thyroid disease), meningitis and subarachnoid hemorrhage (normal pressure hydrocephalus). A history of trauma, seizure disorder, and use of medications (particularly hypnotics, diuretics, anticonvulsants, or psychotropic medications) should be elicited. It is very important to probe the use of alcohol (see Chapter 216). A family history is crucial in identifying those patients with Huntington's disease. Additionally, the physician can form a general impression of the patient's psychologic state from the initial interview.

Physical examination. Assessment begins with a mental status examination to confirm the presence of dementia. The complex faculties that constitute intellect are usually divided into testable, although not necessarily anatomically or pathologically exclusive, functions. Specific states which are not dementias (such as amnesias, aphasias, and agnosias) should be identified as well with these tests.

Immediate and remote memory are tested, as are reading, writing, calculating ability, and constructional capacity. Patients should be asked to recall a short story, to remember three items, to reproduce simple drawings, and to recite a list of digits. Ability to interpret proverbs or to discern similarities among objects offers insight into higher cortical functions. Judgment can be ascertained by presenting the patient with decision-requiring situations ("finding a stamped letter" or "seeing a fire in a theater").

Next, the physician should undertake specific neurologic and medical evaluation. Stigmata of alcoholism (see Chapter 216), renal disease (see Chapter 135), or other systemic processes should be sought. Frontal lobe signs such as grasp and suck should be elicited. Cranial nerve examination should be directed toward discovery of papilledema, visual field cut, optic atrophy, or abnormal pupillary reaction. Extraocular movements can be limited in supranuclear palsy. Nystagmus may indicate recent drug ingestion or the presence of brain stem disease (see Table 157–1). The motor examination should record the presence of abnormal movements and focal deficits. Parkinsonian facies, gait, and tremor, (see Chapter 161) may be encountered. Involuntary movements should be noted, such as tardive dyskinesias, tremors, asterixis, chorea, and myoclonus (see Chapter 156). Sensory examination may reveal parietal lobe disease with inattention to stimuli presented bilaterally, or evidence of peripheral neuropathy or combined system disease (B_{12} deficiency). Gait should be observed carefully; the small, rigid steps of frontal lobe gait apraxia can be distinguished from a wide-based cerebellar gait (alcohol being a major offender) or the "marche à petits pas" of Parkinson's disease.

Laboratory studies. In most cases, the need for further studies is reasonably limited and involves few invasive procedures. The history and physical examination should limit the differential possibilities. The following guidelines outline evaluation, starting with the least invasive, least specific tests and progressing to the most invasive and specific ones. Baseline evaluation should include blood tests for electrolytes, urea nitrogen, thyroid function, syphilis, and complete blood count. The need for additional blood tests is dictated by history and physical examination findings and may include B_{12}, calcium, liver function studies, and toxic screen. A routine chest radiograph should be obtained if none has been performed recently.

At this point, the physician should select specific tests based on a knowledge of their yield in different situations. *Skull radiographs* may demonstrate an old (or new) skull fracture, which may be responsible for a seizure disorder or strengthen suspicion of alcohol ingestion. Calcium present in a subdural hematoma or tumor may be demonstrated (though these lesions are better seen with computerized tomography). *Electroencephalogram* (EEG) may be normal, even in advanced cases of dementia; nonspecific slowing of the baseline rhythm is common. Occasionally, the EEG may raise suspicions of a particular etiology: focal, delta slowing is seen with tumor; unilateral attenuation of voltage suggests subdural hematoma; excessive beta activity is consistent with drug ingestion; a seizure disorder may be demonstrated. Finally, Creutzfeldt-Jakob disease has a highly specific EEG pattern.

Lumbar puncture is frequently inconclusive, but is indicated to confirm normal pressure, to diagnose tertiary syphilis, or to reveal neoplastic invasion of the leptomeninges. Sugar, protein, cell count, gamma globulin, and serology for syphilis should be obtained.

Computerized axial tomography (CT scan) can answer many questions posed by the presence of dementia. Subdural hematomas and intracranial tumors can be readily identified. Huntington's disease is suggested by caudate nucleus atrophy. The CT scan can also distinguish between normal pressure hydrocephalus (NPH) and Alzheimer's disease or senile dementia. In the former, enlarged ventricles and little or no cortical atrophy are seen, while in the latter pronounced cortical atrophy is present as well as ventricular enlargement. The degree of cortical atrophy in NPH is not clearly correlated with response to shunting, and a neurologic opinion should be sought. Prospective studies of clinical course, CT scan, and response to shunt procedures are in progress.

Arteriography is not indicated in the primary evaluation of a dementia; it is best reserved for confirming intracranial tumor or a vascular lesion. Similarly, *brain biopsy* is a method of last resort indicated to confirm the diagnosis of herpes simplex encephalitis and occasionally to explain a subacute dementing process in a patient with atypical features of Alzheimer's or Creutzfeldt-Jakob disease.

For most patients, the workup can be accomplished by the internist. It consists of some screening blood work, a chest film, and, depending on precise circumstances, an EEG, an LP, and a CT scan. This requires about 3 days in the hospital, although the entire evaluation can be accomplished on an outpatient basis. Consultation with a neurologist should be sought for advice on interpretation of CT scans for normal pressure hydrocephalus or if focal neurologic signs are present.

No patient with progressive decline in mental faculties, particularly if he is under age 65, should be presumed to be the victim of an incurable process without evaluation. Careful history, physical examination, and a simple laboratory workup disclose the not infrequent patient whose course can be altered significantly.

SYMPTOMATIC MANAGEMENT AND COUNSELING

The successful management of the patient with deteriorating intellectual function depends on identification of a metabolic or surgically correctable abnormality. Most dementias, including Alzheimer's disease, are not amenable to existing pharmacologic therapy. There is no evidence to support the use of the widely promoted vasodilators to increase cerebral perfusion. The use of sedative and psychotropic agents in the confused patient should be avoided unless extreme agitation hampers care. Haloperidol may be a useful first choice for sedation. Recent studies suggest that acetylcholine may be diminished in the brains of demented patients and dietary repletion with choline (usually in the form of lecithin) is being studied, but results are not yet clear; use of lecithin should be considered experimental.

The physician's primary contribution is adequate instruction of the patient and his family. The goal should be to maintain the highest level of function possible, and this can often be achieved by promotion of an orderly home life. The physician can help the family obtain nursing or homemaker support or arrange admission to a day-care facility. Maintenance at home requires that the patient not have access to potentially dangerous household appliances. Establishment of a familiar routine through the use of calendars, television, newspapers, and frequent attempts at orientation may also help.

ANNOTATED BIBLIOGRAPHY

Freemon, F.R.: Evaluation of patients with progressive intellectual deterioration. Arch. Neurol., *33*:658, 1976. *(A more general hospital series but comparable to that in Marsden, Harrison reference.)*

Hachinski, V.C., Lassen, N.A., and Marshall, J.: Multi-infarct dementia. A cause of mental deterioration in the elderly. Lancet, *2*:207, 1974. *(Describes this syndrome, clearly differentiating it from Alzheimer's disease.)*

Katazman, R., and Karasu, T.B.: Differential diagnosis of dementia. In Fields, W. (ed.): Neurological and Sensory Disorders in the Elderly. New York: Stratton Intercontinental Medical Book Corporation, 1975, p. 1030. *(Clinically oriented discussion.)*

Marsden, C.D., and Harrison, M.J.G.: Outcome of investigation of patients with presenile dementia. Br. Med. J., 2:249, 1972. *(Specialized hospital with referral population; demonstrates relatively high incidence treatable causes of dementia. However, fails to define "cerebrovascular dementia.")*

Ojemann, R.G., et al.: Further experience with the syndrome of 'normal' pressure hydrocephalus. J. Neurosurg, *31*:270, 1969.

Stein, S.C., et al.: Normal pressure hydrocephalus: Predicting the results of cerebrospinal fluid shunting. J. Neurosurg., *41*:463, 1974. *(Although the CT scan is being used more frequently for this purpose, the RISA scan is still essential, and norms for "allowable" cortical atrophy are not yet firm.)*

Strub, R.L., and Black, F.W., The Mental Status Examination in Neurology, Philadelphia: F.A. Davis, 1977. *(Detailed description of the components of the examination.)*

Traub, R.D., Gajdusek, D.C., and Gibbs, C.J., Transmissible virus dementias. The relation of transmissible spongiform encephalopathy to C-J disease, aging, dementia, and cerebral function. *In* Smith, L.W., and Kinsbourne, M. (eds.): Aging and Dementia. New York: Spectrum, 1977, p. 91. *(Specialized but fascinating new discovery.)*

Weiss, J.: The clinical use of psychological tests. *In* Nicoli, A.N., (ed.): Harvard Guide to Modern Psychiatry, Cambridge: Harvard University Press, 1978, p. 41. *(Concise discussion of the use of these tests in distinguishing depression from dementia.)*

Wells, C.E., (ed.): Dementia. Contemporary Neurology Series, ed. 2. Philadelphia: F.A. Davis, 1977. *(Best, thorough, overall reference.)*

158

Approach to the Patient with Seizures

AMY A. PRUITT, M.D.

Evaluation

The occurence of a convulsion is a dramatic and frightening event; the experience is likely to trigger an immediate visit to the physician by an anxious family and a bewildered patient. The physician will need to plan for prevention of future episodes while orchestrating the diagnostic evaluation. Allaying fears and correcting misconceptions are also important tasks. Although an etiology for the majority of seizures is never found, a convulsion may represent a symptom of treatable underlying disease and deserves full evaluation. In addition, the event needs to be distinguished from other causes of loss of consciousness (see Chapter 18).

PATHOPHYSIOLOGY AND CLINICAL PRESENTATION

A seizure is the result of a sudden abnormal discharge from an area of the brain that, for reasons not entirely understood at present, appears to elude the control of normal inhibitory mechanisms that synchronize cerebral electrical activity. The activity of the initial focus may spread to other parts of the brain. Grand mal seizures and petit mal seizures presumably originate in subcortical structures. Any cerebral irritative lesion, whether vascular (such as previous stroke, arteriovenous malformation, or cortical vein thrombosis), neoplastic, or congenital (cyst or hamartoma) may produce clinical convulsive activity. In the majority of patients with epilepsy, no specific cause is ever determined, and pathologic examination after death reveals no diagnostic changes.

Generalized seizures are designated "major motor" or "absence" (petit mal). The term "major motor" includes both the true grand mal seizure, a convulsion without focal onset, and the other kinds of bilateral tonic-clonic convulsions that begin either as focal sensorimotor symptoms or as temporal lobe convulsions. When the onset is focal, the spread of symptoms may follow the cortical representation of body parts, with symptoms beginning, for example, in toes or fingers and spreading either up the leg or down the arm. Symptoms of temporal lobe epilepsy are legion and include motor automatisms, such as lipsmacking or chewing, olfactory or gustatory hallucinations, and behavioral automatisms. Two-thirds of these patients experience generalized major motor convulsions at some time, and many have a distinctive personality, sometimes with psychotic manifestations. (See Table 158–1 for phenotypic classification of seizures.)

A number of misconceptions about clinical presentation require clarification. First, adults rarely seize with high fever; the presence of a temperature greater than 102°F does not suffice to explain the occurrence of a seizure. Second, seizures are rare during the initial presentation of an embolic stroke. However, 20 to 25 per cent of patients who have had an embolic stroke may have seizures at some time after the event. Vascular lesions that are likely to have epilepsy as a sequela are emobli and cortical vein thrombosis, whereas subarachnoid hemorrhages and lacunar and thrombotic strokes rarely are succeeded by seizure activity. Third, alcohol withdrawal seizures occur between 7 and 48 hours after cessation of drinking, with a peak at 13 to 24 hours. They are preceded by a tremulous state in all patients and followed by delirium tremens in about 30 per cent. Usually, only one or two convulsions occur, and status epilepticus is very rare. Alcohol exacerbates pre-existing epileptic foci. Alcohol withdrawal is more likely to produce seizures in an epileptic patient than in a normal person, and less drinking is needed to precipitate a seizure—an evening or weekend of binge drinking may suffice. Other drugs are associated with seizures, either when they are taken in overdose or when withdrawal occurs. These are summarized in Table 158–2.

Finally, trauma is a common antecedent to seizures. When there is a history of closed head trauma, epilepsy usually develops within 2 years if at all, whereas with open head trauma (penetration of dura) seizures may develop at any time after the original injury.

Table 158-1.   Classification of Seizures

Phenotype	EEG	Etiology*	Prognosis	Drug of Choice in order of preference
Generalized				
Major Motor				
Grand mal	Normal, initially, in 20%; nonspecifically abnormal in 40%	Unknown in 85%	Age-related; overall, 25% seizure-free and off medications at 5 years	Phenytoin or carbamazepine, phenobarbital, sodium valproate
Focal onset (sensory or motor)	Focally abnormal in about 65%	Cause found in 33%	Related to etiology	Phenytoin or carbamazepine, phenobarbital
Temporal lobe onset	See below under partial seizures	Cause found in 50%	May be late result of multiple grand mal seizures; difficult to control	Phenytoin or carbamazepine *and* phenobarbital
Absence				
(petit mal)	80% have pathognomic 3/second spike and wave pattern	Unknown autosomal dominant; normal EEGs in both parents in only 50%	Excellent; absences cease by age 20 in 50% but many continue to have grand mal seizures	Ethosuximide, sodium valproate, phenobarbital, trimethadione
Partial				
Simple (no loss of consciousness) motor or sensory	Focally abnormal in about 66%	Cause found in 33%	Related to etiology	Phenytoin or carbamazepine, phenobarbital,
Complex (TLE with or without loss of consciousness)	Awake; 50% abnormal; asleep; 85% abnormal	Cause found in 50%; trauma, neoplasm	15% seizure-free on medication; psychoses develop in 33% of idiopathic temporal lobe seizures	Phenytoin or carbamazepine *and* phenobarbital,

* These figures antedate widespread use of CT scanning in evaluation.

DIFFERENTIAL DIAGNOSIS

Several conditions may mimic seizures, by either causing acute focal motor deficits or by producing episodic loss of consciousness. Under the former should be considered transient ischemic attacks (either in the carotid or in the vertebrobasilar territory), migraine, and local pathology such as nerve compression. Under the latter are syncopal attacks of any etiology, including transient diminished cerebral perfusion from cardiac arrhythmias, transient ischemic attacks, and severe hypoglycemia, as with an insulin reaction.

The differential diagnosis of conditions responsible for a seizure is based largely on the age of the patient at the time of the first seizure. Idiopathic epilepsy is the most common etiology in children, but becomes increasingly rare in the late teenage and young adult population. Thereafter, an underlying lesion becomes increasingly likely; nevertheless, the infrequency of discovering a definite etiology may sur-prise some physicians. In a large retrospective study of patients with more than one documented seizure of any type, only 23 per cent had a cause that became obvious after thorough investigation and a 10-year follow-up. Only 15 per cent of seizures generalized from the outset had a demonstrable etiology, whereas underlying disorders could be found in almost 30 per cent of seizures with a focal component. In the young adult population (18 to 45), the demonstrated causes were drugs (largely alcohol withdrawal), neoplasm, and trauma. In the older adult population, underlying pathology was divided roughly equally among neoplasm, trauma, and cerebrovascular accident.

WORKUP

The first objective in the workup is to distinguish seizure from other types of acute, transient, or focal neurologic deficits and loss of consciousness (see

Table 158-2. Drugs Commonly Associated with Seizures

DRUGS	OVERDOSE SEIZURES	WITHDRAWAL SEIZURES	DOSE REQUIRED TO INDUCE SEIZURE
Alcohol	−	+	Depends on previous drinking or underlying epilepsy
Meperidine (Demerol)	+	+	2-3 g./day*,†
Propoxyphene (Darvon)	+	+	Variable
Pentazocine (Talwin)	−	−	May precipitate withdrawal from other opiates with as little as 100 mg.
Barbiturates	−	+	>600 mg./day (short-acting),†
Meprobamate (Miltown)	−	+	>1.2 g./day,†
Chlordiazepoxide, diazepam	−	+	Unknown—may have 7-8 day latency period
Phenothiazines, haloperidol	− But myoclonus may occur; may cause seizures in patients with old cortical focus	−	Variable

* Overdose seizure
† Withdrawal seizure
+ = occurs
− = does not occur

Chapters 18, 155, 159). In practice, distinguishing syncope from seizure may be difficult, and there are no definitive criteria. However, presence of aura, anatomic spread of symptoms, incontinence, overt tonic-clonic activity, postictal confusion, and report of a sudden loss of consciousness suggest seizure.

History requires an exact description of events from witnesses as well as from the patient. Questioning should include inquiry into presence of an aura, focal onset, loss of consciousness, and observed injury incurred during the convulsion. The physician should also ask about ingestion of drugs, alcohol consumption, cardiac arrhythmias, mitral or aortic valve disease, and previous malignancy, stroke, or trauma. A family history of convulsions is important to elicit, although idiopathic epilepsy becomes less common with increasing age.

Physical examination. The physician may have the opportunity to perform the neurologic examination shortly after the seizure. A focal residual abnormality, such as paralysis of one arm (Todd's postictal paralysis), may suggest the initial focus even when the witnessed event was generalized. The examination should also include checking for head trauma, papilledema, cartoid disease, cardiac dysrhythmias or valvular problems, and manifestations of alcohol abuse (see Chapter 216).

Laboratory studies. Before embarking on a complex and expensive laboratory workup, one should be aware of the likely diagnostic yield of various procedures. The *skull series* rarely shows anything diagnostic, but films can be inspected for calcification (which sometimes occurs in several intracranial neoplasms, vessels, or congenital anomalies) and for evidence of skull fracture.

Familiarity with the *electroencephalogram* (EEG) is essential for proper evaluation of seizures; the major findings are summarized in Table 158-1. The EEG is always unequivocally normal in fully 20 per cent of patients with purely grand mal seizures. It is nonspecifically abnormal (without localizing value) in another 40 per cent. Either slow waves (described as "theta" or "delta" in EEG terminology) or spikes may be seen between seizures. Slow waves are somewhat more common with tumor, but the exact appearance of the EEG abnormalities provides no definitive clues. The EEG is somewhat more useful when there is a focal component to the convulsion;

appropriate localization of spike activity occurs in about two thirds of cases. The EEG may be of considerable use in detection of temporal lobe epilepsy. The likelihood of detecting the condition is increased by obtaining a *sleep study;* 85 to 90 per cent of patients with temporal lobe epilepsy demonstrate appropriately localized abnormalities on the sleep EEG. The EEG picks up cortical disturbances; abnormalities of deep temporal lobe or diencephalic structures may not be evident on the usual EEG study.

After obtaining the EEG, the physician must decide whether to perform a *lumbar puncture.* Obvious contraindications include evidence of raised intracranial pressure, known tumor with high suspicion of CNS metastases, history compatible with intracranial neoplasm, and bleeding diathesis. If there are no major contraindications, most neurologists recommend performing a lumbar puncture. However, the diagnostic yield is quite low. The cell count is normal in 95 per cent of patients with a first seizure, and sugar and protein concentrations are normal in 90 per cent of CSF fluid samples obtained in these circumstances.

Until recently, a *technetium brain scan* was included in every workup. It is a noninvasive procedure that is easily performed and may reveal serious intracranial pathology, particularly subdural hematomas. However, the availability of *computerized axial tomography* (CT) is likely to represent an improvement in noninvasive procedure. At present, the advantage of CT over previous scanners in determining etiology of seizures is not well documented. One large center reports definite diagnoses in 50 per cent of cases, with 20 per cent of lesions discovered by CT being previously missed by conventional scanning.

Most adults with a first seizure and no history of drug or alcohol abuse should receive CT to detect a resectable tumor or an arteriovenous malformation.

INDICATIONS FOR ADMISSION AND REFERRAL

It may be comforting for the physician confronted with the new onset of seizures to realize that patients with brain tumors usually have some evidence of tumor by history, physical examination, or EEG. In a prospective study of epilepsy in patients older than 50, 100 per cent of patients who were subsequently shown to have a brain tumor had one or more of the following on initial evaluation: history of focal onset, abnormalities on neurologic examination, or abnormal EEG. Not every seizure patient must be referred to a neurologic specialist, but an abnormality in any of the above initial studies should prompt consultation. Further diagnostic or therapeutic studies are indicated for these patients because they are at increased risk for serious underlying pathology.

The patient seen in the office with a first seizure can be sent home if there is a clear history of the use of alcohol or other drugs or withdrawal, provided the patient is medically stable. In these instances, further seizures are unlikely and hospitalization unnecessary. Otherwise, the evaluation of a first seizure is best performed in the hospital where the patient can be stabilized and observed; the frequency and severity of seizures, as well as the severity of the underlying cause, can never be known at first glance.

Longterm Outpatient Management

Long-term management of seizures is directed at the underlying disease, the resulting epilepsy, the side effects of the medications, and the psychiatric and social effects of this chronic illness. In practice, the compromise between freedom from seizures and side effects from medication is not always satisfactory. Although statistics vary according to age at onset and type of seizure, on the average, 25 per cent of patients are seizure-free and no longer taking anticonvulsants at 5 years. Because a correctable underlying etiology is not frequently found in epilepsy, most management involves symptomatic intervention by the physician.

NATURAL HISTORY

The prognosis of idiopathic epilepsy is dependent on both age at onset and type of convulsion (see Table 158–1). In general, patients with petit mal seizures have the best prognosis. These childhood-onset seizures cease by age 20 in over 50 per cent of cases, but many patients then suffer from grand mal convulsions.

Grand mal seizures have a less favorable prognosis. Overall, in addition to the 25 per cent of patients who are seizure-free and off medication after 5 years, about 50 per cent of patients have no further convulsions with anticonvulsants. About the same degree of control of the motor manifestations of temporal lobe epilepsy is achieved, but psychosis develops in up to one-third of these patients. Contrary to some older teachings, control of seizure activity does not lead to worsening of psychiatric disturbances.

PRINCIPLES OF MANAGEMENT

The simplest management strategy is to become familiar with the use of one anticonvulsant as a first-line drug and to administer that drug by whichever route the patient can tolerate best. Although *diazepam* is often used for emergency management, it should never be the first drug for long-term seizure control. For most adults, the drug of choice is *phenytoin* (Dilantin). Intravenous or oral administration of this drug is acceptable, but intramuscular delivery results in unpredictable serum levels. Phenytoin is well-absorbed orally and has a serum half-life of 22 to 30 hours. An initial loading dose must be administered. Table 158–3 gives several loading schedules which result in therapeutic phenytoin levels, and demonstrates that failure to "load" the patient with medication results in a delay of as long as 2 weeks before therapeutic levels are reached.

The usual maintenance dose of phenytoin is 300 mg. per day; blood level determinations are readily available in most laboratories. Therapeutic levels usually range from 8 to 20 mg. per 100 ml. In most patients with epilepsy, phenytoin remains the drug of choice for long-term control. However, the medication has numerous side effects and interactions with other common medications (Table 158–4).

If phenytoin fails to control the seizures, a second drug must be employed. Phenobarbital is the usual choice, and its adminstration should begin with 60 mg. at bedtime or 30 mg. 2 or 3 times a day. Patients may report increased sleepiness with larger doses, but with time they will be able to tolerate necessary dosage increases with acceptable side effects.

The patient who has *recurrent seizures* but says that he is taking his medication poses an important problem. Initial evaluation should include obtaining serum for anticonvulsant levels and persistent questioning to determine patient compliance with the regimen. Recent alcohol ingestion or addition of new medication may affect phenytoin levels (see Table 158–4). It is reasonable to administer 200 to 300 mg. of phenytoin orally or intravenously if the history of compliance is unreliable and there is no nystagmus. Alternatively, the physician may elect to administer a second (or third) drug until laboratory results are known. Consultation with a neurologist is indicated in this situation.

Perhaps the most difficult aspect of epilepsy management is the long-term follow-up of a chronic seizure patient. The first obligation is the insurance of adequate anticonvulsant protection. Often this amounts only to yearly monitoring of anticonvulsant

Table 158–3. Methods of Phenytoin Administration

TIME THERAPEUTIC RANGE REACHED *(after initial dose)*	ROUTE AND RATE OF ADMINISTRATION
20 minutes	1000 mg. IV at 50 mg./min.
4–6 hours	1000 mg. p.o., then 300 mg./day
23–30 hours	300 mg. p.o. q8h × 3 doses; then 300 mg./day
5–15 days (no loading dose)	300 mg./day p.o.

Table 158–4. Phenytoin: Side Effects and Drug Interactions

MAJOR SIDE EFFECTS

Dose-related: nystagmus, ataxia, dysarthria, blurred vision, decrease in measured total T_4

Duration-related: osteomalacia, peripheral neuropathy, anemia, cerebellar degeneration

Idiosyncratic: gingival hypertrophy, acne, hypertrichosis, encepealopathy

Rare, toxic: high, spiking fevers, exfoliative dermatitis, bone marrow depression, pseudo- and actual lymphoma lupus-like syndrome, teratogenesis during first trimester, neonatal coagulation defects

INTERACTIONS WITH COMMONLY PRESCRIBED DRUGS

Increased phenytoin levels with:
  Antimicrobials: chloramphenicol, INH
  Anticoagulants: coumadin
  Amphetamines (but seizure threshold decreased)
  Disulfiram (Antabuse)
  Alcohol: acute ingestion raises phenytoin levels, but see below
  Anti-inflammatory agent: phenylbutazone
  Anticonvulsants: ethosuximide; no consistent effect with simultaneous barbiturate administration
  Sedatives: chlordiazepoxide (librium), diazepam (valium), oxazepam (serax), clorazepam (clonopin)

Decreased phenytoin levels with:
  Alcohol: chronic ingestion

Phenytoin effects on levels of other drugs
  Insulin: may interfere with endogenous insulin release
  Quinidine: decreases quinidine effect at given dose
  Falsely low total T_4

levels. Phenytoin has effects on the hematopoietic system related to duration of its use (Table 158–4), so that another useful yearly screen is a complete blood count to detect the development of megaloblastic anemia. No other routine tests are practical.

The physician will surely be asked when the medication can be stopped. As noted, the majority of patients with epilepsy, either idiopathic or with known etiology, do not achieve complete freedom from seizures when anticonvulsant medication is discontinued. Indeed, only about one-half are totally seizure-free with continuing therapy. This knowledge should temper the physician's willingness to attempt *discontinuation of medication.* Obvious contraindications to attempted withdrawal of medicine are recurrent seizures. Most neurologists would require a seizure-free interval of at least 1 year or, more likely, 2 years. The electroencephalogram is of little help in predicting which patients may successfully be weaned from their medicines. Clearly, a persistently abnormal electroencephalogram would make discontinuation of medication inadvisable.

PATIENT EDUCATION

Perhaps the most important obligation of the physician is his role as counselor, educator, and, sometimes, legal advocate. His is a long-standing relationship with a patient whose chronic disease is surrounded by an enormous amount of superstition, prejudice, and misunderstanding.

In addition to reviewing prognosis with the patient, it is important to emphasize that even if seizures are not entirely controlled, most epileptics are able to lead productive lives. Fifteen to 25 per cent of the nation's 4 million epileptics are unemployed, a figure three to four times higher than the national average. However, the few professions from which people known to suffer seizures are barred are those that require a chauffeur's or pilot's license.

The diagnosis of epilepsy imposes definite restrictions on the patient's life, which makes the certainty of diagnosis in a young, healthy person all the more imperative. *Driving laws* vary from state to state, but, in general, states require a seizure-free interval of at least 1 year before re-application for a driver's license may be made. Continued supervision by a physician is mandatory.

Apart from the impersonal considerations of driving permits and employment, the patient may feel that the diagnosis of epilepsy also bestows a social stigma. He may develop unnecessary fears and needlessly limit his life, because he does not understand his disease. The physician can help by recognizing and responding to his apprehensions and by educating him.

A patient may learn that he can tell when a seizure is about to occur; a headache, feeling of malaise, or another vague symptom may be present. Although such symptoms need not necessitate admission to a hospital, the patient can learn to avoid driving or other potentially dangerous activities at such times. Certain stimulants such as alcohol, coffee, and tobacco precipitate seizures, and the physi-

cian can legitimately recommend abstinence, at least from alcohol. Surgical procedures pose no special threat to the epileptic patient as long as his medications are not discontinued at any time.

There is considerable worry about *inheritance* of seizures. Epilepsy is hereditary, although the precise genetics are not known. One-quarter to one third of patients with idiopathic epilepsy have a family history of seizures. Three per cent of children of patients with idiopathic epilepsy develop seizures. Febrile convulsions also appear to be more common in children who have afflicted relatives. Although approximately one-half of these children will have a subsequent febrile convulsion, only one-quarter have a seizure without a high temperature. Six per cent of the population will at some time have a least a single convulsion, so that the additional risk in children with febrile convulsions is about four times that of the general population.

Families of patients with epilepsy should know the fundamentals of emergency management of seizures. They should be instructed in the positioning that protects the airway and cautioned against insertion of the time-honored tongue blade. It should be emphasized that few seizures last long enough to impair cardiopulmonary function seriously, yet the families should understand the essentials of cardiopulmonary resuscitation.

Familiarity with the primary anticonvulsants and their side effects and sound understanding of the facts of epilepsy will enable the physician to control the physical disabilities of his patient's illness and to dispel the equally disabling fears that arise from this disturbing symptom.

THERAPEUTIC RECOMMENDATIONS

- Establish an etiologic diagnosis and treat the underlying cause, if possible. Symptomatic therapy can start while workup is in progress.
- To prevent further convulsions, begin with phenytoin in a loading dose of approximately 1000 mg. over the first day (see Table 158–3). This is usually done while the patient is hospitalized, but can be done on an outpatient basis. Maintenance dosage of 300 mg. per day can then be started. Adjust the dose to achieve a therapeutic level, in the range of 8 to 20 mg. per 100 ml. in most laboratories.
- If phenytoin is ineffective or if adverse reactions to this drug develop, *add* phenobarbital at 60 mg. before bed.
- If seizures persist, check the serum levels of the an-

ticonvulsants and inquire into alcohol and other drug use; administer additional phenytoin if there is a low level of anticonvulsant or add a second or third agent. This is an indication for referral to a neurologist.

- Once seizures are controlled, continue the medication for at least 1 year; if the patient remains seizure-free, a cautious attempt at tapering the medication can be made.
- Teach the patient how to recognize the warning signals of a seizure and what to do to minimize injury; instruct him in the role of alcohol in precipitating seizures.
- Educate the patient and his family about prognosis, activity, and job precautions; teach airway protection by positioning and caution against the insertion of a tongue blade into the mouth.
- Elicit and discuss all patient questions and apprehensions thoroughly; discourage unnecessary restriction of activity.

ANNOTATED BIBLIOGRAPHY

Drugs for epilepsy, Med. Lett., *21 (6)*:25, 1979. *(Best recent summary.)*

Gastaut, H., and Gaitant, J.L.: Computerized axial tomography in epilepsy. In Penry, J.K., (ed): Epilepsy: The Eighth International Symposium. New York: Raven Press, 1977. *(Best available summary on the use of this "cost-effective" controversial device and its use in this setting. 500 patients.)*

Hauser, W.A., and Kurland, L.T.: The epidemiology of epilepsy in Rochester, Minnesota, 1935 through 1967. Epilepsia, *16*:1, 1975. *(Thorough review of epilepsy in patients of all ages including incidence, types, etiology, and prognosis. 10-year follow-up.)*

Reynolds, E.H.: Chronic antiepileptic toxicity: A review. Epilepsia, *16*:319, 1975. *(Very thorough.)*

Slater, E., and Beard, A.W.: The Interictal behavior syndrome of temporal lobe epilepsy. Br. J. Psychiatry, *109*:95, 1963. *(55 pages of detailed psychiatric and neurological study. There are more recent studies, but this is excellent.)*

Woodbury, D.M., et al.: Antiepileptic Drugs, New York: Raven Press, 1972. *(Detailed review of pharmacology.)*

Woodcock, S., and Cosgrove, S.B.R.: Epilepsy after the age of 50: A 5-year follow-up study. Neurology, *14*:34, 1964. *(Montreal study of 80 patients older than 50. Suffers from lack of CT scanner at the time [PEG used] so results are not entirely applicable now. Definition of cerebrovascular disease is also rather vague.)*

Wolf, S.M.: Controversies in the treatment of febrile convulsions. Neurology, *29*:287, 1979. *(A rational approach to a fairly common problem—summarizes all the previous literature.)*

159

Approach to the Patient with Transient Ischemic Attacks

AMY A. PRUITT, M.D.

Transient ischemic attacks (TIAs) are episodes of temporary, focal cerebral dysfunction due to vascular disease. Onset is rapid (often in less than 1 minute) and, strictly defined, the symptom may last up to 24 hours; however, the vast majority of TIAs last only a few minutes. Clearing is as rapid as onset, and the attack leaves no neurologic deficits.

Recognition of TIAs and differentiation from similar nonvascular events are of critical importance. The symptom may be the initial clue to the presence of significant cerebrovascular disease. Although figures vary, it appears that about one-third of patients with TIAs progress to a completed stroke within 5 years. Unfortunately, clinical criteria that identify patients at greatest risk are not well established. Furthermore, the precise benefit of anticoagulation or endarterectomy in reducing stroke risk is not known. However, the primary physician should be able to recognize the occurrence of a TIA and should keep abreast of the extensive and evolving literature on the subject. In this chapter, the available data are discussed in the context of the practical problem of recognizing patients who require urgent evaluation for potentially operable vascular lesions or anticoagulation therapy.

PATHOPHYSIOLOGY AND CLINICAL PRESENTATION

Investigators have long disagreed about pathogenesis of TIAs. Some suggest that transient lowering of blood pressure in the presence of hemodynamically significant stenosis leads to symptoms, while the majority believe that emboli of platelets and fibrin or of atheromatous material break off from a vessel wall (usually the carotid) and transiently occlude branches of cerebral vessels. TIAs are known to occur on the side of a totally occluded vessel. In this case, small clots are presumed to form on the distal end of the thrombus and then dislodge.

On rare occasions, focal symptoms are caused by cardiac arrhythmias; but, recent studies indicate that blood pressure reduction alone rarely results in focal symptoms unless a stenotic lesion is already present.

In certain rare instances, TIAs may be attributable to steal phenomena (such as subclavian steal) or to hyperviscosity states such as polycythemia. Far more commonly (and more importantly for differential diagnosis) emboli from heart valves with rheumatic disease, mitral valve prolapse or endocarditis may produce recurrent focal neurologic deficits.

TIAs can be divided into those that indicate disease in the carotid circulation and those that point to disease in the vertebrobasilar territory. Symptoms of *carotid disease* include transient paresis (usually in the face and/or arm), paresthesias, dysphasia, or amaurosis fugax (transient monocular blindness). The last symptom is due to occlusion of the ophthalmic artery or branches ipsilateral to the carotid stenosis and classically is described by the patient as a "shade" or "curtain" that descends over the affected eye.

Symptoms of *vertebrobasilar disease* include binocular visual disturbance, vertigo, paresthesias, diplopia, ataxia, dysarthria, light-headedness, generalized weakness, loss of consciousness, and transient global amnesia. Any of these may be an isolated symptom of posterior circulation disease.

One particularly troublesome problem is that of the patient who presents with isolated vertigo. As a symptom of vertebrobasilar insufficiency, this complaint is rather uncommon and more often is attributable to labyrinthine pathology (see Chapter 154).

Dizziness in vertebrobasilar disease is usually not true vertigo and usually is accompanied by other brain stem signs.

Certain clinical features are likely to be associated with carotid or vertebrobasilar disease, but no single feature is a consistently reliable sign. In one series, 95 patients with carotid territory TIAs were evaluated by arteriography. These patients had either tight carotid stenosis (defined as a residual vessel lumen of less than 2 millimeters), carotid occlusion, or normal vessels. Fifty-two patients had transient hemispheric attacks, 33 had amaurosis fugax, and 10 had both. Sixty-seven had recurrent episodes of the same general type. Two clinical features were correlated with the arteriographic state of the artery. First, duration of hemispheric attacks over 60 minutes, whether single or multiple, was significantly associated with a normal carotid (and presumably attacks were due to emboli from the heart). Second, the nonsimultaneous occurrence of both transient hemispheric episodes and transient monocular blindness was correlated with an 80 per cent incidence of carotid disease. No difference between normal and diseased carotid groups was found when the cumulative number of attacks per patient was considered. Similarly, division according to pure ocular or pure hemispheric symptoms did not distinguish the two groups. Future similar studies may reveal other diagnostic and prognostic features of the clinical presentation.

DIFFERENTIAL DIAGNOSIS

Transient focal motor or sensory dysfunction does not have to be of vascular origin. Focal seizures (see Chapter 158 can produce a similar picture, as can the focal aura of migraine, which is not always followed by the diagnostic headache (see Chapter 160). Hyperventilation can produce distal tingling and numbness. Cervical discs can also produce transient focal motor or sensory disturbance, sometimes precipitated by manipulation of the head or neck (see Chapter 141). Carpal tunnel syndrome may present with intermittent (often nocturnal) paresthesias in a median nerve distribution. Meniere's disease presents with episodic vertigo and hearing loss, but without signs and symptoms of brain stem dysfunction (see Chapter 154).

The age group affected by TIAs of vascular origin is similar to that affected by cardiovascular disease, and the risk factors for cerebrovascular disease are similar. In general, the other disorders mentioned above do not usually present a practical problem in differential diagnosis (see Chapter 155).

WORKUP

The goals in evaluating a TIA are to establish the risk for significant vascular disease, to identify those patients whose symptoms dictate intervention, and to provide an adequate explanation for the event, should cerebrovascular disease prove not to be the etiology.

History. Questioning should first confirm that the transient episode is indeed a TIA. There ought to be the rapid onset of temporary focal cerebral dysfunction and equally rapid resolution with complete clearing. Duration of symptoms beyond 24 hours rules out TIA. The onset of headache during resolution of the neurologic deficit is more suggestive of a migrainous episode (see Chapter 160). Careful description of symptoms is needed to distinguish vertebrobasilar involvement from carotid disease. In addition, the frequency of episodes, date of first onset, and presence of hypertension and cardiac disease are important to ascertain. These items of the history may help predict clinical course. Patients with carotid symptoms are more likely to develop a disabling stroke than are those with vertebrobasilar dysfunction; the patient is at greatest risk for stroke in the first few months after onset of TIAs. The presence of hypertension, cardiac disease, or advanced age (greater that 65) increases the risk of subsequent stroke.

Physical examination should be directed to the nervous system and vascular structures. Hypertension, atrial fibrillation, and cardiac murmurs should be noted. Ocular examination involves a search for visible atheromatous plaques in retinal artery branches. Neurologic examination, provided the patient has not had a previous completed stroke, is likely to be normal.

Carotid arteries should be palpated for upstroke and volume and should be auscultated for bruits. The presence of a bruit does not invariably herald significant stenosis (a bruit can be present with hemodynamically insignificant lesions or with complete occlusion), but in as many as 70 to 80 percent of cases, the bruit does identify ipsilateral carotid disease. Palpation of facial and superficial temporal pulses with simultaneous assessment of supratrochlear and su-

praorbital pulses may confirm collateral flow to the latter two vessels by way of the external carotid artery and suggest occlusion of the internal carotid artery. Unfortunately, the vertebrobasilar circulation is not accessible to accurate physical examination.

Laboratory studies. At present, there is no entirely reliable noninvasive test for carotid or vertebrobasilar disease. Newer techniques, such as directional Doppler ultrasonography, thermography, carotid ultrasound, and phonoangiography offer much promise for assessment of the carotid circulation. Nevertheless, *arteriography* remains the definitive diagnostic procedure. Many neuroradiologists advise using the above listed noninvasive tests only in the atypical case to "rule in" doing an arteriogram when symptoms are equivocal, but not to "rule out" doing an arteriogram in an otherwise suspicious case. However, arteriography should be performed only if the physician would proceed to endarterectomy in the case of carotid disease or to anticoagulation in the case of vertebrobasilar disease; i.e., the procedure should lead to a critical management decision.

PRINCIPLES OF MANAGEMENT

The literature of therapeutic options is complex and often confusing. Many studies are not well controlled, and, frequently, study populations are not well defined or well characterized. In a large multicenter controlled study done in Canada, *aspirin* was found to reduce risk of stroke by 31 percent and TIA occurrence by 19 percent; both effects were seen only in men. Other antiplatelet drugs do not seem to enhance the protective effect of aspirin. Aspirin and *warfarin* have not been compared in a well-controlled study, and no study of *warfarin* is as well designed as the recent Canadian trial on efficacy of aspirin in TIAs. Similarly, aspirin, warfarin, and surgery have never been directly compared in a thoroughly evaluated, prospectively randomized series. However, surgical morbidity from endarterectomy has been greatly reduced, and it appears that surgery may be the best treatment for tightly stenotic, symptomatic carotid lesion in a patient who has no contraindication to an operative procedure.

Bearing in mind that optimal therapy for TIAs is not yet clearly defined and the new information will be forthcoming, the following guidelines for management are recommended at the present time:

1. Those under 65 years of age who are good sur-

gical risks and have recurrent TIAs, or TIAs within 2 months of examination, require prompt attention. If adequate radiologic support is available, these patients should have arteriography as soon as possible. Some physicians directly admit such patients to the hospital and immediately place them on intravenous heparin until arteriography can be performed if there is an unavoidable delay. Patients with residual carotid lumens of less than 2 mm or with ulcerated plaques should undergo endarterectomy. The physician should refer surgical candidates to a center where many endarterectomies are done.

2. Those with normal carotid vessels should have thorough cardiac evaluation to rule out an embolic source from the heart. In the absence of atrial fibrillation, valvular heart disease, or carotid disease, the proper treatment (anticoagulation with warfarin or aspirin or other therapy) is not known. While natural history studies suggest that these patients are at risk for future stroke, efficacy of available treatment is unclear. After the results of the American and Canadian aspirin studies became known, it became common to place such patients on aspirin prophylactically. While there is some evidence to recommend this practice, it should be clear that these studies did not address the question of TIA or stroke from noncarotid sources.

3. A sense of urgency is equally appropriate in the evaluation of patients with progressing neurologic deficit or with fixed, mild deficit and continuing TIAs. They, too, may benefit from anticoagulation and endarterectomy.

4. Patients over 65, patients with a single remote event, and patients seen in settings where angiographic and surgical services are unavailable may benefit from prophylactic administration of aspirin, although the proper dose is presently in question. Hypertension and other risk factors should be eliminated. Other antiplatelet agents are being studied (no form of antiplatelet therapy yet has been shown to be effective in women). The physician should consider referring patients who would be operative candidates to a surgical center.

5. The neurologist is frequently asked to offer an opinion on the appropriate management of a carotid bruit noted incidentally during physical examination. If the history is clearly negative for prior TIA, the physician is faced with the uncertainty of the *asymptomatic bruit*. Proposed management ranges from surgical studies which advocate instant arteriography and operation on all such patients to a more conservative recent series which suggests that progression to completed stroke in this population is uncommon and that cardiac disease is the major source of mortality. Most authors report that an initial warning TIA occurred in up to 70 per cent of patients who eventually suffered a completed thrombotic carotid stroke. Thus, the physician is justified in following such a lesion carefully, informing his patient about symptoms signifying a TIA, and minimizing risk factors. Progression of these lesions is currently being studied by noninvasive methods and should offer some helpful guidelines. Many physicians would place the patient with an asymptomatic bruit on aspirin. As the sensitivity, specificity, and predictive value of noninvasive tests are established, the natural history should be better understood, and more effective guideline for stroke prophylaxis may soon be available.

ANNOTATED BIBLIOGRAPHY

Ackerman, R.H.: The relative effectiveness of six noninvasive tests for carotid disease. Neurology, *26*:379, 1976. *(Concise summary of a new and important area of diagnosis.)*

Brust, J.C.M.: Transient ischemic attacks: natural history and anticoagulation. Neurology, *27*:701, 1977. *(Excellent review of all previously published studies with critical analysis of their conflicting results.)*

The Canadian Cooperative Stroke Study Group: A randomized trial of aspirin and sulfinpyrazone in threatened stroke. N. Engl. J. Med., *299*:53, 1978. *(Our best available evidence on the subject.)*

Duncan, G.W., et al.: Concomitants of atherosclerotid carotid artery stenosis. Stroke, *8(6)*:665, 1977. *(Shows carotid disease following same risk factors as Framingham study established for cardiac disease.)*

Genton, E.G., et al.: Cerebral ischema: The role of thrombosis and of antithromobtic therapy. Stroke, *8(1)*:150, 1977. *(A critical overview.)*

Pessin, M.S., et al.: Clinical and angiographic features of carotid transient ischemic attacks. N. Engl. J. Med. *296*:358, 1977. *(Discussed in this chapter in detail. Provides useful clinical guidelines for evaluation.)*

Sandok, B.A.: Guidelines for the management of transient ischemic attacks. Mayo Clin. Proc., *53*:605, 1978. *(A reasonable compromise.)*

160
Management of Migraine

Migraine afflicts about 5 to 10 per cent of the adult population. It is a cause of considerable misery. Although there is no cure for migraine, it usually does respond to medical therapy, which can reduce the frequency and severity of attacks. The primary physician should be able to effectively treat the patient with migraine while avoiding inappropriate use of medication that could be harmful if taken chronically (a risk that is substantial due to the condition's chronic, recurrent nature).

CLINICAL PRESENTATION AND COURSE

There are several forms of migraine. *Classic migraine* accounts for 10 to 15 per cent of cases. It is characterized by a prodrome of transient visual, motor, or sensory disturbances (e.g., scintillating scotomata, zig-zag patterns, hemianopsia, paresthesias, hemiparesis, difficulty speaking) followed by onset of a hemicranial throbbing headache, nausea, photophobia, and sensitivity to noise. Typically the aura resolves as the headache begins. *Common migraine* occurs in 80 per cent of patients with migraine. It differs from the classic variety in that there is no prodrome; sometimes the headache is bilateral or shifts sides. Nausea, photophobia and related symptoms usually accompany the headache. Classic migraine may produce a prodrome without headache; this can lead to considerable diagnostic confusion, for there may be only a transient sensory or motor deficit. Since migraine is generally a self-limited disorder, neurologic dysfunction that lasts longer than 24 to 36 hours should suggest another diagnosis.

The list of reported precipitants of migraine includes fatigue, hunger, changes in the weather, menstrual period, emotional stress, alcohol, oral contraceptives, and certain foods. Cheese, nuts, avocados, and chocolate have been known to cause attacks in certain patients. Food cured with nitrates or flavored with monosodium glutamate has also brought on attacks. In over 50 per cent of cases, there is a family history. Many patients were troubled by motion sickness or cyclic vomiting during childhood. All age groups are affected, but attacks usually begin before the third decade and subside by the fifth. Migraine occurs in women about four times as often as in men and may begin or terminate during menopause. It often subsides during pregnancy, but occasionally it may actually worsen during this time.

PRINCIPLES OF MANAGEMENT

There is no cure for migraine, but prophylaxis and symptomatic treatment are reasonably effective. Although the disease is self-limited, attacks may continue for decades, and chronic exposure to some of the drugs used in prophylaxis and treatment may be damaging or addicting. Consequently, design of a long-term management program requires attention to safety as well as efficacy.

Prophylaxis. Prevention of attacks involves nonpharmacologic measures as well as drug treatment. Since migraine may be precipitated by emotional stress or psychological conflict, it is important to investigate family and social circumstances in designing a program of prevention. Regular exercise (e.g., jogging) or relaxation techniques (e.g., meditation or yoga) may significantly decrease the frequency and severity of headaches. These activities help reduce the impact of stress. Many patients prefer to try them before attempting other forms of therapy.

Some patients bothered by migraine are overly competitive, very aggressive, and feel considerable need to succeed. They often harbor repressed hostility toward parents or other loved ones. An analysis of the circumstances associated with attacks may provide a clue to the presence of these factors. Therapy for such patients should include helping them to express their feelings and deal with these issues. Although extensive psychotherapy may not reduce attacks, it is worth trying to determine areas of stress and search with the patient for ways to resolve them.

Drug therapy should be added when nonpharmacologic measures do not suffice. *Propranolol* has been shown to reduce the frequency and severity of attacks in double-blind crossover studies and is FDA-approved for prevention of common migraine attacks. About two-thirds of patients benefit from propranolol, and one-third achieve a 50 per cent or greater reduction in number of attacks; one-third report no benefit or an increase in severity. Most studies are short-term trials; there have been no long-term trials using propranolol, nor comparative studies with methysergide, the other established drug for migraine prophylaxis. The initial propranolol dose is 80 mg. per day in divided doses; the typical maintenance dose is 160 to 240 mg. per day. Beta blockade does not need to be achieved in order to attain a prophylactic effect. Asthma, heart failure, and heart block are the major contraindications.

Tricyclic antidepressants have been found capable of reducing the frequency of migrainous attacks, especially when depression is a prominent problem, but also when there are few depressive symptoms reported. *Antianxiety agents* may contribute to the prophylactic effort when acute situational stress and marked anxiety appear to be responsible for episodes. The efficacy of the popular combination drug Fiorinal is probably due to its barbiturate component, because it additionally contains only aspirin, phenacetin, and caffeine.

Methysergide, a serotonin antagonist, has been relegated to a second-line position in migraine prophylaxis because of its association with retroperitoneal, pleuropulmonary and valvular fibrosis when used for prolonged, uninterrupted periods. Because of its potentially serious side effects, methysergide should be prescribed under close supervision and only after simpler measures have proven inadequate. However, the drug is effective; 60 to 80 per cent of patients who take methysergide achieve at least a 50 per cent or greater reduction in frequency of headaches. An initial dose of 1 mg. should be given; the dose is then gradually increased over a 2-week period to a maximum of 6 mg. per day. After a reduction in episodes of migraine has been achieved, the daily amount should be tapered to the minimum effective dose. Methysergide should be withheld for 1 month after every 6-month course of treatment to reduce the likelihood of fibrotic complications, which may develop silently. If therapy is uninterrupted, a yearly intravenous pyelogram should be obtained to detect any early signs of ureteral obstruction from retroperitoneal fibrosis. Upon initial administration, about 30 per cent of patients experience nausea, vomiting, indigestion, myalgias, insomnia, restlessness, or feelings of depersonalization; about 10 per cent cannot tolerate the drug for these reasons. Because the drug produces vasoconstriction, methysergide is relatively contraindicated in patients with peripheral vascular disease, coronary artery disease, and severe hypertension. Active peptic ulcer disease, arteritis, liver or renal failure, and pregnancy are other relative contraindications.

Treatment of an acute attack. Some patients with migraine find that attacks can be relieved by simple *physical measures* such as hot or cold packs or temporal massage. Dimming the lights and lying down in a quiet room also help to lessen the discomfort. Biofeedback techniques are under study.

Ergotamine tartrate is the drug most effect for acute attacks. It has been found to constrict the arteries of the scalp, and it is therefore believed to counteract the vasodilatation phase of the migraine headache. Complete or partial relief from the headache occurs in about 70 per cent of patients. To be effective, ergotamine must be taken at the first sign of an attack, e.g., during the prodromal phase of classic migraine. The lack of a prodrome in common migraine means there is often little advance warning, and this may limit ergotamine's usefulness.

The initial dose of ergotamine is 2 mg. sublingually. There is some evidence to suggest that the sublingual form is faster acting and more effective than the oral route. Because of nausea and vomiting, some patients prefer to use a rectal suppository preparation of ergotamine. The dose should be repeated every half hour if there is no relief, until a maximum of 6 to 8 mg. is taken. Further doses are generally not helpful and may lead to toxicity.

Ergotamine is reasonably safe when used properly. Serious reactions occur in only 0.1 per cent of patients. Adverse effects include nausea, vomiting, myalgias, paresthesias, chest discomfort, peripheral ischemia, angina, rebound headache, and dependency. Dependency and rebound headaches are managed by discontinuing the drug and controlling the headache with other medications.

Ergotamine is contraindicated in patients with vascular disease such as Raynaud's syndrome, coronary artery disease, thromboangiitis obliterans, thrombophlebitis, and severe atherosclerosis. The drug should not be taken during pregnancy because it causes uterine contractions as well as vasoconstriction.

Analgesics are required when the headache is well established and unresponsive to ergotamine. Control of mild headache may be obtained with 600 mg. of *aspirin* or *acetaminophen* every 4 hours. The combination preparation Midrin, containing acetaminophen, 325 mg., dichloralphenazone, 100 mg., and the vasoconstrictor isometheptene mucate, 65 mg., has been found, in controlled studies, to be superior to acetaminophen alone. The dose of this preparation is 2 capsules at the onset of the headache, followed by 1 capsule every hour until relief occurs, up to 5 capsules per 12 hours. Adverse reactions are chiefly transient dizziness and skin rash. *Narcotics* may be needed for very severe headaches but should be used sparingly. Codeine sulfate, 30 to 60 mg. every 4 to 6 hours, usually will suffice.

Fiorinal is a very popular drug for migraine; it is an aspirin-phenacetin-caffeine preparation combined with a small dose of barbiturate. Long-term use of Fiorinal exposes the patient to the risk of a large cumulative dose of phenacetin; over 10 years, the intake can reach 2 to 3 kg., which has been associated with development of interstitial nephritis. The drug should be prescribed with caution if used at all on a chronic basis.

Photophobia responds to treatment of the headache, but nausea may persist, requiring separate antiemetic therapy. *Prochlorperazine,* 10 mg. orally every 6 hours, or 25 mg. rectally every 12 hours, is indicated if incapacitating nausea and vomiting are present. At times, the nausea may be worsened by ergotamine intake; if ergotamine has been effective and its continued use is desired, addition of prochlorperazine may be helpful.

PATIENT EDUCATION

The importance of careful instruction in the use of medications for prophylaxis and treatment of migraine cannot be overemphasized, because efficacy and safety depend on correct usage. Migraine is a problem that may last for decades, and it is essential to establish good habits related to drug use early on so that complications due to chronic misuse can be avoided. For example, the patient on methysergide must be informed of the need to cease the drug for a full month after every 6 consecutive months of use in order to avoid fibrotic complications. Ergotamine is not likely to be effective unless taken at the first sign of migraine. Fiorinal must not be used indefinitely because of the danger of phenacetin-induced renal damage.

THERAPEUTIC RECOMMENDATIONS
Prophylaxis
- Identify any precipitating factors such as situational stress or psychological conflict and attend to them directly (see Chapter 214). Relaxation techniques and regular exercise may help reduce the impact of stress.
- Begin propranolol, 80 mg. per day in divided doses, if attacks are frequent and severe enough to interfere with the patient's life. Increase the daily dose until a reduction in severity or number of episodes is noted or a dose of 240 mg. per day is reached.
- If propranolol is effective, continue therapy on a daily basis for 6 months, then taper and watch for recurrence.
- If propranolol is ineffective and prophylaxis is definitely needed, begin methysergide, 2 mg. daily, and increase dose to 6 mg. per day over the next 2 weeks. If there is no improvement, stop the drug. If improvement is apparent, taper to the minimum effective dose. Do not use methysergide for more than 4 to 6 months. There must be a medication-free interval of 4 weeks after every 6-month course of treatment to prevent fibrotic complications.
- Consider a tricyclic antidepressant (see Chapter 215) for prophylaxis if depression is accompanied by migraine, or if other agents fail to achieve reduction in frequency or severity of attacks.

Treatment of Acute Attacks
- Begin ergotamine tartrate, 2 mg. sublingually, at the first sign of migraine.
- Repeat every half hour until relief is obtained or a maximum of 6 to 8 mg. has been taken.
- If the headache is severe, well-established, and unresponsive to ergotamine, treat the attack with codeine sulfate, 30 to 60 mg. every 4 hours.
- If the headache is mild, aspirin, 600 mg. every 4 hours, or acetaminophen, 600 mg. every 4 hours, should suffice.
- Avoid chronic use of phenacetin-containing compounds (e.g., Fiorinal).
- Treat incapacitating nausea and vomiting with prochlorperazine suppositories, 25 mg. rectally every 12 hours, or tablets, 10 mg. orally every 6 hours.

ANNOTATED BIBLIOGRAPHY

Elkind, A.H., *et al.:* Silent retroperitoneal fibrosis associated with methysergide therapy. JAMA, *206*:5, 1968. *(Documents this important complication of long-term methysergide therapy.)*

Feuerstein, M., and Adams, H.: Cephalic vasomotor feedback in modification of migraine headache. Biofeedback self-regul, *2*:241, 1977. *(Describes some of the new biofeedback techniques for control of migraine.)*

Graham, J.R.: Methysergide for prevention of headache. N. Engl. J. Med., *270*:67, 1964. *(Classic paper on the effectiveness of the drug for prophylaxis.)*

Waters, W.E.: Controlled clinical trial of ergotamine tartrate. Br. Med. J., *1*:325, 1970. *(Casts some doubt on the efficacy of oral administration of ergot and argues for sublingual or rectal route.)*

Wideroe, T.E., and Vigander, R.: Propranolol in the treatment of migraine. Br. Med. J. *2*:699, 1974. *(A double-blind crossover trial using 30 patients demonstrated significant reduction in mean frequency of migraine attacks when propranolol was used prophylactically.)*

Ziegler, D.K.: Migraine: diagnostic and therapeutic aspects. Postgrad. Med., *56*:169, 1974. *(A terse review of the topic with 23 references.)*

161

Management of Parkinson's Disease

AMY A. PRUITT, M.D.

The development of improved drug therapy for Parkinson's disease has brought new hope and relief to thousands suffering from this immobilizing condition. Proper treatment requires careful timing and skillful utilization of drugs, because there are important difficulties associated with pharmacologic therapy. The agents used for Parkinson's disease often cause drug-drug interactions and produce substantial side effects (including some that resemble symptoms of the disease). Moreover, drug efficacy declines over time, and therapeutic response may be blunted by improper timing or inappropriate selection of antiparkinsonian agents.

The frequency of Parkinson's disease, its ability to interfere with daily activity and independent functioning, and the availability of drug therapy make it important for the primary physician to know the details of management.

CLINICAL PRESENTATION AND COURSE

Tremor is the most obvious initial finding, but it is absent in 20 per cent of patients. Parkinson's disease may begin insidiously with vague, aching pain in the limbs, neck, or back and with decreased axial dexterity before tremor is noted. Other early subtle symptoms are decreases in the caliber of handwriting and the volume of the voice; both reflect disturbances in extrapyramidal motor function. More disabling are rigidity and bradykinesia, which can interfere with daily activity. Distressing episodes of frozen rigidity, sudden loss of postural control, and immobile facies that may be mistaken for depression can result.

Before the introduction of levodopa (L-dopa), the disease had a fairly predictable course. At 5 years from onset, 60 per cent of patients were severely disabled, and at 10 years, nearly 80 per cent were. The rate of progression varied widely. Mortality was three times that of an age-matched population. Death rarely was a direct result of parkinsonism; rather, it was a consequence of immobility (aspiration pneumonia, urinary tract infections) or of trauma. Trauma has actually become more frequent as patients gain mobility but continue to have poor postural control.

L-dopa produces a marked improvement in functional capacity, although treatment does not alter the underlying pathologic process. However, by preventing complications that result from immobility, levodopa does extend the life span of severely affected patients. Over a period of 5 years of therapy, one-third of the 85 per cent of patients who initially respond to treatment retain their benefit, one-third lose some of the response, and one-third lose all initial benefit and are considerably worse than they were when treatment began.

PRINCIPLES OF MANAGEMENT

Dopamine and acetylcholine are neurotransmitters. The normally high concentration of dopamine in the basal ganglia has been found to be depleted in parkinsonian patients. Clinically, these patients appear to have excessive cholinergic activity. These findings have led to the notion of treating Parkinson's disease by either dopaminergic repletion or cholinergic antagonism.

Anticholinergic agents were the mainstay of parkinsonian therapy for more than a century, and they have remained important even with the introduction of levodopa because more than half of the patients who have benefited from levodopa note additional improvement when anticholinergic agents are added. Moreover, levodopa response decreases after the first few years of therapy (regardless of the extent of initial improvement or the severity of the disease), making it necessary to employ a second drug.

One commonly used anticholinergic is trihexyphenidyl (Artane), which resembles the belladonna alkaloids. Adverse effects include blurred vision, urinary retention, and drying of mucous membranes. Similar agents are benztropine (Cogentin) and some antihistamines with weak anticholinergic effect, such as diphenhydramine (Benadryl).

Amantadine, initially used for prophylaxis of influenza A, is believed to act by releasing dopamine from nigrostriatal terminals that are still intact. Amantadine acts maximally within a few days but loses efficacy within 6 to 8 weeks of continuous treatment. Side effects are minimal, although macular degeneration and livido reticularis of the legs have appeared infrequently.

Levodopa has been in common use for a full decade and is now available by itself or in combination with the dopa-decarboxylase inhibitor carbidopa. L-dopa is rapidly absorbed after oral administration, reaches peak effect at 30 minutes to 2 hours, and has a half-life of 1 to 3 hours. The rate of absorption is decreased by eating a protein-rich meal. When used alone, only 1 per cent of an L-dopa dose eventually reaches the brain, but the addition of a peripheral dopa-decarboxylase inhibitor ensures greater delivery to the central nervous system.

Therapeutic efficacy is impressive. Over three-quarters of patients show some response to levodopa. All symptoms diminish, but bradykinesia and rigidity improve more than does tremor.

Adverse reactions are many. Nausea, vomiting, anorexia, hypotension, dyskinesias, and hallucinations can be quite disturbing. Recently defined problems include declining efficacy, a distressing "on-off" phenomenon with sudden fluctuations in disability, and deterioration of intellectual function. Decarboxylase inhibitors have decreased the early gastrointestinal side effects but have led to increased incidence of dyskinetic and psychiatric reactions.

Regardless of duration of disease, the best results with levodopa are obtained in the first 3 years after initiation of therapy. With time there is a declining threshold for the development of adverse central side effects; this may necessitate a decrease in daily dose.

The phenomenon has been explained as a kind of denervation hypersensitivity of dopamine-depleted terminals. On the other hand, an increasing dose of medication is required over time to forestall the inevitable disappearance of responsiveness. Decline in effect is believed related to a reduction in dopaminergic receptor sites or to the depletion of the dopa-converting enzyme that is required to form the active metabolite when levodopa is administered orally. A progressive dementia has been noted in rare cases in patients on prolonged levodopa therapy. Although this symptom has come to be recognized as part of the disease process itself, levodopa clearly has played a direct causative role in some reported cases. Other psychiatric symptoms, including nightmares, hallucinations, and increased sexual drive, are being seen more frequently because higher doses of levodopa are delivered centrally by the combination preparations. The disturbing "on-off" phenomenon, which lacks a plausible biochemical explanation, may limit therapy in young patients with otherwise good response to levodopa. Paradoxically, increased mobility has in some instances led to increased disability as a result of sudden falls by previously rigid patients.

The physician is able to offer the parkinsonian patient much benefit, but one is still quite limited by the toxicity of treatments. The goal of therapy is to maintain the patient at a maximal or at least tolerable level of function with minimal medication. Initiation of L-dopa therapy should be delayed as long as possible, because *regardless of the initial severity of the disease or the initial benefit from the drug, levodopa's efficacy decreases with time.* The patient and physician must tolerate many of the early signs of parkinsonism, which are sufficient to prompt medical consultation, but, aside from provoking psychological discomfort, are not threatening. Clearly, this philosophy must be individualized; the violinist with a tremor is much more drastically disabled by his symptoms than is a retired businessman.

Attempts to abolish all evidence of parkinsonism often necessitate use of doses of levodopa that produce intolerable side effects. The appearance of dyskinesias may require a decrease in dose and a compromise between parkinsonism and dyskinesia, allowing some signs of the original disease to reemerge. For practical purposes, the target symptom of most importance is rigidity. A reasonable therapeutic end point is mobilization of the patient; complete abolition of all parkinsonian symptoms may not be feasible.

Initiating therapy. Each newly diagnosed patient should be evaluated for extent of disability at home and at work, including the effect of the illness on social interactions. Mild tremor that is well tolerated need not be treated; follow-up visits at regular intervals will suffice. If symptoms are more disturbing, one can prescribe an anticholinergic agent such as trihexyphenidyl (Artane), beginning with 2 mg. once or twice a day; an alternative is to start amantadine, at 200 mg. per day.

Finally, L-dopa, the most potent currently available treatment, should be started when patients need immediate symptom relief or are quite advanced at the time of presentation. If early minor signs are treated with levodopa, maximal benefit at a later, more symptomatic time may be impaired. During the initial "induction" phase, treatment is started at a subtherapeutic level with, usually, one of the combination dopa-decarboxylase-levodopa preparations. Treatment may be started with 1 tablet containing 10 mg. carbidopa/100 mg. levodopa (Sinemet) three times a day after meals; 1 tablet may be added every 2 to 4 days. The daily dose is increased gradually to minimize gastrointestinal side effects. Patients who have been taking large doses of levodopa may be switched to Sinemet by decreasing the total daily levodopa dose by about 50 to 75 per cent and using the larger size combination tablet (25 mg. carbidopa/250 mg. levodopa).

Several practical concerns inevitably arise. A protein meal, while decreasing gastrointestinal toxicity, also descreases absorption. Nevertheless, it is reasonable to give the medication with meals to minimize GI upset. Pyridoxine enhances activation of dopa-decarboxylase, and, in the amounts present in many common multivitamin preparations, may decrease the therapeutic effect of levodopa, although not that of the combination preparations. Phenothiazines and haloperidol worsen parkinsonism, and monoamine oxidase (MAO) inhibitors may interact with levodopa to cause a dangerous elevation of blood pressure.

Maintenance. A maintenance phase follows the establishment of a therapeutic dose schedule. Day-to-day and even hour-to-hour fluctuations in clinical status should not be surprising. The clinical situation may not stabilize for at least 2 months from onset of therapy. The physician commonly receives frequent calls from the patient. The occurrence of gastrointestinal side effects from use of L-dopa often necessitates adjustment in the program; if L-dopa is being used alone, switching to a combination agent may allow for a lowering of the L-dopa intake without a loss of therapeutic effect. If bradykinesia and rigidity appear late in the afternoon, it may be worthwhile to add a 10-mg. carbidopa–100-mg. levodopa combination tablet at 4 p.m. It is sometimes necessary to decrease the evening dose of L-dopa at the expense of some stiffness during the late evening hours in order to minimize the occurrence of vivid nightmares, frequently experienced by some patients.

PATIENT EDUCATION

Patient and family education is essential to the success of therapy. The patient and family should receive careful explanation of the side effects and potential benefits of drugs. The need for trial and error to obtain maximal benefit with minimal side effects must be explained. Therapy can be proposed optimistically. The diminishing efficacy of the drug must be anticipated, but the development of newer agents, such as direct dopaminergic agonists, is in progress and may obviate the problem of decreased sensitivity to levodopa.

THERAPEUTIC RECOMMENDATIONS

- Mild tremors that do not interfere with activity or bother the patient do not require treatment. Those that do can be managed by starting an anticholinergic agent such as trihexyphenidyl 2 mg. once or twice daily; levodopa should not be introduced unless the anticholinergic agent does not suffice or is poorly tolerated.
- Amantadine (200 mg. per day) is immediately effective and may be added early in the course of Parkinson's disease to control both bradykinesia and tremor. Its efficacy is lost over time; thus it should not be used as the sole agent.
- Levodopa should be introduced when symptoms interfere significantly with the patient's life *and* other agents have not provided adequate relief. L-dopa treatment should be initiated utilizing the combination preparation containing 10 mg. carbidopa and 100 mg. levodopa. The starting dose is 1 tablet after each meal, increasing the dose by 1 tablet every 2 to 4 days. This schedule will help to minimize gastrointestinal side effects and the cumulative dose of levodopa.
- The development of the disabling side effects of L-dopa usually responds to reduction in dose, but the appearance of uncontrollable dyskinesias or the "on-off" phenomenon requires consultation with an experienced neurologist.

ANNOTATED BIBLIOGRAPHY

Bianchine, J.R.: Drug therapy of parkinsonism. N. Engl. J. Med., 295:814, 1976. *(Good, brief review.)*

Fahn, S., and Calne, B.B.: Considerations in the management of parkinsonism. Neurology, 28:5, 1978. *(A sober note of caution about initial treatment with levodopa.)*

Lieberman, A., et al.: Treatment of Parkinson's disease with bromocriptine. N. Engl. J. Med., 295:1400, 1976. *(Encouraging reports of improvement in patients who are levodopa nonresponders.)*

Marsden, C.D., and Parles, J.D.: Success and problems of long-term levodopa therapy in Parkinson's disease. Lancet, 1:345, 1977. *(Reviews reasons for failure of levodopa therapy against the background of the natural history of Parkinson's disease.)*

New drugs for Parkinson's disease. Medical Letter, 18:117, 1976. *(Discusses Sinemet and bromocriptine.)*.

Sweet, R.D., and McDowell, F.H.: Five years of treatment of Parkinson's disease with L-dopa. Ann. Intern. Med., 83:456, 1975. *(A large case series with lucid discussion of the state of the art.)*

Weiner, W.T., and Bergen, D.: Prevention and management of the side effects of levodopa. *In* Klawans, H.L., (ed.) Clinical Neuropharmacology. vol. 2. pages 1–23. New York, Raven Press, 1977. *(A detailed, rather biochemical explanation of side effects with some practical management suggestions.)*

162

Management of Bell's Palsy
AMY A. PRUITT, M.D.

Bell's palsy is an idiopathic paralysis of the facial muscles innervated by the seventh cranial nerve. The condition encompasses 80 per cent of all facial palsies. Satisfactory explanations for the condition are lacking, although viral infection and ischemia with subsequent edema of the facial nerve and adjacent structures have been invoked. Other causes of facial paralysis involve injury to the facial nerve and include bacterial infection (from a source in the ear), herpes zoster, diabetes mellitus, sarcoidosis, Guillain-Barré syndrome, tumor (acoustic neuroma, pontine glioma, neurofibroma, cholesteatoma) and trauma (fracture of the temporal bone).

The primary physician should be able to distinguish Bell's palsy from other, more ominous causes of facial palsy and temper therapeutic intervention by knowledge of the disease's self-limited course and good prognosis.

CLINICAL PRESENTATION AND COURSE

The distinction between Bell's palsy and other facial paralyses usually is not difficult. The onset of Bell's palsy is acute, involving the peripheral seventh nerve. There are no rashes, signs of trauma or sarcoidosis, history of diabetes, or evidence of ear infection. The patient appears with drooping face and mouth and occasionally with drooling. Maximal deficit develops over a few hours. The condition is almost always unilateral and in two-thirds of the cases may be accompanied by pain in or behind the ear. Fever, tinnitus, and mild hearing diminution may be present during the first few hours.

Voluntary and involuntary motor responses are lost. Upper and lower parts of the face are affected, distinguishing this peripheral facial nerve lesion from a central supranuclear one, in which only lower facial muscles are affected. The palpebral fissure appears widened and the forehead smooth. Bell's phenomenon (the normal upward deviation of the eye with lid closure) is prominent because of orbicularis oculi weakness. The corneal reflex may be decreased on the involved side. Lacrimation is only rarely defective and, depending on the level of the injury, loss or perversion of taste on the anterior two-thirds of the tongue or hyperacusis may be noted.

Seventy-five to 90 per cent of cases recover to a cosmetically acceptable level without treatment. Recovery is best in children, while poor prognosis has been associated with increasing age, hyperacusis, diminished taste, and severity of the initial motor deficit. Prognosis can be predicted by electromyographic (EMG) testing of the involved muscles at 14 to 18 days from onset. If EMG shows no signs of nerve degeneration by this time, there is usually notable clinical improvement, and recovery is almost uniformly complete. If, however, there is EMG evidence of degeneration, recovery may require several months and be less than total. It should be remembered that even though nerve conduction may remain abnormal in up to 20 per cent of cases, the resulting motor function is usually satisfactory from the patient's point of view. The upper face, involved earliest as the disease develops, is the first to recover.

Complications of Bell's palsy result from abnormal regeneration of damaged nerve fibers. Lacrimation with eating or "crocodile tears" result when autonomic fibers regrow and connect with salivary glands instead of lacrimal ducts. Abnormal movements may occur if regenerating motor fibers innervate inappropriate muscles. Contracture of the involved site may be noted during voluntary movement. Seven per cent of patients experience recurrent facial paralysis.

PRINCIPLES OF MANAGEMENT

Of greatest practical importance during the acute stage of the illness is the prevention of injury to the cornea, which is left exposed by weakness of the orbicularis muscle. When the lid is weak, methylcellulose drops should be prescribed for used twice a day and at bedtime; in addition, the lid may need to be taped shut at night.

The prognosis for most cases of Bell's palsy is good. Often little or no treatment is necessary. However, if paralysis is severe and the patient is seen within a few days of onset, a short course of corticosteroid therapy will increase the chances for maximal recovery. One study reported full facial recovery in 88 per cent of the group treated with prednisone and in 64 per cent of the untreated control group. Another study found a decrease in the frequency of chronic autonomic dysfunction (from 10 per cent to 1 per cent) when prednisone was used early in the course of illness. Associated ear pain diminished more quickly when steroids were used. Nevertheless, the benefits from use of steroids are often difficult to demonstrate, because the disease has such a good prognosis. Steroid therapy seems to make a difference only in cases with poor prognostic signs.

Other treatments have been used. Based on the theory that nerve swelling contributes to the deficit, surgical decompression has been tried, but without much success. Some patients have been followed with EMG stimulation of the muscles in order to hasten particularly stubborn paralyses. The possible role of EMG stimulation in management is unclear; it has not been subjected to controlled study.

THERAPEUTIC RECOMMENDATIONS AND INDICATIONS FOR REFERRAL

- Ascertain that the condition is indeed Bell's palsy. Check for involvement of other cranial nerves and ear infection. Examine for zosteriform lesions on the tympanic membrane, in the external auditory canal, and behind the ear.
- Explain the benign nature and good prognosis of the condition and caution the patient about corneal abrasion. Prescribe use of methylcellulose eyedrops twice a day and at sleep with taping of the especially weak lid. Tarsorrhaphy may be considered when severe lid weakness exists.
- If the palsy is complete, the patient is seen within 3 or 4 days of onset, and there is no important contraindication to corticosteroid use, a short course of prednisone may be prescribed on the following schedule: 60 mg. for 10 days, 40 mg. for 2 days, 30 mg. for 2 days, 10 mg. for 1 day, and 5 mg. for 2 days. If postauricular pain recurs when the dose is tapered, the immediately preceding dose may be reinstituted.
- In the 10 per cent of patients who do not achieve acceptable recovery, autografting with a portion of the greater auricular nerve may provide reasonable cosmetic results and afford lasting protection of the eye. Patients in this category should be referred to an otolaryngologist or to a neurosurgeon.

ANNOTATED BIBLIOGRAPHY

Adour, K.D., et al.: Prednisone treatment for idiopathic facial paralysis (Bell's palsy). N. Engl. J. Med., *287*:1268, 1972. *(Controlled part of this study stopped when authors felt pain relief and recovery clearly aided by prednisone. However, results for both groups very good.)*

Hauser, W.D., et al.: Incidence and prognosis of Bell's palsy in the population of Rochester, Minnesota. Mayo Clin. Proc., *46*:258, 1971. *(Gives natural history and establishes excellent prognosis.)*

Wolf, S.H., et al.: Treatment of Bell's palsy with prednisone. A prospective, randomized study. Neurology, *28*:158, 1978. *(There was incomplete recovery in 16 per cent [mild in 14 per cent]. No diabetics included.)*

163
Management of Tic Douloureux (Trigeminal Neuralgia)

Tic douloureux is among the most excruciating of pain syndromes seen in office practice. There are 15,000 new cases annually in the U.S.; mostly, patients are middle-aged or elderly. Some have found the pain so intolerable that they consider suicide. The primary physician needs to know how to use available medical therapies and when to send the patient for neurosurgical consultation.

CLINICAL PRESENTATION AND NATURAL HISTORY

The illness is characterized by paroxysms of unilateral lancinating facial pain involving the jaw, gums, lips, or maxillary region (areas corresponding to branches of the trigeminal nerve). Attacks are often precipitated by minor, repeated contact with a trigger zone, setting off brief but fierce pain that usually lasts up to a few minutes. Repeated paroxysms may continue for several weeks, day and night. The disease is unilateral and unaccompanied by demonstrable sensory or motor deficits, which distinguishes it from other causes of trigeminal pain, such as tumor.

The condition can be chronic, although spontaneous remissions are not uncommon. Women are more often affected than men, and incidence rises with age. The etiology of the condition remains unknown. Despite much speculation, there is no definitive evidence linking it to herpes simplex virus. The pathologic lesion found in some electron micrographs appears to be a breakdown of myelin.

PRINCIPLES OF MANAGEMENT

Treatment is symptomatic. Because the condition may be self-limited and agents that give temporary relief are available, drug therapy should be tried before surgery is contemplated. *Carbamazepine* (Tegretol) is the drug of choice; it was initially tried because anticonvulsants were believed to be helpful in causalgic pain. Studies have shown impressive short-term effects; most patients report marked pain relief within 24 to 72 hours on 400 to 600 mg. per day. The maintenance dose ranges from 400 to 800 mg. per day.

Unfortunately, by 3 years, 30 per cent no longer obtain relief from carbamazepine; alternate therapy is needed. Moreover, the incidence of serious side effects (bone marrow suppression, rash, liver injury) is large (5 to 19 per cent), requiring cessation of therapy. Fortunately, marrow suppression is often reversible if the drug is stopped early. Skin rash often precedes other serious side effects; it may be erythematous and pruritic. The onset of a skin rash is an early indication to halt therapy. Annoying side effects include nausea, diarrhea, ataxia, dizziness, and confusion. Neurologic reactions are reported most commonly and affect about 15 per cent of patients. Starting carbamazepine at 200 mg. daily helps to avoid many of the annoying minor side effects. During the first 3 months of therapy, complete blood and platelet counts should be obtained weekly; later the frequency of monitoring can be about once a month. It is advisable to attempt reduction or cessation of carbamazepine therapy at least once every 2 to 3 months.

If carbamazepine alone begins to lose its effectiveness, *phenytoin* can be added. Before carbamazepine was available, phenytoin was used alone with some success. Regarded by many as a second-line agent, it is still preferred by others, since it may be better tolerated and requires less frequent hematologic monitoring (see Chapter 158).

When drug therapy proves inadequate, surgical approaches can be considered. The procedure producing the least deficit with the greatest relief of symptoms is percutaneous electrocoagulation of the preganglionic rootlets that feed the trigger zone. The poorly myelinated pain fibers are destroyed, while the more heavily myelinated touch fibers that supply the relevant zone are spared. The procedure has produced lasting relief in 90 per cent of those treated once; only 5 per cent have experienced undesirable loss of sensation. The late recurrence rate is 10 per cent, and a repeat procedure achieves pain relief in these patients; few need further treatment.

Formerly used treatment methods included alcohol injection or partial section of the sensory root of the fifth nerve. These techniques provided pain relief, but often only for 1 to 2 years, and at the expense of creating unacceptable permanent sensory deficits. Total tooth extraction is an ineffective and erroneous treatment method.

PATIENT EDUCATION

The patient needs to be told that the condition can be controlled and that it is often self-limited. This knowledge can prevent a distraught sufferer from attempting suicide. The physician must keep in mind the anguish these patients may experience; they require close support. Obvious hints, such as avoiding repetitive contacts with the trigger zone, have usually been discovered by the patient, but can be helpful and are worth mentioning. Patients treated with carbamazepine must be taught to recognize the early symptoms and signs of marrow suppression (fever, sore throat, mouth ulcers, petechiae, easy bruising) and instructed to discontinue the drug and report to the physician immediately if these occur.

THERAPEUTIC RECOMMENDATIONS AND INDICATIONS FOR REFERRAL

- Teach the patient to avoid repetitive contact with the trigger zone.
- Begin drug therapy for disabling and frequent episodes of pain, starting with 100 mg. (half a tablet) of carbamazepine twice daily, and increase the dose by 200 mg. per day until control of symptoms is achieved or a dose of 800 mg. per day is reached.
- During the first 3 months of carbamazepine therapy, monitor complete blood count and platelet count weekly; thereafter, monthly checks will suffice.
- Stop drug therapy immediately if any significant fall in count occurs or if skin rash, easy bruising, fever, mouth sores, or petechiae develop.
- If carbamazepine alone is not sufficient to control symptoms, add phenytoin at a dose of 300 mg. per day.
- Avoid use of narcotics, because they are unlikely to be of help for long-term control of pain, and may only lead to drug dependency.
- Refer the patient who cannot be managed by pharmacologic measures to a neurosurgeon skilled in selective percutaneous electrocoagulation of the preganglionic rootlets.

ANNOTATED BIBLIOGRAPHY

Crill, W.E.: Carbamazepine. Ann. Intern. Med., 79:844, 1975. *(A review of the pharmacology and use of this agent. Argues for its use as the first-line of therapy in tic douloureux.)*

Wepsic, J.G.: Tic Douloureux: Etiology, refined treatment. N. Engl. J. Med., 288:680, 1973. *(An editorial arguing against herpes simplex etiology and for selective percutaneous electrocoagulation of preganglionic rootlets.)*

12

Dermatologic Problems

164
Screening for Skin Cancers
ARTHUR J. SOBER, M.D.

Neoplasms of the skin are among the most common cancers in humans. It has been estimated that over 300, 000 new tumors occur annually in the U.S. The majority are basal cell carcinomas, relatively benign, locally mutilating tumors associated with few deaths. Squamous cell carcinoma, the second most common cutaneous malignancy, causes approximately 1500 deaths annually. Malignant melanoma, of which there are 13,600 cases annually, is responsible for 4000 deaths annually. The first two types of tumor derive from the epidermal keratinocytes; the latter develops from the melanocytes along the basal layer of the epidermis.

Screening for these tumors is important because they are relatively easy to diagnose in early stages when cure is possible by simple measures.

EPIDEMIOLOGY AND RISK FACTORS

Basal cell carcinomas are probably the most common malignancy in man. They are distinctly solar-related. In one study of over 800 tumors, approximately 90 per cent of the lesions occurred on the head and neck. The frequency of these lesions is increased in people who work out-of-doors, such as farmers and sailors. Etiologic factors other than solar exposure are responsible for some basal cell carcinomas. For example, the basal cell nevus syndrome is a genetically transmitted autosomal dominant disorder in which multiple basal cell carcinomas occur in rela-

tively young individuals in association with palmer pits, bone cysts, and frontal bossing. Basal cell lesions can develop in persons exposed to arsenic. Scars from radiation dermatitis can also provide sites favorable to development of basal cell tumors. Previously identified disease is also a risk factor. Once a single basal cell carcinoma has developed, there is a 20 per cent chance that a second one will ensue within 1 year; after two have developed, there is a 40 per cent likelihood that a third or more will occur within 1 year.

Squamous cell carcinomas may develop from actinic keratoses and may also occur following arsenic ingestion or in areas of scarring from radiodermatitis. Two-thirds of these tumors occur on sun-exposed surfaces. Those arising in sun-damaged skin usually behave biologically in a less aggressive fashion than those which occur on surfaces not exposed to the sun. It is the latter group that apparently metastasize more frequently.

Malignant melanoma, while far less common than basal cell and squamous cell cancers, accounts for 70 per cent of the deaths caused by tumors of the skin. The incidence of malignant melanoma has been increasing rapidly over the past decade, and in certain areas, such as Canada, its rate of increased incidence is exceeded only by that of carcinoma of the lung. The current annual incidence exceeds those of Hodgkin's disease, carcinoma of the thyroid, and carcinoma of the pharynx and larynx. The sex ratio for melanoma is approximately 1 : 1. A second pri-

657

mary develops in about 2 per cent of patients; 6 to 10 per cent have affected relatives.

Giant hairy nevus is a form of congenital nevus that has been associated with malignant degeneration in 2 to 40 per cent of cases. When melanomas arise in these lesions, they usually do so by age 10. Smaller *pigmented congenital nevi* occur in about 1 per cent of the population. Malignant melanoma occasionally arises in these nevi, but the frequency is unknown.

The risk of developing skin cancer is not equal in all persons. Individuals with fair skin who burn easily on exposure to sun and who tan poorly are especially at risk. Conversely, blacks and dark-skinned whites have a much lower risk. This observation appears to be valid for malignant melanoma, but the association is less convincing than with other forms of skin cancer.

NATURAL HISTORY OF SKIN CANCERS AND EFFECTIVENESS OF THERAPY

Basal cell carcinomas rarely metastasize, but they can be locally invasive and disfiguring; few deaths result. Only about 400 basal cell carcinomas have been reported to have metastasized. This extremely infrequent event usually occurs in patients who have delayed therapy for many years and who have large, locally invasive, eroded lesions.

Several effective forms of therapy exist, all yielding a cure rate of approximately 95 per cent: surgical excision, radiation therapy, dessication and curettage, and cryotherapy with liquid nitrogen applied by special spray apparatus. Treatment of the 5 per cent of basal cell carcinomas which recur presents a greater challenge. The cure rate of a recurrent basal cell carcinoma is about 66 per cent. In the most difficult recurrent and infiltrative basal cell carcinoma, a special form of surgery called Mohs chemosurgery has been developed. In this technique, the tissue is fixed with zinc chloride paste and is examined directly under the microscope to determine whether the tumor has completely been removed. Additional sections of skin are removed until all borders are histopathologically clear of tumor. With the Mohs technique, cure rates of recurrent tumors exceed 90 per cent. The use of 5-fluorouracil has been advocated by some physicians for the treatment of superficial basal cell carcinoma. Experience has not been sufficient to be able to place this modality in relationship to the other forms of therapy which have a clearly established track record, but it may have some role in patients with multiple lesions in whom other techniques cannot be employed.

Squamous cell carcinomas may begin as actinic keratoses, of which perhaps 1 in 1000 eventually undergoes malignant change. There are several effective therapeutic modalities for actinic keratoses. Application of 5-fluorouracil cream or solution twice daily for 2 to 3 weeks will usually result in the destruction of these lesions. Some clinically inapparent lesions will also be destroyed by this therapy. The patient must be warned about the impressive inflammation that occurs when 5-fluorouracil is used. The inflammation can be decreased by the concomitant use of a topical steroid cream. Because 5-fluorouracil also is a photosensitizing agent, treatment in late fall or winter, when solar exposure is diminished, is preferred. Other effective modalities include cryotherapy with liquid nitrogen and light dessication. If a cutaneous horn is present, biopsy of the lesion is warranted to rule out the presence of a squamous cell carcinoma. Actinic keratoses are extremely common and usually present no great threat to life. Treatment is often of cosmetic consequence only.

Bowen's disease or squamous cell carcinoma *in situ* is substantially less common than actinic keratoses. It represents the next grade of neoplasia in the keratinocytic line. Surgical removal of Bowen's disease lesions is probably the most effective treatment. Alternatively, this tumor can be treated satisfactorily by cryotherapy with liquid nitrogen. Five per cent 5-fluorouracil solution applied two to three times daily and covered by a plastic occlusive dressing for 6 weeks may also be employed for treatment of Bowen's disease.

Effective treatment of squamous cell carcinomas includes surgical excision and radiation; the latter is reserved for people over 60.

There are three primary types of *malignant melanomas:* superficial spreading, nodular, and lentigo maligna melanoma. The *superficial spreading type* is the most common in the United States and represents 70 per cent of all malignant melanomas diagnosed. The early lesion exists 1 to 7 years before a nodule develops, indicating that deep penetration has occurred. During this 1 to 7 years, the lesion grows superficially; removal during this time is associated with a 5-year survival rate approaching 100 per cent.

Nodular melanoma has a poorer prognosis. It may arise *de novo* or within a nevus as an invasive tumor from onset. Even with early recognition, metastasis will already have occurred in a certain percentage of patients. This type of tumor can occur on any cutaneous surface, as can the superficial spreading melanoma. Nodular melanoma represents about 15 per cent of all melanomas.

Lentigo maligna melanoma, the third type, represents about 5 per cent of malignant melanomas and occurs on sun-damaged skin of elderly patients. It is the least aggressive of the melanomas and may be present for 5 to 50 years before an invasive nodule develops. Prior to nodule formation, the lesion is termed lentigo maligna. Local excision is satisfactory in the treatment of lentigo maligna; in lentigo maligna melanoma, excision with at least a 1-cm. margin is advocated. Surgical outcome in this type of tumor is almost uniformly favorable, although recurrence is sometimes seen. Nonetheless, it is unusual for a patient to die from disseminated lentigo maligna melanoma.

Systems for determining prognosis now exist so that the extent of surgery can be matched to the degree of severity of the lesion. The most widely used system is that of Clark, in which the anatomic level of invasion of the primary tumor is determined. Four levels of invasion are employed: Level II penetrating into the papillary dermis, Level III filling the papillary dermis, Level IV penetrating into reticular dermis, Level V penetrating into the subcutaneous fat. Five-year survival rates at Massachusetts General Hospital are as follows: Level II, 93 per cent; Level III, 74 per cent; Level IV, 63 per cent; Level V, 39 per cent. Spread to the lymph nodes greatly worsens the prognosis, in that the overall 5-year survival rate is somewhat less than 30 per cent.

Measurement of the thickness of the primary tumor is a sound system for determination of prognosis; tumor thickness is measured with an ocular micrometer on a standard microscope from the granular cell layer down to the deepest tumor cell. This system, along with the anatomic leveling system, has been useful in further refining the prognosis within groups of patients. Lesions smaller than 0.75 mm. have a uniformly favorable prognosis while those greater than 3.00 mm. have a fairly poor prognosis.

At present, wide local excision is recommended for superficial spreading and nodular melanoma with a free margin of 3 to 5 cm. Split thickness skin graft is employed, where necessary, for closure. Recent data suggest that narrower margins may be safely utilized for thin lesions. The usefulness of elective lymph node dissection is still being debated; current evidence suggests that this procedure has no benefit over delaying removal until nodes become clinically involved.

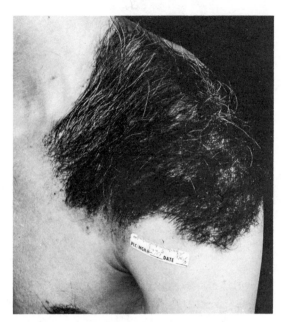

Fig. 164–1. Giant hairy melanocytic nevus.

Nodal dissection is still useful as a staging procedure to identify high-risk patients, enabling meaningful stratification for adjuvant therapy studies.

The treatment of *disseminated melanoma* is at present a difficult and unrewarding problem. The most effective and widely used drug, dimethyl triazenoimidazole carboxamide, has a response rate of approximately 20 per cent. The nitrosoureas such as methyl CCNU are also utilized, and have approximately the same response rate. Even patients who respond usually relapse and die after a few months. At present, combinations of chemotherapy and immunotherapy, such as dimethyl triazenoimidazole carboxamide with BCG, are currently being used and represent an improvement over the use of chemotherapy alone.

Since the prognosis in disseminated melanoma is so poor, attempts are being made to utilize adjuvant therapy postoperatively in patients who are at high risk for recurrence. Recent studies suggest that this may be a useful approach.

Early surgical removal of *giant hairy nevus* (Fig. 164–1) is necessary if development of malignancy is to be prevented. Our current recommendation for treatment of congenital raised, pigmented *melanocytic nevi* is to remove those which have one dimension greater than 1.5 cm.

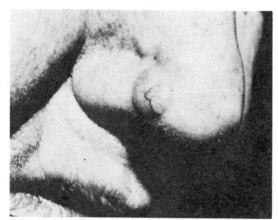

Fig. 164–2.   Nodular basal cell carcinoma. Note telangiectasia.

SCREENING AND DIAGNOSTIC TESTS

Skin cancers are unique in their accessibility and the frequency with which a tissue diagnosis can be made. In the case of *basal cell carcinomas,* the lesion may take several forms. The typical appearance is that of a translucent papule with telangiectasias over the surface (Fig. 164–2) that slowly enlarges and subsequently develops a central ulceration (Fig. 164–3). This lesion has been termed the "rodent ulcer." Basal cell carcinoma may also become pigmented in darker-skinned individuals and be confused with malignant melanoma of the nodular or superficial spreading type. Superficial forms of basal cell carcinoma exist, most commonly, on the back and have the appearance of an erythematous plaque. Usually some papular elements will be present at the border to assist in diagnosis. In a sclerotic form of basal cell carcinoma called the "morphealike" basal cell, nests of tumor cells are interspersed with thick fibrotic bundles. This tumor is more resistant to treatment.

Differential diagnosis of basal cell carcinoma includes dermal nevi and other appendage tumors such as trichoepithelioma. Trichoepithelioma may be clinically indistinguishable from basal cell carcinoma. On histopathologic examination of a basal cell carcinoma, proliferation of basophilic staining cells is seen, usually in nests surrounded by discrete lacunae and located in the upper dermis. This tumor is relatively easy for the pathologist to diagnose microscopically. Because basal cell carcinomas are more frequent in those who have already had one, patients should be followed on an annual basis for early detection of new lesions.

Clinically, *actinic keratoses* appear as flat to slightly raised, scaly erythematous patches, which may be single or multiple and occur predominantly in sun-exposed areas (Fig. 164–4). Often, this lesion is more easily felt (sandpapery) than observed. It appears to go through cycles from macular erythematous lesions through raised scaly lesions. In the later stages a crusted surface, and sometimes even a horn of keratin, develops. Histopathologic examination of these lesions reveals atypical keratinocytes in the basal cell layer of the epidermis.

Bowen's disease usually presents as a chronic, asymptomatic, nonhealing, slowly enlarging erythematous patch usually having a sharp but irregular outline. It may resemble eczematous dermatitis but does not respond to topical steroid therapy (Fig. 164–5). Within the patch, there are generally areas of crusting. The sharp borders, chronicity, and lack of symptoms are clues that suggest the necessity of performing a biopsy. In dark-skinned people, such as some of Mediterranean descent, these lesions may have a brown to blue-grey coloration. Bowen's disease can occur on any part of the skin and on mucocutaneous sites such as the vulva. In the vulvar area, differential diagnosis includes lichen sclerosis et atrophicus, lichen simplex chronicus, squamous cell carcinoma, and, when pigmented, malignant melanoma. On histopathologic examination, atypical keratinocytes are noted throughout the epidermis. There is no invasion of keratinocytes into the dermis.

In the case of *squamous cell carcinoma,* the lesion begins as a flesh-colored, asymptomatic nodule which enlarges and often undergoes ulceration and crusting (Fig. 164–6). The lesion may become quite keratotic and have a thickened surface. A cutaneous

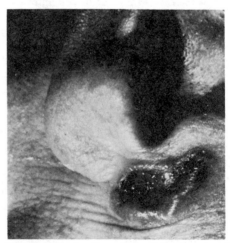

Fig. 164–3.   Basal cell carcinoma—"rodent ulcer."

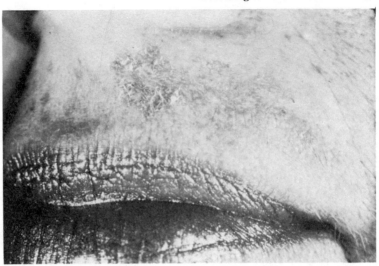

Fig. 164–4. Actinic keratosis on upper lip.

horn may result. Excisional biopsy with close margins is the procedure of choice for the diagnosis of this lesion. Squamous cell carcinoma may sometimes be confused with a benign keratinocytic lesion, which is dome-shaped and exhibits a prominent central plug called a keratoacanthoma (Fig. 164–7). The keratoacanthoma usually exhibits more rapid growth and often regresses spontaneously.

Under the microscope, the squamous cell carcinoma has fingers of atypical keratinocytic cells infiltrating into the dermis. The nuclei are clearly atypical; mitoses are frequently found.

Melanomas share some common characteristics. Hallmarks for clinical recognition of the majority of melanomas include the following features: (1) irregu-

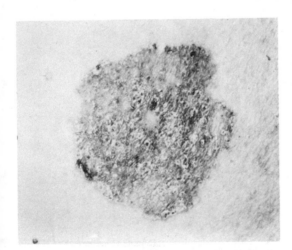

Fig. 164–5. Bowen's disease—squamous cell carcinoma in situ.

larity of the border (sometimes a notch is present; Fig. 164–8), and (2) variegation in the color and pigmentation pattern. Colors in addition to brown and tan, such as red, white, blue, and their admixtures, greys, pinks, and purples, are of great use in distinguishing the overwhelming number of benign pigmented lesions from those that are melanomas. The above characteristics are sometimes found in pigmented basal cell carcinoma and pigmented Bowen's disease. In addition, odd dermal or compound nevi, irritated seborrheic keratoses, and occasionally vascular lesions will be clinically confused with melanoma. The benign blue nevus also shares similar clinical features. Biopsy and histopathologic evaluation by the pathologist are warranted if a lesion meets the criteria noted above.

Each of the different types of melanoma has distinguishing features. *Superficial spreading melanomas* have some irregularity in the border and some alteration in the regularity of pigment pattern and coloration (see Fig. 164–8). *Nodular melanoma,* which arises *de novo* or within nevi as an invasive tumor from the onset, has no radial growth component. It exists as a blue, blue-black, grey nodule of varying size (Fig. 164–9). Most of these lesions are deeply invasive at the time of diagnosis.

The *lentigo maligna* begins as a frecklelike lesion which slowly expands. It has a markedly irregular pigmentation pattern and usually an extremely irregular border. Spontaneous regression may occur; the border may advance on one side while regressing on another, so that the lesion may appear to march across the skin surface. Since about 2 per cent of patients with melanoma incur a second primary, it is

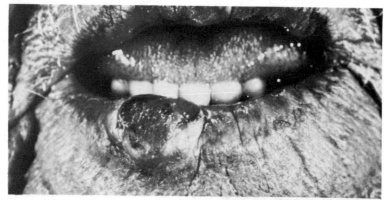

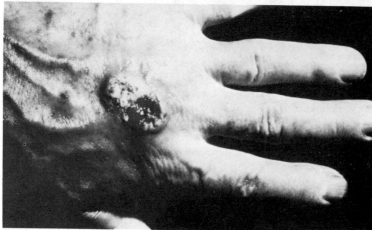

Fig. 164–6. Squamous cell carcinoma in typical locations.

worthwhile to examine the entire skin surface to look for the development of a second tumor upon each encounter. Because a trait favoring the development of melanoma appears to occur in families, family members of patients who have had melanoma should be examined.

Distribution of malignant melanoma across the body surface is not uniform. In both males and females, there is an aggregation on the back, head, and neck. In the female, the lower extremity is heavily affected, but is spared in males, in whom the anterior torso is more likely to be involved. The bra and swim trunk areas are spared in the female, and the swim trunk area and thighs are spared in the male.

CONCLUSIONS AND RECOMMENDATIONS

Screening for skin cancer represents one of the best examples of detection leading to effective treatment. For example, the current 5-year survival rate

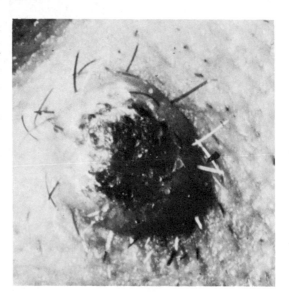

Fig. 164–7. Keratoacanthoma. Note central keratotic plug.

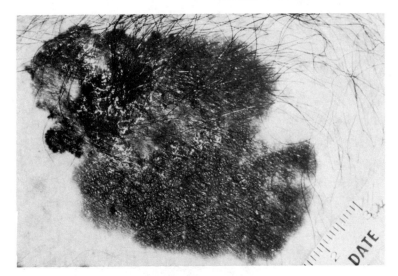

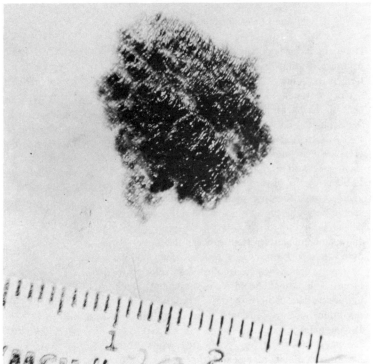

Fig. 164–8. Malignant melanoma of the superficial spreading type. Note irregularity of the border and prominent notch.

for malignant melanoma is 67 per cent, which represents a dramatic increase from the 40 per cent survival rate recorded in 1940. It is estimated that by educating patients and physicians about signs of disease and importance of early diagnosis, the 5-year survival rate for malignant melanoma could approach 85 to 90 per cent.

Every primary physician should be able to recognize the common skin cancers, and his patients should be taught to avoid risk factors and report suspicious lesions. In particular:

- All fair-skinned persons who sunburn easily, and those in whom evidence of solar damage or skin cancer has already developed, should be warned

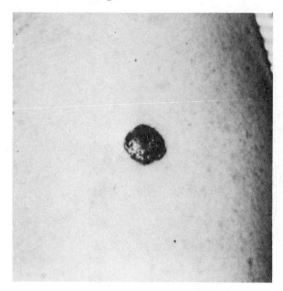

Fig. 164–9. Malignant melanoma, nodular type.

about the hazards of continued high-intensity solar exposure. Rather than suggesting nocturnal activities, it is sufficient to advise that exposure be avoided between 11:00 A.M. and 2:30 P.M.; 70 per cent of the harmful ultraviolet radiation can thus be avoided. The use of sunscreens containing PABA (PreSun, Pabanol) will also serve to decrease the amount of damaging ultraviolet radiation penetrating into the skin.

- Patients with a history of arsenic exposure or previous x-ray therapy with radiation dermatitis should be watched closely for the development of cancer.
- In nonmelanomatous skin cancer, the patient is asked to report any new, slowly growing, nodular or papular lesions which are flesh-colored or translucent. The patient should see a physician if bleeding, ulceration, or horn formation occurs. Areas of maximum solar exposure are at greatest risk.
- In malignant melanoma, the patient is asked to see the physician about any pigmented lesion which has an irregular border or a variation in color, especially blue, grey or black. Any growth in a pigmented lesion should also arouse suspicion.

If any doubt exists, the physician's obligation is either to biopsy the lesion or to refer the patient to an experienced specialist for an opinion. If patients and physicians work together, the incidence of skin cancer and the deaths associated with it can be greatly reduced.

ANNOTATED BIBLIOGRAPHY

Andrade, R., *et al.* (eds.): Cancer of the Skin. Philadelphia: W.B. Saunders, 1976. *(Recent two-volume compendium on all aspects of skin cancer.)*

Clark, W.H. (ed.): Human cutaneous malignant melanomas. Semin. Oncol., *2*:81, 1975. *(Entire issue devoted to melanoma. Covers developmental biology, clinical diagnosis, epidemiology, immunology, surgery and chemotherapy.)*

Epstein, E.H., *et al.*: Mycosis fungoides: Survival, prognostic features, response to therapy, and autopsy findings. Medicine, *51*:61, 1972. *(Comprehensive description of a rare problem.)*

Haynes, H.A.: Primary cancer of skin. *In* Thorn, G.W., *et al.* (eds.): Harrison's Principles of Internal Medicine, ed. 8. New York: McGraw-Hill, 1977, pp. 1795-6. *(Brief discussion of basal cell carcinoma, squamous cell carcinoma and mycosis fungoides [lymphoma].)*

Kopf, A.W., *et al.*: Malignant melanoma: A review. J. Dermatol. Surg. Oncol., *3*:41, 1977. *(Recent comprehensive review.)*

Lever, W.F., and Schaumburg-Lever, G.: Tumors and cysts of the epidermis (Chapter 25), and Tumors of the epidermal appendages (Chapter 26). *In* Histopathology of the Skin, ed. 5. Philadelphia: J.B. Lippincott, 1975. *(Clinical and histopathologic description of cutaneous malignancies.)*

Mihm, M.C., *et al.*: Early detection of primary cutaneous malignant melanoma: A color atlas. N. Engl. J. Med., *289*:989, 1973. *(Eighteen color plates illustrating typical malignant melanomas.)*

Sober, A.J.: Immunology and cutaneous malignant melanoma. Int. J. Dermatol., *15*:1, 1976. *(Review for the general physician of the immunology and immunotherapy of malignant melanoma.)*

Sober, A.J., *et al.*: Early recognition of cutaneous melanoma. JAMA, *242*:2795, 1979. *(Self-assessment approach to the recognition of early lesions in this color atlas.)*

Trozak, D., *et al.*: Metastatic malignant melanoma in prepubertal children. Pediatrics for the Clinician, February 1975. *(Grave indictment of metastatic potential of giant congenital melanocytic nevi.)*

165
Evaluation of Pruritus

Itching (pruritus) is associated with a variety of skin and systemic problems, but it also occurs when there is no underlying disease. Pruritus is particularly common among the elderly. The clinical challenge for the primary physician is to detect any underlying disease, as well as to provide symptomatic relief.

PATHOPHYSIOLOGY AND CLINICAL PRESENTATION

Itching is a cutaneous sensation that arises from a particular pattern of sensory impulses. The sensory receptors are unmyelinated nerve endings located between cells of the epidermis, with higher concentrations in the flexor aspects of the wrist and ankles. The itching sensation is carried by pain fibers in the spinothalamic tracts and is integrated in the thalamus.

Various external stimuli decrease the threshold to itching. These include inflammation, dry skin, and vasodilation. Many chemical mediators of itching have been suggested, including histamine, serotonin, kinins, and prostaglandins. Persons vary in their response to itching. There is a psychological influence on the perception of itching, which explains why a physician may experience itching after attending a patient with scabies or pediculosis.

DIFFERENTIAL DIAGNOSIS

The many conditions that cause itching may be dermatologic, environmental, systemic, or psychological. Dermatologic entities associated with itch include infestation such as pediculosis and scabies, contact dermatitis, urticaria, neurodermatitis, psoriasis, lichen planus, and dermatitis herpetiformis. The most common cause of itching is probably xerosis. Environmental factors that cause itching include sunburn, cats, fiberglass, prickly heat, and overdrying of the skin. Systemic diseases may present or be associated with itching. These include endocrine disorders such as diabetes mellitus, hypo- or hyperthyroidism, and hypercalcemia. Liver disease—particularly obstructive or cholestatic jaundice and,

classically, primary biliary cirrhosis—causes itching. Itching also results from hematologic disorders, including lymphoreticular neoplasm such as lymphoma or mycosis fungoides, polycythemia, particularly after a hot shower, and iron deficiency anemia. Significant uremia is associated with pruritus, as is pregnancy, particularly the last trimester. Allergies to drugs and disorders such as venous stasis, arthropod bites, and parasitic infections may cause itching. Some people experience psychogenic itching, purely a subjective sensation that occurs at night when other stimuli are lacking.

WORKUP

History should focus on trying to determine how severe and widespread the itching is and any symptoms that point to a specific underlying diagnosis. The physician should ask whether itching disturbs sleep, whether it occurs primarily at night, and whether it interferes with daytime activities. If itching does interfere with sleep or activity, treatment is much more imperative. Symptoms should be reviewed for the possibility of associated diseases such as hyperthyroidism, renal failure, liver disease, or drugs.

Physical examination begins with a careful and complete inspection of the skin for evidence of scratching marks, excoriations, or lichenification. The skin should be examined for evidence of inflammation, lice, the interdigital lesions of scabies, or rash suggestive of specific dermatologic diagnosis. The skin, particularly on the legs, chould be examined for scaling and dryness. Lymph nodes should be palpated for enlargement.

Laboratory examination reveals relatively common and treatable conditions. A complete blood count, urinalysis, and blood urea nitrogen test (BUN) constitute an adequate initial screen. If there is no environmental stress, such as winter dryness or obvious skin rash, determination of thyroxine (T_4), calcium, bilirubin levels and obtaining a chest radiograph are justified.

SYMPTOMATIC THERAPY

The patient with itching should be reassured when there is no underlying systemic disease. Many patients may be managed with a conservative therapeutic trial directed at relieving xerosis. Topical approaches include sponging the skin with cool water, substitution of superfatted soaps, humidification of the internal environment, and lubrication before bedtime. The patient should avoid lotions and creams unless they are recommended by the physician. The most effective topical agents available include camphor and phenol, which have an anesthetic quality; menthol, which substitutes a cool sensation for the itch; and hydrocortisone cream or lotion. Calamine lotion is adequate but drying and, therefore, should be limited to weeping lesions. A menthol-phenol combination is useful, but corticosteroid creams or sprays are more effective. If environmental manipulation and topical agents are not effective, then systemic medication must be considered.

The systemic medications that are most used are antihistamines, sedatives, and aspirin. Antihistamines are believed to work by occupying the histamine receptors, but they are specific only for allergically mediated itch. Studies have shown that in most cases antihistamines are no more effective than aspirin. Antihistamines have a sedative quality and can be an effective bedtime medication in patients who have sleep difficulties. The choice of an ideal agent is by trial and error on the basis of the placebo, sedative, and anticholinergic effects of the drug. Good choices include hydroxyzine, an antihistamine with minimal soporific effects; chlorpheniramine, inexpensive in its generic form; and cyproheptadine, effective but more expensive. Because there may be a placebo effect, it might be advisable to start with the cheapest preparation, chlorpheniramine. Sedatives, most commonly diazepam or chlordiazepoxide, are useful for patients who have difficulty sleeping because of the itching. Aspirin, with its low cost and relatively low toxicity, is a useful agent. It has been suggested that its effect is mediated through an anti-inflammatory, antikinin, or prostaglandin-inhibitor effect. Itching due to specific systemic diseases, such as liver obstruction or renal failure, responds to cholestyramine. Dermatologic conditions require specific therapy. Systemic steroids suppress itching but should not be used for symptomatic relief.

PATIENT EDUCATION

All patients with itching can be helped with relatively little risk by several changes in their behavior. They should be told to trim their fingernails and keep them clean to prevent excoriation or infection. It should be noted if vasodilating drugs or foods such as coffee, spices, or alcohol precipitate itching and they should be avoided. Frequent bathing should be avoided because it eliminates the normal oil protection, contributing to dryness. Patients should shower for a short time. The physician should warn against applying lotions or cream except on his recommendation. A simple lubricant can be useful (refer to Chapter 177 for details). Static electricity is known to precipitate itching; therefore, it is sometimes helpful to change one sheet at a time to reduce static electricity. It can also be useful to use Alpha Keri® or other lubricating agents in the rinse cycle when sheets are washed. The physician should advise patients to substitute superfatted soaps for regular soap. They should avoid rough clothing, particularly wool, and use cotton clothing that has been doubly rinsed of detergents. Indoor moisture can be maintained during the winter with humidifiers or by placing bowls of water near the radiator. These measures can be helpful to itching of any etiology and will often reduce or eliminate itching without resort to pharmacologic therapy.

ANNOTATED BIBLIOGRAPHY

Hassar, M., and Weintraub, M.: Treatment of pruritis. Ration. Drug Ther. 9:1 1975. (*A succinct treatment of the subject with an emphasis on therapy.*)

Johnson, S.A.M.: Relieving itching in the geriatric patient. Postgrad. Med. 58:105, 1975. (*A practical paper that recommends small modifications in the external environment to decrease or alleviate itching.*)

Shelley, W.B., and Arthur, R.P.: The neurohistology and neurophysiology of the itch sensation in man. Arch. Dermatol. 76:296, 1957. (*A classic paper on the pathophysiology of itch.*)

Verbov, J.: Itching. Practitioner, 212:854, 1974. (*A good review.*)

Winkelmann, R.K., and Muller, S.A.: Pruritus. Annu. Rev. Med. 15:53, 1964. (*A scholarly review of the literature, emphasizing the prevalence of itching in certain systemic diseases.*)

166
Evaluation of Urticaria
WILLIAM V.R. SHELLOW, M.D.

Urticaria is a usually pruritic eruption of circumscribed wheals on an erythematous base. It is common, with estimates that 10 per cent to 20 per cent of the population experience it at some time. Individual lesions are usually short-lived, but successive crops of lesions may occur. The condition is classified as acute or chronic depending on the duration of the symptoms. Chronic urticaria is defined by persistence of more than 6 to 8 weeks. Establishing a cause for chronic urticaria represents a diagnostic challenge; the primary physician must be capable of evaluating the cause of an urticarial eruption and providing symptomatic treatment.

PATHOPHYSIOLOGY

Urticarial lessions represent a vascular reaction pattern that leads to extravasation of protein-rich fluid from small blood vessels whose permeability has increased. Localized accumulation of fluid produces the characteristic clinical lesions. When extravasation occurs in deep layers of the skin, the cutaneous manifestation is less well circumscribed and is known as "angioedema."

The pathogenesis of urticaria is incompletely understood. It may be precipitated by immunologic or nonimmunologic stimuli, but the cutaneous eruption results from activation of a final common pathway. Mediators, notably histamine, are released from tissue mast cells or circulating basophils. The histamine produces a vascular reaction pattern. Histamine may be released by an innocent-bystander reaction or by activation of the complement enzyme system, which may produce holes in the mast cell membrane allowing histamine to escape. The reaction pattern can be activated by drugs, infection, food allergy, or physical agents such as cold, heat or light. A second pathogenetic mechanism that has been well established results from cutaneous hyperreactivity to acetylcholine, which may be due to inadequate production of cholinesterase. This condition is known as "cholinergic urticaria." In time, better definition of the precipitants of histamine release and probably other mediators of the urticarial reaction will be demonstrated.

DIFFERENTIAL DIAGNOSIS

Urticaria has a long list of possible causes. It may be due to exogenous factors such as inhalants, ingestants, and physical agents, or endogenous sources such as bacterial, fungal, amebic, or parasitic infection. Urticaria is associated with systemic diseases and psychologic stresses.

Common inhalants that produce urticaria include mold, dust, and pollens. *Candida albicans,* which is resident in the gastrointestinal (GI) tract, may have a contributory effect. Aerosols and animal and plant substances are etiologic considerations. Ingestants may cause both acute and chronic urticaria. Food, particularly nuts, chocolate, shellfish, cheese, and berries is an important consideration. Common foods such as milk, eggs, corn, soybean, and wheat rarely may cause chronic urticaria. Drugs and chemicals may be ingested along with foods in the form of artificial colors or preservatives or antioxidants. Penicillin in milk, tartrazine dye in pills, fluoride in drinking water, and even menthol cigarettes have been reported as causes of chronic urticaria. Drugs, including penicillin, aspirin, or barbiturates, may cause urticaria on an allergic basis. Histamine releasers, such as morphine, codeine, thiamine, and pilocarpine, may be urticariagenic agents on a nonallergic basis. It is important to remember that precipitating agents may be absorbed through the conjunctival, vaginal, rectal, or oral mucosa.

Physical agents cause urticaria. Heat is a well-known cause of cholinergic urticaria, while light or cold may produce noncholinergic urticaria. Cold urticaria may be related to cryoglobulinemia, or it may be essential, either familial or acquired. Mechanical stimulation of the skin may give rise to dermographic urticaria.

Endogenous causes of urticaria are predominantly infectious. Bacteria, producing chronic infections such as dental abscesses, sinusitis, cholecystitis, or prostatitis can cause urticaria. Viral infection, particularly mononucleosis, is part of the differential diagnosis. Dermatophytosis and candidiasis are frequent causes of urticaria. *Entamoeba histolytica, Giardia lamblia,* and *Trichomonas vaginalis* may be responsible for urticaria. Parasitic infestations associated with urticaria include strongyloidiasis, ascariasis, uncinariasis, and trichuriasis. Marked eosinophilia may be indicative of parasitosis. Malaria, schistosomiasis, and filariasis may also manifest with chronic urticaria. Systemic diseases that have been associated with urticaria include renal disease, hepatitis, neoplasia, collagen vascular disease, and thyroid disorders. Psychogenic urticaria due to emotional stress must be considered. It should also be noted that two agents may combine to create an urticarial eruption. Hereditary angioedema is a distinct clinical entity with a strong family history and associated GI symptoms.

WORKUP

History. The emphasis of the workup is the history. An exhaustive list of questions may help determine the proximate cause of the urticarial reaction. The physician should ask about recent illness, drug use, and any unusual foods, and he should emphasize drugs, food, and inhalants that have been clearly associated with urticaria. Patients should be encouraged to keep a diary of all foods eaten. They should be screened thoroughly for items of daily use, such as toothpaste, cosmetics, food additives, or birth control pills. The physician should ask about milk products or beer because penicillin in dairy products or yeast in beer may precipitate urticaria. Associated parasympathetic symptoms such as cramps, diarrhea, headache, salivation, or diaphoresis may point to cholinergic urticaria. It should be determined if heat, cold, or light precipitates lesions. A travel history may identify amebic or parasitic infection.

Physical examination is important in evaluating the extent and, occasionally, the etiology of urticaria. Some dermatologists suggest that the clinical appearance is helpful. Bizarre, gyrate hives have been associated with internal malignancy. Lesions without pseudopods suggest allergy. Small lesions with erythematous flares are typical of cholinergic urticaria. The physician should evaluate the extent of urticaria, looking for periorbital or labial swelling and excoriations on the body. He should examine the patient's teeth for tenderness to percussion and palpate for sinus tenderness. He should also palpate for adenopathy, seeking evidence of lymphomas, and examine joints for signs that suggest collagen vascular disease.

Laboratory examination can be selective or exhaustive. It is usually unproductive to seek possible etiologies through laboratory examination without corroborating historical or examination points. There-

fore, a complete blood count, eosinophil count, sedimentation rate, and urinalysis should suffice. The physician should avoid expensive laboratory or radiographic determinations until the clinical evidence points to an underlying etiology.

Several provocative tests can help ascertain the etiology. An ice cube on the skin may induce cold urticaria, and stroking may result in dermographic urticaria. Cholinergic urticaria may be revealed by an intradermal injection of methacholine, 0.1 cc. of a 1:500 dilution. Extensive skin testings for molds, dusts, pollens, or food allergies are difficult to interpret and rarely indicated.

It is sometimes difficult to separate workup from treatment, but a number of therapeutic trials are worth trying in order to identify an etiology. An elimination diet that consists of lamb, rice, string beans, fresh peas, tea, sugar, salt, and rye crackers excludes most common food allergens. A more limited approach is to eliminate dairy products, beer, nuts, shellfish, berries, and food additives. It may be useful to stop all drugs or change preparations or brands to eliminate tartrazine dyes or peculiarities of certain brand-name toothpastes or cosmetics.

The diagnosis of chronic urticaria can be a significant challenge to the physician in terms of both patient and disease management. Some clinicians admit patients for control of diet and long periods of observation. This expensive procedure is notoriously unrewarding because of its expense and the high percentage of patients who remain undiagnosed. A small percentage of patients with chronic urticaria are later found to have an underlying neoplasm or a serious systemic disease, but that is not a universal justification for an extensive workup.

SYMPTOMATIC MANAGEMENT

Antihistamines are the drugs of choice. The most effective agent is hydroxyzine in doses of 10 to 100 mg., four times a day; cyproheptadine, 12 to 20 mg. per day in divided doses, is also very effective. Chlorpheniramine, because of low cost and over-the-counter availability might be tried in doses of 12 to 24 mg. per day. Subcutaneous aqueous epinephrine ameliorates acute attacks, but it is not helpful for chronic urticaria. Acute urticaria may be aborted by parenteral corticosteroids, but in chronic urticaria, corticosteroids that may suppress the eruption are not worth the risks.

Occasionally, therapeutic trials to eliminate common causes of urticaria are worthwhile. Nystatin, 500,000 units, three times a day, may improve the clinical picture by eliminating candida. The association of urticaria with chronic bacterial infection has led to successful resolution with a broad-spectrum antibiotic given for 7 to 10 days. Patients with even asymptomatic trichomonas vaginitis should receive metronidazole, 250 mg., three times a day, for 10 days.

ANNOTATED BIBLIOGRAPHY

Akers, W.A.: Chronic urticaria: Seek at least two causes. Cutis, *10*: 591, 1972. *(An effective demonstration of the multifactorial etiology of chronic urticaria.)*

Akers, W.A., and Naversen, D.M.: Diagnosis of chronic urticaria. Int. J. Dermatol., *17*:616, 1978. *(Scholarly discussion which incorporates a review of the literature from 1971 through 1977; 50 refs.)*

Beakey, J.F.: An allergist looks at urticaria. Cutis, *18*:247, 1976. *(A succinct review, emphasizing the need for careful instruction in elimination diets.)*

Beall, G.N.: Urticarias: A review of clinical and laboratory observations. Medicine (Baltimore), *43*:131, 1964. *(Excellent review, although somewhat dated pathophysiology explanations.)*

Champion, R.W., *et. al.*: Urticaria and angioedema—A review of 554 patients. Br. J. Dermatol., *81*:588, 1969. *(Seventy-nine per cent unknown etiology; atopic history not more frequent; 21% exacerbated by aspirin.)*

Lockshin, N.A., and Hurley, H.: Urticaria as a sign of viral hepatitis. Arch. Dermatol., *105*: 571, 1972. *(An important article that reported the association of urticaria and antigen-antibody reactions in hepatitis.)*

Matthews, K.P.: A current view of urticaria. Med. Clin. North Am., *58*:185, 1974. *(A comprehensive review.)*

Ramsay, C.A.: Solar urticaria. Int. J. Dermatol., *19*:233, 1980. *(Review of the topic.)*

Shapiro, G.G., Bierman, W., and Pierson, W.E.: Urticaria: The final common pathway. Cutis, *13*:957, 1974. *(Concise presentation of the pathophysiology of urticaria.)*

Zamm, A.V.: Chronic urticaria: A practical approach. Cutis, *9*:27, 1972. *(A superb classification of the types of urticaria, with outlines for the workup of chronic urticaria.)*

167
Evaluation of Hyperhidrosis
WILLIAM V.R. SHELLOW, M.D.

Excessive sweating is not an uncommon complaint, but it rarely signifies underlying pathology. Medical consultation may be sought because of abnormal wetness, a change in the pattern or amount of sweating, sweaty palms, stained clothing, or offensive odor. There is much variation in the amount people sweat in response to the physiologic stimuli of heat, emotion, or eating. The interaction of the person, the environment, and his emotions influences the amount of sweating. The primary physician must offer scientific explanation and symptomatic management to the person who complains of excessive sweating.

PATHOPHYSIOLOGY AND CLINICAL PRESENTATION

Sweating helps maintain temperature and fluid and electrolyte homeostasis, particularly under the environmental stresses of heat. There are two kinds of sweat glands, eccrine and apocrine. Cooling results from evaporation of eccrine sweat. Eccrine glands are concentrated on the palms and soles and are present on the face, axillae, and, to a lesser extent, the back and chest. Heat causes sweating on the face, upper chest, and back. Sweating of the palms and soles is a characteristic response to stress. Gustatory sweating occurs on the face, particularly the upper lip, and following ingestion of spiced foods. The eccrine glands have no anatomic relationship to other cutaneous appendages.

Sebaceous and apocrine glands are intimately associated with hair follicles. The apocrine glands are concentrated in the axillae, areolae, groin, and perineum. Apocrine secretion is minuscule drops, viscid, and milky, producing odor after bacteria act upon it.

Eccrine sweating is controlled by neural factors or a reflex. Thermal sweating is governed by the hypothalamus; emotional sweating by the cerebral cortex. The innervation of eccrine glands is anatomically sympathetic, but for reasons that are unexplained the sweat glands are under cholinergic control. Excess sweating may be induced by abnormalities of the autonomic nervous system. Autonomic overactivity of the sweat glands may occur without identifiable cause. Sweating is associated with medical diseases that increase metabolic activity, causing the need for dissipation of heat. Though the eccrine glands are under cholinergic control, epinephrine stimulates excessive sweating.

DIFFERENTIAL DIAGNOSIS

Most cases of excess sweating are due to exaggerated physiologic responses or functional variations of no pathologic consequence. Hyperhidrosis most commonly involves the palms, soles, or axillae. This may be due to an increase in impulses from the central nervous system (CNS), or it may reflect underlying problems with the sweat glands. There is often a relationship to emotional stress, and the problem is disabling when it interferes with work or social interactions. Axillary hyperhidrosis is less common than palmar or plantar, producing the need for frequent clothing changes. The most common pathologic cause of hyperhidrosis is fever. It is well known that during defervescence sweating occurs, particularly at night. Night sweats indicate the possibility of underlying infectious disease. Central neurologic injury from stroke or tumor may produce hyperhidrosis. Peripheral neuropathy associated with the autonomic nerves may produce excess sweating. Medical conditions associated with abnormal sweating include menopause, thyrotoxicosis, and, uncommonly, pheochromocytoma. Parkinson's disease may cause increased sweating and sebaceous activity. Various drugs, such as antipyretics, insulin, meperidine, emetics, alcohol, and pilocarpine may induce sweating. Gustatory sweating, though uncommon, may be due to compensatory diabetic neuropathy, damage to the seventh nerve during parotid surgery, the rare Frey syndrome, or injury to the sympathetic trunk following surgery. Excess sweating due to anxiety or the perception of excess sweating due to functional disorder must always be considered.

WORKUP

History. The workup should identify whether excess sweating is restricted to the axillae, affects the palms and soles, or is more generalized. In patients with axillary hyperhidrosis, the physician should inquire about family history because there is a familial form of this disorder. The physician should determine whether sweating occurs primarily at night and, if so, whether there is fever, fatigue, or any other symptom of a subacute infectious or malignant process. He should inquire about symptoms of thyroid overactivity, and note whether the patient has recently entered menopause. A careful drug history is needed, emphasizing agents that are known to cause excess sweating. The physician should ask whether excess sweating is relatively recent and can be correlated with stress.

Physical examination can identify objective evidence of excess sweating. The patient should be examined for signs of hyperthyroidism. Blood pressure determination is important because if paroxysmal hypertension, flushing, and sweating are present, pheochromocytoma should be considered. The cranial nerves and retina should be examined because of the possibility of CNS disease. There are no mandatory laboratory investigations, but a thyroxine (T_4), blood sugar, or urine vanillylmandelic acid (VMA) should be ordered if there is a clinical indication.

SYMPTOMATIC MANAGEMENT

The primary etiology of excess sweating is usually unknown, and its significance is restricted to the extent of interference with employment or cosmesis. Many therapies have been utilized. Topical therapies include 10 per cent formalin compresses, which can induce allergic sensitization. Buffered glutaraldehyde is effective but stains the skin. Scopolamine and other anticholinergics have been effective, but they may precipitate glaucoma or obstruction from prostatic hypertrophy.

The following steps can be used in symptomatic management:

- Reassure the patient that excess sweating is not due to a pathologic condition.
- For axillary sweating, recommend frequent washing and changes of clothing.
- For excess sweating of the palms or the axillae, the most effective agent currently available is a 20 per cent alcoholic solution of aluminum chloride hexahydrate (Drysol). Apply at bedtime, covered with a plastic wrap or polyethylene gloves. In the morning, wash with soap and water. Clinical improvement in axillary hyperhidrosis may be seen after one to three consecutive treatments per week.
- If topical therapy and reassurance fail, surgery may be considered if hyperhidrosis significantly in-

terferes with occupational or social life. Axillary hyperhidrosis may be cured with surgical extirpation of the eccrine glands in the axillae. Palmar sweating may respond to sympathectomy.

PATIENT EDUCATION

Patient education is crucial to the treatment of excess sweating. Providing the patient with a scientific explanation and firm understanding of sweating is helpful in relieving anxiety. Patients with night sweats should record their temperature so that any significant febrile illness can be identified. The application of topical agents should be well explained and carefully used by patients. Surgical intervention for a problem as minor as hyperhidrosis requires the patient's understanding of the risks and benefits of such a procedure and the active involvement of the primary physician in helping the patient reach a decision.

ANNOTATED BIBLIOGRAPHY

Adar, R., Kurchin, A., and Zweig, A.: Palmar hyperhidrosis and its surgical treatment. A report of 100 cases. Ann. Surg., *186*:34, 1977. *(A report of an 89 per cent success rate in 93 patients who underwent bilateral upper dorsal sympathectomy for palmar hyperhidrosis; a good review of surgical approaches; 40 refs.)*

Bloor, K.: Gustatory sweating and other responses after cervicothoracic sympathectomy. Brain, *92*:137, 1969. *(Incidence as high as 36 per cent. This study showed 29 of 146 patients.)*

Chalmers, J.M., and Keele, C.A.: The nervous and chemical control of sweating. Br. J. Dermatol., *64*:43, 1952. *(Definitive review of the pathophysiology of eccrine sweat production.)*

Cunliffe, W.J., and Tan, S.G.: Hyperhidrosis and hypohidrosis. Practitioner, *216*:149, 1976. *(A good review of differential diagnosis and treatment.)*

Hurley, H.J., and Shelley, W.B.: Axillary hyperhidrosis. Clinical features and local surgical management. Br. J. Dermatol., *78*:127, 1966. *(The surgical technique of removing eccrine sweat glands from the axilla.)*

Hurley, H.J., and Shelley, W.B.: A simple surgical approach to the management of axillary hyperhidrosis. JAMA, *186*:109, 1963. *(Surgical excision of the eccrine glands in the axilla can be used in refractory hyperhidrosis.)*

Levit, F.: Treatment of hyperhidrosis by tap water iontophoresis. Cutis, *26*:193, 1980. *(Use of galvanic generator to control palmar and plantar hyperhidrosis.)*

Shelley, W.B., and Hurley, H.J.: Studies on axillary antiperspirants. Acta Derm. Venereol. (Stockh.), *55*:241, 1975.

168
Evaluation of Purpura

Purpura represents bleeding into the skin. In the office setting, it may be encountered as a complaint related to easy or spontaneous bruising or to a rash. Petechiae (red macules that measure less than 3 mm. in diameter) usually reflect a defect in platelets or vessel walls. Ecchymoses are larger than 3 mm. in diameter and appear with disorders of the clotting system as well as with vascular and platelet problems. Many cases of purpura are caused by unappreciated trauma. Patients who complain of easy or spontaneous bruising need to be evaluated for a bleeding diathesis. In those with petechial rashes, consideration of vasculitis and bacteremia, as well as of disorders of platelets and connective tissue, is required.

PATHOPHYSIOLOGY AND CLINICAL PRESENTATION

Purpura results from a break in small dermal blood vessels and occurs in perfectly normal people in response to significant trauma. The appearance of purpura in multiple sites simultaneolusly or in areas where trauma was trivial or absent suggests a problem in the hemostatic mechanism. The integrity of vessels is maintained by quantitatively and qualitatively adequate platelets and healthy connective tissue. A break in a vessel triggers formation of platelet plug followed by a fibrin clot. Disturbances of platelets present in the skin as petechial lesions, usually in dependent areas. Damage to the capillary endothelium produces a similar clinical picture. Coagulation defects cause delayed but more prolonged blood loss, during which continuous oozing due to inadequate fibrin clot formation results in ecchymoses rather than petechiae.

Platelet disorders are among the most common causes of purpura. *Thrombocytopenic purpura* is not encountered until the platelet count falls below 50,000. The onset and severity of purpura is highly variable; no difficulty may be noted until the platelet count drops well below 10,000, perhaps reflecting the continued integrity of the blood vessel wall in the presence of even a scant population of platelets. Bleeding from other sites may ensue before purpura appears (see Chapter 79).

Defective platelet function is often related to drugs which inhibit adenosine diphosphate (ADP) release, though hereditary thrombocytopathies sometimes account for easy bruising. Aspirin, indomethacin, phenylbutazone and other anti-inflammatory agents block ADP release. The effect can be induced by as little as 600 mg. of aspirin and persists for the life span of the platelets made during the time aspirin is present. Significant bleeding rarely results solely from use of platelet-active drugs, but an underlying bleeding diathesis may be aggravated and hemorrhage precipitated. Platelet function is also impaired in patients with cirrhosis or uremia. Generalized oozing from many sites is sometimes a serious problem in renal failure; the platelet defect can be reversed by dialysis. Platelet function in dysproteinemias may become a problem due to coating with abnormal globins. *Excess platelets*—as in polycythemia vera—may not function normally, and lead to bleeding (see Chapter 78).

Vascular and *connective tissue defects* compromise vessel walls and supportive extravascular structures, leading to easy bruising. Purpura may be caused by pressure applied by clothing or, in elderly patients and those taking corticosteroids, result from trivial trauma. The presentation is usually in the face, neck, dorsum of the hands, forearms and legs; degeneration of dermal collagen is the presumed cause. A variant is the production of stasis or orthostatic purpura, usually occurring in the lower extremities of an elderly patient following a prolonged period of standing. Stasis dermatitis also causes petechial lesions in the legs resulting from a capillaritis. Scurvy compromises the vascular endothelium, and perifollicular purpura develops due to increased capillary fragility. In amyloidosis, deposition of amyloid in the skin and subcutaneous tissue causes fragile vessels with ecchymoses forming when the skin is pinched.

Small vessel vasculitis represents immunologically mediated inflammation and necrosis of arterioles and capillaries. Skin, mucous membranes, brain, lung, heart, kidneys, muscle, and gastrointestinal tract may be affected. Precipitants include drug hypersensitivity reactions (sulfonamides, penicillin, tetracycline, quinidine, guanethidine, phenacetin, phenothiazines, propylthiouracil) and connective tissue diseases such as rheumatoid arthritis, systemic lupus erythematosus and cryoglobulinemia. Petechial papules (palpable purpura) which do not blanch are characteristic of vasculitis and appear in symmetric fashion; dependent areas predominate. Urticaria, vesicles and necrotic ulcerations may also develop. Fever, arthralgias, myalgias, arthritis, pulmonary infiltrates, effusions, pericarditis, peripheral neuropathy, abdominal pain, bleeding and encephalopathy can occur along with the petechial rash. The skin commonly itches, stings or burns. Hematuria and proteinuria are often detected.

Infections which enter the bloodstream may lead to vascular injury and formation of petechiae which sometimes are palpable. Petechial lesions associated with subacute bacterial endocarditis are flat, do not blanch, and appear on the upper chest, neck and extremities in addition to the mucous membranes. In gonococcal and meningococcal septicemias, petechiae develop early, become pustular and then turn hemorrhagic and necrotic. The lower extremities are a common site for the gonococcal lesions, which resolve within 5 to 7 days. The rash of Rocky Mountain spotted fever begins as pink macules on the wrists, soles, ankles, and palms, spreads centripetally, and by the fourth day becomes petechial and papular. Hemorrhagic, ulcerated lesions may follow.

Anticoagulant use, unless excessive, and mild hepatocellular failure do not cause spontaneous bleeding into the skin. Easy bruising following trivial trauma, with formation of ecchymoses, occurs when anticoagulant levels are far beyond therapeutic range or from severe hepatocellular failure. The bleeding is typically oozing and slow to stop. Abuse of these agents is seen in health care personnel. *Coumadin necrosis* is an idiosyncratic hemorrhagic necrosis of unkown etiology which occurs in patients who are in therapeutic range (see Chapter 84).

Autoerythrocyte sensitization is a puzzling form of purpura characterized by spontaneous, painful ecchymoses surrounded by erythema and edema. Headache, nausea and vomiting sometimes accompany the purpura. Intradermal injection of autologous red cells can reproduce the clinical picture. Many patients with this condition have pronounced psychoneurotic complaints.

Purpura simplex is a designation for idiopathic disease. The patient is typically a woman who is in otherwise good health.

DIFFERENTIAL DIAGNOSIS

Purpura can be conveniently divided into thrombocytopenic and nonthrombocytopenic categories (see Chapter 79). Nonthrombocytopenic purpuras are classified according to whether platelet function is defective, abnormalities exist in connective tissue, or vascular integrity has been compromised by degeneration or inflammation. The most common causes of purpura are trauma, benign purpura simplex, senile purpura and drug-induced impairment of platelet function. The extensive list of disorders that must be considered in the patient presenting with petechial or purpuric lesions is presented in Table 168–1.

WORKUP

The workup of the patient complaining of purpuric lesions must emphasize history and physical examination to avoid costly and nonproductive laboratory evaluations. A careful characterization of the site, size and duration of the lesions is essential. Lesions less than 6 cm. in size localized to areas in which trauma is common, such as the thighs, are less likely to be of pathologic significance.

History. A carefully taken history should include inquiry into blood loss from other sites, easy bruisability, and prolonged, heavy bleeding with menstruation, surgery or dental work. The family history is important because there exist numerous hereditary familial purpuric syndromes and a variety of thrombocytopathies, particularly the autosomal dominant von Willebrand's disease. The drug history is essential, focusing on anticoagulants, agents with antiplatelet effects (e.g., aspirin, dipyridamole, phenylbutazone, sulfinpyrazone, indomethacin and the newer anti-inflammatory agents such as ibuprofen, tolectin and naproxen), and drugs which are frequently a source of hypersensitivity reactions (antibiotics, quinidine, phenothiazines).

Associated symptoms—e.g., fever, itching, pleuritic chest pain, abdominal pain, vaginal or penile discharge, myalgias, arthralgias, arthritis, morning stiffness, numbness, paresthesias—provide important diagnostic information. Symptoms of renal disease or hepatocellular failure should be noted.

Physical examination begins with inspection of the skin lesions. Petechiae do not blanch when a glass slide is pressed over them; many nonpurpuric erythematous lesions do. Blanching lesions must not be dismissed too hastily, because telangiectasias and spider angiomas are signs of conditions predisposing to purpura. The size, number and location of purpuric lesions should be recorded, and note made of whether they are palpable or macular, petechial or ecchymotic. Tenderness suggests psychogenic purpura. It is sometimes helpful to circle ecchymoses so that extension or regression may be followed objectively.

A general physical examination is performed, looking for temperature elevation, cushingoid appearance, jaundice, mucosal petechiae, adenopathy, pleural effusion, heart murmur, rub, hepatomegaly, ascites, splenomegaly, purulent vaginal or urethral discharge, joint inflammation, edema, and nuchal rigidity; excessively neurotic behavior may be noted.

The tourniquet test has been used to assess capillary fragility. The test can be performed in the office

Table 168–1.   Important Causes of Purpura

Thrombocytopenic (see Chapter 79)
Nonthrombocytopenic
    Platelet Defects
      1. Nonsteroidal anti-inflammatory agents
      2. Uremia
      3. Thrombocytopathies (hereditary)
      4. Dysproteinemias
      5. Thrombocythemia (polycythemia vera)
    Vascular Defects
      1. Trauma
      2. Venous stasis
      3. Vasculitis (drugs, connective tissue disease, infection)
      4. Amyloidosis
      5. Scurvy
      6. Hereditary hemorrhagic telangiectasia
    Extravascular Support Defects
      1. Age
      2. Cushing's syndrome or corticosteroid use
    Coagulation Defects
      1. Excessive anticoagulant use
      2. Hereditary conditions
      3. Hepatocellular failure
  Idiopathic
      1. Purpura simplex
      2. Erythrocyte autosensitization (psychogenic purpura)
      3. Coumarin necrosis

by inflating the blood pressure cuff to a point half-way between systolic and diastolic blood pressure, maintaining it for 5 minutes, and then releasing it. A positive tourniquet test is demonstrated by 15 or more petechiae in an area the size of a nickel. This test is diagnostic not of thrombocytopenia, but rather of increased capillary fragility. There are some false-positives; petechiae have been demonstrated in 8 per cent of normal individuals.

Laboratory studies. A few tests usually suffice. The peripheral blood smear is studied for presence of platelets. If they are present, significant thrombocytopenia is unlikely. A platelet count can be used to confirm the impression obtained from peripheral smear and to detect any thrombocytosis. A count greater than 800,000 identifies thrombocythemia. A bleeding time is the best screening test for platelet function. The Ivy method is widely used and best performed with a template to ensure an incision 1 mm. deep and 1 cm. long. The cut is made in an avascular area of the forearm while venous return is obstructed with a blood pressure cuff inflated to 40 mm. Hg. Blotting paper is applied to the edge of the incision. A normal result is cessation of blotter-detected oozing by 9 minutes.

Ecchymotic lesions should be evaluated with prothrombin and partial thromboplastin times to be sure there are no defects in the extrinsic or intrinsic coagulation pathways. Patients on oral anticoagulants and those with hepatobiliary disease are also candidates for a PT and PTT.

When palpable purpura is noted, a skin biopsy is needed to confirm vasculitis; it should also be cultured and Gram-stained for organisms. If fever is present in conjunction with petechiae, blood cultures must be obtained. An ANA and rheumatoid factor may be of help, as well.

A stool guaiac test and urinalysis are performed for detection of occult blood loss; in addition, protein and casts are looked for in the urine. In the elderly patient who is at risk for dysproteinemia, a sedimentation rate and serum globin level can be used for screening, and immunoelectrophoresis obtained if these determinations are elevated.

SYMPTOMATIC MANAGEMENT AND PATIENT EDUCATION

Detailed reassurance needs to be given to the patient with no hematologic or systemic abnormality, but only *after* thorough evaluation has been completed. In the elderly patient, supportive explanation that this is a normal concomitant of aging is often helpful. Cessation of drugs that impair platelet function, such as aspirin, indomethacin, phenylbutazone, or newer nonsteroidal anti-inflammatory agents, is advisable but not mandatory. Patients who need these drugs for the treatment of a chronic disease may learn to accept the cosmetic unpleasantness of ecchymoses. Occasionally, otherwise healthy patients buy and take large doses of vitamins C and K in hopes of lessening easy bruisability. Such self-treatment is without any proven efficacy and adds an unnecessary expense. However, the patient with hepatocellular failure may show mild improvement with parenteral vitamin K, provided some synthetic function remains. Patients with thrombocytopenia must pay careful attention to avoiding trauma (see Chapter 79).

INDICATIONS FOR ADMISSION

Any patient with fever and purpura requires prompt hospital admission, since vasculitis and septicemia are possible. The person who gives evidence of bleeding from multiple sites is best hospitalized. Absence of platelets on smear and a very prolonged bleeding time are more safely evaluated in the inpatient setting.

ANNOTATED BIBLIOGRAPHY

Davis, E.: Purpura of the skin: A review of 500 cases. Lancet, 2:160, 1943. *(A good review; includes the mild petechiae and small ecchymoses of purpura simplex.)*

Harker, L.A., and Slichter, S.J.: The bleeding time as a screening test for evaluation of platelet function. N. Engl. J. Med., 287:155, 1972. *(The bleeding time is a useful screening test for evaluating platelet function.)*

Hazard, G.W., et al.: Rocky Mountain spotted fever in the eastern United States. N. Engl. J. Med., 280:57, 1969. *(Describes the clinical syndrome well and documents its occurrence in the east; rash is key to diagnosis.)*

Kramer, J.: Capillary resistance and its relation to bleeding. *In* S.A. Johnson, R.W. Monto, J.W. Rebuck, et al.: Blood Platelets. Boston: Little, Brown, 1961. *(A good description of capillary fragility testing showing that at least 8 per cent of normal individuals have increased capillary fragility.)*

Nalbandian, R.M., Mader, I.J. Barre, H.J.L., *et al.*: Petechiae, ecchymosis, and necrosis of skin induced by coumarin congeners. JAMA, *192*:603, 1965. *(Description of this unusual complication.)*

O'Reilly, R.A., and Aggeler, P.M.: Covert anticoagulant ingestion: Study of 25 patients and review of world literature. Medicine 55:389, 1976. *(A reminder that covert anticoagulant ingestion may occur in patients, particularly those who are paramedical personnel.)*

Ratnoff, O.D., and Agle, D.P.: Psychogenic purpura: A re-evaluation of the syndrome of autoerythrocyte sensitization. Medicine, *47*:476, 1968. *(A careful analysis of this syndrome of painful ecchymoses and a characteristic personality profile.)*

Shuster, A., and Scarboro, H.: Senile purpura. Q. J. Med., *30*:33, 1961. *(Good description of this commonly occurring problem.)*

Soloway, H.B.: Drug-induced bleeding. Am. J. Clin. Path., *61*:622, 1974. *(A comprehensive review by mechanism of drugs that alter hemostasis and may produce purpura.)*

Wallerstein, R.O., and Wallerstein, R.O., Jr.: Scurvy. Semin. Hematol., *13*:211, 1976. *(A review of this uncommon deficiency state showing that hemorrhage may be deep as well as superficial.)*

Weiss, H.J.: Platelets: Physiology and abnormalities of function. N. Engl. J. Med., *293*:531, 580, 1975. *(Reviews platelet function in detail.)*

Zucker, S., Mielke, C.H., Durocher, J.R., *et al.*: Oozing and bruising due to abnormal platelet function (thrombocytopathia). Ann. Intern. Med., *76*: 725, 1972. *(A very good article showing minor platelet dysfunction in patients complaining of purpura.)*

169

Evaluation of Disturbances in Pigmentation
WILLIAM V.R. SHELLOW, M.D.

Disturbances in pigmentation are both conspicuous and common. Patients often complain about general darkening, brown spots, or depigmented areas. Pigmentary alterations may be manifestations of a genetic, endocrine, metabolic, nutritional, infectious, or neoplastic problem. Physical and chemical factors also can be important.

Hypomelanosis or depigmentation may result from genetic loss of melanocytes or destruction by inflammation. Inflammation may be secondary to infection or burns or associated with a variety of immunologically mediated diseases.

PATHOPHYSIOLOGY AND CLINICAL PRESENTATION

Pigmentary changes are caused by melanin being absent, increased, decreased, or abnormally placed or distributed. Hyperpigmentation may result from an increased rate of melanosome production, an increased number of melanosomes transferred to keratinocytes, or a greater size and melanization of the melanosome. Hyperpigmentation is perceived as blue when melanin is located deeply due to the Tyndall phenomenon. The pathophysiologic mechanisms that produce hyperpigmentation through the melanocyte system include elevated adrenocorticotropic hormone (ACTH) which has a melanocyte-stimulating action, ultraviolet radiation, and certain drugs.

DIFFERENTIAL DIAGNOSIS

Hyperpigmentation

The differential diagnosis of hyperpigmentation is organized on the basis of whether the hyperpigmentation is circumscribed or diffuse.

Circumscribed hyperpigmentation includes freckles (ephelides), lentigines, and melasma. *Freckles* are small macular lesions seen on areas exposed to the sun. Freckles may become less dark in adults, but darken after exposure to long-wave ultraviolet radiation.

Lentigines are macular, larger and darker than freckles. Histologically, the two are easily distinguishable. Senile lentigines appear on sun-exposed areas in older patients. They are termed "liver spots" by patients.

Melasma or *chloasma* is a blotchy hyperpigmentation that occurs on the forehead, cheeks, and upper lip, usually in women. Pregnancy, oral contraceptives, and other hormones contribute to their appearance, but exposure to sunlight appears to perpetuate the condition. During pregnancy, a physiologic darkening of the linea alba, pigmented nevi, nipples, and genitalia occurs as a result of melanocyte-stimulating hormone (MSH), and to increased estrogen and progesterone.

Diffuse hyperpigmentation results from increased amounts of melanin in the epidermis. The color may be accentuated in sun-exposed areas, over pressure points or body folds, or in areas of trauma such as new scars. Increased pigmentation occurs in *Addison's disease* owing to increased amounts of MSH and ACTH from the pituitary because of decreased cortisol levels.

Metabolic disease such as Wilson's disease, von Gierke's hemochromatosis, biliary cirrhosis, and porphyria cutanea tarda may be accompanied by diffuse melanosis. On occasion, rheumatoid arthritis, Still's disease, and scleroderma have been associated with hyperpigmentation.

Drugs such as busulfan and cyclophosphamide may produce diffuse melanosis, as can topical nitrogen mustard. Chronic inorganic arsenic poisoning causes diffuse hyperpigmentation with normal or lighter skin areas scattered throughout and colorfully called "rain drops in the dust." Chlorpromazine and antimalarials tend to produce a bluish gray hyperpigmentation. Silver (argyria) and gold (chrysiasis) may accumulate in the skin leading to hyperpigmentation depending upon the dose given.

Diffuse melanosis may be seen during *starvation,* with *hepatic insufficiency, malabsorption syndromes,* and *lymphomas and other malignancies.* Also included in the differential diagnosis are *deficiencies* of vitamins A, C, and B_{12}, niacin, and folic acid.

Postinflammatory hyperpigmentation may occur secondary to a number of precipitants. For example, phytophotodermatitis occurs after contact with photosensitizing agents present in meadow grass, citrus fruits, and edible plants that cause an exaggerated sunburn. Hyperpigmentation follows the acute phase. Skin contact with organic dyes and aromatic compounds may lead to photosensitization followed by hyperpigmentation. Tar, pitch, and oils may induce similar changes.

Physical trauma, friction, and heat may also lead to postinflammatory pigmentary changes, as may inflammatory dermatoses that stimulate melanin formation.

Hypopigmentation

Hypopigmentation may be hereditary or acquired. A hereditary disorder may be associated with a lack or deficiency of melanin. Melanocytes that are deficient or lacking occur in the depigmented areas of partial albinism (piebaldism). A white forelock may be present. In oculocutaneous albinism, melanocytes are normal in number but unable to produce melanin.

Diseases involving abnormal amino acid metabolism, such as phenylketonuria and homocystinuria, have associated hypopigmentation of skin and hair. In tuberous sclerosis, elongated hypopigmented patches are seen. Certain cutaneous diseases lead to loss of melanin into the dermis, lending a gray appearance to the skin.

Vitiligo is a common, acquired disorder of hypopigmentation that may become progressive. Any area of the skin, usually in early adult life, may be the first affected. Lesions may be symmetrical, primarily on exposed skin, on intertriginous areas, over bony prominences, or around orifices. In involved areas, the hair may be white. The border may be sharp and hyperpigmented. Occasionally, vitiligo assumes a segmental or zosteriform pattern. Halo nevi, centrifugal areas of depigmentation that surround a pigmented nevus, accompany one-third of the cases of vitiligo.

Partial repigmentation of vitiligo may occur in sun-exposed areas, but vitiliginous patches may burn because of the lack of protective pigmentation. Vitiligo has been associated with autoimmune diseases such as pernicious anemia, collagen diseases and hypo- and hyperthyroidism. Diabetes mellitus, alopecia areata, male hypogonadism, hypopituitarism, and Cushing's syndrome have been associated with diffuse hypopigmentation.

Depigmentation may be caused by a variety of chemical agents, rubber, antioxidants, germicides, and, most notably, phenolic compounds that interfere with tyrosinase activity. Dermatitis may precede the loss of pigment, and areas remote from the inflamed sites may also lose pigment.

Dermatoses and infections may result in localized areas of pigment loss. Such areas may be more noticeable in dark-skinned persons. Small hypopigmented areas occur on women's legs and may be related to the trauma of shaving. Tinea versicolor, pityriasis alba, and various eczematous conditions may present as areas of hypopigmentation.

WORKUP

Hyperpigmentation

Evaluation of the patient with localized hyperpigmentation requires inspection of the lesions and inquiry about previous dermatoses and the use of oral contraceptives that may produce melasma. The majority of localized hyperpigmented areas are postinflammatory and of only cosmetic concern. Diffuse hyperpigmentation necessitates a careful history that specifies the time of onset and possible sun exposure. A drug history that emphasizes agents known to produce pigmentary changes should be pursued. There should be general review of systems, noting weakness associated with Addison's disease; itching and hepatic dysfunction associated with biliary cirrhosis. The physician should consider the possibility of severe vitamin deficiency or malnutrition. The history should be followed by a physical examination that notes hyperpigmentation in creases and scars, as are characteristic of Addison's disease, and clues to obvious underlying pathology, as may occur with malignancy, hepatic insufficiency, or malabsorption. Laboratory investigation must be based on clinical signs of underlying disease. Biopsy may be indicated when heavy metal deposition or hemosiderosis is a diagnostic consideration.

Hypopigmentation

Hypopigmentation requires a careful history of approximate time of onset and possible exposure to bleaching agents, most notably phenol-containing products. Hypopigmented areas should be scraped, and a KOH wet mount examined microscopically to diagnose tinea versicolor. It may also help differentiate the total depigmentation of vitiligo from partial postinflammatory hypopigmentation. Patients with vitiligo should undergo a careful general review of systems and a physical examination that seeks to identify diseases such as pernicious anemia, thyroid disease, diabetes, or collagen vascular disease known to be associated with the condition.

SYMPTOMATIC THERAPY

Hyperpigmentation

In treating hyperpigmented areas, the chief symptomatic advice is strict avoidance of sunlight.

Topical bleaching with hydroquinone cream may be effective. Strong topical corticosteroid preparations have a pigment-lightening effect, as does retinoic acid.

Hypopigmentation

Hypopigmented areas can usually be masked by appropriate cosmetics, by bleaching normal skin, or by repigmentation with psoralens and ultraviolet radiation. The primary physician must assess the desire for treatment and inform the patient of the alternatives. Treatment should probably be supervised by a dermatologist experienced in using these agents to achieve optimal cosmetic results.

It is important to reassure the patient that there is no systemic disease. The primary physician should advise the patient about cosmetic alternatives and help the patient decide on an appropriate course of treatment.

ANNOTATED BIBLIOGRAPHY

Bleehen, S.S., Pathak, M.A., Hori, Y., and Fitzpatrick, T.B.: Depigmentation of skin with 4-isopropylacatechol, mercaptoamines and other compounds. J. Invest. Dermatol., *50*:103, 1968. *(An investigative screening of 33 compounds to assess depigmenting ability.)*

Cunliffe, W.J., et al.: Vitiligo, thyroid diseases and autoimmunity. Br. J. Dermatol. *80*:135:1968. *(Confirms the association of vitiligo with thyroid disease, pernicious anemia, alopecia areata, and diabetes mellitus.)*

El Mofty, A.M., and El Mofty, M: Vitiligo: A symptom complex. Int. J. Dermatol., *19*:237, 1980. *(Discussion of vitiligo and its association with systemic disease.)*

Kahn, G: Depigmentation caused by phenolic detergent germicides. Arch. Dermatol., *102*:177, 1970. *(Brings attention for the first time to the depigmenting properties of disinfectants used by hospital workers.)*

Lerner, A.B., and Nordlund J.J: Vitiligo! What is it? Is it important?J.A.M.A., *239*:1138, 1978. *(A comprehensive review.)*

Pathak, M.A., Daniels, F., Jr., and Fitzpatrick, T.B.: The presently known distribution of furocoumarins (psoralens) in plants. J. Invest. Dermatol., *39*:225, 1962. *(A scholarly article that lists all plants capable of eliciting phytophotodermatitis.)*

Resnick, S.: Melasma induced by oral contraceptive drugs. J.A.M.A., *199*:601, 1967. *(An important article on a major side effect of oral contraceptive agents—29 percent of 212 patients developed melasma.)*

170

Evaluation of Alopecia
WILLIAM V.R. SHELLOW, M.D.

Alopecia may be described as the lack of hair in areas where it normally grows. The most noticeable area for alopecia to occur is the scalp, but loss of body hair may also occur. Patients may seek medical care for what is perceived as excessive hair loss even when there is no alopecia. Whether the problem is genetically induced male pattern baldness or alopecia as a result of systemic illness, the primary care physician may be the first to whom the problem is presented and must offer the patient a rational approach to diagnosis and treatment.

PATHOPHYSIOLOGY

Hair is a product of keratinocytes in the hair bulb. The hair shaft is made of hard keratin. Synthesis results from mitoses of cells within the hair matrix. The growth of hair is cyclical, with the length of the cycle varying with the location. Scalp hair grows from 3 to 10 years, involutes over 3 months, and rests for another 3 months. In healthy young persons, about 90 per cent of all scalp hairs are in anagen, actively growing. Telogen, or resting hair, accounts for most of the remainder.

Hairs that grow for long periods and rest briefly are most susceptible to interruption of the growth cycle, and variations in the growing-to-resting ratio are most noticeable. The longer the growing period the longer the hair. Scalp hair grows at the rate of approximately 0.35 mm. per day, but there are factors that may affect the rate.

The primary pathogenic mechanisms of hair loss are destruction of the hair matrix by physical agents and infectious or immunologically mediated inflammation. Hair loss may occur secondary to a slowing of hair growth from metabolic diseases, antimetabolites, or other drugs. Physiologic alterations may also produce hair loss by altering the relationship of the growing and resting phases of hair follicles. During pregnancy, fewer hairs are shed, producing fewer telogen hairs. After parturition, the percentage of telogen hairs increases, and there is loss of hair. The process is diffuse and short-lived. This alteration in the relationship of resting hairs to the total may also develop secondary to pharmacologic changes induced by oral contraceptives. Destructive pathogenic mechanisms often produce scarring alopecia while systemic illnesses and drugs usually result in nonscarring alopecia.

DIFFERENTIAL DIAGNOSIS

The standard classification of alopecia is scarring (or cicatricial) and nonscarring (noncicatricial). In the latter, the hair follicles are retained and the process is potentially reversible. In the scarring type, follicles are destroyed and hair never regrows. A few conditions that begin as nonscarring may later scar as a result of chronicity.

Scarring alopecia generally involves significant inflammation. Physical trauma such as burns, radiation, injuries, and chronic traction are often implicated. Traction alopecia usually results from braiding or tight hair rollers. The pattern of hair loss is dependent on the styling. The process is initially reversible but progresses to a scarring phase with chronicity. Hot combs in combination with petrolatum used to straighten hair may result in inflammation with consequent fibrosis and hair loss. Infections—whether they be bacterial, resulting in deep cellulitis; fungal with *Trichophyton schoenleini;* or viral, such as recurrent herpes simplex or herpes zoster—produce inflammatory change and alopecia. Dermatologic processes such as discoid lupus erythematosus, scleroderma, lichen planus, cutaneous neoplasms or granulomas may produce scarring alopecia. Factitial causes and neurotic excoriations must also be considered.

Alopecia is most often nonscarring, with the most common cause being male and female pattern baldness. Male pattern baldness (androgenetic alopecia) is symmetrical, usually beginning in the frontoparietal scalp. The development of male baldness is related to age, genetic predisposition, and the presence of androgenic hormones. The inheritance is probably dominant with incomplete penetrance. The process is permanent with pigmented scalp hairs replaced by fine unpigmented vellus hairs. Female pattern baldness, also androgenetic alopecia, is more diffuse, usually in the central and frontal areas without complete baldness. Age, family tendency, and androgenic hormones are important factors. The presence of a male pattern hair loss in a female should provoke concern about androgen excess.

Nonscarring alopecia often involves systemic disease, medication, or metabolic abnormality. Alopecia areata, a condition of unknown etiology in which hair is rapidly lost, usually in circular patterns, is probably the most common cause of nonscarring alopecia. Alopecia totalis is loss of all scalp hair and alopecia universalis, loss of facial and body hair as well. The course of alopecia areata is unpredictable. Some persons have one episode with one or several bald spots and spontaneous regrowth. Others may develop new areas of baldness and become totally bald. Onset before puberty is associated with a poorer prognosis. Many authors believe that there is an autoimmune mechanism and that there is an association with other autoimmune diseases.

Alopecia may follow infectious diseases with high persistent fevers such as typhoid or pneumonia. Secondary syphilis, superficial folliculitis, and tinea capitis may produce nonscarring alopecia. Medication, notably antineoplastic agents such as 5-fluorouracil, cyclophosphamide, or methotrexate, produce hair loss. Other drugs such as heparin, allopurinol, thiouracil and quinine and hypervitaminosis A have been associated with alopecia.

Oral contraceptives, hyperandrogenism, and pregnancy are known to interfere with the relationship of resting and growing hairs and to produce hair loss. Diffuse hair thinning may occur with thyroid disease and iron deficiency. Less commonly, hypopituitarism and parathyroid disease may produce hair loss. Alopecia is a manifestation of collagen vascular diseases, notably systemic lupus erythematosus and dermatomyositis. Occasional patients have self-induced hair loss, a condition known as trichotillomania. These patients may not be aware that they are plucking hairs, and the condition may indicate significant psychiatric disturbance.

WORKUP

History should identify the date of onset and determine whether the patient is troubled by a specific area of hair loss by the perception of excessive loss. The history may reveal specific physical causes. The physician should ask about the use of curlers, rollers, bleaching, permanent waves, hair straightening, or hot combs, which may produce traction or physical destruction. Febrile illness within the last 6 to 12 weeks may be important. Drug history, noting particularly antimetabolites, colchicine, estrogens, androgens, antithyroid drugs, anticoagulants, or vitamin A, should be pursued. Less common causes that may be revealed by the history include delivery of a baby 3 months before, or recent severe dieting. A family history may suggest probable male or female pattern baldness.

Physical examination is essential to distinguish scarring from nonscarring alopecia. The physician should observe whether the pattern is localized or diffuse and whether the hair loss reveals a genetic pattern or suggests a mechanical cause. The physician should note hirsutism and masculinizing signs in women with baldness. The physician should examine the area surrounding the hair loss for evidence of inflammation, cellulitis, folliculitis, or fungal infection. Also, the physician should note the presence of short broken hairs, which suggest pulling of the hair. It is useful to examine the nails; the presence of Beau's lines may correlate with a systemic process affecting both nail and hair growth.

It is often helpful to collect objective evidence of hair loss in order to distinguish perceived from genuine problems of hair loss. The patient can collect the hairs that he loses daily, count them, place them in an envelope, and note the daily total. It may be found that 100 hairs a day are being lost, and that is within normal limits. Examination of an area of alopecia with a Wood's light may reveal fluorescent fungal infection. The physician should always scrape for microscopic examination and culture any areas of inflammation. Some dermatologists perform telogen counts by removing 100 hairs and counting how many are in the telogen phase. Telogen hair is identified by the presence of a terminal club on the hair shaft. This procedure can separate conditions due to telogen excess from those due to broken hairs, but it may be too time-consuming to be useful to the primary physician.

Laboratory studies. A biopsy may be helpful, particularly in cases of scarring alopecia, both to add histologic evidence to diagnose according to etiology and also to determine areas of activity that might respond to anti-inflammatory therapy. Performance of laboratory tests for systemic disease, such as blood count, serum iron, thyroxine, antinuclear antibody, and others, depends on the history and physical evidence.

SYMPTOMATIC MANAGEMENT

The primary physician can provide the patient with reassurance, advice, and, occasionally, specific therapy. The treatment of alopecia depends on identification of a probable etiology. Patients with the perception of excessive hair loss that is not substantiated by the presence of alopecia and furthermore with a normal hair loss count should be reassured. Patients with hair loss following pregnancy should be reassured with a careful explanation of why it is occurring. Drugs associated with hair loss should be discontinued. Infection, either bacterial or fungal, should be specifically treated. Underlying diseases such as hypo- or hyperthyroidism should be treated, and hair loss will often resolve.

Alopecia areata may respond to specific medical therapy, which should be undertaken by a dermatologist or physician skilled in the technique. A traditional treatment for stimulating new hair growth has been irritation with phenol or ultraviolet light. Topical fluorinated corticosteroids under occlusion may be helpful, and this may be tried by the primary physician. It is often necessary to inject a dilute steroid solution into the scalp, preferably triamcinolone, which appears to be less likely to cause atrophy than other steroids. Small volumes are used, and several injections may be necessary to cover a large area. Systemic corticosteroids have, on occasion, been helpful, but their effectiveness is often lost when the drugs are discontinued, and the risks of chronic therapy outweigh the benefits. They should be used only under exceptional circumstances and only by a dermatologist experienced in treating patients with hair problems.

Patient education can be the most important part of the primary physician's management of the patient with alopecia. Once diagnosis is established or serious diseases excluded, the patient should be reassured. Patients are often concerned whether the hair loss will progress, and the most useful information that can be given is the likelihood of continued or total hair loss. Men with genetic baldness are often reassured to know that there is no systemic disease. Women may be helped by advice on how to restyle hair. Patients are often well aware of the option of wigs and ask the physician about such issues as having their hair woven or having hair transplants. Weaving is a relatively safe procedure performed by nonphysicians. It is successful but must be repeated periodically and thereby becomes expensive and a nuisance. Hair transplants are expensive. The procedure is painful and is usually not covered by insurance. Patients with coarse dark hair are the best candidates for hair transplants. The use of artificial hair implants should be discouraged because they usually fall out or elicit a chronic foreign body reaction. Patients seek advice about shampooing and the treatment of hair. They should be told to avoid alkaline pH shampoo and excessive toweling after washing their hair and that a conditioner may be helpful. It is useful to advise patients that combing is less injurious to hair than brushing and that if one must brush, to gently disentangle the hair from the brush. It is safest to use a natural bristle brush or a nylon brush with rounded edges. Patients should avoid bleaching, permanent waving, straightening, hot combs, or excessive sun exposure. Success in the management of the patient with alopecia is often dependent on the physician's ability to teach the patient to accept the reality of hair loss.

ANNOTATED BIBLIOGRAPHY

Gill, K.A., Jr., and Barter, D.L.: Alopecia totalis: Treatment with fluocinolone acetonide. Arch. Dermatol., *87*:384, 1963. *(Regrowth of hair following steroids under occlusion.)*

Happle, R., Cebulla, K., and Echternacht-Happle, K.: Dinitrochlorobenzene therapy for alopecia areata. Arch. Dermatol, *114*:1629, 1978. *(Eighty-nine per cent of patients treated with DNCB regrew hair using this method.)*

Hanke, C.W., and Bergfeld, W.F.: Fiber implantation for pattern baldness. JAMA, *241*:146, 1979. *(Describes the serious deficiencies associated with this procedure which is probably an unacceptable alternative to baldness.)*

Mehregan, A.H.: Trichotillomania. Arch. Dermatol., *102*:129, 1970. *(Correlation between the clinical and histopathologic features in 16 cases.)*

Muller, S.A., and Winkelmann, R.V.: Alopecia areata: An evaluation of 736 patients. Arch. Dermatol. *88*:290, 1963. *(A comprehensive review of the natural history of this disease.)*

Pinkus, H.: Alopecia: Clinicopathologic correlations. Int. J. Dermatol., *19*:245, 1980. *(Superb review article on all causes of alopecia.)*

Rook, A.: Endocrine influences on hair growth. Br.

Med. J., *1*:609, 1965. *(An informative description of hair physiology and factors that modify it.)*

Weigland, D.A.: Recent developments in alopecias. Int. J. Dermatol., *17*:280, 1978. *(An up-to-date review of selected alopecias; 57 refs.)*

171

Management of Acne
RONALD M. REISNER, M.D.

Acne, the most common of all skin diseases, is a polygenic, multifactorial disease that, depending upon the strictness of its definition, afflicts between 50 and 100 per cent of adolescents in the United States. It ranges in severity from a few scattered whiteheads and blackheads to disfiguring, painful, deep-seated, pus-filled, and bleeding nodulocystic lesions. About 15 per cent of surveyed patients with acne seek medical care; the remainder treat themselves. The primary care physician is in a unique position to identify and treat a high proportion of acne sufferers. Early effective treatment will minimize the physical scarring of the disease and prevent or reduce equally important psychic trauma.

PATHOPHYSIOLOGY AND CLINICAL PRESENTATION

The pathogenesis of acne is proving to be increasingly complex. It involves the interaction of the quantity and kind of sebum produced; enzymatic, immunologic, and chemotactic effects of normal cutaneous microflora; hormonal influences; abnormal keratinization of the sebaceous follicular duct wall; follicular fragility; and host responsiveness.

Acne is a disease of the sebaceous follicles. There are approximately 5,000 sebaceous follicles scattered predominantly over the face and central upper back and chest. The initial event in the pathogenesis of acne is conversion of the loose, easily shed, horny layer of the epithelium lining the follicular duct wall to a self-adhering mass that gradually obstructs the follicular duct. This has been called "retention hyperkeratosis." It takes 1 to 2 months for the accumulated mass of keratin, sebum, and bacteria to reach visible size as a closed comedone or whitehead. Whiteheads may persist or mature by expanding the

opening to communicate freely with the outside. The compact, melanin-rich tip then gives it the name of "blackhead."

Follicular duct walls may rupture, releasing their contents into the surrounding dermis, which provokes a profound inflammatory response, leading to the development of papules, pustules, nodules, and suppurative nodules that are commonly, but mistakenly, termed "cysts." These inflammatory lesions may lead to permanent scarring.

Acne may most conveniently be divided into two categories, obstructive and inflammatory. The former, resulting from the impaction of horny material, bacteria, and sebum in the dilated follicular duct wall, is characterized by closed comedones (whiteheads) and open comedones (blackheads). The latter results from leakage of intrafollicular contents, producing an inflammatory response. Depending upon the level of leakage into the dermis and the amount of material released, lesions vary from small, erythematous papules and superficial pustules to deeper pustules and larger, persistent, or suppurative nodules.

PRINCIPLES OF THERAPY

The goals of therapy are removal of existing lesions and prevention of new ones. The modalities employed depend on the kind of lesion.

A basic principle of therapy is to remove acnegenic agents. Some cosmetics, oils, and creams may be capable of producing comedones, and their use should be stopped. Women should cease taking oral contraceptives with androgenic progestational components such as norethindrone and norgestrel. The physician should inquire about and advise against using acnegenic drugs such as androgens, steroids, iodides, and bromides. It is also important to consider underlying endocrinopathy in the evaluation of an adult with acne of recent onset.

Obstructive acne should be approached by removing closed comedones. Removal is accomplished by atraumatically nicking the covering epidermis with a No. 11 Bard-Parker blade or blood lancet and extracting the contents with a comedone extractor. The expression of open comedones has little influence on future inflammatory lesions, but at the time it does improve the appearance of the skin. After the immediate result of removing existing comedones, the physician should prescribe a comedolytic agent. The two most effective agents available are retinoic acid and benzoyl peroxide. The frequency of application should be adjusted to produce minimally visible erythema and desquamation. Initial therapy may be 5 per cent benzoyl peroxide gel, once or twice daily, followed after several weeks by the addition of 0.05 per cent retinoic acid cream at least 8 hours after the application of benzoyl peroxide. The use or frequency of a more concentrated solution or gel is dictated by the patient's response. The order of therapy may be reversed with retinoic acid started first and benzoyl peroxide added after 3 to 6 weeks.

This combination of agents loosens existing comedones, making extraction easier, and helps prevent formation of new lesions. Retinoic acid thins the outer, horny layer of the epidermis; therefore, the patient must be warned to discontinue other topical medications, avoid excessive cleansing, and minimize sun exposure. Patients should be warned of a possible transient pustular flare when therapy is initiated. Topical agents may be used concomitantly with tetracycline. Benzoyl peroxide and retinoic acid have largely replaced compounds that contain sulfur, salicylic acid, and resorcinol.

Patients with acne may have oily skin, but cleansing measures to remove excess oil do not affect the course of acne. Cleansing may improve what is perceived as a cosmetically undesirable oily appearance, and gentle cleansing methods, such as mild soap and water, are effective and well tolerated. Astringents, generally mixtures of alcohol or acetone and water, may provide a convenient way for removing excessive oil when soap and water are not readily available.

Patients with mild inflammatory acne may be treated with the topical agents used for obstructive lesions. Topical agents increase the rate of resorption of small erythematous papules and thin-roofed pustules. Ultraviolet light, which produces erythema and desquamation also increases the rate of resorption of mild inflammatory lesions. Topical agents and ultra-violet light reduce the life of mild inflammatory lesions to about half of the usual 7 to 10 days.

Severe inflammatory acne—characterized by large, deep papules and pustules and the destructive suppurating, nodular lesions—requires long-term systemic antibiotics. Tetracycline is primarily, or alternatively erythromycin is, effective. They appear to suppress the organism *Propionibacterium acnes,* a normal inhabitant of the follicular canal in humans. This organism may participate in the initiation and aggravation of inflammatory lesions by elaborating enzymes, including lipases, that act on sebum to release potentially irritating free fatty acids. Hyaluronidase, which increases permeability of the follicular duct wall, and protease, which damages the follicular duct wall, increasing the leakage of materials into the surrounding dermis, may also be involved. *P. acnes* produces chemotactic substances for polymorphonuclear leukocytes, which contribute to the initiation and evolution of inflammatory lesions.

Antibiotics prevent the development of new lesions but do not affect existing inflammatory ones. Clinical results are not ordinarily seen before 4 to 6 weeks of therapy, when a decrease in the formation of new lesions should be noted. Existing papulopustular lesions may persist for 7 to 10 days and deep, nodulocystic lesions may remain for months. Extensive experience with antibiotic therapy for two decades, including a recent detailed review of indications and hazards of such therapy by an *ad hoc* committee of the American Academy of Dermatology, has established it as a rational, effective, and remarkably safe means of managing the more destructive forms of acne. The usual regimen is to initiate therapy with tetracycline, 250 mg. to 500 mg. four times a day, for 2 to 4 weeks, gradually reducing the dose according to the response. In some patients, 250 mg. of tetracycline every other day suppresses new eruptions. Therapy should periodically be stopped to determine whether continued antibiotics are necessary. Flares occur between 2 and 4 weeks after discontinuing the antibiotic. Significant contraindications to tetracycline are known hypersensitivity, pregnancy, and age. It should ordinarily not be used before the age of 10 to 12 because of potential permanent staining of the teeth.

Benzoyl peroxide and retinoic acid appear to be synergistic with the antibiotic, possibly by increasing the concentration of tetracycline in the follicular duct. Tetracycline should be given at least 1 hour before or 2 hours after meals, and absorption or patient compliance can be evaluated by examining either the oral mucosa with a Wood's light for greenish yellow fluorescence or the large pores of the nose, which lose their coral red fluorescence as the *P. acnes* population is reduced. An occasional complication of tetracycline is the development of a gram-negative folliculitis with pustules around the nose and mouth and spreading onto the cheek. Culture of the lesions, with identification of the organisms, usually klebsiella or enterobacter, is indicated, and it responds within 2 or 3 days to appropriate antibiotic therapy. Topical antibiotics, particularly 1 per cent or 2 per cent erythromycin or 1 per cent or 2 per cent clindamycin, appear to offer promise for the management of inflammatory acne.

Intralesional corticosteroids may hasten involution of nodulocystic lesions, reducing the risk of permanent scarring. Triamcinolone acetonide 2.0 or 2.5 mg. per cc. in saline, injected with a 30-gauge needle directly into specific lesions, is often remarkably effective. Pseudoatrophy is a danger, and the physician should avoid doses in excess of 20 mg. per week, which may suppress the pituitary-adrenal axis. Some dermatologists prefer to use cryotherapy with liquid nitrogen. This requires experience to avoid excessive freezing and tissue destruction.

There is no evidence that diet has a significant effect on acne. Diuretics, vitamin A, and vaccines, which have been advocated, do not appear to have demonstrable therapeutic value. Radiation therapy is rarely if ever indicated, and administered only by someone expert in its use and cognizant of its risks, after all other modalities have been tried.

Cyclic estrogen-progestin therapy may be considered in highly selected situations with full awareness of and careful monitoring for side effects. Sulfones are reserved for the most severe inflammatory acne conglobata.

THERAPEUTIC RECOMMENDATIONS

- Explanation to the patient is an essential part of treating acne so that understanding and cooperation can be enlisted.
- Eliminate acnegenic drugs, such as steroids or androgens, exposure to oils, and habits such as rubbing the face.
- For obstructive acne, use a combination of benzoyl peroxide, 5 per cent, and retinoic acid, 0.05 per cent, to a point just short of clinically visible erythema.
- In inflammatory acne, prescribe an antibiotic,

most preferably tetracycline, 250 mg. four times a day gradually reducing the dose once control is achieved.
- In acne characterized by large nodules, intralesional steroids or, in the hands of experts, liquid nitrogen may be tried.
- For people with acne scars, dermabrasion should be considered in consultation with a dermatologist. Only someone highly experienced should perform the dermabrasion.

PATIENT EDUCATION

Treatment of acne is generally within the domain of the primary physician. The dermatologist should be consulted if basic topical and antibiotic therapy fails and in cases of severe disfiguring lesions that require techniques such as intralesional steroids or acne surgery. Patient education and cooperation are crucial to the success of therapy. Patients must understand the chronic nature of the process and not be discouraged when lesions continue to appear. Patients who unrealistically expect cure may become increasingly discouraged, uncooperative, and finally angry.

A vast mythology about acne has developed. The patient should be assured that acne has no relationship to diet, masturbation, sexual activity or inactivity, constipation, dirt, or angry feelings. The patient should be helped to gain perspective and discouraged from frequent self-examination in brightly lit mirrors, which often produce a distorted self-image. The patient begins to perceive himself as "acne with a person attached" rather than a person with acne. Describing this process to the patient often brings an answering smile of recognition and is reassuring. Instructions for the use of topical and systemic agents must be precise and carefully followed. The patient should be reminded that therapeutic results are not achieved immediately, and treatment must be continued for 6 to 8 weeks before response is definitely seen.

ANNOTATED BIBLIOGRAPHY

Ad Hoc Committee on Antibiotic Treatment of Acne: Systemic antibiotics for treatment of acne vulgaris—efficacy and safety. Arch. Dermatol., *111*:1630, 1975. (*This authorative report summarizes the indications, side effects and use of systemic antibiotics in the treatment of acne. On balance it concludes that systemic antibiotics, particularly tetracycline, provide a useful and on a risk/benefit basis reasonable modality for the management of selected patients with inflammatory acne.)*

Barranco, V.P., and Jones, D.D.: Effect of oral contraceptives on acne. South. Med. J. *67*:703, 1974. *(A study shows that androgen-dominant oral contraceptives are potentially acnegenic, while estrogen-dominant pills may be beneficial.)*

Bernstein, J.E., and Shalita, A.R.: Topically applied erythromycin in inflammatory acne vulgaris. J. Am. Acad. Dermatol., *2*:318, 1980. *(2% erythromycin evaluated compared to vehicle control in 348 patients.)*

Hurwitz, S.: The combined effect of vitamin A acid and benzoyl peroxide in the treatment of acne. Cutis, *17*:585, 1976. *(Discusses the individual agents and their combined use and concludes in a study of 404 patients with acne that the combination is better tolerated than vitamin A acid alone; the use of systemic antibiotics can be decreased by using this topical therapy; education of the patient and careful follow-up are essential, and significant improvement can be achieved in a relatively short time in a high proportion of patients.)*

Melski, J.W., and Arndt, K.A.: Topical therapy for acne. N. Engl. J. Med., *302*:503, 1980. *(A good review; 34 references.)*

Mills, O.H., and Kligman, A.M.: Acne detergicans. Arch. Dermatol., *111*:65, 1975. *(A description suggesting that obsessive washing may actually produce comedones.)*

Mills, O.H., Marples, R.R., and Kligman, A.M.: Acne vulgaris—Oral therapy with tetracycline and topical therapy with vitamin A. Arch. Dermatol., *106*:200, 1972. *(Three treatments for adolescents with moderately severe acne were compared: 0.05% Vitamin A acid daily alone; demeclocycline hydrochloride 600 mg. a day for the first 3 weeks, and 300 mg. daily thereafter; a combination of the two. Clinical response, free fatty acid concentration and* Propionibacterium acnes *densities all improved most rapidly and to the greatest degree on combined therapy. Described the synergistic use of these two major agents.)*

Peck, G.L., et al.: Prolonged remissions of cystic and conglobate acne with 13-CIS-retinoic acid. N. Engl. J. Med., *300*:329, 1979. *(Discusses in detail the treatment of 14 patients with treatment resistant cystic and conglobate acne with 13 showing complete clearing and one 75 per cent improvement. Discusses this promising new investigational drug.)*

Reisner, R.M.: Current status of retinoic acid and benzoyl peroxide in the treatment of acne. West. J. Med., *130*:158, 1979. *(Reviews the current status of therapy with these agents.)*

Strauss, J.S., Pochi, P.D., and Downing, D.T.: Acne: Perspectives. J. Invest. Dermatol., *62*:321, 1974. *(Pathogenesis of acne is reviewed, showing the relationship between sebaceous glands and the role of follicular keratinization.)*

172

Management of Acne Variants
WILLIAM V.R. SHELLOW, M.D.

Acne-like eruptions occur in adults but are often ignored. Middle-aged women and men may be affected by acne rosacea, younger women by perioral dermatitis, and older people by periorbital comedones. These conditions occasionally cause a patient to seek medical attention, but more often are noted incidentally by an examining physician seeing a patient for another reason. The primary care practitioner's responsibility involves identification of the patient with acne variants and institution of effective therapy.

PATHOPHYSIOLOGY AND CLINICAL PRESENTATION

Acne rosacea is a chronic condition involving the blush area of the face. Persistent erythema is a prominent component and may coexist with telangiectasia. Papules and pustules recur periodically. The condition occurs more commonly in women, but when it occurs in men it tends to be more severe. Presentation may include flushing, telangiectasia, papules, pustules or nodules. Comedones are rarely seen. Rhinophyma, a thick and lobulated overgrowth of connective tissue and sebaceous glands of the nose, may be an associated feature. Ocular complications include blepharitis, conjunctivitis and episcleritis commonly, and iritis and keratitis infrequently.

Perioral dermatitis, a papular erythema around the mouth, chin, upper lip and nasolabial folds, is seen primarily in young women. Eruption is usually bilateral and symmetrical; occasionally papulopustular lesions are widespread.

Periorbital comedones are most frequently seen in older people. The condition is related to senile loss of elasticity of the skin; opened pores favor the accumulation of keratin and sebaceous materials. Senile comedones recur less rapidly than comedones associated with acne vulgaris.

The pathophysiology of all these conditions is incompletely understood. Coffee, alcohol and spicy foods aggravate rosacea, which is also exacerbated upon menopause and during periods of emotional unrest. The follicle mite, *Demodex folliculorum,* is found in abundance in the pilosebaceous follicles of patients with rosacea, but its causative role is questionable.

The cause of perioral dermatitis is unknown, but it may be due to hormonal factors or the use of oily cosmetics. The condition can be replicated by chronic use of fluorinated corticosteroid creams or ointments. An association with the use or discontinuance of oral contraceptives has been noted.

PRINCIPLES OF THERAPY

The principles of therapy involve removal of exacerbating conditions and the use of systemic antibiotics. In rosacea, conditions that lead to flushing or vasodilation should be minimized. Exposure to sunlight, extreme heat or cold, and ingestion of foods known to exacerbate the condition should be interdicted. Topical therapy can be similar to that for acne vulgaris, utilizing agents which enhance the turnover of skin and the restoration of normal skin. Topical agents such as benzoyl peroxide or retanoic acid may be used. The most effective therapy is systemic tetracycline, which may be required for prolonged periods of time. It is most important to cau-

tion against use of fluorinated corticosteroids, which produce an initial response only to result in atrophy of skin and development of permanent telangiectasia.

Perioral dermatitis should be approached by interdicting greasy cosmetics and cold creams. Topical acne preparations which increase turnover of skin have been useful. Fluorinated steroid creams should not be used, but hydrocortisone 1% may provide more rapid resolution of the dermatitis. Topical antibiotic preparations of erythromcyin or clindamycin in an oil-free vehicle are being used instead of systemic antibiotics.

Periorbital comedones may be treated by expression of the blackheads. Redevelopment of blackheads is relatively slow, so that periodic expression at 3- or 4-month intervals is adequate. Retanoic acid applied judiciously is effective in resolving the condition, but compliance may be difficult to obtain in the older population.

THERAPEUTIC RECOMMENDATIONS

Acne Rosacea

- Tetracycline, 250 mg. four times a day, continued for a period of time with gradual reduction in dose down to 250 mg. every other day before it is stopped. Prolonged low-dose treatment may be necessary.
- Fluorinated steroids and foods known to exacerabate the condition should be interdicted.

Perioral Dermatitis

- Treatment should begin with tetracycline, 250 mg. three times a day, gradually reduced over a period of weeks once resolution has occurred.
- Greasy creams and cosmetics should be scrupulously avoided.
- Hydrocortisone cream may occasionally be used.

Periorbital Dermatitis

- Periodically express the blackheads.
- Retin-A may be useful in patients who are concerned about their appearance and capable of compliance.

PATIENT EDUCATION

The major element of patient education is to explain that these conditions are common and treatable. Many patients are bothered by a single pimple, while others can sustain the disfigurement of acne rosacea without concern.

ANNOTATED BIBLIOGRAPHY

Barrie, P.: Rosacea with special reference to its ocular manifestations. Br. J. Dermatol., *65*:458, 1953. *(Discusses the ocular changes associated with rosacea.)*

Epstein, S.: Perioral dermatitis. Cutis, *10*:317, 1972. *(Excellent clinical description with treatment recommendation.)*

Kligman, A.M., and Mill, O.H. Jr.: Acne cosmetica. Arch. Dermatol., *106*:843, 1972. *(A common acne variant seen in adult women is attributable to the long-term use of facial cosmetics.)*

MacDonald, A., and Felwel, M.: Perioral dermatitis: Aetiology and treatment with tetracycline. Br. J. Dermatol., *87*:315, 1972.

Mihan, R., and Ayres, S., Jr.: Perioral dermatitis. Arch. Dermatol., *89*:803, 1964. *(Original description of this condition.)*

Mullanax, M.G., and Kierland, R.R.: Granulomatous rosacea. Arch. Dermatol., *101*:206, 1970. *(Separates this condition from cutaneous tuberculosis.)*

173

Management of Psoriasis
DAVID C. RISH, M.D.

Psoriasis is a chronic proliferative skin disease characterized by discrete erythematous papules and plaques covered with a silvery white scale. The patient may be bothered by itching and occasionally by pain from cracking of the skin on the hands and feet and frequently concerned about the cosmetic disfigurement.

The disease usually has its onset early in adult life but may first appear in childhood or old age. Psoriasis is inherited as a simple autosomal dominant trait with incomplete penetrance or as a polygenic trait. A linkage to tissue types HL-A-13 and W-17 has been reported. An associated inflammatory arthritis commonly of the distal interphalangeal joints, often with juxta-articular destruction of bone, affects about 5 per cent of patients with psoriasis. Psoriasis is common, affecting 1 to 3 per cent of the population of the United States.

The primary physician should be capable of treating mild to moderate cases and understanding all treatment modalities, in order to work with a dermatologist in the care of patients with severe psoriasis.

PATHOPHYSIOLOGY AND CLINICAL PRESENTATION

The epidermal turn-over time for a cell to travel from the basal layer of the epidermis to the surface to be cast off is normally 28 days; in psoriatic skin it is a brief 3 to 4 days. In this shortened time, normal cell maturation and keratinization do not occur. Clinically, this is seen as profuse scaling, histologically increased mitotic activity, immature nucleated cells in the horny layer, a thickened epidermis, and proliferation of subepidermal blood vessels with an inflammatory infiltrate of monocytic cells, accounting for the clinical erythema.

The initiating factor has not been elucidated. Theories about depressed levels of cyclic adenosine monophosphate (AMP) have not been consistently confirmed. A central role for the vasculature with a capillary-stimulating factor or loss of contact inhibition because the carbohydrate lipid complex normally present in epidermal layers is lacking has been proposed. An immunologic pathogenesis has been suggested by the observation of clinical remissions following measles and precipitation of disease by streptococcal infection. The precise etiology, however, remains unknown.

Psoriasis presents as a dermatosis, well-marginated, erythematous, elevated, covered with a thick, silvery scale. Bluntly scraping off the scale reveals punctate bleeding points called Auspitz's sign. The elbows, knees, scalp, and sites of trauma are most commonly involved. Nails often show punctate pitting or collections of subungual keratotic material. Mucous membranes are rarely involved. Pustular lesions may occur particularly on the palms and soles. Variations in size, shape, distribution, and pattern, form the basis of classifications of the disease. Small, discrete papular lesions scattered over the body are characteristic of guttate psoriasis; ring-shaped lesions are called "psoriasis annularis"; merging annular lesions are called "psoriasis gyrata."

PRINCIPLES OF THERAPY

The cardinal principle of therapy is to slow epidermal turnover time and return the skin to a normal appearance. Treatment should suppress cell turnover, remove scales, reduce inflammaion, and control itching. The hazards of treatment must be weighed against the benefits of treating this dermatologic disease.

Topical Therapy

The majority of patients can be maintained on one agent or a combination of topical modalities.

1. *Exposure to sunlight* or artificial ultraviolet light (UVL) induces flattening of lesions. Overexposure may exacerbate psoriasis and should be avoided.
2. *Tar preparations* followed by UVL is a popular treatment (the Goeckerman regimen is a time-tested therapy for psoriasis). Tar enhances the effectiveness of UV rays. Various adjuvants—salicylic acid, sulfur, and steroids—are added to tars to enhance penetration and to decrease epidermal turnover. Tars are messy, difficult to apply, and malodorous; stain clothes and skin; and may induce folliculitis.
3. *Corticosteroids.* Fluorinated corticosteroids in cream, gel, or ointment bases are applied to local lesions. Occlusions with plastic wrap or corticosteroid-impregnated occlusive tape (Cordran®) enhances penetration. Corticosteroid lotions are more suitable for the scalp. Combinations of corticosteroids, coal tar, and UVL are often used.
4. *Intralesional Therapy.* Direct injection of diluted corticosteroids (Kenalog, Celestone) into chronic plaques may produce involution within 7 to 10 days. The dilution and total dose must be chosen carefully to prevent pseudoatrophy at the site of injection.
5. *Antipruritic therapy* with antihistamines can be helpful.

Systemic Therapy

Systemic agents that inhibit DNA synthesis are reserved for patients unresponsive to topical preparations and for whom psoriasis is an economic or social disaster.

1. *Methotrexate,* a folic acid antagonist, inhibits cell replication. Its use requires pretreatment liver biopsy and should be used only by physicians thoroughly familiar with the pharmacology and hazards of the drug.
2. *Mycophenolic Acid.* Oral mycophenolic acid has been shown effective in some cases of psoriasis. Untoward effects include diarrhea, nausea, cramping, soft stools, bone marrow suppression, herpes simplex, herpes zoster, and flulike syndrome. Further studies are needed before mycophenolic acid can be used in psoriasis.
3. *Corticosteroids.* Patients with psoriasis often respond promptly to systemic corticosteroids or adrenocorticotropic hormone (ACTH). Unfortunately, when steroids are discontinued or reduced, the disease is exacerbated. The prolonged use of adrenocorticosteroids is attended by numerous adverse systemic sequelae.
4. *Oral methoxsalen and ultraviolet light (PUVA)* is effective in 80 to 90 per cent of patients with psoriasis. The photoactive drug methoxsalen enhances the efficacy of UVA light. The long-term sequelae of this treatment may include actinic damage, skin cancer, melanoma, and cataracts. Recent reports suggest caution, with findings of increased incidents of basal and squamous cell carcinomas even with short-term follow-up. The treatment should be restricted to centers participating in the nationwide PUVA study.

Psoriasis of the nail responds slowly to therapy because of the long turnover time of the nail. Intralesional injection of corticosteroids into the nail matrix is effective but quite painful.

THERAPEUTIC RECOMMENDATIONS

- The primary physician should be able to treat mild to moderate cases of psoriasis. More extensive lesions require the services of an experienced dermatologist.
- Encourage patients to increase sun exposure but avoid sunburn.
- Fluorinated steroids applied three times a day are

indicated for scattered lesions. Psoriatic lesions of the scalp should be treated with warm mineral oil soaks followed by shampoo and application of fluorinated steroid lotion. Lotion should be used in hairy areas of the body, creams in other locations, and ointments when dryness is a problem.

- Advise the patient to use the steroid sparingly and rub it in well. Inform the patient that purchase of large quantities of steroids will save money.
- Psoriasis of the hands and other areas may be more effectively treated if occlusive dressings are applied after carefully rubbing in steroids. Occlusion should never be applied to ointments.
- Tar baths should be used along with corticosteroids if it is cosmetically acceptable to the patient. Crude tar oils are more messy but more effective. Tar can be used for the treatment of generalized lesions.
- Generalized lesions are effectively treated with tars and UV radiation. This regimen often requires specialized equipment such as an ultraviolet light cabinet, so that it is frequently administered to hospitalized patients or in psoriasis day-care centers.
- Refer patients to dermatologists for the use of more extensive tar and UV radiation or newer therapies, such as psoralen and UVA light, or potentially dangerous systemic therapy, such as methotrexate. The dermatologist must be experienced with these treatment approaches.

PATIENT EDUCATION

The primary physician has a crucial role in patient education. The patient should be encouraged to feel optimistic while being made aware that psoriasis is a chronic disease that requires continuing therapy. Instruction about the recognition of early lesions and the institution of therapy may make management easier. The successful treatment of psoriasis requires cooperation between primary physician and consulting dermatologist. The patient's responsibility for correctly following treatment instructions cannot be overemphasized.

ANNOTATED BIBLIOGRAPHY

Brown, F.S., Burnett, J.W., and Robinson, H.W.: Cutaneous carcinoma following, and long-wave ultraviolet radiation (PUVA) therapy for, psoriasis. J. Am. Acad. Dermatol., 2:393, 1980. *(Multiple basal-cell epitheliomas in 2 patients developed during treatment.)*

Cram, D.L.: Recent advances in pathogenesis and treatment of psoriasis. Journal of Continuing Education in Dermatol., 17:25, 1978. *(A review of the pathophysiology, genetics, and treatment of psoriasis; 91 refs.)*

Cram, D.L., and King, R.I.: Psoriasis day care centers. JAMA, 235:177, 1978. *(A less costly and disruptive approach to the aggressive treatment of psoriasis.)*

Epstein, J.H.: Risks and benefits of the treatment of psoriasis. (Editorial.) N. Engl. J. Med., 300:852, 1979. *(A review of complications associated with PUVA therapy and cautionary note on the importance of patient selection.)*

Goeckerman, W.H.: The treatment of psoriasis. Northwest Med., 24:229, 1925. *(The presentation of tar and sunlight method and the caution that treatment would remain empiric until the cause became known.)*

Hanna, R., Gruber, G.G., Owen, L.G., and Callen, J.P.: Methotrexate in psoriasis. J. Am. Acad. Dermatol., 2:171, 1980. *(Reviews indications, usage and complications of methotrexate therapy.)*

Petrozzi, J.W. and Kligman, A.M.: Photochemotherapy of psoriasis (PUVA) without specialized equipment. Arch. Dermatol., 114:387, 1978. *(Experience with relatively inexpensive equipment modified for PUVA therapy; 58 per cent cleared completely, more than 80 percent improved.)*

Rees, R. B.: Psoriasis: Clinical aspects and management. Cutis, 18:231, 1976. *(A good review of new therapies.)*

Russell, T.J., Schultes, L.M., and Kuban, D.J.: Histocompatibility (HL-A) antigens associated with psoriasis. N. Engl. J. Med., 287:738, 1972. *(A report of increased prevalence of HLA-13 and W-27 in psoriatics.)*

Stern, R.S., Thibodeau, L.A., Kleinerman, R.A., et al.: Cutaneous carcinoma after PUVA treatment of psoriasis. N. Engl. J. Med., 300:809, 1979. *(A 21-year prospective study of 1373 patients treated with PUVA revealed 263 times the expected rate for a matched population. The incidence of squamous cell carcinomas was also notably increased.)*

Thiers, R.: Psoriasis. J. Am. Acad. Dermatol., *3*:101, 1980. *(Reviews theories of pathogenesis and also reviews treatment modalities.)*

Wolff, K., et al.: Photochemotherapy for psoriasis with orally administered methoxsalen. Arch. Dermatol., *112*:943, 1976. *(Oral administration of methoxsalen and UVA light in 91 patients gave complete clearing in 90 per cent of patients.)*

174
Management of Contact Dermatitis
MARVIN J. RAPAPORT, M.D.

Contact dermatitis is a common inflammatory re-action of the skin caused by a primary irritant or an allergen. Irritants include lye, paint remover, solvents and acids. Strong primary irritants produce a reaction in the majority of people. Hundreds of mild irritants such as soaps, mineral oils, polishes and bleaches affect fewer people some of the time. Allergic contact dermatitis is limited to previously sensitized individuals. Common allergens include rubber, nickel, plants, chromates, acrylics, cosmetic preservatives, and topical drugs, particularly antibiotics. Rarely, sensitization may be caused by a chemical antigen plus the ultraviolet portion of sunlight. Contact dermatitis is common, making the primary physician responsible for identification and removal of the contact agent as well as treatment of active inflammation.

PATHOPHYSIOLOGY AND CLINICAL PRESENTATION

The common denominator of contact dermatitis is cutaneous inflammation produced by exogenous agents. Irritants produce a direct toxic effect on the epidermis. Allergic contact dermatitis results from a delayed type of hypersensitivity reaction. It is the cutaneous expression of an acquired alteration in reaction to a contact allergen. The incubation period after initial exposure may be days to weeks, while on reexposure, dermatitis is revealed within 12 to 48 hours. The severity of reaction is dependent on the potency of the provocative agent, its concentration, and the duration of exposure. Factors that contribute to the development and severity of contact dermatitis are friction, pressure, occlusion, previous maceration, extremes of temperature and coexistent dermatologic disease.

Mild irritation produces erythema, microvesiculation and oozing. Stronger irritation leads to blistering, bullae, erosions and ulcers. Repeated exposure will result in a chronic dermatitis causing dryness, thickening and lichenification. Dermatitis having an unusual or artificial distribution and sharp straight margins indicates an external contactant.

PRINCIPLES OF THERAPY

The primary principle of therapy is to confirm that the skin eruption is due to a contact agent. Exposure may occur at home or work, or may be related to a hobby. A history focusing on new exposure to medication, cosmetics, or clothing is essential. Referring to a list of agents known to produce contact dermatitis is more important. Corroboration of the suspected antigenic agents can be achieved by patch testing. Standard antigens are available for such testing; suspected contactants which the patient has encountered may also be used.

If the agent can be identified, specific advice on avoidance should be given. In the absence of a specific allergen or definite irritant, patients should be instructed to decrease exposure to potential irritants within the home such as abrasive soaps, detergents, solvents, bleaches and moist vegetables. It may be helpful to use rubber or plastic gloves, preferably those with thin white cotton liners that absorb sweat and prevent maceration. Washing thoroughly after exposure to any irritants or potential allergen is helpful. Only hypoallergenic cosmetics should be used. Barrier creams may be worthwhile to prevent hand eruptions.

The treatment of acute dermatitis is based on the fundamental principles of all dermatologic therapy. Wet, oozing lesions should be dried. Symptoms that may exacerbate dermatitis such as itching should be treated. Inflammation should be reduced with a potent corticosteroid agent. When possible, therapy should be restricted to topical agents, but systemic medication may be administered if necessary.

The vesicular or exudative lesions of acute dermatitis should be dried by using Burow's solution, in a 1:20 dilution. Old bed sheets, pillowcases, T-shirts or handkerchiefs several layers thick make excellent materials with which to compress; the wet dressings should be applied four to six times a day. In severe or generalized exudative lesions, collodial oatmeal baths will produce a soothing as well as drying effect. If itching is a problem, an antipruritic, particularly at bedtime, can be prescribed. Inflammation should be treated with topical corticosteroids, usually a fluorinated cream, but in lichenified skin an ointment should be used. For bullous contact dermatitis, a short course of high-dose systemic corticosteroids is prescribed. Oral predisone 40 to 60 mg. daily for 5 to 7 days, decreased over a period of 10 to 12 days, will often relieve severe contact dermatitis. Subacute dermatitis with less oozing may be treated primarily with topical corticosteroids. In chronic contact dermatitis, the skin must be rehydrated by soaking it in water; internal moisture is maintained by applying a hydrophobic emollient or topical corticosteroid under occlusion.

THERAPEUTIC RECOMMENDATIONS

- Help patient identify and avoid contactants; interdict all home remedies.
- Advise patient to avoid irritants and use barrier creams or gloves until the irritant is identified.
- Advise patient to wash thoroughly after exposure to any potential antigen.
- Treat exudative lesions with Burow's solution, or in more extensive exudative lesions, collodial oatmeal.
- Apply fluorinated corticosteroids to reduce inflammation; if severe, prescribe occlusion. Use a cream that is paraben-free.
- In generalized bullous contact dermatitis, a short course of 40 to 60 mg. prednisone with rapid tapering is indicated.

- Itching may be reduced with an antihistamine, preferably hydroxyzine, which produces less sedation.

A major problem in managing patients with contact dermatitis is identifying the allergen. The experienced dermatologist knows many possible contactants and methods of exposure. If contact dermatitis returns after repeated treatment, refer to a dermatologist for a more thorough historical investigation. Patients can assist the physician in identifying irritant or allergenic agents by maintaining complete diaries. Patient cooperation in reducing contactants and identifying offending agents is critical to the successful resolution of contact dermatitis.

ANNOTATED BIBLIOGRAPHY

Fisher, A.A.: Highlights of the First International Symposium on Contact Dermatitis. Cutis, *18*:645, 1976. *(Short abstracts of all the newer developments in this field; 35 refs.)*

Jackson, R.T., Nesbitt, L.T., and DeLeo, V.A.: 6-Methylcoumarin photocontact dermatitis. J. Am. Acad. Dermatol. *2*:124, 1980. *(Reports photocontact dermatitis from fragrance in suntan preparations.)*

Kanof, N.B., and Biondi, E.: Routine screening patch test results, 1970-74. Cutis *18*:668, 1976. *(Lists the 10 most prevalent contact allergens for this period.)*

Sinha, S.M., Pasricha, J.S., Sharma, R.C., et al.: Vegetables responsible for contact dermatitis of the hands. Arch. Dermatol. *113*:776, 1977. *(Describes contact dermatitis of the hands in women who prepare meals. Garlic, onion and tomato are common offenders.)*

Storrs, F.J., Mitchell, J.C., and Rasmussen, J.F.: Contact hypersensitivity to Liverwort and the Compositae family of plants. Cutis, *18*:681, 1976. *(Describes another major source of plant dermatitis.)*

175
Management of Eczematous Dermatitis
WILLIAM V.R. SHELLOW, M.D.

Acute and chronic dermatitis constitutes a major portion of cutaneous disease. Eczema is defined clinically by the observable changes in the skin which reflect a common cutaneous reaction to a variety of pathologic processes.

Acute eczematous dermatitis is characterized by erythema, edema, vesiculation, oozing, crusting or scaling; the chronic stage is characterized by excoriation, thickening, hyperpigmentation, and often lichenification. Eczematous dermatitis is common, demanding that the primary care physician render basic therapy. Treatment is often frustrating, and consultation with a dermatologist is frequently required.

PATHOPHYSIOLOGY AND CLINICAL PRESENTATION

Histopathologically, acute dermatitis is characterized by inter- and intracellular edema, with intraepidermal vesicles. In the dermis there is edema, vascular dilatation and perivascular inflammatory cell infiltration. Chronicity causes thickening of the epidermis (acanthosis), capillary proliferation and cellular infiltration with lymphocytes, histiocytes and fibroblasts. The inflammation may be secondary to a variety of pathogenic mechanisms, the most common being contact with an allergic or irritant agent and atopic dermatitis. Eczematous dermatitis of the hands may be due to fungal infection with "id" reaction, contact, household irritants, or the poorly understood abnormal sweating condition referred to as dyshidrosis. Nummular eczema is a morphologically distinct process with coin-shaped lesions. Chronic eczematous change may lead to lichen simplex chronicus. Dermatologic syndromes such as seborrheic or stasis dermatitis may produce eczematous change.

Atopic dermatitis is characterized by intense itching leading to scratching, eczematous change and lichenification. Two-thirds of atopic patients have family members with asthma, hay fever or atopic dermatitis. In adults, the lesions characteristically involve the neck, wrists, the area behind the ears and the antecubital and popliteal flexural areas. Certain fabrics, notably wool, may induce itching. Lesions are exacerbated by extremes of temperature and humidity. Psychological stress may induce flares.

Nummular eczema is a variant recognized by distinctive round lesions located on the external aspects of the extremities, buttocks and posterior aspect of the trunk. The lesions are pruritic; they ooze, crust and may become purulent. The course varies; there may be a few constant lesions or a gradual increase in the number of lesions. The prognosis is good, with eventual clearing, although it may take years.

Chronic dermatitis of the hands or feet may be irritant in nature like "housewives' hands," pustular (chronic pustular eruption), or vesicular (pompholyx or dyshidrosis). These conditions may be acute or chronic. Chronic eczema of the hands presents a diagnostic and therapeutic challenge which may tax the most experienced dermatologist.

Lichen simplex chronicus is a localized neurodermatitis consisting of a circumscribed plaque, thickened skin with increased markings, some scaling and papulation. The occipital region is a common site. Lesions may also be seen on the wrists, thighs or lower aspects of the legs. Women are more frequently affected than are men. The prognosis is variable. If scratching can be stopped, lesions will regress.

PRINCIPLES OF THERAPY

The management of eczema embodies many of the fundamental principles of dermatologic therapy. Precipitants should be eliminated, wet lesions dried, dry lesions hydrated and inflammation treated with steroids. Frustration should be anticipated, and if basic management fails, referral to an experienced dermatologist should be prompt. Acute dermatitis should be treated with drying measures such as Burow's compresses. A search for precipitating factors is mandatory. Topical corticosteroids are always required. Systemic corticosteroids are sometimes used on a short-term basis for generalized or incapacitating dermatitis. Secondary bacterial infection may require systemic antibiotics.

In chronic eczema, identification of irritants is

necessary. Mild irritants include detergents, gasoline, polishes, and many other occupational and household products. Frequent baths or showers, hot water and drying "soaps" should be interdicted. Systemic steroids are contraindicated in chronic eczema. Potent topical agents sometimes used with occlusive dressings may be helpful in chronic eczema.

Emollient creams or ointments are useful to protect the skin and to reduce scaling. Cutaneous hydration may help prevent the eczematous process. Suppression of itching may be important to successful resolution of eczema. Aspirin may be effective, but antihistamines such as cyproheptadine or hydroxyzine are usually required.

THERAPEUTIC RECOMMENDATIONS

- Identify and remove potential contacts, allergens and irritants. Use of rubber gloves with cotton linings may be beneficial.
- Oozing lesions should be dried with Burow's solution compresses applied three to four times a day; colloidal oatmeal baths are indicated for more generalized lesions.
- Patients with dry skin should be managed as described in Chapter 177.
- Fluorinated corticosteroid creams can be used for acute dermatitis. Chronic, lichenified eruptions should be treated with ointments or, if unresponsive, steroid cream under occlusion. In refractory cases, intralesional injection or a diluted triamcinolone solution (2.0 or 2.5 mg. per cc.) given by an experienced physician may be effective.
- Pruritus should be suppressed, if possible, with aspirin or an antihistamine.
- Patient education about the need for chronic therapy cannot be over emphasized. Simple measures

such as clipping fingernails or wearing cotton gloves can reduce secondary excoriation. Early identification of eczematous exacerbations helps facilitate treatment.

ANNOTATED BIBLIOGRAPHY

Dobson, R.L.: Diagnosis and treatment of eczema. JAMA, *235*:2228, 1976. *(A succinct review of classification and principles of treatment.)*

Glickman, F.S., and Silvers, S.H.: Hand eczema and atopy in housewives. Arch. Dermatol., *95*:487, 1967. *(Eighty-two per cent of 50 patients with hand eczema had an atopic history.)*

Rostenberg, A., Jr., and Solomon, L.M.: Infantile eczema and systemic disease. Arch. Dermatol. *98*:41, 1968. *(Discusses eczema as a symptom of underlying systemic disease.)*

Roth, H.L., and Kierland, R.D.: The natural history of atopic dermatitis. Arch Dermatol., *89*:209, 1964. *(Case record review of 492 patients seen at the Mayo Clinic 20 years earlier, with follow-up questionnaire.)*

Schaffer, B., and Beerman, H.: Lichen simplex chronicus and its variant. Arch. Dermatol., *64*:340, 1951. *(The role of psychodynamic mechanisms in this condition.)*

Solomon, L.M., and Beerman, H.: Atopic dermatitis. Am. J. Med. Sci., *252*:478, 1966. *(A scholarly review of the topic.)*

Weidman, A.I., and Sawicty, H.H.: Nummular eczema. Review of the literature: Survey of 516 case records and follow-up of 125 patients. Arch. Dermatol., *73*:58, 1956. *(Review of the literature; 516 cases with 125 follow-ups.)*

176

Management of Seborrheic Dermatitis
WILLIAM V.R. SHELLOW, M.D.

Seborrheic dermatitis is a chronic inflammatory disease that is constitutionally determined but without known cause. Seborrheic dermatitis affects particular areas of the skin, making the condition quite distinctive. It is a benign disorder, but its high preva-

lence and incurability render it a therapeutic challenge. The primary physician must be capable of treating seborrheic dermatitis and educating the patient about chronicity and the need for continued management.

PATHOPHYSIOLOGY AND CLINICAL PRESENTATION

Seborrheic dermatitis presents scaly patches that are occasionally slightly papular, surrounded by minimal to moderate erythema. The borders of the lesions are not well demarcated. The scales may be greasy and appear yellow. The lesion is usually asymptomatic, but pruritus may occur. The scalp is most commonly involved and is distinguished from common dandruff by its association with erythema. More extensive disease involves the forehead at the margin of the hair, eyebrows, nasal folds, and the retroauricular and presternal area. In more severe cases, intertriginous areas, the external ear canal, and the umbilicus are involved. In these areas, there are erythema and exudation, progressing to chronic dermatitis with scaling.

A number of neurologic conditions, notably Parkinson's disease, are associated with oily skin and seborrheic dermatitis. Obesity and endocrinopathies may also be present. Cutaneous diseases such as acne vulgaris, rosacea, or psoriasis may be associated with seborrhea.

The pathogenesis of seborrheic dermatitis is unknown. The anatomic localization correlates with areas of sebaceous gland concentration, although a direct relationship with sebaceous activity has not been established. Empiric data on the bacteriology of people with seborrheic dermatitis have failed to reveal a pathogenic microbiologic mechanism. Seborrheic dermatitis appears to be a constitutional diathesis that may be exacerbated by emotional stress and tension. The mechanism for these exacerbating phenomena is not understood.

PRINCIPLES OF THERAPY

Therapy should remove scaling, reduce oiliness, eliminate redness, and control itching when it is present. Therapy should be guided by the severity, anatomic location, and relative degree of scale, erythema, and oiliness. For most patients, the regular use of an over-the-counter dandruff or antiseborrheic shampoo is usually sufficient. The ingredients in the over-the-counter preparations include sulfur, which is a drying agent; resorcinol, which is anti-inflammatory; salicylic acid or tar, which is keratolytic; and zinc pyrithione or selenium, which decreases the turnover of skin cells. Most preparations contain multiple agents but have one predominant active ingredient. Sebulex, Ionil, and Vanseb contain sulfur and salicylic acid. Zinc pyrithione is found in Head and Shoulders® and Zincon®. Tar, the prominent ingredient in Sebutone®, Pentrax®, and Zetar®, should be used cautiously, if at all, in blond or light gray-haired people because it may change the color of the hair. The patient should use a list of seborrheic agents as a guide to try to find one suitable to his preference for lather, odor, and efficacy. Many patients find that a shampoo works for a period of time then becomes less effective and that a new product must be chosen.

Patients with particularly oily seborrhea may have to shampoo daily. If over-the-counter shampoos have failed, and frequently patients have tried many before reaching the physician, then a 2.5 per cent selenium sulfide shampoo should be prescribed. A recently developed prescription-alternative drug that contains chloroxine, Capitrol®, is effective and may be tried for refractory seborrhea.

The keratolytic component of the over-the-counter preparations removes most scales, but patients with heavy crusting should rub warm mineral oil into the scalp 30 minutes before shampooing. Occasionally, a patient may need to apply a more potent 3 per cent salicylic acid, 3 per cent sulfur and 4 per cent tar cream, known as Pragmatar®, to remove heavy crust. Antiseborrheic scalp preparations that contain salicylic acid and an antibacterial agent may occasionally be useful, but are not necessary to the effective treatment of seborrhea.

The presence of significant erythema requires use of a corticosteroid preparation. In hairy areas, a lotion, spray, or gel may be applied two to four times daily. Creams should be avoided because they cause hair to become matted. Ointments are satisfactory to use at night, but they make the hair greasy, necessitating shampooing again in the morning. On the scalp a fluorinated steroid lotion is acceptable. Mild erythema on glabrous skin should be treated by washing with a mild soap twice a day, followed by application of hydrocortisone cream, 0.5 to 1.0 per cent. Hydrocortisone is relatively inexpensive and has considerably less risk of causing telangiectasia and atrophy; a 1 per cent concentration may be used for erythematous or papular lesions. After initial success, there may be a period of tachyphylaxis, requiring increased concentrations of cream or potent fluorinated steroids. There is considerable danger of telangiectasia with the long-term use of these products, and they should be avoided on the face. Intertriginous seborrheic dermatitis may require Burow's solution compresses for exudative lesions, followed by a fluorinated steroid lotion. Superinfection that requires antimicrobial agents may occur in intertriginous areas.

In selected cases, alleviation of stress with the use of minor tranquilizers may be considered.

THERAPEUTIC RECOMMENDATIONS

- Provide the patient with a list of over-the-counter shampoos to meet personal preferences. For oily hair advise shampooing daily for the first week, decreasing to two to three times a week for maintenance.
- Remove heavy crusts by softening in mineral oil or use a keratolytic agent before shampooing.
- When erythema is present, prescribe a corticosteroid preparation, a fluorinated lotion for the scalp, and hydrocortisone for the face.
- Blepharitis may be treated hygienically, gently rubbing the eyelashes with a coarse washcloth. Occasionally, a steroid-containing eye ointment, such as Metimyd or Blephamide solution, may be used, cautiously, because of the hazard of steroid in the eye.
- Treat exudative intertriginous lesions with drying and a fluorinated topical steroid.
- Patient education is essential. The patient should be taught about the chronic noncurable nature of the disease, its relation to stress, and the need not

to become discouraged. The patient should be cautioned about the deleterious effects of overusing topical steroids. The goal is to suppress inflammation by regular use of an appropriately effective antiseborrheic agent, while cognizant of the chronic nature of the disease.

ANNOTATED BIBLIOGRAPHY

Ingram, J.T.: The seborrheic diathesis. Arch. Dermatol., 76:157, 1967. (Philosophically discusses the various factors that influence seborrheic dermatitis.)

Pachtman, E.A., Vicher, E.E., and Brunner, M.J.: The bacteriologic flora in seborrheic dermatitis. J. Invest. Dermatol., 22:389, 1954. (Numbers of organisms are unrelated to whether particular areas of skin are affected by seborrheic dermatitis.)

Parrish, J.S., and Arndt, K.A.: Seborrhoeic dermatitis of the beard. Br. J. Dermatol., 87:241, 1972. (Facial hirsutism may be accompanied by seborrheic dermatitis. Shaving is not necessary to control the problem.)

Pinkus, H., and Mehregan, A.H.: The primary histologic lesion of seborrheic dermatitis and psoriasis. J. Invest. Dermatol., 46:109, 1966. (Leukocytes and serum are discharged from engorged capillaries in both diseases.)

177
Management of Dry Skin
WILLIAM V.R. SHELLOW, M.D.

Dry skin, or xerosis, commonly seen during the winter months, occurs more often in the elderly. The most common clinical presentation is mild to moderate itching (see Chapter 165). Severe chronically dry skin can become eczematous and may be referred to as "asteatotic eczema." The primary physician must recognize dry skin and use simple measures and effective patient education to relieve the symptom.

PATHOPHYSIOLOGY AND CLINICAL PRESENTATION

Skin is dry because it lacks water. The pathophysiology of cutaneous desiccation may be excessive water loss through the stratum corneum. The lipids that aid retention of water within the stratum corneum diminish with age. Excessive use of soap, detergent, or disinfectants will damage the stratum corneum and increase water loss up to 50 times the normal. Environmental factors such as low humidity, forced air heat, or cold winter winds contribute to dryness. There is an unexplained familial tendency toward the development of dry skin.

Dry skin is characterized by scaling and loss of suppleness and elasticity. The clinical appearance is fine scaling of the lower portions of the legs. In severe xerosis, loss of elasticity leads to cracking and fissuring, producing a superficial appearance of "cracked porcelain" referred to as "erythema craquelé." Itching is a common concomitant and may lead to scratching and excoriation. Occasionally, dry skin is associated with systemic diseases such as hypovitaminosis A, drug reactions, hypothyroidism, or ichthyosis.

PRINCIPLES OF THERAPY

The primary principle of therapy is to restore water. The modalities available include environmental manipulations, modifications in habits, and the judicious use of agents that hold water in the skin. It is important to humidify the external environment, particularly during the winter months. In cold climates, humidification can be economically achieved by leaving pails of water near radiators, but, if necessary, humidifiers may be installed into forced-air heating systems.

It is important to recognize that certain soaps or detergents and frequent bathing dry the skin. A bath is more drying than a brief shower, and many toilet bars that are essentially detergents are extremely dehydrating. The principles to follow are to reduce frequency of bathing to less than once a day; if baths are taken, add a bath oil; avoid detergent soaps, and substitute a well-oilated soap. It is also wise to avoid exposure to mild irritants such as solvents and wool clothing.

The treatment of preexisting dryness requires the addition of water and the application of hydrophobic agents. The physician should instruct patients to soak affected areas several minutes and apply a hydrophobic substance. A variety of agents are available; plain petrolatum is inexpensive and effective, but it is not as pleasant to use as many proprietary preparations. The patient should avoid lanolin-based emollients if he is allergic to wool. Lubriderm and Keri lotions are light, easily applied, but less occlusive than the lanolin substances. Aquaphor and Eucerin are greasier than the above-mentioned lotions and creams. Crisco may be the most economical emollient. The plethora of expensive skin creams do little to retain moisture in the skin. Urea-containing creams are effective because they retain water by osmosis. In severe cases or in order to achieve immediate results, topical corticosteroids, often with occlusive dressing, produce effective and rapid results. Occasionally, oral antipruritic agents such as the antihistamines may be required for severe itching. The physician should emphasize patient education in order to prevent recurrence.

THERAPEUTIC RECOMMENDATIONS

- Instruct the patient on environmental modifications to increase ambient humidity.
- Caution the patient to avoid dehydrating soaps, solvents, or disinfectants.
- Encourage the patient to use bath oils and well oilated soaps. The patient should soak in the tub for 1 to 10 minutes before the bath oil is added.
- Emollients should be used after showering or bathing. Try a variety of agents beginning with the cheapest to find one that is acceptable.
- Lotions or creams that contain from 2 to 20 per cent urea are effective in holding water in the stratum corneum and may be used instead of hydrophobic agents.
- In the presence of eczematous change or for a patient who insists on rapid resolution, topical corticosteroid ointments with or without occlusion may be used.
- The most important aspect of management is patient education. The physician should reinforce the adjustments that prevent the development of dryness.

ANNOTATED BIBLIOGRAPHY

Blank, I.H.: Action of emollient creams and their additives. JAMA, *164*:412, 1959. *(Emollients help to retain water—rather than by aiding as "lubricants.")*

Middleton, J.O.: The effects of temperature on extensibility of isolated corneum and to relation to skin chapping. Br. J. Dermatol., *81*:717, 1969. *(The suppleness of stratum corneum is reduced easily when the temperature is lowered, perhaps a mechanism in chapping.)*

Steigleder, R., and Raab, W.P.: Skin protection afforded by ointments. J. Invest. Dermatol., *38*:129, 1962. *(Various ointments were compared for their barrier ability; white petrolatum proved to be the best.)*

178
Management of Intertrigo
WILLIAM V.R. SHELLOW, M.D.

Intertrigo is a dermatitis that affects the body folds. It is more common in obese people and is exacerbated by warm weather. The areas of involvement are the axillary, inguinal and inframammary folds. The primary physician should be capable of distinguishing intertrigo from other body-fold eruptions such as erythrasma, seborrheic dermatitis, psoriasis, and dermatophyte infections, as well as rendering appropriate treatment.

PATHOPHYSIOLOGY AND CLINICAL PRESENTATION

Intertrigo presents as erythematous exudative inflammation in the body folds. Patients may complain of soreness and itching, and with secondary invasion overt purulence may occur. The principal pathogenic mechanism is mechanical. Heat, moisture, and the retention of sweat produce maceration and irritation, an environment that permits secondary bacterial infection.

The early development of intertrigo is characterized by slight maceration and erythema. The moisture initially comes from eccrine sweat that cannot evaporate in the intertriginous areas. With time, the redness becomes more intense, and the epidermis becomes eroded or even denuded. Subsequent inflammation causes exudation of serous fluid. Increased moisture may lead to bacterial colonization, which accounts for the odor that may be associated with intertrigo. The groin and intergluteal areas may be colonized by gram-negative organisms. Incontinence of urine or feces may add to the maceration.

Intertrigo in the groin must be distinguished from tinea cruris and moniliasis. Tinea cruris is a fungal infection characterized by small, red, scaly patches. The lesions form circinate plaques with scaly or vesicular borders with central clearing. The diagnosis can be confirmed by scraping scales, adding 20 per cent potassium hydroxide solution, and finding hyphae under low microscopic power. Moniliasis produces deep, beefy-red lesions with characteristic satellite vesicopustules outside the border of the primary lesion. Involvement of the scrotum is common, unlike tinea, which usually spares the scrotum.

PRINCIPLES OF THERAPY

The primary principle of therapy is to alter the conditions that cause maceration and irritation when skin is in close apposition. The goal is to promote drying. This can be accomplished by exposing the intertriginous areas to air, possibly adding a fan or electric bulb to promote drying. Addition of a nonmedicated absorbing powder is helpful. Encourage the patient to wear dry, cotton, loose-fitting clothing. Women should wear bras that provide good support. The patient should avoid hot, humid environments and clothing that is made of wool, nylon, or synthetic fibers. Men with groin involvement should be encouraged to wear boxer shorts rather than briefs, and women cotton panties rather than nylon. The physician should forbid ointments and greasy preparations that retain moisture and exacerbate the condition.

There is no evidence that antibacterial soaps are more effective than ordinary toilet soaps. Medicated powders should be banned, but Zeasorb made from corn cobs is useful. Exudative lesions should be treated by the application of Burow's compresses in 1:20 or 1:40 dilutions.

Secondary bacterial infection should be treated. Pustules or scales should be examined microscopically and cultured for evidence of bacteria, candida, or dermatophytes. Therapy with the appropriate antimicrobial agents should be instituted. In uninfected intertrigo, corticosteroids may be added to reduce inflammation. Lotions with an alcohol base are quite drying and may sting. Fluorinated steroids should not be used for prolonged periods because intertriginous striae and atrophy are common complications. Popular preparations such as Vioform-Hydocortisone are effective, but stain clothing yellow. Mycolog has antibacterial, antimonilial, and anti-inflammatory activity, but the preservative ethylenediamine is a sensitizing agent. Hydrocortisone cream is an effective, safe, and cost-saving approach. Topical medication should be used sparingly to avoid retention of moisture. Treat concurrent medical conditions such as diabetes or obesity.

THERAPEUTIC RECOMMENDATIONS

- It is essential in therapy of intertrigo to eliminate precipitating conditions. Carefully dry the area that separates folds with absorbent material, dust with drying powders, and wear loose, absorbent clothing. In exudative lesions, a drying agent such as Burow's solution should be used to compress.
- Treat secondary bacterial or fungal infection with appropriate antibiotics.
- Treat inflammatory areas with topical hydrocortisone, and if necessary, with fluorinated steroids for short periods of time.
- The patient must understand the mechanical effects of skin occluding skin and be encouraged to use support bras, cotton clothing, or sandals to en-

sure adequate aeration of the specifically involved area. The patient should be instructed to look frequently in the intertriginous zone to detect early development of erythema and maceration so that effective therapy can be instituted early. In elderly immobile patients, the physician should educate the family or a friend to inspect intertriginous areas to prevent maceration and secondary infection.

ANNOTATED BIBLIOGRAPHY

Epstein, N.N., Epstein, W.L., and Epstein, J.H.: Atrophic striae in patients with intertrigo. Arch. Dermatol., *87*:450, 1963. *(Calls attention to the hazards of treating intertrigo with potent topical corticosteroids.)*

Sarkany, I., Taplen, D., and Blank, H.: The etiology and treatment of erythrasma. J. Invest. Dermatol., *37*:283, 1961. *(Excellent bacteriologic study of the disease.)*

Sarkany, I., Taplin, D., and Blank, H.: Incidence and bacteriology of erythrasma. Arch. Dermatol., *85*:578, 1962. *(Concise discussion of the disease and its etiology.)*

Smith, M.A., and Waterworth, P.M.: The bacteriology of some cases of intertrigo. Brit. J. Dermatol. *74*:323, 1962. *(Brief discussion of the bacterial flora found in intertriginous areas.)*

179

Management of Corns and Calluses
WILLIAM V.R. SHELLOW, M.D.

Corns and calluses are common and vexing lesions. They may not be a presenting complaint, but the primary care physicians will frequently be asked about them. Calluses can be confused with plantar warts but may be distinguished by the maintenance of normal skin markings, in contrast to verrucae where these markings are interrupted. The primary physician can provide diagnosis, simple therapy, advice on prevention, and referral to a dermatologist or podiatrist when that is indicated.

PATHOPHYSIOLOGY AND CLINICAL PRESENTATION

Corns (helomas or clavi) and calluses (tylomas or tyloses) have a common pathology. Friction and pressure on the skin overlying bony prominences lead to hyperemia, hypertrophy of dermal papillae, and proliferation of keratin. Corns often have a central hard core that is painful when the lesion is pressed. The pressure of shoes on the corn may cause pain when walking. Corns may develop at any joint, but the most common site is over the dorsum of the proximal interphalangeal joint. Hard corns show a translucent avascular core with interruption of normal skin markings. Soft corns appear macerated, resemble dermatophytosis, and are painful. The first and fourth web spaces are favored sites. Persons who do not wear shoes may develop calluses but usually do not develop corns. Calluses do not contain a central core, preserve normal skin markings, and occur preferentially across the metatarsal head area.

PRINCIPLES OF THERAPY

The primary physician's major contribution to therapy is to encourage prevention. The elimination of friction and pressure is the *sine qua non* of prevention. Shoes must fit correctly, and pressure over the toes must be evenly distributed. Softer shoe materials and sandals are often helpful. Stockings must fit properly and should cushion the foot. Keeping the feet dry with powder and changing shoes daily also reduce friction.

Symptomatic relief of calluses can be achieved by paring hyperkeratotic lesions with No. 10 or No. 15 scalpel. Keratin should be shaved off with the blade held parallel to the skin. Repeated strokes of the blade should be made in a direction least likely to cause penetration should the patient move suddenly. Movement from proximal to distal is best. Once a callus is removed, it is essential that previous weight-bearing not be continued, or the callus will return to its previous state.

Patients can treat corns and calluses themselves with intermittent débridement, using keratolytic agents. Salicylic and lactic acid combinations and 40 per cent salicylic acid plasters are used to reduce the thickness of tissue. The patient should cut a piece of 40 per cent salicylic acid plaster smaller than the lesion and apply it to the skin. It may be left overnight or for as long as several days. The dressing should be removed and the foot soaked. The softened and macerated skin is removed with a Buf-Ped or pumice stone. The plaster may be carefully reapplied as often as is necessary, in order to keep the lesions flat and asymptomatic.

A technique recently advocated is the injection of silicone under corns to cushion the skin from underlying bone. The reports of this technique have been successful, but removal from the market of medical-grade silicone fluid makes this technique impractical. The principles of treating soft corns involve reducing excess perspiration. Absorbent lamb's wool, soaking the foot in potassium permanganate, 1:4,000 solution, or silver nitrate cauterization have all been used with success.

Referral to a podiatrist or orthopedic surgeon is indicated when simple measures and advice fail to reduce symptoms or recurrences. Intrinsic bony problems subject the foot to uneven pressure. Pronation, flat feet, and medial and lateral imbalances should be treated. Padding of lesions with felt moleskin or lamb's wool may prevent uneven external pressure. Foam rubber surrounding the lesion will distribute pressure around the lesion rather than directly on it. Latex, plastic, or silicone molds may be individually adapted to prevent localized pressure from producing corns or calluses. Shoes may be constructed by a podiatrist to redistribute weight and pressure. Occasionally, surgical removal of a subjacent bony prominence eliminates the source of abnormal pressure on the skin.

THERAPEUTIC RECOMMENDATION

- Shoes must fit. The physician should advise the patient to avoid tight, pointed-toed shoes, and shoes should be changed frequently. Socks should cushion the sensitive area.
- Corns and calluses may be treated by the patient with proprietary plasters. The physician or patient can apply 40 per cent salicylic acid plaster to the lesion for several days. The lesion may then be pared down by the patient or physician. The physician should instruct the patient never to pull loose skin. Moleskin may be used to protect the tender area after paring. Once the lesions have been removed, the physician should insure that the foot is not subjected to the same pressures that originally produced the corns or calluses. The physician should care for diabetics and others with impaired vascular systems.
- In many cases, patient education and simple office techniques are successful. Refractory or unusual lesions should be referred to a podiatrist or orthopedist for definitive treatment of structural problems. Careful explanation of the objectives is essential to ensuring patient compliance.

ANNOTATED BIBLIOGRAPHY

Balkin, S.W.: Treatment of corns by injectable silicone. Arch. Dermatol., *111*:1143, 1975. *(The use of silicone as a cushion to prevent hyperkeratoses.)*

Gibbs, R.C.: Calluses, corns, warts. Am. Fam. Physician, *3*:92, 1971. *(Succinct and practical treatment of the subject for the primary practitioner.)*

Mann, R.A., and Duvales, H.L.: Intractable plantar keratosis. Orthop. Clin. North Am., *4*:67, 1973. *(Describes surgical techniques for this condition.)*

Montgomery, R.M.: Differential diagnoses of plantar hyperkeratoses. Cutis, *1*:74, 1965. *(A practical discussion of keratotic lesions of the foot.)*

Montgomery, R.M.: Relieving painful feet. Geriatrics, *29*:137, 1974. *(Practical tips useful in the office.)*

Schwartz, N.: A brief discussion on some of the causes of plantar keratoma. J. Am. Podiatry Assoc., *65*:666, 1975.

180

Management of Stasis Dermatitis and Leg Ulcers

WILLIAM F. KIVETT, M.D.

Dermatitis of the lower leg resulting from circulatory disturbances has profound medical, social and economic implications. It has been estimated that nearly half a million Americans have leg ulcers and associated stasis dermatitis. Careful attention to patient education is critical in successful treatment of this often chronic affliction. The primary physician is responsible for early recognition, treatment and prevention of complications. More important, the primary physician can prevent the development of ulcers when medical and surgical conditions predispose patients to this potentially incapacitating and difficult-to-manage problem.

PATHOPHYSIOLOGY AND CLINICAL PRESENTATION

Edema and clinical evidence of venous incompetence are common early warnings of stasis dermatitis. These conditions are frequently neglected by the patient. Stasis dermatitis and ulceration are due to increased hydrostatic pressure secondary to incompetent veins or systemic edema. Venous valves degenerate secondary to resolving thrombi, age, or poorly characterized genetic factors that produce venous varicosities. Edema secondary to congestive heart failure, hypoproteinemia, or venous obstruction may exacerbate venous insufficiency. Stasis changes may follow cellulitis, repeated scratching, blunt trauma, purpura, or prolonged nonspecific dermatitis.

Early dermatitis presents as an itchy red-blue erythema just superior to the medial malleolus, a site of natural inadequacy of local nutritive vascular sup-ply and subcutaneous tissue. The inflammation may become scaly, excoriated and oozing and is significantly worsened by scratching. Vesiculation occurs if sensitization reactions to various topical medicaments or to local infection by bacteria resident on the skin are superimposed. A widespread autosensitization inflammatory reaction ("id") may occur. Persistent venous and arteriolar engorgement leads to diapedesis of disintegrating red blood cells through the skin, resulting in nonpalpable brown, patchy hemosiderin deposits. Fibrotic change and atrophy of hair and local glands may ensue.

Ulcerations develop after stasis changes persist and remain unimproved. The progression to necrosis may be rapid, resulting from trauma, or gradual, secondary to prolonged devitalization by capillary hypertension, lymphatic sclerosis, collagen alteration, hypoxia and impaired exchange of nutrients. Clinically, stasis ulcers are sharply marginated, superficial, noninflamed, mildly painful and slow to heal. Leg ulcers develop from insults other than stasis dermatitis. Mycotic or treponemal infection, organic disease of large or small arteries, hemoglobinopathies such as sickle cell anemia, neuropathies such as diabetes, vasculitides, or vasospastic disorders are associated with leg ulcers.

PRINCIPLES OF THERAPY

The cardinal principle is to treat stasis dermatitis before ulcers develop and to treat ulcers promptly and aggressively to prevent intractability or complications. Treatment of stasis dermatitis begins with correction of edema (see Chapter 16) induced by systemic diseases such as congestive heart failure (see Chapter 27) or renal insufficiency (see Chapter 135). Reduction of venous pressure is critical for relief of stasis changes and ulceration. The physician should recommend weight loss in the obese, advise against prolonged standing, and encourage periods of elevation of the legs above the level of chest during the course of the day. The physiologic consequences of dependency and prolonged standing may be reversed with the use of external compressive dressings or stockings. A variety of commercial stockings are available, and the choice should be based on convenience and comfort. The compressive dressing should be applied in the morning before the patient arises from the supine position (see Chapter 30).

Care of the skin is essential to the prevention of breakdown and eventual ulceration. Dry skin should be treated with nightly washing and application of a hydrophilic substance. Active dermatitis or pruritus should be vigorously controlled with a steroid preparation. Areas of capillary damage with extravasation of fluid and blistering should be kept clean and dry with compresses soaked in Burow's solution applied several times a day. Over-the-counter medicaments and careless application of tape or dressings should be scrupulously avoided.

Preulcerative conditions such as blanching and hyperemia should be identified, and such areas should be protected from pressure or trauma. Once ulceration occurs, the principles are to keep the area scrupulously clean, prevent infection, and encourage development of granulation tissue. The ulcer should be kept clean by frequent application of wet to dry dressings with physiologic or hypertonic saline solution. Counterpressure of a dressing applied to the ulcer can be used to absorb wound discharge and control incompetent perforated veins frequently present beneath the ulcer. Reduction of venous pressure by elevation or compressive dressings should be emphasized. Bed rest with elevation may be necessary.

Adjunctive measures in the management of ulcers are controversial. Exposure of ulcers to sunlight is not necessary; it may induce release of histamine-like substances that promote further inflammation, extravasation of fluid and edema. Numerous topical and systemic agents that have been advocated as adjuvants in the treatment of ulcers are largely without clear indication. Topical antibiotics, elements, and simple compounds such as zinc, gold and titanium, dried blood plasma, and a variety of topical enzymes that chemically debride and clean have been advocated. None of these expensive agents have any clear

benefits, and their use should be restricted to hard-to-manage ulcers that are being treated by experienced clinicians. The use of systemic agents to promote healing, including oral zinc or vitamin C, is unsupported. When there is evidence of cellulitis or frank purulence, systemic antibiotics are indicated.

The general principles of ulcer treatment apply to lesions of arterial, neurotrophic, vasculitic or decubitus origin as well as to stasis ulcers. Identification of the underlying cause of the ulcer allows specific adjunctive measures. In treating decubitus ulcers, pressure on the skin should be avoided. Arterial ulcers should be treated with elevation of the head of the bed. Use of special shoes may avoid repeated trauma in neuropathic patients such as diabetics; vasculitic ulcers may respond to treatment of the primary disease. In all cases, failure of ulcers to resolve requires surgical consultation for consideration of intervention related to the underlying etiology or skin grafting.

THERAPEUTIC RECOMMENDATIONS

- In all patients with stasis changes, avoidance of dependency by rest, elevation and compressive dressings is essential.
- Pruritus should be treated with topical corticosteroids. Steroid ointments are helpful in dry, scaly areas, while creams are indicated in wet dermatitis.
- Avoid topical antibiotic ointments and adhesive tape.
- In difficult cases, weekly application of a zinc oxide paste (Unna) boot after a period of leg elevation may be useful.
- Acute exudative dermatitis should be kept dry and clean with wet compresses of cool water or Burow's solution in a 1:40 dilution three times a day.

Adjunctive measures indicated in stasis ulceration:

- Rigorous adherence to bed rest, elevation and, if the patient must walk, compressive dressings should be used.
- A wet to dry dressing is applied four times a day to the ulcer.
- Observe for purulence extension or periulcer erythema. Bacterial contamination must be investigated with aerobic and anaerobic cultures. Systemic antibiotics may be necessary.
- Radiologic study of the area of persistent ulcers may reveal an unsuspected osteomyelitis.
- Failure to obtain healing with good management and a compliant patient suggests the need for sur-

gical consultation (see Chapter 30). In carefully se-lected cases of stasis dermatitis and ulceration, high vein ligations and strippings performed by an experienced peripheral vascular surgeon may be beneficial. Excision and skin grafting may be indi-cated in selected patients. Patient education aimed at reducing edema, identifying preulcerative le-sions, and treating ulcers early is essential to mini-mizing the complications of stasis dermatitis.

ANNOTATED BIBLIOGRAPHY

Farber, E., and Batts, E.: Pathologic physiology of stasis syndrome. Arch. Dermatol. Syphilol., 70:653, 1954. *(Classic thorough analysis of clini-cal and histopathologic findings in the stasis syndrome.)*

Foley, J., et al.: Anticoagulant therapy of cryoglobu-linemic ulcers in a case of Sjögren's Syndrome. JAMA, 176:149, 1961. *(Description of clinical effects of coumadin on recurrent infected leg ul-cers secondary to cryoglobulinemia.)*

Lynch, P., and Epstein, S. (eds.): Burckhardt's Atlas and Manual of Dermatology and Venerealogy. Baltimore: Williams & Wilkins, 1977, p. 70. *(Ini-tial changes of stasis dermatitis lead to cracking of skin, exposure of nerve endings and further pruritic changes.)*

181

Management of Cellulitis
ELLIE J.C. GOLDSTEIN, M.D.

Cellulitis represents infection of the skin involv-ing the deeper subcutaneous layers. In an outpatient practice, older patients commonly present with red-ness and swelling of the lower extremities, and the differentiation of cellulitis from changes due to vas-cular insufficiency and phlebitis needs to be made. Once cellulitis is identified, the primary physician has to decide who can be managed at home on oral antibiotics and who requires hospitalization.

PATHOPHYSIOLOGY AND CLINICAL PRESENTATION

Any process which causes a break in the integrity of the skin will allow normal skin flora to gain access to the underlying subcutaneous tissue and initiate an inflammatory response; trauma, stasis ulceration, is-chemia and most causes of chronic edema are com-mon precipitants. Contiguous or hematogenous spread from other sites is uncommon, but does occur.

Any condition which impairs host response may predispose to cellulitis caused by opportunistic organ-isms such as gram-negative bacteria. The organisms producing cellulitis are often the normal inhabitants of the skin: the streptococci and, less frequently, *Staphylococcus aureus.* Cellulitis in the perineum may be caused by enteric aerobic and anaerobic bac-teria. Injury to mucosal surfaces predisposes to infec-tion with unusual organisms. Once the connective tis-sue is involved, the infection spread occurs along fascial planes. Staphylococci produce disease through their ability to multiply and through the production of extracellular enzymes, including alpha- and beta-hemolysin, leukocidin, coagulase, hyaluronidase and lipases. Streptococci also produce more than 20 ex-tracellular enzymes. Recent studies have emphasized the role of anaerobes in diabetic foot ulcers, abscess-es and traumatic wounds.

Cellulitis presents with local redness, heat, swell-ing and tenderness coming on over a few days. Fever, chills, or rigors are manifestations of potential bac-teremia. The clinical presentation does not allow de-lineation of the specific microbial etiology. Red streaks extending proximally in conjunction with tender lymph nodes indicate an associated lymphan-gitis. Crepitus indicates gas production and suggests anaerobic involvement.

WORKUP

Cellulitis first needs to be distinguished from oth-er causes of focal erythema, swelling and tenderness. Superficial thrombophlebitis may present very simi-larly, but the inflammatory response is usually cen-tered in the involved vein, which is tender and palpa-ble. The dependent rubor of arterial insufficiency is generalized, nontender and associated with diminish-ed or absent pulses and a cold extremity. Erythema nodosum differs clinically from cellulitis in that the lesions are typically multiple, exquisitely tender, and often pretibial in location. It should be remembered that cellulitis may occur concurrently with phlebitis or arterial insufficiency.

History. Once it is established that cellulitis is present, predisposing factors should be identified. Inquiry into history of diabetes, congestive failure, recent trauma, leg edema, claudication, previous infection and loss of sensation is helpful. A history of fever with rigors suggests bacteremia.

Physical examination should include a careful check for elevated temperature, lymphangitic streaking, proximal lymphadenopathy, heart murmur, peripheral edema, diminished peripheral pulses, skin atrophy or ulceration, and loss of sensation. Marking the borders of the lesion with an indelible pen allows assessment of progression. The presence of a discharge, crepitus or foul odor is important; the latter are suggestive of anaerobic infection.

Laboratory studies begin with a complete blood count and differential. When rigors, fever, heart murmur or lymphangitic spread is present, two blood cultures should be obtained. Most cellulitis is due to streptococci or staphylococci and, therefore, culture of the cellulitis area is not routinely performed. Moreover, it is difficult to culture the offending organism from unbroken skin, and there is no evidence that aspiration from the advancing margin is superior to aspiration from any other part of the skin. Culture is indicated in patients who have open, weeping wounds or infection in unusual areas such as the perineum; in such cases, anaerobic and aerobic cultures should be planted.

PRINCIPLES OF MANAGEMENT

The need for hospital admission must be considered. Hospitalization is required in patients who are compromised hosts or in whom cellulitis is rapidly progressive or recurrent. Cellulitis of the orbit, face or perineum, or elsewhere when accompanied by fever and lymphangitis, in most safely treated in an inpatient setting. When the patient appears unreliable and unable to care for himself at home, admission is indicated.

The majority of patients, however, may be treated as outpatients with oral antibiotics and supportive measures. Patients who are afebrile and in whom adenopathy and lymphangitis are absent may not even require antibiotics, but cellulitis is usually treated with antibiotics. The drugs of choice are either penicillin or a penicillinase-resistant semisynthetic penicillin preparation. There is little definitive evidence on which to base antibiotic selection. The high prevalence of streptococci, the sensitivity of some community-acquired staphylococci to penicillin, and the low cost of penicillin suggest that a reasonable approach is to start patients on penicillin and monitor them carefully. If after 48 hours the patient is still febrile or not improving, a penicillinase-resistant preparation can be substituted. Antibiotic therapy should continue for 7 to 14 days, depending on rate of clinical resolution. Infections of the perineum, face, or hands and those in a compromised host should be treated in consultation with an infectious disease specialist.

In patients with open wounds, the risk of tetanus should be considered. If a booster has not been obtained within 5 years, it should be given. Patients who have not had an initial tetanus series should receive both tetanus toxoid and tetanus immune globulin (see Chapter 4).

Supportive measures, in addition to antibiotics, can be important. These include elevation of the affected part and scrupulous prevention of new trauma. The addition of heat may help in resolution of cellulitis by promoting blood flow to the area. In patients with underlying conditions such as congestive failure, stasis dermatitis or vascular insufficiency, control of edema and maintenance of skin moisturization may be necessary for prevention of recurrent episodes.

THERAPEUTIC RECOMMENDATIONS AND INDICATIONS FOR ADMISSION

- Hospitalize the patient unable to reliably care for himself at home, as well as anyone with high fever, rigors, lymphangitis, rapid progression, compromised host defenses, or involvement of the face, orbit or perineum. Consultation with an infectious disease specialist is advisable.
- If the uncomplicated, mildly ill patient can be followed closely on an ambulatory basis, begin oral therapy with phenoxymethyl penicillin, 500 mg. every 6 hours, and monitor over the next 48 hours. If close contact with the patient is not possible or if inflammation and fever do not resolve within 48 hours, a penicillinase-resistant penicillin, such as dicloxacillin, 500 mg. every 6 hours, should be substituted. In patients allergic to penicillin, erythro-

mycin, 500 mg. every 6 hours, is the drug of choice.

- All patients should receive supportive care, including the application of heat, elevation of the affected part, and strict avoidance of trauma.
- Patients without a recent tetanus booster and with an open wound should be given 0.5 cc. of tetanus toxoid intramuscularly.

PATIENT EDUCATION

The patient should be instructed to remain in bed most of the time, but may have bathroom privileges. If there is leg edema, he should be encouraged to keep the swollen foot elevated and do foot exercises to reduce the possibility of thrombophlebitis. It is crucial to protect the affected area and to insist that the patient not scratch. The importance of taking antibiotic therapy as instructed should be reinforced, as well as the need to take penicillin on an empty stomach. The patient should be asked to record progression and temperature on a daily basis and to call if there is persistent elevation or a failure of resolution of the cellulitic area. The patient needs to know that cellulitis usually resolves within 5 to 7 days and to return promptly for follow-up if improvement is not evident.

ANNOTATED BIBLIOGRAPHY

Finegold, S.M.: Anaerobic Bacteria in Human Disease. New York: Academic Press, 1977, pp. 395-402. *(An excellent discussion and source of references on anaerobic cellulitis, gas gangrene and clostridial myonecrosis.)*

Louie, T.M., Bartlett, J.G, Tally, F.P. *et al.*: Aerobic and anaerobic bacteria in diabetic foot ulcers. Ann. Intern. Med. *85*:461, 1976. *(Twenty diabetic patients were studied using optimal culture techniques. A complex flora of both aerobic and anaerobic bacteria was found which should be considered in the selection of antimicrobial therapy.)*

Meislin, H.W., Lerner, S.A., Graves, M.H., *et al.*: Cutaneous abscesses: Anaerobic and aerobic bacteriology and outpatient management. Ann. Intern. Med., *87*:145, 1977. *(One hundred thirty-five patients were studied, and the microbiologic findings discussed. Primary therapy was felt to be incision and drainage, while use of antibiotics was considered adjunctive or optional.)*

Wannamaker, L.W.: Differences between streptococcal infections of the throat and of the skin. New. Eng. J. Med., *282*:23, 78, 1970. *(A must for basic reading; includes a discussion of nephrogenic serotypes and site of antecedent infection.)*

182

Management of Pyodermas
WILLIAM V.R. SHELLOW, M.D.

Primary cutaneous bacterial infections are usually initiated by a single organism such as coagulase-positive staphylococci or beta-hemolytic streptococci. Primary infection develops on normal skin while secondary infection is defined as a bacterial component superimposed on diseased skin. Cutaneous bacterial infections may be classified according to the depth of the infection and the propensity for scarring. Infection demands prompt recognition by the primary physician and effective antibiotic treatment.

PATHOPHYSIOLOGY AND CLINICAL PRESENTATION

The pathogenic mechanism of pyodermas is infection. The clinical expression of the infection re-

flects the organism, environmental factors, skin appendages, and host resistance. The common pyodermas include impetigo, ecthyma, folliculitis, furunculosis, and erysipelas.

Impetigo is a common lesion caused by staphylococci or beta-hemolytic streptococci. Some observers believe that intense erythema at the base of a pustule suggests streptococcal causation. Impetigo is seen most frequently in children, but it also occurs in adults. Poor hygiene may predispose persons to the development of infection. Impetigo is less highly contagious in adults than among infants.

Impetigo begins as a small erythematous macular lesion that evolves into a vesicle. Vesicles are located beneath the stratum corneum, and the thin-roofed collection of fluid ruptures easily, leaving denuded, oozing areas. The fluid dries and builds up to form a honey-colored crust. New lesions appear in the same location and they coalesce. When the honey-colored crusts are removed, the skin appears raw. Individual lesions usually do not exceed 2 cm. in size. The face is the most common site of involvement. Ordinary lesions do not produce scarring but may leave erythematous marks for a time. Untreated infections may last for weeks.

Ecthyma, usually caused by streptococci, is a deeper version of impetigo. Erosion of the epidermis creates ulcerative, crusted lesions. The heaped-up crust conceals the underlying erosion. Healing is accompanied by some scarring because of the depth of the lesions. The legs are commonly involved, and children are more susceptible. Antecedent conditions include eczema, scabies, arthropod bites, trauma, and hot, humid climates.

Folliculitis is infection of the hair follicles, usually caused by coagulase-positive staphylococci, and may be divided into superficial and deep types. Superficial folliculitis consists of a small pustule pierced by the hair shaft. It may be seen on the scalp or other hairy portions of the body. Occupational exposure to cutting oils, coal tar products, or topical corticosteroids under occlusion may precipitate folliculitis. Rarely, small pustules with surrounding erythema due to *Propionibacterium acnes* may develop around the occiput in males.

Furuncles or *boils* may develop from a preceding folliculitis. They are not seen where there is no hair. The erythematous and tender lesion usually becomes fluctuant after 4 days. A yellowish pointed area may be seen on the surface, and if the lesion ruptures spontaneously, pus and necrotic tissue are extruded. The buttocks, axillae, neck, face, and waist areas are frequent sites of involvement. Systemic factors such as diabetes, malnutrition, obesity, and hematologic disorders predispose persons to furunculosis. Carbuncles are a coalescence of deep furuncles with multiple points of drainage.

Erysipelas, caused by beta-hemolytic streptococci, is characterized by a peripherally spreading, infiltrated, erythematous, sharply circumscribed plaque. The lesion is warm to touch. The face, scalp, hands, and genitals are frequently involved. Rapid evolution of the lesions is seen, and some patients have constitutional symptoms such as fever and malaise. Poor hygiene and lowered resistance promote infection. Trauma may elicit infection, and recurrent erysipelas may lead to brawny edema.

PRINCIPLES OF THERAPY

The principles of therapy are the use of physical measures to enhance resolution and make the skin surface less amenable to colonization by bacteria and to treat infecting agents with antimicrobial drugs. The physical measures employed differ with the pyoderma being treated. Impetigo must be compressed to remove the crust in order to expose the surface where bacteria are present. Furuncles and carbuncles are treated with hot compresses to enhance drainage. Fluctuant lesions may require incision. Exudative lesions require drying compresses to remove detritus and desiccate the lesion. Saline, tap water, or Burow's solution may be applied for 10 to 20 minutes, three to four times a day. Dehydration improves the appearance of the skin and destroys many organisms.

The principle of reducing colonization is particularly important in the treatment of recurrent furunculosis. Frequent cleansing with soap, particularly hexachlorophene-containing detergents, is useful. Nails should be clipped and vigorously scrubbed. Antibiotic cream should be instilled into the anterior nares. Before shaving, the beard should be soaked with hot water for 5 minutes, and blades should be discarded after each use. The razor should be soaked in alcohol. Separate towels, sheets, and clothing should be used, and everything should be laundered and changed frequently. If vigorous reduction of colonization is unsuccessful, consideration should be given for replacement of the pathogenic staphyloccal flora with a less pathogenic strain.

Antibiotics are essential in treating infections. Lesions may be treated on clinical appearance, but microscopic examination of Gram-stained material is a quick and inexpensive way to confirm a diagnosis. Culture and sensitivity are usually not necessary for superficial infections, but are for more destructive lesions or if the patient is not improving. Topical therapy is usually sufficient for impetigo and folliculitis, particularly when it is combined with cleansing and débridement. Most pyodermas are caused by gram-positive organisms and respond to erythromycin or bacitracin. Neomycin is effective, but it should be used sparingly because of potential allergic sensitization. Systemic antibiotic therapy is indicated when there are constitutional symptoms or if the patient is uncooperative.

Glomerulonephritis is an uncommon complication secondary to cutaneous streptococcal infection. There is no evidence that antibiotics prevent postimpetigo glomerulonephritis. When systemic antibiotics are required for streptococcal infections, penicillin is adequate. Erythromycin is effective against both staphylococci and streptococci. Resistant staphylococci must be treated with semisynthetic penicillins.

THERAPEUTIC RECOMMENDATIONS

- Impetigo should be treated with Burow's compresses for 20 minutes, two to four times daily, followed by gentle débridement using a washcloth and cleansing with Phisohex® or Hibiclens®. A topical antibiotic such as erythromycin or a bacitracin-polymyxin combination should be applied lightly to the area after drying. Ointments may be used at night. The lesions should not be covered, and the family should be instructed to avoid using the same towel or washcloth and to keep children away from the patient with impetigo.
- Folliculitis should be treated with débridement and topical antibiotics. Furuncles and carbuncles should be treated with hot compresses until the lesions are fluctuant and spontaneous drainage occurs. Larger lesions may require removal of the core with a 4-mm. biopsy punch to facilitate drainage. Furuncles or carbuncles associated with cellulitis, fever, or located on the face must be treated with systemic antibiotics such as erythromycin, 1 g. a day for 10 days, or a semisynthetic penicillin. Recurrent furunculosis requires a 10- to 14-day course of a systemic antibiotic, combined with removal of bacteria from potential sources such as the skin, nares, nails, razor or other fomites. Aggressive hygienic measures and occasionally replacement with nonpathogenic staphylococcus can resolve recurrent furunculosis. Erysipelas should be treated with cool compresses and penicillin G.
- A primary consideration in the therapy of all pyodermas is patient education. Aggressive and regular use of cleansing and débridement are essential to the successful resolution of the infection.

ANNOTATED BIBLIOGRAPHY

Dillon, H.C., Jr.: Impetigo contagiosa: Suppurative and non-suppurative complications. Am. J. Dis. Child., *115*:530, 1968. *(Excellent discussion of clinical epidemiologic and bacteriologic characteristics of impetigo in 497 children.)*

Dillon, H.C., Jr.: The treatment of streptococcal skin infections. J. Pediat., *76*:676, 1970. *(Intramuscular benzathine penicillin G was the drug of choice for these pyodermas.)*

Dillon, H.C., Jr., et al.: Epidemiology of impetigo and acute glomerulonephritis. Results of serologic typing of group A streptococci. Am. J. Epidemiol., *86*:710, 1967. *(Certain strains of streptococci causing impetigo are nephritogenic.)*

Duncan, W.C., Dodge, B.G., and Knox, J.M.: Prevention of superficial pyogenic skin infections. Arch. Dermatol., *99*:465, 1969. *(The regular use of an antibacterial soap reduced the incidence of superficial bacterial infections.)*

Maibach, H., Strauss, W.G., and Shinefield, W.: Bacterial interference therapy in the management of recurrent furunculosis. Br. J. Dermatol., *81 [Suppl. 1]*:69, 1969. *(The principles and practice of inducing bacterial interference with staphylococci 502A.)*

Steele, R.W.: Recurrent staphylococcal infection in families. Arch. Dermatol., *116*:189, 1980. *(Controlled study which showed 83% retention of inoculated* S. aureus *organism after 6 months.)*

Storrs, F.J.: Treatment of nonbullous impetigo. Cutis, *16*:886, 1975. *(Brief discussion of the various topical and systemic methods of treating impetigo.)*

Zayhoun, S.T., Uwayda, M.M., and Kurban, A.C.: Topical antibiotics in pyoderma. Br. J. Dermatol., *90*:331, 1974. *(Patients treated with topical gentamicin did no better than those on a placebo cream. Antibacterial soap was used and crusts were removed.)*

183

Management of Superficial Fungal Infections

WILLIAM V.R. SHELLOW, M.D.

Superficial fungal infections are prevalent and easily diagnosed. It is paradoxical that such infections are undiagnosed, or nonfungal dermatoses are incorrectly treated as, fungal infections. The primary physician must be familiar with definitive methods of diagnosis and cost-effective therapy. It is essential that the physician diagnose superficial fungal infection precisely in order to treat specifically. Though neither dangerous nor life-threatening, fungal infections can be irritating and recurrent. Therefore, the primary physician must educate patients on ways to reduce recurrence.

PATHOPHYSIOLOGY AND CLINICAL PRESENTATION

A pathophysiologic consideration that is still incompletely understood is why most people resist these ubiquitous pathogens while others seem unable to rid themselves of infections. Systemic diseases such as diabetes increase susceptibility to Candida infection. Studies suggest that hereditary factors may be involved, but an important factor may be local susceptibility caused by maceration of the skin.

Fungal infection occurs when one of these ubiquitous organisms invades the superficial layers of the skin. Dermatophytes do not invade below the level of keratin because a potent antifungal factor prevents deeper infection. Candidal infection produces inflammatory change through elaboration of an endotoxinlike substance.

Tinea versicolor is characterized by brown, scaly patches that occur on the chest, back, and shoulders. Tinea versicolor, particularly during the summer, may present as hypopigmented areas, often erroneously interpreted as vitiligo. The organism appears to prevent pigment transfer from melanocytes to epidermal cells. The diagnosis can be suspected if scratching a macular area raises a fine and branny scale. Examination of the skin with a Wood's light reveals gold or orange-brown fluorescence. The infection is diagnosed by scraping a scaly lesion and examining it with a drop of 20 per cent potassium hydroxide for characteristic short hyphae and spores, sometimes referred to as "spaghetti and meatballs."

Dermatophytic and candidal infections are scaly, mildly erythematous, with defined margins occurring in characteristic areas of the body which promote the growth of fungi.

Dermatophyte infections are defined by the area of the body that they affect. The most common are tinea cruris, which involves the groin, inner thigh, and sometimes the abdomen and buttocks, and tinea pedis, characterized by blisters and inflammation on the soles and interdigital areas of the feet. Tinea corporis affects the nonhairy portion of the skin, particularly the face, arms, and shoulders. Tinea capitis, or scalp ringworm, occurs almost exclusively in children. Tinea barbae has become relatively uncommon. Onychomycosis is characterized by the accumulation of subungual keratin, which produces a thickened, distorted, and crumbly nail.

Diagnosis requires microscopic examination for hyphae and spores in a potassium hydroxide wetmount. Occasionally, a scraping will have to be planted on Sabouraud agar in order to culture the fungus.

Candida infections of the skin occur principally in intertriginous locations such as the axillae, groin, intergluteal folds, inframammary area, or interdigital web spaces. Crusted involvement of the labial commissures, known as perlèche, and involvement of the glans penis also occur. Lesions are pustular, thin-walled, on a red base, often producing burning and itching. Candidiasis may be clinically suspected as a result of the presence of characteristic satellite pustules outside of the margin of the primary lesion. Diagnosis requires microscopic demonstration of budding spores and pseudohyphae.

PRINCIPLES OF MANAGEMENT

Fungal infections require management of the conditions that predispose to infection and use of specific antifungal agents. The elimination of moisture reduces the likelihood of fungal infection. Inflammatory or weeping lesions should be dried with the application of a desiccating agent such as aluminum acetate, available as Burow's solution. Once predisposing factors have been reduced and the lesions dried, specific antifungal medication is appropriate. There are a host of effective agents available; the physician should prescribe the least expensive effective agent that produces the fewest annoying side effects. The physician must instruct the patient on how to keep the skin dry and on the proper use of the topical antifungal agents, including manner of application, duration of application, and treatment course.

It may be worthwhile to investigate host factors that predispose to fungal infection, such as corticosteroids or coexistent disease, such as diabetes.

MANAGEMENT RECOMMENDATIONS

The etiologic agent *Pityrosporon orbiculare* can effectively be treated by selenium sulfide, sodium thiosulfate, salicylic acid, or one of the antifungal agents such as haloprogin, miconazole, or clotrimazole. For effectiveness, convenience, and least expense, a 2.5 per cent suspension of selenium sulfide applied with a rough washcloth, allowed to remain on affected areas for 10 minutes and repeated daily for 1 week, is the recommended therapy. In refractory cases, the selenium sulfide suspension may be left on the skin overnight. Treatment must be continued for at least 7 days. Sodium thiosulfate may be malodorous, and other topical antifungal agents are four to five times more expensive. Patients who suffer relapse may reduce recurrence by applying selenium sulfide for two consecutive nights monthly for a period of 6 months to a year.

Trichophyton rubrum, Trichophyton mentagrophytes, and Epidermophyton floccosum are the most frequent infecting organisms, but the actual agent is less important than is the establishment of a fungal etiology. Treatment is similarly independent of location; the lesion should be kept dry and clean, and an effective topical agent applied. The patient should dry oozing lesions by applying compresses soaked in Burow's solution one to three times a day, depending on results, and then apply a nonmedicated talcum powder. There are a number of effective anti-fungal agents, but it is not clear that any is distinctly superior. Tolnaftate (Tinactin®) is available over the counter, and many patients have already tried it by the time they seek a physician's counsel. Clotrimazole (Lotrimin®), haloprogin (Halotex®), or miconazole (MicaTin®) may be used. Haloprogin has the disadvantage of being slightly malodorous. All have been demonstrated to be quite effective though expensive. Topical lotions should be applied in the morning, on return from work, and as a cream at night. Refractory cases may be managed by using a combination of two agents, one during the day and a different preparation at night. If lesions persist, it may be necessary to use griseofulvin, a systemic medication. This costly but effective medication (125 mg. twice daily), taken in ultramicrosized form, should be taken for 2 to 3 weeks. Before using this toxic systemic agent, a dermatologic consultation may be helpful.

Onychomycosis sometimes responds to ultramicrosized griseofulvin, 125 mg., three or four times a day, for as long as it takes for the nail to regrow. Some physicians advocate monthly blood counts because griseofulvin has been associated with leukopenia. It may be necessary to remove the affected nails and then treat with griseofulvin. This rather radical therapy may not effect a cure, and even when cure is obtained, reinfection is common. Men should be counseled to live with their infections, and women have the option of using nail polish to cover cosmetic unsightliness.

Treatment of candidiasis requires meticulous drying of the area, adequate ventilation, and specific therapy. Gentian violet and Castellani's Paint are old and effective, but quite messy. Staining therapies have largely been abandoned. Nystatin is the most specific drug, but clotrimazole is increasingly being used. The creams are applied to the area 2 or 3 times daily. The ointment should generally be avoided because it maintains a moist environment, contributing to maceration. Nystatin is available in combination with steroids and other antimicrobial agents. Combination agents should be avoided because of greater cost and their potential for inducing sensitization. In highly inflamed infection, nystatin in combination with steroid may be useful. In difficult skin infections, daily use of nystatin during the day may be combined with a nighttime application of iodochlorhydroxyquin and hydrocortisone cream. In patients with candidal infections, the physician should consider predisposing factors such as the use of corticosteroids, birth control pills, tetracycline, or other antibiotics. Pregnancy, diabetes, Cushing's syndrome and defects in cellular immunity may predispose to candida.

Candidal paronychia is difficult to treat. Therapy consists of avoiding exposure to water by wearing rubber gloves with cotton gloves underneath whenever contact is unavoidable. Nystatin or Amphoterin B lotion should be applied two to four times daily to the affected area. In highly inflamed conditions, nystatin with steroids may be applied overnight under a fingercot. Nails grow out normally after the paronychia has healed.

Referral to a dermatologist is necessary only when a fungal infection proves refractory to conventional treatment. The primary physician should perform a workup on a patient with a recurring infection, and on rare occasions—when recurrences are frequent and in several locations despite aggressive therapy—a patient will need to be referred for immunologic evaluation.

PATIENT EDUCATION

At the time of the first incident, patients with fungal infection should be instructed in appropriate measures to prevent recurrence. Dryness is the essential condition that the patient should maintain. This is particularly important in tinea pedis, tinea cruris, and candidal infections. Preventive measures should be taken in areas that have shown a tendency to become infected.

Additionally, the patient should be told to apply powder liberally to naturally moist areas of the body and to wear cotton clothing and loose-fitting underwear. Also, patients with tinea pedis should always wear socks and avoid sneakers and rubber-soled shoes, and the physician should encourage exposure of feet to the air as frequently as possible. Last, people who sweat profusely should change clothing more frequently, shower, and apply nonmedicated talcum powder.

It is important for the physician to instruct the patient carefully in appropriate therapy and length of treatment. Prophylactic measures may reduce recurrences. After treatment for fungal infections, patients do not usually need to return to the physician. Examine patients with tinea versicolor, for continued scaling is evidence of persistent activity. The patient should be advised that depigmentation may persist though the infection has been adequately treated. Patients should be instructed to call at the first sign of recurrence and to institute appropriate drying measures and specific therapy after physician consultation.

ANNOTATED BIBLIOGRAPHY

Albright, S.D., and Hitch, J.M.: Rapid treatment of tinea versicolor with selenium sulfide. Arch. Dermatol., *93*:460, 1966. *(Discussion of various regimens utilizing selenium sulfide.)*

DeVillez, R.L., and Lewis, C.W.: Candidiasis seminar. Cutis, *19*:69, 1977. *(A good review of the epidemiologic, diagnostic and therapeutic considerations in treating Candida.)*

Jones, H.E., Reinhardt, J.H., and Rinaldi, M.G.: A clinical, mycological and immunological survey of dermatophytosis. Arch. Dermatol., *108*:61, 1973. *(An in-depth, scientific discussion of the pathophysiology of dermatophyte infections.)*

Kligman, A.M.: Tinea capitis due to *M. audouini* and *M. canis:* II. Dynamics of the host-parasite relationship. Arch. Dermatol., *71*:313, 1955. *(Elegant and literate description of the subject.)*

Leyden, J.J., and Kligman, A.M.: Interdigital athlete's foot: New concepts in pathogenesis. Postgrad. Med., *61*:113, 1977. *(A review of the role of bacteria and fungi as well as how to prevent this common disease.)*

Lyddon, F.E., Coundersen, K., and Maibach, H.I.: Short-chain fatty acids in the treatment of dermatophytoses. Int. J. Dermatol., *19*:24, 1980. *(Reviews topical antifungal therapy with emphasis on undecylenic acid.)*

Maibach, H.I.: Iodochlorhydroxyquin-hydrocortisone treatment of fungal infections. Arch. Dermatol., *114*:1773, 1978. *(Double-blind investigation proved that the combination was effective in the treatment of cutaneous fungal infections.)*

Maibach, H.I. and Kligman, A.M.: The biology of experimental human cutaneous moniliasis *(Candida albicans)*. Arch. Dermatol., *85*:233, 1962. *(The definitive monograph on the nature of disease produced by* Candida albicans.)

Mandy, S.J., and Garrott, T.C.: Miconazole treatment for severe dermatophytoses. JAMA, *230*:72, 1974. *(A 2 per cent cream compared with placebo is 90 per cent effective, with recurrence in only 1 of 62.)*

Quiñones, C.A.: Tinea versicolor: New topical treatments. Cutis, *25*:386, 1980. *(Use of various imidazole antifungal creams.)*

Sutton, R.L., and Waisman, M.: Dermatoses due to fungi. Cutis, *19*:377, 1977. *(A comprehensive review of all fungal skin infections.)*

Van Dersal, J.V., and Sheppard, R.H. Clotrimazole vs. haloprogin treatment of tinea cruris. Arch. Dermatol., *113*:1233, 1977. *(Discusses the newer topical antifungal agents and their efficacy.)*

Zaias, N.: Onychomycosis. Arch. Dermatol., *105*:263, 1972. *(A lucid discussion of fungal infections of the nails.)*

184

Management of
Cutaneous Herpes Simplex
WILLIAM V.R. SHELLOW, M.D.

Herpes simplex, also known as herpesvirus hominis (HVH), is one of the most ubiquitous viruses that affect man. Most people have been infected by this large DNA virus, although infection is usually subclinical. Primary symptomatic infection by HVH results in distinct but uncommon clinical syndromes, but recurrent cutaneous herpes simplex infection is common and therefore important in office-based practice. Patients may seek medical advice because of recurrent cosmetic concern, burning or irritation. The primary physician must be able to render good advice and supportive treatment.

PATHOPHYSIOLOGY AND CLINICAL PRESENTATION

Entrance into the body by the herpes simplex virus may be unnoticed. Children, usually 2 to 5 years of age, and occasionally adults, demonstrate primary herpes infection syndrome as gingivostomatitis. Painful oral or gingival lesions and localized lymphadenopathy, fever and malaise over a 2- to 3-week period are characteristic. Primary herpetic vulvovaginitis is an increasingly recognized venereally transmitted infection of adolescents and young adults. The infection is characterized by pain, mucosal erosion and soft tissue edema. An unusual form of primary infection results from the implantation of the virus into broken skin, as in medical and dental personnel who come in contact with infected patients. "Herpetic whitlow" is characterized by pain, swelling and erythema of the fingers, with pronounced adenopathy. Wrestlers may incur "herpes gladiatorum"—primary herpes on exposed parts of the body.

The most common presentation is recurrent herpes labialis, often referred to as a cold sore or fever blister. Regardless of whether HVH infection is symptomatic or subclinical, the virus travels up the nerve axon to the regional ganglia. There it may remain in a nonreplicative state during the lifetime of the host, or, in response to various stimuli, viral particles may travel down the endoneural sheath to the skin, producing the characteristic clear grouped vesicles on an erythematous base. After several days, the vesicles become turbid and may coalesce. Crusting supervenes and lasts for another 4 to 8 days, rarely longer. Location on the lips and genitals is common, but herpes simplex lesions may appear on the ear, buttock, shoulder or elsewhere, depending upon the location of the ganglion to which the virus has migrated. Recurrences usually appear within the same dermatomal distribution. Virus is present in the skin for the first 96 hours after the vesicles appear, during which time the disease can be transmitted from person to person. Periodic reactivations of HVH produce self-limited eruptions that last 5 to 14 days. Recurrences at the same site may produce some atrophy or scarring.

Recurrent herpes simplex infections characteristically last from 7 to 10 days; unlike primary infections, they do not have a systemic component. Localized lymphadenopathy may be present, and mild to moderate paresthesias may result from nerve irritation as the virions travel down the nerve from the ganglion. This prodrome of tingling, burning or itching may occur hours to days before the lesion appears.

PRINCIPLES OF THERAPY

Since herpes is a self-limited condition, attention is directed at prevention. Recurrences may be reduced by minimizing precipitants, which include sunlight, colds, fever, menses and psychological stress. Secondary infection can be reduced by topical antibiotic ointments, with or without hydrocortisone, that reduce inflammation.

There is no specific antiviral therapy, nor has any approach to preventing recurrences been established as safe and effective. The physician should allow the infection to run its natural course without causing additional harm. Intralesional injection of corticosteroids, which may accelerate healing but also may cause localized atrophy of the skin, should be avoided. Topical antiviral agents such as idoxuridine and adenine arabinoside work *in vitro* but do not significantly affect cutaneous disease in practice. New vehicles which enhance penetration may make antiviral therapy clinically effective. Photoinactivation of the virus with dyes and visible light has been interdicted as no better than placebo and potentially oncogenic.

Repeated vaccinations with smallpox vaccine are no more effective than placebo and should be interdicted because of the potential side effects. BCG vaccination and therapy with levamisole are no better than placebo. The safety or efficacy of specific vaccines against HVH has not been established. The use of oral type II poliomyelitis vaccine has been reported but is in need of confirmation. Popular treatments such as ether, chloroform, or oral lysine are without documented benefit. Many clinicians advocate early and frequent application of topical corticosteroids to abort progression of the lesions. This empiric approach lacks scientific support, though no evidence exists to show that it is dangerous. Over-the-counter preparations such as Blistex®, Camphophenique® or Anbesol® may provide minimal symptomatic relief but do not affect the course of the eruption. Considering the long history of ineffective therapeutics in this disease, one should remain skeptical about any new remedy suggested.

THERAPEUTIC RECOMMENDATIONS

- The self-limited nature of the problem combined with marginally effective treatments make preventive therapy the preferred approach.
- For symptomatic relief of weeping lesions, drying compresses of Burow's solution are helpful. The astringent effect of wet tea bags may be useful.
- Patients may use over-the-counter preparations they believe are helpful.
- The lesions should be kept clean with drying compresses, and topical antibiotics should be instituted at the first sign of bacterial infection.
- The patient should be reassured about the benign nature of the problem. Patients concerned about keratoconjunctivitis should be assured that cutaneous to ocular infection is not believed to occur. Simple cleanliness and the avoidance of exposure to precipitants such as sunlight should be emphasized. In patients in whom herpes labialis occurs with menses, aspirin taken prior to the onset of each period may prevent the eruption.

ANNOTATED BIBLIOGRAPHY

Barringer, J.R.: Recovery of herpes simplex virus from human sacral ganglion. N. Engl. J. Med., *291*:828, 1974. *(Evidence given for residence of the latent Type II HVH within human sacral sensory ganglia.)*

Bierman, S.M.: The mechanism of recurrent infection by herpes virus hominis. Arch. Derm. atol., *112*:1459, 1976. *(An excellent short review of the reasons for the recurrence of herpes simplex infection.)*

Curry, S.S.: Cutaneous herpes simplex infections and their treatment. Cutis, *26*:41, 1980. *(Excellent up-to-date review with 61 references.)*

Felber, T.D., Smith, E.B., Knox, J.M., et al.: Photodynamic inactivation of herpes simplex: Report of a clinical trial. JAMA, *223*:289, 1973. *(Theoretical basis for heterocyclic dye and light therapy.)*

Myers, M.G., Oxman, M.N., Clark J.E., et al.: Failure of neutral red photodynamic inactivation in recurrent herpes simplex virus infections. N. Engl. J. Med., *293*:945, 1975. *(Discusses potential oncogenicity of photodynamically inactivated HVH.)*

Nahmias, A.J., and Roizman, B: Infection with herpes simplex viruses 1 and 2. N. Engl. J. Med., *289*:667; 719; 781, 1973. *(A most comprehensive three-part discussion of HVH infection including its role in carcinogenesis, 234 refs.)*

Notkins, A. L., Bankowski, R.A., Baron, S., et al.: Workshop on the treatment and prevention of herpes simplex virus infections. J. Infect. Dis., *127*:117, 1973. *(Epidemiologic statistics and suggested areas for research.)*

Sabin, A.B.: Misery of recurrent herpes: What to do. N. Engl. J. Med., *293*:986, 1975. *(Recommendations of topical ether therapy.)*

Spruance, S.L., Overall, J.C., Kern, E.R., et al.: The natural history of recurrent herpes simplex labialis: Implications for antiviral therapy. N. Engl. J. Med., *297*:69, 1977. *(Recent observations on untreated herpetic lesions of the lip, and the difficulties in studying antiviral medications.)*

185
Management of Herpes Zoster
WILLIAM V.R. SHELLOW, M.D.

Herpes zoster (shingles) is a common viral cutaneous eruption. It presents with radicular pain followed by the appearance of grouped vesicles on an erythematous base in a dermatomal distribution. Incidence increases with age. No seasonal variations are seen, nor is it correlated with outbreaks of varicella. The primary physician must be able to recognize zoster, make the patient more comfortable, and prevent complications.

PATHOPHYSIOLOGY AND CLINICAL PRESENTATION

Zoster represents a recrudescence of infection by the varicella-zoster virus. The virus apparently lies dormant in a nerve ganglion in a genomic state until reactivation occurs later in life. Few patients have an associated disease, though leukemia, Hodgkin's disease and other lymphomas are sometimes present. Some patients describe feeling "run down" or being emotionally distressed before the development of clinical lesions. Nerve root changes consist of necrotization and sometimes cyst formation.

Zoster may present with dermatomal pain, itch, or tenderness that precedes cutaneous lesions by 1 to 7 days, rarely longer. The cutaneous eruption is characterized by tense vesicles that arise on an erythematous base and are distributed along a dermatome. They become pustular within a few days, followed by crusting and healing over a 14 to 18-day period. The crust may be dark, almost black. Depending upon the depth of lesions, residual scarring and atrophy, or merely transient erythema, may be seen. Malaise, low-grade fever and adenopathy may accompany the eruption. The most commonly affected dermatomes are C2, L2, and the opthalmic branch of the trigeminal nerve. The course is related to the time new vesicles develop; several days of vesicle development leads to a two and a half week course; development of new vesicles over a week predicts a more prolonged course.

Complications include infection, uveitis, postherpetic neuralgia, and dissemination. Vesicles on the tip of the nose indicate nasociliary involvement and intraocular inflammation. Patients over 50 years of age may suffer persistent postherpetic neuralgia. The pain may be intractable, requiring extreme procedures such as posterior rhizotomy or cordotomy.

Generalized or disseminated zoster is serious and is usually limited to patients with immune systems impaired by lymphoproliferative disease or immunosuppressive drugs. In localized zoster, clinical lesions usually do not cross the midline of the body. The presence of more than ten lesions outside a dermatomal distribution suggests early generalized zoster. Zoster encephalitis and pneumonitis have a high mortality rate and may complicate the widespread vesicular eruption.

Diagnosis is suggested by the typical dermatomal rash. A positive Tzanck preparation demonstrating multinucleated giant cells is supportive evidence of zoster, and the diagnosis may be confirmed by viral cultures or rising complement fixation titers.

PRINCIPLES OF THERAPY

The goals of therapy are to dry the vesicles, relieve pain, and prevent secondary infection and other complications. Lesions may be kept clean and dry by the application of wet to dry cool compresses soaked with Burow's solution three to four times a day. Purulence suggests secondary infection, which may be treated with topical antibiotics. Spreading erythema may indicate cellulitis and the need for systemic therapy. Little evidence exists to support one or another agent, so that a number of broad-spectrum low allergenic preparations would be acceptable. There are no certain data to support prophylactic antibiotics.

Pain relief is extremely important. Analgesia can usually be achieved with a mild agent, but one should not hesitate to use codeine and, rarely, stronger narcotics, if necessary. The physician should begin therapy with aspirin or acetaminophen and add codeine 30 to 60 mg. if pain is unrelieved. The pain of thoracic zoster may be reduced by splinting the affected area with tight wrappings, as would be used for fractured ribs. The lesions should be covered with cotton and then wrapped with an elastic bandage. Malaise reflecting viremia may accompany zoster and should be treated with rest and limitation of activity. Severe local pain may be ameliorated with intralesional injections of triamcinolone 2 mg. per cc. in lidocaine. This solution, injected under each group of lesions along the dermatome, provides effective analgesia. Systemic corticosteroid therapy for zoster has received attention. There is little evidence to suggest that pain or the rate of healing is affected by steroids during the first weeks of the eruption, but the duration and incidence of postherpetic neuralgia appears to be reduced by systemic steroids. There is no evidence that corticosteroid therapy produces generalization of the eruption. Corticosteroids can be administered orally or by IM injection. Steroids should be restricted to patients over 60 who are at risk for postherpetic neuralgia and should be used only in the absence of contraindications.

Treatment of complications of zoster has proven difficult. The presence of lesions at the tip of the nose is an indication for ophthalmologic consultation. Postherpetic neuralgia can be one of the most disabling and frustrating conditions. Conventional analgesics usually fail and the physician must tread lightly with narcotics to avoid the potential problem of addiction. Success has been reported with the use of repeated injections of triamcinolone acetonide into symptomatic areas, intercostal nerve block or sympathetic ganglion block. The block must be repeated daily until symptoms subside. Some clinicians have also found that chlorprothixine (Taractan) in doses of 25 to 50 mg. three to four times daily relieves the pain.

THERAPEUTIC RECOMMENDATIONS

- Lesions can be dried with Burow's solution made by adding one or two packages of powder to a half liter of cool water. A soft cloth, such as an old sheet, pillowcase or T-shirt, soaked in solution and wrung out slightly is applied to the affected area for 30 minutes. The cloth is remoistened as it dries. These soothing compresses may be used two to four times daily.
- Cortisporin cream or ointment should be applied to the lesions two or three times per day if signs of infection are present.
- Codeine 30 to 60 mg. with aspirin or acetaminophen should be given to control pain. Severe pain may require narcotics, natural or synthetic.
- Prednisone 60 mg. a day for a week, tapered over the next 2 weeks, can be prescribed. Triamcinolone

40 mg. intramuscularly into the buttock at the first visit may be given to patients over 60 years of age in the hope of reducing the incidence of postherpetic neuralgia.

- Involvement of the tip of the nose or presence of visual symptoms requires an ophthalmologic consultation for diagnosis and treatment of uveitis.
- Patients should rest in bed when symptoms are severe.
- The patient should be told that zoster is a self-limited illness and that it does not recur. Instruct the affected individual to avoid contact with infants and severely ill or immunosuppressed patients.

ANNOTATED BIBLIOGRAPHY

Blank, H., Eaglestein, W.H., and Goldfaden, G.L.: Zoster, a recrudescence of V-Z virus infection. Postgrad. Med. J., *46*:653, 1970. *(Succinct overview of herpes zoster—Pathophysiology and clinical manifestation.)*

Burgoon, C.F., and Burgoon, J.S.: The natural history of herpes zoster. JAMA, *164*:265, 1957. *(Discussion of the course of herpes zoster in 206 unselected cases. Complications developed in 16.9 per cent; about half of these were cases of postherpetic neuralgia.)*

Eaglestein, W.H., Katz, R., and Brown, J.S.: The effects of early corticosteroid therapy on the skin eruption and pain of herpes zoster. JAMA, *211*:1681, 1970. *(The duration of postherpetic neuralgia [pain lasting more than 8 weeks] was decreased by oral triamcinolone therapy begun early in the disease course.)*

Epstein, E.: Triamcinolone-procaine in the treatment of zoster and postzoster neuralgia. Calif. Med., *115*:6, 1971. *(Describes the techniques of sublesional injection and the results derived.)*

Goffinet, D.R., Glatstein, E.J., and Merigan, T.C.: Herpes zostervaricella infections and lymphoma. Ann. Intern. Med., *76*:235, 1972. *(11.4 per cent of 1,130 patients with lymphoma had associated Z-V infection.)*

Gold, E.: Serologic and virus isolation studies of patients with varicella or herpes zoster infection. N. Engl. J. Med., *274*:181, 1966. *(Virologic techniques of isolating the V-Z virus from both diseases. Disease course not correlated with specific antibody production.)*

Schimpff, S., Serpick, A., Stoler, B., et al.: Varicella-zoster infection in patients with cancer. Ann. Intern. Med., 76:241, 1972. *(Discusses the association of V-Z infection and malignancy. Of 37 patients, 12 had dissemination.)*

Taub, A.: Relief of postherpetic neuralgia with psychotropic drugs. J. Neurosurg., 39:235, 1973. *(Guidance for treatment of the difficult problem.)*

Thiers, B.: Herpes-varicella-zoster. J. Am. Acad. Dermatol., 2:443, 1980. *(Discussion of the recent therapies including interferon.)*

Vonderheid, E.C., and van Voorst Vader, P.C.: Herpes zoster-varicella in cutaneous T-cell lymphomas. Arch. Dermatol., 116:408, 1980. *(Overall frequency was 12% in 221 patients with T-cell lymphoma.)*

186
Management of Warts
ROBERT M. MILLER, M.D.

Warts are epidermal tumors caused by a papova-type DNA virus. They are transmitted by direct contact or autoinoculation, and are more commonly found in young people. Warts disappear naturally, presumably by an immunologic mechanism. Approximately two-thirds of warts will disappear within 2 years; however, if the source of the virus, the wart, is not removed, new ones will appear. The primary physician must distinguish warts from other skin lesions and be able to remove them.

PATHOPHYSIOLOGY, CLINICAL PRESENTATION AND COURSE

The pathophysiology of warts is viral infection. It was thought that a single virus caused many different warts, but it now appears that various warts are caused by slightly different viruses. The virus is not easily cultured; therefore, its properties have not been well elucidated.

Warts have a varied morphology, but a few forms are common. The *verruca vulgaris,* or common wart, a flesh-colored papule with a characteristic hyperkeratotic surface, may appear anywhere on the skin, particularly elbows, knees, and periungual areas. *Verruca plana,* the flat wart, which is smaller and has a smoother surface than *verruca vulgaris,* is often found in great numbers on the face but may occur anywhere. *Filiform warts* are threadlike and few in number. *Condylomata acuminata* grow on warm moist surfaces, may become large and have a cauliflower appearance, and are often, but not always, venereal. They can be transferred by the patient's own hands. *Verruca plantaris,* or plantar wart, defined by location, acquires its appearance from being pressed into the foot by the weight of the patient. Plantar warts may occur as a single lesion or in a mosaic pattern in which the warts are grouped closely together like tiles. A mosaic pattern may also occur in other locations. Superficial thrombosed vessels seen as black dots occur in almost all warts. Warts are generally asymptomatic; patients consult the physician because of cosmetic concerns. Plantar warts acting as a foreign body may be painful; condylomata acuminata may become friable and cause discomfort, and periungual lesions may develop fissures.

Because the varied morphology makes diagnosis equivocal, the differential diagnosis must be considered. Multiple facial warts must be differentiated from trichoepitheliomas, syringomas, and sarcoidosis. Condylomata acuminata must be differentiated from condylomata lata or squamous cell carcinomas. When in doubt, a serological test for syphilis and/or biopsy is indicated. Verruca vulgaris should be differentiated from squamous cell carcinoma, molluscum contagiosum, dermatofibroma, corns and calluses. If the lesion is pared with a scapel, skin lines or markings are found in corns and calluses but are lost in warts. Plantar warts have a friable verrucous surface and, often, black dots. The black dots raise the question of malignant melanoma. If the diagnosis is not absolutely certain, a dermatologist should be consulted or the lesion should be biopsied (Biopsies should be done judiciously because scars may occur.)

PRINCIPLES OF THERAPY

Once the diagnosis is established, a decision of whether and how to treat must be made. Because warts often disappear spontaneously and treatment may cause scarring, it is sometimes preferable not to treat. Multiple facial and plantar warts often present this problem. Although warts may disappear, they may also worsen.

The treatment decision depends on location of the warts and available modalities. Warts are an epidermal phenomen only, so the dermis need not be invaded. Destruction of the dermis may lead to scarring. Only minimal scarring should be expected or accepted. Treatment should embrace this fundamental principle.

Liquid nitrogen causes a separation of the wart-containing epidermis from the dermis at the dermo-epidermal junction. A bulla results, and the wart comes off with the blister top after several weeks. The treatment is quick and can be used on several warts in one office visit. Although it is somewhat painful, local anesthetics are not necessary. Liquid nitrogen is less effective on large warts.

Light electrodesiccation or chemical cautery with mono-, bi-, or trichloracetic acid can be used successfully in weekly or fortnightly treatments, especially on multiple warts. Curettage with or without electrodesiccation is effective for small numbers of warts. It should be used cautiously on plantar warts because painful incapacitating scars may result. Correction of orthopedic defects or use of prescription shoes may reduce symptoms and prevent recurrences.

Twenty-five per cent podophyllin in tincture of benzoin applied every 2 weeks to condylomata acuminata on mucous membranes can be effective. It should be washed off 1 to 4 hours after application to prevent undue pain from the ensuing inflammatory reaction.

Topical 5-fluorouracil applied twice daily to multiple flat facial warts may be used by experienced clinicians. Therapy should be stopped or decreased when inflammation develops. Cantharidin, a blistering agent, is painless when applied and therefore can often be used in children. Within 24 to 48 hours, however, a painful blister usually develops. Daily 10% formaldehyde or 25% glutaraldehyde swabs can be used for plantar warts, but sensitization is a potential problem. Salicylic acid 40% plaster used repeatedly is probably the preferred approach to plantar warts. To date, no vaccine has been proven effective beyond a placebo effect.

THERAPEUTIC RECOMMENDATIONS

• The primary physician must observe the basic principle that warts are benign and treatment must not be overly aggressive so as to cause permanent scar-

ring. One should apply simple and safe treatments. Failure of response to benign modalities will necessitate referral to a dermatologist.
• In general, therapy with liquid nitrogen is simple and benign and the best therapy for most warts on skin surfaces. If liquid nitrogen is unavailable, a drop of cantharidin under an occlusive bandage for 24 hours is a good alternative.
• Condylomata acuminata in the vagina or on the glans penis may be treated by applying podophyllin lightly, emphasizing to the patient to wash the podophyllin off after 1 to 4 hours.
• Flat warts may be treated with keratolytic preparations of 6% salicylic acid in a gel marketed as Keralyt.®
• Plantar warts should be treated with 40% salicylic acid plaster cut to the size and shape of the wart, applied for 24 hours, followed by paring down the wart. The procedure should be repeated every other day with biweekly follow-up. If this is unsuccessful, referral to a dermatologist is indicated. Correction of orthopedic defects must also be considered.

PATIENT EDUCATION

In the absence of a vaccine, prevention involves eliminating the viral reservoir in the host. This can be done by removing present warts, diminishing direct contact with warts in other people, and avoiding spread. In many children and some adults, spread occurs by biting the warts and exposing the virus to oral tissue and other parts of the body.

The need to treat each wart must be emphasized to the patient to prevent recurrence and spread. The patient should examine himself for recurrence of warts and return to the physician before treatment is made more difficult by the appearance of multiple lesions. Although over-the-counter preparations usually contain salicylic acid and may be effective, the patient should be encouraged not to treat himself but to visit the physician if response is not rapid and complete.

ANNOTATED BIBLIOGRAPHY

Caravati, C.M., et al.: Onychodystrophies secondary to liquid nitrogen cryotherapy. Arch. Dermatol., 100:441, 1969. (Nail dystrophy followed liquid nitrogen treatment of warts in 2 patients.)

Massing, A.M., and Epstein, W.L.: Natural history of warts. Arch. Dermatol., 87:306, 1963. (One thousand children with warts were observed for 2 years. Without treatment, there was an increase in the total number of verrucae.)

Mendelson, C.G., and Kligman, A.M.: Isolation of wart virus in tissue culture: Successful reinoculation into humans. Arch. Dermatol., *83*:559, 1961. *(Reinoculation of viral particles into humans and passage through tissue culture.)*

Pringle, W.M., and Helms, D.C.: Treatment of plantar warts by blunt dissection. Arch. Dermatol., *108*:79, 1973. *(Describes removal of plantar warts by blunt dissection; 85 per cent cure after one procedure.)*

Sanders, B.B., and Stretcher, G.S.: Warts: Diagnosis and treatment. JAMA, *235*:2859, 1976. *(A review emphasizing the design of treatment regimens based on the specific wart being treated.)*

Saul, A., Sanz, R., and Gomez, M.: Treatment of multiple viral warts with levamisole. Int. J. Dermatol., *19*:342, 1980. *(No better than placebo therapy in 77 patients; 32 with cellular immune deficiency.)*

187

Management of Scabies and Pediculosis

RICHARD M. SALIT, M.D.

Man is subject to attack by innumerable species of arthropods. Reactions vary from potentially lethal spider and scorpion bites to the annoying effects of mites and flies. Positive identification of the attacker is possible if it is captured or commonly recognized. In many cases, the organism can be deduced by careful history-taking. Food mites may cause dermatitis in warehouse workers and housewives, while poultry workers may come in contact with bird mites. The primary physician should be familiar with common offenders and be prepared to treat mite and lice infestations.

PATHOPHYSIOLOGY AND CLINICAL PRESENTATION

Scabies is a dermatosis caused by an infestation with *Sarcoptes scabiei* var. *hominis.* The disease has a worldwide distribution and occurs in cyclical pandemics. Scabies is transmitted by close personal contact and affects all social and economic groups.

The cardinal symptom of scabies is itching, frequently most severe at night. The typical patient presents with burrows, grouped papules or nodules, characteristically on the webs of the fingers, wrists, elbows, knees, axillary folds, umbilicus and thighs. In women, the nipples may be involved, while genital lesions are common in men. Eczematous areas are often seen, and pustules or crusts may develop secondary to infection. The diagnostic burrow is a direct result of the female mite's tunneling into the epidermis to lay eggs. Burrows are a few millimeters long and best seen on the extremities. The burrow can be unroofed and scraped with a scapel blade. Scraped

material is placed on a microscope slide and a drop of mineral oil added. Positive identification of scabies depends upon demonstrating adult mites, ova or feces. When mites cannot be identified, diagnosis may be made on clinical evidence.

Scabetic symptoms are, in part, an allergic reaction to the mite or its products. Pruritus usually develops 2 to 4 weeks after primary infestation. The patient may be infested with only a few mites but have hundreds of nonspecific lesions.

Lice may affect the entire body, especially the head and pubic area. All forms of infestation cause itching and should be considered in the differential diagnosis of pruritic dermatoses. Lice feed on blood and can survive only a week or two away from a host.

Body and head lice are variants of *Pediculus humanus.* These are elongate insects transmitted by shared clothing, combs or even furniture. Poor personal hygiene facilitates infestation. The head louse typically infests the temporal and occipital aspects of the scalp. Eggs (nits) become firmly attached to hairs. Isolation of nits or an adult louse confirms the diagnosis. The body louse usually lives and lays eggs in clothing, usually in seams; nits are rarely attached to body hairs. *Phthirus pubis,* the pubic or crab louse, has a rounded body and crablike claws. Although usually found in the pubic area, it can infest any hairy area, including the eyelashes.

The cardinal symptom of infestation is pruritus, produced when the lice inject saliva, digestive juices and fecal material into the skin. Adult lice may be difficult to isolate; the diagnosis is made by detection of nits attached to hair shafts. Spotty bluish discolorations of the skin, termed *maculae caeruleae,* are sometimes seen in areas of infestation. Unexplained pyoderma of the scalp or cervical or occipital adenopathy should raise suspicion of pediculosis capitis. Extensive infestations can result in skin irritation and eczema. Secondary bacterial infection is not uncommon.

PRINCIPLES OF THERAPY

Treatment is aimed at killing the mites or lice and assuaging hypersensitivity manifestations. Since scabies is usually spread by intimate personal contact, family members and sexual contacts should be treated. The long asymptomatic period between infestation and symptoms emphasizes the importance of treating contacts. The patient should be examined for signs of secondary bacterial infection and treated with antibiotics if necessary. Postscabetic glomerulonephritis is a rare complication.

Mites and ova are killed by proper use of a scabicide. The choice of agent depends on efficacy and potential toxicity. The scabicide should be applied from the neck down with emphasis on the hands and flexural creases. Patient compliance should be emphasized; incorrect use may not effect a cure, while overuse may lead to local irritation and possible systemic toxicity secondary to excessive absorption. A good principle to observe is to limit the quantity of scabicide prescribed. Gamma benzene hexachloride (GBH) is a commonly used, effective scabicide, but has been reported to cause central nervous system toxicity and aplastic anemia. Topical and systemic steroids and antihistamines may be needed to treat cases of severe pruritus.

Management of lice requires the use of a pediculicide and the disinfection of clothing, bedding and grooming aids. The method of application is adapted to the primary site of involvement. Bacterial infection requires antibiotic therapy. Severely irritated skin may be treated with soothing compresses and topical corticosteroids. The cardinal principle of therapy is to treat the reservoir by disinfecting common sources of infestation. Lice living in clothing may be killed by heat or pesticides; boiling, dry cleaning or ironing are all acceptable approaches. Nits remaining attached to the hair should be removed with a fine-toothed comb. In order to prevent reinfestation and epidemics, family, roommates, and sexual contacts should all be examined and treated.

THERAPEUTIC RECOMMENDATIONS

- The treatment of choice for scabies is 1% gamma benzene hexachloride (GBH) lotion or cream (Kwell, Gamene) applied to the entire body from the neck down; 60 to 120 ml. is required for the average adult. It should be left on for approximately 12 hours and then washed off.
- Crotamiton (Eurax) is an alternative scabicide and should be thoroughly applied from the neck down and reapplied after 24 hours. It should be washed off 24 hours after the last application.
- Clothing and bed linen should be changed, laundered or dry cleaned.
- If resistance or reinfestation is suspected, a second course of treatment with GBH or crotamiton may be given.
- Pediculosis capitis is treated with GBH (Kwell) shampoo. The shampoo is lathered into the hair and left on for 5 minutes. Adherent nits can be removed by careful use of a fine-toothed comb or judicious trimming. Rarely, repeat treatment is necessary.
- Pediculosis corporis and pubis respond to GBH lotion or cream applied to affected areas and left on for 12 to 24 hours. Occasionally, a second application is required 4 to 7 days later. Lice infesting the eyelashes can be treated with an anticholinesterase ointment such as phospholine iodide or physostigmine. Severe involvement may require ophthalmologic consultation.
- Residual irritation and pruritus may be treated with a corticosteroid cream or lotion applied two to three times a day.
- Prevention of reinfestation by treating contacts and disinfecting clothing and other common sources of infestation is essential. The patient must be given detailed instructions in the use of gamma benzene hydrochloride in order to prevent irritation and systemic toxicity. Family, roommates and sexual contacts should be considered for treatment to prevent reinfection.

ANNOTATED BIBLIOGRAPHY

FDA Drug Bulletin, 6:28, 1976. *(Highlights potential toxicity associated with improper use of insecticides.)*

Nielsen, A.O., and Secher, L. Pediculosis pubis in a patient treated with topical steroids. Cutis, 25:655, 1980. *(Generalized infestation which was not pruritus due to use of corticosteroid cream.)*

Orkin, M., Epstein, E., and Maibach, H.: Treatment of today's scabies and pediculosis. JAMA, 236:1136, 1976. *(Excellent review with emphasis on management.)*

188
Management of Animal and Human Bites
ELLIE J.C. GOLDSTEIN, M.D.

Animal bites are common, and patients frequently present to the primary physician for information and therapy. Human bites are less frequent but potentially more serious. Clenched-fist injuries result from striking the mouth. Patients may appear shortly after injury concerned about rabies, tetanus, or repair of a disfiguring tear. They may delay seeking medical care only to present later with infection. The primary physician must provide first aid and tetanus prophylaxis, decide when antibiotics are necessary, and be able to estimate the risk of rabies.

PATHOPHYSIOLOGY AND CLINICAL PRESENTATIONS

Bite wounds produce a break in the skin, allowing inoculation by bacteria that normally inhabit the skin and oral cavity. Once the protective barrier of the skin is compromised, conditions favoring infection have been established. The risk of infection increases the longer the wound is left unattended. The infecting organisms are usually the normal flora of the oral mucosa. *Pasteurella multocida* is a frequent etiologic agent, present in 50 per cent of animal oral cavities and in 20 per cent of animal bite wounds. Bites from animals who ingest feces may become infected with enteric organisms. In humans, the mouth flora is more abundant than in most animals and includes *Strep. viridans,* bacteroides species, anaerobic diphtheroids, vibrios, fusobacteria and spirochetes. Wounds may also be infected by skin flora such as a streptococcus, staphylococcus or *Eikenella corrodens*. Human bites are responsible for most bite wound infections because of the heavy inoculum of bacteria usually received.

Bites initially thought to be trivial may become infected hours or days later. Cat bites occasionally lead to severe cellulitis, and an occasional patient presents with cat scratch fever.

The most serious bite wounds are caused by clenched-fist injuries. Damage occurs when the tendons and other tissues of the exterior area of the finger are stretched to full length, the skin is broken, and the tendon and possibly the joint are exposed. As the fingers are straightened, the damaged parts relax, and infecting organisms are carried into the tissues, producing infection in wounds that initially appear minor. If the joint capsule is penetrated, the risk of osteomyelitis is increased.

PRINCIPLES OF THERAPY

Principles of therapy include characterization of the injury, vigorous cleansing, tetanus prophylaxis, and appropriate antibiotics. It is important to elicit a history of the circumstances surrounding the injury. If an animal bite occurred, the type of animal and the animal's behavior need to be detailed, as well as whether the animal has been vaccinated and whether the attack was provoked or unprovoked.

Since 1967, there have been only one or two cases of rabies in man each year in the United States. There have been no cases of rabies in man in New York or Los Angeles for many years. In 1976, 3,073 animals in the United States were reported to have rabies—114 dogs, 159 cattle, 187 foxes, 174 raccoons, 725 bats, and 1,466 skunks. Rabies is of concern if the attack is unprovoked, occurs in a rural setting, or involves a bat, a skunk or an animal which is behaving in a peculiar manner. The local health department should be notified for follow-up and statistical reasons. It is unlikely that the patient will need treatment for rabies. When a person is bitten by a pet, the animal should be watched at home by the owner for 2 weeks and reported to the local health department.

It is important to determine if the patient has had an initial series of tetanus shots and a booster within the past 5 years. Those who have not had an initial series should be given both tetanus toxoid and tetanus immune globulin (see Chapter 4). In those who have had the initial series but no recent booster, 0.5 cc. of tetanus toxoid intramuscularly should be administered. Most minor puncture wounds from animal bites may be cleansed with soap and water and treated expectantly without antibiotics.

Therapy of tear wounds is problematic. There have not been controlled trials of closure vs. nonclosure, with or without antibiotics. The principles of therapy are to trim loose edges and cleanse and debride the wound. After leaving the wound open for 24 to 48 hours, the edges can be approximated with Steri-strips or sutured, and phenoxymethyl penicillin, 250 mg. four times a day, can be given for 3 to 5 days. Secondary closures may be done when it is apparent that no infection is present. Facial wounds should be closed and antibiotics given. It may be useful to refer these patients to a plastic surgeon.

Patients may present after 24 hours with infection. Principles of treatment include débridement, drainage, cleansing, delayed closure of the wound and institution of appropriate antibiotic therapy. Penicillin is the drug of choice because it is effective against *P. multocida,* some staphylococci, streptococci, anaerobes and *E. corrodens.* In penicillin-allergic patients, either tetracycline or erythromycin may be used.

Human bites are usually located on an extremity; wounds of the hand are more serious than those located elsewhere. The same principles of cleansing, drainage and débridement apply. Human bites should not be closed primarily, though edges may be approximated if the tear is severe. Antibiotics should be instituted as soon as wound cultures are taken. Penicillin and penicillinase-resistant penicillin should be administered pending culture results to cover oral anaerobes and gram-positive cocci, particularly *Staph. aureus.* In one series, 44 per cent of wounds grew *Staph. aureus.* Infrequently, a penicillin-resistant gram-negative organism may be present, necessitating a change in antibiotic regimen. Tetanus toxoid 0.5 cc. should be administered to all those previously immunized who have not had a booster in the previous 5 years. Follow-up is essential, because of the potential delayed presentation of serious infection.

Clenched-fist injuries usually require specialized care. Radiographs should be taken to rule out fractures and to provide a baseline for future assessment of osteomyelitis. Extension and flexion of digits should be carefully checked and sensation tested. The third metacarpophalangeal joint is most frequently affected. The integrity of the joint capsule needs to be determined; this should be done by an experienced surgeon. If the capsule is intact, the hand is cleaned, débrided, immobilized and elevated. Penicillin and a penicillinase-resistant penicillin are started and tetanus toxoid administered. Patients seen within 8 hours of injury with intact joint capsules may be managed as outpatients with careful follow-up. Those with torn capsules need to be admitted for surgery and treatment with intravenous antibiotics. Patients who present after 8 hours should be admitted for observation whether the capsule is intact or interrupted.

THERAPEUTIC RECOMMENDATIONS AND PATIENT EDUCATION

- Clean all wounds vigorously with soap and water.
- Immunize against tetanus with 0.5 cc. of tetanus toxoid intramuscularly in those who have previously been immunized but have not had a booster in the past 5 years.
- Animal puncture wounds which are small and clean require no other treatment.
- Treat fresh, uninfected tear wounds with cleansing, débridement and phenoxymethyl penicillin (250 mg. four times a day), followed by secondary closure in 24 to 48 hours if there are no signs of infection.
- Treat infected animal bite wounds with débridement, drainage and cleansing. Culture the wound, delay wound closure until infection subsides, and begin phenoxymethyl penicillin 500 mg. four times daily, *plus* a penicillinase-resistant semisynthetic penicillin—e.g., dicloxacillin, 500 mg. four times a day—and treat for 7 to 10 days, pending culture results. If the patient is allergic to penicillin, substitute erythromycin 500 mg. four times a day for initial antibiotic therapy.
- Treat *all* human bites initially with *both* penicillin and a penicillinase-resistant agent, as above. Delay closure of the wound.
- Refer clenched-fist injuries to a hand surgeon.
- Instruct the patient to watch the wound for signs of infection, such as redness, warmth, swelling or purulent exudate.

ANNOTATED BIBLIOGRAPHY

Baile, W.E., Stowe, E.C., and Schmitt, A.M.: Aerobic bacterial flora of oral and nasal fluids of canines with reference to bacteria associated with bite. J. Clin. Microbiol., 7:223, 1978. *(Aerobic oral and nasal flora of 50 dogs was determined. P. multocida, II-j, EF-4 and Staph. aureus were all recovered, with high incidence. No anaerobic work was done.)*

Callahorn, M.L.: Treatment of common dog bites. JACEP, 7:83, 1978. *(A retrospective study of 106 patients demonstrated an increased risk of infection in patients older than 50, who delayed seeking treatment and had puncture wounds located on the upper extremities.)*

Chuinard R.G., and D'Ambrosia, R.D.: Human bite infections of the hand. J. Bone Joint Surg. 59:416, 1977. *(Forty-two patients were studied retrospectively, and another 59 prospectively. Recommend early and aggressive surgical management and stress the need for determination of capsule integrity.)*

Francis D.P., Holmes, M.A., and Brandon, G.: *Pasteurella multocida* infection after domestic animal bites and scratches. JAMA, 233:42, 1975. *(A retrospective study attempting to define the role of* P. multocida.)

Goldstein, E.J.C., Caffee, H.H., Price, J.E., *et al.*: Human bite infections. Lancet 2:1290, 1977. *(Stresses the need for accurate and complete microbiology and recommends the use of both peni-*

cillin and a penicillinase-resistant penicillin as initial empiric therapy.)

Goldstein, E.J.C., Citron, D.M., Miller, T.A., *et al.*: Infections following clenched fist injury: A new perspective. J. Hand Surg. 3:455, 1978. *(Uses optimal microbiological methods. Notes significant number of anaerobes (9/16) and* Eikenella corrodens *(5/15) isolated in wounds. Both penicillin and a penicillinase-resistant penicillin are recommended as initial empiric therapy.)*

Mann, R.J., Hoffeld, T.A., and Farmer, C.B.: Human bites of the hand: Twenty years of experience. J. Hand Surg. 2:97, 1977. *(One hundred thirty-six patients over 20 years were studied retrospectively, and another 38 patients were studied prospectively.* Strep. viridans *was the most frequent aerobic pathogen; 44 per cent of wounds had* Staph. aureus. *The use of penicillinase-resistant penicillin is recommended.)*

189
Management of Minor Burns

Accidental minor burns are common; the majority of the estimated two million burn victims can be treated as outpatients. The primary physician will frequently be asked to give advice about immediate care and should render definitive treatment for localized partial thickness burns.

PATHOPHYSIOLOGY AND CLINICAL PRESENTATION

Burns represent direct thermal injury to the cells of the skin and underlying structures. The clinical presentation is dependent on the degree of damage, which is a direct function of the intensity and duration of exposure to heat. The skin in *first degree burns* is painful, red and swollen; it blanches with pressure and shows little or no edema. Ultraviolet radiation, scalding, low intensity exposure to steam or contact with a hot object are common causes. Complete recovery usually occurs within a week, often with peeling and sometimes with postinflammatory hyperpigmentation. *Second degree burns* present as painful red blisters or broken epidermis exposing a weeping edematous surface. They are most often caused by scalds or brief exposure to a flame. Recovery requires 2 to 3 weeks; sometimes scarring occurs.

Third degree burns usually result from prolonged contact with steam, hot objects or flames. They present with ulceration, tissue necrosis, and are painless because nerve tissue in the area has been destroyed.

PRINCIPLES OF THERAPY

The first object is to document the depth of injury and ascertain the area involved. Outpatient management should be limited to patients with partial thickness burns that involve less than 5 to 10 per cent of the body and spare the face, perineum, hands and feet. Feasibility of outpatient management is determined not only by the extent of the burn but also by the patient's reliability and the support available at home.

The goals of therapy are to reduce inflammation, prevent infection, relieve pain and promote healing. First aid to minor burns involves immediate application of ice packs or cold compresses of water, milk, or oatmeal. Cold reduces discomfort, edema, and hyperemia and may diminish the extent of injury. The application of cold should continue until the burn is pain-free. Superficial burns require no medication or dressing.

Chemical burns should be placed under running

water for at least 15 to 30 minutes before cleansing or debridement is started. Patients complaining of pain or displaying anxiety should be given an analgesic or a sedative prior to manipulation of the injured area.

If the skin is broken by a second degree burn, it is important to protect the wound so that healing may occur without infection. This involves gently washing the area of the burn with water and a mild antiseptic soap, such as one containing hexachlorophene. Washing is followed by gentle irrigation with sterile isotonic saline and application of a sterile occlusive dressing. Dressings are prepared by applying a nonadherent fine mesh gauze soaked in sterile saline to the burn, and covering this with a bulky dressing that allows drainage into but not through it. The patient should be examined in two days for pain, adenopathy or fever, and the dressing should be checked. If no evidence of infection is noted, the dressing may remain for 5 to 7 days when the area is reexamined to determine the need for a dressing change.

Controversy exists over the prophylactic use of topical antibiotics in minor burns. The evidence from the literature suggests that they have little or no effect. Topical anesthetics provide symptomatic relief but should be avoided because of the risk of sensitization.

Tetanus prophylaxis includes administering tetanus toxoid booster to previously immunized patients. Pain can usually be relieved with aspirin or acetaminophen. Aspirin has the advantage of suppressing inflammation and is particularly helpful in sunburn. In cases of extensive sunburn, a topical corticosteroid lotion or spray may provide symptomatic relief. Systemic corticosteroids do not reduce the edema associated with sunburn and are not indicated.

THERAPEUTIC RECOMMENDATIONS AND INDICATIONS FOR ADMISSION

- For first degree burns, immediately apply cold and maintain until the area is free of pain even after cold is withdrawn.
- If the skin is broken, cleanse with mild soap and water before application of cold water or ice.
- No dressing or emollient or antibiotic is needed for first degree burns, but topical corticosteroid lotion may provide symptomatic relief of extensive sun-

burn. Aspirin, 600 mg. every 4 hours, will provide some analgesia and help limit inflammation.
- Second degree burns with broken skin should be covered by a wet sterile saline compress, and a topical antibiotic cream (e.g., Neospirin) should be applied if the wound appears infected.
- Any patient with a second degree burn involving more than 5 to 10 per cent of body surface or involving face, hands or feet should be admitted.

PATIENT EDUCATION

Patient education is extremely important to the successful resolution of a burn. The patient should be carefully instructed to keep the wound clear and watch for signs of infection. Following healing of the burn, the new epithelial layer may tend to dry and crack; this can be reduced by applying lanolin-containing creams for 4 to 8 weeks following healing. Patients with a healed burn should avoid prolonged exposure to direct sunlight for at least 6 months, as well as constricting clothing and strong soaps. The need to tan gradually should be stressed, and the patient should be encouraged to use a sunscreen containing para-aminobenzoic acid to help prevent severe sunburn in the future.

ANNOTATED BIBLIOGRAPHY

Moncrief, J.A.: Burns. N. Engl. J. Med., *288*:444, 1973. *(A comprehensive review, with only part directed to ambulatory management.)*

Moncrief, J.A.: Burns. I. Assessment. II. Initial treatment. JAMA, *242*:72, 1979. *(A current review focusing on emergency management.)*

Nance, F.C., Lewis, V.L., Jr., Hines, J.L., *et al.*: Aggressive outpatient care of burns. J. Trauma, *12*:144, 1972. *(An approach for the emergency physician.)*

Shuck, J.M.: Outpatient management of the burned patient. Surg. Clin. North Am., *58*:1107, 1978. *(A practical and well-reasoned approach to treating burns.)*

Sorenson, B.: First aid in burn injuries: Treatment at home with cold water. Mod. Treat., *4*:1199, 1967. *(The rationale behind using cold water as an initial treatment.)*

13

Ophthalmologic Problems

190
Screening for Glaucoma

Glaucoma affects more than one million Americans and is the cause of 12 per cent of the cases of blindness in the United States. It is a disease marked by ischemic damage of the optic nerve, in most cases primarily caused or aggravated by abnormally high intraocular pressure. Strictly speaking, the disease process is neither preventable nor curable, but clinicians agree that blindness can be prevented if the patient is identified early and the intraocular pressure is controlled.

Secondary glaucoma is associated with ocular inflammation, trauma or neoplasm and often occurs in patients already under the care of an ophthalmologist. Angle-closure glaucoma is a symptomatic disease; patients present with eye pain or headache associated with decreased visual acuity during an attack. Primary open-angle glaucoma, by far the most prevalent type, is the most insidious cause of blindness. Detection of the asymptomatic patient who may be developing irreversible loss of vision depends on routine glaucoma screening by the primary care provider.

EPIDEMIOLOGY AND RISK FACTORS

The prevalence of glaucoma in populations of adults over age 40 is about 2 per cent. Prevalence increases with age and may be greater in non-white populations. Rates as high as 6.4 per cent have been reported in medical clinics.

Elevated intraocular pressure can be considered the principal risk factor for glaucoma. While the mean level of intraocular pressure in adult populations is 15 mm. Hg, both the mean and the standard deviation increase with age.

There is a genetic predisposition to development of primary open-angle glaucoma; the prevalence among siblings and offspring of patients is approximately 10 per cent. There is no clear-cut sex predilection. Diabetes is a major risk factor for glaucoma, the incidence of which is increased two- to threefold among diabetics. Individuals with a high degree of myopia are also at increased risk for open-angle glaucoma.

NATURAL HISTORY OF GLAUCOMA AND EFFECTIVENESS OF EARLY THERAPY

Glaucoma is not simply blindness due to elevated intraocular pressure. Visual deficits in the glaucomatous eye result from an imbalance between the vascular supply of the optic nerve and the level of intraocular pressure. Vascular supply is the immediate precursor of nerve damage and loss of vision. Ocular hypertension increases vascular resistance and aggravates any level of insufficiency. However, the relationship between intraocular pressure and glaucomatous field defect in an individual eye is uncertain; there is great variability among individuals in ability to tolerate elevated intraocular pressure for varying periods of time without losing vision. The mean duration of high intraocular pressure before development of field defects has been estimated to be 18 years. The incidence of glaucomatous field defects among patients with ocular hypertension has been shown to be about 1 per cent per year of follow-up.

Visual field loss due to glaucoma is irreversible. The disease process cannot be arrested in an absolute sense, regardless of the stage at which therapy is instituted. Glaucoma is controlled by medical or surgical therapy; in either case the objective is simply to lower intraocular pressure. The clinical consensus is that the optic nerve is more vulnerable to any increase in intraocular pressure once damage has occurred. Lower pressure must be maintained to prevent progression in more advanced cases. Several studies support this impression, but it has never been tested with controlled investigation.

SCREENING METHODS

Tonometry. For the primary physician who is not an ophthalmologist, Schiotz tonometry is the most feasible method for measuring intraocular pressure. Applanation tonometry is generally agreed to be both more accurate and precise, but the equipment is expensive and the technique demands considerable skill. Newer tonometers using an air jet to measure pressure are not available to most primary physicians.

While measurement error using the Schiotz tonometer can be significant, the uncertain relationship between intraocular pressure and glaucoma is a more important problem in tonometric screening. Within limits, the physician chooses the sensitivity and specificity of tonometric screening by his choice of the level of intraocular pressure used as an indication for referral. Referring patients with modestly elevated pressures will result in a fairly sensitive but nonspecific screen. One study found a sensitivity of about 70 per cent and a specificity of 80 per cent, for a referral level of 21.9 mm. Hg. Raising the referral level to 25.8 mm. Hg increased specificity to 95 per cent, but at a cost of reduction in sensitivity to 50 per cent.

Ophthalmoscopy. Fundoscopic changes, in particular changes in the contour of the optic cup, provide the first definitive evidence of glaucoma. The optic cup is the depressed area in the center of the optic disc. The usual cup has a round, regular contour; the cup in early glaucoma becomes notched on the superotemporal or inferotemporal rim. Later changes include increase in the depth and width of the physiologic cup, nasal displacement of the central retinal vessels, and progressive pallor of the optic nerve head.

There is disagreement about the value of ophthalmoscopy in detecting early glaucoma; while some authors feel that it is equal to tonometry in detecting definite glaucoma, at least one study has demonstrated unacceptably low sensitivity and specificity. However, characteristic changes, particularly when asymmetrical, should prompt referral.

Visual field testing. Since glaucoma cannot be distinguished from ocular hypertension without demonstration of visual field loss, visual field testing is an ultimately necessary diagnostic test for suspected cases. In early glaucoma, field loss is subtle, usually involving enlargement of the blind spot and a localized narrowing of peripheral vision, most often in the supranasal quadrant. Simple confrontation testing of visual fields is not sensitive enough to detect early changes. In most settings, formal visual field testing requires referral and is too expensive and time-consuming for routine screening; it can be appropriately reserved as a specific diagnostic test applied to patients suspected of having glaucoma.

CONCLUSIONS AND RECOMMENDATIONS

- Glaucoma is highly prevalent in the adult population. It is a major cause of blindness.
- Risk factors for primary open-angle glaucoma include elevated intraocular pressure, age, family history, diabetes mellitus, and myopia.
- Clinical consensus holds that treatment early in the course of the disease is more effective and more likely to prevent visual loss. Such early treatment depends on detection of the asymptomatic patient.
- Schiotz tonometry is a feasible method of screening for the primary physician. The sensitivity and specificity of the procedure depend on the choice of a cutoff point for referral. High false-positive rates should be expected with low cutoffs; high false-negative rates with higher levels.
- Schiotz tonometry should be performed on all individuals over 40 years of age. Individuals with persistently elevated levels (greater than 21.9 mm. Hg) should be referred for visual field examination and examination by an ophthalmologist.
- There are little data on which to base recommendations regarding the frequency of tonometric screening. The apparently long duration of elevated intraocular pressure before development of visual field deficits indicates that pressure measurement every 3 to 5 years is sufficient after a stable baseline is established for the individual patient.

- Fundoscopic examination cannot be considered a sensitive or specific screening procedure. However, characteristic changes in the optic cup or retinal vessels should prompt ophthalmologic referral.

ANNOTATED BIBLIOGRAPHY

Anderson, D.R.: The management of elevated intra-ocular pressure with normal optic discs and visual fields. I. Therapeutic approach based on high-risk factors. Surv. Ophthalmol., *21*:479, 1977. *(Excellent review of relationship between ocular hypertension and glaucoma.)*

Kitazawa, Y., *et al.*: Untreated ocular hypertension. Arch. Ophthalmol., *95*:1180, 1977. *(Seven of 75 ocular hypertensives followed a minimum of 9 years developed typical glaucomatous visual field defects. Early clinical findings were not helpful in predicting course.)*

McDonald, J.E., and Johnson, M.O.: Glaucoma screening in offices of general practitioners and internists: A study of 10,000 patients. Am. J. Ophthalmol., *59*:875, 1965. *(The authors found a 2.4 per cent prevalence of glaucoma by encouraging internists to screen their private patients.)*

Packer, H., *et al.*: Frequency of glaucoma in three population groups. JAMA, *188*:123, 1964. *(Reports a 6.4 per cent prevalence of glaucoma in a medical clinic population that was 88 per cent black and had a mean age of 61 years.)*

Packer, H., *et al.*: Efficiency of screening tests for glaucoma. JAMA, *192*:693, 1965. *(Provides estimates of sensitivity and specificity for tonometric screening over a range of possible cutoff points.)*

Perkins, E.S.: The Bedford glaucoma survey. I. Long-term follow-up of borderline cases. Br. J. Ophthalmol., *57*:179, 1973. *(Four per cent of 141 patients followed for 5 to 7 years because of ocular hypertension, suspicious discs, or a positive family history developed glaucoma.)*

Pollack, I.R.: The challenge of glaucoma screening. Surv. Ophthalmol., *13*:4, 1968. *(An extensive review recognizing problems with available screening methods. Recommends age-specific screening levels: age 20-39, 21 mm. Hg; 40-59, 22 mm. Hg; 60-79, 24 mm. Hg.)*

Schwartz, J.T.: Influence of small systematic errors on the results of tonometric screening. Am. J. Ophthalmol., *60*:409, 1965. *(Points out that a consistent measurement error of 2 mm. Hg can increase or decrease the number of patients referred by 60 per cent.)*

191

Evaluation of the Red Eye
ROGER F. STEINERT, M.D.

The red eye is the most common eye problem encountered by the primary care physician. Most cases represent benign self-limited disorders which can be expeditiously diagnosed and treated by the primary physician; however, because redness of the eye may signal serious disease which threatens vision, the physician must be aware of the differential diagnosis and able to conduct a proper initial evaluation.

PATHOPHYSIOLOGY AND CLINICAL PRESENTATION

Redness of the eye and the periocular tissues reflects inflammation and/or hemorrhage. Causes of inflammation include bacterial, viral, chlamydial, and fungal infections, allergic responses, immune disorders, elevated intraocular pressure, environmental and pharmacologic irritants, foreign bodies, and trauma. Hemorrhage may be due to laceration, contusion, coagulopathy, or concomitant infection. The pattern of conjunctival injection provides important clues in differential diagnosis. Corneal or intraocular inflammation produces "ciliary flush," dilatation of the fine capillaries around the corneal border. Larger, deep episcleral vessels may also be engorged. Primary conjunctivitis induces diffuse vessel engorgement on the palpebral as well as bulbar conjunctiva, without a ciliary flush. The clinical presentations of various causes of red eye are quite distinctive. Those of conjunctivitis, corneal disease, iritis and acute glaucoma are summarized in Table 191-1.

Table 191-1.   The Red Eye

| | CONJUNCTIVITIS | | | CORNEAL INJURY | | | ACUTE |
	Bacterial	Viral	Allergic	OR INFECTION	IRITIS	GLAUCOMA	
Vision	−	−	−	↓ − ↓↓	↓		↓↓
Pain	−	−	−	+	+		+++
Photophobia	−	±	−	+	++		−
Foreign body sensation	−	±	±	+	−		−
Itch	±	±	++	−	−		−
Tearing	+	++	+ or ++	++	+		−
Discharge	mucopur-ulent	mucoid	−	−	−		−
Preauricular adenopathy	−	+	−	•	−		−
Pupils	−	−	−	NL or small†	small		mid-dilated and fixed
Conjunctival hyperemia	diffuse	diffuse	diffuse	diffuse and ciliary flush	ciliary flush		diffuse and ciliary flush
Cornea	clear	sometimes faint punctate staining or infil-trates	clear	depends on disorder	lightly cloudy		steamy
Intraocular pressure	−	−	−	−‡	NL or ↓		↑↑

* In herpes keratitis.
† Indicates secondary iritis.
‡ Very low in perforating trauma.

Blepharitis connotes redness of the lid margins with scaling and crusting. Examination of the lid margin may reveal inspissated sebaceous material. Staphylococcal blepharitis causes dry scales, lash loss, and sometimes conjunctivitis and corneal limbal infiltrates. Seborrheic blepharitis is associated with greasy scales and less redness. Blepharitis tends to be chronic with acute flare-ups, and is more common in fair-skinned people.

Hordeolum is an acute staphylococcal infection of the meibomian glands (internal hordeolum) or of the glands of Zeis or Moll around the lashes (external hordeolum or sty). It may present as diffuse redness, tenderness, and edema, localized only by an inspissated meibomian gland. An internal hordeolum may point either to the skin or conjunctival side of the lid, while an external hordeolum always points to the skin. Hordeolum may produce a diffuse superficial lid infection known as "preseptal cellulitis."

A *chalazion* is a sterile granulomatous inflammation of the meibomian gland, which may be tender and mildly inflamed or a quiet, discrete mass.

Acute dacryocystitis is a tender, warm, localized infection of the tear ducts over the lateral nose; purulent material may be expressed from the tear duct upon the application of pressure.

Orbital cellulitis is usually caused by gram-positive organisms which enter the orbit either directly or through venous channels from the sinuses. It presents as swollen, red eyelids with chemosis, exophthalmos, pain, fever, and leukocytosis.

Paresis of the third, fourth, and sixth cranial nerves, or the ophthalmic division of the fifth, suggests *cavernous sinus thrombosis.*

Hypersensitivity to eye medications may cause erythema of the external lids, especially at the lateral canthus. *Angioneurotic edema* of the lids may occur bilaterally as an allergic response to a systemic allergen, often food, or unilaterally secondary to exposure to local allergens such as topical chemicals, poison ivy, and insect bites; it develops rapidly and resolves in 1 to 2 days. Edema without erythema suggests allergy.

Conjunctivitis is probably the most common cause of a red eye. Discharge, lids frequently stuck together in the morning, and absence of photophobia and visual loss is the usual clinical presentation. Distinguishing the cause of conjunctivitis may be impossible without slit lamp examination or culture.

Bacterial conjunctivitis is characterized by a mucopurulent discharge and usually occurs unilaterally without preauricular adenopathy. Pneumococcus is most commonly the infectious agent in temperate zones, and *Hemophilus aegyptius* in tropical climates. Grossly purulent conjunctivitis suggests *Neisseria infection,* which may scar the cornea or lead to systemic dissemination. Chronic conjunctivitis is often due to *Staph. aureus* or *Moraxella lacunata.* Concomitant sterile marginal corneal ulcers are common with chronic staph infection. *Chlamydial conjunctivitis,* transmitted from the genitourinary tract, occurs as bilateral "inclusion conjunctivitis" in sexually active young adults. Exudate is profuse, and preauricular adenopathy common.

Trachoma is the leading cause of blindness worldwide, but is rare in the United States except in American Indians in the Southwest.

Viral conjunctivitis is characterized by watery, sometimes mucoid discharge, often beginning in one eye but spreading to the other eye several days later. Preauricular adenopathy is common. It may be associated with fever and pharyngitis (pharyngoconjunctival fever), particularly in children. Epidemic keratoconjunctivitis (EKC) is a highly contagious adenoviral infection which may be accompanied by a superficial punctate keratitis in the first week and subepithelial infiltrates in the second week, with some diminution of vision. Pseudomembranes or scarring of the conjunctiva may occur and sometimes are painful.

Bilateral itching and clear tears characterize *allergic conjunctivitis,* which may be associated with seasonal allergies and atopic dermatitis. Vernal keratoconjunctivitis is a chronic recurrent hypersensitivity reaction which may lead to the formation of corneal ulcers. Bilateral *sterile conjunctival inflammation* occurs in acne rosacea, Reiter's syndrome, and Stevens-Johnson syndrome.

Hemorrhage in the lids or forehead, either spontaneous or traumatic, may rapidly dissect along the tissue planes of the lids and cause an impressive generalized ecchymosis, greatly alarming the patient.

Subconjunctival hemorrhage is distinctive in appearance. In most cases the bleeding occurs secondary to trauma. The patient may be unaware of the minor trauma involved. In patients receiving anticoagulant medications, spontaneous subconjunctival hemorrhage may be a sign of overdosage. Massive subconjunctival hemorrhage accompanied by proptosis and limited extraocular movements, usually after trauma, signals orbital hemorrhage which may compromise the optic nerve and retinal circulation. Subconjunctival hemorrhage may occur in EKC.

A *foreign body* on the conjunctiva under either the upper or lower lid may result in copious tearing, conjunctival injection, and a sensation that a foreign body is present; or it may be well tolerated, the eye remaining white and quiet.

Episcleritis is usually a benign inflammation of superficial episcleral vessels, while *scleritis,* often associated with rheumatoid arthritis and other immune disorders, is a potentially destructive inflammation of deep episcleral vessels and the sclera itself. Fortunately, scleritis is rare. An experienced observer is required to make the diagnosis.

Keratitis presents with a perilimbal ciliary flush, accompanied by clear tears and photophobia. Corneal ulcers detected by fluorescein staining may be sterile or caused by bacteria, viruses, or fungi. Particularly distinctive is the "dendritic" figure of herpes simplex keratitis, in which the epithelium stains in a fine, branching pattern. Herpes simplex and zoster may also cause broader, "geographic" defects. *Staph. aureus* may cause a sterile infiltrate in the corneal limbus.

Corneal abrasions stain with fluorescein but have no infiltrate unless untreated for several days. *Hyphema* indicates severe trauma and requires ophthalmologic consultation. *Recurrent erosion* presents as an epithelial defect at the site of an abrasion which occurred months or years before and which was often caused by organic material (e.g., tree branch, fingernail). It may also occur in corneal dystrophies. In both instances, it is due to a defect in epithelial adherence to the underlying stroma. A *corneal foreign body* may cause tearing and hyperemia with little sensation of a foreign body. This is particularly true of rust rings left by ferrous foreign bodies. Dry eyes can cause intense reactions secondary to superficial keratitis, as does contact lens overwear (corneal hypoxia) and ultraviolet keratitis. *Corneal laceration* with perforation is suggested by a shallow or absent anterior chamber, markedly decreased intraocular pressure, and eccentric pupil with iris prolapse into the wound.

Uveitis refers to inflammation of the uveal tract, including the iris, ciliary body, and choroid. The diagnosis is suggested by pain, photophobia, redness, and ciliary flush. Iritis may be unilateral or bilateral; if unilateral, the pupil is smaller than that of the other eye because of spasm. Flashlight examination suggests a slightly cloudy anterior chamber. Slit lamp examination discloses cells in the anterior chamber and "flare," representing increased aqueous humor protein. Inflammatory cells, called "keratic precipitates," may collect in clusters on the posterior cornea.

Table 191-2. Some Important Causes of Red Eye

A. Conjunctivitis

1. Infection (bacterial, viral, chlamydial)
2. Allergy
3. Autoimmunity
4. Irritation

B. Keratitis

1. Herpes simplex
2. Adenovirus
3. Herpes zoster
4. Keratoconjunctivitis sicca
5. Exposure keratopathy
6. Chemical trauma
7. Corneal ulceration (with or without concomitant infection)

C. Iritis

1. Primary iritis
2. Secondary iritis (infection, trauma)
3. Systemic diseases

D. Diseases of the Eyelid, Sclera and Conjunctivae

1. Blepharitis
2. Chalazion
3. Hordeolum
4. Dacryocystitis
5. Pinguecula
6. Pterygium
7. Episcleritis
8. Scleritis

E. Acute Glaucoma

F. Subconjunctival Hemorrhage

Iritis and uveitis are associated with a large number of systemic and ocular disesases, but are often idiopathic. Ankylosing spondylitis, celiac disease, granulomatous colitis, tuberculosis, sarcoidosis, and juvenile rheumatoid arthritis are sometimes associated with iritis and uveitis. The HLA-B27 tissue antigen is strongly associated with iritis, often accompanied by ankylosing spondylitis or Behçet's disease. Secondary iritis occurs in response to blunt trauma or corneal inflammation.

Acute glaucoma is an ocular emergency which presents as a painful, red eye with prominent ciliary flush. The pupil is mid-dilated and fixed, and the cornea is cloudy secondary to edema. Intraocular pressure is above 40 and may reach 70 to 80. The patient reports cloudy vision, colored rings around lights (due to corneal edema), and unilateral headache, often accompanied by nausea and vomiting, occasionally leading the physician to consider an acute abdomen. Acute glaucoma is usually due to closure in eyes with narrow angles, but may be due to inflammatory cells or red blood cells in the anterior chamber, neovascularization of the iris (rubeosis iridis), or peripheral anterior synechiae.

DIFFERENTIAL DIAGNOSIS

The causes of red eye can be divided into the catagories of conjunctivitis, keratitis, iritis, acute glaucoma, hemorrhage and focal lesions (see Table 191-2). Differentiation can usually be made on clinical grounds (see Table 191-1).

WORKUP

History is directed toward ascertaining duration of redness, rapidity of onset, the patient's activity at the time, and degree and quality of symptoms. Ophthalmologic history and medications should be noted. Key symptoms include visual changes, pain, itching, crusting in the morning, tearing, mucoid or purulent discharge, photophobia, and foreign body sensation. While usually helpful, the history can be misleading, as viral conjunctivitis may be accompanied by itching or a foreign body sensation, or the patient may ascribe the symptoms of herpes simplex keratitis to a "chemical in the eye" because she first noted the symptoms after a home hair permanent.

Examination. Accurate measurement of visual acuity, preferably at a distance, is essential. If it is abnormal, it is important to check for uncorrected optical abnormality by use of a pinhole. Any patient with reduced vision which is not readily explained should be evaluated by an ophthalmologist promptly. Mucus and tearing may reduce vision one or two lines at most. Corneal lesions may further reduce vision, with only partial improvement on pinhole testing; a central epithelial abrasion typically maintains vision at about 20/100 or better. Preauricular nodes should be palpated. A complete examination of the eye and fundus is important. The lid margins should be inspected for crusting, ulceration, inspissations, and masses, and the conjunctiva for distribution of redness, ciliary flush, foreign bodies (including lid eversion) and, if a slit lamp is available, follicles and papillae. Corneal clarity is noted with a flashlight and a direct ophthalmoscope set at about +15 diopters can be used to magnify corneal details. A blue filter should be used to detect lesions which stain with fluorescein. A slit lamp examination is helpful, but not mandatory. Corneal examination with fluorescein staining is essential to detect corneal infections. Intraocular pressure should be determined if glaucoma is suspected. Depth of the anterior chamber of the other eye can be assessed by a flashlight shined parallel to the iris (coronal plane) from the temporal side. A shallow anterior chamber is usually convex and will cast a shadow on the nasal iris.

Laboratory studies are usually the responsibility of an ophthalmologist. The primary practitioner may attempt conjunctival smears, which show polymorphonuclear leukocytes in acute bacterial conjunctivitis, lymphocytes in viral or late bacterial conjunctivitis, and eosinopils in allergic reactions. This is time-consuming and generally not necessary. Purulent discharges should be cultured on blood agar and, if *Neisseria* is suspected, chocolate agar; Gram stain may reveal gram-negative diplococci in such cases. Scrapings for inclusion bodies in suspected chlamydial or viral disease are usually unrewarding, and scraping and culture of an infected corneal ulcer requires an ophthalmologist.

White blood and differential count are indicated in suspected cellulitis. Clotting studies for subconjunctival hemorrhage are not indicated unless other evidence of coagulopathy is present or the patient is being treated with anticoagulants.

PRINCIPLES OF MANAGEMENT AND THERAPEUTIC RECOMMENDATIONS

Blepharitis usually responds to aggressive lid hygiene therapy. The patient can dilute Johnson's Baby Shampoo 50:50 with water and, using a cotton ball, scrub the lids well with the eyes closed. After rinsing with water, a hot compress is applied to the closed lids for 10 to 20 minutes, followed by instillation of erythromycin or bacitracin ophthalmic ointment in the inferior fornix. If this procedure is followed three to four times daily, most cases will improve or resolve. Normal lids can be maintained by nightly lid hygiene and warm compresses. A hordeolum may respond to this treatment or, like chalazia, may require incision and curettage by an ophthalmologist.

Cellulitis of the lid, unless severe, responds to the above topical treatment plus oral antibiotics. Erythromycin 250-500 mg. PO t.i.d. is effective for resistant cases, but is costly. Warm compresses and oral antibiotics are also indicated for acute dacryocystitis, but persistent localized abscess requires incision and drainage by an ophthalmologist. Orbital cellulitis and cavernous sinus thrombosis require hospitalization and intravenous therapy.

Mild hypersensitivity reactions of the lids respond rapidly to discontinuation of the offending agent and application of cool compresses. Systemic antihistamines are useful in moderate reactions, and steroids in severe reactions.

Cool compresses and ice packs applied early may minimize lid *ecchymoses*; later, warm compresses speed resolution. In cases of *bacterial conjunctivitis*, erythromycin ophthalmic ointment four times daily is usually an effective antimicrobial treatment for the conjunctivitis. Bacitracin ophthalmic ointment and sodium sulfacetamide are alternative medications. *Neisseria* requires systemic penicillin therapy. Bacterial conjunctivitis improves in several days; viral conjunctivitis may take several weeks. Viral conjunctivitis is quite contagious, and live virus is shed in the tears for up to 2 weeks; the patient should be instructed regarding personal hygiene. Cases which worsen or fail to respond should be reevaluated by an ophthalmologist. A nonophthalmologist should never prescribe topical steroid or steroid-antibiotic combination drops, as infection may be worsened and a corneal ulcer may rapidly perforate.

Allergic conjunctivitis in seasonal allergies is relieved by cool compresses and decongestant-antihistamine drops (Vasocon-A, Albalon-A) four times a day, as well as oral antihistamines. Long-term use of these drops is not recommended, as marked rebound vasodilation may develop. Severe allergic conditions may require steroid therapy instituted by an ophthalmologist.

Subconjunctival hemorrhage usually requires only reassurance; compresses (initially cool, then warm) and erythromycin ophthalmic ointment may reduce discomfort in cases with marked swelling.

Conjunctival foreign bodies are usually easily removed with a cotton swab or fine forceps; erythromycin ointment t.i.d. for 2 days is adequate for healing.

Corneal ulcers require intensive emergency evaluation and treatment by an ophthalmologist. Patients with typical herpes simplex dendritic keratitis may be started on idoxuridine or vidarabine ointment five times daily and erythromycin ointment twice daily if an ophthalmologist is not available. *Corneal abrasions* heal rapidly with erythromycin ointment and a tight sterile patch that prevents lid motion for 24 to 48 hours. If the initial abrasion was sizable (roughly 25 per cent of the cornea or more), healing should be checked after removal of the patch. Lesions of this size also require cycloplegia for relief of painful secondary iritis during healing (see iritis treatment). After reepithelialization occurs, ointment applied three times daily for 4 days helps complete the healing process. Cases involving *foreign bodies* and rust rings are treated like abrasions once the body has been removed. Foreign bodies may be irrigated and then removed with a cotton swab, a sterile "golf stick," or an 18-gauge needle with a syringe as a handle. Rust on the surface is easily debrided, but scraping is prohibited as it will damage Bowman's membrane and cause permanent scarring. Left untreated, rust may be irritating, but will surface and slough in 1 or 2 weeks. *Contact lens overwear* and *ultraviolet keratitis* respond to brief cycloplegia, erythromycin ointment, and sterile pressure patching for 24 hours. The associated pain often requires codeine.

Suspected *corneal laceration* and *perforation* is an ophthalmic emergency. A protective metal shield ("Fox shield") should be placed over the eye; no medication should be instilled.

An ophthalmologist must evaluate and treat *primary iritis,* but initial cycloplegia by tropicamide 1% q.i.d. or cyclopentolate 1% q.i.d. will prevent posterior synechia formation and relieve pain. *Secondary iritis* may be treated with these medications or, in an eye which will be patched for 1 or 2 days, several drops of scopolamine 0.25% will provide longer cycloplegia. The nonophthalmologist should avoid atropine, as its effects persist for 1 to 2 weeks.

Acute glaucoma should be treated by immediate administration of acetazolamide 500 mg. IV and glycerol 120 cc. orally in orange juice. Pilocarpine 2% should be begun with instillation as frequently as every 15 minutes to break the attack. Immediate attention by an ophthalmologist is necessary, because the only definitive treatment is surgery.

ANNOTATED BIBLIOGRAPHY

Drugs for bacterial conjunctivitis. Medical Letter, *18*:70, 1976. *(A succinct, critical review of topical agents; external infections with gonococci, C.* trachomatis *and* Pseudomonas *require systemic as well as topical treatment. Caution is suggested in the use of topical corticosteroids. A table of suggested treatments for the major organisms involved in bacterial conjunctivitis is presented.)*

Jones, E.L.R.: The red eye. Practitioner *219*:59, 1977. *(An excellent review that divides the red eye into those where vision is affected, watery eyes where vision is not affected, and red sticky eyes where vision is not affected. A flow chart is presented.)*

Leibowitz, H.M., Pratt, M.V., Flagstad, I.J., *et al.*: Human conjunctivitis: Diagnostic evaluation. Arch. Ophthalmol., *94*:1747, 1976. *(A diagnostic approach is presented showing little correlation between clinical signs and ultimate etiologic diagnosis.)*

Perkins, R.E., Kundsin, R.B., Pratt, M.V., *et al.*: Bacteriology of normal and infected conjunctiva. J. Clin. Microbiol., *1*:147, 1975. *(A careful bacteriologic study that showed that anaerobic organisms may be responsible for many cases of chronic conjunctivitis.)*

Smolen, G., and Okumoto, M.: Staphylococcal blepharitis. Arch. Ophthalmol. *95*:812, 1977. *(A review of this very common cause of red eye, emphasizing detailed treatment.)*

Vaughan, D., and Asbury, T: General Ophthalmology (Ed. 8). Los Altos: Lange, 1977. *(A practical and inexpensive reference with photographs and details.)*

192

Evaluation of Impaired Vision
CLAUDIA U. RICHTER, M.D.

Patients with decreasing or blurred vision often refer themselves directly to an eye specialist, but at times complain first to their primary physicians. Sudden visual loss is a medical emergency. Gradual diminution of sight raises the specter of eventual blindness and loss of ability to function independent-

ly. Paradoxically, some elderly patients may not volunteer that their vision is decreasing because they consider it a natural consequence of aging. As a result, the primary physician should screen elderly patients for treatable causes of decreased vision. In addition, one needs to be capable of distinguishing visual impairment due to the refractive error from cataracts, glaucoma, and retinal disease in order to provide proper initial care and institute appropriate referrals.

PATHOPHYSIOLOGY AND CLINICAL PRESENTATION

Vision becomes impaired when there is opacification of transparent ocular media, damage to the photoreceptor cells of the retina, or a lesion of the optic nerve, its radiations, or the visual cortex. Anatomic orientation provides a framework for considering the pathophysiology of visual difficulties.

Some patients complain of sudden visual loss only to find that their eyelids are closed by swelling due to trauma, insect bites, cellulitis or angioneurotic edema. Acute blepharospasm, often secondary to the pain of a corneal abrasion, also occurs.

Refractive error remains the most common cause of decreased visual acuity. It results from inability of the eye to focus light precisely on the retina, and may be due to an abnormality in the cornea, lens or size of the globe. Myopic patients commonly present during their late teens and early twenties. Patients in their forties may report decreased visual acuity, but in fact simply cannot accommodate to near distances and require reading glasses. Early cataracts can produce an increased myopia before they opacify and block transmission of light. Uncontrolled diabetes mellitus produces swelling of the lens and changes in refractive error which resolve with control of blood sugar. Some drugs, e.g., sulfonamides and anticholinergic agents, may cause blurred vision.

The cornea is the major refracting surface of the eye, and any change in it can lead to visual disturbances. Acutely, corneal abrasion, herpes simplex virus keratitis, or ulcer may cause decreased vision. Acute angle-closure glaucoma causes sudden visual loss by producing corneal edema. Corneal dystrophies or degenerations result in a more gradual reduction in visual acuity, often progressing over a period of years.

Disease of the anterior chamber rarely compromises vision, except in the case of hyphema, usually secondary to trauma, which may extend into the path of light transmission.

Cataracts, i.e., opacifications of the lens, are a leading cause of gradual vision loss in older patients. The classic history is a painless, slow deterioration of eyesight. However, a traumatic cataract may develop over a period of hours to days.

Vitreous opacification occurs most often from hemorrhage, rarely from inflammation or infection. Hemorrhage all too often complicates proliferative diabetic retinopathy. Hypertension, sickle cell retinopathy, trauma, and other less common retinal diseases are other causes of vitreous hemorrhage. A vitreous floater occasionally may be called a blind spot by the patient.

Glaucoma leads to visual loss when left undetected and untreated. Prolonged elevated intraocular pressure in chronic open-angle glaucoma results in damage to nerve fibers at the optic disc and visual field defects. Four types of visual field defects occur: a paracentral scotoma occurring along the distribution of the arcuate nerve fiber bundle, arcuate scotomata, sector-shaped defects, and nasal steps. Before glaucomatous changes progress, central vision remains intact. However, if the glaucoma is untreated or inadequately treated, even central vision is lost and the eye is blind. Acute angle-closure glaucoma produces a red eye, fixed pupil, hazy cornea, eye pain, and acute impairment of vision. Acute angle-closure glaucoma accounts for less than 5 per cent of all glaucoma cases. Most visual loss due to untreated glaucoma is gradual and progressive.

The retina may be compromised by degeneration, inflammation, trauma, detachment, or ischemia. *Senile macular degeneration* occurs in pateints over age 55 and is presently the leading cause of legal blindness in England. The disease, which results from a variety of macular changes related to aging, has diverse clinical manifestations. Central vision is decreased, while peripheral vision remains intact. Fundoscopic examination may show macular drusen, loss of the foveal reflex, atrophy of the macular retinal pigment epithelium resulting in prominent choroidal vessels, or a central fibrous scar. Attempts at treatment have been disappointing, but photocoagulation offers hope for some patients in whom the changes do not directly affect the fovea.

Central serous retinopathy is an idiopathic, spontaneous detachment of the retina in the macular area. Patients range in age from 20 to 50. Again, central vision is reduced, but recovery is usually spontaneous within a few months.

Inflammation of the retina and choroid, as with histoplasmosis or toxoplasmosis, can lead to loss of central vision when the macula is involved.

Trauma may cause retinal edema resulting in decreased visual acuity when it occurs in the macular region. This edema usually resolves within a few days.

Retinal detachment is heralded by flashing lights,

which indicate traction on the retina, and vitreous floaters, i.e., condensed vitreous or a small hemorrhage. The patient may notice a visual field defect progressing like a shade being drawn or may report suddenly blurred vision. In some cases, the patient notes no change in visual acuity. The retina appears ballooned forward with undulating folds.

The vasculature of the retina or optic nerve may become compromised, leading to sudden visual loss. The vascular diseases involving the arteries are central retinal artery occlusion, giant cell arteritis, and anterior ischemic optic neuropathy. The most important to recognize promptly is *central retinal artery occlusion.* The history is one of sudden, painless loss of ability to perceive light or hand movements. The patient may have had previous episodes of amaurosis fugax. Ophthalmoscopy reveals a pale optic disc, attenuated arterioles, "box car" veins, hazy edematous retina, and a cherry-red spot in the macula. Occasionally, an embolus may be seen in one of the retinal vessels. The most common source is an atheromatous plaque in the ipsilateral carotid artery. A Marcus Gunn pupil will often be present.

Giant cell or *temporal arteritis,* an inflammation of the medium and large arteries in elderly people, may cause sudden visual loss. These patients may have had premonitory visual symptoms similar to amaurosis fugax. They may also have symptoms of polymyalgia rheumatica (see Chapter 150). The fundus examination may reveal a swollen optic disc, a normal optic disc, or a central retinal artery occlusion.

Anterior ischemic optic neuropathy is the disease produced by ischemia or infarction of the anterior portion of the optic nerve. The patient notes a sudden visual field defect, usually involving superior or inferior visual field and the macula. The optic disc initially appears edematous, sometimes just one portion, with a few flame-shaped hemorrhages. Optic atrophy follows the disc edema. Thrombosis of an arteriosclerotic vessel is the most common etiology. Some evidence exists that the visual prognosis is improved if corticosteroids are used early, while the optic disc edema is still present.

Central or branch *retinal vein occlusions* cause a sudden painless decrease in visual acuity. In central retinal vein occlusion, ophthalmoscopy reveals a classic "blood and thunder" fundus. The veins are tortuous and dilated. The retina is edematous and covered with flame-shaped hemorrhages. The optic disc margin is blurred. The fundus changes in branch retinal vein occlusion are similar, but limited to the distribution of the involved vein. The decreased visual acuity

is due to macular edema and retinal ischemia. In central retinal vein occlusion, 20 per cent of patients have preexisting chronic open-angle glaucoma, and 50 per cent of men have preexisting hypertension. In branch retinal vein occlusion, 75 per cent of all patients have preexisting hypertension.

Optic neuritis, the primary inflammation of the optic nerve, presents with a relatively acute impairment of vision. Most often it is caused by multiple sclerosis or is idiopathic. Clinically, there is relatively acute impairment of vision progressing over hours to days, typically unilateral, with pain on eye motion and improved visual function in the second to third week. Examination reveals a Marcus Gunn pupil, globe tenderness, visual field defects, and changes in color perception.

Infiltrative or compressive lesions of the optic nerve, such as pituitary adenomas, meningiomas, gliomas, or internal carotid artery aneurysms, cause gradual, relentless field cuts and visual loss. It is unusual for lesions posterior to the optic chiasm to present with decreased visual acuity because of the decussation of fibers in the optic chiasm. Unilateral lesions, such as a brain tumor or a cerebrovascular accident, may cause a homonymous hemianopsia or related visual field defects. However, bilateral CNS lesions may cause profound visual loss.

Many patients complain of blurred vision at night. Rarely, these patients may be found to have true *night blindness* caused by retinitis pigmentosa or vitamin A deficiency. More commonly, no etiology is found; slight decrease in visual acuity at night is common and normal.

Systemic diseases may involve the retina and cause decreased vision. Hypertension, diabetes mellitus, anemia, Waldenström's macroglobulinemia, and systemic lupus erythematosus are examples. Also, hysterical patients and malingerers may present with complaints of visual loss, but opticokinetic reflexes are not lost.

WORKUP

History is most important in evaluating a complaint of sudden visual loss. It is necessary to determine the length and pattern of visual loss; whether visual function has improved, deteriorated or remained the same during the disease course; whether visual loss is bilateral or unilateral, painful or painless. The presence of premonitory symptoms is often helpful. Acute loss is suggestive of a vascular event or retinal detachment. Preceding episodes of amaurosis fugax indicate central retinal artery occlusion or giant cell arteritis. The presence of flashes of light and vitreous floaters may precede a retinal detachment. Progressive visual loss points to a chronic disturbance, such as glaucoma, cataract or macular degeneration. Previous episodes of decreased visual acuity with halos around lights and pain indicate angle-closure glaucoma. An associated sensation of a foreign body indicates a corneal abrasion or herpes simplex keratitis. Pain on eye movement and globe tenderness are associated with retrobulbar optic neuritis. The presence of other diseases such as diabetes, hypertension, heart disease or sickle cell anemia may be contributory. A history of trauma is also important.

Examination. Vision should be tested one eye at a time. If the patient complains of pain, a topical anesthetic such as proparacaine can be used to allow examination. If the lids are tightly swollen, it may be necessary to pry them apart forcibly. A Snellen eye chart with its standardized letter sizes is most convenient for vision testing. If one is not available, any printed material can be used. One notes the size of the smallest print the patient can read and the distance at which he can read it. The patient should wear his glasses when distance or reading is tested. If the patient cannot read the largest letters, the distance at which he can accurately count fingers or identify hand motions is noted. If targets cannot be seen, it is important to determine whether or not the eye can perceive light. Next, vision is rechecked with the patient looking through a pinhole to eliminate any residual refractive error he may have.

The pupils should be examined carefully, noting the size, direct and consensual reactions to light, and the presence of a Marcus Gunn pupil (positive swinging flashlight test). A Marcus Gunn pupil may be found in optic neuritis, central retinal artery occlusion, giant cell arteritis, and large vitreous hemorrhages. A fixed pupil in conjunction with a red eye is indicative of acute angle-closure glaucoma.

The examination of the conjunctiva will reveal whether the eye is red and inflamed or white and quiet. With the exception of trauma, acute glaucoma, and infection, the diseases which may cause sudden visual loss do not cause a red eye. The cornea normally is clear with a crisp light reflex and no fluorescein stain. If a tonometer is available, the intraocular tension should be measured.

Ophthalmoscopy is the most important step in arriving at a diagnosis. One notes first whether the fundus can be visualized or if a dense cataract or vitreous opacity is present. If the fundus can be visualized, the optic disc is observed for loss of sharp disc margins. The macula is examined, looking for a cherry-red spot (seen in central retinal artery occlusion), hemorrhages, and scars. The vessels are examined, with attention paid to the caliber and the presence or absence of emboli. In patients over 50 with sudden visual loss, the erythrocyte sedimentation rate should be determined to check for temporal arteritis.

If a patient is a malingerer, the examination of the eye will be normal. It may be necessary to attempt to trick the patient in order to make a diagnosis of hysterical blindness. An easy way is to test opticokinetic responses, one eye at a time. In order to have normal opticokinetic responses, the eye must be able to fixate on the test object. A newspaper is a useful test object; normal opticokinetic responses with headlines correlate with 20/200 vision, the stock market pages with 20/20.

MANAGEMENT

Patients with sudden visual loss are appropriately referred for ophthalmologic consultation. If an ophthalmologist is not immediately available, there are appropriate emergency measures.

If a central retinal artery occlusion exists which is less than 24 hours old, and preferably less than 4 hours old according to the history, it is reasonable to attempt heroic measures to salvage vision. The principle is to lower the intraocular pressure to encourage the embolus to break apart and move distally. First, one can gently massage the globe with the fingers to attempt to dislodge the embolus. Have the patient breathe a mixture of 5% CO_2 and 95% O_2 to cause the retinal vessels to vasodilate and to deliver a high pO_2 to any viable retinal cells. If this mixture is not available, have the patient breathe into a paper bag. Next, give the patient 500 mg. intravenous acetazolamide to decrease the production of aqueous humor.

If the physician suspects giant cell arteritis, the patient should be started at once on 60 mg. of prednisone a day. Some vision may be salvaged in the affected eye, but, more important, the other eye may be protected (see Chapter 150).

Acute angle-closure glaucoma should be treated at once with topical pilocarpine in *both* eyes and acetazolamide 500 mg. intravenously. The pilocarpine acts therapeutically in the involved eye and prophylactically in the uninvolved eye. Pain medication and antiemetics are in order. If available, osmotic agents such as intravenous mannitol or oral glycerol should be used. All patients with acute angle-closure glaucoma need a peripheral iridectomy to prevent further attacks.

Visual blurring from erratically controlled diabetes will improve when swings in the blood sugar are minimized.

INDICATIONS FOR REFERRAL

All patients with acute loss of vision should be seen immediately by the ophthalmologist. Those with refractive errors can be sent to optometrists. Individuals suspected of having glaucoma, macular degeneration, or retinal vein occlusions, as well as those in whom the cause of impaired vision is unclear, should have early ophthalmologic consultation. Referral for cataracts can wait until some visual loss is noted by the patient.

ANNOTATED BIBLIOGRAPHY

Chisolm, I.A.: Gradual visual loss. Practitioner, *219*:64, 1977. *(A good review with clear branching logic.)*

Cohen, D.N.: Temporal arteritis: Improvement in visual prognosis and management with repeat biopsies. Trans. Am. Acad. Opthalmol Otolaryngol., *77*:74, 1973. *(A prospective study of 14 patients with histologically confirmed temporal arteritis.)*

Cullen, J.F., and Coleiro, J.A.: Ophthalmic complications of giant cell arteritis. Surv. Ophthalmol., *20*:247, 1976. *(An excellent review of temporal arteritis and its visual manifestations.)*

Editorial: Senile disciform macular degeneration. Br. Med. J., *1*:1444, 1979. *(A succinct update on this common and frustrating cause of visual loss; 18 refs.)*

Gass, J.D.R.: Drusen and disciform macular detachment and degeneration. Arch. Ophthalmol., *90*:206, 1973. *(A follow-up study of 200 patients with macular drusen to determine the cause of central visual loss.)*

Hayreh, S.S.: Central retinal vein occlusion: Differential diagnosis and management. Trans. Am. Acad. Ophthalmol. Otolaryngol., *83*:OP379, 1977. *(An excellent discussion of the different clinical presentations and of the inadequacy of therapy.)*

Karjalainen, K.: Occlusion of the central retinal artery and retinal branch arterioles. Acta Ophthalmol., *109*:1, 1971. *(A long, detailed discussion of 175 patients with retinal arterial occlusion, covering final vision, associated diseases and ocular complications.)*

Kornzweig, A.L.: Visual loss in the elderly. Hosp. Pract., *12*:51, 1977. *(A paper on ocular and systemic causes of visual loss.)*

Lessel, S.: Optic neuropathies. N. Engl. J. Med., *299*:533, 1978. *(A superb review of the characteristics and differentiation of ischemic, compressive and inflammatory optic nerve disorders.)*

Sanders, M.O.: Sudden visual loss. Practitioner, *219*:43, 1977. *(A straightforward review emphasizing differential diagnosis.)*

193
Evaluation of Eye Pain

Pain in the eye is most often produced by conditions that do not threaten vision. However, at times the discomfort may be due to corneal or intraocular pathology that is capable of compromising eyesight. The first responsibility of the primary physician is to promptly determine if there is an immediate threat to vision that requires urgent therapy or quick referral to the ophthalmologist; minor problems can be treated symptomatically in the office.

PATHOPHYSIOLOGY AND CLINICAL PRESENTATION

The pain-sensitive structures of the eye include the cornea, conjunctiva, lid, sclera, and uveal tract. Pathology confined to the vitreous, retina, or optic nerve is rarely a source of pain.

Cornea. The cornea is densely innervated by pain fibers, so that even a minor injury may result in considerable discomfort. Pain arises from exposure of nerve endings in the epithelium; the patient complains of a burning or foreign body sensation. Reflex lacrimation may accompany the discomfort. *Keratitis* (inflammation of the cornea) occurs with trauma, infection, exposure, vascular disease, or decreased lacrimation. Cellular infiltration and loss of corneal luster ensue. If blood vessels invade the normally avascular corneal stroma, vision may become cloudy. Severe pain is a prominent symptom; movement of the lid typically exacerbates symptoms. Fluorescein stain reveals the epithelial defects quite well and allows identification with a penlight.

Conjunctiva. Conjunctival disease causes less severe discomfort than corneal injury and does not pose a threat to vision unless the disease process extends to the cornea. Mild burning, itching, or a foreign body sensation is commonly noted. In *conjunctivitis* (see Chapter 191), the eye appears injected and exudation may occur. Patients often complain that the eyelids feel stuck together in the morning upon arising. At times, a thick exudate may develop and transiently cloud vision; blinking the eyelids a number of times in rapid succession is usually sufficient to clear the material. Infectious and allergic causes of conjunctivitis are the major sources of bilateral involvement; toxic, mechanical, and chemical injuries are commonly responsible for unilateral disease.

Eyelid. Inflammation of the eyelid is also capable of producing a foreign body sensation, often in association with redness, swelling, and tenderness of the lid.

Sclera. Compared to disease of the eyelids, scleral problems are more likely to cause dull, deep pain. If the condition involves the anterior sclera, it may be readily visible as an area of redness. The blood supply to the sclera is not extensive and its metabolism is relatively inactive; consequently, inflammatory conditions of the sclera tend to be rather torpid; many are associated with connective tissue disease.

Intraocular structures. Intraocular pathology can sometimes produce pain in the eye. *Acute anterior uveitis* is characterized by pain, photophobia, excessive tearing, and a constricted pupil; vision may become compromised if an exudate forms in the anterior chamber of the eye. Some degree of injection is usually present at the limbus, but its detection may require a slit lamp; in severe cases the eye may appear grossly reddened. An acutely painful red eye may also be the presentation of *acute angle-closure glaucoma.* Often the patient gives a history of mild intermittent episodes of blurred vision preceding the onset of an attack of throbbing pain, nausea, vomiting, and decreased visual acuity; halos about lights are sometimes noted. A fixed, midposition pupil, redness, and a hazy cornea may be present. *Retrobulbar optic neuritis* (inflammation of the optic nerve behind the eye) may cause pain, especially if inflammation spreads to the contiguous extraocular muscles. Most cases are idiopathic, but 10 to 15 per cent are associated with multiple sclerosis. Symptoms include pain on eye movement, abnormal color vision, and some loss of central vision. In most instances, the optic disc appears normal, but occasionally there is edema. A central scotoma may be found.

Orbital structures. Inflammation of the orbit can be a source of eye pain in conjunction with redness and swelling. Tumor or pseudotumor of the orbit may also produce orbital pain. Displacement of the globe is the most obvious finding, and diplopia may result.

Other sources. Mild headache referred to the orbit is seen with refractive error, ocular muscle imbalance, sinusitis (see Chapter 209), and other causes of nonocular headache (see Chapter 153). However, severe aches in the eye cannot be attributed to refractive error, nor can aches about the eye that are noted on awakening in the morning.

DIFFERENTIAL DIAGNOSIS

Extraocular causes of eye pain include diseases of the lid, conjunctiva, cornea, and sclera. Common lid conditions are hordeolum (a small abscess of the lid), acute dacryocystitis, cellulitis, and chalazion. Incipient herpes zoster involving the ophthalmic branch of the fifth nerve may cause eye pain. Conjunctival irritation related to prolonged sun exposure, pollution, occupational irritants, aerosol propellants, wind, dust or lack of sleep, as well as that due to viral or bacterial infection, is an important source of eye discomfort. Episcleritis and scleritis can present with severe pain. The most common causes of corneal pain are abrasions, foreign bodies, ulcers, ingrown lashes, contact lens abuse, excessive exposure to sun or other forms of ultraviolet radiation, and viral or bacterial infection.

The important intraocular conditions that produce eye pain may compromise vision and include acute angle-closure glaucoma, acute anterior uveitis, and retrobulbar optic neuritis. The list of conditions associated with anterior uveitis includes the collagen diseases, sarcoidosis, and inflammatory bowel disease; however, most cases are idiopathic. Any orbital tumor or inflammatory process may cause eye pain.

Pain may be referred to the eye from the sinuses, teeth, or other cranial structures.

WORKUP

The initial task is to be sure that there is no threat to vision. Most intraocular conditions that cause eye pain may compromise vision and should be carefully checked for, as should corneal injuries.

History. The quality of the pain needs to be considered. Deep pain is suggestive of an intraocular problem; a foreign body sensation makes it likely that the problem is on the surface of the eye. The patient should be asked about any change in visual acuity or color vision, because any report of deteriorating vision requires urgent ophthalmologic consultation. A history of diplopia and displacement of the eye raises the possibility of an orbital problem. Ascertaining the aggravating and alleviating factors can aid diagnosis. Pain exacerbated by lid movement and relieved by cessation of lid motion is very suggestive of a foreign body or corneal lesion. Pain worsened by eye motion may be due to retrobulbar optic neuritis, especially if accompanied by loss of central vision and a normal appearing optic disc. Photophobia is often prominent in acute anterior uveitis. Localization of a extraocular lesion by history is often difficult, because most of the time the foreign body sensation is felt in the outer portion of the upper lid, regardless of the lesion's location. In considering causes of conjunctival irritation, it is important to ask about occupational exposures, trauma, sun and other forms of ultraviolet radiation (e.g. arc welding), as well as foreign body contact. History of sinusitis and headaches should be noted.

Physical examination. An ophthalmoscope, penlight, ability to perform lid eversion, and use of fluorescein stain can be very helpful for assessment. First, visual acuity, color vision, and extraocular movements should be tested and recorded. The eye, lid, and conjunctiva are inspected for masses and redness, the pupil for reactivity, the cornea for clarity, and the fundus for any abnormalities of the disc. A cloudy cornea in conjunction with a fixed, midposition pupil is consistent with acute glaucoma; the eye may be red. A constricted pupil in the presence of an eye that is tearing excessively suggests anterior uveitis; in severe cases, the eye also may be reddened

and the anterior chamber hazy. Finding a central scotoma should raise suspicion of retrobulbar neuritis; a normal appearing disc supports the diagnosis. The upper lid should be inverted to check for a foreign body or chalazion. The penlight can then be used to survey the cornea for gross injury; examination is facilitated by use of a small hand lens. The iris ought to be examined for evidence of dilated vessels around the limbus; this ciliary flush is characteristic of intraocular inflammation and occurs in anterior uveitis. Often the flush cannot be seen without the aid of a slit lamp.

All but very small lesions can be detected without the use of a slit lamp if fluorescein and a cobalt blue filtered light are employed in the eye examination. Because of the ease of *Pseudomonas* contamination of the fluorescein, it must be instilled by means of either a single-dose container or sterile fluorescein strips wetted with sterile saline. The strip is touched to the inferior cul de sac while the patient looks upward; the patient is then asked to blink once. The fluorescein stains into denuded areas of corneal epithelium, producing a bright green color when viewed by normal light. The intensity of staining is enhanced if the eye is illuminated with a cobalt blue light. Among the lesions that can be identified by fluorescein staining are the dendritic ulcers of herpes keratitis, abrasions, small foreign bodies, and punctate defects due to irradiation.

If pain is not clearly related to the external eye or adnexa, the intraocular pressure should be measured (see Chapter 190) to rule out glaucoma.

INDICATIONS FOR REFERRAL

The suspicion or detection of intraocular inflammation, acute glaucoma, retrobulbar optic neuritis, keratitis, an orbital problem or any other lesion that impairs vision or has not responded within 48 hours to conservative therapy is an indication for referral to the ophthalmologist. Foreign bodies that cannot be removed by irrigation or a cotton swab also require referral, unless the primary physician is comfortable using a sterile 25-gauge needle to remove a foreign body from the surface of the eye.

SYMPTOMATIC MANAGEMENT

Foreign bodies. Removal should first be attempted by means of *irrigation,* particularly for foreign bodies on the cornea. Sterile saline is directed at the area by means of a syringe with the needle removed;

the objective is to try to float the material off the surface. If irrigation fails, no further attempt should be made by the nonophthalmologist to remove the foreign body if it is firmly embedded in the cornea; use of a dry cotton-tipped applicator will only remove much normal corneal epithelium. However, foreign bodies on the conjunctiva can often be safely removed by employing a cotton applicator or a 25-gauge needle. Following removal of a corneal foreign body, an antibiotic solution is instilled and the eye is patched to immobilize the lids and prevent discomfort from blinking. *Patching* is accomplished by having the patient close both eyes tightly, placing the patch over the closed lid, and taping from the brow to the cheek bone.

Corneal abrasions (see Chapter 191). The patient can be made much more comfortable by tightly patching the eyelids closed. Sometimes antibiotics are employed, but are not necessary unless infection is feared. Erythromycin ointment is commonly used, with a small amount placed on the lower lid before patching.

Conjunctivitis. See Chapter 191.

Acute angle-closure glaucoma. If an ophthalmologist is not immediately available and the patient is thought to have this form of glaucoma, emergency treatment should be started. The intraocular pressure can be brought down with oral administration of 100 gm. of glycerin mixed with an equal volume of water or fruit juice; unfortunately there is often subsequent vomiting. Pilocarpine 4% is applied to both eyes and may be repeated as often as every 15 minutes. Simultaneously, acetazolamide, 500 mg., should be given intravenously, if possible.

ANNOTATED BIBLIOGRAPHY

Chandler, P.A., and Grant, W.M.: Glaucoma. Philadelphia: Lea and Febiger, 1979. *(A thorough treatise emphasizing clinical aspects.)*

Newell, F.S., and Ernest, J.T.: Ophthalmology: Principles and concepts. St. Louis: C.V. Mosby, 1978. *(Chapter 15 provides a clear and clinically oriented discussion of uveitis.)*

Paton, D., and Goldberg, M.F.: Management of Ocular Injuries. Philadelphia: W.B. Saunders, 1976. *(A detailed but very practical account of important eye injuries; although meant for the ophthalmologist, there is much of value for the primary physician, including instructions on removal of foreign bodies and eye patching.)*

Records, R.E.: Primary care of ocular emergencies: Traumatic injuries. Postgrad. Med., *65*(5):143, 1979. *(A terse but helpful guide to common injuries; well illustrated.)*

Schwartz, B.: The glaucomas. N. Engl. J. Med., *299*:182, 1978. *(A brief summary of the mechanisms, presentations, and therapy of the glaucomas.)*

194
Evaluation of Dry Eye
DAVID A. GREENBERG, O.D., M.P.H.

Dry eye is a common symptomatic problem that may occur in association with a variety of systemic conditions. The primary physician must decide whether referral is indicated, determine if systemic disease exists, and decide on symptomatic therapy.

PATHOPHYSIOLOGY AND CLINICAL PRESENTATION

The tear film functions as a wetting agent, preventing damage to corneal and conjunctival epithelium; as a smooth primary refracting surface; as an inhibitor of microorganisms by mechanical flushing and chemical protection with lysozyme and gamma globulin; and as a lubricant. The tear film is composed of three layers. The superficial oily layer formed by the meibomian glands retards evaporation, maintains corneal thickness, and traps foreign debris. The intermediate aqueous layer derived from the main and accessory lacrimal glands contains bactericidal lysozyme and plays a role in corneal nutrition. The deep mucinous layer, formed by conjunctival goblet cells, is in direct contact with corneal and conjunctival epithelium, and it functions as a wetting agent to stabilize the tear film.

Normal tear secretion consists of constant tearing from accessory lacrimal glands and reflex tearing from the main lacrimal gland. Corneal dry spots occur in normal persons after blinking; rehydration is accomplished by another blink. A dry eye may result from aqueous hyposecretion or abnormal mucin production, which causes premature breakup of tear film. The primary dimunition in tear production by the main and accessory lacrimal glands is known as keratoconjunctivitis sicca. Decrements in tear secretion may be physiological, accompanying old age, or result from drugs that inhibit tear secretion or from neurogenic abnormalities. Also, various systemic diseases may result in lymphocytic infiltration or destruction of the glands that secrete the components of tear film and thus produce dry eye. Local change in corneal or conjunctival tissue is known as xerosis and represents the second major pathogenic mechanism of dry eye. Xerosis may occur secondary to infectious, inflammatory, surgical or traumatic damage to the corneal or conjunctival tissue.

Patients with dry eye will rarely present with that complaint. The clinical presentation that suggests dry eye is grittiness, itching, burning, soreness, difficulty in moving the eyelids, or the sensation of a foreign body in the eye. Ironically, a number of patients with dry eye seek treatment for excessive tearing. Rarely, patients present with corneal ulcers and a red eye.

DIFFERENTIAL DIAGNOSIS

The most common cause of keratoconjunctivitis sicca is the generalized diminution of lacrimal secretion associated with old age. This physiological alteration is often exacerbated by the desiccating effect of a cold dry wind, which probably accounts for the majority of complaints associated with dry eye. Systemic diseases associated with keratoconjunctivitis sicca include Sjögren's syndrome, rheumatoid arthritis, sarcoidosis, Hodgkin's disease, systemic lupus erythematosus, scleroderma, and Mikulicz's syndrome of dacryoadenitis and parotitis. It is also seen as a side effect of anticholinergic drugs such as atropine and antihistamines. It may also result from neurogenic hyposecretion, associated with such uncommon conditions as basal skull fracture or the Ramsay Hunt syndrome. Dry eye secondary to xerosis is somewhat less common. The causes include trachoma of the upper lid, erythema multiforme of the lower lid, Reiter's syndrome, benign mucosal pemphigoid, chemical irritation, dermatitis herpetiformis, and hypovitaminosis A. Mechanical causes of dry eye include exposure keratitis, which causes aqueous layer evaporation, possibly due to exophthalmos, deficient lid closure, ectropion, or absence of blinking.

WORKUP

History. The workup should begin by noting the duration and frequency of symptoms as well as whether they appear to be associated with cold, dry, or windy environments. Symptoms of keratoconjunctivitis sicca are usually more pronounced as the day progresses and are frequently exacerbated by tobacco smoke. The physician should ask if tears are produced with crying and about associated dry mouth. Patients should also be questioned about the presence of symptoms associated with collagen vascular diseases, such as arthritis, and about prior ocular disease, infection, or surgery. A drug history is helpful.

Examination. Following the measurement of visual acuity, examination should focus on the conjunctiva, cornea, and eyelids. The dry eye most commonly appears grossly normal. Physical findings may include an enlarged lacrimal gland, thick yellow mucous strands in the lower fornix, hyperemic and edematous bulbar conjunctiva, or an abnormal corneal light reflex. Abnormal corneal sensitivity reflex may indicate a neuroparalytic keratitis or facial nerve palsy. It is mandatory to check for completeness of lid closure as well as position of eyelashes. The skin and joints should be examined as indicated.

The Schirmer I test is a useful simple screening procedure for assessment of tear production. False-positives and false-negatives occur 20 per cent of the time. The test is performed by placing a 5-mm. corner of folded Schirmer paper between the middle and temporal thirds of the lower lid margin for 5 minutes. The eye should be kept open, but blinking should not be prevented. Light should be subdued to reduce reflex tearing. Normal secretion is wetting in excess of 15 mm. of paper after 5 minutes. Dampening of less than 10 mm. indicates a deficiency.

Applying a topical anesthetic to the eye before performing a Schirmer test will eliminate reflex secretion and measure only basal secretion. This is known as a Schirmer II test, which correlates more significantly with the presence of pathology when secretion is less than 3 mm.

An ophthalmologist should be consulted by patients who do not respond to simple symptomatic measures within 2 weeks. The ophthalmologist may examine the eye with a slit lamp after applying rose bengal stain. The time it takes for the tear film to break up may also be measured. Rarely, conjunctival biopsy, lysozyme activity, or quantitative mucus assays may be helpful in specific cases.

SYMPTOMATIC MANAGEMENT

As long as there are no signs of ocular disease, the primary physician may attempt symptomatic relief. A 2-week trial of one of the many commercially available artificial tear substitutes is recommended. Methylcellulose (Visculose®, 0.5% or 1%), polyvinyl alcohol (Liquifilm Tears®, 1.4%, or Liquifilm Forte, 3%), and hydroxypropyl methylcellulose, 1% (Ultra Tears, Tears Naturale, and Adsorbotear) have all been successfully used. Although there is no ideal tear substitute, polyvinyl alcohol appears to be the most retentive ocular wetting agent. Patients with Stevens-Johnson syndrome, benign mucosal pemphigoid, or hypovitaminosis A require a mucoid tear substitute, sometimes in combination with a hydrophilic contact lens. Topical application of 1 or 2 drops, four times a day, is a useful starting dosage. The patient may increase the frequency of application to as often as hourly in order to achieve comfort. A bland ointment may be used at night. Toxicity is uncommon, but topical sensitivity or corneal epithelial damage may occur. Topical steroids or antibiotics should not be used unless they are specifically indicated. Ophthalmologic consultation should be obtained if there is no response to this symptomatic regimen after 2 weeks.

The ophthalmologist may prescribe protective goggles, ocular inserts with continuous secretion, or soft contact lenses. Surgical procedures, such as closure of the puncta, tarsorrhaphy or parotid-duct transplants, are occasionally indicated. Instruction in the use of artificial tears is important. It may be necessary for the patient to use the drops as frequently as every 15 minutes in some cases. The patient should be instructed to seek immediate ophthalmologic attention in the event of a red eye, visual disturbance, or eye pain.

ANNOTATED BIBLIOGRAPHY

Barsam, P.C., *et al.*: Treatment of the dry eye and related problems. Ann. Ophthalmol., *4*:122, 1972. *(A series demonstrating subjective relief of symptoms in patients with idiopathic ocular discomfort and dry eye using an artificial tear substitute.)*

Baum, J.L.: Keratoconjunctivitis sicca. Trans. Am. Acad. Ophthalmol. Otolaryngol., *81*:519, 1976. *(A scholarly review of the current understanding of the dry eye syndrome.)*

Holly, F.J., and Lemp, M.A.: Tear physiology and dry eyes. Surv. Ophthalmol., *22*:69, 1977. *(The ultimate review.)*

Jones, D.B.: Prospects in the management of tear deficiency states. Trans. Am. Acad. Ophthalmol. Otolaryngol., *83*:OP692, 1977. *(A superb review with a comprehensive table listing the causes by mechanism.)*

Moutsopoulos, H.M., *et al.*: Differences in the clinical manifestations of sicca syndrome in the presence and absence of rheumatoid arthritis. Am. J. Med., *66*:733, 1979. *(An article suggesting that the sicca syndrome in the absence of rheumatologic disease may represent a distinct pathology with specific systemic effects.)*

Sjögren, H., and Block, K.J.: Keratoconjunctivitis sicca and Sjogren's syndrome. Surv. Ophthalmol., *16*:143, 1971. *(A comprehensive review of the ocular consequences of Sjögren's syndrome.)*

Wright, P.: The dry eye. Practitioner, *214*:631, 1975. *(A terse review focusing on the components of the ideal tear replacement drop.)*

195

Evaluation of Excessive Tearing
DAVID A. GREENBERG, O.D., M.P.H.

The presence of watery eyes reflects an increased production of tears or a decreased ability to drain them. Patients complain of watery eyes or may actually describe tears overflowing and running down their cheeks, a condition called epiphora. The primary physician must decide whether structural pathology exists or if reassurance is the appropriate treatment.

PATHOPHYSIOLOGY AND CLINICAL PRESENTATION

Overproduction of tears may be a reflex response to dry eye, to environmental irritants, or to emotion. The second important pathogenic mechanism of watery eyes is an abnormal lacrimal system. The lacrimal drainage system consists of upper and lower puncta that drain through upper and lower canaliculi which may form a common canaliculus and enter the lacimal sac. The sac empties into the inferior meatus of the nose by way of the nasolacrimal duct. Obstruction of the drainage system or loss of the appropriate anatomic relationship of the puncta and globe causes watery eyes. The patient with reflex hypersecretion frequently experiences the symptom on cold or windy days. The patient with dry eye may express the condition as tired eyes associated with excess tearing. The patient with viral conjunctivitis, allergy or a foreign body may complain of excessive tearing. The clinical presentation of these entities is discussed in more detail in Chapter 191.

Ectropion causes epiphora because the punctum is no longer in apposition to the globe. This condition is far more common in the elderly and is characterized by a sagging lower lid. The lacrimal passage may be obstructed by a stone, laceration, burn, surgery, atresia, acute or chronic inflammation. The most common entity is dacryocystitis, which presents as a warm, slightly tender mass in the region of the lacrimal sac. Digital pressure may express purulent material from the puncta. Impairment of drainage may occasionally occur as an adverse consequence of glaucoma or topical antiviral medications.

DIFFERENTIAL DIAGNOSIS

The most common causes of watery eye are senile ectropion or increased physiological tearing. These problems are more common in the elderly. Excessive moisture may be the complaint in a patient who has an inflammatory process such as keratitis, blepharitis or conjunctivitis.

Obstruction in the drainage system most commonly results from dacryocystitis. The puncta may be obstructed by a myriad of causes: tumors, burns, erythema multiforme, or redundant skin. The lacrimal passage may be obstructed by a stone, laceration, burn, surgery, senile atresia, or infection of the lacrimal duct. The puncta may be rendered ineffective by ectropion, sagging of the lower lid. Excessive tearing accompanies facial palsies but is rarely the primary complaint.

WORKUP

History. The physician should determine if tears actually run down the cheek and, if so, how frequent-

ly. Overflowing tears in the absence of environmental irritants suggests structural pathology. Watery eyes noted upon exposure to cold, air conditioning, or a dry environment may be due to an exaggerated perception of physiological tearing.

External examination of the eye. The physician should examine the puncta for patency. A basic test for patency may be performed by instilling fluorescein dye in the eye and inserting a cotton-tipped applicator into the interior meatus. Staining of the cotton swab indicates patency; nonstaining, obstruction. The physician should observe whether the lid is in close apposition to the globe. He should note inflammation of the conjunctiva or around the puncta. If the lacrimal sac is inflamed, the physician should gently express fluid for culture. Obstruction generally requires ophthalmologic consultation for more precise diagnosis and therapy.

The perception of watery eyes may reflect pseudoepiphora secondary to the sicca complex; therefore, it is advisable to inquire about rheumatoid arthritis or dry mouth and perform a Schirmer test (see Chapter 194) after instillation of proparacaine to block reflex tearing. Watering may be a response to denuded corneal epithelium. After the conjunctival sac is touched with a fluorescein strip, the eye is examined with a bright cobalt-blue light to reveal whether there is corneal disease that requires ophthalmologic care.

SYMPTOMATIC MANAGEMENT

Watery eyes pose no danger to the patient if there is no infection. Symptomatic management requires that the physician reassure the patient and recommend that excess tears periodically be dried. Keratoconjunctivitis sicca should be treated with a tear substitute (see Chapter 194). Conjunctivitis should be treated as outlined in Chapter 191. Dacryocystitis usually responds to warm compresses and erythromycin ophthalmic ointment q.i.d. and erythromycin 250 mg. three times daily for 10 days. Culture results and the clinical course may dictate a change in antibiotic. Unresponsive lesions must be drained by an ophthalmologist.

Concerned or disabled patients should be referred to an ophthalmologist who may probe and irrigate the lacrimal system and perform dye flow studies and a dacryocystorhinogram. Surgery may be indicated to repair ectropion, punctual stenosis, canalicular obstruction, or nasolacrimal obstruction if epiphora is convincingly troublesome or if chronic, recurrent infection ensues. The primary physician should explain that there is no danger associated with epiphora and that surgery is available. Discussion with patient may help determine whether referral is advisable.

ANNOTATED BIBLIOGRAPHY

Jones, L.T., and Linn, M.L.: The diagnosis of the causes of epiphora. Am. J. Ophthalmol., *67*:751, 1969. *(A good discussion of basic and more sophisticated tests to determine the existence of lacrimal obstruction.)*

196
Evaluation of Flashing Lights and Scotomata

Patients, particularly the elderly, may complain of flashing lights (photopsia) or spots, or the problem may be revealed during a review of symptoms. "Floaters" or flashes may be a benign annoyance or herald a vitreous or retinal detachment that requires treatment by an ophthalmologist. Patients may be disturbed by spots because they fear they will enlarge. The primary physician needs to know when lights or spots presage serious pathology and to supply the patient with an accurate explanation of the symptoms when there is no underlying disease.

PATHOPHYSIOLOGY

Flashing lights are a subjective phenomenon commonly produced by mechanical stimulation of the retina. The stimulation may simply be rubbing the eyes, or it may be blunt trauma. Advancing age causes the vitreous to liquefy, which reduces its stability, thereby increasing the tendency for movement to produce retinal traction. As the vitreous loses its gel structure, fine fibers, membranes, and cellular aggregates may become visible. A patient who wakes from sleep and looks around stimulates the retina and may produce Moore's lightning flashes. The mechanism is traction of a partially liquefied vitreous of the retina. The pathophysiology of flashing lights that precede migraine headaches is not known, but probably reflects ischemia due to vascular constriction.

Spots before the eyes, dots of filament that move with the eye, are usually caused by opacities that cast shadows on the retina. The perception of spots is increased by bright illumination and by greater proximity of the opacities to the retina and the visual axis. Vitreous opacities characteristically float across the field. Numerous vitreous opacities may cause diffraction of light and a reduction in visual acuity.

The opacities may be embryonic remnants of hyaloid vessels called "muscae volitantes," soaps from degenerating fibrils, that cause a condition called "asteroid hyalitis," cholesterol crystals called "synchysis scintillans," inflammatory particles, or foreign bodies. Also, retinal tears secondary to vitreous detachment may release pigment debris of the blood which causes spots.

DIFFERENTIAL DIAGNOSIS

The differential diagnosis of flashing lights includes, succinctly, migraine prodrome, benign mechanical stimulation, retinal breaks without separation, and vitreal or retinal detachment. Meniere's disease, sinus or dental infection, central retinal vein thrombosis, and tumors of the chiasm, temporal lobe, or visual cortex all may be associated with light flashes. Intermittent angle-closure glaucoma may be accompanied by flashing light or halos around lights. The physician must always consider digitalis toxicity, particularly if the lights are yellow.

Spots are due to vitreal material, inflammatory posterior eye disease, or impending vitreal or retinal detachment. Lens opacities may cause fixed floaters. Occasionally, an anemic patient will complain of black spots.

WORKUP

History. The essential decision is to determine whether the flashes or spots reflect impending vitreal or retinal detachment. The history should establish whether flashes occur upon waking from sleep or rubbing the eyes. A sudden shower of flashing lights raises the suspicion of retinal tear or detachment.

In evaluating spots, the physician should record the acuteness, number, and size and whether they float across the field of vision or are stationary. A sudden shower of spots in the periphery suggests hole formation. A moderately large floater that appears suddenly suggests vitreous detachment. Benign spots are often first noted in bright sunlight.

Physical examination should include thorough ophthalmoscopy to detect retinal detachment, evidence of chorioretinitis or lens opacities. Confrontation field tests should be performed to detect a loss that accompanies a detached retina (however, many detachments will not produce field loss). Aphakic or highly myopic patients are more susceptible to detachment. It is often necessary to have an ophthalmologist perform a complete examination with indirect ophthalmoscopy and scleral depression to identify early retinal or vitreal detachment.

SYMPTOMATIC MANAGEMENT AND PATIENT EDUCATION

There is no therapy for flashes or spots. Flashes that occur in situations easily attributed to mechanical stimulation require reassurance and scientific explanation. Light flashes in association with sinus or dental infection, migraine headache, or Meniere's disease should be explained as part of the underlying pathologic process.

A sudden shower of persistent flashes or spots requires urgent referral to an ophthalmologist. Referral is even more urgent if a field loss is detected.

Elderly patients with chronic spots or flashes that may accompany ongoing syneresis should have complete indirect ophthalmoscopy, but it is not urgent. Light flashes may signify retinal breaks, but it is uncertain how often breaks progress to detachment. Patients with spots or flashes need an explanation and a warning to go to an ophthalmologist without delay if they experience a sudden shower of lights or spots.

ANNOTATED BIBLIOGRAPHY

Aring, C.D.: The scintillating scotoma. JAMA, *220*:519, 1972. *(A review of flashing lights in migraine syndrome.)*

Berens, C., *et al.*: Moore's lightning streaks. Trans. Am. Ophthalmol., *52*:35, 1954. *(A series of 36 patients: 7 retinal detachments, 3 choroidal tumors, 1 central retinal vein thrombosis, 14 associated with sinus disease, 2 with dental infection, and 1 with tonsillitis. Three patients had chorioretinitis.)*

Jaffe, N.S.: Complications of acute posterior vitreous detachment. Arch. Ophthalmol., *79*:568, 1968. *(Flashes of light are associated with acute posterior vitreous detachment.)*

Moore, F.: Subjective "lightning flashes." Am. J. Ophthalmol., *23*:1255, 1940. *(A classic article.)*

Morris, P.H., Scheie, H.G., and Aminlari, A.: Light flashes as a clue to retinal disease. Arch. Ophthalmol., *91*:179, 1974. *(One hundred patients complaining of light flashes were studied: 23 per cent had demonstrable vitreoretinal disease; of these, 16 per cent had retinal breaks or holes.)*

197
Evaluation of Exophthalmos

Exophthalmos, or protrusion of the eye, may be a clue to a significant systemic or local disease or simply a misinterpretation of normal physiognomy. The primary physician must recognize exophthalmos and evaluate possible endocrine, systemic or neoplastic causes to decide whether further workup or referral is indicated.

PATHOPHYSIOLOGY AND CLINICAL PRESENTATION

Exophthalmos frequently presents asymptomatically as a perception, on the part of the patient or physician, of bulging eyes. The protrusion of the globe may lead to disturbances in vision or ocular motility. The chief etiology mechanisms of exophthalmos are inflammation, mass lesions, and vascular abnormality. The most common cause of exophthalmos is Graves' disease. The pathology of Graves' ophthalmopathy involves an inflammatory infiltrate of lymphocytes, mucopolysaccharides, and water behind the globe. The mechanism is probably autoimmunity involving thyroglobulin, antithyroglobulin antibodies, and sensitized lymphocytes. Extraocular muscle membranes may also be affected.

Patients with infiltrative ophthalmopathy frequently have symptoms of eye pain, lacrimation, photophobia, blurring of vision or double vision. Blurred vision may be due to lacrimation, imperfect fusion, compression of optic nerve or exposure keratopathy. Hyperthyroidism of any etiology produces proptosis by sympathetic stimulation of the levator palpebrae muscle. Lid lag, thyroid stare or lid retraction are signs of thyroid disease, while lid edema, chemosis or impairment of extraocular muscle function suggest Graves' infiltrative ophthalmopathy. Inflammatory processes due to infection in the orbit, periorbital areas or adjacent structures, such as the sinuses, may produce signs and symptoms of infiltrative ophthalmopathy. Neoplasms, such as primary orbital lesions, hematopoietic malignancies, or solid tumors metastatic to the orbit, produce exophthalmos by the effect of their mass. Neoplastic lesions characteristically present with exophthalmos, impaired ocular motility, and disturbances in visual acuity. In one series, 56 per cent had decreased visual acuity, 30 per cent muscle dysfunction and 14 per cent pupil abnormalities. Vascular abnormalities such as carotid cavernous fistulas or hemangiomas may push the eye forward. Both neoplastic and vascular lesions present as unilateral exophthalmos. In three combined series of 668 patients with unilateral exophthalmos, 15 per cent had thyroid disease, 8 per cent carotid cavernous fistulas, and 54 per cent tumors, predominantly hemangioma, meningioma, and optic nerve gliomas. Carotid cavernous fistulas present with pulsating exophthalmos.

DIFFERENTIAL DIAGNOSIS

Bilateral endocrine exophthalmos occurs most often in association with thyrotoxicosis and occasionally in Cushing's syndrome, acromegaly and lithium ingestion. Orbital mass lesions are the next most common cause, and these include primary, metastatic, and adjacent carcinoma. Lymphomas, optic gliomas, meningiomas, rhabdomyosarcomas, lacrimalgland epithelial tumors, malignant melanomas, and sinus carcinomas are important neoplastic causes. Inflammation, orbital cellulitis or pseudotumor of the orbit are possible diagnoses. Vascular disorders such as hemangiomas, aneurysms, varices, carotid cavernous sinus fistulas and cavernous sinus thrombosis all must be considered.

Skeletal abnormalities, such as Paget's disease, may produce exophthalmos. Black people normally have orbital prominence and exophthalmometer readings outside of the range defined for whites.

Asymmetry of the orbit, severe myopia in one eye, ptosis or enophthalmos in the opposite eye, facial nerve paresis, and glaucoma may produce the appearance of exophthalmos.

WORKUP

The finding that directs the workup is the presence of either bilateral or unilateral orbital involvement. The differential diagnosis of bilateral involvement is so often thyroid disease that few patients require workup other than thyroid function tests and eye examination. Unilateral orbital involvement has a much longer differential diagnosis that requires evaluation. The physician should search for systemic disease and the ocular complications associated with exophthalmos.

History should determine whether vision has been affected, and the physician should ask about diplopia, pain, excessive lacrimation, photophobia, or a foreign body sensation suggestive of exposure keratopathy. If there are no symptomatic or functional eye problems, workup is less urgent. Obtain old photographs to determine if the apparent problem is really a long-standing anatomic variant. The history should identify recent trauma to the orbit, nasal congestion or discharge, headache, or drug ingestion, particularly lithium. The physician should ascertain whether there are symptoms of hyperthyroidism, such as weight loss, increased appetite, tremulousness, sweating, tachycardia, or excessive anxiety.

Examination should include a general physical assessment as well as a careful eye examination, specifying the degree of exophthalmos, generally with a Hertel exophthalmometer. A normal reading in white patients is generally up to 16 mm.; the range of normal is different for black patients. Asymmetry is particularly significant in defining exophthalmos. The physician should record visual acuity and check extraocular motility for double vision. The cornea should be surveyed for evidence of haziness, suggesting corneal ulcers or edema, and the optic disc should be examined for signs of compression. The physician should measure intraocular pressure. The globe and orbit should be auscultated for bruits and the sinuses examined for tenderness, fluid levels, and abnormal discharge. The physician should perform a physical examination to detect signs of hyperthyroidism, including pretibial edema, which is characteristic of Graves' disease.

Laboratory examination does not have to be extensive. It is the medical doctor's responsibility to rule out hyperthyroidism while determining whether ophthalmologic referral is necessary or urgent. The primary physician not only sees the patient who presents with exophthalmos but also receives a number of patients referred from ophthalmologists in order to rule out hyperthyroidism. The primary physician should obtain thyroid function tests on all patients with exophthalmos. These include tests of thyroxine (T_4) and free T_4 or resin uptake. A T_3 suppression test of autonomy in thyroid function should be performed when other tests are normal. A number of patients are clinically and metabolically euthyroid.

When there is evidence of facial asymmetry, sinus tenderness, or abnormal discharge, the primary physician should obtain sinus films to check for sinusitis or paranasal sinus neoplasms. In unilateral exophthalmos without evidence of hyperthyroidism, radiographs of the orbit should be obtained. Once thyroid disease is excluded, further workup may be conducted by an ophthalmologist experienced in the application of new technologies, such as ultrasonography, orbitography, venography, thermography, radionuclide scanning, and computerized tomographic scanning. The judicious application of these new techniques requires experience and an understanding of the ultimate goals of diagnosis. Some patients require surgical exploration for histologic diagnosis and for the determination of treatment.

SYMPTOMATIC MANAGEMENT

The primary physician must be cognizant of potential ocular complications and give advice about relief of minor symptoms. Periorbital and lid edema may be reduced by elevating the head of the bed and possibly using diuretics. Complaints of a foreign body sensation may be relieved with 1 per cent methylcellulose drops or, if due to faulty coverage of the lid, by tarsorrhaphy or section of Muller's muscle. Simple measures that may help keratopathy are taping the lids at night and using sunglasses to reduce photophobia. Intermittent diplopia may be considerably improved by refraction and prescription of prisms. The physician should treat hyperthyroidism carefully without inducing precipitous hypothyroidism because this may be associated with exacerbation of infiltrative ophthalmopathy. Consultation with an ophthalmologist should be obtained early in the course of evaluating the patient with exophthalmos. Graves' ophthalmopathy involving severe inflammatory changes often requries treatment with steroids or occasionally surgical decompression when corneal or optic nerve compromise is possible. Exophthalmos due to neoplasms may require surgery or radiotherapy, and the treatment of carotid cavernous fistula involves careful vascular surgery to correct the abnormal communication. It is judicious to discontinue lithium in patients with exophthalmos.

Patient education is important because the process may be lengthy, and the patient may be unaware of underlying systemic disease. The primary physician should explain that the eye findings may be indicative of other disease and that evaluation will be slow and methodical. The patient should be assured that vision is rarely permanently affected. The need to recognize the ocular dangers and to apply symptomatic prophylactic therapies must be emphasized.

ANNOTATED BIBLIOGRAPHY

Gorman, C.A.: Management of the patient with Graves' ophthalmopathy. Thyroid Today, *1*:1, 1977. *(Good medically oriented review.)*

Grove, A. S.: Evaluation of exophthalmos. N. Engl. J. Med., *292*:1005, 1975. *(A comprehensive review detailing the various radiographic techniques used in diagnosis.)*

Hamburger, J.I., and Sugar, H.S.: What the internist should know about the ophthalmopathy of Graves' disease. Arch. Intern. Med., *129*:131, 1972. *(A great review focusing on physical findings in exophthalmos.)*

Moss, H.M.: Expanding lesions of the orbit: A clinical study of 230 consecutive cases. Am. J. Ophthalmol., *54*:761, 1962. *(A classic series.)*

O'Neill, P.B.: Passive ocular proptosis. J. Neurol. Neurosurg. Psychiatry, *40*:1198, 1977. *(Two pa-*

tients with oculomotor neuropathy demonstrated passive ocular proptosis.)

Segal, R.L., Rosenblatt, S., and Eliasoph, I.: Endocrine exophthalmos during lithium therapy of manic-depressive disease. N. Engl. J. Med., 289:136, 1974. *(Five of 44 patients [11 per cent] started on lithium developed exophthalmos.)*

Smigiel, M.R., and MacCarty, C.S.: Exophthalmos: The more commonly encountered neurosurgical lesions. Mayo Clin. Proc., 50:345, 1975. *(A good review making the point that 54 per cent of unilateral exophthalmos is caused by tumor.)*

Solomon, D.H.: Identification of subgroups: euthyroid Graves' ophthalmopathy. N. Engl. J. Med., 296:181, 1977. *(A subset of patients with clinically classic Graves' ophthalmopathy but no abnormality in thyroid function.)*

Werner, S.C., Coleman, J., and Franzen, L.A.: Ultrasonographic evidence of a consistent orbital involvement in Graves' disease. N. Engl. J. Med., 290:1447, 1974. *(Consistent involvement in Graves' disease was demonstrated on ultrasonography in 44/77. Involvement was found in extraocular mucus.)*

198
Management of Glaucoma

Ocular hypertension, defined as pressures greater than 21 torr, may occur in as many as 15 per cent of the elderly. The incidence of ocular hypertension increases with age but does not become clinically significant unless it produces field loss or changes in the optic nerve. Elevated pressure occurs six to seven times more often than actual visual disturbances. Epidemiologic data report different prevalence rates based on the definition of the disease. The physician who is not an ophthalmologist will not be responsible for treatment of this disease, but he will identify patients with increased intraocular pressure. It is important for the primary physician to understand the disease, its progression, principles of referral, and systemic effects of therapy.

PATHOPHYSIOLOGY AND CLINICAL PRESENTATION

Glaucoma is characterized by three primary elements: elevated pressure, abnormal cupping or pallor of the optic disc, and loss of visual field. The essential pathophysiological feature is decreased perfusion of the optic nerve, leading to ischemic damage. It has also been suggested that increased pressure leads to direct physical damage of the optic nerve. The pathophysiology of increased intraocular pressure can best be understood in terms of aqueous flow. In front of the lens, the eye is divided into an anterior and posterior chamber. The iris separates these two compartments, which communicate by way of the pupil. The chambers are filled with aqueous humor which then flows through the pupil into the anterior chamber

and leaves the eye through the trabecula, a connective tissue filter at the angle between the iris and the cornea. The fluid enters the canal of Schlemm and then empties into the venous system. The pressure in the eye is maintained by the dynamic equilibrium of aqueous production and outflow. An increase in production or an obstruction to outflow will result in elevated pressure. In primary open-angle glaucoma, obstruction cannot be seen but apparently exists on a microscopic level in the connective tissue meshwork through which the aqueous must drain to reach the venous system. In angle-closure glaucoma, the iris blocks access to the outflow pathway. Secondary causes of obstruction include inflammation, trauma, neoplasm, neovascularization and corticosteroid therapy.

The most common presentation of open-angle glaucoma, which accounts for over 90 per cent of cases, is detection of asymptomatic elevated pressure by a primary physician, an optometrist, or an ophthalmologist. It is frequently called "the silent blinder" in that extensive damage may occur before the patient becomes aware of visual field loss. The patient is usually over 40 and may be diabetic. Occasionally, glaucomatous changes of the optic nerve are noted on routine ophthalmoscopy.

Angle-closure glaucoma presents as a painful red eye. The physical findings include redness, fixed and unreactive pupil in mid-dilation, and, with time, corneal haziness. Occasionally, the principal symptoms of angle-closure glaucoma are nausea and vomiting, and the patient may be thought to have an abdominal disease. The patient with angle closure generally has marked loss of vision and requires emergency treatment. Identification of patients susceptible to angle closure can be accomplished before the episode occurs by inspecting the angle by shining a light perpendicular to it. This is particularly important in patients with a positive family history or episodes of halos or painful blurred vision, especially those occurring in dark environments.

PRINCIPLES OF THERAPY

The objective of treatment of chronic open-angle glaucoma is stabilization of intraocular pressure in a range that will prevent compromise of the optic nerve head and loss of visual field. Therapy involves the use of medications that reduce aqueous production or facilitate drainage. The drugs employed include cholinergic agents, anticholinesterases, sympathomimetics and topical beta-blocking agents. Pilocarpine, the most frequently used parasympathomimetic, acts by contracting the ciliary body and opening the trabecula to facilitate aqueous outflow. Side effects include pinpoint pupil, myopia, spasm of accommodation, and occasionally conjunctival hyperemia. Anticholinesterases act to increase endogenous cholinergic effects and are used to treat patients in whom pilocarpine is not successful. The most commonly used agent is echothiophate iodide (Phospholine iodide). A patient on an anticholinesterase who is treated with succinylcholine may have appreciably prolonged respiratory depression.

Epinephrine is a sympathomimetic drug that works by decreasing aqueous production and, over time, may increase aqueous outflow. It may be used in combination with and is additive in effect to pilocarpine. The ocular side effects of epinephrine include a burning sensation, conjunctival pigmentation, and allergic reactions. With increased doses, systemic effects including tachycardia, palpitations, and elevated blood pressure may be noted.

Timolol, a topical beta-blocker, has recently been introduced into clinical practice. Its advantages over epinephrine and pilocarpine include increased effectiveness in increased numbers of patients with fewer side effects. Also, it is given twice daily, a simpler schedule than either of the other two agents. The primary physician should be alert to the possibility of bradycardia, congestive failure, and asthma, all of which are associated with beta-blockers, although side effects have been uncommon.

Some patients require carbonic anhydrase inhibitors, such as acetazolamide, which can reduce aqueous production. Acetazolamide may be used in combination with epinephrine and can have a variety of systemic effects, including mild metabolic acidosis, paresthesia of the face and extremities, metallic taste, anorexia, nausea, vomiting, diarrhea, and occasionally renal stones.

Surgical intervention should be considered in chronic open-angle glaucoma when maximal medical therapy does not arrest progressive changes to the disc or the visual field. The usual surgical procedure is to create a drainage or filtering route from the anterior chamber into subconjunctival or intrascleral space. Occasionally, cryotherapy of the ciliary body is used to decrease aqueous production. In angle-closure glaucoma, surgery is the treatment of choice; usually peripheral iridectomy is performed to provide communication between the anterior and posterior chambers. Prophylactic surgery is indicated in the unaffected eye. Lasers are being used to create small openings in the iris without resorting to surgery.

THERAPEUTIC RECOMMENDATIONS

Drugs that increase intraocular pressure should be used cautiously. These include systemic and topical steroids, particularly when they are applied to the eye or on the periorbital skin. Many drugs with anticholinergic effects are relatively contraindicated in patients with glaucoma. These agents do not elevate ocular pressure but may precipitate angle closure in patients with shallow angles. Reports on hypotensive optic neuropathy following precipitous lowering of blood pressure suggest that a gradual reduction in blood pressure in consultation with an ophthalmologist is preferable in patients with coincident systemic and ocular hypertension.

Most patients are under treatment with topical pilocarpine. Increasingly, patients are being started with timolol because of its ease of administration and lower incidence of side effects. Acetazolamide (Diamox®) is occasionally necessary, but the primary physician should consider its numerous systemic side effects when evaluating a patient with complaints. Surgery is indicated when progression of disc changes or field defects persists despite maximal medical therapy.

The primary physician must be able to recognize angle-closure glaucoma, institute miotic therapy with pilocarpine, and refer the patient without delay.

PATIENT EDUCATION

A chief responsibility of the primary physician is to educate the patient about the meaning of elevated intraocular pressure and glaucoma. It is not uncommon for patients to be told that they have glaucoma when their condition is merely a reflection of elevated intraocular pressure. Many patients with pressures in the middle 20s do not have glaucoma. Patients may occasionally call their primary physician for reassurance about the side effects of drugs, and the physician should provide an explanation and facilitate consultation with the ophthalmologist. The primary physician's role in the early detection of glaucoma is discussed in Chapter 190.

ANNOTATED BIBLIOGRAPHY

Bulpitt, C.J., Hodes, C., and Evertt, M.G.: Intraocular pressure and systemic blood pressure in the elderly. Br. J. Ophthalmol., 59:717, 1975. (This article reviews some of the data about precipitous changes in systemic blood pressure exacerbating glaucoma.)

Editorial: Medical treatment of open angle glaucoma. Br. Med. J., 1:460, 1978. (A short statement on the many systemic drugs that have been shown useful in the treatment of glaucoma.)

Hayreh, S.: Optic disc changes in glaucoma. Br. J. Ophthalmol., 56:175, 1975. (An excellent review of the optic disc changes which one should detect as a sign of glaucoma.)

Keeney, M.M., et al.: Prevalence of senile cataract, diabetic retinopathy, senile macular degeneration, open angle glaucoma in the Framingham eye study. Am. J. Ophthalmol., 85:28, 1978. (An important landmark in epidemiology of eye disease, including presentation of important data on glaucoma.)

Leske, M.C., and Rosenthal, J.: Epidemiologic aspects of open-angle glaucoma. Am. J. Epidemiol., 109:250, 1979. (A consummate review; 105 refs.)

Schwartz, B.: Current concepts in ophthalmology: The glaucomas. N. Engl. J. Med., 299:182, 1978. (A superb succinct review.)

Zimmerman, T.J., et al.: Timolol maleate: Efficacy and safety. Arch. Ophthalmol., 97:656, 1979. (A randomized double-blind trial of various concentrations of timolol solution revealed it to be a safe and effective ocular hypotensive agent.)

199
Management of Cataracts

Frequently, cataracts that produce no functional disability are identified on routine examination. Clinically, a cataract is an opacification on the crystalline lens that reduces the visual function and eventually affects the patient's way of life. The prevalence of cataracts increases markedly with age. The Framingham study found a prevalence rate of just under 5 per cent in the age group 52 to 64, and a rate of 18 per cent in those 64 to 75. Vision can be improved with eyeglasses, but definitive therapy is surgical. The primary physician should be able to educate the patient about the significance of cataract, allay fears about surgery, and advise about the timing and consequences of operation.

PATHOPHYSIOLOGY AND CLINICAL PRESENTATION

Cataracts may arise from a variety of causes. Occasionally, they are congenital; a few develop during the early years of life, usually in association with specific diseases such as diabetes, Wilson's disease, Down's syndrome, and other metabolic diseases. The majority of cataracts occur in the elderly and reflect senescent change occasionally associated with systemic diseases. The precise mechanism of cataract is uncertain, but a cogent theory implicates the decreasing water content of the lens with advancing age. Soluble protein becomes insoluble, calcium increases, and the concentration of glutathione diminishes. The loss of transparency is an inextricable part of aging. Systemic conditions that contribute to cataracts include familial predisposition, diabetes mellitus, and Paget's disease. Secondary cataracts occur with hypocalcemia, a variety of dermatologic conditions, inflammatory or traumatic ocular disease, and drug therapy, including chlorpromazine, steroids, and ergot.

Senescent cataracts, which constitute 85 per cent of clinically significant cataracts, may be nuclear sclerotic with predominant sclerosis of the lens nucleus, or cortical with spokelike changes, or posterior subcapsular changes. These anatomic entities account for the majority of senescent cataracts. All cataracts are associated with diminution in vision. The majority of patients have a gradual reduction in acuity, while a few describe rather rapid visual loss. Specific visual symptoms are associated with particular types of cataracts. In nuclear sclerosis, a central loss of transparency may be seen, accompanied by yellowish discoloration. The refractive index increases, which improves reading ability but impairs distance vision. Patients with cortical cataracts occasionally have mild acquired farsightedness. Patients may note a yellowing of vision, particularly with nuclear sclerosis, in which the shorter wavelengths of the visual spectrum are selectively absorbed, allowing the longer yellow and red wavelengths to be transmitted.

Patients with posterior subcapsular cataracts may complain of glare, distortion, and halos while driving at night. They suffer decreased distance vision and disproportionate difficulty in reading because the pupil becomes smaller during convergence accommodation reflex activity. Their problems are greatest in bright light when the pupil contracts, permitting light to enter only through the visual axis. They see best in subdued lighting because reflex dilatation of the pupil allows more light to enter. Some patients complain of fixed spots.

PRINCIPLES OF THERAPY

A principle of treating a patient with cataracts is to defer surgery until it is absolutely necessary. Some patients may be less comfortable after cataract surgery, and because of age and varying visual needs, operation may not be indicated. There are many methods of cataract extraction and approaches to correcting aphakic vision. Generally, cataract extraction is indicated when poor vision interferes with job performance or enjoyment of life. Visual disability is directly related to the needs and activities of the patient. Surgery is mandatory when the cataract becomes hypermature, and leaking material stimulates macrophages that obstruct aqueous outflow and precipitate glaucoma. Before surgery is undertaken a complete eye examination is essential in order to detect a concurrent condition that may impair vision or complicate surgery.

There are several surgical approaches to the removal of cataracts: extracapsular removal, intracapsular removal by cryosurgery and phacoemulsification. The extracapsular procedure removes the cataract, leaving the posterior lens capsule in place. This is indicated in pediatric patients and young adults when the vitreous is likely to be attached to the posterior lens capsule.

For all but young patients, the intracapsular method is superior. In this procedure, the entire lens and capsule are removed, most commonly with a cryoextractor, which freezes the lens substance so that it can be removed intact. The lens is delivered as the cryoprobe is removed. It is critical to remove the lens without disturbing the vitreous. Postoperative complications, including retinal detachment, increase dramatically if the vitreous is compromised or lost.

In phacoemulsification procedures, the lens material is broken up by ultrasonic vibrations. It may be used in older patients whose cataracts are more sclerotic. Aspiration and irrigation are performed simultaneously to maintain the structural integrity of the eye.

Three methods of optical correction—eyeglasses, contact lenses, and intraocular implants—are available. Cataract spectacles produce a 25 to 30 per cent magnification, which reduces peripheral vision and produces severe spatial distortion. Patients with monocular aphakia may no longer be able to use both eyes. However, if they see adequately with one good eye and have no special need for binocular or stereoscopic vision, it is often wise to postpone cataract extraction. Contact lenses magnify only 5 to 10 per cent, which usually allows fusion, enabling the patient to be comfortable despite monocular aphakia. The limiting factor is the aged patient's ability to master the insertion and removal of contact lenses.

Intraocular lens implantation represents a controversial advance. The advantages include only 1 to 3 per cent magnification between the two eyes; the need to manipulate contact lenses is eliminated. Reading glasses may still be needed. Disadvantages include a greater risk of complications and lack of well-documented experience with more than 20 years follow-up. Intraocular implants may allow elderly patients to see without a prolonged period of adaptation. They do not appear to be indicated in younger patients who are capable of manipulating contact lenses. Research aimed at perfecting implants and developing continuous-wear contact lenses is underway.

THERAPEUTIC RECOMMENDATIONS

The decision to perform cataract surgery is complicated by the patient's individual needs and the surgeon's skill. N.S. Jaffe, an ophthalmologist writing in the New England Journal of Medicine, suggested, "The surgeon must assess the needs of his patients and not yield to pressure from information disseminated by the media, demands of the patient, or the temptations of economic reward." Frequently, patients ask primary care physicians for advice on cataract extraction. The primary physician can help the patient by presenting information about cataract surgery and postoperative prognosis.

It must be explained that the quality of vision enjoyed in earlier years cannot be restored and that a period of adjustment is required. Removal of the cataractous lens sacrifices the variable focusing mechanism of the eye. The use of fixed-focus spectacles reduces peripheral vision and occasionally makes objects appear closer than they really are, requiring proprioceptive readjustment. Technological advances in lens design have alleviated some of these problems, and contact lenses provide nearly a full field of vision and reduce size distortion. A great number of patients wear contact lenses successfully, but instruction is essential. The values and risks of intraocular removal and implantation should be explained. Complications associated with cataract extraction, including vitreous loss, often lead to retinal detachment, intraocular hemorrhage, cystoid maculopathy, or postoperative infection. Significant complications may occur in as many as 5 per cent of cases.

The primary physician should help the patient understand that surgical correction is an imperfect solution. When vision is good in one eye and there are no particular social or economic constraints, it may be preferable to defer surgery; careful refraction may improve vision sufficiently. The primary physician should not advise cataract surgery in patients who have a limited life expectancy. Following surgery, it may take several months for the patient to adjust to the aphakia unless he has had an intraocular lens implant. Some patients adapt rapidly and others never do.

It is important to choose an ophthalmologist carefully. The ophthalmologist must be trained in the particular procedures that he uses, and his surgical conscience must be of the highest caliber. It is also essential that the ophthalmologist appreciate the need for careful refraction and visual rehabilitation after the operation; even a procedure that succeeds technically may worsen the patient's already inadequate vision if care and attention conclude with the final suture.

ANNOTATED BIBLIOGRAPHY

Blodi, F.C.: A surgical storm. Arch. Ophthalmol., 96:427, 1978. (A discussion of the issues surrounding cataract surgery.)

Jaffe, N.S.: Current concepts in ophthalmology: Cataract surgery—A modern attitude toward a technological explosion. N. Engl. J. Med., 299:235, 1978. (A remarkably useful article presenting both substantive information about cataract surgery and an intelligent discussion of when to operate.)

Jaffe, N.S., et al.: A comparison of 500 Binkhorst implants with 500 routine intracapsular cataract extractions. Am. J. Ophthalmol., 85:24, 1978. (A good review of the techniques emphasizing the more recent lens implant technique.)

Kahn, H.A., Leibowitz, H.M., Ganley, J.P., et al.: The Framingham eye study outline and major prevalence findings. Am. J. Epidemiol., 106:17, 1977. (Findings of an 18 per cent prevalance of cataracts in those 65 to 74 which are similar to other epidemiologic studies from Edinburgh and New York City.)

Paton, D., and Craig, K.A.: Cataracts development, diagnosis. Management Clinical Symposia, 26:1, 1974. (This is an excellent review of all aspects of cataracts, including illustrations that help both the physician and patient understand the cataractous process.)

200
Management of
Diabetic Ophthalmopathy

Various ocular problems are associated with diabetes, including refractive changes, cataracts, glaucoma, ophthalmoplegia and retinopathy. Diabetic retinopathy is a leading cause of blindness in the United States. Its incidence has increased dramatically since the introduction of insulin and the consequent increases in long-term survival of diabetics. The prevalence of retinopathy increases with age and with duration of diabetes, and is somewhat greater in women. The primary physician caring for diabetic patients must decide when referral to an ophthalmologist is indicated.

PATHOPHYSIOLOGY AND CLINICAL PRESENTATION

Diabetic retinopathy is diagnosed by ophthalmoscopic examination. There are two forms of retinopathy: background and proliferative. Background retinopathy usually begins at the posterior pole of the fundus. The earliest change is venous dilatation and tortuosity which may be difficult to detect without fundus photographs for comparison.

The characteristic findings of background retinopathy include microaneurysm, exudates, hemorrhages and edema. Globular, fusiform or general dilatation of capillaries is thought to be secondary to degeneration of intramural pericytes. The basement membranes of capillaries are abnormally thickened and contain lipid fibrin, platelets and red cells. The pathogenesis of these changes is uncertain. Circular hemorrhages occur near the posterior pole of the fundus. Diabetic exudates are usually "hard," sharply defined, shiny, irregular, often in the area of the macula. Soft exudates, often called cotton wool spots, are nerve layer infarcts resulting from capillary closure. Retinal edema occurs from serum leakage through retinal blood vessels. Background retinopathy is usually asymptomatic unless exudates or retinal edema occurs around the macula. Patients with macula edema may complain of blurred vision.

Proliferative retinopathy is much more significant and is characterized by neovascularization on the ret-ina or into the vitreous cavity, at the disc, where there is no internal limiting membrane, or peripherally, where large vessels course close to the surface. The proliferative vessels are tiny, delicate, irregular, and often enveloped by fibrous tissue; they sometimes develop a fanlike appearance. The danger of neovascularization results from fragile vessels having a tendency to bleed. Contraction of the fibrous tissue around new vessels may lead to retinal traction or detachment.

Proliferative retinopathy usually presents as a physical finding, but hemorrhage into the vitreous may produce specks or cobwebs. An occasional patient will present with the flashing lights and visual loss because of vitreal bleeding or retinal detachment.

The theorized etiology of proliferative retinopathy is a response to retinal tissue hypoxia. The unresolved question is why retinal hypoxia develops. Theories proposed include increased platelet aggregation slowing blood flow, decreased 2, 3, diphosphoglycerate causing decreased oxygen delivery, and failure of blood supply. Identification of the precise defect may allow more specific and effective treatment.

Background retinopathy is related to the length of time the patient has diabetes, but is not highly correlated with severity. Proliferative retinopathy when it occurs tends to be more severe in the adult-onset diabetic. Proliferative retinopathic blindness occurs within 5 years of diagnosis in 30 to 40 per cent of younger patients and in 40 to 60 per cent of older patients. It is thought that retinopathy rarely exists without nephropathy. It is not possible to predict whether or when proliferative change will develop or bleeding will occur in an individual patient.

PRINCIPLES OF TREATMENT

Promising treatments for proliferative diabetic retinopathy have recently been developed. That strict control of hyperglycemia prevents or retards retinopathy has remained a controversy without resolution. There is no secure evidence that rigid maintenance of euglycemia is effective (see Chapter 98). Other medical approaches to managing diabetic retinopathy have also been tried. Improvement of hemorrhages has been noted in patients on clofibrate and low-fat diets, particularly when cholesterol levels were reduced. Aspirin has been tried because of its antiplatelet activity, but its usefulness has not been established. A retrospective study has shown less retinopathy in nonsmoking diabetics than in those who smoke.

The major therapeutic modality is photocoagulation, which burns areas of the retina, rendering them nonviable and incapable of initiating proliferative change. Xenon, red ruby and green argon lasers have been used. The green light of the argon laser is absorbed by hemoglobin and pigment epithelium, giving it a selectivity that allows its use in delicate areas. Panretinal photocoagulation is the most commonly employed treatment. The theory is that destroying hypoxic retinal tissue reduces its potential for initiating neovascularization. New vessels have been observed to regress after photocoagulation. Direct photocoagulation is sometimes used, but the risk of hemorrhage is greater. Patients with macular edema may benefit from photocoagulation. The adverse consequences of photocoagulation include a slight reduction in visual acuity, inadvertent burn of the fovea, hemorrhage and angle-closure glaucoma. In a 2-year follow-up of a multicenter trial, 61 per cent fewer eyes became blind in the group treated with photocoagulation.

The fortuitous discovery that hypophysectomy arrested the development of retinopathy led to its brief use. Hypophysectomy is reserved for selected young diabetics with fulminant retinopathy. Vitrectomy is a new surgical procedure for evacuating hemorrhagic or fibrous tissue in the vitreous that has not been reabsorbed over a long time. It is advisable to wait for hemorrhage to resolve (usually for 1 year) and to establish the viability of the retina before subjecting a patient to vitrectomy.

THERAPEUTIC RECOMMENDATIONS AND PATIENT EDUCATION

The decision about whether and how to treat diabetic retinopathy should be made by a retinal specialist. The timing of referral is the responsibility of the primary physician. It is important to examine the fundus through dilated pupils on a regular basis every 6 months or every year. Treatment of concurrent hypertension should be diligent, because high blood pressure may exacerbate retinopathy. Referral

should be made to an ophthalmologist skilled in retinal disease when:

1. A diabetic patient reports a change of vision
2. The physician observes evidence of background or proliferative retinopathy
3. Neovascularization is found in the area of the iris
4. The physician is unable to examine the fundus clearly

Patient education about the nature and prognosis of diabetic retinopathy and continued support by the primary physician are important in management. The physician should explain that most diabetic patients do not lose their vision but that regular examinations and prompt reporting of decreased vision or symptoms such as spots, cobwebs or flashing lights are essential. The patient with proliferative changes is instructed to sleep with his head elevated to lower blood pressure in the eyes, and if possible, to avoid straining while defecating, sneezing, coughing, or vomiting. Cigarette smoking will accelerate retinopathy and should be interdicted. The primary physician must consider all aspects of the patient's well-being, utilizing family and community resources to begin rehabilitation and modification in life-style in anticipation of blindness. Emotional and psychological support is a fundamental aspect of caring for the person with diabetic eye disease.

ANNOTATED BIBLIOGRAPHY

Ashikaga, T., Borodic, G., and Sims, E.A.H.: Multiple daily insulin injections in the treatment of diabetic retinopathy. Diabetes, *27*:592, 1978. *(A reanalysis of the Job study, pointing out its methodologic defects.)*

Diabetic Retinopathy Study Research Group, The: Preliminary reports on effects of photocoagulation therapy: The diabetic retinopathy. Am. J. Ophthalmol., *81*:383, 1976. *(A report that indicates a promising role for photocoagulation.)*

Diabetic Retinopathy Study Research Group, The: Photocoagulation treatment of proliferative diabetic retinopathy: The second report of Diabetic Retinopathy Study findings. Ophthal., *85*:82, 1978. *(A later report that indicates a promising role for photocoagulation.)*

Kahn, H.A., and Bradley, R.F.: Prevalence of diabetic retinopathy. Age, sex, and duration of diabetes. Br. J. Ophthalmol., *59*:345, 1975. *(Comprehensive epidemiology.)*

Knowler, W.C., Bennett, P.H., Ballintine, E.J.: Increased incidence of retinopathy in diabetics with elevated blood pressure. N. Engl. J. Med., *302*:645, 1980. *(Twice the number of exudates in diabetics with systolic blood pressures greater than 145.)*

Kohner, E.M.: Diabetic retinopathy. Clinical Endocrinol. Metab., 6:345, 1977. *(A solid review.)*

Kohner, E.M., Hamilton, A.M., and Joplin, G.F., *et al.*: Florid retinopathy and its response to treatment by photocoagulation or pituitary ablation. Diabetes, 25:104, 1976. *(A report of 34 patients with rare florid retinopathy showing dramatically better results with pituitary ablation.)*

Job, D., Eschwage, E., Gugot-Argenton, C., *et al.*: Effect of multiple daily insulin injections on the course of diabetic retinopathy. Diabetes, 25:463, 1976. *(A cohort of 42 randomly assigned patients who were treated with once-daily multiple injections, followed for a mean of 3 years, showed benefit in delaying retinal changes in divided insulin injections.)*

L'Esperance, F.A., Jr.: Diabetic retinopathy. Med. Clin. North Am., *62*: 767, 1978. *(A superb comprehensive review; 97 refs.)*

Morse, P.H., and Duncan, T.G.: Ophthalmologic management of diabetic retinopathy. N. Engl. J. Med., *295*:87, 1976. *(A straightforward exposition on the current treatment of diabetic retinopathy.)*

Paetkau, M.E., Boyd, T.A.S., Winship, B., *et al.*: Cigarette smoking and diabetic retinopathy. Diabetes, *26*:46, 1977. *(A sample of 181 diabetics was analyzed, showing that proliferative retinopathy rose with increasing tobacco consumption.)*

Palmberg, P.F.: Diabetic retinopathy. Diabetes, *26*:703, 1977. *(A concise review; 79 refs.)*

Shafer, D.M.: Vitrectomy. (Editorial). N. Engl. J. Med., *295*:836, 1976. *(A review of vitrectomy which is reserved for eyes with unresolving vitreous hemorrhage.)*

Treatment of diabetic retinopathy. Medical Letter, *18*:107, 1976. *(A terse review of the treatment of diabetic retinopathy concluding that photocoagulation is useful in many patients and vitrectomy may be of benefit in selected patients.)*

14

Ear, Nose, and Throat Problems

201
Screening for Oral Cancer
JOHN P. KELLY, D.M.D., M.D.

Cancer arising in the oral cavity will affect nearly 25,000 new patients this year in the United States, representing 5 per cent of new cancer cases in males and 2 per cent in females. Over 8,000 deaths result from oral cancer yearly, the death rates for both men and women being unchanged over the past 25 years. Depite the ready accessibility of the oral cavity to inspection by physicians, dentists and patients themselves, 50 per cent of total cancers already have metastasized at the time of diagnosis.

Pain is the most common symptom which leads the patient to seek medical attention, but the early stages of oral carcinoma are notoriously painless. Hence, careful examination on a routine basis will enable more patients to be diagnosed in the early stages of their disease when treatment can be most effective.

EPIDEMIOLOGY

The peak incidence of oral carcinoma is in the sixth decade for women and is equally frequent in each decade after the age of 50 for men. However, the appearance of the disease in the third and fourth decades is not rare, and must not be overlooked.

Exposure to tobacco in all its forms is highly correlated with the risk of development of oral cancers. Unlike cancers of the lung and larynx, which are related to cigarette smoking, malignancies of the mouth are associated with use of, cigars, pipes, and chewing tobacco as well as cigarettes. Among non-smokers, cancers of the tongue and buccal mucosa are seen more frequently than are lesions of the floor of the mouth or other oral sites.

The most common form of oral cancer is that of the lower lip. Chronic exposure to the ultraviolet rays of the sun appears to play a significant causal role. Squamous cell or epidermoid carcinoma of the lower lip has high incidence among fair-skinned people residing in sunny climates and in those whose occupations subject them to prolonged exposure to the sun. On the other hand, such cancers are rare among blacks, probably because of pigmentary protection against actinic radiation.

An epidemiologic association between alcohol consumption and oral carcinoma has long been recognized. However, no direct correlation can be made, because most heavy users of alcohol are also users of tobacco products. It has been suggested that alcohol may chronically irritate the oral tissues, facilitating the carcinogenic properties of tobacco products, or that the nutritional deficiencies associated with alcoholism predispose the oral mucosa to malignant change.

Cancer of the tongue is highly correlated with the atrophic glossitis seen with tertiary syphillis. Mucosal atrophy from other causes is also associated with an increased incidence of oral cancers. Most notably, chronic iron deficiency leading to Plummer-Vinson

751

syndrome is known to alter mucosal tissues and this change may be related to the increased incidence of oral carcinoma.

Chronic irritation of the oral mucosa by ill-fitting dentures, poorly restored teeth, or particularly spicy diets has often been mentioned as contributing to the development of oral carcinoma. However, there are no epidemiologic data to support this view.

The precise etiology of oral cancer is unknown. The etiology factors mentioned above probably act as cocarcinogens, effecting malignant change in concert with some primary agent not yet elucidated.

NATURAL HISTORY

The 5-year survival rate for localized oral cancer is over 67 per cent, but only 30 per cent of patients with metastatic disease survive for 5 years. When untreated, oral carcinoma metastasizes to the regional lymph nodes of the neck, ultimately leading to respiratory embarrassment or involvement of the great vessels.

Ipsilateral node involvement is most common, but metastasis to the contralateral side—especially from primary lesions of the tongue or floor of the mouth—occurs with such frequency that treatment for control of metastasic disease is very difficult. Hence, early diagnosis and control of the primary site is essential. The lungs are the most frequently involved sites of extranodal metastasis.

Local recurrence is seen, although many such recurrences may, in fact, be new primary sites of disease. The appearance of multiple separate cancers within the oral cavity has led to use of the term "field cancerization" to characterize the susceptibility of the entire oral mucosa to malignant change in affected patients.

SCREENING AND DIAGNOSTIC TESTS

The challenge to primary care health providers is to recognize malignancies of the oral cavity in their earliest stages. Lesions which show deep ulceration and fungating borders are easily recognized and the patient can readily be referred for treatment, but the greatest hope for control of the disease exists prior to the appearance of the grossly invasive lesion.

Thorough examination of the tissues of the oral cavity, both by inspection and by palpation, must be included in the routine evaluation of every patient. Recognition of the normal appearance of the mucosa

in contrast with either atrophic or hyperplastic tissue serves as a baseline. Similarly, familiarity with normal anatomic structures, such as the circumvallate papillae of the tongue and the lingual tonsils, is necessary in order to differentiate such structures from neoplasms.

For many years, the term *leukoplakia* was used as a clinicopathologic term signifying a premalignant or frankly carcinomatous lesion. More appropriately, however, the term is now employed to indicate the development of a "white patch" on the oral mucosa. Causes of such lesions (which can result from a variety of etiologies), include hyperkeratosis, ectopic sebaceous glands in the buccal mucosa, leukoedema, chemical burns (most commonly, from aspirin), lichen planus, candidiasis, or pemphigus vulgaris, as well as malignancies.

Recently, the diagnostic significance of *erythroplasia* has been stressed. The appearance of a red, hyperplastic area of mucosa is highly suggestive of an early carcinoma. While most cancer screening protocols have emphasized a search for white lesions, the predominant color in premalignant or early lesions is red, not white, In fact, while some white lesions may only be "premalignant," the red lesions must be considered to be true malignancies unless proven otherwise by biopsy.

The oral mucosa may show pigmented lesions of black, blue or brown color. Benign conditions such as vascular malformations, heavy metal ingestion, amalgam tattooing, pigmented nevi and the pigmentations associated with such systemic conditions as neurofibromatosis, intestinal polyposis and Addison's disease, must be differented from the blue-black lesion of malignant melanoma. Biopsy is essential if this diagnosis is suggested by the appearance of the lesion.

Initial evaluation of a suspicious lesion begins with eliciting appropriate historical data in order to eliminate such relatively harmless lesions as the acute aspirin burn. Irritative lesions can be identified by removing or repairing jagged teeth and poorly fitting or protruding dental prostheses and following the clinical healing of the mucosal wound. In any patient with a suspicious lesion, use of a noxious agent such as tobacco must be eliminated at the outset.

Any red or white lesion which persists for 2 weeks after initial recognition and elimination of irritating agents demands further investigation. Many authors have suggested the use of exfoliative cytology or in vivo staining with toluidine blue for screening purposes, but neither of these procedures yields unequivocal results and, even if they are positive, biopsy will be necessary for confirmation of the diagnosis.

Hence, referral of the patient to an oral and maxillo-facial surgeon for biopsy is preferable as the definitive diagnostic maneuver. High-risk patients, specifically those with histories of smoking and drinking, should be referred for biopsy promptly, as should any patient with a deeply ulcerative or fungating lesion.

Any swelling beneath a normal-appearing oral mucosa must be evaluated by an appropriate specialist for diagnosis or treatment. Such lesions are commonly benign and are the result of infection, bony exostosis, or mucous retention phenomena, but they may represent neoplasms of the minor salivary glands or other submucosal structures.

RECOMMENDATIONS

- A thorough visual and manual examination of the oral cavity should be a part of every patient's evaluation; red or white mucosal patches are sought.
- A high index of suspicion must be maintained for patients with a history of smoking, drinking and heavy exposure to sunlight.
- Atrophic or hyperplastic patches on the oral mucosa must be viewed with suspicion, particularly if they are red or white (erythroplasia or leukoplakia) and last more than 2 weeks after cessation of smoking, drinking and exposure to irritants.

- Referral for definitive biopsy is indicated for persistent lesions.

ANNOTATED BIBLIOGRAPHY

Baker, H.W., Rickles, N.H., et al.: Oral Cancer. New York: American Cancer Society, 1973. (A well-illustrated booklet on the diagnosis, treatment and rehabilitation of the oral cancer patient.)

Ballard, B.R., Suess, G.R., et al.: Squamous cell carcinoma of the floor of the mouth. Oral Surg., 45:568, 1978. (A good review of the epidemiology, clinical staging and prognosis of 100 recently treated patients.)

Mashberg, A.: Erythroplasia: The earliest sign of asymptomatic oral cancer. J. Am. Dent. Assoc., 96:615, 1978. (A significant recent contribution to the literature with good illustration and description of the early malignant lesion.)

Rubin, P.: Cancer of the Head and Neck. New York: American Cancer Society, 1972. (A comprehensive collection of JAMA reprints from the series on Current Cancer Concepts. An excellent basic reference.)

202
Evaluation of Impaired Hearing

It is estimated that approximately 10 per cent of the United States population has a hearing problem. People with seriously impaired hearing often become withdrawn or appear confused. Subtle hearing loss may go unrecognized. Patients with hearing loss can often be greatly helped, particularly if loss is due to a conduction problem. The primary physician has the responsibility to detect hearing loss, to search for a remedial etiology, and to decide when referral to an otolaryngologist is indicated.

PATHOPHYSIOLOGY AND CLINICAL PRESENTATION

Impaired hearing may result from an interference with the conduction of sound, its conversion to electrical impulses, or its transmission through the nervous system. Hearing involves an acoustic stage during which sound waves cause the tympanic membrane to vibrate. Ossicles amplify the sound, causing the footplate of the stapes to rock the oval window, transmitting sound waves to the perilymph of the inner ear. The perilymph protects the cochlear duct which contains endolymph. Deformation of the endolymph stimulates the hair cells, converting sound waves to neural impulses which are conveyed to the temporal lobes. Interference with mechanical reception or amplification of sound, as occurs with disease of the auditory canal, tympanic membrane or ossicles, creates conductive hearing loss. Degeneration or destruction of hair cells or the acoustic nerve produces sensorineural hearing loss.

Conductive hearing loss presents with diminution of volume, particularly for low tones and vowels.

There is often a history of previous ear disease. The Weber test demonstrates better hearing in the conductively deaf ear. The Rinne test shows that bone conduction is better than air conduction. The physical examination may reveal a specific etiology, such as obstruction of the auditory canal by impacted cerumen or a foreign body, scarring or perforation of the drum due to chronic otitis, or ongoing otitis media with effusion.

Otosclerosis, a surgically remediable cause of conductive hearing loss, is a sclerotic disease of the bony labyrinth and stapes commonly presenting in the second or third decade of life. The condition is inherited in an autosomal dominant fashion with varying clinical expressivity. The incidence is 3 to 5 per 1000 adults, with a female predominance. In postmortem studies, the condition is found in 10 per cent of the white population. Tinnitus commonly accompanies the slow progressive loss of hearing.

Sensorineural hearing loss characteristically produces impairment of high tone perception. Patients may complain that they can hear people speaking but have difficulty deciphering words because discrimination is poor. Shouting may only exacerbate the problem. The patient with high frequency loss may have difficulty hearing doorbells, telephones, or a ticking watch. Air conduction is better than bone conduction. Tinnitus is often reported.

Presbycusis or hearing loss associated with aging is believed due to degeneration and atrophy of the ganglion cells in the cochlea. It is the most common cause of diminished hearing in the elderly. The hearing loss is typically bilateral and gradual in onset. It begins with loss of high frequencies and progresses slowly. Eventually, middle and low frequency sounds also become hard to perceive.

Noise-induced hearing loss is of major epidemiologic and economic significance. Chronic exposure to sound levels in excess of 85 to 90 decibels causes hearing loss in the frequency range around 4000 cycles per second. The patient may be unaware of the problem because the speech frequencies (500, 1000, and 2000 cycles per second) are initially unaffected. The first stage of noise-induced hearing loss is referred to as temporary threshold shift, in which there is a reversible decrease in sensitivity to sound with a rise in threshold for sound perception. If exposure to loud noise is reduced at this stage, hearing returns to its previous level. If exposure persists, a permanent threshold shift ensues.

Drug-induced hearing impairment has become more frequent due to the increased use of agents which are ototoxic. The aminoglycoside antibiotics are the most potent of the common offending agents; ethacrynic acid, quinidine, furosemide and salicylates are of lesser importance. Fortunately, salicylate toxicity is completely reversible. Among the aminoglycosides, dihydrostreptomycin, neomycin and kanamycin are the most ototoxic.

Meniere's disease produces a fluctuating unilateral low frequency impairment, often in conjunction with tinnitus and vertigo. Later, hearing of higher frequencies may be lost. Recruitment of loudness (an abnormally rapid increase in loudness) is common. Superficially resembling Meniere's disease is *acoustic neuroma,* a rare but important cause of diminished hearing. Tinnitus usually precedes hearing loss, and vertigo follows its onset. Unlike Meniere's disease, the hearing problem does not wax and wane. The patient's ability to discriminate is poor and out of proportion to the impairment in pure tone perception.

Sudden deafness of the sensorineural variety can be due to head trauma or can appear without obvious cause or warning. The idiopathic variety is usually profound, unilateral and can be permanent. Complete recovery occurs in 25 to 30 per cent of cases, and partial improvement is seen in a similar percentage. Etiology is unclear, but viral infection and vascular mechanisms have been implicated, though not well documented.

Injury to the internal ear or eighth nerve will in-

Table 202–1.   Common and Important Causes of Impaired Hearing

CONDUCTIVE	SENSORINEURAL
Impacted cerumen	Presbycusis
Foreign body	Acoustic trauma
Occlusive edema of the auditory canal	Drugs (aminoglycosides, loop
Otosclerosis	diuretics, quinidine, aspirin)
Chronic otitis media	Meniere's disease
Perforation of the tympanic membrane	Acoustic neuroma
	Hypothyroidism (mild loss)
	Idiopathic sudden deafness
	Congenital syphilis
	Diabetes

duce sensorineural loss. Skull fracture, meningitis, otitis media, scarlet fever and mumps are major etiologic factors.

Congenital syphilis may produce sensorineural hearing loss with onset in adult life. One or both ears may be affected; the course can be variable, with remissions and exacerbations. Vertigo is sometimes present as well.

DIFFERENTIAL DIAGNOSIS

The causes of hearing loss can be grouped according to whether the problem is conductive or sensorineural in etiology (Table 202–1). The categorization is of practical use because the conductive defects lend themselves to correction in many instances.

WORKUP

History. Evaluation of the patient with hearing loss should focus on detection of a correctable lesion; this search is aided by identifying whether the impairment is conductive or sensorineural. History is of some help. Conduction disease often results in loss of low frequency hearing when sensorineural problems cause high frequency hearing loss, it is worth trying to find out the sounds or situations in which the patient has most trouble hearing. Difficulty deciphering spoken words suggests sensorineural disease. Inquiry into drug use is essential, focusing on aminoglycosides, quinine derivatives, salicylates, and the diuretics—furosemide and ethacrynic acid. A history of otitis or head trauma should be noted. Inquiry into acoustic trauma is important, especially the details of occupational exposure.

Physical examination. Rinne and *Weber tests* will separate most sensorineural cases from those due to conduction problems. A tuning fork which vibrates at a frequency of 512 cycles per second is adequate; the 128-cycle tuning fork used for testing vibratory sensation is not. Testing should be done near the threshold of perception. A common technique is to test by a gentle tap of the fork on the knuckle to provide sufficient but not excessive intensity.

The normal response to a vibrating fork placed midline on the skull is equal loudness in both ears as the vibration activates the cochlear fluid. When the vibrating fork is placed on the mastoid process, it is heard for a period of time and then dies away; it is heard again if the same fork is promptly moved without any reactivation to the external auditory meatus.

Normal patients will hear sound conducted by air for about twice as long as a sound conducted by bone, due to the greater efficiency of the middle ear apparatus.

In the Weber test, the tuning fork is placed anywhere in the midline of the skull. The sound will be heard more clearly in the ear with a conduction defect, because ambient noise is blocked out. If there is a sensorineural loss in one ear, sound will be better perceived in the other.

In the Rinne test, sound by air conduction is normally heard for twice as long as sound by bone conduction. With a marked conductive loss, the reverse is found. With lesser degrees of conductive impairment, the ratio is closer to 1:1. The normal ratio is preserved in patients with sensorineural loss, but hearing via both bone and air conduction is reduced.

In the *Schwabach test,* the examiner's hearing by bone conduction is compared to the patient's. The vibrating tuning fork is alternatively placed on the mastoid process of examiner and patient. If the examiner's hearing is normal, he will perceive the sound for a longer time than the patient with a sensorineural deficit and for a shorter time than the patient with a conduction problem.

Other simple hearing tests can be performed in the office and are of qualitative use. The *watch tick* is an easy though crude method of detecting high frequency impairment. *Whispering* from 2 feet after full exhalation is another rough means of gauging capacity to hear. The best words to use are familiar bisyllabic ones in which one syllable is clearly accented over the other (e.g., snowball, cowboy). Patients with sensorineural loss hear a spoken voice much better than a whisper, even if the whisper is loud, because they have impairment of high-frequency hearing.

Physical examination of the ear includes inspection of the external auditory canal for obstruction by impacted cerumen, foreign body, or external otitis. Removal of the foreign body and retesting will identify its contribution to hearing loss. Otoscopic examination of the tympanic membrane should include a check for inflammation, perforation, and scarring. Pneumatic otoscopy assesses tympanic membrane mobility, which if reduced, will impair hearing.

Cranial nerve examination is essential, especially if vertigo is an associated symptom (see Chapter 154).

Laboratory studies. An *audiogram* is an essential component of the evaluation of patients with clinically significant hearing impairment. The pattern of hearing loss has considerable diagnostic and therapeutic importance. Interpretation requires an otolaryngologist or audiologist; the test should probably be obtained prior to the time of a patient's referral. Skull films with polytome views of the internal auditory meatus are needed when an acoustic neuroma is suspected.

SYMPTOMATIC MANAGEMENT AND INDICATIONS FOR REFERRAL

The primary physician's role in the treatment of hearing loss is relatively limited. Maneuvers that are available include removal of impacted cerumen, cessation of ototoxic drugs, treatment of otitis media (see Chapter 208), advising patients exposed to occupational noise to use earplugs and avoid further acoustic trauma, and identification and correction of metabolic abnormalities.

Referral to an otolaryngologist for further evaluation and treatment is indicated when a conductive etiology or acoustic neuroma is suspected or simple symptomatic measures do not suffice and the hearing impairment is disabling. The otolaryngologist needs to determine whether the patient is a candidate for medical or surgical therapy and whether a hearing aid is appropriate.

ANNOTATED BIBLIOGRAPHY

Heffler, A.J.: Hearing loss due to noise exposure. Otolaryngol. Clin. N. Am., *11*:723, 1978. *(A good review of this increasingly important cause of hearing loss.)*

Meyerhoff, W.L., and Paparella, M.M.; Diagnosing the cause of hearing loss. Geriatrics, *33*(2):95, 1978. *(Provides a practical approach to the assessment of hearing loss in adults, with emphasis on problems seen in the elderly.)*

Quick, C.A.: Chemical and drug effects on the inner ear. *In* Paparella, M.M., and Shumrick, D.A. (eds.): Otolaryngology: Ear. Philadelphia: W.B. Saunders, 1973, Vol. 2, p. 391. *(An excellent discussion of ototoxic agents.)*

203
Approach to Epistaxis

Most spontaneous nosebleeds are self-limited; however, when a patient presents for medical care, the bleeding is usually brisk or episodes are becoming frequent. Severe or recurrent bleeding necessitates evaluations for a bleeding diathesis and important nasal pathology. The immediate therapeutic objective is control of bleeding.

PATHOPHYSIOLOGY AND CLINICAL PRESENTATION

The primary mechanism of epistaxis is disruption of the nasal mucosa, which may be caused by inflammation, neoplasia or trauma. Uncommonly, nosebleeds are associated with disorders of coagulation or platelet function. The most frequent site of nasal hemorrhage is Kiesselbach's venous plexus, on the anterior inferior aspect of the nasal septum. The posterior aspect of the nose is supplied by the sphenopalatine branch of the maxillary artery, which derives from the external carotid system. Blood vessels become increasingly vulnerable to trauma and bleeding with age, because vessel musculature atrophies and scleroses. Nosebleeds are frequently precipitated by the combination of dryness due to low-humidity heating, inflammation from an upper respiratory infection, and the trauma induced by blowing the nose.

Nosebleeds are commonly attributed to hypertension, but epidemiologic studies reveal that few hypertensives present with nosebleeds, and few nosebleeds are attributable to hypertension.

Active *anterior epistaxis* usually presents as moderate continuous bleeding from the front of the nose when the patient is in the upright position. There is often a history of recurrent episodes of bleeding controlled by pressure on the anterior nares. *Posterior epistaxis* tends to be massive and uncontrolled, with blood flowing into the pharynx; it should be suspected when an anterior pack fails to control hemorrhage. Posterior hemorrhage is more common in the elderly and after nasal trauma.

DIFFERENTIAL DIAGNOSIS

The differential diagnosis of nosebleeds can be divided into local and systemic disorders. The local causes are most commonly inflammatory or traumatic. The most notable inflammatory lesions are upper respiratory infections, allergies, and chronic sinusitis. Trauma may be induced by habitual picking, constant rubbing, or forceful blowing of the nose. Chronic occupational exposure to volatile chemical irritants and repeated nasal use of cocaine are becoming increasingly frequent. Local vascular lesions include angiomas and hereditary hemorrhagic telangiectasia. More than 90 per cent of bleeds are related to local irritation; most occur in the absence of a specific underlying anatomic lesion.

Nosebleeds occasionally occur during the course of certain infectious diseases such as chickenpox and influenza. The patient with an underlying hematologic disease, a clotting problem, or a disorder of platelet function may present with bleeding from the nose.

WORKUP

History. One should inquire into previous episodes of epistaxis and the site, direction, duration and frequency of bleeding. History ought to include discussion of habits which may lead to mucosal injury, such as chronic cocaine use, repeated nose blowing or habitual picking. Of much practical importance is an assessment of the patient's environment; in centrally heated homes, the indoor environment can be very dry in winter, with humidity falling to less than 10 per cent. Detailed inquiry into occupational exposure to chemicals, dust, or other irritants may provide therapeutically important information. One should ask about easy bruising, hematuria, melena, heavy periods, family history of bleeding disorders, and use of oral anticoagulants and drugs with antiplatelet effects (e.g., aspirin).

Physical examination should be performed with the patient in the sitting position. If severe blood loss is suspected, one should check pulse and blood pressure supine and standing for postural change. Any clots obscuring vision of the nasal mucosa can be removed by suction or by having the patient blow his nose. The nasal mucosa is examined to locate the site of bleeding, assess the condition of the mucosa, and

detect any underlying lesions. Anterior sites of bleeding are readily visible on inspection; posterior sites are not. The patient with posterior epistaxis will swallow blood as it flows down into the posterior pharynx. Evidence of a bleeding disorder is checked for by examining the skin for petechiae, purpura and telangiectasias (see Chapter 168).

Laboratory studies. A hematocrit should be obtained in patients who have had substantial or repeated bleeding. If evidence of a more generalized bleeding problem is present, prothrombin time, partial thromboplastin time, platelet count, and bleeding time should be ascertained.

SYMPTOMATIC MANAGEMENT AND INDICATIONS FOR REFERRAL

Every physician should be capable of rendering initial treatment to a patient with a severe nosebleed. The patient should sit upright to reduce venous pressure and facilitate expectoration of accumulated blood. Firm, continuous pressure is applied to both sides of the nose superior to the nasal alar cartilage. Pressure sustained for 10 to 15 minutes will stop many anterior nosebleeds. Applying ice to the overlying skin may help by inducing vasoconstriction. However, many patients who present to the physician have already tried these measures without success.

When bleeding persists from an anterior site despite pressure, cotton balls are soaked in 1:1000 epinephrine and inserted into the bleeding nostril. Pressure is applied for several minutes. The ball is removed, and the patient is observed for rebleeding. If this maneuver fails, the nose must be packed. *Anterior packing* is accomplished by layering Vaseline-impregnated gauze strips from the nasal floor toward the nasal roof, extending most of the length of the nasal cavity. Unilateral packing on the side of the bleeding should be attempted first, but packing should be bilateral if bleeding continues. Patients with anterior packs may be treated as outpatients with instructions to sit upright most of the day and elevate the head 30° at night. The pack may be removed in 2 to 3 days.

Failure to stop bleeding with the use of epinephrine and/or an anterior pack is an indication for referral to an otolaryngologist or a surgeon capable of rendering definitive care, usually with a posterior pack. Hospitalization is required for elderly, debilitated, anemic people and those requiring posterior packing.

Definitive treatment of recurrent bleeding or a severe episode often requires *cauterization.* If the bleeding is from Kiesselbach's plexus, and therefore easily accessible, the primary physician can cauterize the area with a silver nitrate stick. This is accomplished by first applying a topical anesthetic, such as 4% cocaine, to the area, followed by use of a silver nitrate stick, which is held gently against the disrupted mucosa for 15 to 20 seconds, until crusting forms. The crust will fall off over time, and the mucosa will be healed. Referral to an otolaryngologist for electrocauterization may be necessary.

Recurrent minor epistaxis from an unidentified source may be due to chronic sinusitis or to a nasopharyngeal or paranasal sinus tumor; it requires consultation with an otolaryngologist. Epistaxis due to facial trauma should be managed by the surgeon. Patients who habitually pick their noses and have crusting and local trauma can be treated by packing the nose with cotton balls covered wtith an antibiotic ointment (e.g., Neosporin). These are left in place for 7 to 10 days and then removed. Healing is achieved and the stimulus to pick is reduced.

PATIENT EDUCATION

Is is important to explain the etiology of the nosebleed and to instruct the patient on prevention and first aid.

- Reassure the patient when the nosebleed is purely a local phenomenon; many people attribute nosebleeds to hypertension and fear cerebral hemorrhage.
- Instruct the patient on the need to avoid traumatizing the mucosa. Specifically, warn against habitual nose picking, constant rubbing with a handkerchief, and excessively forceful blowing.
- Explain the importance of humidifying the home environment. This may be done by keeping a few windows partially open, by placing containers of water near radiators or stoves, or by installing a humidifier. Occasionally, patients may benefit from use of a water-based lubricant applied to the rims of the nostrils in order to maintain mucosal moisture; however, this does involve a very small risk of lipoid pneumonia, and should be avoided in children and the elderly.
- Instruct patients in first aid methods, such as sitting upright, applying ice, and maintaining pressure for 15 to 20 minutes.

ANNOTATED BIBLIOGRAPHY

Hallberg, O.E.: Severe nosebleed and its treatment, JAMA, *148*:355, 1952. *(A classic article that is still very useful.)*

Lingeman, R.A.: Epistaxis. Am. J. Fam. Phys., *14*(6):78, 1976. *(A brief, practical article that clearly illustrates methods for nasal packing.)*

204
Evaluation of Facial Pain and Swelling
JOHN P. KELLY, D.M.D., M.D.

The primary care physician often encounters patients whose presenting complaint of facial pain or swelling is related to the masticatory apparatus (teeth, gums, jaws, muscles) or salivary glands. Dental decay is the most prevalent disease in the United States and a major cause of conditions leading to facial pain and swelling. Because symptoms may be referred to nondental structures and because an odontogenic infection may involve areas of the head and neck seemingly unrelated to the teeth, the patient may first seek the advice of a physician rather than of a dentist. Prompt recognition and effective initial treatment may well prevent development of a serious complication such as abscess formation.

PATHOPHYSIOLOGY AND CLINICAL PRESENTATION

Odontogenic infection. Dental decay is a multifactorial disease that encompasses dietary factors (most notably, refined carbohydrates), environmental factors (such as availability of fluoride ion during the production of the enamel of the teeth) and various host factors (not the least of which is the patient's oral hygiene habits). Oral bacteria utilize dietary carbohydrates to form plaque on the enamel of the teeth; susceptible enamel is then decalcified, resulting in a "cavity" or carious lesion.

In its initial stages, *decay* is asymptomatic. However, when the dentin beneath the enamel is exposed, the patient may complain of aching pain when the affected tooth comes into contact with hot, cold or sweet substances. The frequent finding of referred pain may make localization of the offending tooth difficult and is one reason why a patient may first consult his physician rather than his dentist.

Progressive decay of the tooth will result in *inflammation of the pulp* (pulpitis); the symptoms will be unchanged until the dental pulp becomes necrotic and, eventually, suppurative. The cardinal symptom then is deep, throbbing pain on exposure to hot foods or drinks; the pain is abruptly relieved by ice or cold water. This symptom complex is quite distinct from the paroxysmal, lancinating pain of trigeminal neuralgia, which has no relationship to extremes of temperature, but which may be related to eating because of the presence of trigger zones in the oral cavity (see Chapter 163).

Simple dental decay, pulpitis and pulpal necrosis all are recognized by pain and by clinical and radiographic examination. They are not associated with fever, swelling or leukocytosis. However, when the infection of the pulp spreads beyond the confines of the tooth to involve the periodontal ligament and the adjacent alveolar bone, an acute *alveolar abscess* may ensue. In this condition, the affected tooth is tender to percussion or to masticatory forces and is mobile. The adjacent soft tissues begin to show the classic signs of acute inflammation: edema, erythema, heat and tenderness. The location of the involved tooth will determine the location of the swelling. Abscessed maxillary teeth will produce labial or infraorbital edema; an infected mandibular tooth will produce submandibular edema. Lymphadenopathy of the cervical chain can be seen in either maxillary or mandibular infection. Fever, leukocytosis and dehydration are frequent concomitants of the acute alveolar abscess with facial cellulitis.

Spread of the infection along the fascial planes of the head and neck can result in life-threatening complications, such as cavernous sinus thrombosis, meningitis or mediastinitis. Such devastating complications were once quite common; they are still seen today, even with the availability of antibiotics.

A typical history obtained from a patient with a *facial cellulitis* reveals a previous episode of toothache with pain suggestive of pulpitis, which may regress spontaneously. An asymptomatic period, corresponding to pulpal necrosis, then precedes the onset of swelling and pain when the necrotic pulp becomes infected and the process spreads to adjacent anatomic structures.

Periodontal infection. Acute bacterial infection of the periodontal tissues is most often localized to the gingiva or mucosa adjacent to the involved tooth. The typical patient will complain of a "gum boil," and examination will reveal a discreet fluctuant swelling which may drain easily on manual palpation.

In the late adolescent years, infection of the soft tissue surrounding erupting third molars or wisdom teeth (periocoronitis) is common. Low-grade, chronic infection may be accompanied by symptoms described as "teething;" acute infection will result in pain, swelling and difficulty in opening the mouth (trismus) as the adjacent masticator space becomes involved.

Salivary gland swelling. Acute infection of the major salivary glands (parotid, submandibular and sublingual) may be either viral or bacterial. *Viral parotitis* (mumps) is a disease well known to family practitioners, occurring most frequently in school-age children and appearing either unilaterally or bilaterally. The efficacy of immunization programs should make this disease a relative rarity in the future. Viral lymphadenopathy in the preauricular area, such as that seen in infectious mononucleosis and in "cat scratch" fever, may masquerade as parotid swelling and must be considered.

Sialadenitis, bacterial infection of the salivary glands, commonly affects a single gland. The infection is generally an ascending infection in which bacteria gain access to a gland made susceptible to infection by stasis of saliva. Obstruction of the salivary duct by a stone or mucinous plug is the usual inciting event, but any low-flow state can lead to sialadenitis. The condition is frequently seen in elderly, debilitated or postoperative patients, in whom dehydration may lead to decreased salivary flow and consequent infection. The parotid gland is the usual target organ for this infectious process and involvement is more often unilateral than bilateral. Purulent drainage can be obtained from the duct orifice. Previous episodes of parotitis or congenital abnormality of the acinar structure of the parotid gland may produce sialoangiectasis, which facilitates pooling and stasis of saliva within the gland and increases the patient's susceptibility to episodes of acute infection.

Noninfectious salivary swelling is a component of a number of *systemic conditions,* including diabetes mellitus, uremia, Laennec's cirrhosis, chronic alcoholism and malnutrition. A toxic reaction to a variety of drugs, such as iodine, mercury and guanethidine, causes a painless bilateral parotid gland

Table 204-1.   Important Causes of Facial Pain or Swelling

CAUSE OF PAIN	SYMPTOMS
Odontogenic pain	
Caries	Hot, cold, or sweet sensitive; brief
Pulpitis	Hot and cold aggravate; prolonged; more severe; radiation of pain
Periapical abscess	Heat aggravates, cold relieves; sensitivity to percussion; mobility of tooth
Alveolar abscess	Swelling, malaise
Nonodontogenic pain	
Neuralgia	Lancinating pain; trigger zone
Myalgia	Trismus or pain on opening; deviation of jaw to affected side; tender muscle
Referred	Angina
Salivary Pain and Swelling	
Viral infection (mumps)	
Bacterial infection	
Obstructed flow	
Chemical, metabolic agents	
Lymphoproliferative diseases	
Autoimmune diseases (Sjögren's syndrome)	
Tumors	
Lymphadenopathy	
Masseter hypertrophy	

swelling. A specific triad of keratoconjunctivitis sicca, salivary gland swelling and rheumatoid arthritis is known as *Sjögren's syndrome.* Since its original description with rheumatoid arthritis, the syndrome has also bee related to other chronic autoimmune connective tissue disorders, such as systemic lupus erythematosus (SLE) and polyarteritis nodosa. The diagnosis of Sjögren's syndrome may be made initially without apparent systemic disease and may be the stimulus for further workup to detect the presence of rheumatoid disease. Development of lymphoma in a patient with long-standing Sjögren's syndrome has been recently recognized and must be considered.

Infiltration of both major and minor salivary glands by lymphoproliferative processes is an important consideration in the differential diagnosis of salivary swelling. Lymphomas, tuberculosis and sarcoidosis (uveoparotid fever) have all been first diagnosed from salivary gland enlargement.

DIFFERENTIAL DIAGNOSIS

The causes of facial pain or swelling can be divided into odontogenic, nonodontogenic, and salivary gland etiologies (Table 204-1).

WORKUP

History. Evaluation of facial pain and swelling requires thorough consideration of the pain's onset, severity, quality, location, radiation, aggravating or ameliorating factors, and duration. The various stages of dental infection can be characterized by specific pain histories. For example, pain brought on by contact with hot, cold, or sweet substances is indicative of dental caries, whereas aggravation by heat and relief by cold suggests a periapical abscess. If fever and swelling ensue, an alveolar abscess must be considered. Lancinating pain precipitated by contact with a trigger zone is typical of trigeminal neuralgia; it can be distinguished by history from abscess formation because symptoms are unrelated to the temperature of the contacting substance, and swelling is absent.

In the patient who complains of salivary gland enlargement, it is important to inquire about site(s) of involvement, presence of fever or tenderness, history of chronic illness, malignancy, toxin or drug exposure, and symptoms of rheumatologic disease or sicca syndrome (dry eyes, dry mouth). Unilateral painful swelling of acute onset suggests sialadenitis, especially when seen in an elderly, debilitated, or postoperative patient. A unilaterally enlarged, painless parotid may be due to tumor, particularly if there is a history of progressive increase in size and extension beyond the gland. Bilateral involvement requires consideration of lymphoma and sarcoidosis as well as Sjögren's syndrome (which is bilateral in about half of cases).

It is important to keep in mind that episodic jaw pain may be due to angina (see Chapter 14).

Physical examination. A semisitting position will usually allow both patient comfort and examiner access. While a flashlight can be used, a lighting fixture that can illuminate the oral cavity and leave the examiner with both hands free is preferable.

Inspection of the mouth for fractured, decayed or heavily restored teeth and for heavy deposits of debris and calculus ("tartar") on the teeth and gingiva requires little experience and will direct the examiner's attention to odontogenic disease as a likely source of the pain or swelling. A dental mirror or a short-handled laryngoscopy mirror serves as a better retractor than does a wooden tongue blade. Palpation of the teeth to determine tenderness or mobility will help to identify an abscessed tooth. The soft tissues should be palpated to detect the presence of indurated or fluctuant swelling adjacent to a suspicious tooth. Tenderness to percussion of a tooth, using a short, sharp tap with the dental mirror handle, is diagnostic of an abscessed tooth. The salivary glands are palpated bimanually intraorally and extraorally; the salivary duct orifices should be observed for salivary flow or purulent drainage during palpation of the individual glands. Cervical lymph nodes should be checked for enlargement and tenderness.

Laboratory studies. Suspicion of dental caries can be confirmed by X-ray, as can abscess formation. Most other conditions produce few radiologic changes. White blood count in the potentially toxic patient or blood sugar in the diabetic patient may aid in subsequent management. Suspicion of Sjögren's syndrome can be confirmed by lip biopsy. It is important to obtain any purulent drainage for Gram stain, culture, and sensitivity testing.

INDICATIONS FOR REFERRAL

Early recognition of dental decay and gingival inflammation with consequent referral to a general dentist for complete evaluation and treatment is the most effective means of preventing infection. In the patient with valvular heart disease, full dental evaluation on a periodic basis is mandatory and is particularly indicated prior to consideration of a valvular prosthesis so that potential sources of dental sepsis may be eliminated. Adequate antibiotic prophylaxis for subacute bacterial endocarditis must be provided for such patients at the time dental procedures are performed (see Chapter 11).

When physical examination indicates no other source of facial pain, referral for dental evaluation is indicated. Abscess formation necessitates prompt referral for definitive drainage. When the patient's clinical appearance demonstrates involvement of deep fascial spaces, as evidenced by fever, trismus, elevation of the tongue, ophthalmoplegia, etc., referral to an oral surgeon and admission to the hospital for parenteral antibiotics are urgent.

The patient with acute salivary swelling should be seen by an oral surgeon for radiographic examination, by which sialoliths causing obstruction are sought. Gentle dilatation of the duct may help to relieve the obstruction; in some cases, surgery is necessary to remove the stone. Sialography, or examination of the salivary system with radiographic contrast injections, is contraindicated in the acute period of infection.

When salivary swelling is chronic in nature, no antibiotics are indicated. Sialography is highly diagnostic in this group of patients. If the differential diagnosis includes Sjögren's syndrome, sarcoidosis, or lymphoma, a biopsy of one of the minor salivary glands of the lower lip will usually confirm the diagnosis, without necessitating a more complex parotid biopsy.

SYMPTOMATIC MANAGEMENT

While awaiting dental evaluation, the very uncomfortable patient may require strong analgesia (e.g., codeine sulfate, 30 mg. every 4 to 6 hours). Penicillin remains the primary antibiotic of choice in treatment of odontogenic infection. Initiation of an oral penicillin-VK regimen of 250 mg. every 6 hours is appropriate at the first recognition of swelling associated with an infected tooth or periodontal tissue. Antibiotics are not indicated in the absence of swelling. Erythromycin is the preferred drug for the patient allergic to penicillin. Referral of the patient to an oral surgeon for definitive drainage of the infection at the earliest opportunity is indicated and should be made simultaneously with the prescribing of antibiotics.

Acute swelling of a salivary gland, accompanied by purulent or inspissated saliva from the involved duct, requires antibiotic treatment. Stimulation of salivary flow with sour candies and warm compresses is a helpful local measure. The submandibular gland tends to be infected with the same flora as is found in odontogenic infections. Hence, penicillin is the drug of choice for submandibular sialadenitis. Acute bacterial parotitis, on the other hand, is associated with staphylococcal species, and one of the penicillinase-resistant antibiotics, such as dicloxacillin, is preferred. Antiobiotic treatment for other infections which may have preceded the onset of the salivary infection can alter the oral flora and produce infection of the salivary system by unusual organisms, such as *E. coli.* Thus, culturing of the purulent saliva is suggested.

ANNOTATED BIBLIOGRAPHY

American Heart Association: Prevention of bacterial endocarditis. Circulation, *56*:139, 1977. *(The rationale and current prophylaxis recommendations for dental treatment of patients with valvular heart disease.)*

Chow, A.W., Roser, S.M., and Brady, F.A.: Orofacial odontogenic infections. Ann. Intern. Med., *88*:392, 1978. *(A comprehensive review of pertinent oral microbiology, surgical anatomy of the spread of infection and the signs and symptoms of patients with odontogenic infection.)*

Guralnick, W.C., Dinoff, R.B., and Galbadini, J.: Tender parotid swelling in a dehydrated patient, J. Oral Surg. *26*:669, 1968. *(A good differential diagnosis of salivary gland swelling.)*

205
Evaluation of Hoarseness

Hoarseness is a symptom of laryngeal disease. The majority of acute episodes are self-limited and due to viral upper respiratory tract infection; however, acute laryngeal edema must be considered. The patient who is bothered by persistent hoarseness requires careful assessment, because carcinoma of the larynx, damage to the recurrent laryngeal nerve from tumor, or another serious etiology may be responsible.

PATHOPHYSIOLOGY AND CLINICAL PRESENTATION

Vocal quality is determined by complex factors, including the distance between the vocal cords, the tenseness of the cords, and the rapidity of vibration. Hoarseness results from interference with normal apposition of the vocal cords. Inflammatory, traumatic, and neoplastic lesions might alter the relationship between the vocal cords.

Acute laryngitis is the most common cause of hoarseness. It is usually secondary to viral infection; voice abuse, foreign body, excessive smoking, and inhalation of irritant gases are other important precipitants. Acute laryngitis may present with hoarseness, inability to project the voice, or, sometimes, complete loss of the voice. Laryngitis due to infection is frequently accompanied by a scratchy throat, nonpro-

ductive cough, and low-grade fever; the patient often has mild pain which is aggravated by talking, but he rarely has difficulty breathing. Acute laryngitis is identified by its relatively rapid onset and its temporal relationship to a causal factor, such as infection or voice abuse.

In *chronic laryngitis,* recurrent or persistent hoarseness is the chief symptom. Inability to use the voice for prolonged periods is common. Hoarseness is often accompanied by a nonproductive cough; pain is absent or minimal. The condition develops as a consequence of repeated episodes of acute laryngitis and recurrent exposure to an aggravating factor, such as smoking, allergy, or voice overuse. Formerly, tuberculosis and syphilis were commonly responsible for chronic laryngitis but are rarely involved today.

Laryngeal edema can present as hoarseness that may rapidly progress to dyspnea, a serious development. Angioneurotic edema, infection and direct injury are sources of acute edema. Radiation and tumor may produce edema that develops more slowly.

Leukoplakia of the vocal cords results from persistent irritation of the larynx; smoking is a particularly common cause. Hoarseness is the chief symptom; pain is absent. Leukoplakia appears as whitish, patchy membrane on the cords; often hyperkeratosis is evident on histologic examination.

Contact ulcers are granulomatous lesions caused by trauma. They usually occur in men who forcefully bring the arytenoid cartilages together. The patient complains of pain and slight hoarseness.

Vocal cord paralysis can produce a hoarse, breathy voice. In unilateral cord paralysis, the presence of hoarseness depends on the position of the paralyzed cord. Sometimes there is an initial loss of voice range and a progression to hoarseness over time. In bilateral vocal cord paralysis the predominant symptom is dyspnea on exertion; the quality of the voice is relatively intact, though weak. Vocal cord paralysis can develop secondary to a central or peripheral lesion. Central causes of hoarseness include multiple sclerosis and basilar insufficiency in the area of the nucleus ambiguous; multiple neurologic deficits result. Peripheral lesions result from compromise of the nerve along its course to the larynx. Paralysis may be caused by nerve injury during thyroidectomy or other neck surgery. Neoplasms of the thyroid, esophagus, and apex of the lung may disrupt the nerve. Occasionally an aortic aneurysm, a dilated left atrium, or a rapidly enlarging hilar lymph node is capable of producing nerve compression on the left side. Approximately 16 to 30 per cent of cases of vocal cord paralysis are idiopathic.

Laryngeal carcinoma may present with hoarseness as an early manifestation, especially if the neoplasm involves the free edge of the vocal cord. Pain is relatively uncommon. Tumors of the larynx extrinsic to the cords often do not produce symptoms early in the course of the disease. Pain, due to ulceration, is common and felt as a burning discomfort that occurs when the patient drinks hot liquids or citrus juices. Hoarseness is a late symptom. Hoarseness is also a presentation of *benign tumors* of the larynx.

Hoarseness can be a symptom of various systemic disorders. *Rheumatoid arthritis* may involve the cricoarytenoid joint, presenting with pain referred to the ear, dysphagia, and hoarseness. In marked *hypo-*

Table 205–1.   Important Causes of Hoarseness

ACUTE HOARSENESS	CHRONIC HOARSENESS
Acute laryngitis	**Chronic laryngitis**
Viral infection	Chronic or recurrent vocal abuse
Vocal abuse	Smoking
Toxic fumes	Allergy
	Persistent irritant exposure
Laryngeal edema, acute	**Carcinoma of the larynx**
Angioneurotic edema	Intrinsic to the vocal cords
Infection	Extrinsic to the vocal cords
Direct injury	**Vocal cord lesions**
	Polyps
	Leukoplakia
	Contact ulcer and granuloma
	Vocal nodule
	Benign tumors
	Vocal cord paralysis
	Laryngeal nerve injury (tumor, neck surgery, aortic aneurysm)
	Brain stem lesion
	Vocal cord trauma
	Chronic intubation
	Systemic disorders
	Hypothyroidism
	Rheumatoid arthritis
	Virilization
	Psychogenic

thyroidism, hoarseness related to atrophy or myxede-matous infiltration of the vocal cords develops. Other infiltrative diseases, such as sarcoid and amyloid, may produce hoarseness and, rarely, obstruction. It is important to remember that hoarseness developing in a woman may be a sign of *virilization,* and therefore should be considered in the context of other mascu-linizing changes.

DIFFERENTIAL DIAGNOSIS

The causes of hoarseness are best considered in terms of acute and chronic etiologies (see Table 205–1).

WORKUP

History. The evaluation of hoarseness depends on the chronicity of the condition. One needs to de-termine whether the onset was sudden or gradual and the course self-limited or progressive. Difficulty in breathing or stridor suggests obstruction and is an in-dication for emergency hospital admission. It is help-ful to find out if hoarseness is exacerbated by talk-ing; also whether the voice completely disappeared and, if so, for how long. Any recent upper respiratory tract infection, sore throat, fever, chills, sputum or myalgias should be noted, as well as excessive voice use. Exposure to dust, fire, smoke, or irritant fumes should be documented, as should tobacco and alcohol intake. A history of neck mass, neck surgery, intuba-tion, or lung tumor may provide important clues to etiology. Symptoms of hypothyroidism (see Chapter 100) are worth checking for when the etiology is not readily evident.

Physical examination. The primary physician should examine the oropharynx and palpate the thy-roid and cervical lymph nodes. Direct visualization of the larynx can be accomplished by indirect mirror laryngoscopy, which many primary physicians are capable of doing, and should be an essential part of every evaluation of hoarseness. The advent of fiber-optic laryngosocopy may make it easier for a larger number of primary care physicians to adequately ex-amine the larynx.

INDICATIONS FOR REFERRAL

If the primary care physician does not feel com-petent to visualize the vocal cords, a decision must be made about whether to refer the patient to an oto-laryngologist. Hoarseness of greater than 3 weeks duration, particularly when there has not been a his-tory of an acute infectious process, requires referral; any patient with concurrent dyspnea should be im-mediately hospitalized. In those who have a resolving process and are at low risk for malignancy (young, nonsmoker, nondrinker), a complete otolaryngologic examination may be deferred.

SYMPTOMATIC MANAGEMENT AND PATIENT EDUCATION

Acute hoarseness. Symptomatic management of the patient with acute hoarseness includes voice rest, humidification, and removal of irritants, such as fumes, gases or cigarettes. It is important to instruct the patient to completely rest his voice, because par-tial voice rest is often difficult to accomplish. Aerosol therapy, such as a steamy shower or a vaporizer, is particularly helpful in acute inflammatory processes.

Chronic hoarseness. The patient whose difficulty is due to recurrent voice abuse can benefit from a few simple suggestions. Proper modulation of voice, reduction of tone, and avoidance of excessive voice use are helpful, particularly for people involved in public speaking or performing. Occasionally it is beneficial to try vocal therapy to direct the patient to proper use of the voice. It is essential that irritants be avoided, the major offender being cigarette smoke. Avoidance of irritants and limitation of vocal abuse will make recurrence and chronicity less likely and reduce the chances of developing nodules, polyps, or leukoplakia.

ANNOTATED BIBLIOGRAPHY

DeWeese, D.D., and Saunders, W.H.: Textbook of Otolaryngology, ed. 5. St. Louis: C.V. Mosby, 1977. *(Chapters 6, 7, and 8 provide good discus-sions of the conditions that can present as hoarseness.)*

206
Evaluation of Smell and Taste Disturbances

Impairment of taste and smell, in addition to being intrinsically unpleasant, are annoying because they interfere with the ability to derive pleasure from food. Moreover, a diminished ability to detect noxious agents in the environment leaves the patient vulnerable to them. Patients may complain of total loss, attenuation or perversion of these senses. Problems of smell are often reported as alterations of taste because much of the awareness of taste is olfactory. The primary physician should be capable of recognizing taste and smell disturbances that are manifestations of serious illness requiring detailed evaluation, as well as simple forms in which symptomatic relief will suffice.

PATHOPHYSIOLOGY AND CLINICAL PRESENTATION

Smell. The olfactory area is located high in the nasal vault above the superior turbinate. The neurons of the first cranial nerve penetrate the cribriform plate and travel to the cortex at the base of the frontal lobe on top of the cribriform plate. The most common mechanism of anosmia or hyposmia is *nasal obstruction* that prevents air from reaching olfactory areas high in the nose. Food is tasteless while the problem persists. In most instances, such as those related to the common cold or allergic rhinitis, the process is fully reversible, but sometimes more lasting damage is done. *Chronic infection* may lead to partial replacement of olfactory mucosa with respiratory epithelium. *Influenza* is known for its ability to cause permanent destruction of the nasal receptors; the onset is often acute. Another mechanism of acute anosmia is *head trauma,* in which the nerve filaments coming through the cribriform plate are damaged.

More gradual onset of reduced smell is typical of an expanding *mass lesion* at the base of the frontal lobe; meningiomas and aneurysms of the anterior cerebral circulation are the most important sources of this problem. Upward extension of a mass lesion into the frontal lobe is manifested by lack of initiative, personality change and forgetfulness; posterior extension may involve the optic chiasm.

Perversion of smell (parosmia) can result from local nasal pathology such as *empyema* of the nasal sinuses, or *ozena,* a chronic rhinitis of unkown etiology causing thick greenish discharge and crusting (see Chapter 212); *Klebsiella* and *Pseudomonas* are often cultured from the discharge. *Olfactory hallucinations* are central in origin and may present as the aura of a seizure; the responsible lesion is typically found in the area of the uncus. *Olfactory delusions* are reported by schizophrenic patients while their sense of smell remains intact.

Many disorders of smell are of unknown cause. The mechanisms of reduced smell associated with *hypothyroidism, hypogonadism,* and *hepatitis* are not understood. A recent subject of speculation has been the influence of various trace metals, particularly copper and zinc, on the production and treatment of smell disorders.

Taste. The tongue, seventh and ninth cranial nerves and the hippocampal region of the cerebral cortex make up the taste apparatus. The front of the tongue detects sweet and salty tastes, the sides sense sour tastes, and the large papillae in the back detect bitter tastes. The pharynx also has the ability to sense taste. The taste buds are concentrated in the anterior two thirds of the tongue, which is innervated by the chorda tympani branch of the seventh cranial nerve. The posterior third of the tongue and palate are supplied by the glossopharyngeal nerve.

The most frequent source of diminished fine taste is impairment of smell. In addition, the taste buds may be directly injured by alcohol and smoking. The common observation that food tastes better after these habits are terminated is due to improvement in both the olfactory receptors and the taste buds. Age is associated with a decrease in taste buds. Diseases and drugs that dry the mouth, e.g., Sjögren's syndrome and tricyclic antidepressants, reduce the threshold for taste. Chorda tympani and seventh nerve lesions are rarely bilateral and therefore do not produce a complete loss of taste. Cerebral mass lesions usually do not involve the hippocampal gyrus. Depression, endocrinopathies and a host of drugs are associated with complaints of altered taste. The

Table 206–1. Some Important Causes of Impaired Taste

A. Disturbances in smell

B. Injury to taste buds

    1. Age
    2. Smoking
    3. Hot liquids
    4. Dental disease
    5. Sjögren's disease
    6. Idiopathic conditions

C. Cranial nerve lesions (seventh or ninth, partial loss only)

    1. ear surgery
    2. Bell's palsy
    3. Ramsay-Hunt syndrome (herpes zoster infection of the geniculate ganglion)
    4. Cholesteatoma
    5. Cerebellopontine angle tumors (advanced disease)

D. Central lesions

    1. Head trauma
    2. Tumors (very rare)

E. Psychiatric disorders

    1. Depression

F. Drugs

    1. Griseofulvin
    2. Imipramine
    3. Clofibrate
    4. Lithium
    5. Thiamazole
    6. Acetazolamide
    7. Metronidazole
    8. Penicillamine
    9. Iron
    10. Tetracycline

G. Metabolic-endocrine problems

    1. Hypogonadism
    2. Uremia
    3. Hypothyroidism
    4. Hepatitis
    5. Pregnancy

mechanisms are unknown, but in many instances the primary disturbance seems to be in part an alteration of smell.

DIFFERENTIAL DIAGNOSIS

Most of the conditions which disrupt taste are annoying but not life-threatening (Table 206–1). However, a disturbance in the sense of smell may be a sign of more serious illness (Table 206–2).

WORKUP

Smell

History. A primary objective is to distinguish local nasal pathology from a central or cranial nerve lesion. History of head trauma, worsening headaches, olfactory hallucinations, change in personality, unexplained forgetfulness, visual disturbances, gradual onset or steady progression of symptoms suggests disease beyond the nasal cavity. History of head congestion, nasal discharge, allergies, sinus problems, influenza, chemical exposure, or a recent cold suggests the nose as the source of difficulty. Inquiry into symptoms of hepatitis (see Chapter 70) and hypothyroidism (see Chapter 100) may uncover an endocrine-metabolic etiology. A careful psychiatric history is needed when there is description of abnormal smells in the absence of any other pathology.

Physical examination. One can document the disorder by challenging each nostril with a representative sample of each primary odor: pungent, floral, mint, and putrid. Smell is most accurately assessed by the use of chemicals, such as pyridine, garlic-like

Table 206–2. Causes of Disturbances in Smell

A. Nasal

    1. Upper respiratory tract infection
    2. Polyps
    3. Ozena
    4. Chronic sinusitis
    5. Allergic rhinitis
    6. Influenza and other virus
    7. Chemical injury, e.g., tar, formaldehyde

B. Cranial Nerve

    1. Trauma
    2. Meningioma
    3. Cerebral aneurysm

C. Cerebral Cortex

    1. Seizure disorder
    2. Meningioma
    3. Aneurysm
    4. Schizophrenia

D. Metabolic-Endocrine

    1. Hypothyroidism
    2. Hypogonadism
    3. Liver disease

odor, nitrobenzene, bitter almond, thiophene, and burnt rubber odor. Kits are available which contain these substances. Ammonia, which will produce a response by irritation even in the absence of olfactory powers, should be avoided.

On physical examination, the head is assessed for trauma and the nares are inspected for polyps, deviated septum, mucosal inflammation, and discharge. The sinuses are transilluminated to look for evidence of sinusitis. Fundi are checked for blurring of the disc margins, and the visual fields are tested by confrontation for evidence of optic chiasm compression. The skin, thyroid, and ankle jerks are examined for signs of hypothyroidism (see Chapter 100), and the hair, voice, muscles and testes for hypogonadism. Any jaundice, hepatomegaly, ascites or asterixis should be noted.

Laboratory studies. Sinus films should be reserved for patients with clinical evidence of sinusitis. Routine skull x-rays are of low yield; only if there is a history of recent head trauma or there are signs on physical examination of a cerebral mass is a skull film worthwhile, in which case fracture or shift of pineal to one side is sought. Far more sensitive for detection of an intracranial mass lesion is computerized tomography (CT). CT will be needed if the presence of an intracranial lesion is strongly suspected. Liver, thyroid function, and gonadotropin tests are useful only when there are relevant findings on history and physical examination, not in otherwise asymptomatic individuals with impaired smell.

Taste

History. The initial objective of the evaluation is to localize the problem. Intracranial disease is distinctly rare, so assessment can be concentrated on disease in the mouth, in the area of chorda tympani, and seventh nerve. Alcohol abuse, smoking, dental disease, and severe mouth dryness suggest a buccal cavity source. Facial palsy, herpes zoster rash about the ear, recent ear surgery, hearing problems, vertigo and tinnitus are clues to diseases which may injure the seventh nerve. Drug use and concurrent metabolic or endocrinologic problems (see Table 206–1 and above) deserve exploration. Isolated reduction in taste requires inquiry into smell impairment and concurrent depression. Dry eyes in conjunction with dry mouth suggests Sjögren's syndrome, especially if rheumatoid arthritis is present.

Physical examination. Careful examination of the nose, ears, oral cavity, tongue and teeth is essen-tial. The condition of the gums and teeth is worth noting. Taste should be assessed by challenging the withdrawn tongue with sweet, salty, bitter and sour stimuli on each side and asking the patient to indicate what he tastes. Lateralizing the defect suggests a lesion of the seventh nerve. Examination of the cranial nerves needs to concentrate on testing of olfaction, hearing and facial motor functions.

Laboratory studies. If history or physical examination suggests hypothyroidism, a TSH level should be obtained; likewise a BUN and creatinine if renal disease is suspected. Sjögren's syndrome can be confirmed by lip biopsy (see Chapter 204). Suspicion of a cerebellopontine angle tumor is an indication for CT scan.

SYMPTOMATIC MANAGEMENT

Smell. Local nasal pathology is often self-limited, but when chronic sinusitis or allergic rhinitis persists, definitive therapy is indicated (see Chapter 209 and 212). Avoidance of toxic fumes (e.g., formaldehyde) and removal of nasal polyps should also help. When influenza has caused sudden, complete and permanent loss of smell, little can be done. Ozena sometimes requires local or even systemic antibiotic therapy; saline irrigations to remove obstructing crusts are helpful (see Chapter 212). Correction of hypothyroidism improves smell. A literature has developed suggesting that zinc salts will restore normal olfaction and taste, though a recent double-blind controlled trial showed zinc to be no better than placebo.

Taste. Regardless of the cause of reduced taste, the patient should be encouraged to stop smoking and reduce alcohol consumption; often the development of a disability such as altered taste is sufficient motivation to get the patient to stop (see Chapter 49). If possible, medications which may impair taste should be stopped or reduced to determine what contribution, if any, they make to the taste disturbance. Any dental disease of consequence should be corrected. The same pertains to hypothyroidism (see Chapter 100). Concurrent depression may respond to a tricyclic antidepressant, but the drug may impair taste by causing a dry mouth (see Chapter 215); forewarning the patient can prevent side effects from becoming an unpleasant surprise. Disease related to the brain stem, chorda tympani and inner ear requires referral for treatment.

INDICATIONS FOR REFERRAL

Olfactory hallucinations, change in personality, visual field defects, and impairment of memory in conjunction with disorders of smell, and multiple cranial nerve defects, vertigo and tinnitus in conjunction with altered taste, are indications for neurologic consultation. Patients with ozena, nasal polyps, deviated nasal septum, refractory sinusitis or a chorda tympani lesion may benefit from evaluation by the otolaryngologist.

ANNOTATED BIBLIOGRAPHY

Henkin, R.I., *et al.*: The molecular basis of taste and its disorders. Ann. Intern. Med., *71*:791, 1969. *(A comprehensive review of the pathophysiology of taste disorders.)*

Henkin, R.I., *et al.*: Idiopathic hypogeusia with dysgeusia, hyposmia and dysosmia: A new syndrome. JAMA, *217*:434, 1971. *(A report of 35 patients presenting with an apparently new syndrome. Pathologic changes in taste buds were observed on electromicroscopy.)*

Henkin, R.I., et al.: Abnormalities of taste and smell in Sjögren's syndrome. Ann. Intern. Med., *76*:375, 1972. *(An important cause to consider.)*

Henkin, R.I., *et al.*: A double-blind study of the effects of sulfate on taste and smell dysfunction. Am. J. Med. Sci., *272*, 1976. *(Zinc and placebo were equally effective.)*

McConnell, R.J., *et al.*: Defects of taste and smell in patients with hypothyroidism. Am. J. Med., *59*: 254, 1975. *(A study of 18 unselected patients, 9 who were aware of alteration in taste, and 7 of alteration in sense of smell.)*

Rollin, H.: Drug-related gustatory disorders. Ann. Otol. Rhinol. Laryngol., *87*:1, 1978. *(A review of drugs that alter taste.)*

Schecter, P.J., *et al.*: Abnormalities of taste and smell after head trauma. J. Neurol. Neurosurg. Psychiatry, *37*:802, 1974. *(Decreased taste and smell acuity were studied in 29 patients after head trauma.)*

Smith, F.R., Dell, R.B., *et al.*: Disordered gustatory function in liver disease. Gastroenterology, *70*:568; 1976. *(A common complication and probably a contributor to anorexia.)*

207
Evaluation of Tinnitus

Tinnitus is an important but nonspecific symptom of otologic disease. "Ringing," "buzzing" or "roaring" are terms used to decribe the sensation, which can be annoying and a source of concern. The occurrence of tinnitus requires assessment for a serious or treatable otologic problem. In the absence of a specifically treatable etiology, it is still important to provide the patient with some symptomatic relief, especially at night.

PATHOPHYSIOLOGY AND CLINICAL PRESENTATION

The pathophysiology of tinnitus remains very poorly understood. Research on the problem is often limited to studies of therapeutic responses to empirical treatments. The most that can be said with certainty is that tinnitus is usually a manifestation of disease in the ear, eighth nerve, or central auditory apparatus; it is often accompanied by hearing loss.

External and middle ear conditions. Tinnitus due to such problems as impacted cerumen, perforation of the tympanic membrane, and fluid in the middle ear is commonly low-pitched, intermittent, and accompanied by muffled hearing and a change in the sound of one's own voice. In otosclerosis, tinnitus is constant, but may disappear as the disease progresses. Acute otitis media (see Chapter 208) sometimes produces a pulsating type of tinnitus that resolves as inflammation subsides.

Inner ear and eighth nerve disease. Presbycusis and acoustic trauma can give rise to a high-pitched tinnitus that is near the frequency of greatest hearing loss. Transient tinnitus that follows acute acoustic trauma is a forerunner of hearing loss and a warning sign to avoid repeated exposure. Ototoxic drugs, such as the aminoglycoside antibiotics, may produce high-pitched tinnitus and hearing loss that often persist after cessation of drug use. Salicylates are frequently responsible for reversible, dose-related tinnitus. Meniere's disease results in transient, low-pitched tinnitus that varies with the intensity of the condition's other symptoms, often worsening when vertigo and hearing loss are imminent. Acoustic neuroma produces a similar set of symptoms, but the clinical course is progressive, with tinnitus frequently preceding other symptoms (see Chapter 154).

Other sources. Tinnitus cerebri is described as a roaring in the head and is believed to be vascular or neurologic in origin. A vascular aneurysm with an audible bruit, palatal myoclonus with audible muscle contraction, and an unusually patent eustachian tube that transmits respiratory sounds are examples of "objective" tinnitus, i.e., the sounds can be heard by the examiner. When ambient noise is reduced, most people will notice some head sounds. These may be due to the rushing of blood (severest in aortic insufficiency) or contraction of auditory muscles. Loss of hearing due to conduction defect accentuates the problem. Depressed and neurotic individuals have less tolerance for these normal head sounds and complain of them when in quiet settings. The ability to withstand tinnitus is also subject to much individual variation; tolerance is lessened by fatigue and emotional upset.

DIFFERENTIAL DIAGNOSIS

Most tinnitus results from the same conditions that cause hearing loss, whether conductive or sensorineural, peripheral or central. Important etiologies are listed in Chapter 202 (see Table 202–1). Subjective complaints of ear or head noise in the absence of otologic pathology may be a concomitant of psychogenic disease. Objective tinnitus suggests cerebrovascular pathology, palatal myoclonus, or a patulous eustacian tube.

There are few data on the frequency of the various etiologies responsible for tinnitus. Of interest is the fact that reports from otologic practice list as many as 50 per cent of cases as being of unknown etiology.

WORKUP

The diagnostic assessment of tinnitus follows the same pattern as that for hearing loss (see Chapter 202).

History. The quality of the tinnitus in unfortunately of limited use for diagnosis, though some conditions are more likely than others to be associated with tinnitus of a certain pitch. Any association of the sound with respiration, drug use, vertigo, noise trauma, or ear infection should be checked for. When the problem is present only at night, it suggests increased awareness of normal head sounds. Most patients with tinnitus of otologic origin have an associated hearing defect or soon develop one, whereas those without other signs of ear disease may have a vascular lesion or an accentuated awareness of normal head noises.

Physical examination ought to include inspection of the external ear and tympanic membrane for cerumen impacted, foreign bodies, perforation, and signs of otitis media (see Chapter 208). Weber and Rinne testing should be performed to determine if there is sensorineural or conductive hearing loss (see Chapter 202). The cranial nerves are examined for evidence of brain stem damage, a sign of an advanced acoutic neuroma. Testing for nystagmus (see Chapter 154) is worthwhile if vertigo is reported. The skull should be auscultated for a bruit if the origin of the problem remains obscure.

Laboratory studies. An audiogram can help to identify and localize an otologic lesion. If acoustic neuroma is suspected because of progressive worsening of hearing loss, vertigo, and tinnitus, an audiogram can provide further evidence for the condition. A positive audiogram is an indication to proceed with futher workup that might include polytomes of the internal auditory meatus and computerized tomography; definitive diagnosis may require posterior fossa myelography.

INDICATIONS FOR REFERRAL

Referral is essential when a conductive hearing loss is discovered, because many of these losses are correctable. Suspicion of an acoustic neuroma is also an indication for consultation, especially before embarking on an expensive workup. Referral to the otolaryngologist may be necessary to satisfy the anxious patient that everything has been explored and that there is no serious or correctable underlying condition.

SYMPTOMATIC MANAGEMENT AND PATIENT EDUCATION

The patient with a lesion that cannot be cured will still want relief from the annoyance of the tinnitus. Drugs of all types have been tried, including nicotinic acid, vasodilators, and tranquilizers. None has proven superior to placebo. The symptom is most troublesome at night and in quiet rooms. Use of a clock radio at night that shuts off after a half-hour of playing background music often allows the patient to fall asleep. Keeping a radio on during the day when the patient has to work in a quiet room is helpful. Many devices are promoted that one wears like a hearing aid to help mask tinnitus; but they are of questionable value.

ANNOTATED BIBLIOGRAPHY

Fowler, E.P.: Head noises in normal and disordered ears. Arch. Otolaryngol., *39:* 498, 1944. *(A classic article on the causes of tinnitus.)*

Michel, R.G., *et al.*: A practical approach to the treatment of subjective tinnitus. Eye, Ear, Nose, Throat Monthly, *55:*96, 1976. *(A paper that describes supportive therapy and the use of masking devices.)*

Myers, E., and Berstein, J.: Salicylate ototoxicity. Arch Otolaryngol., *82:*483, 1965. *(A clinical and experimental study documenting reversibility of aspirin ototoxicity.)*

Pulec, J.L., Hodell, S.F., and Anthony, P.F.: Tinnitus: Diagnosis and treatment, Ann. Otolaryngol., *87:*821, 1978. *(A study of 64 patients from an otologic practice, with emphasis on use of hearing aids and/or tinnitus maskers to relieve the symptoms.)*

Vernon, J.: Attempts to relieve tinnitus. J. Am. Audiol. Soc., *2:*124, 1977. *(An extensive and excellent review of measures that have been employed to treat tinnitus.)*

208
Approach to the Patient with Otitis
HARVEY B. SIMON, M.D.

Not infrequently a patient presents complaining of ear pain or purulent discharge. Inspection of the ear often reveals signs of otitis media or external otitis. The primary care provider should know how to recognize and treat these common conditions so that only refractory or complicated cases need to be referred.

PATHOPHYSIOLOGY AND CLINICAL PRESENTATION

Although *acute otitis media* is an extremely common problem in early childhood, its incidence declines with increasing age, and it is an uncommon infection in adults. Purulent otitis media results when bacteria ascend from the nasopharynx to the normally sterile middle ear. Abnormal eustacian tube reflux or obstruction caused by viral nasopharyngitis are considered important in the pathogenesis of acute otitis media. Pain, fever and hearing loss are the classic presenting complaints. Tympanic membrane perforation and otorrhea may occur.

The most common cause of otitis media is the *Pneumococcus.* While *H. influenzae* was once considered important only in young children, a recent study identified these organisms in 36 per cent of patients with otitis media between 5 and 9 years of age. Other organisms implicated in some patients include streptococci, *Neisseria catarrhalis,* and *Staph. epidermidis.* Gram-negative bacilli and *Staph. aureus* can cause acute otitis in neonates. Viruses and Mycoplasma are not etiologically important. Anaerobic bacteria have recently been implicated in some cases.

The prognosis for acute otitis media is excellent. Chronic serious otitis, hearing loss, and recurrent purulent otitis are the most common difficulties encountered in the antibiotic era. In the past, acute suppurative mastoiditis was the most common sequela of acute otitis, and purulent labyrnthitis, meningitis, lateral sinus thrombosis and brain abscess were disasterous, if less common, complications.

Serous otitis media is a noninfectious variant in which fever and pain are absent. Clear fluid is present in the middle ear, the tympanic membrane remains retracted, and bony landmarks are intact. It often follows eustacian tube obstruction.

Chronic otitis media is seen in all age groups and results from neglected or recurrent acute otitis media. Pain and fever are usually absent, but can occur during sporadic flare-ups in activity. Diminished hearing and foul otorrhea are the major symptoms.

Physical examination discloses perforation of the tympanic membrane. Central perforations of the pars tensa are associated with benign disease, but marginal or peripheral perforations may be associated with invasive cholesteatomas. X-rays may reveal sclerosis of the mastoid air cells and bone destruction. A great variety of organisms can be cultured from the drainage in cases of chronic otitis media, including staphylococci, streptococci, *Pseudomonas aeruginosa* and enteric gram-negative bacilli.

External otitis is a common, generally benign inflammatory condition usually precipitated by excessive moisture in or trauma to the external auditory canal. Patients complain of pruritus or pain, which may be severe. Crusting, inflammation and discharge in the canal are typical findings. The pain, which results from movements of the external ear helps distinguish otitis externa from otitis media. A broad range of organisms including gram-positive cocci, gram-negative bacilli, and fungi can cause otitis externa.

DIAGNOSIS

The cornerstone of the clinical diagnosis of acute purulent otitis media is the finding of a bulging tympanic membrane with impaired mobility and obscuration of the bony landmarks. The other diagnostic possibility is a serous otitis media, in which fever and pain are absent and, although fluid is present in the middle ear, the tympanic membrane is usually retracted and the bony landmarks are preserved. Cultures of the nasopharynx are not helpful in defining the etiology of acute otitis media. Needle aspiration of the middle ear can be used to confirm the diagnosis and to identify the causative organism; however, this is rarely necessary in clinical practice because the bacteriology of acute otitis media is relatively well defined and the response to antibiotics is easy to monitor.

In chronic otitis media, a perforated drum and discharge strongly support the diagnosis. Pain, erythema and discharge in the external auditory canal are diagnostic of otitis externa.

PRINCIPLES OF MANAGEMENT AND THERAPEUTIC RECOMMENDATIONS

The therapy of *acute otitis media* includes use of analgesics, decongestants and antibiotics. Ampicillin is generally the drug of choice in the pedriatic age group, while penicillin may suffice in adults. Unfortunately, ampicillin-resistant strains of *H. influenzae*

have now been implicated in 2.4 to 8 per cent of all cases of otitis media. When such organisms have been isolated or when patients fail to respond to ampicillin or are penicillin-allergic, combinations of erythromycin and sulfisoxazole or trimethoprim and sulfamethoxazole have proved excellent alternatives. Sulfisoxazole may be useful in the chemoprophylaxis of recurrent otitis in children. Myringotomy does not hasten recovery but is indicated in patients with intractable pain, progressive deafness, or early mastoiditis, and in those who have had a poor response to medical therapy.

In *chronic otitis,* antibiotics are generally of little benefit and surgery is required in advanced cases. Without therapy, chronic otitis media can cause the same intracranial suppurative complication as acute otitis media.

Treatment of *otitis externa* is carried out topically; eardrops containing polymyxin and neomycin produce excellent results. Two drops are applied three times daily for a week. True cellulitis of the external ear requiring systemic antibiotics may develop in some patients. Malignant otitis externa is a rare but life-threatening infection in diabetics caused by *Pseudomonas aeruginosa;* prompt hospitalization and parenteral antibiotics are required.

INDICATIONS FOR REFERRAL

An otolaryngologist should be consulted if acute otitis media fails to respond to medical therapy or if complications such as tympanic membrane perforation, recurrent acute otitis, serous otitis or chronic otitis media develop.

PATIENT EDUCATION

The pain of acute otitis media almost always impels the patient to seek prompt medical attention, so little education or encouragement is required. Patients with recurrent external otitis can learn to recognize symptoms and treat themselves. Patients who have active external otitis or chronic otitis media with perforation of the eardrum should be instructed to avoid swimming; ear plugs usually do not suffice to keep out water.

ANNOTATED BIBLIOGRAPHY

Brook, I., Anthony, B.F., and Finegold, S.M. Aerobic and anaerobic bacteriology of acute otitis media in children. J. Pediatr., *92*:13, 1978. *(A bacteriologic study of 62 children with acute otitis* media. Pneumococci and H. influenzae *were isolated from 57 per cent; a wide group of organisms occurred in the remainder of cases.)*

Cameron, G.G., Pomachac, A.C., and Johnston, M.T.: Comparative efficacy of ampicillin and trimethoprim-sulfamethoxazole in otitis media. CMA J., *112*:87S, 1975. *(A study of 79 children with acute otitis media demonstrating the equal efficacy of ampicillin and trimethoprim-sulfamethoxazole.)*

Rowe, D.S.: Acute suppurative otitis media. Pediatrics, *56*:285, 1975. *(An excellent clinical review of the pathogenesis, diagnosis and therapy of acute otitis media.)*

Schwartz, R., et al.: Acute purulent otitis media in children older than 5 years. JAMA, *238*:1032, 1977. *(H. influenzae was identified as the cause of acute otitis media in 36 per cent of 58 children with otitis between the ages of 5 and 9.)*

Schwartz, R., et al.: The increasing incidence of ampicillin-resistant *Hemophilus influenzae*. JAMA, *239*:320, 1978. *(A study of 625 children with otitis. Overall, 8 per cent of those infections were caused by ampicillin-resistant strains of H. influenzae.)*

Tilles, J.G., et al.: Acute otitis media in children. N. Engl. J. Med., *277*:613, 1967. *(Only 2 viruses and no mycoplasms were recorded in 90 cases of acute otitis media.)*

Zaky, D.A., et al.: Malignant external otitis: A severe form of otitis in diabetic patients. Am. J. Med., *61*:298, 1976. *(A report of 2 cases of malignant otitis externa with a review of the recent literature.)*

209
Approach to the Patient with Sinusitis
HARVEY B. SIMON, M.D.

While infections of the paranasal sinuses are common, they tend to be overdiagnosed by patient and physician alike. Often a frontal headache or congested sensation is attributed to "sinus trouble" and self-medicated with over-the-counter decongestants. Individuals with allergic or vasomotor rhinitis may present seeking treatment for their "sinus condition." The primary physician should be able to distinguish true sinusitis from other causes of nasal congestion, treat uncomplicated cases, and recognize complications.

PATHOPHYSIOLOGY AND CLINICAL PRESENTATION

True sinusitis may be acute or chronic. *Acute purulent sinusitis* is characterized by nasal congestion, purulent nasal discharge, facial pain (that typically increases when the patient stoops forward), and, often, fever and other constitutional symptoms. Viral, allergic or vasomotor rhinitis are frequent antecedent events. The presence of nasal polyps or deviation of the nasal septum may also predispose the patient to purulent sinusitis by obstructing sinus drainage. Other contributing factors may include rapid changes in altitude, trauma, intranasal foreign bodies or tumors, and, occasionally a systemic process such as cystic fibrosis or Kartagener's syndrome (situs inversus, bronchiectasis and sinusitis).

The sinuses may be involved singly or, more often, in combination. Maxillary and frontal sinusitis are common in adults; ethmoiditis is more common in children. The signs and symptoms of sinusitis depends upon which sinuses are involved. *Frontal sinusitis* produces pain and tenderness over the lower forehead and purulent drainage from the middle meatus of the nasal turbinates. *Maxillary sinusitis* produces pain and tenderness over the cheeks; in addition, pain is often referred to the teeth, and the hard palate may be edematous in severe cases. Purulent drainage is present in the middle meatus. Patients with *ethmoid sinusitis* complain of retro-orbital pain, and may have tenderness and even erythema over the upper lateral aspect of the nose. Drainage from the anterior ethmoid cells occurs through the middle meatus, while drainage from the posterior cells is through the superior meatus. Isolated *sphenoid sinusitis* is uncommon, but can present as pain over the occiput or vertex, with purulent drainage from the superior meatus.

Symptoms of *chronic sinusitis* include nasal congestion and discharge, but pain and headache are usually mild or absent, and fever is uncommon.

Because of technical difficulties in obtaining valid cultures, the bacteriology of sinusitis has been incompletely defined. The most common pathogens in acute sinusitis are pneumococci, streptococci, and *Hemophilus influenzae*. Although some studies report the isolation of *Staph. aureus* from significant numbers of patients with acute sinusitis, these studies have been based on nasal cultures and probably reflect nasal contamination rather than a true etiology. In contrast, small numbers of *Staph. aureus* were recovered in one study from operative cultures in 18 per cent of patients with chronic sinusitis. In the same study, heavy growths of anaerobic organisms were isolated in 28 per cent of patients with chronic sinusitis; anaerobic streptococci and *Bacteroides* species predominated. The importance of anaerobes in chronic sinusitis is reflected by the predominace of anaerobes in brain abscesses of sinus origin. Viruses have been considered rare causes of sinusitis, but may be etiologically important in some patients. Rarely, fungi such as *mucor, Rhizopus* or *Aspergillus* species can produce invasive sinusitis in poorly controlled diabetics or leukemics.

Complications of sinusitis have become uncommon in the antibiotic era but can be life-threatening. Frontal sinusitis can lead to osteomyelitis of the frontal bones, especially in children. Patients present with headache, fever, and a characteristic doughy edema over the involved bone, which is termed "Pott's puffy tumor." The organisms involved are the same as those responsible for the underlying sinusitis except that *Staph. aureus* is more common. Osteomyelitis of the maxilla is an infrequent complication of maxillary sinusitis.

Because the orbit is surrounded on three sides by paranasal sinuses, orbital infection can result from sinusitis. This is most frequently a complication of ethmoid sinusitis due to direct extension of infection through the lamina papyracea. *Orbital cellulitis* usually begins with edema of the eyelids and rapidly progresses to ptosis, proptosis, chemosis and diminished extraocular movements. Patients are usually febrile and acutely ill. Pressure on the optic nerve can lead to visual loss which can be permanent, and retrograde spread of infection can lead to intracranial infection.

Retrograde extension of infection along venous channels from the orbit, ethmoid or frontal sinuses, or nose can produce septic *cavernous sinus thrombophlebitis*. These patients are highly febrile and appear "toxic." Lid edema, proptosis, and chemosis are present, but unlike uncomplicated orbital cellulitis, third, fourth, and sixth cranial nerve palsies are prominent, the pupil may be fixed and dilated, and fundoscopic examination may reveal venous engorgement and papilledema. Although the process is usually unilateral at first, spread across the anterior and posterior intercavernous sinuses results in bilateral involvement. Patients may exhibit alterations of consciousness.

Finally, sinusitis can lead to intracranial suppuration either by direct spread through bone or via venous channels. A great variety of syndromes can result, including epidural abscess, subdural empyema, meningitis, and brain abscess. Clinical findings vary greatly, ranging from subtle personality changes with frontal lobe abscesses to headache, symptoms of elevated intracranial pressure, alterations of consciousness, visual symptoms, focal neurologic deficits, seizures, and ultimately, coma and death.

DIFFERENTIAL DIAGNOSIS

The common cold and allergic or vasomotor rhinitis (see Chapter 212) are by far the most common causes of "sinus" symptoms, but polyps, tumors, cysts, foreign bodies, and vasculitides such as Wegener's granulomatosis occasionally produce symptoms resembling sinusitis.

WORKUP

History is checked for presence of a purulent nasal discharge and frontal, maxillary, retro-orbital or vertex pain which worsens on bending forward. Risk factors such as nasal polyps, deviated nasal septum, trauma, foreign bodies and rapid changes in altitude are inquired about. Special attention is paid to toxic symptoms of high fever and rigors in association with complaints suggestive of extension of infection, such as edema of the eyelids and diplopia.

Physical examination may reveal a purulent discharge draining from one of the turbinates. The diagnosis of sinusitis can be confirmed by the finding of opacity on transillumination of the frontal or maxillary sinuses and tenderness to percussion.

Laboratory studies. Confirmation of the diagnosis can also be achieved by radiographic findings of mucosal thickening, sinus opacification, or air fluid levels. Bone erosion can be present in chronic sinusitis. Nasal cultures correlate poorly with actual sinus fluid and cannot be relied upon.

directed against both staphylococci and gram-negative rods. Surgical drainage may be urgently needed.

PRINCIPLES OF MANAGEMENT AND THERAPEUTIC RECOMMENDATIONS

The patient with acute sinusitis can be made more comfortable by employing local application of heat. Decongestants are of paramount importance. Pseudoephedrine can be administered by mouth and by nasal spray. The danger of "rebound" following short-term use of nasal spray has probably been exaggerated. Patients should be instructed to spray each nostril once, and then wait a minute to allow the anterior nasal mucosa to shrink; a repeat spray will then reach the upper and posterior mucosa including the nasal turbinates and sinus ostea. This procedure can be repeated every 4 hours for several days if needed. Antihistamines may provide additional decongestion if there is an allergic component to the problem. Steroid are not necessary in most patients, and may be harmful.

Most patients with acute sinusitis respond well to decongestants and analgesics without the use of antibiotics. There is little controlled data to support the use of antibiotics in acute sinusitis, much less to dictate the choice of drugs. Nevertheless, many physicians administer ampicillin, penicillin, cloxacillin, or erythromycin in conjunction with decongestants. Antibiotics should be used in "toxic" patients, in those who fail to respond to decongestants, and in those with complications. Surgical intervention should be avoided in acute sinusitis unless patients fail to respond to medical therapy and complications are present. Sinus irrigation or surgical drainage may be necessary in chronic sinusitis.

INDICATIONS FOR ADMISSION AND REFERRAL

Any patient who appears toxic or has clinical evidence suggestive of extension to the orbit, bone, brain, or cavernous sinus requires urgent admission for emergency assessment and high-dose intravenous antibiotics. Warning symptoms include high fever, rigors, lid edema, diplopia, pupillary abnormalities, ptosis, and palsies of extraocular movements. The patient should be seen by both an otolaryngologist and infectious disease consultant. Antibiotic coverage is

PATIENT EDUCATION

Patients should understand that nasal congestion and frontal headaches are much more commonly caused by viral "URI"'s and allergic or vasomotor rhinitis than by true sinusitis. Nevertheless, decongestants are indicated in all of these conditions to promote sinus drainage and prevent purulent sinusitis. The patient with recurrent symptoms should learn to recognize them and begin decongestant therapy, but the decision to begin antibiotics should be reserved by the physician.

ANNOTATED BIBLIOGRAPHY

Axelson, A., and Brorson, J.E.: The correlation between bacteriological findings in the nose and maxillary sinus in acute maxillary sinusitis. Laryngoscope, *83*:2003, 1973. *(A Swedish study which shows that nasal cultures correlate poorly with cultures obtained by sinus puncture. Staphylococci were common nasal contaminants but were rarely recovered from the sinus tap. Pneumococci and H. influenzae were the most common causes of sinusitis.)*

Evans, F.W., et al.: Sinusitis of the maxillary antrum. N. Engl. J. Med., *293*:735, 1975. *(An intensive study of 24 patients with maxillary sinusitis. Opacity on transillumination and marked mucosal edema on x-ray were suggestive of purulent sinusitis.)*

Frederick, J., and Braude, A.I.: Anaerobic infection of the paranasal sinuses. N. Engl. J. Med., *290*:290, 1974. *(A heavy growth of anaerobic bacteria in pure culture was obtained in 23 of 83 surgical specimens from patients with chronic sinusitis.)*

Price, C.D., Hameroff, S.B., and Richards, R.D.: Cavernous sinus thrombosis and orbital cellulitis. Southern Med. J., *64*:1243, 1971. *(A study of 9 patients with orbital cellulitis and four with cavernous sinus thrombosis, showing clinical differentiation of these two serious complications of sinusitis.)*

210
Approach to the Patient with Pharyngitis
HARVEY B. SIMON, M.D.

A wide variety of organisms may be responsible for pharyngitis, but the differential diagnosis usually comes down to determining whether the cause is viral or streptococcal. The differentiation is important because acute rheumatic fever is a preventable complication of *Strep. pyogenes* infection. Unfortunately, in most cases clinical features are not distinctive enough to separate viral from streptococcal pharyngitis.

The objectives of management should be to maximize the chances that a patient with streptococcal infection will be identified and treated and to minimize unnecessary use of antibiotics, delay of therapy, inconvenience, and expense. The strategy for achieving these goals has been the subject of recent study and much unresolved debate. Determining the best approach to the sore throat remains a surprisingly complex problem; the primary physician needs to know the advantages and shortcomings of available alternatives.

PATHOPHYSIOLOGY AND CLINICAL PRESENTATION

Respiratory viruses and group A beta-hemolytic streptococci account for the majority of sore throats in adults. A host of other bacteria, viruses, fungi, and spirochetes have also been identified as etiologic agents. Trauma, inhaltion of irritant gases, and dehydration are among the noninfectious causes of sore throat.

Streptococcal pharyngitis accounts for about 10 to 15 per cent of sore throats in adults who are subjected to throat culture. The onset of discomfort is typically acute, with difficulty swallowing often noted. Pharyngeal erythema, exudate, cervical adenopathy, and fever greater than 101°F (38.3°C) are common. Children with "strep throat" exhibit exudate and high fever with greater frequency than do adults with the same disease. Cough, rhinorrhea, and other symptoms of upper respiratory infection are reported in less than 25 per cent. About one-quarter of adult patients give a history of recent exposure to streptococcal infection. The pharyngitis is self-limited; symptoms usually resolve within 7 to 10 days.

Peritonsillar cellulitis and *abscess formation* are important suppurative complications of streptococcal pharyngitis. The peritonsillar tissue and then the tonsils become edematous and inflamed; abscess formation may ensue unless antibiotic therapy is instituted. One or both tonsils may be involved. A grayish-white exudate forms on the tonsils; high fever, rigors, and leukocytosis are associated symptoms. Other suppurative complications include retropharyngeal and parapharyngeal space infections. Scarlet fever is a rare complication in adults, due to infection with a toxigenic strain of *Strep. pyogenes.*

Acute rheumatic fever is the most important non-suppurative complication of group A beta-hemolytic streptococcal infection. It appears most frequently among children aged 5 to 15 and, in general, parallels the frequency and severity of streptococcal infection. About 15 per cent of hospitalized patients with rheumatic fever are over the age of 18. The chances of developing rheumatic fever increase with length of time that the organism persists in the pharynx and with the intensity of the immunologic response. *Acute glomerulonephritis* is another non-suppurative complication. Unlike rheumatic fever, it does not seem to be preventable by means of antibiotic therapy.

OTHER STREPTOCOCCI. Groups C and G streptococci can cause pharyngitis, but with far less frequency than group A organisms. Suppurative complications are rare and rheumatic fever and glomerulonephritis never follow.

Viruses. Respiratory viruses are the most common causes of sore throat. Pharyngitis can be the only manifestation of illness or may be accompanied by conjunctivitis, cough, sputum production, rhinitis and systemic symptoms. Pharyngeal erythema, exudates, tonsillar enlargement, and cervical adenopathy are often present, but with less frequency than in streptococcal disease.

Ebstein Barr virus is the agent responsible for *infectious mononucleosis* and, as such, is sometimes a cause of sore throat. Prodromal symptoms of mononucleosis include malaise, headache, and fatigue foilwed by fever, sore throat, and cervical lymphadenopathy. Sore throat is the most common feature; the pharynx shows hyperplasia of lymphoid tissue, erythema, and edema. About half of patients develop tonsillar exudates. Petechiae at the junction of the hard and soft palate occur in about a third of patients and are highly suggestive of the diagnosis of mononucleosis. Both anterior and posterior cervical adenopathy may develop; generalized lymphadenopathy often follows. Splenomegaly is noted in about half of cases, and hepatomegaly and tenderness are present in about 10 per cent; clinical hepatitis sometimes ensues. A faint, maculopapular rash and transient supraorbital edema occasionally appear.

Other causes of pharyngitis include *herpes simplex* and *Coxsackie A* virus. Herpes infection is typically in the form of a stomatitis that involves the buccal mucosa and tongue as well as the pharynx; vesicles and small ulcers develop. Coxsackie A infection is characterized by vesicles and ulcers on the tonsillar pillars and soft palate.

Other organisms. In patients engaging in orogenital sexual activity, *gonococci* can lead to sore throat, pharyngeal exudate, and lymphadenopathy, or just asymptomatic colonization of the pharynx. In rare instances, bacteremia may result. *Hemophilus influenzae* is a rare cause of pharyngitis in adults, but the infection can be extremely painful; epiglottis is a life-threatening complication that occurs mostly in children. Outbreaks of diphtheria, which is caused by *Corynebacterium diphtheriae*, have taken place in unimmunized populations. The infection is characterized by development of an adherent whitish-blue pharyngeal exudate ("pseudomembrane") that covers the pharynx and causes bleeding if removal is attempted.

About 5 to 15 per cent of healthy people harbor *meningococci* in the pharynx. Although sore throat may be a prodromal symptom of meningococcemia, isolated pharyngitis due to meningococcal infection is very rare; most instances of meningococcal recovery from the pharynx represent asymptomatic colonization.

Although numerous other bacterial species can be cultured from the pharynx in both symptomatic and asymptomatic individuals, they do not cause pharyngitis except under most unusual circumstances. In particular, it should be emphasized that while pneumococci and staphylococci commonly reside in the nasopharynx and can cause severe disease in other parts of the repiratory tract, they do not cause pharyngitis. However, mixed infections with normal mouth flora do occur in debilitated patients.

Fusobacteria and *spirochetes* can cause gingivitis ("trenchmouth") or necrotic tonsillar ulcers ("Vincent's angina"). Patients present with foul breath, pain, pharyngeal exudate, and a dirty gray membranous inflammation which bleeds easily. A similar combination of bacteria and spirochetes can produce an extremely serious invasive gangrene of the mouth known as cancrum oris; this process occurs only in malnourished infants or patients with advanced malignancy and immunosuppression, and is fortunately rare. *Treponema pallidum* can cause pharyngitis as part of primary or secondary syphilis. The diagnosis requires a high index of suspicion and serology.

Other organisms. Among other organisms that can cause pharyngitis, *M. tuberculosis* is very rare. While most forms of fungal pharyngitis are also rare *Candida albicans*, present in the normal mouth flora, can produce pharyngitis if antibiotics or debilitating illnesses upset microbial interactions and host defenses. Oropharyngeal moniliasis (thrush) can be painful and is characterized by a cheesy, white exudate which can be scraped off to demonstrate yeast forms by smear and culture. Finally, while *Mycoplasma pneumoniae* is a cause of pharyngitis in both children and adults, this diagnosis is rarely made in the absence of pneumonitis.

WORKUP

History. As with many other upper repiratory tract infections, the signs and symptoms of pharyngitis do not usually enable the physician to establish an etiologic diagnosis. However, questions concerning family members with documented strep throats, orogenital sexual contact, concurrent steroid or immunosuppressive therapy, and previous history of rheumatic fever are appropriate.

Physical examination of the pharynx is useful for identifying a less common cause of pharyngitis such as thrush, characterized by its white cheesy exudate; gingivitis or necrotic tonsillar ulcers suggest fusobacteria and spirochetes. Associated physical findings, such as a viral exanthem, conjunctivitis, petechiae, generalized lymphadenopathy, splenomegaly, or hepatic tenderness, may provide important clues to etiology.

Laboratory studies. While *throat culture* remains the most reliable and practical means of diagnosing streptococcal pharyngitis, the test is not needed in every case of sore throat. Patients at very high risk of rheumatic fever (i.e., those with a history of rheumatic fever and those in a closed population that is currently experiencing an epidemic of streptococcal pharyngitis) can be managed without dependence on culture results. In other circumstances, the need for a throat culture is more pressing because the clinical assessment of the likelihood of strep infection is very crude; most clinical data are, at best, only suggestive. But, those with recent household exposure, fever greater than 101°F, pharyngeal exudate, cervical adenopathy, and absence of cough probably could forego culturing and be treated directly. Culturing and treating in a few days if the culture is positive is quite safe. Because delay of a day or two in initiating therapy does not increase the risk of rheumatic fever, and because treatment does not shorten the clinical course of pharyngitis, antibiotics can be withheld until culture results are ready. Available techniques for office plating and culturing of pharyngeal specimens are inexpensive and reliable when performed correctly. Proper technique for culturing the throat includes swabbing the tonsils and posterior pharynx. Patients with no clinical evidence of streptococcal infection, and with typical symptoms and signs of viral upper respiratory infection, do not need a throat culture; the incidence of streptococcal infection in this group has been found to be less than 5 per cent.

Although the throat culture remains the standard for identification of streptococcal pharyngitis, it has some shortcomings. Not all patients with positive cultures have infection; it has been estimated that the carrier rate is as high as 20 to 30 per cent. This represents colonization rather than true infection. There is some evidence to suggest that patients with cultures showing less than 10 colonies per plate are either colonized or have very mild infection that is not likely to lead to serious sequelae. Definitive identification of significant infection with risk of rheumatic fever necessitates serologic testing for an antibody response. Such testing is of little practical use because results do not become available in time to be of help. Some researchers have looked into the use the *Gram stain* to aid in prompt identification of patients with streptococcal infection. Although reports from one group are very enthusiastic, others have found large numbers of false-positive and false-negative results when readings are carried out by inexperienced individuals.

In sum, despite the frequency of sore throat and the risk of resultant rheumatic fever, no firm guidelines are available for selection of patients in whom throat cultures are indicated. Even when the culture is positive for group A strep, there is at present, no clinically proven method to distinguish between the carrier state and active infection without waiting for the results of serologic tests.

Viral pharyngitis due to respiratory pathogens is essentially a clinical diagnosis and requires no laboratory investigation. On the other hand, the patient with sore throat and diffuse lymphadenopathy, splenomegaly or pharyngeal petechiae deserves evaluation for infectious mononucleosis. A *heterophile* should be obtained, provided there is no prior history of infectious mononucleosis (prior infection renders the patient immune to the virus). It is important to recognize that it may take as long as 3 weeks for the heterophile to become positive, and, therefore, a negative result in a patient suspected of having mononucleosis is indication for having a repeat test in a few weeks.

The patient with a history of orogenital contact should be cultured for gonococcal infection (see Chapter 113). Some cultures for gonococci will grow out meningococci, which in most instances represents a carrier state. Suspected candidal infection can be confirmed by scraping off the exudate and examining a wet prep.

PRINCIPLES OF MANAGEMENT AND THERAPEUTIC RECOMMENDATIONS

The rationale for treating group A streptococcal infection is to prevent rheumatic fever, suppurative complications such as peritonsillar or retropharyngeal abscess, and the spread of streptococcal infection. Treatment does not shorten the course of the pharyngitis.

Rheumatic fever can be prevented by prompt eradication of *Strep. pyogenes* from the throat. The attack rate for rheumatic fever is reduced by over 90 per cent if antibiotic therapy is instituted within a week of the onset of sore throat. However, the efficacy of prophylactic therapy is substantially reduced if there is a marked delay in initiating treatment. Starting antibiotics 2 weeks after sore throat is first noted is associated with a reduction in attack rate of only 67 per cent, and delaying treatment until 3 weeks into the illness provides no more than a 40 reduction in attack rate.

To be effective, antibiotic therapy must completely eradicate the streptococcus from the pharynx. This can be achieved by a single intramuscular injection of 1.2 million units of benzathine penicillin or a 10-day course of oral penicillin V, 250 mg. four times per day. The advantages of the intramuscular route are the certainty of full treatment and convenience; its major disadvantage is a five- to tenfold increase in the incidence of serious allergic reactions to penicillin. In the patient allergic to penicillin, oral erythromycin, 250 mg. four times daily for 10 days, is an effective alternate. Treatment of asymptomatic individuals who have small numbers of group A streptococci on throat culture is probably unnecessary, except in very high-risk patients who have a prior history of rheumatic fever; however most of these patients should already be on prophylactic therapy (see Chapter 12).

The meningococcal carrier state sometimes presents a therapeutic dilemma, in terms of both selecting patients who actually need treatment and choosing antibiotics. Carriers should be treated only when there is evidence of active meningococcal disease in household or dormitory contacts. Penicillin will not eradicate the meningococcal carrier state, and since many strains are now sulfonamide-resistant, either minocycline or rifampin must be used.

In gonococcal pharyngitis, the usual penicillin and tetracycline regimens are effective (see Chapter 133), but spectinomycin is not. In the case of diphtheria, antitoxin is necessary to prevent myocarditis and peripheral neuritis, and is the mainstay of therapy. Both erythromycin and penicillin are effective in eliminating the organism from the upper respiratory tract.

Necrotizing pharyngitis due to fusobacterial infection responds to penicillin and good nutrition. *Candida* infections require gargling with oral nystatin suspension; the frequent administration of large doses may be necessary. Viral sore throats are treated symptomatically. Voice rest, humidification, and lozenges or hard candy provide some relief; saline gargling and aspirin or acetaminophen also help to some extent.

PATIENT EDUCATION

Many patients insist on antibiotic therapy for a sore throat, often because they think they will obtain symptomatic relief more rapidly from such treatment. Much of the unnecessary antibiotic exposure associated with management of pharyngitis is probably due as much to patient insistence as to the physician's desire to do something. When the etiology is viral, patients ought to be informed that antibiotics are not indicated. On the other hand, the patient who proves to have group A streptococcal infection should be carefully instructed on the importance of completing a full 10-day course of antibiotic therapy; otherwise, many patients will stop taking the medication when symptoms resolve.

ANNOTATED BIBLIOGRAPHY

Bisno, A.L.: Diagnosis of streptococcal pharyngitis. Ann. Intern. Med., 90:426, 1979. (*An editorial reviewing the difficulties of diagnosing the cause of sore throat, with particular critique of the use of the Gram stain.*)

Crawford, G., Brancato, F., and Holmes, K.K.: Streptococcal pharyngitis: Diagnosis by Gram stain. Ann. Intern. Med., 90:293, 1979. (*A study that argues for the use of Gram stain as a reliable and accurate method for early diagnosis.*)

Glezen, W.P., et al.: Group A streptococci, mycoplasmas, and viruses associated with acute pharyngitis. JAMA, 202:119, 1967. (*A clinical study of the various etiologies of acute pharyngitis.*)

McCloskey, R.V., et al.: The 1970 epidemic of diphtheria in San Antonio. Ann. Intern. Med., 75:495, 1971. (*An overview of 201 patients with diphtheria in a single epidemic.*)

Peter, G., and Smith, A.L.: Group A streptococcal infections of the skin and pharynx. N. Engl. J. Med., 297:311, 1977. (*An authoritative review of the biology of the group A streptococcus with an up-to-date discussion of streptococcal pharyngitis.*)

Tompkins, R.K., Burnes, D.C., and Cable, W.E.: An analysis of the cost-effectiveness of pharyngitis management and acute rheumatic fever prevention. Ann. Intern. Med., 86:481, 1977. (*An examination of various strategies for workup and treatment of sore throat.*)

Walsh, B.T., Bookheim, W.W., Johnson, R.C., and Tompkins, R.K.: Recognition of streptococcal pharyngitis in adults. Arch. Intern. Med., *135*:1493, 1975. *(Attempts to identify a cluster of clinical findings that suggest an increased likelihood of streptococcal infection.)*

Wannamaker, L.W.: Perplexity and precision in the diagnosis of streptococcal pharyngitis. Am. J. Dis. Child., *124*:352, 1972. *(A forthright account*

of the surprising number of uncertainties and controversies surrounding this common problem.)

Weisner, P.J., Tronen, E., Bonin, P., et al.: Clinical spectrum of pharyngeal gonococcal infection. N. Engl. J. Med., *288*:181, 1973. *(A comprehensive study of patients in a venereal disease clinic, describing the incidence, clinical features and therapy of gonococcal pharyngitis.)*

211

Approach to Hiccup

Hiccup is usually a transient, innocuous symptom, but when persistent it may become an exhausting and disabling problem. Intractable hiccup has been attributed to a host of metabolic, peridiaphragmatic, neurologic, and psychogenic conditions, but many cases are of unknown etiology. The primary physician should be able to offer the exasperated patient symptomatic relief while conducting a judicious evaluation to determine the source of difficulty.

PATHOPHYSIOLOGY AND CLINICAL PRESENTATIONS

No useful function has been found for the hiccup, which occurs as a result of synchronous clonic spasm of intercostal muscles and diaphragm that causes sudden inspiration followed by prompt closure of the glottis and inhibition of respiratory activity. It is believed to be a reflex. There is debate about whether it is centrally mediated. The afferent pathway is from T-10 to T-12, and the efferent limb is along the phrenic nerve. During the hiccup, the glottis is closed. Some investigators believe the hiccup is related more to gastrointestinal than to respiratory function. Current understanding of pathophysiology does not yet permit an explanation of how the presumptive etiologies operate to produce the hiccup, though the classic explanation is that it is due to stimulation of the phrenic nerve.

It is often unclear whether the reported causes of hiccup are etiologies or only associations. In a series of 220 cases seen at the Mayo Clinic men outnumbered women by 5 to 1, and most were in their 60s. Over 90 per cent of the women had no concurrent illness other than an emotional problem, whereas only 7 per cent of men were labeled as having a psycho-

genic disorder. About 20 per cent of men who experienced hiccup did so after undergoing intra-abdominal, intrathoracic, or neurologic surgery. About 25 per cent had a diaphragmatic hernia, another 20 per cent had cerebrovascular disease or another CNS problem, 5 per cent had a metabolic illness, and in 10 per cent no associated disease or psychiatric problem was identified.

DIFFERENTIAL DIAGNOSIS

The causes of hiccup typically listed are clinical associations and cannot be considered proven etiologies (Table 211–1).

WORKUP

Persistent hiccup that proves refractory to simple measures is an indication for further investigation. Extensive workup is usually not very productive, but a check for a previously unsuspected metabolic or subdiaphragmatic process is sometimes rewarding.

History. Questioning should include inquiry into recent abdominal, thoracic, or neurologic surgery, abdominal pain (especially that which radiates to the tip of the shoulder or is worsened by respiration), prior renal disease, excess consumption of alcohol, fever, cough, diabetes, and emotional problems. Also of help is reviewing the various methods that the patient has tried for relief of symptoms. Any neurologic complaints should be noted.

Physical examination should include a temperature determination, percussion of the lungs for evidence of reduced diaphragmatic excursion, and aus-

Table 211-1.   Conditions Associated with Hiccup*

A. Diaphragmatic Irritation/Gastrointestinal Disease

 1. Pericarditis
 2. Tumor
 3. Subdiaphragmatic abscess
 4. Pneumonia
 5. Pleuritis
 6. Myocardial infarction
 7. Hiatus hernia
 8. Peritonitis
 9. Gastric dilatation
10. Pancreatitis
11. Biliary tract disease

B. Metabolic Disturbances

 1. Uremia
 2. Diabetes
 3. Alcoholism

C. CNS Disease

 1. Tumor
 2. Infection
 3. Surgery

D. Psychogenic Disease

 1. Hysteria
 2. Anorexia nervosa
 3. Anxiety

* These are not proven etiologies.

cultation for signs of an infiltrate, effusion, or pleuritis. The abdomen is examined for distention, organomegaly, upper abdominal tenderness, and signs of peritonitis. A careful neurologic examination is needed if there is a history of neurologic difficulties.

Laboratory studies. If a peridiaphragmatic process is suspected, a chest film followed by fluoroscopy may reveal an effusion or a paralyzed hemidiaphragm indicative of a subdiaphragmatic condition. A BUN and creatinine are worth obtaining if there is suspicion of a metabolic etiology. A costly gastrointestinal workup that includes barium studies is not indicated, unless there is definite clinical evidence of an intra-abdominal problem. Watchful waiting is often appropriate if the workup is unrevealing.

SYMPTOMATIC THERAPY AND INDICATION FOR REFERRAL

The plethora of drugs, folk medicines and bizarre maneuvers that have been suggested for relief of hic-cup attests to the absence of a universally effective therapy. The common denominator in the myriad of treatments is interruption of respiration. The popular approaches of breath-holding or rebreathing into a paper bag to raise CO_2 reduce the amplitude but not the frequency of hiccups. Swallowing a teaspoonful of sugar, which is thought to overload the afferent limb of the hiccup reflex and counteract the original stimulus, has been reported to be effective. Inserting a catheter to stimulate the pharynx opposite C2-3 is believed to interrupt the afferent pathway; its success rate is quite impressive.

At the onset of hiccups, the patient can be instructed to try a simple measure such as swallowing dry granulated sugar or stimulating the nasopharynx with a Q-tip; one of these often suffices. If both fail, pharyngeal stimulation with a catheter can be carried out in the office.

Many drugs have been employed in the therapy of hiccups; most are without inpressive results. Drugs which have been tried include antidepressants, amphetamines, diazepam, haloperidol, phenytoin, and barbiturates. Chlorpromazine, 50 mg. IV, is probably the most effective pharmacologic treatment. The oral and intramuscular routes have not been found to be as effective. Metoclopramide, 10 mg. every six hours for 10 days, has also been reported to stop hiccups; the relapse rate associated with its use is low.

In the rare patient whose hiccups prove intractable to mechanical and pharmacologic interventions, anesthesiologic and surgical consultations should be obtained for consideration of a phrenic nerve procedure to abolish the symptom.

ANNOTATED BIBLIOGRAPHY

Editorial: Hiccup. Br. Med. J., *1*:235, 1971. *(A terse review of pathophysiology and the significance of the hiccup.)*

Engleman, E.G., Lankton, J., and Leakton, B.: Granulated sugar as treatment for hiccups in conscious patients. N. Engl. J. Med., *285*:1489, 1971. *(A letter reported successful relief of hiccups in 19/20 patients following swallowing a teaspoon of ordinary dry, white sugar.)*

Salem, M.R., *et al.*: Treatment of hiccups by pharyngeal stimulation in anesthetized and conscious subjects. JAMA, *202*:321, 1967. *(Therapeutic success in 84/86 patients by introduction of a catheter through the nose and stimulating the pharynx at the level of C2-3. The suggested mechanism is inhibition of afferent impulses transmitted through the vagi.)*

Samuels, L.: Hiccup: A ten-year review of anatomy, etiology, and treatment. Can. Med. Assoc. J., 67:315, 1952. *(The classic hiccup paper with differential diagnosis.)*

Souadjian, J.V. *et al.*: Intractable hiccup: Etiologic factors in 220 patients. Postgrad. Med., *43*:72, 1968. *(A review of 220 patients from the Mayo Clinic presenting probable causes and arguing for a psychogenic etiology in 92 per cent of females in the series.)*

Williamson, B.W.A., and MacIntyre, J.M.C.: Management of intractable hiccup. Br. Med. J., 2:501, 1977. *(A succinct review of therapeutic approaches, finding chlorpromazine and metoclopramide the most effective drugs; 39 refs.)*

212
Approach to the Patient with Chronic Nasal Congestion and Discharge

It is estimated that 15 to 20 per cent of the population suffers from recurrent or chronic nasal problems. Allergic rhinitis accounts for many such cases, but vasomotor rhinitis, mechanical obstruction, certain drugs, and abuse of decongestants are also responsible for symptoms in many people. These conditions cause a great deal of discomfort and absenteeism, and result in the expenditure of many millions of dollars for therapy. The primary physician needs to be able to distinguish an allergic etiology from one due to obstruction, inflammation or vasomotor instability. Moreover, one must know the proper uses of antihistamines, decongestants and topical corticosteroids as well as the indications for skin testing and referral to the allergist or ENT specialist.

PATHOPHYSIOLOGY AND CLINICAL PRESENTATION

Allergic rhinitis is due to IgE-mediated release of histamine, slow-reacting substance, bradykinin and other mediators from mast cells in the nasal mucosa, resulting in nasal congestion and rhinitis. The reaction develops in response to inhalation of allergen that forms antigen-IgE complexes on receptors in the nasal mucosa. The condition is *seasonal* when the antigen is a pollen ("hay fever") and *perennial* when the allergens are dusts, molds, or animal danders. Patients with seasonal allergic rhinitis outnumber those with perennial complaints by a ratio of about 10 to 1. It is not unusual for an individual to be allergic to a number of antigens and to show increased sensitivity to chemical irritants as well. The incidence of allergy among patients with normal parents is about 10 per cent; incidence rise to 25 per cent if one parent is allergic, and to 60 per cent if both are.

In some instances, the patient has all the earmarks of perennial allergic rhinitis but no evidence of IgE mediation, and skin tests for inhaled allergens are negative. Such patients have been designated as having *nonallergic rhinitis,* even though their nasal secretions often contain large numbers of eosinophils and they respond to corticosteroids.

Onset of allergic rhinitis is usually during childhood, but may occur at any age; childhood cases frequently continue into adulthood. Some patients have asthma, but there is no evidence that allergic rhinitis predisposes to development of asthma. However, there is an increased incidence of recurrent upper respiratory infections and sinusitis. Patients often improve with time.

Nasal congestion, sneezing, and profuse watery discharge dominate the initial clinical presentation. Itching of the nose, throat, and eyes is common, as is postnasal drip and tearing. Often the nasal mucosa appears pale and edematous. Symptoms typically vary over the course of the day; they are most severe in the morning, lessen in the afternoon, and worsen again by evening.

Vasomotor rhinitis may mimic perennial allergic rhinitis and is felt by some clinicians to be a diagnosis of exclusion when no allergen is identified. Others consider the condition a readily distinguishable entity characterized by a normal appearing nasal mucosa and persistent nasal stuffiness without itching, that is worsened by changes in ambient temperature and humidity. Although congestion is the most prominent symptom, a discharge may also be present. Sneezing is relatively absent. The pathophysiology is poorly understood but believed to involve abnormal autonomic responsiveness and vascular dilatation of the submucosal vessels. IgE levels are normal and the number of eosinophils in nasal secretions is usually, but not always, normal. Abnormal autonomic reactivity is felt to account for the nasal stuffiness or rhinorrhea sometimes occurring with *emotional upset* and *sexual arousal*.

Drugs. Overuse of topical alpha-adrenergic *nasal decongestants* (rhinitis medicamentosa) can result in a worsening of symptoms. Response to these agents becomes blunted (tachyphylaxis), leading to increased use, often on an hourly basis. As soon as the vasoconstrictor effect subsides, nasal stuffiness returns worse than ever, presumably due to marked reflex vasodilatation. The nasal mucosa appears erythematous. The problem resolves in 2 to 3 weeks if topical decongestants are stopped. Agents with adrenergic blocking activity can aggravate preexisting rhinitis and cause mild nasal congestion even in normal patients. *Reserpine* and *guanethidine* are the major offenders.

Hormonal etiologies. *Hypothyroidism* and *pregnancy* may cause the turbinates to become pale and edematous, leading to nasal congestion. Hypothyroidism may otherwise be subclinical save for the chronic nasal obstruction. Symptoms resolve with correction of the hypothyroidism or with delivery.

Mechanical obstruction. Unilateral congestion and discharge are characteristic of mechanical obstruction due to tumor, polyp or deviated septum. *Neoplasm* is rare but is suggested by a blood-tinged discharge. *Polyps* occur in association with allergic and vasomotor rhinitis, chronic sinusitis, aspirin-induced asthma, cystic fibrosis and reserpine use. The mechanism of formation is unknown. Polyps move freely since they are pedunculated and nontender, and appear as soft, pale gray, smooth structures. Patients with asthma and nasal polyps are often hypersensitive to aspirin. Polyps do not regress spontaneously and may become large or multiple, causing considerable obstruction. A *deviated septum* is sometimes the source of obstructive symptoms. Most are not traumatic in origin and develop during growth. Associated sinus occlusion is rare.

Obstruction due to crusting is seen with *atrophic rhinitis*. The condition is of unknown etiology, appears mostly in women, and is characterized by dry atrophic nasal turbinates, mucosal crusts and a foul or fetid greenish discharge referred to as ozena. The purulent discharge is believed due to secondary infection.

Chronic inflammatory disease. A number of serious chronic inflammatory conditions may cause obstruction. *Midline granuloma* is an uncommon illness of unknown etiology that causes ulcerative destruction of upper respiratory tract structures. It oftens presents as nasal stuffiness, crusting and granulations, but progresses steadily as ulcerations form in the nasal septum and elsewhere. The majority of patients are over 50 and many have histories of allergic rhinitis. *Wegener's granulomatosis* may have a similar insidious presentation with nasal obstruction, rhinorrhea or chronic sinusitis. Necrotizing granulomatous lesions and vasculitis are found in the upper and lower airway. Middle-aged men and women are equally affected. *Sarcoidosis* may present as bilateral nasal obstruction.

Table 212–1.   Important Causes of Chronic or Recurrent Nasal Congestion

A. Allergic

  1. Seasonal allergic rhinitis (pollens)
  2. Perennial allergic rhinitis (dusts, molds)

B. Vasomotor

  1. Idiopathic (vasomotor rhinitis)
  2. Abuse of nose drops
  3. Drugs (reserpine, guanethidine, prazosin)
  4. Psychological stimulation (anger, sexual arousal)

C. Mechanical

  1. Polyps
  2. Tumor
  3. Deviated septum
  4. Crusting (as in atrophic rhinitis)
  5. Hypertrophied turbinates (chronic vasomotor rhinitis)
  6. Foreign body (usually in children)

D. Chronic Inflammatory

  1. Sarcoidosis
  2. Wegener's granulomatosis
  3. Midline granuloma

E. Infectious

  1. Atrophic rhinitis (secondary infection)

F. Hormonal

  1. Pregnancy
  2. Hypothyroidism

DIFFERENTIAL DIAGNOSIS

The causes of nasal congestion and discharge can be organized pathophysiologically and are listed in table 212–1.

WORKUP

Although it is important to rule out mechanical obstruction, chronic inflammatory disease, and drug-induced illness, the usual diagnostic problem is to distinguish between allergic and vasomotor disease.

History should focus on timing of symptoms and aggravating and alleviating factors. Nasal congestion that coincides with periods of pollenation is virtually diagnostic of seasonal allergic rhinitis. Continuous waxing and waning of symptoms throughout the year, with exacerbations during the hay fever season, suggests a combination of perennial and seasonal allergic disease.

When symptoms occur chronically without respect to seasons, one may be dealing with vasomotor rhinitis, perennial allergy, mechanical obstruction or a chronic inflammatory condition. Perennial rhinitis is a possibility when the patient reports frequent "colds."

Patients bothered by dusts are generally atopic, whereas those whose symptoms are aggravated by quick changes in temperature, emotion, or drugs fall into the vasomotor category. Use of antihypertensive agents and topical nasal decongestants needs to be explored, as does exposure to fur-bearing animals, feathers, other possible sources of animal danders, or chemical irritants. Pollutants are often more irritating to allergic patients, but may also cause symptoms in nonatopic people.

Symptoms accompanying nasal congestion sometimes provide useful diagnostic clues. Fever and a purulent nasal discharge are evidence of an infectious etiology. A cold is the most likely cause of acute discharge, but chronic discharge that is fetid, foul-smelling and accompanied by crusting indicates secondary infection as in atrophic rhinitis, Wegener's granulomatosis or midline granuloma. Bloody discharge and unilateral obstruction suggest tumor. Mechanical obstructions are often unilateral as well. The presence of asthma or aspirin sensitivity increases the likelihood of nasal polyps. Sneezing, postnasal drip and itching are nonspecific and of little help in distinguishing among etiologies. When the cause is obscure, exploration of hypothyroid symptoms and or possible pregnancy may provide explanations.

Epidemiologic data need to be considered. Onset in childhood is typical of allergic disease, but onset of symptoms during adulthood does not rule out atopy. When chronic progressive nasal congestion develops in a middle-aged patient, particularly a woman, one must consider atrophic rhinitis or one of the necrotizing inflammatory diseases. The allergy histories of the patient's parents should be ascertained.

Physical examination includes inspection of the nasal mucous membranes for color, atrophy, edema, crusting and discharge; the presence of polyps, erosions, and septal perforations or deviations should be noted. A nasal speculum markedly improves visualization of the nasal cavity and ought to be used in every examination. Some findings are nonspecific. For example, a pale boggy appearance to the mucosa is allegedly a classic sign of allergic disease, but erythema sometimes occurs in allergy and certainly does not rule it out. Transillumination and percussion of the sinuses, pharyngeal examination for erythema and discharge, a look in the ears for evidence of otitis, cervical node examination for adenopathy, and auscultation of the chest for wheezes complete the physical examination.

Laboratory studies. When the differentiation between allergic and nonallergic disease is difficult to make on the basis of clinical findings, *skin testing* might prove helpful. Preparations of commonly inhaled allergens (dusts, molds, animal danders, and local pollens) are injected into the skin to see if there is an immediate wheal and flare reaction. A positive skin test only indicates atopy. Correlation with history and physical examination is needed to establish an etiologic role for the antigen. Antihistamines must be omitted for 12 to 24 hours before testing to avoid a false-negative result. A common cause of false-positive testing is the presence of dermographism; because 15 to 20 per cent of the population exhibits dermographism, a saline control injection should be given along with injections of allergens.

Other studies are available for detection of an allergic etiology, but are not as inexpensive, easily performed, or necessarily more sensitive than skin testing; moreover, results of some tests take over a week to become available. Determination of *total IgE* is helpful if the level is markedly elevated, but some cases of allergic rhinitis are not associated with high serum concentrations. Thus a normal result is not useful for diagnosis. The same is true for the *total eosinophil count.* A count at the time of an exaceration that is in excess of 500 cells per mm^3 is suggestive of an allergic etiology. The absence of peripheral eosinophilia does not rule out allergic rhinitis. Smears of nasal secretions for eosinophils should be done but are of limited specificity, because eosinphils may be present in substantial numbers in both vasomotor and allergic rhinitis. The smears can be of use when infection is in question, because neutrophils should be in abundance.

Purulent discharges not associated with an obvious cold are worth culturing. Sinus films should be obtained if fever, facial asymmetry, opacification or tenderness suggests an accompanying sinusitis (see Chapter 209).

PRINCIPLES OF MANAGEMENT AND PATIENT EDUCATION

Allergic rhinitis. The basic approach to relief of symptoms begins with *avoidance of known allergens.* Patients with allergic seasonal rhinitis can be advised to avoid long walks in the woods during the pollination period and to stay indoors with the windows closed when symptoms are severe and the pollen count is high (e.g., hot windy sunny days). Some patients find air conditioners helpful, but the machine's filter does little to remove pollen from the air. The air conditioner simply makes it more tolerable to stay indoors with the windows closed on a hot day. The hot air vent on the air conditioner should be kept closed to avoid the intake of pollinated air. If ragweed is a problem, daisies, dahlias and chrysanthemums should not be kept indoors. Preventing accumulation of excess dust in the bedroom and avoiding irritants such as tobacco smoke, chemical vapors and strong perfumes lessen symptoms.

Control of perennial allergic rhinitis requires particular attention to allergens in the home, but recommendations should be practical. Cleaning the house and especially the bedroom with a damp mop two to three times a week will reduce dust. Feather pillows should be replaced by Dacron or polyester ones, and mattresses should be covered with an elastic fabric casing. Areas where mold can collect, such as piles of old newspapers or furniture in a damp basement, should be cleaned up. A dehumidifier may prevent mold growth. Throwing out carpets and draperies is excessive, but new furnishings made of synthetic fabrics are preferable to cotton and wool to minimize dust collection. Humidification of air in winter also helps keep down dusts. Patients allergic to molds should avoid having African violets and geraniums in

the home. No new fur-bearing pets should be obtained; most pets usually have to be removed from the home entirely if symptoms are disabling. Simply keeping the pet out of the bedroom does not help sufficiently, because the dander circulates in the air throughout the house.

When history provides ready identification of allergens, there is little need for skin testing, but if drastic environmental measures are being contemplated, documentation of the specific allergens is worthwhile.

Antihistamines and *oral decongestants* work best after environmental measures have been maximized. The best antihistamines for starting therapy are the Class 3 agents, typified by *chlorpheniramine,* because they are potent but least sedating. A typical regimen of chlorpheniramine is 4 mg. every 4 to 6 hours as needed. Fortunately, symptoms usually subside during the middle of the day, allowing a morning and nighttime dose to be sufficient. If drowsiness or nasal congestion are major problems, a sympathomimetic can be added. Long-acting preparations are available for use before bed. *Phenylpropanolamine* is essentially an alpha adrenergic agent; *ephedrine* and *pseudoephedrine* have a combination of alpha and beta effects. All are effective decongestants, but those with beta properties are preferred by some when drowsiness is a problem. A typical regimen is use of pseudoephedrine, 60 mg. every 4 to 6 hours; lower doses may suffice in mild cases. Empirical trials of various antihistamines and decongestants are often necessary to select the best agent(s) and dose(s). Combination preparations are convenient if the fixed doses match the doses needed; these preparations should not be used as initial therapy.

Topical decongestant sprays have a limited role because of the risks of tachyphylaxis and rebound nasal congestion. They are best used for keeping the eustachian tubes patent in patients who ride in airplanes. An application of *phenylephrine* (Neo-Synephrine) or *oxymetazoline* (Afrin) every 3 to 4 hours while patient is airborne should suffice, especially when preceded by an oral decongestant an hour before flight time. Rebound congestion occurs if sprays are used repeatedly for more than 4 or 5 days in a row.

Topical corticosteroids such as *beclomethasone* aerosol have been proven effective in double-blind studies without causing adrenal suppression when used in therapeutic doses (less than 20 inhalations, 1 mg., per day). Both seasonal and perennial allergic rhinitis seem to respond well to beclomethasone. Steroid therapy should be considered when antihistamines and decongestants do not adequately control symptoms.

Cromolyn sodium (see Chapter 45) has been found effective in double-blind crossover studies of patients with allergic rhinitis. The agent is administered either as an inhaled powder or as a dissolved liquid. At present, the agent is not FDA-approved for nasal use and consequently no nasal inhalers are available in the United States. Cromolyn works by preventing degranulation of mast cells and is used prophylactically. Patients with very high IgE levels are most responsive. The literature should be followed for further data on the use of the drug in allergic rhinitis; it probably will be worthy of consideration when other forms of drug therapy fail to alleviate symptoms.

Immunotherapy is indicated as a last resort. Small doses of allergen are administered parenterally over many weeks to stimulate production of blocking antibodies. The therapy should be considered as an adjunct to other forms of treatment, because it usually does not suffice by itself. Patients require skin testing to identify the responsible antigen(s) and a long series of visits for injections. Patient inconvenience and cost are high, while responses are often not dramatic. However, a patient with allergic rhinitis on a full medical regimen who is still inadequately controlled should be referred to the allergist for skin testing and consideration of immunotherapy.

Vasomotor rhinitis. This condition is difficult to treat. Avoidance of tobacco smoke, rapid changes in temperature or humidity, and irritant chemical vapors is helpful. Humidification of the home in winter is also worthwhile. Cessation of nasal spray use is essential; altering antihypertensive medications may be needed. A mild adrenergic agent with some alpha activity (e.g., pseudoephedrine) sometimes provides partial improvement. Addition of an antihistamine may give some extra relief, but is ineffective by itself.

Immunotherapy and steroids are of no proven benefit.

INDICATIONS FOR REFERRAL

The patient should be referred to an otolaryngologist for removal of polyps or foreign bodies, for management of a suspected tumor, necrotizing inflammatory condition or atrophic rhinitis, and for correction of deviated septa. An allergist can be of help when an allergic etiology cannot be distinguished from vasomotor rhinitis, when the antigen(s) must be identified for management purposes, and when immunotherapy is contemplated.

ANNOTATED BIBLIOGRAPHY

Broder, I., *et al.*: Epidemiology of asthma and allergic rhinitis in a total community, Tecumseh, Michigan. IV. Natural history. J. Allergy Clin. Immunol., *54*:100, 1974. *(Demonstrates that asthma is neither a common accompaniment nor a consequence of allergic rhinitis; also showed that the remission rate for perennial allergic rhinitis was 5 to 10 per cent over 4 years of follow-up.)*

Seebohm, P.M.: Allergic and nonallergic rhinitis. *In* Middleton, E., and Ellis, E. (eds.): Allergy: Principles and Practice. St. Louis; C.V. Mosby, 1978, p. 868. *(An excellent critical summary of these conditions, with emphasis on clinically relevant data.)*

Slavin, R.G. Diagnostic tests in clinical allergy. Post Grad. Med., *67*:(3):72, 1980. *(Critical review of skin testing and other techniques used to detect allergic rhinitis.)*

213

Management of Aphthous Stomatitis
WILLIAM V. R. SHELLOW, M.D.

Aphthous stomatitis (canker sores) is a common recurrent condition involving painful ulcers of the oral mucosa. About 20 per cent of the population is affected at one time or other; prevalence is high among upper middle class individuals. The lesions can be very painful, and the primary physician should be capable of providing symptomatic relief.

PATHOPHYSIOLOGY, CLINICAL PRESENTATION AND COURSE

The etiology of aphthous stomatitis has not been established, although there is some evidence for an immunologic pathogenesis. For example, aphthous stomatitis is associated with diseases presumed to be caused by immune mechanisms, such as Crohn's disease and chronic ulcerative colitis. Moreover, exposure to oral epithelial antigens or cross-reacting microbial antigens leads to elevated levels of IgA and production of hemagglutinating antibodies to oral mucosa. Lymphocytes from affected patients cause cytotoxic changes in tissue cultures of oral epithelium. Low titers of antimucosal antibodies have been found in the sera of patients with aphthous stomatitis.

Although the condition seems to involve injury, other factors may be important. For example, an association of aphthous stomatitis with nutritional deficiences of iron, folate and B12 has also been found; lesions clear with correction of the deficiency. Infection seems to play a contributing role; after mucosal breakdown has occurred, the lesions are invaded by mouth flora and become secondarily infected. Emotional stress can precipitate an attack.

Aphthous stomatitis develops in four clinical stages.

1. *Premonitory*—tingling, burning or hyperesthetic sensation, lasting up to 24 hours
2. *Preulcerative*—lasting from 18 hours to 3 days, characterized by moderately painful erythematous macules or papules with erythematous halos
3. *Ulcerative*—lasting 1 to 16 days, characterized by painful discrete ulcers covered by gray yellow membrane with a dusky erythematous halo. Pain ceases during this stage.
4. *Healing*—usually without scarring, averages 2 weeks (range ½ to 5 weeks).

Aphthous ulcers are classified according to size. The majority are "minor," that is, are less than 1 cm. in diameter and appear in crops of four or five. "Major" lesions are greater than 1 cm., solitary, indolent, and heal with scarring. Minor lesions heal without scarring within 7 to 10 days. Lesions are painful and may occur anywhere within the oral cavity. In two-thirds of patients, recurrent lesions do not develop, but in one-third, recurrences continue for up to 40 years.

PRINCIPLES OF THERAPY

Aphthous stomatitis is a difficult problem to treat. The goals of therapy are to provide acute relief and prevent recurrence. *Tetracycline liquid* used as a mouthwash has been the most effective symptomatic therapy. *Carbamide peroxide gel* is an oxidizing agent which releases oxygen on contact with the oral mucosa. It has some bactericidal effect against many mouth organisms and is a mild debriding agent. In the presence of extremely painful lesions, use of *topical anesthetic agents* (e.g., viscous lidocaine) before meals may allow the patient to eat. Avoidance of abrasive foods also helps.

Immunologically targeted therapies have been tried. *Corticosteroids* should be helpful, but the physical environment within the oral cavity makes topical use difficult. Vehicles that help the steroid component cling to the mucous membrane (e.g., Orabase) slows the release of the active ingredient. In cases associated with severe pain, intralesional corticosteroids may be tried by a clinican experienced in their use. *Levamisole,* which stimulates immune response, has been reported efficacious in about two-thirds of cases, but the unknown long-term safety of this antihelmintic agent limits its use.

Women with a definite premenstrual flare may be helped by estrogen-dominated oral contraceptives.

Identification and correction of an existing deficiency of folate, B_{12}, or iron may cure aphthous stomatitis. For lesions precipitated by emotional stress, judicious use of tranquilizers is reasonable. Chemical cauterization by means of silver nitrate sticks ($AgNo_3$) is used by some practitioners to treat acute lesions, but is fraught with the possibility of destroying normal tissue and should not be used by inexperienced physicians. Avoidance of local trauma to the oral mucosa and maintenance of good oral hygiene and nutrition are important supplements to therapy.

THERAPEUTIC RECOMMENDATIONS AND PATIENT EDUCATION

- Any deficiency of iron, B_{12}, or folate should be identified and corrected.
- Tetracycline, 250-mg. capsules, dissolved in a teaspoonful of warm water can be used as a mouthwash three or four times a day. The solution should be expectorated.
- Oxygen-liberating agents such as carbamide peroxide gel have a temporary soothing effect and may supplement tetracycline.
- Viscous lidocaine, 1 teaspoonful, retained in the mouth for several minutes and then expectorated, may allow patients with intense pain to eat.
- Patients should avoid stressful situations as much as possible, and diazepam may be taken before bedtime for a brief period (see Chapter 214).
- Patient education ought to stress good mouth hygiene. The use of a fluoride toothpaste sometimes helps. Patients can be advised to avoid food with sharp surfaces, salt, and talking while chewing and to use a soft-bristled toothbrush. It may be comforting for the patient to know that the condition is self-limited, though the possibility of recurrence should also be explained.

ANNOTATED BIBLIOGRAPHY

Cooke, B.E.D.: Recurrent oral ulceration. Br. J. Dermatol., *81*:159, 1969. *(Classification of the various types of recurrent aphthous lesions.)*

Lehner, T.: Immunologic aspects of recurrent oral ulcers. Oral Surg., *33*:80, 1972. *(Discusses the various immunologic changes which have been described in recurrent aphthous stomatitis.)*

Olson, J. A., Nelms, C., Silverman, S., and Spitler, L.E.: Levamisole, a new treatment for recurrent aphthous stomatitis. Oral Surg., *41*:588, 1976. *(The use of levamisole in the treatment of this condition. Open trial in 50 patients: 6 per cent remission, 56 per cent improvement, 38 per cent no change.)*

Sircus, W., Church, R., and Kelleher, J.: Recurrent aphthous ulceration of the mouth. A study of the natural history, history, aetiology and treatment. Q. J. Med., *26*:235, 1957. *(An investigation of the natural history and factors which affect course.)*

Stanely, H.R.: Aphthous lesions. Oral Surg., *33*:407, 1972. *(Description of the various stages of aphthous lesions and their duration.)*

15

Psychiatric and Behavioral Problems

214

Approach to the Patient with Anxiety

ARTHUR J. BARSKY, III, M.D.

Anxiety is a common precipitant of bodily complaints and accounts for a substantial proportion of the symptoms encountered in office practice. It may be a manifestation of unresolved psychological conflict, a normal response to the threat of illness, a reaction to situational stress, or a symptom of a medical problem. Many anxious patients concentrate on their physical complaints, convinced that there is a serious medical cause. Psychologically minded patients are likely to attribute their symptoms to emotional factors, but still may come to the physician for reassurance.

The primary physician needs to be expert in clinically distinguishing bodily complaints due to anxiety from those which originate from an underlying medical problem, without resorting to elaborate and expensive testing (see Chapters 14, 20, 53, 58, 95, 153, 154, 156). Unfortunately, many patients are subjected to much unnecessary laboratory workup, sometimes at their own insistence. On the other hand, it is equally important to avoid dismissing the patient's symptoms after only a cursory history and physical examination; patients are all too often sent home with a tranquilizer prescription and perfunctory reassurance that "it's only nerves."

Although recognition of anxiety is relatively straightforward, the identification of its etiology requires a thorough consideration of the patient's psychosocial status. Defining the source of anxiety is essential to designing a safe and effective treatment plan and avoiding excessive tranquilizer use, a problem that has reached major proportions nationally.

PSYCHOPATHOPHYSIOLOGY AND CLINICAL PRESENTATION

Anxiety ranges from a vague sense of uneasiness to one of imminent danger or dread. It may include cognitive and somatic symptoms as well as the characteristic affect. Thinking is accelerated and concentration is difficult. Anxious patients have a heightened self-awareness and an exaggerated startle response. They usually admit to feeling nervous and may report difficulty falling asleep (see Chapter 200). Restlessness, a quavering voice, bitten fingernails, garrulousness, tremor, tics, and excessive sweating are often noticeable. Physical complaints are common; even minor bodily sensations may become a source of concern. Autonomic activity is increased. Sympathetic discharge can cause palpitations, flushing, and sweating; blurred vision may develop if pupillary dilatation becomes marked. In the bowel, autonomic influences may contribute to nausea, vomiting, diarrhea, or abdominal pain. With acute attacks of severe anxiety, the patient may begin to hyperventilate, which can cause the pCO_2 to fall and result in light-headedness and paresthesias, including circumoral numbness and tingling.

Situational anxiety is a normal reaction to illness and other environmental threats and stresses, whether emotional or physical. It is usually self-limited, resolving as the stress subsides. In *post-traumatic anxiety,* survivors of unanticipated and tragic events have recurrent nightmares, restlessness, and frequent reexperiencing of the tragedy. These patients become socially withdrawn and experience profound feelings of inadequacy.

Psychopathologic anxiety includes anxiety neurosis, prepsychotic terror, and agitated depression. *Anxiety neurosis* often reflects unresolved internal psychological conflict over such issues as aggression or sexuality. It includes both chronic, free-floating anxiety and recurrent anxiety attacks with sharply defined onset and spontaneous termination. These attacks occur without forewarning, last from minutes to hours, and leave the patient exhausted. *Prepsychotic terror* is intense, incessant anxiety with personality disintegration, hallucinations, and delusions. *Agitated depressions* (see Chapter 215) are characterized by marked restlessness and anxiety, constant worry, and preoccupation with depressive thoughts; neurovegetative signs are often present. Many such patients are middle-aged or elderly and seem to suffer from an endogenous involutional type of depression.

Medical and pharmacologic etiologies. Anxiety is a prominent symptom of conditions associated with catecholamine excess, such as pheochromocytoma (see Chapter 20), hyperthyroidism (see Chapter 99), hypoglycemia (see Chapter 95), and acute hypoxia. The use of cocaine, amphetamines, hallucinogens, caffeine, exogenous thyroxine, corticosteroids (see Chapter 101) and, in the elderly, barbiturates may cause the patient to feel anxious. Anxiety may be severe during the withdrawal syndrome that follows discontinuation of any addicting agent.

DIFFERENTIAL DIAGNOSIS

Anxiety may have a situational, intrapsychic, or medical cause. It may be a normal reaction to the threat posed by illness, financial problems, family conflict, job stress, or similar situational difficulties. If the patient survives an unexpected tragedy, post-traumatic anxiety may ensue. Anxiety neurosis, agitated depression, and prepsychotic terror constitute the most common intrapsychic etiologies. Pheochromocytoma, thyrotoxicosis, hypoglycemia, acute hypoxia, stimulant drug use, and drug withdrawal are among the responsible medical conditions.

WORKUP

The first task is to determine whether the anxiety is a normal reaction to stress or is a manifestation of either psychiatric or medical illness. The distinction can be based upon the duration, intensity, and precipitants of the patient's anxiety and the degree of functional impairment.

For most patients, the visit to the doctor is in itself anxiety-provoking. Prompt resolution of nervousness during the course of the visit is characteristic of this normal situational anxiety. However, persistence of anxiety and excessive concern about a multitude of minor bodily sensations suggest underlying psychopathology. Moreover, if the anxiety seems abnormally intense, disabling, and unrelated to environmental stress, the physician is obligated to search for psychological and medical precipitants.

The patient needs to be encouraged to provide a detailed psychosocial history, including an account of interpersonal relationships and any troubling emotional experiences. Questioning is most effective if done in a sympathetic, nonjudgmental, facilitative manner; interrogation often meets with resistance. Patients who are most concerned about bodily symptoms may be reluctant to talk about "nonmedical" issues, unless the rationale for doing so is made clear and they are assured of a full medical assessment. Otherwise, they are likely to feel that the evaluation is incomplete and that their physical complaints are not being taken seriously.

A report of discrete, paroxysmal anxiety attacks that occur without discernible cause is indicative of neurotic anxiety. The patient who presents with chronic nervousness, insomnia, fatigue, irritability, timidity, multiple somatic complaints, and an occasional anxiety attack is likely to have a chronic variant of neurotic anxiety. The presence of other neurotic symptoms (phobias, compulsions, or obsessions), supports the diagnosis; these should be looked for. Anxiety appearing in conjunction with symptoms of depression (see Chapter 215) is indicative of an agitated depression. Acute anxiety may represent the presychotic terror preceding frank psychosis when the patient's thinking is becoming disordered or there is evidence of acute personality disintegration. The patient should be asked about hallucinations and delusions.

In investigating possible medical causes of anxiety, it is essential to check into drug use and the possibility of withdrawal. A nonjudgmental approach is helpful to obtaining an accurate account. Cocaine, amphetamines, hallucinogens, high-dose steroids, and even alcohol and large doses of caffeine can in themselves provoke anxiety. Serum drug levels may be useful to confirm suspicions when the history is incomplete. If the patient has serious heart or lung disease, it is important to consider the possibility of acute hypoxia; agitation is a nonspecific clue but should not be mistaken for psychogenic anxiety. An arterial blood gas determination may be necessary. Anxiety is not a symptom of chronic hypoxia. Hypertension and sympathetic overactivity in conjunction with anxiety are suggestive of a pheochromocytoma; a 24-hour urine collection for metanephrines and VMA is reasonable for screening (see Chapter 20). All anxious patients should be routinely checked for symptoms and signs of hyperthyroidism, but measurements of free thyroxine and total T_3 are necessary only if clinical suspicion is strong. In the diabetic patient, assessment of blood sugar at the time symptoms occur may uncover an insulin reaction. A history of head trauma and loss of consciousness may be important, because anxiety is sometimes a component of a postconcussion syndrome.

Symptoms associated with anxiety may mimic those due to other conditions. When headache (see Chapter 153), abdominal pain (see Chapter 53), shortness of breath (see Chapter 36), dizziness (see Chapter 154), diarrhea (see Chapter 58), palpitations (see Chapter 20), or chest pain (see Chapter 14) is encountered, a thorough medical assessment is necessary. To dismiss a symptom as anxiety-induced without careful workup is potentially dangerous. Fortunately, the history and physical examination are usually sufficient to rule out most underlying organic illnesses.

Although anxiety-provoked symptoms often resemble those due to medical illness, they sometimes have features that are rather characteristic of an underlying anxiety state. For example, chest discomfort that is described as "tightness" lasting hours to days, unrelated to exertion or meals, and unrelieved by nitroglycerin is suggestive of anxiety (of course, anxiety may also precipitate true angina). Shortness of breath at rest that feels like an inability to breathe in enough air, and is accompanied by paresthesias or light-headedness is typical of anxiety-induced dyspnea; sighing and frequent shallow respirations are observed, along with a perfectly normal cardiopulmonary examination and the absence of cyanosis. A headache of the muscle contraction or migrainous variety (see Chapter 153) may be a manifestation of anxiety. Palpitations that are regular in rhythm, normal in rate, and noted mostly at night in a patient with a normal physical examination most likely represent little more than an increased awareness of one's heartbeat. (However, anxiety may trigger a host of dysrhythmias, especially in patients with underlying cardiac disease). Chronic abdominal discomfort that does not disturb sleep (although the patient may awaken for other reasons), occurs independently of meals or the acid peptic cycle, is unresponsive to antacid therapy, and is unaccompanied by change in bowel habits, weight loss, abnormal physical findings or guaiac positivity is very likely to be functional in origin. Barium studies of the upper and lower gastrointestinal tracts usually prove to be unremarkable, but are commonly ordered to reassure both patient and physician. "Dizziness" that is actually a sensation of lightheadedness, unrelated to posture or position, and sometimes accompanied by shortness of breath and paresthesias is indicative of anxiety. Voluntary hyperventilation can be used to reproduce symptoms for diagnostic purposes.

PRINCIPLES OF MANAGEMENT

The patient with symptoms due to anxiety needs meaningful reassurance and empathic support. At times, these efforts need to be supplemented by drug therapy to alleviate bothersome symptoms. The all too common practice of readily prescribing a tranquilizer after superficial evaluation and perfunctory reassurance is ineffective; it often leads to patient dissatisfaction and visits to other physicians for the same complaints. Quickly dismissing symptoms as anxiety-induced usually does little to reduce concern.

Reassurance and support. For reassurance to be effective, it must incorporate a number of important components: eliciting a detailed description of symptoms and their meaning to the patient, performing a thorough physical examination, obtaining necessary and, sometimes, requested laboratory tests, detailing the differential diagnosis, and finally indicating how the data support the diagnosis of anxiety and not the more worrisome conditions that the patient fears. Most patients find it particularly comforting to know that their symptoms are comprehensible, transient, and of no serious consequence. The omission of any step in the sequence can compromise the effort. Perfunctory reassurance is likely to be counterproductive.

The development of a trusting and supportive doctor-patient relationship is central to effective treatment. Eliciting concerns, perceptions, thoughts, and feelings facilitates understanding the patient's experience and conveys a sense of interest. The patient begins to feel that the physician understands and cares. This helps to foster the growth of a therapeutic relationship. When situational anxiety develops in anticipation of a stressful event, the physician can help the patient to prepare realistically for the challenge. If the problem is an anxiety neurosis, supportive psychotherapy aimed at a gentle exploration and discussion of the patient's psychological concerns may prove beneficial. The patient with agitated depression might benefit from expressing his feelings and discussing important losses.

Pharmacologic treatment. All too often tranquilizers are dispensed in lieu of talking to the patient. Drug therapy is most effective when used to supplement the doctor-patient relationship. Properly employed, an antianxiety agent may sufficiently lessen anxiety and its attendant symptoms to facilitate discussion of underlying problems and fears. When drug therapy is abused, attention may be deflected from important psychosocial issues or even from significant medical data. Antianxiety agents work best in patients whose stress is situational. Chronic anxiety neurosis is more refractory, but short-term drug therapy can be helpful during exacerbations. Agitated depression may require a tricyclic antidepressant with sedative action (see Chapter 215).

The benzodiazepines are the preferred class of tranquilizers for use in management of anxiety. Compared to barbiturates, antihistamines, and propanediols, benzodiazepines are more effective and less toxic. Their relatively low lethality when taken in excessive amounts, minor side effects (beyond drowsiness and impaired coordination), few important drug-drug interactions, and low (albeit real) addiction potential at therapeutic doses make them reasonably safe, especially for short-term use. Nevertheless, it is important to remember that their depressant effect on the central nervous system (CNS) is synergistic with that of alcohol and other CNS depressants, making suicide possible when overdoses are taken in combination with other agents.

Onset of antianxiety activity is rapid with benzo-diazepines that are well absorbed. Initially, these effects may be brief due to extensive redistribution throughout the body. Chronic administration can lead to considerable tissue accumulation if drug elimination is slow or metabolites are active. Benzodiazepines are metabolized by the liver; some undergo desmethylation and oxidation, while others are simply conjugated. Those which are conjugated (oxazepam and lorazepam) have a relatively short half-life (Table 214–1) and little tendency to accumulate in the body; multiple doses are required each day. Those which are desmethylated and oxidized (e.g., diazepam and chlordiazepoxide) have metabolites that are biologically active and thus are long-acting (Table 214–1). Daily use of a long-acting benzodiazepine for more than a week or two can result in considerable drug accumulation, with effects persisting for days to weeks after cessation of therapy. Old age and hepatic insufficiency impair drug metabolism and also prolong the effect of a given dose.

Although some benzodiazepines have been promoted for particular problems (e.g., for difficulty sleeping; see Chapter 220), there is no evidence that one is particularly more effective than another for anxiety or sleep. Selection of a given agent should be based on desired duration of action and cost (chlordiazepoxide is now available generically and sells for about a quarter to a third the price of brand name preparations for an equivalent dose). There is no reason to simultaneously use one benzodiazepine for anxiety and another for sleep; excessive doses may result (see Chapter 220).

Several potential problems associated with benzodiazepine use must be kept in mind. First, prescribing a medication for situational stress carries with it a strong covert communication to the patient that a drug can be used in place of a more direct solution to a problem of daily life. Second, because the agents

Table 214–1. Pharmacokinetic Properties of Benzodiazepine Antianxiety Agents

DRUG	ELIMINATION HALF-LIFE (Range in Hours)	NUMBER OF CLINICALLY IMPORTANT ACTIVE METABOLITES	EFFECTIVE DURATION OF CLINICAL ACTION (Due to Parent Drug and Metabolites)
Chlordiaze-poxide	5–30	2–3	Long
Diazepam	20–50	1	Long
Prazepam	36–200	1	Long
Oxazepam	5–10	None	Short
Lorazepam	10–20	None	Intermediate

Adapted from Greenblatt, D.J., and Shader, R.I.: South. Med. J., *71* (Suppl. 2):2, 1978.

are less effective when used in the absence of supportive therapy, there is the danger of the patient's taking excessively large doses to achieve an adequate effect when the drug is used in lieu of a therapeutic doctor-patient relationship. Third, tolerance to the sedative effects of benzodiazepines begins rather early, and there is some addiction potential, although it remains to be more clearly defined. Psychological dependence is probably very widespread, but genuine physiological addiction is uncommon. Duration of therapy and doses required for development of dependence are subjects of ongoing research. At the present time, most authorities favor intermittent use of benzodiazepines at times when anxiety is particularly disabling. A treatment schedule that utilizes several doses each day is reasonable only for the first week or two of therapy; thereafter, a bedtime dose usually suffices if daily therapy is necessary. Tranquilizer therapy should never be continued indefinitely. The need for periodic reassessment of benzodiazepine treatment cannot be overemphasized. Review of its indications and efficacy is essential for avoidance of unnecessary drug use and its attendant complications.

Behavioral techniques can be used for patients with discrete recurrent anxiety attacks, for those troubled by chronic long-standing anxiety, and for those whose anxiety is a reaction to an identifiable environmental stimulus. Relaxation is taught as systematic voluntary muscle relaxation in conjunction with a focusing of attention upon a single thought or bodily process such as breathing. The objective is to enable the patient to induce this state of relaxation whenever he feels anxiety arising or whenever he is confronted with an anxiety-provoking situation.

Referral is indicated for troublesome anxiety neurosis and for agitated depression that does not respond readily to support and drug therapy. Prepsychotic terror is a psychiatric emergency.

PATIENT EDUCATION

The taking of benzodiazepines and other tranquilizers has become so engrained in our society that a great deal of patient education is essential to ensure proper use. It should be made clear that intermittent use is preferable to daily intake on a chronic basis, that psychological and even physiological dependence are possible, that the effects of medication may last long after intake is stopped, and that drug therapy is no substitute for resolving problems that

produce excessive stress. This position can be reinforced by prescribing only a limited amount of medication per unit of time and authorizing no refills. Those patients who rely on tranquilizers to get through the day—they are probably psychologically addicted—will protest such action and try to badger the physician into dispensing more medication. Such patients may be managed with a firm but negotiated approach (see Chapter 1) to reduction of drug use, in which doctor and patient mutually construct and agree to a schedule for diminished tranquilizer intake. The patient usually feels relieved knowing that support is not going to be withdrawn and that medication will be available (albeit in less copious quantities) on a predictable basis.

THERAPEUTIC RECOMMENDATIONS AND INDICATIONS FOR REFERRAL

Situational Anxiety

- Establish a therapeutic alliance with the patient, with emphasis on being supportive and nonjudgmental.
- If the anxiety is based on a fear of illness, take the time to provide thorough and meaningful reassurance.
- In situations in which anxiety develops in anticipation of a recognizable environmental stress, strive to prepare the patient for the situation; preparation includes rehearsing the details of the situation, discussing the feared and desired consequences, and gathering as much information as possible about the challenge.
- If the above procedures are ineffective and the patient frequently confronts the anxiety-provoking stimulus, try relaxation techniques.
- A short course of benzodiazepine therapy can be helpful in treating severe transitory anxiety that is clearly related to situational stress. Therapy can begin with a dose every 6 to 8 hours (e.g., chlordiazepoxide, 5 mg. every 6 to 8 hours), reduced to a single dose before bed as soon as symptoms improve or after a week of three-times-a-day therapy. Need for daily use beyond 2 to 4 weeks requires reassessment.

Anxiety Neurosis

- Begin with evaluation of conflicts in the patient's life.
- Provide supportive counseling, along with gentle

exploration and discussion of the patient's psychological concerns.

- Antianxiety agents are of very limited use in these chronic conditions, and, if used at all, should be taken only intermittently.
- If the patient has recurrent acute anxiety attacks, behavioral relaxation techniques may be helpful.
- If the acute anxiety attacks are accompanied by hyperventilation, instruct the patient to observe his breathing pattern when he is anxious and to breathe into a paper bag or to slow respirations consciously.
- If the patient does not respond, psychiatric referral is indicated. If the patient is particularly bothered by anxiety attacks, the psychiatrist may consider the use of an antidepressant. The patient's prognosis in psychotherapy depends less upon the severity of the symptoms than upon motivation.

Depression

- Encourage discussion of the patient's losses and facilitate the expression of grief (see Chapter 215).
- In anxious depressions, it is necessary to decide whether to treat the anxiety or the depression first. If the depression is more prominent and accompanied by neurovegetative signs, initial treatment with a tricyclic antidepressant is indicated (see Chapter 215). Amitriptyline or doxepin may be the tricyclic of choice, because each is quite sedating. If anxiety and agitation are very prominent and accompanied by the suggestion of prepsychotic or psychotic thinking, treatment may be initiated with an antipsychotic agent, and the antidepressant added later if needed.
- If the patient does not show adequate response to the above measures, obtain a psychiatric consultation.

Prepsychotic Terror

- This is a psychiatric emergency necessitating the immediate initiation of antipsychotic medication and consideration of hospitalization. Refer for psychiatric help.

Medical Conditions

- Hyperthyroidism: see Chapter 99.
- Pheochromocytoma: refer for surgical therapy.
- Insulin reaction, hypoglycemia: see Chapters 95 and 98.

- Acute hypoxia: oxygen therapy (provided the patient does not have chronic obstructive lung disease); arrange for immediate hospitalization.

ANNOTATED BIBLIOGRAPHY

Choice of a benzodiazepine for treatment of anxiety or insomnia. Medical Letter, *19*(12):49, 1977. *(For treating anxiety or insomnia, these consultants believe that chlordiazepoxide is as effective as any other benzodiazepine, with the added advantage of its availability as an inexpensive generic drug.)*

Detre, T.P., and Jarecki, H.G.: Modern Psychiatric Treatment. Philadelphia: J.B. Lippincott, 1971. *(One of the best short textbooks.)*

Enelow, A.J., and Swisher, S.: Interviewing and Patient Care. New York: Oxford University Press, 1972. *(Helps the physician understand the anxiety that arises from fearing one is sick and encountering the physician; suggests how to manage such anxiety in the interview.)*

Granville-Grossman, K.: Recent Advances in Clinical Psychiatry. London: J. & A. Churchill, 1971. *(The biological and descriptive approach to anxiety, particularly its causes, manifestations, and pathophysiology.)*

Greenblatt, D.J., and Shader, R.I.: Benzodiazepines. N. Engl. J. Med., *291*:1011, 1974; *291*:1239, 1974. *(Thorough review of basic and applied pharmacology.)*

Greenblatt, D.J., and Shader, R.I.: Pharmacokinetic understanding of antianxiety drug therapy. South. Med. J., *71* (Suppl. 2):2, 1978. *(A clinically useful review of the metabolism of the benzodiazepines; helpful for deciding on selection of a particular agent.)*

Marks, I., and Lader, M.: Anxiety states (anxiety neurosis): A review. J. Nerv. Ment. Dis., *156*:3, 1973. *(Good survey of the literature on anxiety neurosis.)*

Nemiah, J.C.: Anxiety neurosis. *In* Freedman, A.M., et al. (eds.): Comprehensive Textbook of Psychiatry, ed. 2. Baltimore: Williams & Wilkins, 1975. *(The psychodynamic conceptualization of anxiety, its causes, significance, and importance in psychological conflict.)*

Shader, R.I., and Greenblatt, D.J.: The psychopharmacologic treatment of anxiety states. *In* Shader,

R.I. (ed.): Manual of Psychiatric Therapeutics. Boston: Little, Brown, 1975. *(Concise, clinically relevant, and current; this survey includes a general discussion of the different types of anxiety.)*

Wolpe, J.: Psychotherapy by Reciprocal Inhibition. Palo Alto: Stanford University Press, 1958. *(The classic behavioral text, which includes techniques of relaxation.)*

Woodruff, R.A., Goodwin, D.W., and Guze, S.B.: Psychiatric Diagnosis. New York: Oxford University Press, 1974. *(The descriptive approach to anxiety neurosis.)*

215

Approach to the Patient with Depression

ARTHUR J. BARSKY, III, M.D.

Office medical practice abounds with depressed patients who present with bodily complaints. The primary physician must be familiar with depression's many somatic manifestations, know how to distinguish them from those due to organic illness, and be capable of carrying out supportive and pharmacologic therapies.

PSYCHOPATHOPHYSIOLOGY AND CLINICAL PRESENTATION

There is considerable evidence supporting a biochemical basis for many types of depression. For example, drugs with antidepressant activity are known to alter the brain's metabolism of serotonin and catecholamines. Moreover, agents that have been found to precipitate clinical depression (e.g., reserpine) are known to deplete central nervous system stores of catecholamines. Current research is directed at further elucidating the role of biogenic amines within the limbic system and other parts of the brain.

Depression is a syndrome with affective, cognitive, behavioral, and physical components. The patient feels sad, worthless, guilty, hopeless, and ineffective. Emotional attachments, sources of gratification, and interests seem to wither away. Thinking is slow and indecisive; thoughts are few, barren, and full of self-deprecation. The patient has difficulty concentrating. Recurrent ideas of death and suicide characterize severe cases. Patients appear listless or, on occasion, agitated. The depressed patient finds it difficult to initiate action and to finish a task. Crying spells are common but not universal. Constitutional symptoms—anorexia, early morning awakening, diminished sexual drive, fatigue, and diurnal mood swings—are frequent; these symptoms are termed the neurovegetative cluster. There may also be a potpourri of other physical complaints, including chronic headache and refractory forms of abdominal or low back pain.

One or several of the manifestations of depression may be much more severe than the others; depressive affect may be subtle or even lacking. For example, the patient may complain only of boredom and listlessness. Loss of hope is particularly characteristic, and behavioral manifestations may be the most noteworthy findings in early phases of the illness; routine work becomes overwhelming, minor problems become major, and simple tasks are uncompleted. The depressed person may begin to drink heavily for the first time in his life. Alternatively, the picture may be dominated by chronic somatic complaints; fatigue, difficulty sleeping, impotence, headache, chest tightness, abdominal pain, constipation, and back pain.

In the elderly, depression may mimic dementia. The apathetic, withdrawn, uncooperative aged person who appears forgetful, unkempt, inattentive, and confused may actually be depressed rather than demented (see Chapter 157). At times, both states may occur simultaneously.

There are many types of depression, and there is currently no universally agreed upon classification. *Endogenous depression* refers to circumscribed depressive episodes accompanied by neurovegetative symptoms, occurring in individuals who functioned normally before the episode. There is no clear precipitating event, and the depression has an autonomous quality, in that it does not improve with any favorable changes in the patient's life or environment (such as a family reconciliation or a vacation). When these episodes are recurrent, with periods of complete recovery in between, the patient is said to be suffering from a *primary affective disorder*. If there are only bouts of depression, it is termed *unipolar affective disorder,* and if manic swings occur, the illness is termed *bipolar affective disorder.*

In other patients, chronic and more nearly constant depressive symptoms, evoked by relatively minor stresses, seem to be an integral part of the personality. These people are chronically dissatisfied, self-pitying, irritable, complaining, dependent, pessimistic, and malcontented. They are said to have *characterological depression.*

Middle-aged and elderly patients may have endogenous depressions characterized more by anxiety, agitation, and restlessness than by psychomotor retardation. They are tormented by recurrent worries, suffer from guilt and self-reproach, and display paranoid and hypochondriacal thinking. These are refered to as *agitated or involutional depressions.*

The most common type of depression seems to be reactive, in that it temporally follows, and appears clearly related to a significant life stress or a loss, such as the loss of an important person, a lifelong goal, self-esteem, ability, or health. These *situational* or *reactive depressions* are often self-limited and are usually not accompanied by persistent suicidal thoughts or marked neurovegetative signs; some capacity for enjoyment, at least in certain situations, remains preserved. *Pathological grief reactions* may be considered as one type of reactive depression. Because the patient is unable to mourn normally, there ensues the onset of depressive symptoms.

Depression may be *secondary to a medical illness.* Here depression may even be the first, or major, manifestation of an underlying neoplastic, infectious, metabolic, or neurologic condition.

DIFFERENTIAL DIAGNOSIS

Depression may occur alone or in conjunction with another psychiatric or medical problem. Among the first type are the primary affective disorders and characterological, involutional, and reactive depressions. Important psychiatric conditions that accompany depression are chronic alcoholism, schizophrenia, and dementia. Any disabling or disfiguring medical illness can precipitate reactive depression. In addition, some medical disorders seem specifically to produce mental changes, with depression being one of their characteristic manifestations. These include chronic infections (tuberculosis, brucellosis, mononucleosis, and hepatitis), occult malignancies, endocrine disorders (hypercalcemia, hypothyroidism, and Cushing's disease), metabolic disorders (uremia, liver failure), and neurologic conditions such as stroke, tumor, Parkinson's disease, and multiple sclerosis. Drugs such as reserpine, methyldopa, corticosteroids, oral contraceptives, L-dopa, and sedatives can cause depression; withdrawal from steroids and stimulants may have a similar effect (see Chapter 101).

WORKUP

Depression is protean in its manifestations, and may be so subtle as to be easily overlooked. It is important to keep in mind that its presence may mask other conditions and certainly does not rule out the possibility of organic illness. A thorough history and physical examination are always in order and essential to assessment. Depressed patients who consult primary care physicians often focus on their physical complaints. The first task for the physician is to distinguish the complaints due to depression from those due to an underlying medical condition. A helpful clue to depression is the presence of the characteristic neurovegetative symptoms, especially fatigue, early morning awakening, and alteration of appetite. The presence of multiple bodily complaints involving many organ systems also suggests depression. In addition, a complaint which persists for years without demonstrable pathology may be a sign of chronic depression. Loss of hope is characteristic; even patients with very severe medical problems rarely experience complete loss of hope. Depression should also be considered when the patient seems to feel that he deserves to be sick, or that he is not worth treating.

Psychological data are crucial. The physician should explore the patient's mood, sense of worth, interest and involvement in his environment, and feelings about the future. Does the patient seem to have a negative and critical attitude toward himself? Direct questions about thoughts of death and suicide are mandatory and may be lifesaving. Checking for significant losses and defeats in the patient's life, such as illness, career setbacks, or deaths of family members is most important.

The physician should keep in mind that depression may be one of the early manifestations of a systemic or serious illness. Inquiry is needed about fever, weight loss, adenopathy, change in bowel habits, persistent cough, easy bruising, unexplained or enlarging mass, etc. In addition, drug history ought to be reviewed for use of such agents as reserpine, methyldopa, corticosteroids, barbiturates, amphetamines, L-dopa, and bromides.

Once depression has been identified, it is necessary to estimate its clinical significance. Duration is an important factor: depression that lasts more than 2 months without some clear improvement is a cause for concern. Most normal grief reactions begin to improve after 1 or perhaps 2 months and are predominantly resolved after 6 months. The more severe depressions obliterate the patient's capacity for enjoyment; neither old friends, favorite pasttimes, nor work or other sources of satisfaction give pleasure. Depressions are more serious when they produce significant functional impairment in the social, family or occupational sphere. Psychotic thinking and suicidal thoughts are important signs of severity.

Assessment of the quality and nature of social supports and the family environment is very important because of their central role in the outpatient management of the depressed patient. A complete and thorough physical examination is essential. Not only does it help to rule out an underlying medical cause, it also provides the personal attention and physical contact these patients often lack. The patient's grooming, dress, mood, and interactions can be particularly revealing. The examination should include a check for fever, pallor, adenopathy, organomegaly, breast, abdominal and rectal masses, and signs of thyroid disease, hepatitis, and chronic infection.

When there is no evidence on history or physical examination of a medical condition responsible for the symptoms, it is unlikely that extensive laboratory investigations will be fruitful. However, a few simple tests are indicated which help distinguish other causes of generalized fatigue from depression (see Chapter 5); these include a complete blood count, BUN, serum calcium, erythrocyte sedimentation rate, blood sugar, and thyroid indices.

An all-too-common error in the evaluation of these patients is the substitution of extensive laboratory testing and radiographic procedures for careful history and physical examination. A few additional moments spent talking with and examining the patient may obviate much laboratory testing and have an impressive effect on accuracy of diagnosis.

PRINCIPLES OF MANAGEMENT

The majority of depressions respond to therapy or resolve spontaneously. Although these can be life-threatening disorders, their prognosis has improved dramatically with the advent of antidepressants. Nevertheless, the doctor-patient relationship still remains a primary therapeutic modality. In order to understand the patient and facilitate formation of an alliance, the physician must be willing to listen to the patient's feelings of sadness, guilt, and despair.

The potential for suicide should always be assessed. If the patient does not volunteer the necessary information, the physician needs to inquire specifically about thoughts, impulses, plans, and attempts. Detailed discussion will usually produce sufficient information to estimate how close the patient is to a successful suicide attempt. If the patient has plans for suicide, hospitalization is urgent.

Treatment combines psychological clarification and support, social and environmental interventions, and medication. The specific course of therapy is partially dictated by the type of depression that has been diagnosed. When another psychiatric disorder is present, the treatment must be modified accordingly. When there is a presumed medical etiology, it should be attended to directly. The primary care physician can manage the majority of depressions. Psychiatric consultation or referral is indicated when the patient appears psychotic, has a history of mania, or is suicidal. If, after treatment by the primary physician, the depression does not improve or recurs, psychiatric consultation or referral is similarly indicated.

Supportive therapy. The physician needs to provide reassurance and to function as an accepting, understanding, empathic, yet firm figure. A detailed explanation of the diagnosis can be very beneficial to the fearful patient. For some patients, it is a relief to learn that their distressing symptoms constitute a known, understandable, and treatable clinical entity. The patient can be reassured that most depressions are self-limited and eminently treatable and that recovery is usually complete. However, after an acute episode has resolved, the patient ought to be informed that depressions can recur in some individuals and that it is important to contact the physician at the first suspicion of a recurrence. While conveying hope and optimism, the physician should take care not to dismiss the patient's painful losses and negative feelings as invalid or untrue. Identifying the specific activities, relationships, or interests from which the patient derived his sense of value and self-esteem in the past and encouraging participation in them again, where practicable, can help start the rebuilding process. Attempts should be made to decrease brooding, self-pity, and inactivity; simple concrete tasks or projects with clear, easily attainable, and immediate goals are useful. The patient's attempts to maintain social, vocational, and recreational activities need to be supported. Visiting friends, becoming involved in church or community activities, and substituting some new goals for a recently lost objective are often constructive. The physician should be careful, however, not to set up expectations that the patient cannot meet, lest these then constitute further proof to the patient of his incompetence and worthlessness.

Social and environmental intervention. It is particularly important to involve the family and friends in the treatment plan. Mobilization of social support helps to demonstrate concern and caring, and counteracts the patient's painfully low self-esteem and his notions that no one could care about him. Additionally, social support counters isolation and loneliness and provides some monitoring of the patient's progress and suicide potential. Family members and friends can also help assure that the patient takes his medication and keeps follow-up appointments. In addition, the physician should look for and try to modify specific factors in the environment which are distressing the patient and reinforcing the depression. For example, if job pressures are troublesome, it may be worth speaking with the patient's supervisor at work to alter temporarily the patient's responsibilities or schedule.

Antidepressant medication is most effective in endogenous depressive episodes that are accompanied by the cluster of neurovegetative symptoms. These medications are helpful when the patient's depression is insensitive to any favorable changes in his life, but are not very effective in depressions which are chronic and characterological. The presence or absence of an environmental precipitant is not a predictor of antidepressant response. The *tricyclic antidepressants* are generally the agents of choice; the *monoamine oxidase inhibitors* are reserved for special situations.

Arriving at the proper tricyclic dosage for each patient involves some trial and error and is determined empirically by that individual's clinical response and tolerance to side effects. As much as a thirtyfold difference in serum levels has been demonstrated among patients given the same dose. This appears to be due to individual variation in hepatic microsomal activity, and to the high lipid solubility of these compounds. Standard practice is to start a healthy average-sized adult with 50 mg. amitriptyline, or its equivalent, taken at bedtime. Because of the long half-lives of the tricyclic antidepressants, once-daily dosage achieves adequate serum levels. The dose is then built slowly over about 7 to 10 days to 150 mg. at bedtime This regimen minimizes the discomfort of side effects. In the elderly, one-third to

one-half the standard dose may suffice; increments should be made more slowly. A before bedtime schedule fosters compliance and capitalizes upon the hypnotic effect while minimizing the other uncomfortable side effects. Many of the symptoms of depression, such as constipation, dry mouth, and lassitude, may mimic the minor side effects of these agents and thus should not be used as an indication to discontinue therapy. Full clinical effect of the tricyclic takes between 1 and 4 weeks to become evident. A full trial consists of 4 to 6 weeks at the upper limits of the therapeutic dose range, which is 300 mg. of amitriptyline or its equivalent. A common error is to conclude that tricyclic therapy is ineffective after employing too small a dose for too short a period of time.

Tricyclics differ mainly in their sedative and anticholinergic side effects. Selection of a particular tricyclic agent is based upon the patient's past history and the side effects which the physician may wish to maximize or minimize in the particular case. The best predictor of a positive response to a particular tricyclic is a history of having responded to that agent in the past. Barring that, side effects are the major determinants of selection (Table 215–1). The depressed patient who is anxious, agitated, and troubled by insomnia may benefit from an agent that has considerable sedative activity, such as amitriptyline or doxepin. Conversely, a retarded and withdrawn patient may do best with a less sedating agent such as desipramine. Some patients initially complain of a bothersome groggy or drowsy feeling during the day; they should be cautioned about driving and told that their usual amount of alcohol will worsen the problems.

As a class, tricyclics are relatively strong anticholinergics. Amitriptyline is the most active, followed by imipramine and then doxepin and desipramine. Difficulty in visual accommodation, dry mouth, mild tachycardia, constipation, and urinary hesitancy are common. In men, urinary retention may result when there is prostatic hypertrophy. An anticholinergic, toxic, confusional delirium may be induced, particu-

Table 215–1. Tricyclic Antidepressant Side Effects

DRUG	SEDATIVE ACTIVITY	ANTICHOLINGERGIC ACTIVITY
Amitriptyline	High	High
Imipramine	Moderate	Moderate
Doxepin	High	Moderate
Desipramine	Low	Low

larly in the elderly. If anticholinergic effects are to be avoided, desipramine or doxepin, which have relatively less anticholinergic activity, may be tried. This is particularly important in the elderly (in whom these agents must be used cautiously), since they may be very sensitive to their anticholinergic action.

There are a number of other potentially adverse effects. Fine tremor and subtle memory deficits may develop. In patients with bipolar disease, there is a danger that mania may be precipitated by tricyclic use. In unrecognized psychotic depressions, the tricyclics may unmask the underlying psychosis; an antipsychotic is a more appropriate first drug. Cardiac side effects include orthostatic hypotension (a particular concern in the aged), an array of dysrhythmias (e.g., premature ventricular contractions, supraventricular tachycardias), and reversible electrocardiographic changes (T-wave abnormalities). Allergic reactions such as urticaria, maculopapular rashes, and photosensitivity, and agranulocytosis are rare.

These agents must be used with caution in patients with glaucoma, preexisting cardiac arrhythmias, conduction disturbances, recent myocardial infarction, and prostatic hypertrophy. It also should be borne in mind that tricyclics antagonize the action of guanethidine and clonidine.

When depression has remitted, maintenance of tricyclic therapy is continued for roughly 6 to 8 months before attempts are made to reduce the dosage and cease the medication. The dosage may be reduced over 4 to 6 weeks while a careful watch is maintained for the reemergence of symptoms. Should this occur, the dose is increased to the original level, and withdrawal is attempted after a few more months of therapy. Long-term maintenance is appropriate in some patients with recurrent depressive episodes; a psychiatric consultation is helpful in making this decision.

The patient who fails to respond to tricyclic therapy should be referred for psychiatric consultation. The possible approaches to further treatment include psychotherapy, a trial of a different tricyclic or a monoamine oxidase inhibitor, and electroconvulsive therapy. Selection of a particular modality is based on the type of depression and the seriousness and urgency of the clinical situation.

Chronic tricyclic use has not been associated with dependence or tolerance. However, the therapeutic range of the tricyclics is relatively narrow, and ingestion of amounts over 1 gram is very toxic; ingestion of amounts as low as 1.5 grams (i.e., a 7- to 10-day supply) can be fatal. The physician must always be aware of his patient's suicide potential, and until he knows the patient well, it is prudent to prescribe no more than 1 week's supply at a time.

The not uncommon practice of adding a minor tranquilizer, such as diazepam, for anxiety should not be routine; use of a sedating tricyclic may be more effective and simpler. If the patient evidences any psychotic thinking, an antipsychotic is indicated along with the tricyclic.

PATIENT EDUCATION

Compliance with a tricyclic regimen can be a problem for depressed patients, necessitating much education and close support. The sedative and anticholinergic effects are sometimes poorly tolerated by these patients, who have a very low threshold for bodily complaints. They stop their medications after only a few days of therapy because they feel drowsy or light-headed and notice no improvement in their depression or neurovegetative symptoms. To avoid poor compliance, the physician should discuss with the patient prior to onset of therapy the side effects to be expected (e.g., dry mouth, mild constipation, mild drowsiness) in the initial phases as well as the fact that it may take a few weeks before improvement is noted. The importance of taking the medication on a daily rather than p.r.n. basis also deserves emphasis. Many depressed patients are too preoccupied to remember all that is discussed during the office visit; written instructions can be very helpful. Checking with the patient by phone a week after initiation of antidepressant treatment provides needed support, helps to ensure compliance, and can prevent premature discontinuation of therapy.

THERAPEUTIC RECOMMENDATIONS

- Assess potential for suicide and arrange immediate hospitalization for the patient who admits to having made specific plans for suicide.
- For the nonsuicidal patient who has some social supports, begin with supportive therapy and social and environmental interventions.
- Begin a tricyclic antidepressant for the patient with neurovegetative symptoms.
- Select a tricyclic agent on the basis of its sedative and anticholinergic side effects and the patient's response to any previous tricyclic therapy.
- Starting dose should be approximately one-third to one-quarter the average therapeutic dose (e.g., 50

mg. of amitriptyline) and should be given at bedtime.

- Explain to the patient the expected side effects and reassure him that most tend to abate with time.
- Increase dose by 25 to 50 mg. every 2 or 4 days (more slowly in the elderly) until the dose is in the therapeutic range (for amitriptyline, this is 150 to 300 mg. daily). If side effects are troublesome, build up to therapeutic levels slowly; it may take several weeks. Doses for elderly patients should be one-third to one-half the regular amount.
- Perform a 4- to 6-week trial of the agent at the upper limit of the dose range before concluding that tricyclic therapy is ineffective. If it is, refer the patient for psychiatric consultation.
- Prescribe no more than a week's supply of the tricyclic at a time if there is any risk of suicide.
- Maintain therapy for at least 6 months after the depression has cleared, and then taper gradually.

ANNOTATED BIBLIOGRAPHY

Bladessarini, R.J.: Chemotherapy. *In* Nicholi, A.M. (ed.): The Harvard Guide to Psychiatry. Cambridge: Harvard University Press, 1978. *(Authoritative review by one of the leading researchers in the field.)*

Burgess, A.M., and Lazare, A.: The Bereaved. *In* Community Mental Health Target Populations. Englewood Cliffs: Prentice-Hall, Inc., 1976. *(The diagnosis and management of normal and pathological grief.)*

Freud, S.: Mourning and melancholia. *In* Strachey, J. (ed.): Complete works of Sigmund Freud. Standard edition. London: Hogarth Press, 1958. *(The psychoanalytic distinctions between grief and depression.)*

Glassman, A.H., and Perel, J.M.: The clinical pharmacology of imipramine. Arch. Gen. Psychiatry, 28:649, 1973. *(Imipramine considered as an example of all tricyclic antidepressants in discussion of pharmacodynamics; marked individual variability of blood levels stressed.)*

Hollister, L.E.: Treatment of depression with drugs. Ann. Intern. Med., 89:78, 1978. *(Up-to-date review of antidepressant agents.)*

Klerman, G.L.: Affective disorders. *In* Nicholi, A.M. (ed.): The Harvard Guide to Modern Psychiatry. Cambridge: Harvard University Press, 1978. *(Clear conceptualization of the topic, as well as comprehensive overall discussion.)*

Poe, R.O., Lowell, F.M., and Fox, H.M.: Depression. JAMA, 195:345, 1966. *(Depression found in one-half of all psychiatric consultations in a general hospital; its varied manifestations are presented.)*

Sachar, E.J.: Evaluating depression in the medical patient. *In* Strain, J.J., and Grossman, S. (eds.): Psychological Care of the Medically Ill: A Primer in Liaison Psychiatry. New York: Appleton-Century-Crofts, 1975. *(A nice review of approach to evaluation.)*

Schildkraut, J.J., and Klein, D.F.: The classification and treatment of depressive disorders. *In* Shader, R.I. (ed.): Manual of Psychiatric Therapies. Boston: Little, Brown, 1976. *(Practical review that includes the biochemical aspects of depression.)*

Woodruff, R.A., Goodwin, D.W., and Guze, S.B.: Affective disorders. *In* Psychiatric Diagnosis. New York: Oxford University Press, 1974. *(What is definitely known about the clinical course, family history, and presentations of primary affective disorders.)*

216

Approach to the Patient with Excessive Alcohol Consumption

ARTHUR J. BARSKY, III, M.D.

Alcoholism is a chronic behavioral disorder, defined not by the amount of alcohol consumed but by the development of tolerance, physiological dependence, alcohol-associated physical illness, or disruption of social functioning in a person who drinks regularly. The alcoholic characteristically drinks in spite of strong negative consequences, be they social, vocational, legal, medical or psychological. Twelve per cent of the population drink heavily; i.e., these people drink almost every day and become intoxicated several times a month. Two to 5 per cent of the population meet the criteria for alcoholism, men outnumbering women by approximately 5 to 1.

Evidence of heavy alcohol consumption is sometimes noted during a routine history and physical examination. Most of the time the patient refuses to admit that excessive drinking is a problem and denies any loss of control; occasionally a patient identifies drinking as a means of coping with stress.

The primary physician must assess the significance of alcohol consumption and help the patient to recognize the problem and obtain treatment.

PSYCHOPATHOPHYSIOLOGY AND CLINICAL PRESENTATION

Research has sought to identify social, psychological, and biological precipitants of alcoholism. Several social factors have been found that increase the risk of developing alcoholism; these include family history of alcoholism or of rigid abstinence, alcoholism or abstinence in the spouse, divorced parents or severe parental discord, heavy smoking and position as the last child of a large family. Among women, family history of depression is a very important additional risk factor.

Psychological stimuli that can lead to alcoholism include depression and personality disorders. The depressed patient uses alcohol as an anesthetic against feelings of loss. New onset of heavy drinking in a patient over age 45 is very suggestive of an underlying depression. In the patient with a character disorder, basic needs have never been fulfilled; this leads to dependence on alcohol.

Debate continues about whether alcoholics differ from other people in their biochemical or physiological response to the metabolism of alcohol. Research on this subject is in progress and should be carefully followed for new developments.

Alcoholism usually presents in one of three forms. The first is a subtle presentation; the patient exhibits a pattern of heavy, frequent, but controlled drinking. Overt intoxication is uncommon, and cessation of drinking does not precipitate a withdrawal syndrome. Such people are able to abstain, but often appear to drink heavily in reaction to definable environmental stress. Their level of social and psychological function is close to what it was before they began to drink heavily. Although they do not meet the strict criteria for alcoholism, they can be considered prealcoholic because they have an increased risk of developing a more severe drinking problem.

A second presentation involves those who have lost control over their drinking. Once they begin to drink, they are unable to stop. They often manifest minor physiological withdrawal symptoms upon cessation. These patients sneak drinks, gulp them, drink alone, and drink without eating. They show diminished social and psychological functioning, miss work frequently, avoid social interactions, and exhibit remorse, resentment, and anxiety.

A third presentation occurs among the most severely affected. Alcohol and its procurement are the organizing principles and prime preoccupations of the lives of these people. They feel compelled to drink without cessation and without enjoyment, are intoxicated for long periods, and have major withdrawal symptoms. There is personality disintegration, intellectual impoverishment, and physical deterioration.

Medical sequelae occur in several organ systems. The amount and duration of alcohol consumption necessary to produce tissue damage varies from patient to patient; nutritional status is an important factor. The risk of developing an alcohol-related complication increases considerably in patients who drink in excess over a period of 5 to 10 years. Patients may present with neurologic symptoms such as numbness and tingling in the extremities secondary to peripheral neuropathy, or difficulty with gait due to cerebellar degeneration. If thiamine deficiency becomes severe, a Wernicke-Korsakoff syndrome may develop. Head trauma is particularly common among alcoholics. Alcoholic cardiomyopathy is an important and potentially reversible complication that is manifested by cardiomegaly and congestive heart failure. Upper gastrointestinal problems include abdominal pain, pancreatitis, gastritis or gastric ulceration, and bleeding due to varices or injury to the gastric mucosa. Fatty infiltration and micronodular cirrhosis are classic hepatic consequences of alcoholism. Binge drinking may result in alcoholic hepatitis. Anemia and thrombocytopenia are complications of hypersplenism and folate deficiency.

The characteristic long-term psychological sequelae include diminished cognitive function, untrustworthiness, impaired judgment, anxiety, and severe depression. Sexual dysfunction is very common and linked to both psychological and physiological impairments (see Chapter 217). The possibility of suicide must be respected, for the suicide rate among alcoholics is five times that of the general population.

Social consequences include lowered social and occupational competence, marital separation, divorce, accidents, and legal violations.

DIFFERENTIAL DIAGNOSIS

A number of psychiatric disorders may coexist with alcoholism and often contribute to the drinking behavior. Alcoholism is common among sociopaths and those with personality disorders in which dependency is a prominent feature. Depressed patients are particularly prone to heavy drinking.

Intoxication with alcohol resembles intoxication due to other central nervous system depressants, and the two frequently coexist. A high proportion of suicide attempts utilizing sleeping pills or tranquilizers are made by people who are intoxicated with alcohol. Clinical withdrawal from alcohol is similar to that from sedatives, hypnotics, and tranquilizers; in addition, cross-tolerance and cross-dependence exist between alcohol and other central nervous system depressants.

WORKUP

Evaluation of the patient who drinks heavily requires a nonjudgmental and supportive approach; it is important to avoid accusation and anger. In assessing the seriousness of the patient's drinking, the physician should focus on the consequences of excessive consumption and not on the actual quantities consumed or the applicability of the label "alcoholism," both of which may provoke argument. The objective is to ascertain whether and to what extent drinking is destructive to the patient's life. The loss of control over drinking and the inability to cut back in spite of adverse consequences are important subjects of inquiry. If there is a history of excessive alcohol consumption but no apparent physical or psychological sequelae, the physician should withhold judgment and observe the patient over time. Nevertheless, the patient should be directly confronted about heavy intake and evaluated for an underlying depression (see Chapter 215) or character disorder.

Problem drinking can be identified clinically when a person answers affirmatively to three or more of the following questions: (1) Have you ever thought you should cut down on your drinking? (2) Have you ever been annoyed at others' complaints about your drinking? (3) Have you ever felt guilty about your drinking? (4) Do you ever take morning "eye openers"?

The evaluation of a chronic drinker should include a careful search for evidence of important medical sequelae such as hepatic insufficiency, gastrointestinal bleeding, cirrhosis, peripheral neuropathy, cerebellar degeneration, memory disturbances, head trauma, cardiomyopathy, and malnutrition. Laboratory evaluation ought to include a stool guaiac test, complete blood count, examination of a blood smear, serum albumin, transaminase, and prothrombin time. When there is abdominal pain, a serum amylase test should be included (see Chapters 53 and 72). If symptoms of heart failure are present, a chest x-ray is indicated (see Chapter 27).

CLINICAL COURSE

Alcoholism is a chronic and relapsing disorder whose course, even with treatment, is periodically marked by the resumption of drinking. Within 6 to 12 months of cessation, a majority of patients will have returned to alcohol on at least one occasion. It is not clear that this initial relapse indicates a poor long-term prognosis. The course of untreated alcoholism is extremely variable and unpredictable. The outcome may range from spontaneous remission to precipitous decline that culminates in the classic "skid row" personality, which accounts for only 3 to 5 per cent of all alcoholics. Treatment seems to be more effective than is generally assumed. When abstinence is the criterion of successful outcome, treatment success rates approach 45 to 50 per cent. There is an additional group of alcoholics who recover function yet continue to drink in a controlled fashion in accord with social norms.

PRINCIPLES OF MANAGEMENT

Regardless of the severity of alcoholism, the doctor-patient relationship remains central to any therapeutic program. The physician needs to convey an interest in the entire person, not just in the drinking problem. The alcoholic is usually depressed and pessimistic and has painfully little self-esteem; he anticipates the scorn of others. Since alcoholism is a chronic and relapsing disorder, a temporary return to drinking need not be considered a treatment failure. It is important to avoid responding to the patient with unwarranted anger or excessive pessimism. A successful therapeutic relationship is dependent upon the physician's remaining an accepting, consistently available, concerned, and supportive figure in the patient's life.

As soon as the physician has evidence of excessive alcohol consumption, it must be promptly shared with the patient. Two common mistakes are to collude with the patient in denying that there is a problem and to force the patient to accept a diagnosis prematurely that he cannot yet acknowledge.

The interview should center upon the destructive consequences of the drinking (medical, marital, vocational, financial, legal, etc.) and the need to lessen them. If alcohol is being used to counter stress or psychological problems, physician and patient can begin to jointly explore less destructive ways to deal with them. The focus thus continues to be upon identifying specific undesired experiences and consequences, and then upon devising therapeutic interventions for them.

Treatment strategies can be divided into those that are appropriate for the heavy controlled drinker; for the addicted drinker who manifests social, psychological, or physical disability; and for the severely deteriorated alcoholic.

The Heavy Controlled Drinker

The heavy controlled drinker may be managed entirely by the primary physician. A strong alliance between doctor and patient is crucial to success. Helping the patient maintain the therapeutic effort involves a number of steps:

1. Mutually agreeing upon explicit treatment goals. These goals initially emphasize restraint from drinking, but later may include exploration of the psychological desire for alcohol.
2. Understanding the painful psychological experience that causes the patient to anesthetize himself with alcohol; i.e., determining the precipitating and perpetuating psychological and social factors.
3. Elaborating specific plans to decrease drinking. These may include such measures as cessation of drinking by other family members, removal of all alcohol from the home, and avoidance of social occasions at which alcohol is served.
4. Involving important figures in the patient's life in the therapeutic effort. This should be done only after it has been discussed with the patient and agreed to. This can give the patient tangible evidence that he is not alone and that others do indeed care. Family members need to see the ways that they may inadvertently foster the patient's continued drinking so that they do not hinder recovery.
5. Supplementing therapeutic efforts with selective drug therapy. When drinking results from de-

pression, it may be necessary to utilize a tricyclic antidepressant; a trial should be considered (see Chapter 215). The patient who drinks in response to situational stress may benefit from using a benzodiazepine instead of alcohol (see Chapter 214). The reduction in anxiety often facilitates other therapeutic efforts. Minor tremulousness due to mild withdrawal symptoms also responds well to benzodiazepines. Both anxiety and mild withdrawal can be treated with doses given three or four times for up to 1 week. After 1 week, the dose needs to be reduced, owing to accumulation of the drug.

The Addicted Drinker

Though the primary care physician remains crucial in the treatment of addicted drinkers, this group of patients requires approaches that are more specialized and more intensive. Certain specialized alcohol treatment programs can be helpful. *Alcoholics Anonymous* is the most widely known. Sessions are held in a group format to help the patient improve his social skills, to provide personal support and acceptance, and to foster a sense of self-worth by means of helping others. The group encourages the person to come to view himself more honestly. Those who are most likely to succeed in these situations have sufficient psychological and social skills to tolerate group treatment, and share socioeconomic status, ethnic background, and religious beliefs with the rest of the group.

Disulfiram (Antabuse) is helpful when a patient strongly wants to remain in a state of enforced sobriety so that supportive and psychotherapeutic treatment can be applied to the greatest advantage. Without proper motivation and supportive therapy, the drug in itself is no cure for alcoholism. The drug causes acetaldehyde accumulation when alcohol is consumed. The resultant symptoms include nausea, vomiting, sweating, thirst, throbbing headache, chest pain, marked uneasiness, weakness, and vertigo. There can be blurred vision and confusion. In severe reactions, there may be respiratory depression, hypotension, and arrhythmias. The intensity of the reaction is proportional to the amount of disulfiram and alcohol ingested.

Disulfiram therapy is contraindicated in patients who are intoxicated or have atheroslerotic heart disease, diabetes, cirrhosis, organic brain syndrome, or a psychosis. It interferes with metabolism of phenytoin and can potentiate its effect. The patient must be fully informed of disulfiram's effects when alcohol is taken, and that the effect can even occur 4 to 14 days after disulfiram has been discontinued. Even the small amounts of alcohol found in cough syrups, vinegars, and sauces can produce a disulfiram-alcohol reaction.

During the initial 1 to 2 weeks of treatment, a daily single dose of up to 500 mg. is given. The average maintenance dose is 125 to 250 mg. per day. Some patients experience a sedative effect from the drug; in such instances the drug can be given before bed. Administration should never begin until the patient has abstained completely from alcohol for at least 24 hours, and preferably several days or more. The patient should carry a card that indicates that he is receiving disulfiram and that describes the symptoms likely to occur if alcohol is taken. Since disulfiram may cause hepatic dysfunction, a baseline transaminase level should be obtained, followed by another transaminase in 2 weeks. Patients with hepatic insufficiency should not use disulfiram. Adverse reactions to the drug include rashes, unpleasant taste in the mouth, organic brain syndrome, and neuropathies.

Recently, *behavioral treatment* modalities have been employed in treating this group of addicted drinkers. Behaviorists treat alcoholism by studying the drinking behavior itself in terms of the factors that seem to reward it and those that seem to discourage it. The therapist then seeks to devise a drinking schedule that emphasizes new rewards for controlled drinking or conditioned avoidance techniques that discourage uncontrolled drinking. Early treatment results are encouraging.

The Severely Deteriorated Alcoholic

Severely deteriorated alcoholics are unfortunate people who require the most all-encompassing and intensive of care. Hospitalization, or at least partial inpatient treatment, is an important part of the program. The patient is removed from the environmental stresses that lead to the drinking. An attempt is made to establish a significant therapeutic relationship. Social support, vocational training and recreational outlets are provided. The behavioral and pharmacologic modalities mentioned above are used with these patients as well. Prolonged outpatient followup is important to success. The primary physician can play an important role in providing coordinated and continuous care for these patients over the course of treatment and followup.

ANNOTATED BIBLIOGRAPHY

American Medical Assocation: Manual on Alcoholism. Chicago: American Medical Association, 1968. *(Practical discussion, including the kind of material that could be presented to patients whom the clinician is counseling.)*

Chafetz, ME: Alcoholism and alcoholic psychoses. *In* Freedman, A.M., *et al.* (eds.): Comprehensive Textbook of Psychiatry, 2. ed. Baltimore: Williams & Wilkins, 1975. *(Excellent, comprehensive review of the entire topic.)*

Franks, C.M.: Behavior therapy, the principles of conditioning and the treatment of the alcoholic. J. Stud. Alcohol, 24:511, 1963. *(Good example of the behavioral conceptualization of the problem.)*

Gerrein, J.R., Rosenberg, C.M., and Manohar, V.: Disulfuram maintenance in outpatient treatment of alcoholism. Arch. Gen. Psychiatry, 25:545, 1973. *(Details of disulfiram treatment.)*

Knight, R.P.: The psychodynamics of chronic alcoholism. J. Nerv. Ment. Dis. 86:538, 1937. *(A classic example of the psychodynamic approach to the problem.)*

National Council on Alcoholism: Criteria for the diagnosis of alcoholism, A.M.J. Psychiatry *129*: 127, 1972. *(Excellent discussion of the definitional problems and clinical features.)*

Pattison, E.M.: Nonabstinent drinking goals in the treatment of alcoholism. Arch. Gen. Psychiatry *33*:923, 1976. *(Simple abstinence does not correlate well with improvement in other areas of adjustment, and it may well be that less than total abstinence is compatible with rehabilitation.)*

Pittman, D.J. and Snyder, D.R. (eds.): Society, Culture and Drinking Patterns. New York: John Wiley & Sons, 1962. *(Collection of many papers on the social and cultural influences on drinking and alcoholism.)*

Sellers, E. and Kalant, H.: Alcohol intoxication and withdrawal. N. Engl. J. Med. *294*:757, 1976. *(Straightforward, up-to-date statement of the medical approach.)*

Tiebout, H.M.: Psychology and treatment of alcoholism. J. Stud. Alcohol, *7*:214, 1946. *(Good example of the intrapsychic conceptualization of the problem and treatment.)*

217

Approach to the Patient with Sexual Dysfunction

ARTHUR J. BARSKY, III, M.D.

Sexual function is a sensitive indicator of psychological and physical health. Approximately 10 per cent of medical outpatients experience significant sexual dysfunction, but often the problem goes unrecognized, because the physician and patient do not discuss the topic. Successful diagnosis and treatment require that the physician be able to elicit the patient's concerns in a comfortable, understanding and supportive manner. Many patients are embarrassed to raise the issue, but often desperately search for some clue that the physician is willing to listen and to help with omnipresent sexual doubts, fears and difficulties.

The term sexual dysfunction encompasses a wide range of problems, which include impotence, premature ejaculation, retarded ejaculation, frigidity, inability to achieve orgasm, dyspareunia and vaginismus. Each disorder is classified as "primary," when there has never been a period of satisfactory sexual function, or "secondary," when the difficulty follows a period of adequate function.

DEFINITIONS

Defining sexual problems in functional terms helps to facilitate diagnosis. *Impotence* denotes the inability to maintain an erection sufficient to engage in intercourse. *Premature ejaculation* refers to ejaculation which persistently occurs before or immediately after penetration. Arbitrarily, the term is applied when in over 50 per cent of instances the patient is unable to delay ejaculation until his female partner has achieved orgasm. *Retarded ejaculation* is the persistent failure to ejaculate in the presence of a satisfactory erection.

The distinction between enjoyment of sexual intercourse and orgasmic ability is particularly important in women. *Frigidity* implies a lack of sexual interest and erotic feeling; the term has lost favor due to its derogatory connotation, and some authors now prefer *excitement phase dysfunction*. The historic controversy over the issue of frigidity stemmed from

mistakenly equating it with inability to experience orgasm. The term *orgasmic dysfunction* denotes the absence of orgasms, even though the woman may enjoy sexual intercourse and have normal sexual desire. *Dyspareunia* is painful intercourse. *Vaginismus* is involuntary spasm of the vagina and pelvic musculature with adduction of the thighs, preventing penile insertion.

PSYCHOLOGICAL MECHANISMS AND CLINICAL PRESENTATIONS

Sexual problems may have a physiological as well as a psychological basis (see Chapters 110 and 128). Three broad categories of psychological difficulty may result in sexual dysfunction. The first category involves formative experiences early in life. These include the general family orientation toward sexual activity and sexual identity, and any sexually traumatic occurrences. A second group encompasses current emotional stresses, tensions and intrapsychic conflicts, which can be compounded by inadequate or inaccurate sexual knowledge. Interpersonal conflicts are a third source of difficulty, in which sexual partners are at odds over nonsexual as well as sexual issues. Interpersonal problems may also be a consequence of sexual dysfunction rather than a cause.

Once established and regardless of the source, any sexual disorder is likely to induce a vicious, self-perpetuating cycle: the sexual difficulty generates anxiety, guilt, shame and fear of failure, all of which in turn make sex even less satisfactory. Moreover, concerns related to sexual competence and the safety of engaging in sex that routinely arise in the context of serious physical illness may trigger sexual dysfunction.

There is no one-to-one correlation between underlying psychological mechanisms and clinical presentation. Many different causes can produce similar clinical pictures, and similar psychological difficulties may manifest themselves as different sexual dysfunctions.

The anxiety which surrounds any sexual problem may be somatized. Thus patients with psychological concerns about sexuality may present clinically with bodily complaints, such as headache, low back pain, generalized pelvic pain, and vulvar pruritus, which have no apparent medical cause.

Impotence. The sporadic occurrence of impotence is normal. It is considered clinically significant only when erection fails to occur in 25 to 50 per cent of coital attempts. While 1.5 per cent of men are impotent at age 40, the percentage rises to 25 per cent at age 70 and 55 per cent at 75. The converse is of equal importance—namely, that almost half of 75-year-old men are able to achieve satisfactory intercourse.

Mild, transient impotence is seen in normal people who (1) lose their confidence following a traumatic sexual experience, (2) feel guilty, depressed, anxious, or angry with their partner, (3) fear discovery of their sexual activity, (4) fear failure to perform, or (5) fear exerting themselves after an illness. Prolonged impotence and primary impotence are more likely to reflect physical illness (see Chapter 128) or severe psychological problems, such as fears of intimacy and trust, an ambivalent sexual identity, or feelings of aggression and hostility toward women. The person raised in an environment where sex was regarded as sinful and dirty may be troubled by much anxiety and guilt.

Premature ejaculation is most common in men whose partners have difficulty achieving orgasm. It is one of the most common male sexual disorders and is occasionally experienced by normal men. If it occurs for a prolonged period and remains untreated, the patient may go on to become impotent. Premature ejaculation is usually psychological in origin and is often related to anxieties about sexual inadequacy or to fears of castration. It is also commonly seen when premarital sexual activity requires rapid completion of the sex act. Once premature ejaculation occurs, it can easily be reinforced by the partner's negative response.

Retarded ejaculation occasionally has a physical basis (see Chapter 128), but primary retarded ejaculation generally tends to reflect deep-seated psychological difficulties. It usually occurs in men with low self-esteem and with fears of being overwhelmed or abandoned by women, or of competing with them. It also may stem from unconscious conflicts about female genitals or pregnancy. Secondary retarded ejaculation is often a manifestation of troubled relations between patient and partner; there may be loss of physical attractiveness, feelings of hostility, inability to produce orgasm in the partner, or disagreement about having a child.

Retrograde ejaculation reflects a physical disturbance of sphincter activity (see Chapter 128).

Excitement phase dysfuntion. Women who have never felt sexual desire are rare. Primary excitement phase dysfunction occurs when there is severe neurotic conflict, latent homosexuality, gender confusion or social naiveté. Causes of secondary excitement phase dysfunction include depression, deterioration of interpersonal relationships, medications, pelvic pathology and pregnancy (see Chapter 110).

Orgasmic dysfunction is often seen in women with normal sex drives who enjoy fulfilling sexual intercourse, but who simply are not orgasmic. True aversion to all sexual activity is extremely rare, while some degree of orgasmic dysfunction is experienced at one time or another by most women. The problem is most common in the first few years of sexual activity; the capacity for orgasm seems to increase with experience. It is important to remember that most postmenopausal and elderly women, like aging men, retain their desire and capacity for gratifying sexual intercourse, though sexual responsiveness may be slower and perhaps of diminished intensity. Primary orgasmic dysfunction stems from intrapsychic conflict, sociocultural forces or early experiences. Such women have learned when younger that sex is dirty, sinful or only for the pleasure of the man. Alternatively, orgasms may be unconsciously equated with loss of control, selfishness or hostility. Secondary orgasmic dysfunction is common and may reflect interpersonal discord, depression or underlying organic illness. Conflicts with the partner often originate outside the sexual sphere, and the patient may feel angry or rejected. Depression may produce orgasmic dysfunction as part of a general reduction in libido.

Dyspareunia. is most often a consequence of difficulty achieving adequate vaginal lubrication or the existence of underlying pelvic pathology (see Chapter 110). When dyspareunia has a psychological origin, the causes are similar to those of orgasmic dysfunction, though a recent traumatic experience such as rape may also be responsible. When untreated, dyspareunia can lead to vaginismus.

Vaginismus. The causes of vaginismus are similar to those of dyspareunia. Patients with primary vaginismus frequently have had little sexual experience and harbor misunderstandings about their own sexual anatomy and physiology, leading to fears of penetration. If patients with primary vaginismus do have psychological conflicts, they often center around dangers and fears of sexuality and the penis. Secondary vaginismus is often a consequence of pelvic pathology or dyspareunia. If long-standing, it may contribute to the development of impotence in the male partner.

WORKUP

Assessment of the patient's problem has to be done with empathy and respect in order to foster honesty and trust. Inquiry into sexual values, ideas, and behavior is important, but useful only if done in a nonjudgmental fashion. A thorough description of the sexual difficulty and interpersonal circumstances surrounding it is essential. Questioning needs to cover not only the historical facts, but also the patient's level of understanding and feelings about them. The specific language chosen by the physician to discuss the problem should reflect the patient's level of understanding. It is sometimes beneficial to reassure the reticent, anxious patient of the confidentiality of the doctor-patient communication.

A thorough sexual history should include the age when the patient developed secondary sexual characteristics and acquired sexual knowledge, past and present masturbatory practices, previous capacity for sexual activity, and adolescent sexual experiences. Preferences as to activities and partners should be explored, including both homosexual and heterosexual experiences. Women ought to be questioned about menarche, pregnancies, abortions, and method and use of contraception.

Once a clear description of the sexual problem is obtained, the task is to determine if the dysfunction is predominantly medical or psychological in origin. Although over 90 per cent of sexual dysfunction encountered in ambulatory patients has a psychological etiology, it is obviously essential not to overlook an important medical problem (e.g., diabetes). Consequently, a thorough medical history and physical examination are mandatory (see Chapters 110 and 128).

History provides much of the information necessary to identify a psychological etiology. For example, the patient who performs satisfactorily in certain situations (e.g., during intercourse with a particular partner, masturbation, or oral or manual stimulation) clearly has a disorder of functional origin. The same is true of the impotent patient who reports normal erections on awakening from sleep. A psychological etiology is likely when the history contains a common psychosocial precipitant, such as interpersonal difficulty, and when, in the absence of medical illness, there are concurrent changes in sexual appetite as well as sexual function.

PRINCIPLES AND TECHNIQUES OF TREATMENT

Explicit sexual education is an important first step in improving many sexual disorders. *Directive sexual therapy* is indicated if a psychological basis for the dysfunction is discovered, or if adequate treatment of an underlying medical condition fails to fully alleviate the difficulty. Directive therapy focuses upon communication between the patient and partner, treating the problem in sexual function as a reflection of covert and unexpressed interpersonal conflicts. Treatment attempts to improve communication between partners and to reestablish trust, affection and acceptance—a climate in which sexual contentment is more likely to occur. The open expression of feelings, preferences, disagreements and wishes is encouraged. Deeply rooted neurotic conflicts require psychotherapy, but many cases may be dealt with effectively by directive techniques.

Directive treatment also aims at reducing performance fears and minimizing the tendency to assume the spectator role, which occur soon after sexual dysfunction begins and can perpetuate the disorder. The partners may not be aware of the degree to which they have become spectators of their own sexual experiences and are thus unable to participate spontaneously in sensual enjoyment. The physician can work to help them see the ways in which they have come to focus only on the sexual problem and to trace with them the repercussions which the disorder has had in their relationship.

Directive sex therapy involves prescription of a graduated series of specific exercises which enhance the experience of sensual pleasure and sexual arousal, increase the communicative aspect of sex, and diminish performance anxiety. By prescribing specific exercises and prohibiting other sexual activities, the therapist lifts from the patient the responsibility to perform. Exercises are conducted at specific prearranged times when the couple is free from other responsibilities and is sure not to be disturbed or interrupted. The goal of each exercise is not to overcome the particular sexual dysfunction but rather to discover what is most pleasurable and stimulating, to improve mutual guidance, and to gradually rebuild confidence. Early exercises allow only nongenital caressing; subsequent sessions move from inclusion of sexual foreplay and genital stimulation to mutual masturbation, nongenital penetration, insertion of the penis without movement, intercourse, and finally intercourse with orgasm. The couple is not allowed to progress from one stage to the next until they have had pleasurable success without anxiety at the preceding one.

Specific techniques and exercises are utilized depending upon the particular sexual disorder. In premature ejaculation, the "squeeze" technique is employed. The woman is instructed to apply pressure with her fingers around the coronal ridge of her partner's penis just prior to ejaculatory inevitability. This diminishes the urge to ejaculate, and periods of arousal and stimulation are then alternated with periods of squeezing. Gradually the man experiences longer periods of erection without ejaculation. In the treatment of orgasmic dysfunction, particular emphasis is placed upon instructing the woman in techniques of self-stimulation. The earliest exercises may involve only the woman, as she masturbates and shares what she has learned with her partner for him to use when they begin to engage in two-party sex play. In dyspareunia, the stage of intromission is gradually negotiated in many small steps, and the couple is instructed to use copious amounts of artificial lubricant. The treatment of vaginismus often includes the use of graduated dilators. These are inserted by the woman or by the physician in the partner's presence, thereby removing him from the role of aggressor or intruder while the woman discovers her own sexuality. Intercourse is attempted only after complete comfort with the largest dilator has been attained.

The efficacy of directive sex therapy appears to be high. Most outcome studies report extremely favorable results, but some caution is warranted in interpreting them since the patients treated are often carefully selected and highly motivated. Failure, when it does occur, is often in the form of protestations by the couple that they are unable to carry out the therapeutic exercises prescribed. Such behavior is often an indication that a deeper psychiatric or intramarital difficulty is present and that psychiatric referral should be considered.

INDICATIONS FOR REFERRAL

Directive sexual therapy can be undertaken by the primary care physician, or the couple may be referred to a psychiatrist interested in sexual therapy, or to a sexual dysfunction clinic. Referral is definitely indicated when (1) severe underlying psychopathology is suspected, (2) marital discord is very serious, (3) directive sexual therapy has failed, or (4) the couple proves unwilling or unable to cooperate with the directive sexual therapy undertaken by the primary care physician.

PATIENT EDUCATION

Sexual dysfunction often stems in part from inadequate or inaccurate knowledge of sexual practice, anatomy and physiology; sex education should not be overlooked. Such education should include the reassuring information that occasional sexual dysfunction, particularly in periods of stress, is very common, self-limited, and not pathologic. Educational sessions are best conducted with both partners present because mutual understanding and communication improve as each learns not only about the self, but about the other as well.

ANNOTATED BIBLIOGRAPHY

Aaron, R.: Male contributions to female frigidity. Medical Aspects of Human Sexuality, 5:42, 1971. *(The spouse's sexual problems may be a major cause of the woman's frigidity.)*

Green, R.: Human Sexuality: A Health Practitioners Text. Baltimore: Williams and Wilkins, 1975. *(Good for use in counseling patients.)*

Labby, D.: Sexual concommitants of disease and illness. Postgrad. Med., 58:103, 1975. *(Reviews the impact of common illness on sexual function.)*

Levine, S., and Rosenthal, M.: Marital sexual dysfunction: Female dysfunctions. Ann. Intern. Med., 86:588, 1977. *(Proposes clinically useful classification system and provides good review of the literature; 78 refs.)*

Masters, W.H., and Johnson, V.E.: Principles of the new sex therapy. Am. J. Psychiat., 133:538, 1976. *(Authoritative discussion.)*

Solberg, D., Butler, J., and Wagner, N.: Sexual behavior in pregnancy. N. Engl. J. Med., 288:1098, 1973. *(Third trimester is frequently accompanied by loss of libido and capacity for orgasm.)*

Wright, J., et al.: The treatment of sexual dysfunction. Arch. Gen. Psychiat., 34:881, 1977. *(Reviews efficacy.)*

218

Approach to the Somatizing Patient

ARTHUR J. BARSKY, III, M.D.

The somatizing patient presents with bodily complaints or disability out of proportion to any demonstrable organic pathology. Included in this category are anxious and depressed patients, hypochondriacs, chronic pain patients, and malingerers. These people are among the most frustrating and troublesome encountered in office practice, but they can be evaluated and managed successfully. Attention to the causative psychological disorder helps to render symptoms understandable, enables the physician to distinguish them from those due to organic pathology, and facilitates management.

PSYCHOLOGICAL MECHANISMS AND CLINICAL PRESENTATIONS

Anxiety (see Chapter 214). Individuals suffering from *chronic anxiety* focus on and become alarmed by normal bodily sensations. They report headache, gastrointestinal disturbance, or musculoskeletal pain. *Acute anxiety* can have somatic manifestations; individuals complain of palpitations, chest pain, tachycardia, dyspnea, choking sensations, diarrhea, cramps, dizziness, and fainting.

Depression (see Chapter 215). Depression's neurovegetative symptoms may overshadow the characteristic affective, cognitive, and behavioral changes. As many as one half of somatizing ambulatory medical patients over age 40 are depressed. The chief complaint may be headache, constipation, weakness, fatigue, abdominal pain, insomnia, anorexia or weight loss. Depressed patients worry about and focus attention upon their bodies; a positive review of systems, chronic pain, or complaints involving multiple organ systems typify the clinical presentation, and symptoms recur with the periodicity characteristic of depressions.

Personality disturbances exist in a considerable number of somatizers. The terms "crock," chronic pain patient, hypochondriac, and chronic complainer refer to patients whose symptoms, illness, role as patient, and pursuit of medical care have become a way of life. For them, illness and medical treatment are means of relating to and manipulating other people, a way of dealing with stress, and a mechanism for the expression and management of psychological needs and conflicts. These patients have multiple somatic symptoms of functional origin accompanied by a fear of these symptoms and an intense preoccupation with their bodies and the possibility of disease. Their symptoms shift and fluctuate over time; they are nonspecific, diffuse, and similar to the transient sensations felt by healthy individuals. Worry about being ill is remarkably persistent, and it is not assuaged by reassurance after thorough medical evaluation. At times, they may have genuine medical problems, but their suffering, disability and medical care needs are typically in excess of any objective pathology. By their reports, medical care has been disappointing, failing to provide a cure or even relief of symptoms.

When interviewed, they talk mainly about their illnesses and medical care; one hears little about friends, work or hobbies. They often seem more concerned with establishing the authenticity of their complaints than with obtaining relief. They adamantly refuse to consider the possibility of an emotional cause for their symptoms (in contrast to most patients with demonstrable physical disease, who are willing to consider the possibility).

In attempting to understand these patients, some authorities have emphasized the unconscious meaning and gratification derived from pain and discomfort. Illness and suffering may be welcomed by the "guilty" individual unconsciously seeking atonement and expiation. Bodily complaints may be assumed by the deprived and needy person who has known care and attention only when sick or in pain. Anger and hostility are also involved; they feel cheated and wronged, and thus seek to express recrimination, blame, and reproach by belaboring others with their suffering. The importance of dependency has also been noted. Suffering and illness are ways to express and gratify yearnings for attention, contact and comfort.

Chronic complainers gain self-esteem and a sense

of identity from their ability to endure suffering, survive misfortune, and tolerate discomfort. Their requests for relief and cure can be understood as attempts to be respected for their ability to endure and survive rather than as a true desire to end discomfort.

Postconcussion syndrome is a self-limited condition which follows mild to moderate head trauma. A variety of somatic symptoms (headache, dizziness) accompany emotional ones (sleeplessness, irritability). An underlying depression is often the source of the problem; it becomes exacerbated by the traumatic event.

Hysterical conversion reactions represent internal conflict and emotional distress unconsciously converted into, and expressed as, physical rather than mental symptoms. Symptoms are either sensory or neuromuscular, i.e., weakness, paralysis, ataxia blindness, aphasia, deafness, anesthesia, pain, paresthesias, or seizures. The process is unconscious and not objectively provable, but there is often a prior history of similar reactions, emotional stress prior to onset, apparent symbolic meaning to the symptom (e.g., "heartache" following the loss of a loved one; blindness after viewing a horrifying event), inappropriate lack of concern about the symptom ("la belle indifference"), secondary gain, and the presence of other significant psychopathology.

Compensation (or accident) neurosis is marked by a wide range of somatic symptoms of undetermined cause that follow an accident in which there is litigation pending. The patient is not consciously aware of any relationship between the symptoms and the legal proceedings, yet the condition subsides when the litigation is concluded.

Somatic delusions are seen in schizophrenia, severe affective disorders, and organic brain syndromes. These are false, fixed ideas which are often vivid, bizarre, or extraordinary. Unlike hypochondriacal concerns, they do not fluctuate. The individual may believe some extraordinary change has occurred in his body; for example, that his organs are shriveling up, that body parts are deformed or missing, or that foreign objects are inside an orifice or organ.

Malingering is relatively rare outside situations in which illness confers some benefit. Symptoms are exaggerated, and the subject's description of them may vary with each interview. When the patient is unaware that he is being observed, he may relax the simulation and thus betray himself. Such individuals are frequently sociopaths or drug addicts; some may have worked in a medically related field.

DIFFERENTIAL DIAGNOSIS

The differential diagnosis of somatizing includes anxiety, depression, postconcussion syndrome, conversion reaction, compensation neurosis, hypochondriacal personality disturbance, schizophrenia, and malingering. Multiple sclerosis and polymyalgia rheumatica (see Chapter 150) are among the medical conditions sometimes mistaken for somatization.

WORKUP

Differentiating psychologically induced symptoms from those of organic disease is not always easy (see Chapters 214 and 215), but the quality, timing and precipitants of symptoms, as well as the patient's response to illness, attitude and choice of words can be of considerable help. Once a psychogenic etiology is suspected on the basis of the clinical presentation, evaluation should proceed to better define the underlying psychopathology.

Attention is first directed to the symptoms. A complaint whose charateristics are anatomically and physiologically nonsensical is very likely to be psychogenic in origin. For example, psychogenic sensory complaints often cross the midline or involve a combination of sensory modalities that is neurologically impossible. Multiple complaints involving many organ systems and many parts of the body suggest depression. Hysterical seizures do not involve incontinence or tongue-biting, and the hysterically blind exhibit a withdrawal or startle reflex when a hand is flashed before the face. Psychogenic aphonia may be differentiated from true aphasia in that the ability to read and write is unimpaired in the former. With hysterical paralysis of the upper extremity, the patient's arm avoids the face after being held above it and released. In hysterical paralysis of one lower extremity, attempts to move the afflicted leg do not invoke contraction of the other leg, as is the case in neurologic disease.

Psychogenic pain is typically unaffected by activity or by the passage of time, and the patient often seems more concerned with the physician's accepting the authenticity of his pain than with relieving it. The presence of a significant psychogenic component to a symptom can be suspected when it is exactly like a symptom that afflicted someone important to the patient.

The patient's description may provide important evidence of a psychological cause. Excessively vague, diffuse, and inconsistent descriptions as well as overly detailed, vivid and elaborate ones are very suggestive. Psychological factors may be revealed in the choice of words (e.g., "pain in the neck," or "not having a leg to stand on").

Timing and relation to prior events may be helpful clues. Although both physical and psychological illness can be precipitated by stress, the onset of psychogenic complaints is often closely associated with significant emotional stress, such as the loss of a loved one, or the onset of a major interpersonal conflict or sexual problem. Functional complaints are also prone to occur on the anniversary of a psychologically meaningful event, such as the death of a loved one.

The attitude of the patient toward the symptom should be noted. When the patient is unconcerned, inappropriately calm, or more concerned with establishing the authenticity of his symptoms than with obtaining relief, one should suspect a strong emotional component. Patients with psychogenic complaints who unconsciously derive considerable gain from their illness are often reluctant to consider an emotional cause for their symptoms.

The workup of the somatizing patient needs to include inquiry into possible precipitants and response to illness. History is searched for ongoing psychological stress, pending litigation, prior medical complaints without a demonstrable physical cause, depression, anxiety, prior psychosis, and recent head trauma. Details of previous medical care experiences can be revealing. A history of consulting many physicians for the same complaints, or of the immediate replacement of a treated symptom with a new one, help in the diagnosis of psychogenic illness.

It is important to determine if illness, discomfort and disability have become important parts of the patient's personality and to what extent they are used to deal with emotional discomfort, interpersonal difficulties, and environmental stress. Does the patient see himself as the suffering unfortunate one whose life is filled with disappointment, "bad luck," and defeat, as well as with illness? Expressions of anger and hostility may be indirect, as in cynicism, sarcasm, and uncooperativeness. The individual feels deprived and put upon and is likely to recriminate, accuse and blame. Finally, excessive dependence upon others

may be a feature of his personality. One senses an overpowering desire for care, attention, sympathy and human contact. The patient's attitude to the physician may have a clinging and hungry quality.

In addition to information about the patient's personality, other psychologically relevant data are helpful for diagnosis and sound management. What personal significance does he attach to his symptoms or to the suspected illness? Are there possible secondary gains, such as (1) receiving sympathy, attention and support (including financial support) from family and friends, (2) being excused from duties, challenges, and responsibilities (e.g., competing for a promotion at work, having to care for children), and (3) achieving the ability to influence and manipulate others because he is sick.

A thorough physical examination and a careful mental status examination are essential; not only may unexpected evidence of organic illness turn up, but a normal examination is a prerequisite for effective reassurance and the avoidance of unnecessary laboratory testing. Unless there is evidence that is strongly suggestive of organic pathology, elaborate and, particularly, invasive studies should be avoided. Performing a noninvasive test to help provide reassurance can be constructive, but radiologic and biochemical hunting expeditions may only add to confusion and expense. The likelihood of a false-positive result is high (see Chapter 2).

PRINCIPLES OF MANAGEMENT

Support. Management must be directed at the underlying psychopathology as well as at the presenting bodily complaints. The first step is to put the complaint in perspective, while recognizing that the patient has come because of physical symptoms. When the results of the workup are presented, the reality of the symptoms should not be denied, nor should it be implied that they are imaginary. The patient can be told that serious, damaging organic disease has been ruled out and that stress can amplify real bodily sensations and disrupt normal function. It is important to avoid making the patient feel foolish because there is "nothing wrong." The presence of symptoms is an indication of considerable distress, which the patient should be encouraged to discuss. The patient needs to know that the relationship with his physician will not terminate because the medical workup is negative. Additional visits should be scheduled to provide time to further discuss personal and situational problems on a regular basis. By offering the patient a long-term relationship that is not contingent upon organic symptoms, one may remove a major stimulus for their development. Refractory cases may benefit from referral to a psychiatrist.

Drug therapy. Nonspecific attempts to suppress somatization pharmacologically should be avoided. All too often, patients are told that their symptoms are due to their "nerves" and sent away with a prescription for a minor tranquilizer. Such an approach to therapy usually fails, and it often alienates the patient. It is especially important to recognize depression because of its high prevalence, subtle manifestations, and good response to therapy. The neurovegetative symptoms of depression respond well to antidepressant medication (see Chapter 215). Anxiety neurosis may be helped by the use of a benzodiazepine (see Chapter 214); schizophrenia, by a phenothiazine. The postconcussion syndrome is self-limited, resolving within 6 to 24 months.

Personality disorders. The primary care physician can manage the majority of somatizing patients having personality disturbances, because the best treatment is supportive. Medical intervention should be minimized whenever possible; in particular, major diagnostic workups involving expensive and invasive tests, especially for equivocal or questionable findings, should be avoided, as should pain medication and tranquilizers. Even though medication is often requested, these patients generally do not respond to it and tend to be especially prone to development of troublesome side effects and adverse reactions.

The patient's need to remain disabled, distressed and symptomatic must be recognized. The physician must not expect cure, because the patient loses no time in reporting that he is no better, and perhaps is worse. To avoid struggles, the patient, especially if hostile and angry, should be involved as much as possible in therapeutic and diagnostic decisions. The physician ought to make it clear that his role is to help the patient tolerate discomfort rather than to eliminate it. Therapeutic suggestions should be made with the implication that although they may be of some palliative value, they will probably not help dramatically.

The patient's self-esteem needs bolstering. Acknowledging his strength to endure suffering, tolerate discomfort, and survive hardship and misfortune is particularly gratifying to him. These qualities are the ones the patient values most in himself and are the source of what little self-esteem he has.

Conversion reactions. There are two aspects to the treatment of hysterical conversion reactions: symptom removal and management of the internal conflict to avoid the development of bodily complaints. The first is done through the use of suggestion—hysterical patients are exceptionally suggestive—and education. The patient should be assured that the disorder is self-limited and that the symptoms will gradually improve and finally vanish. Conversion symptoms are likely to recur, however, unless psychotherapy is arranged to alter the psychological forces at work.

Compensation neurosis. The best treatment for compensation neurosis is settlement of litigation. Interim therapy includes encouraging the patient not to stop work, minimizing medical treatment of the injury, and stressing its favorable prognosis. Litigation should be completed as soon as possible.

Malingering. Malingering is generally resistant to treatment. Diagnostic and therapeutic procedures should be avoided whenever possible because they reinforce pathologic behavior. Any abnormal laboratory tests or physical findings are suspect.

INDICATIONS FOR REFERRAL

Most somatizing patients can be well managed by the primary physician. Referral is indicated when a patient has accepted a psychological explanation of his symptoms and wants to see a psychiatrist, when a conversion reaction, anxiety neurosis or psychosis is present, or when the primary physician has such a negative reaction to the patient with a personality disorder that he cannot serve him well.

TREATMENT RECOMMENDATIONS

- Explain the results of the medical workup without denying the reality of the patient's discomfort.
- Encourage discussion of psychosocial problems and set up a regular schedule of appointments for further elaboration and supportive therapy. Make it clear to the patient that he need not have physical symptoms to see the doctor. Avoid p.r.n. appointments.

- Treat the underlying psychological problem specifically; do not attempt the nonspecific suppression of symptoms with tranquilizers.
- Do not try to remove or cure symptoms in the patient with a somatizing personality disorder. Acknowledge the suffering and provide support. Avoid the use of medication and the extensive workup of vague symptoms. Make adaptation to chronic discomfort the goal of care.

ANNOTATED BIBLIOGRAPHY

Drossman, D.A.: The problem patient. Ann. Intern. Med., 88:366, 1978. (Presents an approach that is useful clinically.)

Engel, G.L.: "Psychogenic" pain and the pain-prone patient. Am. J. Med., 26:899, 1959. (This article makes the psychology of many types of somatizing comprehensible.)

Kenyon, F.E.: Hypochondriasis: A survey of some historical, clinical, and social aspects. Br. J. Med. Psychol., 38:117, 1965. (An exhaustive survey of the literature.)

Kreitman, N., Sainsbury, P., Pearce, K., and Costain, W.R.: Hypochondriasis and depression in outpatients at a general hospital. Br. J. Psychiatry, 111:607, 1965. (Differences between somatizing and nonsomatizing depressed patients, including poorer interpersonal relationships, poorer sexual adjustment, more chronic medical illness, and less depressive affect.)

Lipsitt, D.R.: Medical and psychological characteristics of "crocks." Psychiatry Med., 1:15, 1970. (How to understand and manage the chronic somatizer.)

Lowy, F.H.: Management of the persistent somatizer. Int. J. Psychiatry Med., 6:227, 1975. (Though written for the psychiatrist, the article is still helpful for the internist.)

McKegney, F.P.: The incidence and characteristics of patients with conversion reactions. I. A general hospital consultation service sample. Am. J. Psychiatry, 124:542, 1967. (An example of much of the research in this area, including difficulties in sampling methods and control groups.)

Raskin, M., Talbott, J.A., Meyerson, A.T.: Diagnosed conversion reactions. JAMA, 197:530, 1966. (The most helpful clues in distinguishing conversion symptoms from organic symptoms are a prior history of functional symptoms, a significant emotional precipitant, and some evidence that the symptom solves a conflict.)

Ziegler, F.J., and Imboden, J.B.: Contemporary conversion reactions. Arch. Gen. Psychiatry, 6:279, 1962. (Conversion reactions are unconscious attempts to take the sick role as a defense against a range of unpleasant emotions.)

219

Approach to the Angry Patient
ARTHUR J. BARSKY, III, M.D.

Patients often become angry in response to the suffering and disability caused by disease, adverse life events, or the psychological threats intrinsic to being a patient. When faced with an angry patient, the primary physician needs to be able to recognize the source of the patient's anger, prevent it from interfering with therapeutic efforts, and help the patient to cope.

PSYCHOLOGICAL MECHANISMS

People become angry when they feel threatened or when their wishes and aims are frustrated. Illness often leads to anger since it presents the threat of disfigurement, pain, lost opportunity, abandonment, and even death. Some patients are particularly enraged by the helplessness, lack of control, and enforced passivity that disease confers.

Other patients are uncomfortable in the doctor-patient relationship because it represents the threat of dependence upon the physician—of allowing someone powerful to take control of, take care of, and be responsible for them. They use anger to defend themselves against the intimacy, closeness, and warmth that develop with the doctor in the course of receiving medical care. Anger, then, can be an unconscious attempt to drive the physician away and allay the threat of dependency or intimacy which is inherent in the doctor-patient relationship.

Patients commonly express to their clinicians anger derived from threats and stresses they have encountered elsewhere in their lives. In such instances, the animosity and hostility seem inappropriate to the situation and out of proportion to any provocation the doctor can think of. This usually occurs when patients are in conflict with people important to them to whom they cannot express their anger, such as an employer or a spouse.

Other patients appear to have a personality and life-style permeated by a quick temper, chronic resentments and dissatisfactions. The physician is little more than a screen onto which they project hostility garnered elsewhere. Globally angry patients may have a borderline personality organization. Both in their relationships to the physician and in the other aspects of their lives, they seem to be generally abusive, uncooperative, and ungrateful people. These patients have long histories of relating to physicians and others in a dependent and demanding fashion, exhibiting hostility toward and devaluation of the very people upon whom they depend so desperately. Their anger expresses their sense that people are menacing and unsympathetic; it also reflects their disappointment at having been let down and not having received the help they feel they need and deserve.

RECOGNIZING THE ANGRY PATIENT

Anger may be expressed verbally in direct statements which convey demands, annoyance, and resentment, as well as in personal histories of temper outbursts and undirected violence (e.g., slamming doors). It may be expressed more obliquely through cynicism, sarcasm, negativism, and behavior which, while superficially compliant, innocent and cooperative, is actually obstructive. Anger may be evidenced by behavior as well as words, e.g., failure to adhere to a medical regimen, keep appointments, or quit self-destructive health habits. Helpful nonverbal clues may be observed during the interview. The angry patient clenches his fists and jaws or knits his forehead in a frown. The palpebral fissures are narrowed, lips compressed, and nostrils widened. Gestures and gait may be explosive. Finally, the interviewer's own subjective, emotional response to the patient during the interview may convey important diagnostic information. Whenever the interviewer is aware of being irritated or bored with the patient, he should question himself as to whether these feelings are an unconscious response to anger and hostility.

It is important not only to recognize that the patient is angry, but also to learn what he is angry about. During the interview, the physician should note the subject matter that brings out irritation, annoyance, or hostility. The themes which seem to evoke anger are obvious and important clues to issues that are troubling the patient.

The globally angry patient with a borderline personality organization can be recognized by a few clinical characteristics: (1) interpersonal relationships are either superficial or very dependent and manipulative; (2) emotions are intense and labile, and extreme emptiness and anger are predominant; (3) social and intellectual skills may be well developed, but the patient's life is marked by lack of fulfillment and frequent failures; (4) impulsive, manipulative and self-destructive behavior is present; and (5) past history may include brief psychotic episodes.

PRINCIPLES OF MANAGEMENT

Once the physician has recognized that the patient is angry and has defined any specific threats or frustrations that are fueling the anger, he can proceed to acknowledge the patient's feelings and reassure him that they will not destroy their relationship. This often helps bring about a more open give-and-take discussion between the doctor and patient. The physician need not agree that the patient's feeling is justified, but he should acknowledge its existence by explicitly presenting the patient with his observations and the reasons for concluding that the patient is angry. Such discussion can introduce an atmosphere of frankness, honesty and sensitivity into the therapeutic relationship. The physician conveys the sense that he is not afraid of the patient's feelings and that he will respond not by rejecting but by helping the patient.

If the patient's hostility interferes with communication, the therapeutic program, or optimal coping with illness, the doctor should point this out. The physician needs to indicate that while he recognizes the patient's anger and his right to have it, it nonetheless represents a problem because it is self-destructive, interfering with therapy and recovery. One need not be bullied by the globally angry patient; it is possible and necessary to set limits on the patient's behavior while making it clear that there will be no counterattack in retribution.

By defining the specific frustrations and threats,

the physician should be able to approach the patient more effectively. For the patient who is angry about being ill, detailed investigation of exact fears and sources of despair is helpful. For the patient who is angry about having to be a patient, the doctor may be able to structure their relationship so as to minimize those aspects which most threaten the patient. If the patient most fears dependency, the physician should assume a somewhat cool, reserved, and proper stance, while still conveying his support and sympathy. Finally, if the anger seems to be displaced upon the physician from some other situation or relationship, this may be pointed out, without specifically encouraging the direct and immediate venting of the hostility upon its actual source.

The physician should take care that he does not react with his own hostility to the angry and provacative patient. Maintaining an objective perspective on the situation will help the physician to recognize when anger is not a criticism of him but rather is a response to the inner torment of threats and frustrated wishes. By doing so, one is in a good position to work with the angry patient, to preserve the therapeutic relationship, to help the patient, and to get on with the business of optimal medical care.

ANNOTATED BIBLIOGRAPHY

Adler, G.: Valuing and devaluing in the psychotherapeutic process. Arch. Gen. Psychiatry, *22*:454, 1970. *(Psychiatric patients express hostility toward their psychiatrists as protection against wishes for nurturance, against envy, against low self-esteem, and as a focal point for rage coming from elsewhere in their lives.)*

Groves, J.E.: Taking care of the hateful patient. N. Engl. J. Med., *298*:883, 1978. *(Discussion includes the physician's own emotional responses to patients, and the ways to use these responses constructively.)*

Gunderson, J., and Singer, M.: Defining borderline patients. Am. J. Psychol., *132*:1, 1975. *(An excellent review identifying basic characteristics of such patients, including intense, often hostile, affect; 87 refs.)*

Kahana, R.J., and Bibring, G.L.: Personality types in medical management. *In* Zinberg, N. (ed.): Psychiatry and Medical Practice in a General Hospital. New York: International University Press, 1965. *(Though not dealing specifically with the angry patient, this is an excellent discussion of the emotional meaning that illness holds for particular personality types.)*

220
Approach to the Patient with Insomnia
ARTHUR J. BARSKY, III, M.D.

Data from population surveys indicate that over 30 per cent of people have occasional trouble falling or staying asleep, while an additional 15 per cent have frequent difficulty. Insomnia affects patients of all ages; it is a particularly troublesome problem in the elderly. There is no precise definition of insomnia because the range of normal sleep requirements is very wide. Moreover, sleep laboratory studies indicate that the quality of sleep may be just as important as the quantity. Nevertheless, if the patient falls asleep within 30 minutes and obtains at least 6 hours of restful sleep per night, it is unlikely that he will complain of serious insomnia.

Most patients with insomnia try a host of techniques, home remedies, and nonprescription drugs before seeking medical help. They frequently come to the primary physician requesting prescription medication for sleep while overlooking the cause of their sleeplessness. The primary physician needs to be skilled in the assessment and therapy of insomnia, not only because the problem is extremely common and a cause of considerable misery, but also because it is an important precipitant of excessive drug use. Almost a billion dollars are spent each year in the United States on medication for sleep.

PATHOPHYSIOLOGY AND CLINICAL PRESENTATION

Normal sleep can be divided physiologically into two major categories: rapid eye movement (REM) sleep and non-REM sleep. *REM sleep* is characterized by flaccid voluntary musculature, increased cardiovascular and respiratory activity, and rapid synchronous nonpatterned eye movements. There is striking neurophysiological activity in the cortical centers that receive and integrate sensory input. Most dream activity occurs during this phase. *Non-REM sleep* has four phases. Stage 1 occurs as the person begins to fall asleep and shows a low amplitude, fast-frequency electroencephalogram (EEG) pattern. Stages 2 through 4 show progressive slowing of the EEG and an increase of amplitude of wave patterns. Muscular and cardiovascular activity are decreased, and little dreaming occurs.

Normal sleep follows a patterned cycle. It begins with a period of non-REM sleep of increasing depth, which is followed by a period of REM sleep usually lasting 10 to 25 minutes. The cycle repeats itself roughly every 90 minutes throughout the night. The length of each REM period increases as the night progresses, except in the elderly, in whom this increase does not occur. Approximately four to six cycles of REM sleep occur each night.

Sleep physiology is altered in the insomniac. Poor sleepers spend more time in Stage 2 and less in Stage 4 than people with no complaints. Surprisingly, the percentage of REM sleep is unchanged. Poor sleepers have a high level of physiological activity during the night; there are increases in heart rate, peripheral vasocontriction, and rectal temperature. The degree of abnormality varies considerably from night to night.

Insomniacs who chronically use hyponotics have a marked diminution of REM sleep and almost complete absence of Stages 3 and 4. When they undergo gradual withdrawal from drugs, there is a rebound phenomenon characterized by a marked increase in REM sleep, intense dreams, and even some nightmares. Stages 3 and 4 slowly return to normal, without a rebound phenomenon. During withdrawal from hypnotics, there is no worsening of insomnia when reduction in dose is gradual.

The chronic use of all *hypnotics* over weeks and months almost always exacerbates the insomnia for which they were originally taken. This effect is probably due to the development of tolerance and dependence and to the distortion of the sleep cycle. In addition, the precipitous withdrawal of hypnotics and minor tranquilizers also worsens insomnia and produces nightmares. Thus, when the chronic hypnotic user suddenly stops his medication, he finds his insomnia actually worsens, and he resumes the medication. *Stimulants,* including over-the-counter preparations, cocaine, amphetamines, and the caffeine in soft drinks as well as in coffee and tea, can be important factors in the cause of insomnia. Over-the-counter medications often contain scopolamine and an antihistamine. Their anticholinergic properties can produce an atropinelike confusional state and worsen the sleeplessness.

Almost any *physical disorder* involving pain, itching, or discomfort can cause difficulty sleeping. Several disorders seem to cause insomnia specifically, including respiratory insufficiency, renal failure, congestive heart failure, and hyperthyroidism. Hyperthyroidism produces marked increases in Stages 3 and 4. With treatment, the sleep pattern slowly returns to normal as the patient becomes euthyroid. Some conditions may be exacerbated by sleep. Nocturnal angina may be precipitated by increased myocardial oxygen demands that occur during REM sleep. In patients with duodenal ulcer, there is a marked increase in acid secretion during REM periods; this may account for the nocturnal pain that is so frequently reported.

Any *stressful experience* (e.g., occupational pressures, marital crises, the death of a relative, physical discomfort) can produce insomnia. In addition, frustration and tension following deliberate attempts to force oneself to fall asleep engender a vicious cycle in which trying harder simply increases arousal and wakefulness. This can lead to insomnia becoming a *conditioned* or *learned response* to the act of going to bed. Insomnia may develop if the ritual of going to bed becomes associated with sleeplessness, frustration, and anxiety which may originally have been due to a temporary situational stress, emotional upset, or brief medical illness. The patient notes that he cannot fall asleep in his own bed, but is able to sleep well in other places, e.g., on the living-room sofa or in a hotel.

The patient with insomnia of psychogenic origin may complain of difficulty falling asleep or staying asleep, of waking too early, or any combination of these. Most cases are short-term and parallel acute situational stress. Patients with *depression* report early morning awakening and the inability to fall back into a sound sleep, whereas anxiety tends to produce difficulty falling asleep. Patients who suffer from mania actually enjoy their sleeplessness. Patients with long-standing psychological problems or *alcoholism* report being plagued by years of poor sleep that is fragmented and shallow.

Finally, some individuals suffer from *idiopathic insomnia.* This diagnosis should not be made on the basis of the history alone, as self-reporting of sleep patterns is notoriously unreliable. Thus, if a sleep laboratory is available, it is helpful in establishing this diagnosis. Roughly, about 10 to 15 per cent of insomniacs suffer from idiopathic insomnia.

DIFFERENTIAL DIAGNOSIS

Insomnia may be secondary to situational stress, medical illness, hypnotic or stimulant abuse or withdrawal, an underlying psychiatric disorder, or a behavioral problem (Table 220–1). An etiology is usually found when a careful workup is performed.

Table 220–1.   Causes of Insomnia

A. Medical illness
  1. Any physical illness accompanied by discomfort or pain
  2. Specific disorders: e.g., respiratory disease, renal insufficiency, hyperthyroidism, congestive heart failure
B. Medication use, dependence, or withdrawal
  1. Long-term use of any hypnotic or sedative
  2. Precipitous withdrawal of any hypnotic or sedative
  3. Use of stimulants
C. Psychiatric illness
  1. Depression
  2. Anxiety
  3. Mania
  4. Alcoholism
  5. Schizophrenia
D. Behavioral and situational causes
  1. Life stress
  2. Preoccupation with falling asleep
  3. Sleeplessness as a learned behavior
E. Idiopathic

WORKUP

Most cases of insomnia can be diagnosed by history alone, although many purported insomniacs actually demonstrate adequate sleep when they are observed in a sleep laboratory. It is important to define the pattern of sleep and its effects. How long it takes the patient to fall asleep, how long he stays asleep, and how rested he feels in the morning need to be determined. Since subjective recall of sleep is often unreliable, the use of a diary may be helpful. Difficulty falling asleep has to be distinguished from early morning awakening. The former is characteristic of insomnia due to anxiety, physical discomfort, preoccupation with attempts to fall asleep, stimulant abuse, situational stress, and chronic hypnotic use.

Early morning awakening strongly suggests the presence of an underlying depression. The distinction is important because the conditions are treated differently. When sleep is fragmented—i.e., when the night is punctuated by periods of wakefulness—it is possible the problem involves chronic alcohol abuse or hypnotic withdrawal.

The circumstances surrounding the onset of insomnia require elaboration, including any concurrent situational stresses, medical illnesses, and drug use. A complete drug history is crucial. Duration of use, any recent cessation, and doses of over-the-counter remedies, as well as prescription medications, need to be detailed, with particular attention paid to hypnotics, tranquilizers, and stimulants. Often overlooked is stimulant use. The amount of caffeine consumed per day may be astronomical and unappreciated by the patient. Not only are tea and coffee important sources, but caffeine is put into many soft drinks of both cola and noncola varieties. Amphetamine abuse is common among people having jobs that require long periods of wakefulness, e.g., long-distance truck drivers. Recent termination of chronic hypnotic, sedative, or stimulant use may be the precipitant of insomnia. Previous attempts to discontinue medication and the results of these attempts should be covered. Patients who report difficulty sleeping in their own bed but not elsewhere are likely to have developed a learned conditioned response following a situational stress or medical problem.

Since psychiatric illness is a primary cause of chronic insomnia, the patient should be evaluated for anxiety (see Chapter 214), depression (see Chapter 215), mania, schizophrenia, and alcoholism (see Chapter 216). A careful medical history and complete physical examination are needed to search for evidence of an underlying medical illness that may be a source of discomfort or anxiety. In addition, the patient ought to be questioned and checked for symptoms and signs of congestive heart failure (see Chapter 27) and chronic lung disease (see Chapter 44), both of which may be worsened by the act of lying down to sleep, as well as for evidence of hyperthyroidism (see Chapter 99) and renal insufficiency (see Chapter 135), which can be subtle causes of sleep disturbance. Laboratory evaluation beyond that suggested by history and physical examination is of limited usefulness, but when drug abuse is in question, obtaining a serum or urine level of the drug might be very informative. Referral to a sleep laboratory, if one is available, is indicated when the etiology remains unknown, treatment is unsuccessful, and the patient is incapacitated.

PRINCIPLES OF MANAGEMENT

To be effective, treatment has to be specific. Superficial evaluation followed by uncritical prescribing of hypnotics produces poor results, unnecessary expense, and potentially serious drug-induced morbidity. When a medical illness is causing sleeplessness, it should be treated specifically rather than attempting to suppress insomnia with heavy doses of hypnotics or sedatives. For example, the restless patient with severe pulmonary disease may be placed in grave jeopardy by the use of a hypnotic, which could depress his already tenuous respiratory drive.

If there is an underlying emotional problem, it should be attended to directly, even though the patient may be reluctant to discuss his feelings and may focus upon somatic complaints. When the problem is anxiety, short-term use of a benzodiazepine (see Chapter 214) may provide symptomatic relief and help the patient to establish an effective relationship with the physician, thus facilitating treatment of the underlying difficulty. Unfortunately, many patients stop short of further therapy once their symptoms are relieved; however, their symptoms tend to return within a short period of time, even with continued use of sleep medication.

Insomnia due to situational stress is usually self-limited but can be treated with a short-term course of a benzodiazepine. With the exception of the benzodiazepines, none of the hypnotics has been shown to be effective for longer than 10 to 14 consecutive days of therapy. Beyond this period, tolerance and dependence appear, rendering the drugs ineffective. The safety and efficacy of long-term use of the benzodiazepines for sleep are currently under investigation. Some degree of tolerance and dependence (particularly psychological) seems to occur; guidelines for chronic use remain to be established. Flurazepam (Dalmane) has been heavily promoted for sleep, but it is no more effective for sleep than the other benzodiazepines. In fact, it is less rapidly absorbed than some other drugs in this class. Chlordiazepoxide, which is now available generically, can be prescribed for sleep at a fraction of the cost of flurazepam and other brand name benzodiazepines.

All hypnotics suppress REM sleep and deep sleep; the benzodiazepines do so as well, but to a lesser degree than other hypnotics. When benzodiazepines are taken alone, the hazards of overdose are small and less than those of other medications for sleep. However, most overdoses of benzodiazepines involve mixtures of drugs, and the combination of a benzodiazepine and other depressants can definitely be lethal.

All hypnotics, including the benzodiazepines, distort the sleep cycle. The best means of treating insomniacs who have been using a hypnotic chronically is to gradually withdraw the agent. Slow tapering is necessary because sudden withdrawal worsens insomnia and produces anxiety, nightmares, and a rebound phenomenon in which the percentage of REM sleep is increased. A commonly used regimen is to omit one full dose per week, slowing to one half of the nighttime dose in the final stages. Once drug use is terminated, sleep usually improves.

Treatment of the elderly patient is a particular problem. The elderly are especially sensitive to the sedating action of the hypnotics and frequently report residual drowsiness the next morning. They occasionally respond to hypnotics with a paradoxical effect characterized by excitement, agitation, and confusion. If a patient is already mildly demented, the hypnotic will often increase disorientation, confusion, and difficulty thinking. In instances when it is absolutely necessary to prescribe a hypnotic, a small dose of an antipsychotic (e.g., haloperidol) may be more effective than the usual types of sleeping medications.

Sleeplessness that has become a conditioned response, perpetuated by continuing unsuccessful attempts to fall asleep, can be treated behaviorally. Behavior therapy requires that the patient rigidly adhere to certain rules which aim to reestablish the association of bed with sleep, rather than the more recent association of bed with wakefulness. For example, the patient must not use the bed for any activity (e.g., eating, reading, watching television) other than sleeping. In addition, the patient should go to bed only when sleepy and not before. If unable to fall asleep within 15 minutes, the patient should go into another room and occupy himself with some other activity until feeling sleepy again. It is recommended that the patient arise at the same time each morning, regardless of how many hours of sleep were obtained during the night.

For the first few nights the patient may find these rules difficult and may need encouragement from the physician that with time things will in fact improve.

PATIENT EDUCATION

Regardless of the cause of sleeplessness, some practical suggestions are generally helpful in management. Establishing a regular pattern for sleeping and waking is crucial. The particular hours chosen for sleep are less important than the regularity with which they are observed. Daytime naps should be avoided. Regular physical exercise improves nocturnal sleep; however, if the patient exercises immediately before bedtime, the exercise may actually increase the time it takes to fall asleep. Constancy of the physical environment is also important; the absolute amounts of noise, light, motion, and temperature are not as crucial as the fact that they remain the same during the night and from night to night. Since hunger may disturb sleep, a light bedtime snack may be helpful.

THERAPEUTIC RECOMMENDATIONS

- If the insomnia is due to a behavioral or situational cause, use practical behavioral suggestions. If they are not sufficient, begin a benzodiazepine (e.g., chlordiazepoxide, 5 to 10 mg. before bed) for a limited period. Attempt to resolve situational stresses.
- If depression is responsible for the sleep disorder, begin a tricyclic antidepressant which has sedating action (e.g., amitriptyline, 50 mg. before bed) (see Chapter 215).
- If anxiety neurosis is the cause of insomnia, begin therapy with a benzodiazepine (see Chapter 214).
- Schizophrenia and mania also require specific psychopharmacologic treatment, utilizing phenothiazines and lithium, respectively.
- If the patient has significant medical disease, direct treatment at alleviating the underlying condition. If insomnia persists, employ behavior techniques and consider short-term use of a benzodiazepine (e.g., chlordiazepoxide, 5 to 10 mg. before bed).
- Hypnotics must be used in lower doses and with great care in the elderly. If there is already organic brain disease, a low dose of an antipsychotic may be preferable.
- Avoid employing one benzodiazepine for anxiety and another one for sleep; excessive benzodiazepine intake may result.

ANNOTATED BIBLIOGRAPHY

Choice of a benzodiazepine for treatment of anxiety or insomnia. Medical Letter, *19*:49, 1977. *(Other benzodiazepines are as effective as flurazepam for sleep; chlordiazepoxide is the least expensive.)*

Dement, W.E., and Guilleminault, C.: Sleep disorders: The state of the art. Hosp. Pract., *8*:51, 1973. *(A practical discussion of the general clinical approach to sleep disorders.)*

F.D.A. Drug Bulletin, *8*:5, 1978. *(All hypnotics, even flurazepam, distort the sleep cycle.)*

Hartmann, E.: The Functions of Sleep. New Haven: Yale University Press, 1973. *(Comprehensive discussion of the physiology and biochemistry of normal and abnormal sleep.)*

Hauri, P.: The Sleep Disorders. Kalamazoo, Michigan: The Upjohn Co., 1977. *(Covers the differential diagnosis of insomnia as well, including the estimate that only 10 to 15 per cent is primary insomnia.)*

Jouvet, M.: Biogenic amines and the states of sleep. Science, *163*:32, 1969. *(Excellent example of the research in this field, illustrating the closeness of theoretical research and understanding the clinical entities.)*

Kales, A., et al.: Chronic hypnotic use: Ineffectiveness, drug withdrawal, insomnia and hypnotic drug dependence. J.A.M.A., *227*:513, 1974. *(The best discussion of the common insomnia due to hypnotic dependence.)*

Kales, A., and Kales, J.: Sleep disorders. N. Engl. J. Med., *290*:487, 1974. *(Excellent survey of the general field, including some discussion of sleep physiology.)*

Williams, R.I., Karacan, I., and Hursch, C.J.: Electroencephalography of Human Sleep: Clinical Applications. New York: John Wiley & Sons, 1974. *(Mainly for the reader interested in pursuing the physiology of sleep, but includes estimates on prevalence of various sleep complaints.)*

221
Approach to the Patient with Obesity
FREDERICK G. GUGGENHEIM, M.D.

One feeds on lard, and yet is leane;
And I but fasting with a bean,
Grow fat and smooth: The reason is
Jove prospers my meat, more than his.
                              Robert Herrick, 1627

A substantial proportion of the U.S. population suffers from obesity. The U.S. Public Health Service reports that between 25 and 45 per cent of adults over age 30 are obese, i.e., they are at least 20 per cent over ideal body weight. Obesity costs billions of dollars annually when medical complications, lost wages, and expenditures for weight reduction efforts are taken into account. Just as important, obesity produces untold psychic pain and physical discomfort.

The incidence of obesity varies within particular groups; it is more common in females than in males, more common in lower socioeconomic groups than in upper income groups, and more common in recently arrived immigrants than in second or third generation groups. The vast majority of cases are unrelated to underlying endocrinologic, neurologic, or metabolic disease, but obesity is an important contributing factor to medical problems. For example, in a series of 524 patients presenting to an outpatient obesity clinic at a city hospital, a medical etiology was detected upon careful workup in fewer than 10 percent, but almost 50 per cent had one or more of the following diseases as a consequence of obesity: diabetes, osteoarthritis, hypertension, gout, and hyperlipidemia. The risk of having one of these conditions was found to be proportional to the degree of obesity and was significantly greater than that for a control group matched for age and sex.

Until a decade ago, most treatment programs for obesity were considered unsatisfactory by both physicians and patients; success rates after 1 to 2 years of follow up were less than 20 per cent; usually, weight gain recurred. However, the incorporation of behavior techniques into dietary programs seems to have improved results. To properly manage the obese patient, the primary physician must understand and identify the factors contributing to obesity, be cognizant of the popular diets and nonprescription drugs used by patients and aware of their complications, and know how to design a simple, safe, and effective weight reduction program. In addition, one needs to understand the methods and efficacy of the various self-help and commercial group programs available in the community and how to make the best use of the dietitian's services.

PATHOPHYSIOLOGY AND CLINICAL PRESENTATION

In the simplest sense, obesity results when intake of food exceeds caloric needs. But why this happens is usually far from clear, inasmuch as the mechanisms responsible for alteration of appetite and caloric needs and stimulation of excessive food intake are not well understood. The hypothalamus plays a role in the regulation of appetite. Destructive lesions of the ventromedial nucleus lead to appetite arousal, including hyperphagia. A lateral but less well-defined region of the hypothalamus seems to be responsible for integration of food-selecting behavior; injury to this region can result in aphagia and inactivity in other spheres.

A small fraction of obese patients have an identifiable genetic, neurologic or endocrinologic disorder. More often, psychological, developmental, dietary, exertional, socio-occupational, and pharmacologic factors operate and interact in a complex fashion to precipitate weight gain. There is no definitive evidence that obese people utilize food more efficiently than slender people, contrary to popular belief. But some obese patients have demonstrated a physiological resistance to slimming, and some slender normal volunteers have shown a resistance to experimental fattening.

Psychological factors frequently contribute to the onset and perpetuation of obesity. In many, obesity results from overeating as a pattern of coping with emotional turmoil during important events. Loss often prompts overeating, be it loss of a significant person, body part or function. Sometimes it is not the loss itself that causes the problem, but rather the threat of separation or rejection. The other major setting for "compensatory" eating is frustration, such as that due to anger at a spouse in the context of a dependent-hostile relationship. In either loss or frustration, eating becomes a defense to ward off the pangs of anxiety, depression or even self-destructive tendencies. Other people lose their appetite when they are angry, tense or blue. There is no known explanation of why some people develop reactive hyperphagia while others react to stress with anorexia. Indeed, considerable research has been unable to determine any particular personality organization or cluster of psychological defense mechanisms clearly linked to obesity.

Despite the negative medical and societal responses to obesity and the poor self-image associated with it, many obese people have difficulty keeping weight off. Often this is because of emotional problems that arise during such efforts. Weight reduction can precipitate severe depression or even psychosis, especially in people with a history of childhood-onset obesity or weight-loss-induced depression. Those with the night-eating syndrome, characterized by insomnia, massive late evening "refrigerator raids," and morning anorexia, also experience particular emotional distress when trying to reform their eating behavior. Usually there are coinciding social stresses as well. Indeed, because of the rigors of weight reduction, people undergoing considerable situational distress should be prompted to defer weight reduction programs until their psychosocial situation has stabilized.

Having survived the pitfalls and potential complications of weight reduction, the formerly obese person faces new problems. Many now find that previously unsatisfactory, though stable, relationships begin to fall apart when their morbid image is shed. Moreover, new sexual demands may be encountered by people who previously had avoided such demands by remaining fat and physically unattractive. Some obese women have prominent fantasies of promiscuity and fear they would "act out" sexually should they lose weight and become physically attractive. In sum, loss of obesity poses new psychological and interpersonal challenges which may be resisted and lead to compromise of efforts for change.

Developmental obesity refers to excessive weight gain that begins in childhood as a result of prenatal influences, constitutional and environmental factors, and, probably most important, rearing practices. Although fat children can in themselves pose many problems for their parents, most often it is the parents who have deep-seated psychological conflicts

long antedating the child's overeating and overweight. Paradoxically, the more specialists an obese child is taken to for treatment, the less likely he is to lose weight and the more neurotic the parents are likely to be. Obesity that begins in early childhood is associated with changes in fat cell numbers and composition, body image distortion, and refractoriness to later weight reduction (often because of a striking depression that accompanies weight loss).

Dietary causes of obesity involve both unwise preferences for calorie-rich food and purely elective indulgence in gluttony (this latter condition is rarely seen in clinical practice today). The proportion of patients whose obesity has a purely dietary basis has probably been exaggerated, since neither education nor shame has been particularly effective in the treatment of this disorder. If dietary indescretion by itself were so important, obesity should respond to simple restrictive measures. Another factor in dietary obesity involves the schedule of eating. There is some evidence that those who eat once daily, particularly before going to bed, may be more prone to accumulate adipose tissue.

Inactivity The contribution of decreased physical activity to the initiation, propagation, and maintenance of obesity is unclear, but available evidence suggests a role. It has been noted that obese people exercise and move about less than do nonobese people. The athlete who stops running a mile a day and does not reduce his caloric intake can gain 11 to 22 pounds in a year.

Socio-occupational obesity is commonplace. Excess weight occurs far more frequently among people in lower socioeconomic classes (one in three) than among those in upper socioeconomic classes (one in twenty). Whether this difference represents dietary preference, socially motivated behavior, or interactional factors is unclear. In certain occupations, e.g., wrestling, obesity is a help, not a hindrance. In former times, corpulence was a sign of prosperity and cultivated by bankers and businessmen.

Pharmacologic agents have been shown in many instances to stimulate food intake, especially of carbohydrate-rich products. For example, amitriptyline (Elavil), the tricyclic antidepressant, often produces the "blind munchies" several weeks to months after the patient has begun to recover from depression. Antipsychotic agents such as chlorpromazine, thioridazine, trifluoperazine, and haloperidol have been associated with considerable weight gain. Among the antipruritic agents, cyproheptadine (Periactin) has produced significant increases in appetite and weight gain, which also may occur when a patient is initially placed on corticosteroids.

Endocrine disturbances are more often the result rather than the cause of excess weight. However, hypothyroidism has been found to account for up to 5 per cent of cases in some series (see Chapter 100). Cushing's syndrome is a rare cause and is usually accompanied by characteristic features of truncal obesity and peripheral muscle wasting. Stein-Leventhal syndrome—polycystic ovaries, absent menses and moderate hirsutism (see Chapter 107)—often goes unrecognized as an endocrinologic form of obesity; the precise mechanism of the obesity is unknown. Eunichism and hyperinsulin states may also be associated with obesity.

Neurologic causes of obesity are usually not cryptic; they mostly result from hypothalamic injury, as occurs with craniopharyngiomas, encephalitis or trauma. Visual field defects or headaches are usually present. Two rare types of neurologic disease without obvious central nervous system symptoms have been described. Kleine-Levin syndrome consists of periodic hyperphagia and hypersomnia. A second syndrome is characterized by preoccupation with food and electroencephalographic abnormalities which respond to phenytoin.

A purely genetic cause of obesity is not often seen in general practice. This type of obesity is usually associated with rare autosomal recessive traits and mental retardation.

WORKUP

Gross obesity is easy to recognize, but errors in making a diagnosis of mild to moderate obesity may be frequent. Using standard height/weight charts to determine obesity has inherent problems. Standard charts usually list "ideal" or desired weights, which are based on actuarial data indicating weights associated with lowest mortality (Table 221–1). These charts measure body mass rather than the percentage of adipose tissue (which is the better criterion for determing the obese state). The person having a significant percentage of lean body mass, such as a physical laborer, may well exceed "ideal body weight," yet not be obese.

More sophisticated methods for determining obesity, e.g., total body radioactive potassium-40 densitometry, are for research purposes only and are impractical in clinical practice. Skinfold thickness,

particularly triceps measurement, provides an additional objective measurement of adipose tissue, but its use is best suited for surveying a population rather than for following an individual patient.

Brief workup for an underlying endocrinologic or neurologic cause should be carried out because of its implications for treatment. One needs to ask questions about cold intolerance, hoarseness, change in skin and hair texture, amenorrhea, hirsutism, easy bruising, weakness, drug use, visual disturbances, and headaches. In the physical examination, it is important to check for moon facies, hirsutism, dry, thickened skin, coarse hair, truncal obesity, pigmented striae, goiter, adnexal masses, lack of secondary sex characteristics, delayed relaxation of ankle jerks, and visual field deficits. Evaluation should include assessment for consequences of obesity, such as symptoms and signs of hypertension (see Chapter 13), diabetes (see Chapter 98), and osteoarthritis (see Chapter 103).

Table 221–1. Optimal Weights,* in Pounds, for Adults Aged 25 and Over (Light Clothing)

HEIGHT (in shoes)	SMALL FRAME	MEDIUM FRAME	LARGE FRAME
Men			
5 ft. 2 in.	112–120	118–129	126–141
5 3	115–123	121–133	129–144
5 4	118–126	124–136	132–148
5 5	121–129	127–139	135–152
5 6	124–133	130–143	138–156
5 7	128–137	134–147	142–161
5 8	132–141	138–152	147–166
5 9	136–145	142–156	151–170
5 10	140–150	146–160	155–174
5 11	144–154	150–165	159–179
6 0	148–158	154–170	164–184
6 1	152–162	158–175	168–189
6 2	156–167	162–180	173–194
6 3	160–171	167–185	178–199
6 4	164–175	172–190	182–204
Women			
4 10 in.	92–98	96–107	104–119
4 11	94–101	98–110	106–122
5 0	96–104	101–113	109–125
5 1	99–107	104–116	112–128
5 2	102–110	107–119	115–131
5 3	105–113	110–122	118–134
5 4	108–116	113–126	121–138
5 5	111–119	116–130	125–142
5 6	114–123	120–135	129–146
5 7	118–127	124–139	133–150
5 8	122–131	128–143	137–154
5 9	126–135	132–147	141–158
5 10	130–140	136–151	145–163
5 11	134–144	140–155	149–168
6 0	138–148	144–159	153–173

* Weights associated with the lowest mortality rates (derived from actuarial data)

Laboratory testing is probably more productive for detecting the metabolic consequences of obesity than for revealing etiology. Two-hour postprandial glucose, cholesterol, fasting triglyceride, and uric acid tests are sufficient to detect common metabolic abnormalities resulting from excess weight. Thyroid stimulating hormore (TSH) is the most sensitive indicator of primary hypothyroidism and worth ordering if there is a clinical suspicion based on history or physical examination. Laboratory testing for Cushing's syndrome is of low yield unless symptoms or signs are suggestive. An overnight 1 mg. dexamethasone suppression test is a reasonable screening procedure. When a mass lesion in the region of the sella turcica is suspected, tomography is much more sensitive than simple skull films for detection of sellar enlargement.

PRINCIPLES OF MANAGEMENT

Treatment of any underlying medical etiology takes priority over other forms of therapy and may in itself suffice. For the vast majority of obese patients without a definite medical cause, there are no absolute guidelines for selection of a treatment modality. Most patients with a considerable degree of obesity have been on a long odyssey in search of help. They have tried many types of interventions and have talked with other obese people to find out the pros and cons of different techniques. Nevertheless, the physician can help select a weight reduction method by having a thorough understanding of the patient's psychological and social barriers to weight reduction and a knowledge of available methods, community resources, patient's preference, and degree and type of inconvenience, deprivation and invasiveness the patient is willing to tolerate.

Patients seeing the physician for the first time about their obesity, whether it is of recent onset or long-standing, sometimes respond to simple measures such as dietary and exercise counseling. Since the decision to lose weight may be part of a complex decision to improve the conduct of one's life, the physician should be aware that the patient may be asking by his visit for permission to make environmental or life-style changes, or to resolve some nagging conflicts in a close relationship.

Techniques of Weight Reduction

The methods available for weight reduction include exercise, diet, behavior modification, self-help groups, fasting, drug therapy and surgery.

Exercise facilitates weight reduction by increasing expenditure of calories, enhancing one's sense of well-being, improving appearance, and, at times, altering appetite. Aerobic or isotonic exercises such as swimming, jogging, walking and cycling lead to lowered food intake, while anaerobic or isometric activities such as calesthenics and weight lifting often stimulate appetite. The amount of weight which can be lost by exercise alone is modest when food intake is kept constant. An additional 3,500 calories must be expended to eliminate 1 pound of fat. Jogging 1 mile a day for one year will result in a loss of only 11 to 22 pounds in an average individual, provided there is no increase in food intake. Only about 100 extra calories are consumed in each jogging session of 10 to 15 minutes or in walking 25 to 30 minutes. For the patient who is mildly to moderately overweight, an aerobic exercise program should be constructed. Even if the amount of weight loss is not impressive, the improvement in muscle tone and loss of fat can lead to better physical appearance, self-image and conditioning.

Diet. Weight reduction usually requires control of food intake. A gradual reduction in weight can be achieved by limiting the number of calories ingested per day to about 500 fewer than are expended. This will provide for a loss of about 1 to 2 pounds per week. The number of calories permitted can be calculated by multiplying the patient's ideal weight by 13. Ideal weights are based on height and frame (see Table 221–1). If a patient should weigh 150 pounds, 1950 calories are permitted. The diet should contain a balanced distribution of fats, carbohydrates and proteins and adequate provision for necessary vitamins and minerals (see Chapter 222).

At times, the patient will want to achieve a more rapid and striking degree of weight loss; a caloric deficit of 1000 calories per day can be prescribed and maintained for a number of weeks or even months. As long as the total number of calories consumed is above 1200, the diet is usually well tolerated for prolonged periods. A daily 1000-calorie reduction will produce a 7000-calorie deficit in 7 days and a loss of 2 pounds of fatty tissue weekly, plus some added weight reduction due to fluid loss.

With any diet for weight reduction, two phases of weight loss are observed: first, a phase of rapid weight loss due mostly to a net loss of fluid. After 2 or 3 weeks fluid losses diminish and the patient enters a phase of slower weight loss reflecting the catabolism of fat. Patients often become discouraged when they enter the slower phase. Some individuals tend to adjust to caloric restriction by unknowingly diminishing their energy expenditures; some form of physical activity is essential to any weight reduction program.

The multiplicity of diets and their adherents testifies to the inherent difficulty in controlling food intake. Numerous methods have been devised to help limit consumption of calories. These include special diets and commercial programs (see Chapter 222) as well as self-help groups and behavioral modification.

Self-help groups are frequently resorted to, especially by the chronically obese and others who seek the benefit of group support. One such group, pioneered by Alcoholics Anonymous, is TOPS (Take Off Pounds Sensibly), a 25-year-old organization that has enrolled more than 300,000 members in 12,000 chapters in different parts of the U.S. This organization stresses a buddy system, gentle competition, and group support. Middle class, gregarious women seem to do well in TOPS. TOPS, like most other programs for treatment of obesity, has a high dropout rate.

Overeaters Anonymous (OA) is more recent and enlarging organization for wieght control. This group program also models itself after Alcoholics Anonymous, having 12 steps, 12 traditions, and a view of obesity as a condition in which compulsive urges to eat overwhelm the person. The program emphasizes the need for a spiritual component, a recognition of the need for guidance without reference to any specific deity. OA often works very well with people who have a belief in God, although no formal religious background or affiliation is needed. Overeaters Anonymous does not provide a specific diet for its members, but it does have a suggested meal plan which includes a balanced deficit calorie diet. Members are encouraged to follow any diet that works for them. One major attraction of this group is the absense of fees or dues. The support system is extended beyond the meetings by pairing new members with more experienced members, who act as advisers. Before eating in the morning, the new member phones in his/her meal plan for the day. This serves as a commitment and a daily food record, in addition to providing a daily contact for motivation.

Follow-up studies on these organizations are incomplete, but their results seem to be no worse than those of more traditional techniques; 25 per cent of patients entering programs lose up to 20 pounds, but no more than 5 per cent lose as many as 40 pounds.

Behavior modification has come into prominence as a method of weight reduction since the best results ever recorded in outpatient treatment of obesity were reported in 1967. Behavioral treatment is directed toward the mildly to moderately obese. Operant conditioning techniques appear to be somewhat more effective than aversive techniques, in which a noxious stimulus is paired with food. Experimental data have shown that obese patients are more prone to respond to external cues than are control subjects of normal weight. Each individual has a pattern of eating behavior; the stimuli that trigger a complex system of response chains may be situational, physiological, or emotional. The aim of the behavioral approach is to substitute an alternative eating behavior that is practical and leads to decreased caloric intake.

Four general principles are utilized:

1. Description of the behavior to be controlled (e.g., patients are instructed to keep records of all eating behaviors, including daily weight, time and place of eating, stimuli preceding eating that the individual is aware of, and description of surroundings)
2. Modification and control of stimuli
3. Development of techniques to control the act of eating (e.g., decreasing speed of eating by counting mouthfuls)
4. Prompt reinforcement of behaviors that delay and control eating

Patients are advised to eat only in one room (cue elimination), to have company while eating (cue supervision), to develop methods of making diet food attractive (cue strengthening), to arrange for deviations of the diet, and to arrange for positive feedback if they comply with exercise diet programs. Distracting activities like watching television or reading while eating are discouraged. Eating behavior is made to be associated with highly specific stimuli.

Group programs utilizing behavioral techniques have been developed. Studies have shown that members of behavior modification groups achieve greater weight reductions than individuals treated with traditional methods, including supportive psychotherapy, instruction in nutrition and dieting, and use of appetite suppressants upon demand. The results are encouraging, but few carefully controlled studies are available. Long-term follow-up studies may suggest that the really significant role of behavior modification is in helping people maintain weight loss regardless of how it was achieved.

Fasting is employed as a drastic form of dietary control and is used in efforts to bring about a significant, rapid weight reduction in those with morbid or refractory obesity. Many patients find that after the first three days, this procedure becomes fairly easy to tolerate, since the resulting ketosis acts as an appetite suppressant (see Chapter 222). However, the basic outcome represents only wieght loss, not a change in the individual's eating habits, life-style or emotional adjustments. There is no evidence that fasting alone results in anything more than a temporary weight loss. Indeed, many insurance companies will not pay for medical hospitalization for this procedure.

Pharmacologic treatment is commonly requested by patients who have trouble controlling their food intake. *Amphetamines* and amphetaminelike drugs have been the most widely used agents for appetite suppression, but they can produce bothersome side effects such as sleep disturbances, nervousness and diarrhea, not to mention their potential for addiction and development of tolerance. Weight loss is at best temporary, even with continued use, since eating habits are usually not altered. Prolonged use may lead to fatigue and depression. The role of amphetamines and amphetaminelike agents in weight reduction is debatable; if used at all, these agents should be prescribed for a brief period to supplement other efforts.

Phenylpropanolamine is a sympathomimetic commonly used as a nasal decongestant and widely promoted as an active weight-reducing agent. It is found in many over-the-counter weight loss preparations. There is no published evidence demonstrating its efficacy for weight control. The same is true of *benzocaine,* a topical anesthetic also used in many nonprescription diet pills.

When drugs with appetite-stimulating effects are being used in treatment of severe psychiatric disorder, such as schizophrenia or endogenous depression, the substitution of molindone for other neuroleptics and of desipramine or protriptyline for amitriptyline can lessen drug-initiated excessive eating.

In the rare instance of abnormal food preoccupation and binge eating in association with electroencephalographic abnormalities, phenytoin may alleviate the problem. More commonly, binge eaters have primitive, impulsive characters, often diagnosed as borderline states. With successful psychotherapy, these regressive episodes tend to disappear as more healthy defenses and a less chaotic life-style emerge.

Surgical treatment has been developed for control of morbid obesity (defined as weight that is at least twice ideal weight). Over the past 25 years, a variety of surgical procedures have been developed, replacing the basically useless adiposectomy. The *ileojejunal bypass,* a technically straightforward pro-

cedure, is still in use in many centers. In this operation, an end-to-end anastomosis is formed between proximal jejunum and distal ileum, the jejunum being transected 30 cm. distal to the ligament of Treitz and the ileum 15 cm. proximal to the ileocecal valve, thus markedly decreasing the area available for absorption of fats and other nutrients.

Selection criteria for the operation, as well as for other drastic surgical procedures for obesity, include:

1. Weight either 100 pounds in excess or twice the ideal body weight
2. Failure to achieve and maintain significant weight loss with less drastic procedures
3. High motivation to have the procedure on the part of both patient and significant other(s)
4. Absence of untreated psychosis, severe depression, or alcoholism
5. Ability to cooperate fully with physicians in follow-up
6. Lack of masochistic or other type of severe characterologic pathology
7. Age under 50
8. Absence of arteriosclerotic heart disease
9. Absence of active liver or kidney disease
10. Adequate financial support, should repeated hospitalization be needed

Although these factors are not absolute criteria for every case, they weigh heavily in the decision to accept the patient for surgery. If the pickwickian syndrome is present, the patient should first go on an inhospital fast until the pCO_2 comes back to normal.

Following the ileojejunal bypass, the average patient may expect to lose one-third of body weight, but there are many variations in response. Weight loss is quite precipitous in the early weeks after the operation. By 3 months, the weight curve begins to flatten until a plateau finally occurs 1 to 3 years postoperatively as the small intestine begins to hypertrophy and take on additional absorptive function. Five to 20 per cent of patients undergoing an ileojejunal bypass do not achieve adequate weight loss.

Reanastomosis may be required when (1) diarrhea, triggered by food ingestion, becomes intolerable; (2) weakness accompanying extreme weight loss becomes profound; (3) liver function deteriorates due to fatty infiltration; or (4) severe arthritis occurs directly attributable to the metabolic abnormalities of the ileojejunal bypass. In addition, renal stone formation, cholecystitis, alopecia and peripheral neuropathy can be precipitated.

Only about one-half of the patients who undergo ileojejunal bypass have a reasonably satisfactory outcome. Indeed, so disappointing are these results that the *gastric bypass,* a technically much more demanding procedure, has become the surgical procedure of choice because it is associated with fewer long-term complications. The gastric bypass is in some ways similar to the Billroth II gastrojejunostomy. In the gastric bypass, nothing is resected, but 85 to 95 per cent of the stomach is excluded from direct contact with ingested food. A 12-mm. opening is achieved between the 10 to 15 per cent of proximal stomach and the jejunum to produce a relatively narrow food passageway that promotes early satiety. The weight losses resulting from ileojejunal and gastric bypass do not differ markedly, and now a majority of surgeons doing bypasses prefer the gastric bypass.

Both types of surgical bypasses are often accompanied by long-term normalization of eating habits. A few ileojejunal bypass patients can "outeat" the operation, and a few gastric bypass patients can "nibble through" the bypass and gain weight. Generally, gastric bypass patients adapt to their limited intake capacity; weight loss proceeds at a steady, gradual rate for 6 to 18 months. Although there are considerable problems in the immediate postoperative phase when the gastric bypass is performed by an inexperienced surgeon, long-term complications occur in fewer than 20 per cent of cases, and are usually limited to nausea and vomiting, which typically occur only after overindulgence. Rarely, stomal ulcers occur.

Two other surgical procedures deserve note. Truncal vagotomy is also associated with long-term decreased food intake, lack of appetite and change in food preference. Little information is available yet on how effective this simple procedure is in comparison to bypass procedures. Jaw wiring, by contrast, produces only transient, though dramatic, weight loss and is probably as useless as adiposectomy for treatment of obesity, since no long-term changes in eating habits occur.

ANNOTATED BIBLIOGRAPHY

A nasal decongestant and a local anesthetic for weight control? Medical Letter, *21*:65, 1979. *(Argues that there is no substantive evidence to support the use of phenylpropanolamine or benzocaine for weight reduction. These agents are found in widely advertised over-the-counter diet pills.)*

Blackburn, G.: The liquid protein controversy: A closer look at the facts. Obes. Bariat. Med., *7*:25, 1978. *(The author pioneered protein-sparing modified fasts.)*

Bray, G. A.: The varieties of obesity. *In* Bray, G., and Bethune, J. (eds.): Treatment and Management of Obesity. New York: Harper and Row, 1974. *(A small, very readable soft-covered book that is a sensible introduction to obesity from a biopsychosocial perspective.)*

Bray, G.A., *et al.*: Evaluation of the obese patient. JAMA, *235*:2008, 1976. *(Describes the utility of laboratory tests for evaluation of the obese patient.)*

Bruch, H.: Eating Disorders. New York: Basic Books, 1973. *(The author has had the broadest experience in obesity from a psychoanalytic perspective.)*

Bullen, B., Reed, R., and Mayer, J.: Physical activity of obese and nonobese adolescent girls appraised by motion picture sampling. Am. J. Clin. Nutr., *14*:211, 1964. *(Obese subjects were far less active, even when engaged in sports.)*

Drenick, E.: Contraindications to long-term fasting. JAMA, *188*:88, 1964. *(Psychiatric observations in starvation-induced depressions.)*

Garb, J., and Stunkard, A.: A further assessment of the effectiveness of TOPS in the control of obesity. Arch. Intern. Med., *134*:716, 1974. *(The program was found to be effective for many subjects in lower socioeconomic groups.)*

Green, R., and Rau, J.: Treatment of compulsive eating disturbances with anticonvulsant medications. Am. J. Psychiatry, *131*:428, 1974. *(The first of several studies showing that phenytoin helps some food-preoccupied binge eaters.)*

Guggenheim, F.: Basic considerations in the treatment of obesity. Med. Clin. North Am., *61*:781, 1977. *(A comprehensive current review of obesity from the internist's and psychiatrist's viewpoint.)*

Harger, B., Miller, J., and Thomas, J.: The caloric cost of running,. JAMA, *228*:482, 1974. *(The table translates weight, duration of exercise and speed of running into caloric expenditure.)*

Heil, G., and Ross, S.: Chemical agents affecting appetite. *In* Bray, G., and Bethune, J. (eds.): Obesity in Perspective: Part II. New York: Harper and Row, 1975, p. 81. *(A review of anorexic agents in obesity.)*

Sandstead, H.: Jejunoileal shunt in morbid obesity. *In* Bray, G., and Bethune, J. (eds): Obesity in Perspective: Part II. New York: Harper and

Row, 1975, p. 459. *(A description of a previously used operative procedure.)*

Schachter, S.: Obesity and eating. Science, *161*:751, 1968. *(The externality of obese patients is demonstrated in some ingenious and landmark experiments.)*

Skinner, B.: Contingencies of Reinforcement: A Theoretical Analysis. New York: Appleton Century Crofts, 1969. *(The author is the father of behavior modification.)*

Solomon, N.: The study and treatment of the obese patient. Hosp. Pract., *14*:90, 1969. *(An outpatient medical evaluation of the obese patient who comes to an obesity clinic.)*

Stuart, R.: Behavioral control of overeating. Behav. Res. Ther. *5*:357, 1967. *(The first documented report of weight loss from behavior modification using operant conditioning.)*

Stuart, R.: Act thin, stay thin. New York: W.W. Norton, 1978. *(A sensible readable book for motivated intelligent patients.)*

Stunkard, A.: The pain of obesity. Palo Alto: Bull Publishing, 1976. *(An informal, readable book of patients' experiences by the psychiatrist with the widest experience in the field.)*

Stunkard, A.: Obesity and the social environment. Current status, future prospects. Ann. N.Y. Acad. Sci., *300*:298, 1977. *(An important review of the present and future aspects of obesity and the social system.)*

Stunkard, A.: Behavioral treatment of obesity. Failure to maintain weight loss. *In* Stuart, R. (ed.): Behavioral Self-Management Strategies: Techniques and Outcomes. Brunner New York: Brunner/Mazel, 1977. *(Dr. Stunkard's chapter in this remarkable book emphasizes the need for long-term follow-up treatments for obesity, and he discusses some reasons for failure to maintain weight loss with behavioral techniques.)*

Stunkard, A., Grace, W., and Wolff, H.: The night-eating syndrome. Am. J. Med., *19*:78, 1955. *(An important observation.)*

Weiss, A.: Characteristics of successful weight reducers. A brief review of predictor variables. Addict. Behav., *2*:193, 1977. *(Patients with adult onset obesity who are self-reinforcing and well-adjusted have the best prognosis.)*

222

Dietary Programs for Weight Control

The vast array of diets touted for weight reduction attests to the fact that no single program has proved to be uniquely effective. Dietary fads crowd the lay literature, and many people bring questions about them to their doctors. The primary physician must be familiar with the rationale, efficacy, side effects and complications of the more popular diets and commercial diet programs in order to advise the patient adequately and help in the choice of a safe and practical program for loss.

HIGH PROTEIN, KETOGENIC DIETS

High protein diets have had a cyclic history of public appeal and currently abound in the popular press. The common factor among these diets is the exclusion of a specific macronutrient, usually carbohydrate, leading to the development of ketosis which produces some degree of appetite suppression. Most include caloric restricions as well, which are important if not central to their efficacy.

Stillman's Quick Weight Loss Diet is among the most popular of the high-protein diets. The program is also referred to as the high-protein/water diet. It prescribes eating lean foods composed mainly of protein and drinking 3 or more liters of water per day. Only lean meat, poultry, lean fish, eggs and low-fat cheese are permitted in unlimited quantities. One is instructed to drink 6 to 8 glasses of noncaloric fluids each day in order to facilitate ketone excretion; to take a small quantity of orange juice for fatigue; and to use a daily multiple vitamin.

Stillman's rationale for the diet is based on a food's specific dynamic action (SDA). Calories are wasted as heat, rather than preserved in the form of ATP. In the case of protein, the specific dynamic effect amounts to approximately 20 per cent of the energy value of the food ingested; for carbohydrate the figure is 6 per cent and for lipid 4 per cent. The theoretical calorie deficit from SDA in Stillman's diet program is only 330 kilocalories per day, not even one-tenth of the deficit needed to comprise a 1-pound weight loss of fat tissue. The initial rapid weight loss that occurs with Stillman's diet is due to the water and electrolyte loss resulting from low carbohydrate feedings. An additional contribution to weight loss is the coincident calorie restriction (approximately 1500 Kcal per day) which occurs as a consequence of the complete exclusion of carbohydrate. In addition, ketosis may induce appetite suppression.

Atkins and West promote a high-fat, high-protein diet, in addition to an initial exclusion of carbohydrates. The dieter is permitted to ingest unlimited amounts of food in a fat-to-protein ratio of 40:60 per cent of total calories. Ketosis is usually established within the first week. During the second week, carbohydrate is added at the rate of 5 grams per day, until no more can be added without reversing ketosis. While the diet rigidly restricts carbohydrate intake (usually less than 50 grams per day), some suggested meals include chicken salad, bacon and eggs and fried fish.

Atkins states that the obese are carbohydrate intolerant and that restriction of carbohydrate rather than calories is the key to weight loss. He states that carbohydrate restriction triggers secretion of an alleged "fat mobilizing hormone," which he claims promotes utilization of fat stores. He points also to the loss of energy via urinary ketones and acetone excretion through expiration.

Atkins and West have received considerable criticism, including an investigation by the U.S. Senate Committee on Nutrition and Human Needs (1973). It is noted that Atkins ignores the first law of thermodynamics, in addition to having insufficient evidence to back the existence of a "fat mobilizing hormone." Moreover, the amount of calories lost through ketone excretion could rarely exceed 100 Kcal per day, hardly sufficient to account for the dramatic weight loss claimed by Atkins. Apart from the transient changes in water loss, no evidence exists that shows that weight loss is more rapid with ketogenic diets than with balanced diets of equal energy value.

In addition to the questionable basis for the program, potential complications are associated with it. The diet ignores epidemiologic evidence linking high-cholesterol, high-saturated fat intake with increased risk of coronary disease. In addition, there is no effort to ensure the copious fluid intake needed to promote safe ketone excretion.

Neither Stillman nor Atkins addresses the initially rapid water and eletrolyte losses and attendant risks of hypokalemia and postural hypotension that occur with ketogenic diets. Postural hypotension is not uncommon in the minimally obese subject. No attention is given to the potential for acute gouty attacks resulting from competition of ketoacids and uric acid for renal tubular excretion (see Chapter 146). Constipation, a problem with many dieters, is exacerbated by these regimens, due to the absence of bulky low-calorie vegetables and fruits prescribed in balanced deficit calorie diets.

The *Scarsdale Medical Diet* is another popular high-protein, low-carbohydrate, low-fat diet. It averages about 1000 calories per day; 43 per cent of calories are from protein, 22.5 per cent from fat, and 35.5 per cent from carbohydrates. It is claimed that the diet induces mild ketosis, which helps suppress appetite. Specific menus to be used over a 2-week period are provided; no substitutions are permitted. After 14 days, the user is instructed to go off the diet and onto a maintenance program that requires avoidance of concentrated carbohydrate and excess fat. After 2 weeks on the maintenance program, the patient is allowed to go back on the diet for further weight loss. Although reference is made to the importance of initiating behavioral changes, only perfunctory instruction is given, such as exhortations to chew food thoroughly and not to overeat. The importance of exercise is only briefly considered.

PROTEIN-SPARING MODIFIED FAST (PSMF)

The use of high-biologic value protein supplements during fasting to maintain nitrogen balance was initially developed as a research effort for treatment of critically ill hospitalized patients. The concept was later adopted by nonresearchers and popularized as an intensive weight reduction program for outpatients. The basic idea is to provide small amounts of high quality protein during a modified fast to prevent utilization of body protein for caloric needs, as occurs in strict fasting.

The researchers who initially developed the approach do not advise unsupervised widespread use of the PSMF program, but those who promote the program urge use of liquid protein preparations, which they market. The preparation is usually a protein hydrolysate made from animal hide. Liquid protein products are classified as food and are available without prescription. Some of the brand names include Prolinn, Gro-Lean, Super Pro-Gest, LPP, EMF, and T-Amino Predigested Animal Liquid Protein. A protein-sparing modified fast involves feedings of protein hydrolysates, or lean, edible animal protein, at a level of 1.0 to 1.5 gm. of protein per kg. of ideal body weight. Dieters exist on 300 to 700 calories of the liquid protein substance mixed in low-calorie fluids, in addition to a wide assortment of vitamins and minerals. Advocates claim dramatic results with a minimum of temptation to the dieter.

The poorly supervised PSMF, especially with the use of protein hydrolysates, has some obvious deficiencies. Many of the hydrolysates are made from protein of poor biologic quality and need to be fortified with tryptophan, one of the limiting essential amino acids. The use of low-biologic value protein is contrary to the basic concept of nitrogen sparing. Additional deficiencies of potassium, phosphorus, calcium and magnesium may be present in poorly supplemented regimens, since these minerals are not usually found in adequate quantities in standard vitamin-mineral preparations.

The FDA has reported on ten deaths in women following PSMF using liquid protein products. Additional deaths have been cited in patients using liquid protein under medically supervised PSMF. It appears that cardiac arrhythmias were the major cause of death, and a prospective study documented onset of serious arrhythmias in some patients. At the present time, unsupervised PSMF diets utilizing liquid protein should be discouraged. Another flaw in a do-it-yourself PSMF or in a casually supervised program is the absence of any attempt to alter behavior in order to sustain weight loss. As with other weight loss programs, weight maintenance is the limiting factor in long-term success.

COMMERCIAL WEIGHT LOSS PROGRAMS

Weight Loss Clinic provides an eclectic, supervised program of weight control. Behavioral techniques are incorporated. The basic diet is approximately 500 kilocalories per day, derived from usual food sources (lean animal protein, fruit, and vegetables), with a daily nutrient distribution of 45 to 70 grams of protein, 15 to 25 grams of fat, and 15 to 30 grams of carbohydrate. Variations from the standard are made upon physicians' requests. Excluded from the clinic program are people with insulin-dependent diabetes or chronic liver or pancreatic disease; screening is performed by registered nurses.

The program is divided into three phases: active weight loss, stabilization, and weight maintenance. During active weight loss, participants are required to visit the clinic office three to five times per week to check weight, food records, blood pressure, and urinary ketones. Multiple vitamin and mineral supplements are provided on the premises. Stabilization involves slow refeeding to prevent rapid fluid accumulation due to increased carbohydrate intake and to determine precisely maintenance caloric needs. The maintenance phase consists primarily of weight checks and reinforcement by clinic personnel.

The positive aspects of this program include frequent individual follow-up and some instruction in calorie counting and behavior modification. In addition, the financial commitment probably increases client motivation and expectations. Problems with the Weight Loss Clinic program include its expense, which is usually several hundred dollars, and the questionable ability of the personnel to carry through with the behavior modification component within the 10 to 15 minutes allotted to patients for daily visits. Clinic personnel consist of registered nurses and technicians who are not formally trained in behavior modification techniques.

In addition, the diet plan may not provide adequate protein for maintaining lean body mass in individuals with larger frames. The upper limit of protein intake on the standard diet plan is 70 grams of protein per day. This provides only 1 gram of protein per kilogram for a 70-kilogram person, which is slightly less than amounts recommended by some investigators to spare nitrogen losses. It is possible for clients with specific food preferences to consume consistently less than 2 grams of potassium per day, thought to be the necessary intake during PSMF. Finally, the vitamin-mineral supplement (prepared exclusively for Weight Loss Clinic) contains more than adequate (according to 1974 RDA) amounts of vitamins A, C, D, E, thiamine, riboflavin and pyridoxine, but inadequate amounts of calcium, phosphorus, iodine, iron, magnesium and zinc. The capsules also contain methylcellulose, a bulk-producing agent.

Since this program is relatively new, long-term success rates and complications have not yet been ascertained. With a more careful assessment of individual nutrient needs, use of an intensified behavior modification component and better provision of necessary minerals, this program might be reasonable for selected obese patients who require close follow-up and support.

Weight Watchers is a commercial, international corporation with a membership of approximately one-half million. While the contact person is a nonprofessional (a successful Weight Watcher), the corporation employs a medical director, a nutrition director and psychological director. The diet utilized is a balanced deficit calorie diet with a nutrient distribution of 25 per cent protein, 40 per cent carbohydrate, and 35 per cent fat, with a polyunsaturated-to-saturated-fat ratio of 2:1. The focus of the diet is three meals and snacks from the prescribed food allowances, for a total of 1200 calories per day for females and 1500 to 1600 calories per day for males. A program for adolescents is also available. The dietary program has recently been supplemented by an exercise program.

The Weight Watchers program is divided into three phases: active weight loss, a plateau or leveling period, and a maintenance plan. The plateau or leveling plan is more restrictive (lower carbohydrate content) than the plan for the weight loss phase, in an effort to "rid the body of accumulated water weight." The maintenance plan runs for 8 weeks, during which restricted foods are readded to the diet in a portion-controlled fashion.

Weight Watchers provides members with a wide variety of printed recipes and weekly meal plans. The program also includes a series of behavior modification modules, called Personal Action Plans, that help members analyze their eating habits. This approach is probably of value to the person who needs group support and is willing to conform to the rules of limiting food intake based on Weight Watchers' decisions of "legal and illegal," some of which appear to be arbitrary.

That a significant number of Weight Watchers' clients are "repeaters" clearly indicates that the program has not solved the more difficult problem of weight maintenance. The recidivism rate is probably a direct reflection of the neglect of individual lifestyles and lack of personalized behavioral teaching. It appears to be difficult to extinguish individual feeding cues in a group atmosphere. The group leaders receive training in conforming to the highly stylized Weight Watchers program but are not specifically taught how to employ behavior modification techniques.

Diet Workshop addresses the problem of obesity eclectically in four areas: diet, general nutritional education, exercise, and behavior modification. The program includes a balanced deficit calorie diet of 1200 calories per day for females and 1500 to 1600 calories for males. Reduction diets are also available for patients with secondary therapeutic concerns such as hypertension or elevated serum lipids.

The program involves individual counseling as well as group participation. The emphasis of the nutrition education is on low-calorie cooking. The exer-cise component suggests activities to strengthen specific muscles. As with Weight Watchers, Diet Workshop uses former clients as instructors; medical and nutritional advisers are employed at the national level. There are no statistics available regarding success rates. Compared to Weight Watchers, Diet Workshop may appeal to a wider population since it offers some individual counseling, which may help the client resolve conflicts related to specific food preferences and life-styles.

In summary, most commercial weight loss programs function as support systems for the obese client. In addition to group support and motivation, their success is based on peer pressure and a certain amount of competitive spirit. The success of these groups should not be ignored. One chapter of a certain commercial program has reported success rates equal to those cited in professional literature. In the past, it appeared that induction of new members probably equaled the attrition rate. Perhaps the recent incorporation of some behavior modification components into the majority of programs will reduce the number of clients in whom weight loss is only temporary.

CONCLUSIONS

- A balanced deficit calorie diet in conjunction with behavioral teaching to facilitate maintenance of weight loss is probably the safest and most reasonable weight reduction program.
- The unsupervised protein-sparing modified fast should be discouraged, especially when based on use of liquid protein preparations.
- The popular high protein diets are based on unfounded assumptions and probably exert most of their effect by ketosis-induced appetite suppression, calorie restriction and water loss due to limitation of carbohydrate.
- The majority of commercial weight loss programs serve as support systems. Patients requiring such support may benefit from them.
- Dietary programs which do not attempt to achieve a permanent change in the patient's eating behavior are unlikely to provide long-term benefit.

ANNOTATED BIBLIOGRAPHY

Bistrian, B.R.: Clinical use of a protein-sparing modified fast. JAMA, *240*:229, 1978. (*A practical and detailed discussion of the program; the author suggests that it be used only with informed consent, but does feel that it may have a place under carefully supervised conditions.)*

Felig, P.: Four questions about protein diets. N. Engl. J. Med., *298*:1025, 1978. *(A critique of liquid protein diets that urges that they be used only for investigative purposes.)*

Lantigua, R.A., *et al.:* Cardiac arrhythmias associated with a liquid protein diet for the treatment of obesity. N. Engl. J. Med., *303*:735, 1980. *(A pro-spective study demonstrating onset of serious arrhythmias in some patients subjected to liquid protein diets.)*

Protein-sparing diets. Medical Letter, *19*:69, 1977. *(Warns of their adverse effects and argues against their use.)*

Stunkard, A., and Penick, S.: Behavior modification in the treatment of obesity. Arch. Gen. Psychiatry, *36*:801, 1979. *(Excellent summary by one of the authorities in the field.)*

Index